A Practical Guide to Pediatric Emergency Medicine: Caring for Children in the Emergency Department

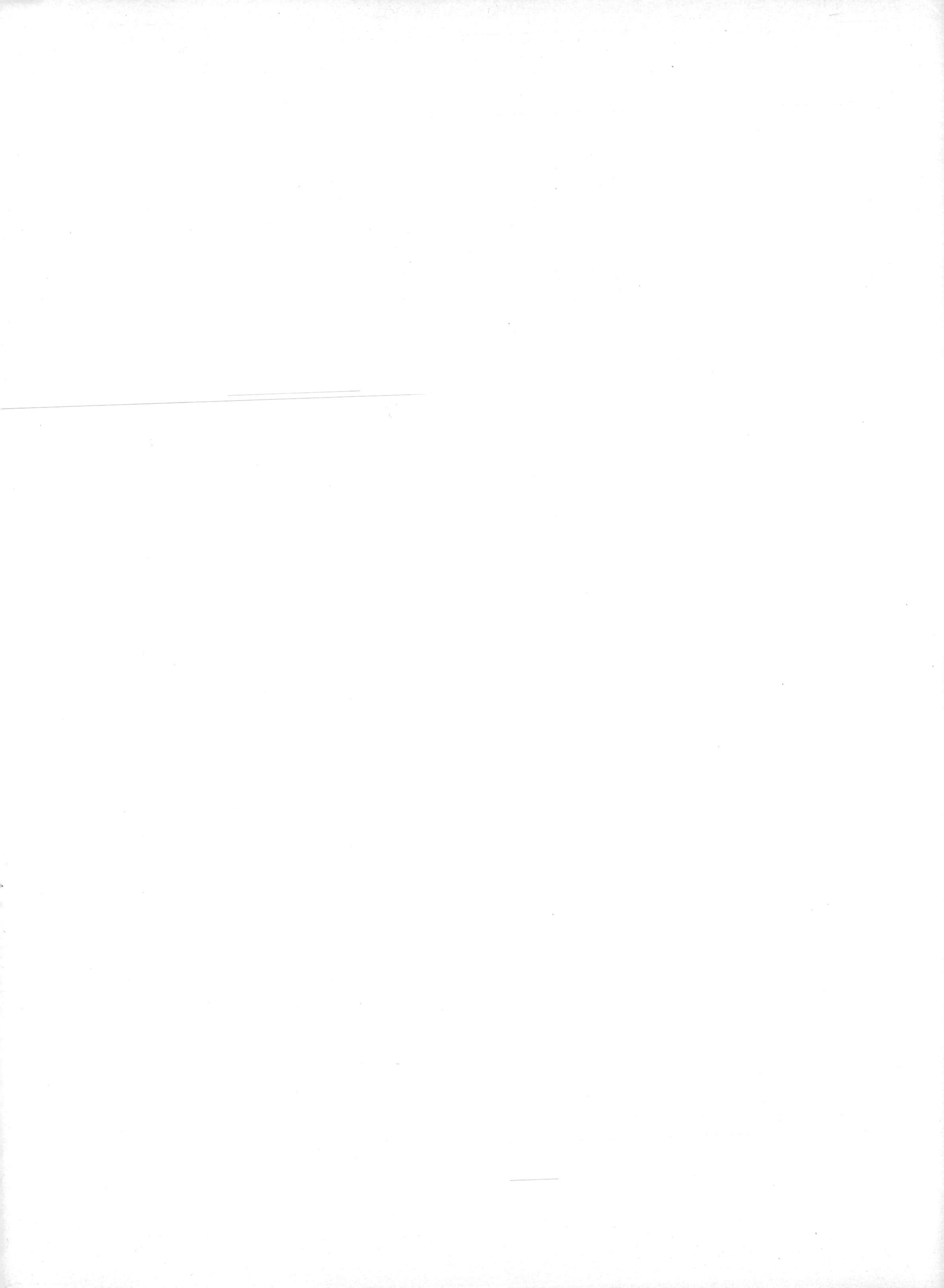

A Practical Guide to Pediatric Emergency Medicine: Caring for Children in the Emergency Department

---

Edited by:

N. Ewen Amieva-Wang

Associate Editors

Jamie Shandro

Aparajita Sohoni

Bernhard Fassl

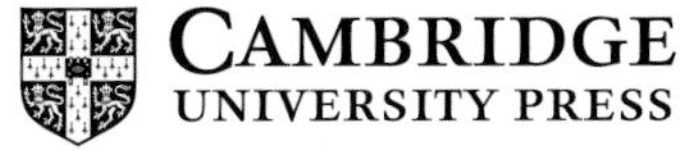

CAMBRIDGE UNIVERSITY PRESS
Cambridge, New York, Melbourne, Madrid, Cape Town,
Singapore, São Paulo, Delhi, Tokyo, Mexico City

Cambridge University Press
The Edinburgh Building, Cambridge CB2 8RU, UK

Published in the United States of America by
Cambridge University Press, New York

www.cambridge.org
Information on this title: www.cambridge.org/9780521700085

First published 2011

Printed in the United Kingdom at the University Press, Cambridge

A catalog record for this publication is available from the British Library

Library of Congress Cataloging-in-Publication Data

A practical guide to pediatric emergency medicine : caring for children in the emergency department / edited by
N. Ewen Amieva-Wang ; associate editors, Jamie Shandro, Aparajita Sohoni, Bernhard Fassl.
p. ; cm.
Includes bibliographical references and index.
ISBN 978-0-521-70008-5 (pbk.)
1. Pediatric emergencies–Handbooks, manuals, etc. 2. Critical care I. Amieva-Wang, N. Ewen, 1964–
[DNLM: 1. Emergencies–Handbooks. 2. Child. 3. Critical Care–methods–Handbooks. 4. Emergency Treatment–methods–Handbooks. 5. Infant. WS 39]
RJ370.P73 2010
618.92′0025–dc22

2010036372

ISBN 978-0-521-70008-5 Paperback

With love and thanks to Adrian, for being my biggest supporter; to my family, for being my role models; and to my friends, for making it so much fun

Aparajita Sohoni

To Hans, Nina and Margot, with gratitude and love.

Jamie Shandro

Dedications to the brewmaster of Wasatch Brewery for malt and hop support during the editing process...

Bernhard Fassl

To my family, especially to Ana Sofia, Lucia and Manuel. You are my wisdom, light and meaning. Although this book took time away from you, it is all for you

To my co-editors, expert reviewers, and collaborators, without whom this "good idea" would never have become a reality

N. Ewen Amieva-Wang

Contents

Section 4 – Dental emergencies

Expert reviewer: Brian Su-Chieh Liu

Section 5 – Dermatology

Section 6 – Ear, nose, and throat

Expert reviewer: Anna Messner

Section 7 – Endocrine emergencies

Expert reviewers: Darrell M. Wilson and Nikta Forghani

Section 8 – Environmental emergencies

Section 9 – Fluids and electrolytes

Expert reviewers: Steven Alexander and Nikta Forghani

Section 17 – Ophthalmology

Section 18 – Psychiatric emergencies

Expert reviewer: Shashank V. Joshi

Section 19 – Renal emergencies

Expert reviewers: Steven Alexander and Paul C. Grimm

Section 20 – Respiratory emergencies

Section 21 – Social and emotional emergencies

Expert reviewer: Tonya Chaffee

Section 22 – Toxicology

Section 23 – Trauma

Expert reviewers: James Holmes Jr., Michael S. B. Edwards, and William A. Kennedy II

Contributors

Steven Alexander MD
Division Chief and Professor of Pediatrics & Nephrology,
Lucile Packard Children's Hospital at Stanford,
Stanford University School of Medicine,
Stanford, CA, USA

N. Ewen Amieva-Wang MD
Associate Professor, Division of Emergency Medicine,
Stanford University School of Medicine,
Stanford, CA, USA

James P. Andrus MD
Associate Professor,
Pediatric Intensive Care,
Lucile Packard Children's Hospital at Stanford,
Stanford University School of Medicine,
Stanford, CA, USA

Sandra Leigh Bardas BSP
Clinical Pharmacist,
Division of Emergency Medicine,
Stanford University Hospital & Clinics,
Stanford, CA, USA

Barbie J. Barrett MD
Clinical Associate Professor,
Division of Emergency Medicine,
Stanford University School of Medicine
and Mills-Peninsula Health Services,
Burlingame, CA, USA

David R. Berk MD
Assistant Professor,
Department of Internal Medicine and Pediatrics,
Divisions of Dermatology,
Washington University School of Medicine,
St. Louis Children's Hospital,
St. Louis, MO, USA

Daniel Bernstein MD
Chief, Pediatric Cardiology,
Packard Children's Hospital,
Professor of Pediatrics
Stanford University, CA, USA

Rebecca Blankenburg MD MPH
Clinical Assistant Professor, Pediatrics,
Lucile Packard Children's Hospital at Stanford,
Stanford University School of Medicine,
Palo Alto, CA, USA

Chioma Agbo Boukai MD
Clinical Fellow,
Department of Emergency Medicine,
Brigham & Women's Hospital and
Massachusetts General Hospital,
Boston, MA, USA

Richard N. Bradley MD
Associate Professor, Emergency Medicine,
Center for Translational Injury Research,
The University of Texas Medical School at Houston,
Houston, TX, USA

Beau Briese MD
Division of Emergency Medicine,
Stanford University School of Medicine,
Palo Alto, CA, USA

Yi-Mei Chng MD
Clinical Instructor,
Division of Emergency Medicine,
Stanford University School of Medicine,
Stanford, CA, USA

Alice Chiao MD
Clinical Instructor,
Division of Emergency Medicine,
Stanford University School of Medicine,
Stanford, CA, USA

Benjamin R. Cohen MD
The Johns Hopkins University School of Medicine,
Baltimore, MD, USA

Clinton J. Coil MD MPH
Assistant Clinical Professor of Medicine,
David Geffen School of Medicine,
Harbor–UCLA Medical Center,
Torrance, CA, USA

Patrick Coleman MD
Department of Emergency Medicine,
Northwestern University Feinberg School of Medicine,
Chicago, IL, USA

Benjamin Constance MD
Division of Emergency Medicine,
Stanford/Kaiser Emergency Medicine Residency,
Palo Alto, CA, USA

Stephanie Cooper MD
Assistant Professor,
Division of Emergency Medicine,
University of Washington Medical Center,
Seattle, WA, USA

Ginny Curtin RN MS PNP
Pediatric Nurse Practitioner,
Otolaryngology, Head & Neck Surgery,
Lucile Packard Children's Hospital at Stanford,
Stanford, CA, USA

Barbara Dahl MD
Department of Emergency Medicine,
Jordan Valley Medical Center,
West Jordan, UT, USA

Ann Dahlberg MD
Fellow, Pediatric Hematology/Oncology,
Seattle Children's Hospital,
Seattle, WA, USA

Jonathan E. Davis MD
Associate Professor,
Department of Emergency Medicine,
Georgetown University Hospital &
Washington Hospital Center,
Washington, DC, USA

Melissa S. DeFreest MD
Clinical Instructor, Emergency Medicine,
Oregon Health and Science University,
Eugene, and Sacred Heart Medical Center,
Springfield, OR, USA

Eva Delgado MD
Division of Emergency Medicine,
Children's Hospital & Research Center Oakland,
Oakland, CA, USA

Luigi DiStefano MD
Division of Emergency Medicine,
Stanford University School of Medicine,
Palo Alto, CA, USA

Sean Donahue DO ABFM
Emergency Medicine, Memorial Hospital,
Colorado Springs, CO, USA

Stephanie J. Doniger MD
Director of Emergency Ultrasound,
Division of Emergency Medicine,
Children's Hospital & Research Center Oakland,
Oakland, CA, USA

Joan Hwang Dunlop MD
Clinical Assistant Professor of Pediatrics,
George Washington University School of Medicine;
Clinical Associate of Emergency Medicine,
Children's National Medical Center,
Washington, DC, USA

Ram S. Duriseti MD PhD
Clinical Assistant Professor,
Division of Emergency Medicine,
Stanford University School of Medicine,
Palo Alto, CA, USA

Laura Edgerley-Gibb MD
Division of Emergency Medicine,
Stanford University School of Medicine,
Palo Alto, CA, USA

William Eidenmuller MD
Emergency Medicine Physician,
Sutter Emergency Medical Associates,
Memorial Medical Center,
Modesto, CA, USA

Betsy Encarnacion MD
Department of Obstetrics,
Gynecology & Reproductive Sciences,
University of California,
San Francisco, CA, USA

Bernhard Fassl MD
Assistant Professor,
Pediatric Inpatient Medicine,
University of Utah School of Medicine,
Salt Lake City, UT, USA

Nikta Forghani MD
Clinical Instructor, Pediatric Endocrinology,
CHOC Children's University of California,
Irvine Orange, CA, USA

Tammy Foster MD
Emergency Medicine Physician,
Mills-Peninsula Health Services,
Burlingame, CA, USA

Douglas Fredrick MD
Clinical Professor, Ophthalmology,
Lucile Packard Children's Hospital at Stanford,
Stanford University School of Medicine,
Stanford, CA, USA

Renata C. Gallagher MD PhD
Assistant Professor,
Clinical Genetics and Metabolism,
Department of Pediatrics,
University of Colorado Denver,
Aurora, CO, USA

Cynthia Galvan MD
Department of Emergency Medicine,
Northwestern University Feinberg School of Medicine,
Chicago, IL, USA

Daniel Garza MD
Assistant Professor,
Division of Emergency Medicine & Sports Medicine,
Stanford University School of Medicine,
Stanford, CA, USA

Medley O'Keefe Gatewood MD
Assistant Professor,
Division of Emergency Medicine,
University of Washington Medical Center,
Seattle, WA, USA

Gregory H. Gilbert MD
Clinical Assistant Professor,
Division of Emergency Medicine,
Stanford University School of Medicine,
Palo Alto, CA, USA

Michael A. Gisondi MD
Assistant Professor,
Emergency Medicine,
Northwestern University Feinberg School of Medicine,
Chicago, IL, USA

Bertil Glader MD PhD
Professor,
Pediatric Hematology/Oncology,
Lucile Packard Children's Hospital at Stanford,
Stanford University School of Medicine,
Palo Alto, CA, USA

Carol L. Greene MD
Professor of Pediatrics,
University of Maryland School of Medicine,
Baltimore, ML, USA

Rebecca Gudeman JD MPA
Senior Attorney,
National Center for Youth Law,
Oakland, CA, USA

Bo Yoon Ha MD
Chief, Pediatric Radiology,
Santa Clara Valley Medical Center,
San Jose, CA, USA

Noel C. Hastings MD
Resident Physician,
UC Davis Health System,
Sacramento, CA, USA

Robert Hilt MD
Assistant Professor,
Department of Psychiatry & Behavioral Sciences,
University of Washington,
Seattle, WA, USA

Renee Y. Hsia MD MSc
Assistant Professor of Emergency Medicine,
Department of Emergency Medicine,
San Francisco General Hospital & Trauma Center,
San Francisco, CA, USA

William T. Hurley MD
Assistant Professor,
Division of Emergency Medicine,
University of Washington Medical Center,
Seattle, WA, USA

Bryce Inman MD
Department of Emergency Medicine,
Loma Linda University Medical Center,
Loma Linda, CA, USA

Kathleen Ann Jobe MD
Associate Professor, Division of Emergency Medicine,
University of Washington Medical Center,
Seattle, WA, USA

Tyler Johnston BA MS
Department of Orthopedic Surgery,
Sports Medicine Center,
Stanford University School of Medicine,
Stanford, CA, USA

David Kammer MD
Department of Emergency Medicine,
Carolinas Medical Center,
Charlotte, NC, USA

Laura W. Kates MD
Department of Emergency Medicine,
San Francisco General Hospital,
San Francisco, CA, USA

Judith R. Klein MD
Assistant Professor of Emergency Medicine,
Department of Emergency Medicine,
UCSF – San Francisco General Hospital,
San Francisco, CA, USA

Edward Klofas MD
Clinical Associate Professor,
Division of Emergency Medicine,
Stanford University School of Medicine,
Stanford, CA, USA

Zita Konik MD
Division of Emergency Medicine,
Stanford University School of Medicine,
Stanford, CA, USA

Anita Kulkarni MD
Emergency Medicine Physician,
Kaiser Santa Clara Medical Center,
Santa Clara, CA, USA

Amy B. Kunihiro MD
Emergency Medicine Physician,
Kaiser Redwood City, Santa Clara, CA, USA

Patrick M. Lank MD
Department of Emergency Medicine,
Northwestern University Feinberg School of Medicine,
Chicago, IL, USA

Katrina A. Leone MD
Department of Emergency Medicine,
Northwestern University Feinberg School of Medicine,
Chicago, IL, USA

Joel T. Levis MD PhD
Emergency Medicine Physician,
Kaiser Santa Clara Medical Center,
Santa Clara, CA, USA

Ingrid T. Lim MD
Kaiser Permanente,
San Francisco Medical Center,
Assistant Clinical Professor,
Department of Emergency
University of California, San Francisco
San Francisco, CA, USA

Stephen J. Liu MD
Associate Medical Director, Emergency Services,
California Hospital Medical Center,
Los Angeles, CA, USA

Brian Su-Chieh Liu DDS MS
Pediatric Dentist,
Palo Alto, CA, USA

Swaminatha V. Mahadevan MD
Associate Professor,
Division of Emergency Medicine,
Stanford University School of Medicine,
Palo Alto, CA, USA

Millicent Marmer BA
Albany Medical College,
Albany, NY, USA

Nicole Marsico MD
Clinical Instructor Pediatrics,
Lucile Packard Children's Hospital at Stanford,
Stanford University School of Medicine,
Stanford, CA, USA

Danielle M. McCarthy MD
Department of Emergency Medicine,
Northwestern University Feinberg School of Medicine,
Chicago, IL, USA

Alison K. Meadows MD
Department of Pediatric Cardiology,
University of California,
San Francisco, CA, USA

Marcela P. Mendenhall MD
Instructor Pediatrics,
Children's Hospital Denver,
University of Colorado Health Sciences Center,
Denver, CO, USA

Anna Messner MD
Professor,
Otolaryngology, Head & Neck Surgery,
Lucile Packard Children's Hospital at Stanford,
Stanford University School of Medicine,
Palo Alto, CA, USA

Kirsten E. Mewaldt MD
Emergency Medicine Physician,
California Hospital Medical Center,
Los Angeles, CA, USA

Steven H. Mitchell MD
Acting Assistant Professor of Medicine,
University of Washington School of Medicine,
Seattle, WA, USA

Claudia R. Morris MD
Division of Emergency Medicine,
Children's Hospital & Research Center Oakland,
Oakland, CA, USA

Nancy Murphy MD
Associate Professor,
Department of Pediatrics,
University of Utah School of Medicine,
Salt Lake City, UT, USA

Beverley Newman MD
Associate Professor,
Radiology,

Lucile Packard Children's Hospital at Stanford,
Stanford University School of Medicine,
Stanford, CA, USA

Carolyn Nguyen PharmD
Clinical Pharmacist,
Division of Emergency Medicine,
Stanford University Hospital and Clinics,
Palo Alto, CA, USA

Robert L. Norris MD
Professor,
Chief, Division of Emergency Medicine,
Stanford University School of Medicine,
Stanford, CA, USA

Colleen O'Connor MS, CCLS
Child Life Specialist,
Division of Emergency Medicine,
Stanford University Hospital and Clinics,
Stanford, CA, USA

J. Grace Park DO MPH
Assistant Professor,
Division of Pediatric Emergency Medicine,
University of New Mexico,
Albuquerque, NM, USA

Ketan H. Patel MD
Attending Physician,
Bronx-Lebanon Hospital,
Bronx, NY, USA

Amritha Raghunathan MD
Attending Physician,
Department of Emergency Medicine,
Kaiser Santa Clara Medical Center,
Santa Clara, CA, USA

Naresh Ramarajan MD
Departments of Emergency Medicine
and Internal Medicine,
UCLA David Geffen School of Medicine,
Los Angeles, CA, USA

Jennifer R. Reid MD
Assistant Profesor,
Pediatric Emergency Medicine,
University of Washington School of Medicine,
Seattle, WA, USA

Jay Riva-Cambrin MD FRCSC
Assistant Professor of Neurosurgery,
Department of Neurosurgery,
University of Utah and Primary Children's
Medical Center,
Salt Lake City, UT, USA

Alan F. Rope MD
Associate Professor of Pediatrics,
Division of Medical Genetics,
University of Utah School of Medicine,
Salt Lake City, UT, USA

Heather Ross Ogle MD
Senior Clinical Instructor of Emergency Medicine,
Department of Emergency Medicine,
University of Colorado School of Medicine,
Exempla St. Joseph Hospital,
Denver, CO

David H. Salzman MD
Department of Emergency Medicine,
Northwestern University Feinberg School of Medicine,
Chicago, IL, USA

Kimberly Schertzer MD
Clinical Instructor,
Division of Emergency Medicine,
Stanford University School of Medicine,
Palo Alto, CA, USA

Donald H. Schreiber MD
Associate Professor,
Divison of Emergency Medicine,
Stanford University School of Medicine,
Stanford, CA, USA

Bill Schroeder DO
Clinical Instructor,
Division of Emergency Medicine,
Stanford University School of Medicine,
Palo Alto, CA, USA

Sangeeta Kaur Gill Schroeder MD
Clinical Instructor Pediatrics,
Lucile Packard Children's Hospital at Stanford,
Stanford University School of Medicine,
Stanford, CA, USA

Jamie Shandro MD MPH
Assistant Professor, Division of Emergency Medicine,
University of Washington School of Medicine,
Harborview Medical Center,
Seattle, WA, USA

Erik Shraga MD
Emergency Medicine Physician,
Mills-Peninsula Health Services,
Burlingame, CA, USA

Tamara D. Simon MD MSPH
Assistant Professor,
Pediatric Inpatient Medicine,

University of Utah School of Medicine,
Salt Lake City, UT, USA

Rebecca Smith-Coggins MD
Professor,
Division of Emergency Medicine,
Stanford University School of Medicine,
Palo Alto, CA, USA

Aparajita Sohoni MD
Attending Physician,
Alameda County Medical Center,
Oakland, CA, USA

Pimwan Sookplung MD
Prasat Neurological Institute,
Bangkok, Thailand

Matthew Strehlow MD
Clinical Assistant Professor,
Division of Emergency Medicine,
Stanford University School of Medicine,
Stanford, CA, USA

George Sternbach MD
Clinical Professor,
Division of Emergency Medicine,
Stanford University School of Medicine,
Stanford, CA, USA

Bryan L. Stone MD
Associate Professor,
Pediatrics,
University of Utah School of Medicine,
Salt Lake City, UT, USA

Gannon Sungar BA
College of Osteopathic Medicine,
Touro University-California,
Vallejo, CA, USA

Chere Taylor LASW
Stanford University Hospital and Clinics,
Stanford, CA, USA

David A. Townes MD MPH
Associate Professor,
Emergency Medicine,
University of Washington Medical Center,
Seattle, WA, USA

Claire Turchi MD
Clinical Instructor,
Division of Emergency Medicine,
Stanford University School of Medicine,
Palo Alto, CA, USA

Irma T. Ugalde MD
Pediatric Emergency Department Fellow,
UT Southwestern Medical Center,
Children's Medical Center,
Dallas, TX, USA

Theresa M. van der Vlugt MA MD
Emergency Physician,
Inova Fairfax Hospital and
Inova Fairfax Hospital for Children,
Falls Church, VA, USA; and Northwest Emergency
Physicians of Teamhealth, Bellingham, WA, USA

Monica S. Vavilala MD
Associate Professor,
Anesthesiology & Pain Medicine,
Pediatrics, and Neurological Surgery,
University of Washington/Harborview Medical Center,
Seattle, WA, USA

Pichaya Waitayawinyu MD
Assistant Professor, Anesthesiology,
Siriraj Hospital/Mahidol University,
Bangkok, Thailand

Eric C. Walter MD
Kaiser Permanente Northwest and Northwest
Permanente, PC Portland, OR, USA

Emily Wessler MD
Clinical Instructor, Pediatric Cardiology,
Lucile Packard Children's Hospital at Stanford,
Stanford University School of Medicine,
Palo Alto, CA, USA

Darrell M. Wilson MD
Professor, & Cheif,
Pediatric Endocrinology & Diabetes,
Lucile Packard Children's Hospital at Stanford,
Stanford University School of Medicine,
Stanford, CA, USA

Cynthia J. Wong MD
Assistant Professor, Nephrology,
Lucile Packard Children's Hospital at Stanford,
Stanford University School of Medicine,
Stanford, CA, USA

Wendy B. Wong MD
Clinical Assistant Professor,
Pediatric Hematology/Oncology,
Lucile Packard Children's Hospital at Stanford,
Stanford University School of Medicine,
Palo Alto, CA, USA

Teresa S. Wu MD
Director of Emergency Medicine Ultrasound,
and Co-Director of Simulation-Based
Training Program,
Maricopa Medical Center,
Phoenix, AZ, USA

Sophia Yen MD MPH
Clinical Instructor, Adolescent Medicine,
Lucile Packard Children's Hospital at Stanford,
Stanford University School of Medicine,
Stanford, CA, USA

Andrew S. Zeft MD MPH
Assistant Professor,
Pediatric Immunology and Rheumatology,
University of Utah School of Medicine,
Salt Lake City, UT, USA

Expert reviewers

Steven Alexander MD
Division Chief,
Professor of Pediatrics & Nephrology,
Lucile Packard Children's Hospital at Stanford,
Stanford University School of Medicine,
Stanford, CA, USA

Manuel Amieva MD PhD
Assistant Professor,
Pediatric Infectious Diseases,
Lucile Packard Children's Hospital at Stanford,
Stanford University School of Medicine,
Stanford, CA, USA

James P. Andrus MD
Associate Professor,
Pediatric Intensive Care,
Lucile Packard Children's Hospital at Stanford,
Stanford University School of Medicine,
Stanford, CA, USA

Dorsey M. Bass MD
Associate Professor,
Pediatric Gastroenterology,
Lucile Packard Children's Hospital at Stanford,
Stanford University School of Medicine,
Stanford, CA, USA

Tonya Chaffee MD MPH
Associate Clinical Professor, Pediatrics,
University of California,
San Francisco, CA, USA

Gary V. Dahl MD
Professor,
Department of Hematology & Oncology,
Lucille Packard Children's Hospital at Stanford,
Stanford University School of Medicine,
Stanford, CA, USA

Anne M. Dubin MD
Associate Professor,
Pediatric Cardiology,
Lucile Packard Children's Hospital at Stanford,
Stanford University School of Medicine,
Stanford, CA, USA

Michael S. B. Edwards MD
Professor,
Pediatric Neurosurgery,
Lucile Packard Children's Hospital at Stanford,
Stanford University School of Medicine,
Stanford, CA, USA

Nikta Forghani MD
Clinical Instructor, Pediatric Endocrinology,
University of California,
Irvine, Orange, CA, USA

Hayley A. Gans MD
Associate Professor,
Pediatric Infectious Diseases,
Lucile Packard Children's Hospital at Stanford,
Stanford University School of Medicine,
Stanford, CA, USA

Bertil Glader MD PhD
Professor,
Pediatric Hematology/Oncology,
Lucile Packard Children's Hospital at Stanford,
Stanford University School of Medicine,
Stanford, CA, USA

Paul C. Grimm MD
Professor,
Pediatrics-Nephrology,
Lucile Packard Children's Hospital at Stanford,
Stanford University School of Medicine,
Stanford, CA, USA

Arun Gupta MD
Clinical Assistant Professor, Neonatology,
Lucile Packard Children's Hospital at Stanford,
Stanford University School of Medicine,
Stanford, CA, USA

Kathleen M. Gutierrez MD
Assistant Professor,
Pediatric Infectious Disease,
Lucile Packard Children's Hospital at Stanford,
Stanford University School of Medicine,
Stanford, CA, USA

Jin S. Hahn MD
Professor of Neurology,
Neurological Sciences,
Pediatrics and Neurosurgery,
Lucile Packard Children's Hospital at Stanford,
Stanford University School of Medicine,
Stanford, CA, USA

Andrew Man-Lap Ho MD PhD
Division of Orthopedic Surgery,
Sacramento Veterans Affairs Medical Center,
Mather, CA, USA

James Holmes Jr. MD MPH
Professor,
Emergency Medicine,
UC Davis School of Medicine,
Sacramento, CA, USA

Shashank V. Joshi MD
Assistant Professor,
Psychiatry and Behavioral Medicine,
Stanford University School of Medicine,
Stanford, CA, USA

William A. Kennedy II MD
Associate Professor,
Department of Urology,
Lucile Packard Children's Hospital at Stanford,
Stanford University School of Medicine,
Stanford, CA, USA

Janice Lowe MD
Clinical Professor,
Pediatrics,
Lucille Packard Children's Hospital at Stanford,
Stanford University School of Medicine,
Stanford, CA, USA

Brian Su-Chieh Lui DDS MS
Pediatric Dentist,
Palo Alto, CA, USA

Anna Messner MD
Professor,
Otolaryngology, Head & Neck Surgery,
Lucile Packard Children's Hospital at Stanford,
Stanford University School of Medicine,
Palo Alto, CA, USA

Claudia Mueller MD
Assistant Professor, Pediatric Surgery,
Lucile Packard Children's Hospital at Stanford,
Stanford University School of Medicine,
Stanford, CA, USA

Anand Rajani MD
Fellow, Neonatology,
Lucile Packard Children's Hospital at Stanford,
Stanford University School of Medicine,
Stanford, CA, USA

Emily Wessler MD
Clinical Instructor, Pediatric Cardiology,
Lucile Packard Children's Hospital at Stanford,
Stanford University School of Medicine,
Stanford, CA, USA

Darrell M. Wilson MD
Professor,
Pediatric Endocrinology & Diabetes,
Lucile Packard Children's Hospital at Stanford,
Stanford University School of Medicine,
Stanford, CA, USA

Wendy B. Wong MD
Clinical Assistant Professor,
Pediatric Hematology/Oncology,
Lucile Packard Children's Hospital at Stanford,
Stanford University School of Medicine,
Stanford, CA, USA

Sophia Yen MD MPH
Clinical Instructor,
Adolescent Medicine,
Lucile Packard Children's Hospital at Stanford,
Stanford University School of Medicine,
Stanford, CA, USA

Foreword

Let's face it; it is tough evaluating and managing children in the emergency department (ED). Often the patients cannot provide a history of illness or injury, and there are potential congenital issues which can complicate evaluation and management. Also, the types of conditions they present with change with age, growth and development. Having trained as an emergency physician and seeing adult and pediatric patients over the last 27 years of my career I can say that "A Practical Guide to Pediatric Emergency Medicine" is a welcome addition to the reference texts in pediatric emergency medicine. It provides practical information that builds on what an emergency physician already knows about the care of children. The book starts out with a wonderful quick summary of many of the common pediatric specific diseases/conditions affecting children in an easy to read set of tables. Dr. Ewen Wang and colleagues then cover the breadth of pediatric emergency medicine in the book's well illustrated 29 sections, but does so with an approach that is refreshing. The authors focus on the unique conditions that affect children and provide much needed practical advice for management in children in the ED. Expert reviews of each of the sections provide enhanced content that boosts the depth as well as the practical knowledge found in each chapter. For example – in the cardiology section, readers will learn tips and techniques in reading a pediatric ECG, learn about congenital heart disease and the complications of repairs of those lesions, and even learn about the special issues with children post heart transplant. My favorite feature is "The Tutorials" which cover much needed procedural education in diverse aspects of care, such as needle cricothyrotomy and jet ventilation, mechanical ventilation management, intraosseous and umbilical vein catheter placement, fluid and electrolyte management, eFAST and FAST for trauma, ultrasound guided procedures, pediatric radiology interpretation, and splinting to name a few; it even has a discussion on practical aspects of care of the "gizmos" such as VP-shunt (obstruction/infection), G-and J-tubes (leakage, wound infection, hemorrhage, dislodgement, and obstruction), trachesotomy tubes (displacement and obstruction), and genitourinary/gastrointestinal conduits. It contains just the right amount of information to manage patients in the ED, and also provides tutorials on important aspects of outpatient care (e.g. management of outpatient asthma from the emergency department) that will assist the ED physician in bridging care of the patient to the next follow-up visit.

Cambridge University Press and Drs Wang, Shandro, Sohoni and Fassl have succeeded in producing a different kind of textbook; one that works for the practicing "ER" doctor.

Bravo!

Enjoy reading and using in your practice "A Practical Guide to Pediatric Emergency Medicine".

Marianne Gausche-Hill, MD, FACEP, FAAP
Professor of Medicine,
David Geffen School of Medicine at UCLA
Director of EMS and Pediatric Emergency Medicine Fellowships
Harbor-UCLA Medical Center,
Department of Emergency Medicine
Torrance, CA

Preface

This manual is written for the emergency medicine practitioner who cares for children as well as adults. It is not designed to replace any of the many definitive references in emergency medicine or pediatric emergency medicine but rather to fit a special niche focusing on those who juggle the balance of caring for children alongside adults.

For the physician who takes care of adults and children simultaneously in an emergency department (ED) setting, it can be challenging to change medical perspective as one switches patient rooms. For example, the differential diagnosis and workup for a neonate with a seizure is very different to that for a 40 year old with the same chief complaint. Additionally, there are unusual but pediatric specific conditions, such as Kawasaki disease and Henoch–Schönlein purpura, whose constellation of symptoms may elude the emergency medicine provider. This can result in a diagnosis being missed. Given the range of ages, developmental stages, sizes, and vital signs included in the pediatric realm of emergency medicine, it might be handy to have a reference that can remind the physician of age-based differential diagnoses and specifically highlights differences between children and adults.

In this age of medical and technological advancements, children are also surviving previously lethal congenital anomalies and inherited conditions. Populations of "children with special health care needs" have distinct medical issues and technological needs, which are constantly evolving. The emergency provider must be trained and equipped to recognize urgent and emergent medical problems in children with inborn errors of metabolism, congenital heart disease repair, or other chronic illnesses. Similarly, children who are recipients of advances in technology, be it tracheostomies, home ventilators, or gastrostromy tubes, may come in with equipment problems or malfunctions that must be identified and treated.

This manual is not meant to be a definitive reference for pediatric emergency medicine. Rather, a basic knowledge of emergency medicine is assumed to allow emphasis on areas where children and adults differ. Each chapter emphasizes the age-based differential diagnosis and areas where treatment of a disease entity differs from an adult. There are also at the end of each chapter a list of pearls and pitfalls. The manual includes many high-quality photographs, diagrams, and figures. The dermatology and infectious disease sections, which compare common childhood rashes graphically and visually, are unique.

There are special sections on specific pediatric populations: neonates, adolescents, and children with special health care needs, including children with cerebral palsy or genetic diseases, children graduating from the neonatal intensive care unit, and technology-dependent children.

Tutorials in pediatric imaging, pediatric ECG interpretation, procedural sedation, and procedures offer in-depth study of pediatric-specific skills. We hope that this manual provides a resource for busy practitioners caring for both children and adults, reminding us of the many ways in which children are unique and the specific considerations we must have when caring for children in our EDs.

Ten ways children are different from adults.

1. Kids are smaller and they grow
2. Kids metamorphose from aquatic to terrestrial creatures in an instant (sometimes in the ED)
3. Child's equipment is first use; congenital anomalies manifest in early childhood.
4. Kids have a different anatomy from adults
5. Kids have a different physiology than adults
6. Kids are infected by different bugs at different ages
7. Kids act like kids
8. Kids speak a different language
9. Kids usually belong to an adult
10. In general, we are kinder to children.

Acknowledgements

We would like to acknowledge the entire Emergency Medicine Division faculty at Stanford for their unwavering belief and confidence in our vision. We would particularly like to thank Drs. Robert Norris, Bernard Dannenberg (EW) and Chris Maloney (BF) for their unconditional support and encouragement. Several colleagues and friends went beyond the call of duty to offer advice; write chapters; and to locate experts, photographs, and contributors, including Drs. Paul Auerbach, Gus Garmel, Mike Gisondi, S. V. Mahadevan, and Matthew Strehlow.

We want to acknowledge our expert reviewers, including Drs. Anand Rajani and James P. Andrus (neonatal and pediatric critical care), Anne Dubin and Emily Wessler (cardiology), Su-Chieh Brian Liu (dental), Anna Messner (ENT), Darrell M. Wilson (endocrine), Steven Alexander (FEN and renal), Dorsey Bass and Claudia Mueller (gastroenterology), Janice Lowe and Arun Gupta (general pediatrics), Bertil E. Glader and Gary V. Dahl (hematology and oncology), Hayley Gans (immunology), Kathleen M. Gutierrez and Manuel Amieva (infectious disease), Andrew Man-Lap Ho (hand), Jin Hahn (neurology), Tonya Chaffee (child abuse), Shashank Joshi (psychiatry), James Holmes (trauma), Michael S. B. Edwards (neurosurgery), and William A. Kennedy II (renal, genitourinal trauma, and urology). All these subspecialists were "curb-sided" shamelessly to review each subspecialty chapter. We are grateful to all of our contributors, particularly the subspecialists and experts who do not usually write from an EM perspective.

We want to give special thanks to Dr. Marianne Gausche-Hill for writing the Preface and Raymond Johnson for reviewing the book. Manuel Amieva went out of his way to take photographs for the cover and to create its design. Others who contributed invaluable images include Drs. Hans Kersten, S. V. Mahadevan, Paul Matz, Mehran Mosley, Steven Shpall, and Anne Strehlow. Dr. Inger Olson contributed vital pediatric electrocardiographs to the text. I want to thank Logical Images and especially Heidi Halton who cheerfully and rapidly provided the last 11 images needed to complete the book. Chris Gralappe, Lynne Larson, and Chris Miles added clarity to the book with their crisp and clear illustrations. Colleen Acosta retrieved, copied and edited images.

We are indebted to Kelly Lazkani, and Dolly Kagawa for their generous and invaluable administrative assistance in the USA. Without the hard and painstakingly detailed work of Katherine Tengco, Nisha Doshi, Joanna Chamberlin, and Caroline Mowatt at CUP, this book would never have become a reality. The careful copyediting of Jane Ward transformed this mass of text into a book. The indexing skills of Jeanette Dennison has made accessing the information in this text possible. We are also indebted to the professionalism, dedication and perspective of Nicholas Dunton and Deborah Russell, our editors at Cambridge University Press.

Abbreviations

AAP	American Academy of Pediatrics
ABC	airways, breathing, and circulation
ACE	angiotensin-converting enzyme
ACTH	adrenocorticotropic hormone
AIDS	acquired immunodeficiency syndrome
ALOC	altered level of consciousness
ALT	alanine transaminase (aminotransferase)
AST	aspartate transaminase (aminotransferase)
BID	twice daily
bpm	beats per minute
BUN	blood urea nitrogen
CBC	complete blood count
CDC	US Centers for Disease Control and Prevention
CMV	cytomegalovirus
CNS	central nervous system
CRP	C-reactive protein
CSF	cerebrospinal fluid
CT	computed tomography
ECG	electrocardiography/electrocardiogram
ED	emergency department
ENT	ear, nose, and throat
EP	emergency physician
ESR	erythrocyte sedimentation rate
FDA	US Food and Drug Administration
GI	gastrointestinal
HIV	human immunodeficiency virus
HSV	herpes simplex virus
ICU	intensive care unit
IM	intramuscular
INR	international normalized ratio
IO	intraosseous
IV	intravenous
LFT	liver function test
max.	maximum
min.	minimum
MRI	magnetic resonance imaging
NSAIDs	non-steroidal anti-inflammatory drugs
$PaCO_2$	arterial partial pressure carbon dioxide
PaO_2	arterial partial pressure oxygen
PCR	polymerase chain reaction
PO	oral
PT	prothrombin time
PTT	partial thromboplastin time
q.	every
QID	four times a day
QTc	corrected QT interval
RLQ	right lower quadrant
RUQ	right upper quadrant
SC	subcutaneous (administration route)
TID	three times a day
ULN	upper limit of normal
WBC	white blood cell count
WHO	World Health Organization

Pediatric-specific disease

N. Ewen Amieva-Wang

There is a small but important subset of disorders that are pediatric specific. The physician who cares for adults and children must keep these more unusual diagnoses within the differential when caring for children. Some of these disorders are secondary to differences in susceptibility to infection, and physiologic and anatomic development. Neonates and young children can also have congenital disease manifesting with first use of malformed anatomy (e.g., tracheoesophageal fistula), time (e.g., ductal-dependent congenital heart disease), and stress (e.g., inborn error of metabolism).

Tables 1 and 2 are not meant to be a comprehensive list of pediatric-specific disorders, more a list of the more "common" diseases, as well as the organ system they affect, the age range, and symptoms.

Table 1 Neonatal disease

Disease	Organ system	Age range	Symptoms	Comments
Choanal atresia (bilateral; p. 000)	Respiratory	From birth	Cyanosis with feeding; resolution with crying	Neonate is an obligate mouth breather
Tracheo-esophageal fistula	Respiratory/GI	From birth	Choking with feeds	Symptoms depend on location and extent of fistula
Vascular sling/ web	Respiratory	4–8 months (variable)	Inspiratory stridor	Can be asymptomatic until mild upper respiratory disease; misdiagnosed as croup
Congenital heart disease: ductal-dependent lesion ?tet spell?	Circulatory	<1 week	Shock, cyanosis, respiratory distress	Timing will depend on severity of lesion
Necrotizing enterocolitis	GI	Weeks	Abdominal distention, discomfort, and shock	Although usually occurs in premature infants, up to 10% of cases occurs in term neonates
Pyloric stenosis	GI	2–5 weeks	Projectile vomiting of milk (no bile)	Classically occurs in first-born males, can be familial
Intestinal malrotation ± volvulus	GI	50% diagnosed in first month of life; majority in first year	Vomiting of bile, abdominal distention, and ultimately shock	Must be diagnosis of exclusion in a vomiting neonate
Intussusception	GI	3 months to 3 years; often after mild viral infection	Abdominal pain (colicky), distension and later currant-jelly stools, shock; can manifest with altered level of consciousness	Most common cause of intestinal obstruction in children Thought secondary to Peyer's patch hyperplasia; if diagnosed in adult, should prompt workup for malignancy

Table 1 *(cont.)*

Disease	Organ system	Age range	Symptoms	Comments
Neonatal herpes	ID	<6 weeks	Severe sepsis (<1 week); skin and mucous membrane disease (2–4 weeks); herpes encephalitis (2–3 weeks)	Perinatal infection; acquired maternal infection may not be apparent Sepsis and encephalitis can manifest without skin lesions Skin and mucous membrane disease can be controlled with radiotherapy
Opthalmalgia neonatorum	ID/eyes	2–4 weeks	Purulent conjunctivitis	*Neisseria meningitidis* ophthalmic infection can cause blindness
Congenital adrenal hyperplasia	Endocrine	2–4 weeks	Vomiting, dehydration, shock Virilized female genitalia	
Kernicterus	Hematological/ neurological	Neonates	Untreated severe jaundice	Guidelines for phototherapy depend on risk factors of neonate as well as age and bilirubin level

GI, gastrointestinal; ID, infectious disease.

Table 2 Pediatric-specific disease

Disease	Organ system	Age range	Symptoms	Comments
Laryngotracheal bronchitis	Respiratory/ID	3 months to 6 years	Inspiratory stridor/barking	Usually outgrown by age 5 years
Popsickle panniculitis	Dermatological	Infants/ toddlers	Tender plaques or nodules on cold exposed areas	Resolve in months; no treatment
Infant botulism	ID	<1 year	Hypotonia, constipation, respiratory insufficiency	High index of suspicion necessary Exposure usually respiratory
Kawasaki disease	Immune/ID	6 months	Generalized inflammation with fever, rash (non-vessinular), non-purulent conjunctivitis, mouth changes, extremity changes, lymphadenopathy	Atypical Kawasaki disease can occur outside typical age range Most common form of acquired heart disease in children
Hemolytic uremic syndrome	Immune/renal	Peak incidence in children <5 years	Microangiopathic hemolytic anemia, thrombocytopenia, and AKI	Similar pathophysiology to TTP in adults Kidney disease more common in children whereas neurologic disease is more common in adults
Henoch–Schönlein purpura	Immune/ dermatological/ GI	2–6 years	Abdominal pain, palpable purpura, arthritis, renal involvement	Most common systemic vasculitis in children
Cerebral edema associated with diabetic ketoacidosis	Endocrine	<18 years	Cerebral edema with severe diabetic ketoacidosis	Occurs in ~1% of diabetic ketoacidosis and causes the majority of deaths from diabetic ketoacidosis
Acute cerebellar ataxia	Neurological	Toddlers	Isolated ataxia after viral prodrome	Self-limited disease; diagnosis of exclusion
Febrile seizure	Neurological	6 months to 6 years	Seizure when febrile	Strong familial history; risk of epilspsy is <5%

Table 2 *(cont.)*

Disease	Organ system	Age range	Symptoms	Comments
Torus, greenstick fractures, Salter–Harris (physeal) fractures	Musculoskeletal	Prior to closure of the physis	Pain and sometimes deformity	Usually good prognosis; can be difficult to reduce greenstick fractures
Avulsion fractures	Musculoskeletal	Adolescents	Severe pain with activity	
Apophyseal injury (tibeal apophysitis (Osgood–Schlatter disease), calcaneal apophysitis (Sever's disease))	Musculoskeletal	10–15 years of age with increased activity, overuse	Pain with activity	Treated with rest and reduced activity
Physeal, epiphyseal, injury; slipped capital femoral epiphysis	Musculoskeletal	Classically large boys 10–16 years of age	Pain in hip or knee; onset can be insidious and chronic	Non-weight bearing and possible surgical fixation
"Toddlers fracture," spiral fracture of distal tibula	Musculoskeletal	Toddler	Refusal to bear weight, limp	Manage with immobilization even if fracture not visualized
Legg–Calvé–Perthes disease (avascular necrosis of hip)	Musculoskeletal	4–12 years of age	Pain in hip or knee; onset can be insidious and chronic	Non-weight bearing and possible surgical fixation
Nursemaid's elbow (radial head subluxation)	Musculoskeletal	<6 years of age, with traction of the elbow	Refusal to move the forearm; no apparent pain at rest	Can recur with repeated traction

AKI, acute kidney injury; ID, infectious diseases; TTP, thrombotic thrombocytopenic purpura.

Section 1

Resuscitation

Expert reviewers: James P. Andrus and Anand Rajani

Chapter 1 Airway, breathing, and ventilation

N. Ewen Amieva-Wang

Introduction

While resuscitation concepts and priorities are the same for children and adults, the situation of a pediatric code is quite different. An acute life-threatening medical emergency in a child is usually unexpected and a child can often be resuscitated with the expectation of full recovery. Appropriate airway management is vital since hypoxia is the most common cause of cardiac arrest in children. Pragmatically, the need for varying sized equipment and weight-based dosing can cause confusion, delay, and mistakes.

This section will discuss the anatomic and physiologic differences between the pediatric and adult airway and apply these to principles of airway management. We discuss rapid sequence intubation (RSI) and rescue airway measures as well as special pediatric cases that may present airway management difficulties.

Assessment of respiratory status

A child may be too young to declare shortness of breath. Pediatric vital signs should be compared with age-related normal values. Pulse oximetry is a fifth vital sign and useful in monitoring oxygenation, not ventilation. Capnography is being increasingly used to identify situations of decreased ventilation.

Observation is the most accurate method to identify respiratory distress. Tachypnea is the initial compensatory mechanism for preserving minute ventilation. Chest rise or abdominal excursions also reveal the adequacy of the patient's respirations. Snoring or stridor indicates upper airway obstruction; wheezes indicate lower airway obstruction. Retractions (supraclavicular, subcostal, or abdominal), as well as grunting and nasal flaring can be subtle but significant signs of increased work of breathing. Overall general appearance – posture, level of alertness or responsiveness – and indications from other organ systems such as the central nervous system (CNS) (lethargy, agitation, or other altered mental status) and skin (pallor, cyanosis, or delayed capillary refill) will contribute to recognition of respiratory distress and impending respiratory failure in a child.

The pediatric airway

Anatomy

The pediatric airway is usually a different, rather than a difficult, airway. The differences are most pronounced in infants, and decrease with growth so that the airway in an 8-year-old child is considered similar to an adult's airway (Fig. 1.1). These anatomical differences result in different management techniques (Table 1.1).

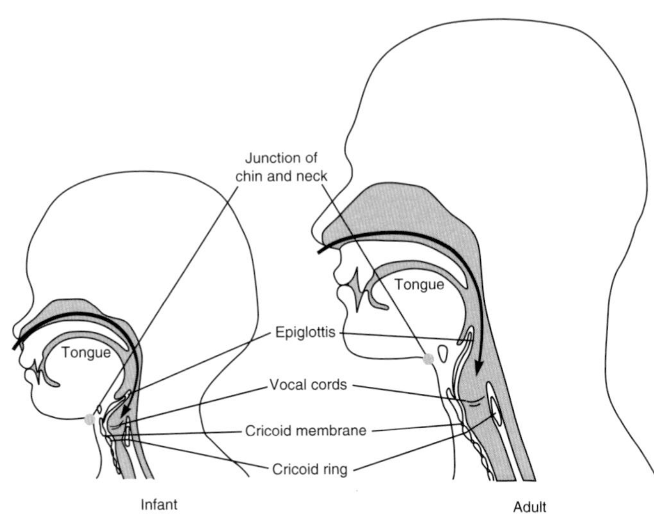

Figure 1.1 Anatomic airway differences between children and adults. Features that are distinct to the child are: higher, more anterior position for the glottic opening in a child (note the relationship of the vocal cords to the chin–neck junction); relatively larger tongue in the infant, which lies between the mouth and glottic opening; relatively larger and more floppy epiglottis in the child; cricoid ring is the narrowest portion of the pediatric airway whereas the vocal cords are in the adult; position and size of the cricothyroid membrane differs between infant and adult; sharper, more difficult angle for blind nasotracheal intubation in the child; larger relative size of the occiput in the infant. (Reproduced with permission from Walls RM, Murphy MF, Luten RC, *et al. Manual of Emergency Airway Management*, 3rd edn. Philadelphia, PA: Lippincott Williams & Wilkins, 2008.)

A Practical Guide to Pediatric Emergency Medicine: Caring for Children in the Emergency Department, ed. N. Ewen Amieva-Wang (associate eds. Jamie Shandro, Aparajita Sohoni, and Bernhard Fassl). Published by Cambridge University Press.

Table 1.1. Unique characteristics of pediatric airway anatomy and its consequences in airway management

Pediatric anatomic feature	Airway management significance	Airway management adjustment
Large head, short neck	Neutral cervical spine position/sniffing position difficult to achieve	Shoulder roll or elevation of head
Nares smaller; infants up to 6 months of age are obligate nasal breathers	Small nares cause increased resistance to airflow particularly when narrowed by secretions	Avoid accidental compression of nares with bag-valve mask, which can cause significant respiratory obstruction
Small mouth, large soft tissue structures	Less space for laryngoscope blade and airway visualization	Use of smaller straight laryngoscope blade
Large tongue	Most common cause of airway obstruction is the tongue	Use of chin lift maneuvers and airway adjuncts (nasopharyngeal, oropharyngeal)
Large adenoids	Potential for bleeding and soft tissue obstruction	Blind nasotracheal intubation contraindicated in children <9 years Oropharyngeal airway should not be initially inserted upside down and turned
Anterior and cephalad airway	Acute angle between epiglottis and anterior glottic opening makes nasotracheal intubation difficult	Alignment of different airway axes is often better accomplished with a straight blade than a curved blade
Long floppy epiglottis	Epiglottis can block visualization of the airway	Straight blade, with a narrower tip can be used to lift it out of the way
Cricoid ring is narrowest part of pediatric airway	Failure to get good compliance and seal with uncuffed endotracheal tube	Gently inflated cuffed endotracheal tube can be used to decrease air leak and improve ventilation
Pediatric airway smaller and shorter and delicate	Pediatric airway more prone to obstruction, compression; right main stem intubation and tube dislodgement are more common	Vigilance with tube placement and confirmation, particularly with transfer of child
Chest wall pliability	Children can have increased lung parenchymal damage with few outward signs	Increased index of suspicion for lung injury in the setting of trauma
Diaphragm is the main muscle of breathing	Abdominal trauma and distention can cause or contribute to severe respiratory compromise	Placement of nasogastric and orogastric tubes with airway management as bag-valve mask can cause abdominal distention
Small cricothyroid membrane	Cricothyroidotomy contraindicated in children <8 years of age	Needle cricothyroidotomy can be used as an airway rescue technique

The oropharyngeal soft tissues are proportionately larger and have less tone in children than in adults, resulting in less space for manipulation inside the child's mouth. The tongue is the main cause of airway obstruction in the child. During infancy, the larynx is at the level of C1 and descends to the level of C4–C5 in the adult. This, coupled with the child's more anterior airway, changes the axes needed for alignment of the oropharynx and larynx during direct laryngoscopic intubation (Fig. 1.2). In an infant, the straight laryngoscope blade is better able to align these axes, and is also thinner and fits better into the mouth. The thinner tip of the straight blade also helps to elevate the floppy epiglottis out of the visual field.

The tongue is the main cause of airway obstruction in a child. If unable to use a bag-valve mask (BVM), use naso- and or oropharyngeal airways as adjuncts.

The narrowest portion of the pediatric airway is the cricoid cartilage, while the adult airway narrows at the level of the cords and then widens. Historically, uncuffed endotracheal tubes (ETT) have been recommended in children <8 years of age. Recently, ETT with uninflated or lightly inflated cuffs as well as new cuffed ETTs developed for children are more frequently recommended for pediatric intubation, particularly during resuscitation.

The large infant occiput can cause passive flexion of the cervical spine and subsequent compression of the pharyngeal airway. Consequently, an infant must be kept in the "sniffing position" to maintain cervical spine protection and open the airway (Fig. 1.2B). Overextension of the neck should be avoided to ensure optimal visualization of the cords. Since the child's vocal cords are more antero-caudally angled than in an adult, the vocal cords can be difficult to visualize during intubation if the child's head is not in an anatomical position. The pediatric trachea is smaller in diameter and length, and is more pliable and compressible than the adult airway. The infant's trachea is approximately 5 cm long and grows to 7 cm by 18 months. Failure to take the

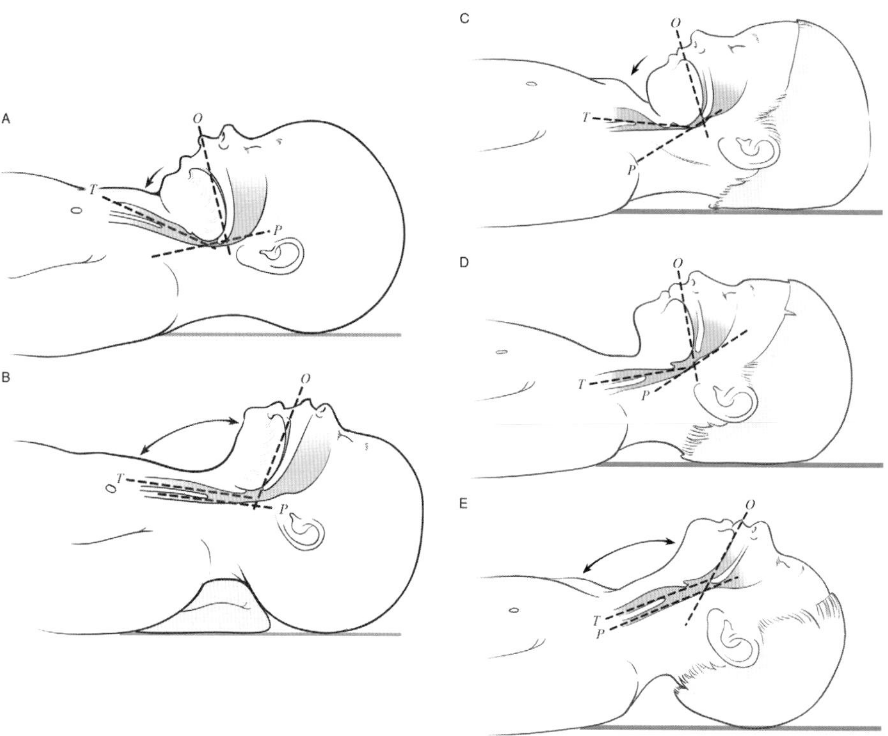

Figure 1.2 Comparison of infant and child positioning for ventilation and endotracheal intubation. (A) Incorrect infant positioning with neck flexion. (B) Correct infant positioning (also known as sniffing position) with oral (O), pharyngeal (P) and tracheal (T) axes aligned. (C) Incorrect child positioning with neck flexion and divergent axes. (D) Improved positioning with increased alignment of the pharyngeal and tracheal axes. (E) Increased extension causes maximal alignment of the axes. (Copyright Chris Gralapp.)

short length of an infant's trachea into account can result in right main-stem intubation, tube dislodgement, or mechanical barotrauma. The angle between the epiglottis and the larynx is more acute than in the adult patient and is difficult to maneuver. Blind nasotracheal intubation is contraindicated in young children because manipulation can cause trauma and bleeding of the oropharyngeal soft tissues. Cricothyroidotomy is contraindicated in children <8 years of age because the cricothyroid membrane is very small, difficult to palpate and incise (Fig. 1.3).

The diaphragm and abdominal wall musculature – the major respiratory muscles in a child – are underdeveloped and fatigue more quickly than in adults. Abdominal trauma or distention can impede these muscles and cause respiratory distress. Crying and BVM can lead to stomach inflation and increases the risk of aspiration while decreasing tidal volume. It is important to place a nasogastric or orogastric tube after definitive airway management.

Physiology

Children have smaller lung volumes and higher oxygen demands than adults. They also deplete their respiratory reserves more quickly than in adults. Hypoxia is poorly tolerated because of their baseline increased metabolic rate and increased cerebral blood flow. Children also have increased oral secretions and vagal tone compared with adults. Historically, this has led to the dictum of pretreatment with atropine to avoid bradycardia with laryngeal manipulation. Recent evidence has questioned this practice and atropine may not be required for all pediatric patients.

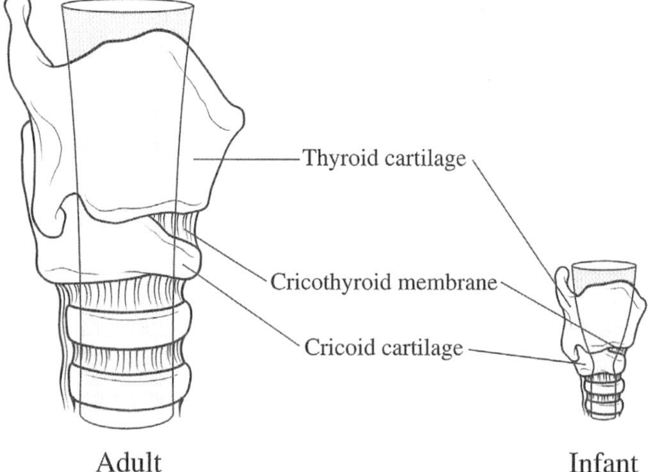

Figure 1.3 Comparison of infant and adult airway shape. The narrowest portion of the pediatric airway is the cricoid ring, whereas in the adult the narrowest portion is the vocal cords. The pediatric airway is funnel shaped but the adult is cylindrical. (Reproduced with permission Walls RM, Murphy MF, Luten RC, *et al. Manual of Emergency Airway Management*, 3rd edn. Philadelphia, PA: Lippincott Williams & Wilkins, 2008.)

Equipment

Medication dosing for children has been fraught with error, and color-coded, length-based resuscitation systems have been demonstrated to decrease medication errors as well as increase response time in emergency situations.

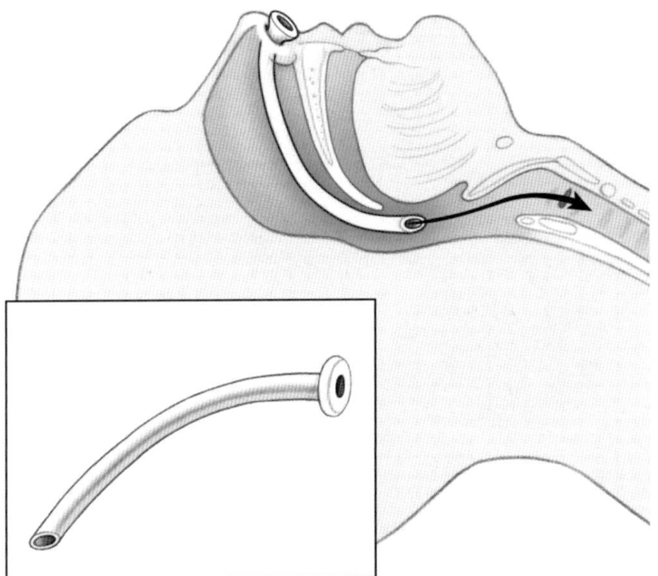

Figure 1.4 Nasopharyngeal airway. (Copyright Chris Gralapp; reproduced with permission from Mahadevan SV, Garmel GM. *An Introduction to Clinical Emergency Medicine.* Cambridge, UK: Cambridge University Press, 2005.)

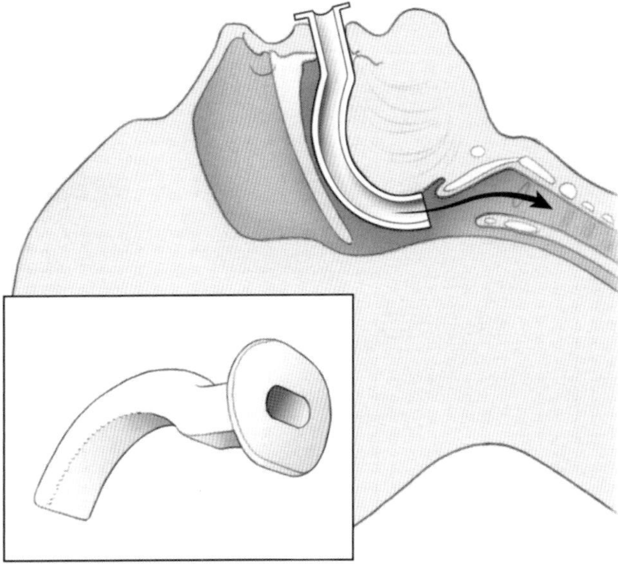

Figure 1.5 Oropharyngeal airway. (Copyright Chris Gralapp; reproduced with permission from Mahadevan and Garmel, 2005.)

Oxygen delivery adjuncts

Nasal cannula

Nasal cannula is acceptable for children who require minimal oxygen supplementation. The concentration of oxygen delivered can be unpredictable, and high flow can be upsetting to young children. A flow rate of <3–5 l/min is usually tolerated. Nasal prongs should be trimmed in small children.

Oxygen face mask

Oxygen flow rates should be set at 10 l/min to deliver 30–60% oxygen concentration and to prevent rebreathing of exhaled gas.

Non-rebreather oxygen mask

The non-rebreather masks are attached to a reservoir bag with an oxygen source. Most systems have a one-way valve to the reservoir bag to prevent exhaled gas from entering the reservoir. The oxygen flow rate should be 6–10 l/min (greater than the child's minute volume) and the reservoir bag must be larger than the patient's tidal volume and should stay inflated. Non-rebreather masks can deliver 60–90% oxygen concentration.

Airway adjuncts

Nasal airway

The nasal airway is for children who are conscious or semiconscious with a partially obstructed airway. An appropriately sized nasopharyngeal airway extends from the tip of the nose to the tragus of the ear, with the outside diameter smaller than the inner diameter of the nostril (Fig. 1.4).

Oral airway

The oral airway is used in unconscious children with airway obstruction. It is contraindicated in conscious children since it can trigger a gag reflex. An appropriately sized oral airway extends from the incisors to just anterior to the angle of the mandible. If the oral airway is too small, the tongue can be pushed into the pharynx, thus increasing airway obstruction. Place the oral airway by depressing the tongue with a tongue blade. (Fig. 1.5).

Ventilation assistance

Bag-valve mask

The BVM consists of a mask, valve, and bag that entrains room air between valve and mask but should be attached to an oxygen reservoir. The masks should be transparent and extend from the bridge of the nose to just under the mouth without compressing the eyes or extending over the edge of the chin. The BVMs used in the ED are usually self-inflating.

Laryngeal mask airways

The laryngeal mask airways can be used as a life-saving bridge to a definitive airway in children who cannot be ventilated effectively with the BVM; however, they do not provide protection from aspiration.

Intubation equipment

The ETT size can be calculated using the following formula:

uncuffed tracheal tube size (mm) $=$ (Age in years $+$ 16)/4

cuffed tracheal tube size (mm) $=$ Age in years $+$ 16/3

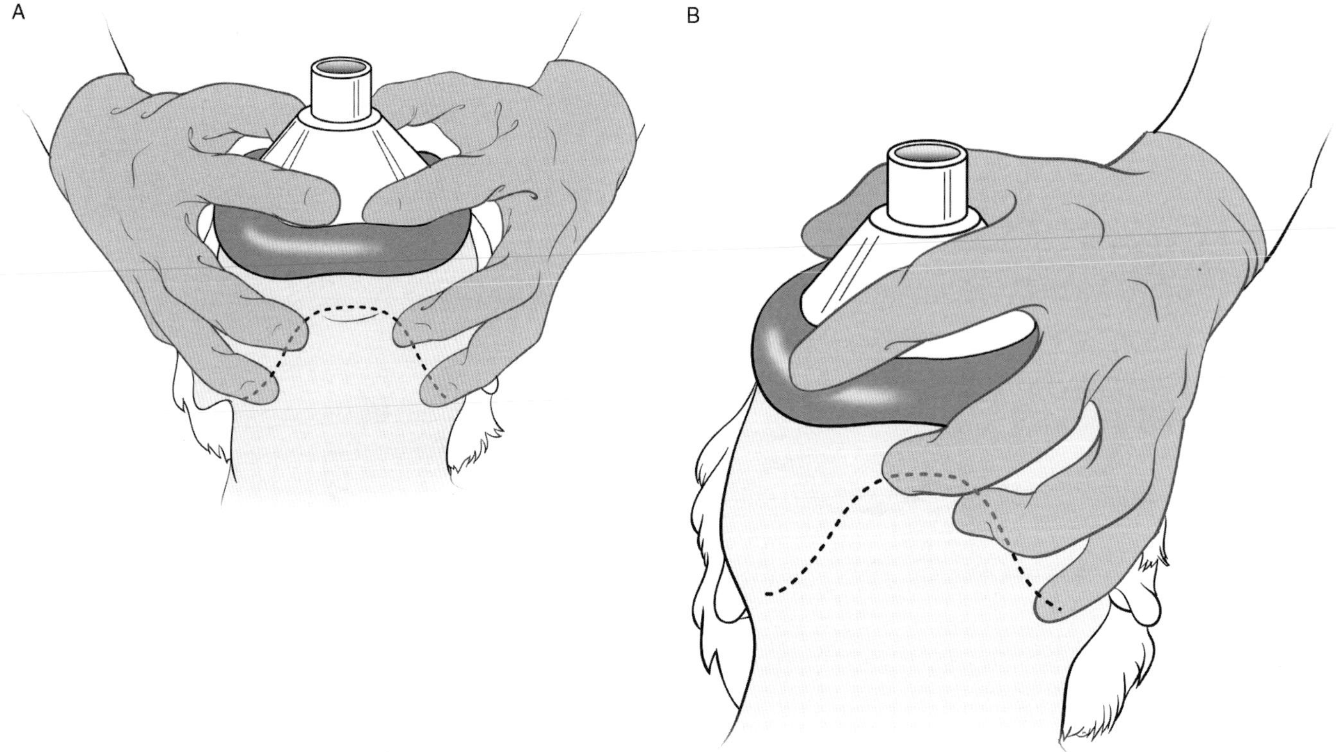

Figure 1.6 The EC technique for use of a bag-valve mask. The thumb and index finger form a "C" shape over the mask, with the third, fourth and fifth digits forming an "E" along the jaw line. (A) Two-handed technique. (B) One-handed technique. (Copyright Chris Gralapp.)

Most ETT have a mark that indicates the length at which the tube should have passed the vocal cords. The appropriate ETT depth of insertion can be calculated by the formula:

$$\text{ETT depth (cm)} = 3 \times \text{ ETT size}$$

Laryngoscope blades

Straight blades are easier to insert in the child's small mouth and can lift the relatively large and floppy epiglottis of infants. However, it can be difficult to retract the large, sometimes slippery tongue with the thinner, straight blade. Although the curved laryngoscope blade is larger and bulkier than the straight blade, it retracts the tongue more easily and may be useful in pediatric populations when the tongue is larger than usual.

Suction devices

Yankauer suction is necessary to clear anticipated and unanticipated blood and secretions.

Breathing and ventilation

If spontaneous ventilation and breathing are not adequate, children need assistance. Well-performed BVM ventilation can be life-saving and can temporize a situation until intubation is possible. The majority of children can be ventilated effectively with BVM, although complications include gastric distention and aspiration.

Because of the relative size of an adult's hand to a child's neck, it can be easy to accidentally cause further obstruction of the airway by applying pressure to the child's neck. The optimal method to hold the mask is to place the index finger on the mask, the middle finger on the chin, and the ring and little finger on the bony angle of the mandible (EC method) (Fig. 1.6).

Self-inflating BVM devices will not deliver oxygen unless squeezed. Tidal volumes set from 5–8 ml/kg in infants and children will mimic spontaneous breathing. Although most BVM devices have a pop-off valve to limit the amount of pressure that can be exerted manually on the child's airway, the potential for iatrogenic bronchoalveolar injury or pneumothorax from overexuberant ventilation exists. If BVM ventilation cannot be achieved, the airway should be repositioned. If jaw thrust or chin lift are not successful in relieving the airway obstruction (Figs. 1.7 and 1.8), an airway adjunct such as an oral and or nasal airway may be key in achieving successful BVM ventilation.

Intubation

The overall goal of emergency airway management is the same for children as for adults: (1) to supply supplementary oxygen, (2) to support ventilation, (3) to provide a secure patent

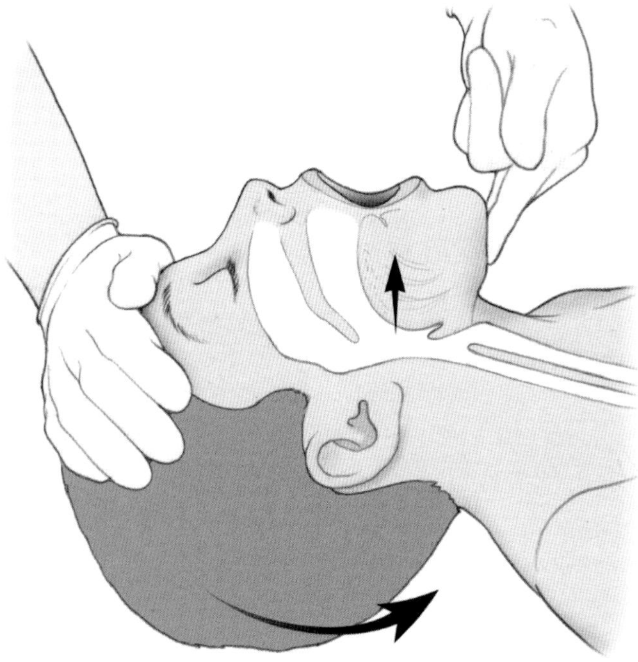

Figure 1.7 Head tilt with chin lift. This maneuver should not be used in trauma situations. (Copyright Chris Gralapp; reproduced with permission from Mahadevan SV, Garmel GM. *An Introduction to Clinical Emergency Medicine.* Cambridge, UK: Cambridge University Press, 2005.)

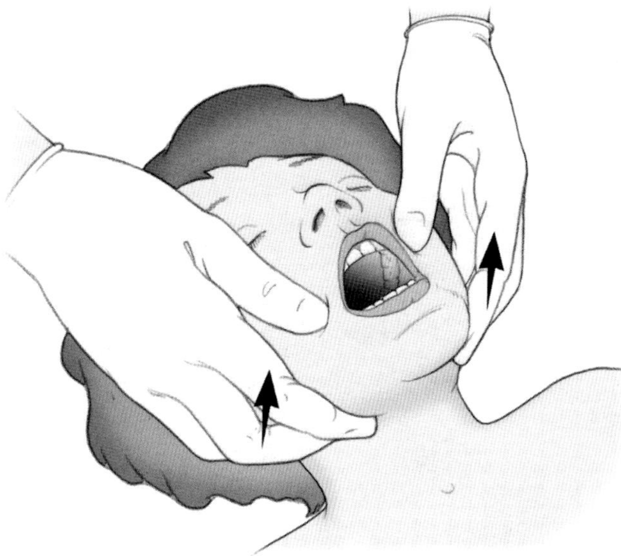

Figure 1.8 Jaw thrust without head tilt. (Copyright Chris Gralapp; reproduced with permission from Mahadevan SV, Garmel GM. *An Introduction to Clinical Emergency Medicine.* Cambridge, UK: Cambridge University Press, 2005.)

airway, and (4) to prevent aspiration. Definitive airway management, usually achieved by endotracheal intubation, is indicated for airway protection, to decrease the work of breathing, or for respiratory failure.

Positioning

The airway should be optimized by placing the child's head in the sniffing position while maintaining neutral alignment of the cervical spine. Often, a shoulder roll for an infant, or pillow for a child <2 years of age, is helpful for positioning. A chin lift or jaw thrust maneuver combined with bimanual in-line spinal immobilization may be necessary to maintain an unobstructed airway in a trauma victim.

A systematic protocol, RSI, uses sedatives and neuromuscular blocking agents to increase chances of a successful intubation and decrease risks of aspiration, while avoiding elevated intracranial pressure for head injured patients There are 10 steps in RSI.

1. Brief history
2. Preparation
3. Monitoring
4. Preoxygenation
5. Premedication
6. Cricoid pressure $\pm$ assisted ventilation
7. Sedation
8. Paralysis
9. Intubation
10. Confirmation of tube placement.

Major differences between pediatric and adult RSI occur at the steps of preoxygenation and premedication (Table 1.2). Preoxygenation consists of the patient breathing 100% oxygen spontaneously for 5 min. During this time, all nitrogen should be effectively displaced from the lungs, providing the patient with an oxygen reserve. While the adult patient can tolerate up to 5 min of apnea without developing hypoxia, children can tolerate only 2–3 min before developing hypoxia.

Pharmacy for RSI involves a choice of premedications, sedatives, and paralytics depending on the clinical situation. Areas of historical controversy in pediatric RSI include the use of atropine as a premedication, the use of etomidate as an RSI sedative, and the use of succinylcholine (suxamethonium) as a paralytic agent. The addition of adjunctive agents should be critically considered, since each additional agent adds time and complexity to RSI.

Medications for rapid sequence intubation

Premedications

Anticholinergic drugs

Atropine (0.01–0.02 mg/kg IV; minimum 0.1 mg; maximum 1 mg) has been recommended in the past to prevent bradycardia resulting from vagal stimulation. Recent literature suggests that there is a decreased role for atropine in advanced airway management. Atropine can increase arrhythmias as well as obscure the physician's ability to identify physiologic responses to pain, hypoxia, and shock. Currently, it is recommended to use atropine in children <1 year of age. Any patient

Table 1.2. Rapid sequence intubation: modifications for children

Phase of RSI	Pediatric modification
History and anatomic assessment (AMPLE)	
Preparation	Use length-based system for equipment organization and size determination and medication dosages
Monitoring	Pediatric size EZCap
Preoxygenation	8 vital capacity breaths with high-flow oxygen can be used if 5 min of preoxygenation not available; children will tolerate only 2–3 min of apnea
Premedication	Avoid bradycardia: in general, it is the authors' opinion that premedication can increase the complexity and the time required for RSI, thus defeating its main rationale Atropine 0.01–0.02 mg/kg if a second dose of succinylcholine is given
Assisted ventilation and cricoid pressure	
Sedation	Etomidate 0.3 mg/kg: least cardiovascular effects Ketamine 1–4 mg/kg: contraindicated with increased ICP, but good to maintain blood pressure Thiopental 0.5–4 mg/kg: can cause hypotension
Paralysis	Depolarizing neuromuscular blockade: succinylcholine 1–2 mg/kg Non-depolarizing neuromuscular blockade: rocuronium 0.6–1.2 mg/kg, vecuronium 0.1–0.2 mg/kg
Intubation	
Confirmation of endotracheal tube placement	End-tidal CO_2, O_2 saturation EZCap: purple, unsuccessful; tan, questionable; yellow: successful Historically uncuffed tubes were used to avoid mucosal damage; however, use of cuffed ETT decreases air leak

ICP, intracranial pressure; RSI, rapid sequence intubation.

who receives a second dose of succinylcholine should receive atropine, as should any patient with bradycardia.

Defasciculating agents

The procedure of using 1/10th the dose of a non-depolarizing muscle relaxant 1–3 min before succinylcholine administration to decrease muscle fasciculation is not necessary in children 5 years or younger.

Sedatives

Etomidate (amidate; 0.2–0.3 mg/kg IV) is an imidazole hypnotic agent. It does not cause hypotension or increased intracranial pressure, making it the ideal sedative for the multitrauma patient with or without head trauma. Recent studies have demonstrated that etomidate is safe for children and does not cause clinically significant adrenocorticoid suppression or hypotension. Side effects include clinically insignificant vomiting and myoclonic jerking. Etomidate is not approved by the US Food and Drug Administration (FDA) in children <10 years of age despite the growing amount of data to support its utility and safety in children.

Paralytics

Paralytics are essential in creating the optimal intubation conditions, although clinicians seem to use paralytics less frequently with children than adults. There is a consensus that succinylcholine is the most reliable and rapid paralytic available for RSI.

Succinylcholine (suxamethonium [Anectine, Quelicin]; 1.5–2 mg/kg IV) is the classic depolarizing agent. Its onset is rapid (30–60 s) and its duration is short (5–10 min). Maximum dose should be used to avoid complications associated with repeat dosing. Succinylcholine has been demonstrated in studies to cause bradycardia; however, it is unclear if the etiology of the bradycardia stems from the medication itself or from the vagal response to intubation. Succinylcholine can cause a rise in intracranial pressure (ICP) or intraocular pressure (IOP); however, the clinical significance is controversial.

Complications of succinylcholine use include case reports of asystole, malignant hyperthermia, and hyperkalemia. Succinylcholine can increase serum potassium by approximately 0.5–1.0 mEq/l by two mechanisms. The first is potassium leak with muscle depolarization. Therefore, succinylcholine is contraindicated in patients with potential hyperkalemia, including patients with renal failure or a significant burn or crush injury greater than 48 h old. Succinylcholine can also cause hyperkalemia by receptor stimulation in patients, with upregulation of acetylcholine receptors and subsequent exaggerated release of potassium. This mechanism of hyperkalemia could occur in patients with spinal cord injury and neuromuscular diseases with wasting, such as muscular dystrophy.

Rocuronium (Zemuron; 1.0 to 1.2 mg/kg IV) is a non-depolarizing neuromuscular blocker with the shortest onset of all the non-depolarizing agents. The onset of rocuronium is comparable to succinylcholine (60–90 s), with a duration of action of 30–45 min. It is an effective agent for RSI when succinylcholine is contraindicated. Its actions can also be potentially reversed although the reversal agent is not yet FDA approved. Disadvantages are its longer duration.

Intubation

Children with any kind of upper respiratory infection or with repeated attempts at intubation may require an ETT of smaller diameter than expected. Any single intubation attempt should last no longer than 30 s in order to prevent hypoxemia. The steps of RSI and modifications for children are shown in Table 1.2.

Preparation is key to the success of intubation. All equipment should be laid out with smaller and larger half sizes. (The physician should have a secondary plan in the case of a difficult airway.) The ETT cuff should be checked with a syringe attached and stylet in place. End-tidal carbon dioxide and Yankauer suction should be available. The BVM should be connected to oxygen and providing 100% blow by oxygen. The child should be preoxygenated. The RSI medications should be given by the nurse with simultaneous cricoid pressure placed by the intubating practitioner. At the time of medication onset, the laryngoscope should be inserted on the right side of the mouth and then moved to the midline. While the straight blade is usually inserted into the vallecula, it can also be used to lift the epiglottis out of the way. Suctioning and adjustment of position should be used to get a view of the vocal cords (often if just tissue is in the field of view, the laryngoscope is too deep). Adjunct personnel can take over cricoid pressure when the intubating physician indicates that the cords can be seen, then hand over the ETT. The ETT should be advanced just beyond the vocal cords and the cuff should be inflated.

Visualization of the ETT passing through the vocal cords and confirmation of proper placement by auscultation over the lung fields and epigastrium are the initial confirmation signs of successful endotracheal intubation. Disposable capnographic devices and end-tidal carbon dioxide monitors are becoming standard to confirm endotracheal intubation.

Airway rescue procedures

If RSI is initiated and the patient cannot be endotracheally intubated, oxygenation and ventilation must be performed immediately until the airway is secured by other means. Most patients can be ventilated with BVM until the neuromuscular blocker has worn off. However, a nasogastric tube should be placed to decompress the stomach and avoid gastric distention and regurgitation.

The Laryngeal Mask Airway (LMA) is an alternative to BVM that effectively seals off the hypopharynx from the airway until a definitive airway can be obtained. The LMA is a tube with an inflatable silicon cuff on the distal end (Fig. 1.9). The insertion procedure is illustrated in Figs. 1.10 and 1.11):

1. The appropriately sized cuff is fully deflated.
2. The LMA is blindly inserted into the mouth with opening facing anteriorly.
3. The LMA should be inserted by sliding the mask along the hard palate until resistance is encountered at the level of the upper esophageal sphincter. The mask is then inflated (the tube often moves outward). The blackline along the tubing should be midline and against the lip. The LMA should be secured with tape.

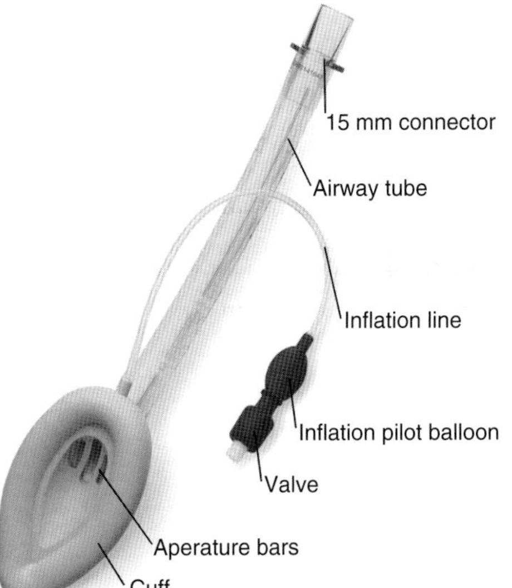

Figure 1.9 The Laryngeal Mask Airway. The mask has a soft cuff that is deflated before insertion. (Courtesy of LMA North America, Inc.)

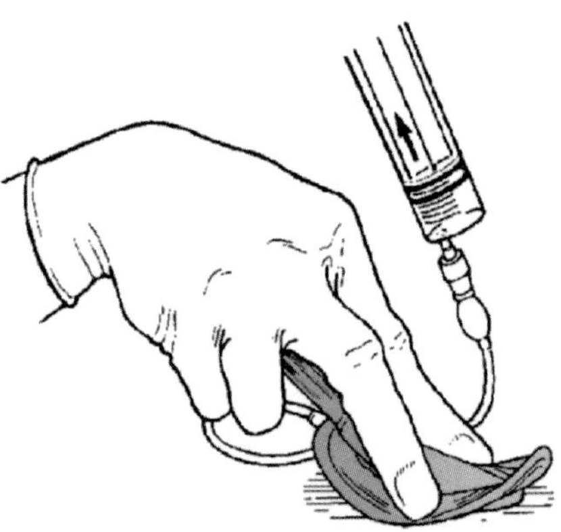

Figure 1.10 Prior to insertion of the Laryngeal Mask Airway, the cuff should be tightly deflated so that it forms a smooth wedge shape without any wrinkles. This can be accomplished by compressing the mask top between finger and thumb to achieve the correct shape. Alternatively, the mask can be properly deflated by using two index fingers and placing the mask against a solid surface. (Courtesy of LMA North America, Inc.)

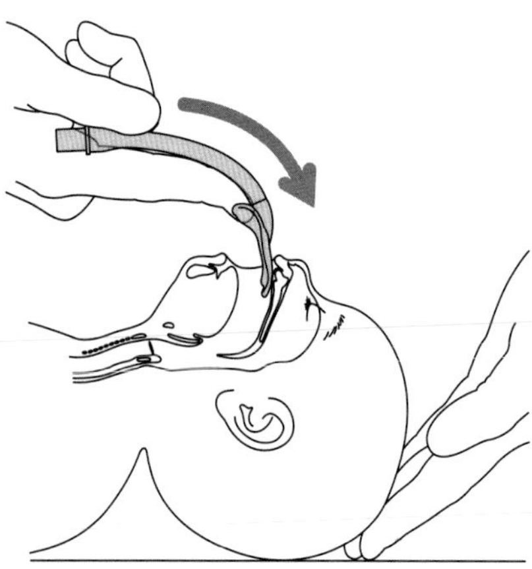

1 Press the mask up against the hard palate

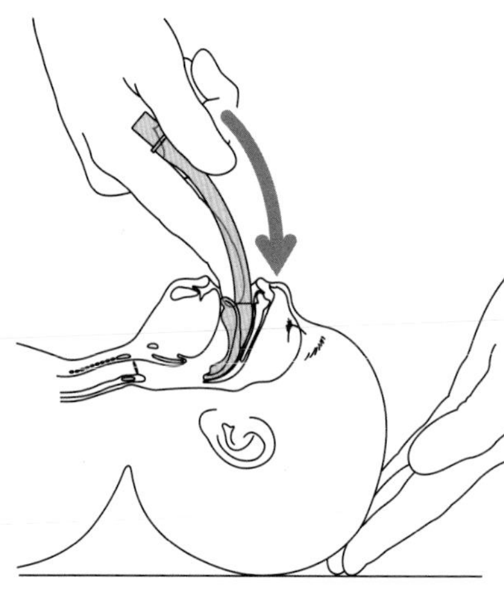

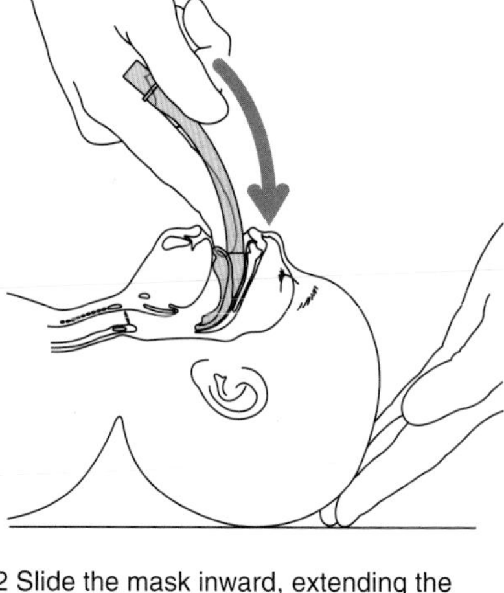

2 Slide the mask inward, extending the index finger

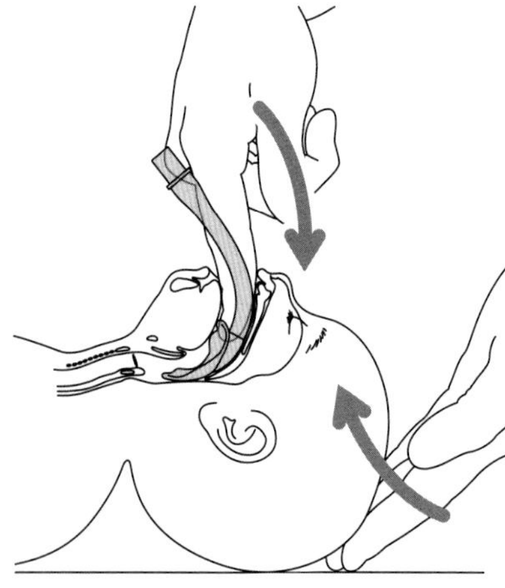

3 Press the finger toward the other hand, which exerts counter-pressure

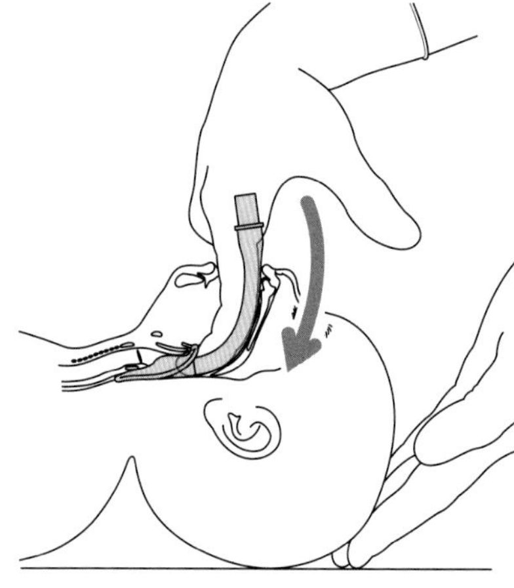

4 Advance the LMA cuff into the hypopharynx until resistance is felt

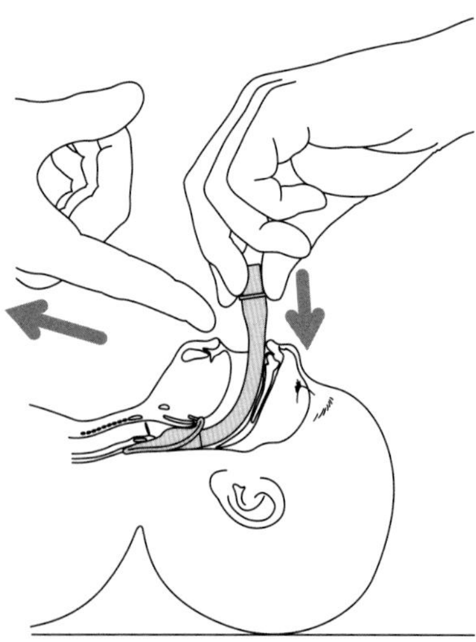

5 Hold the outer end of the airway tube while removing the index finger

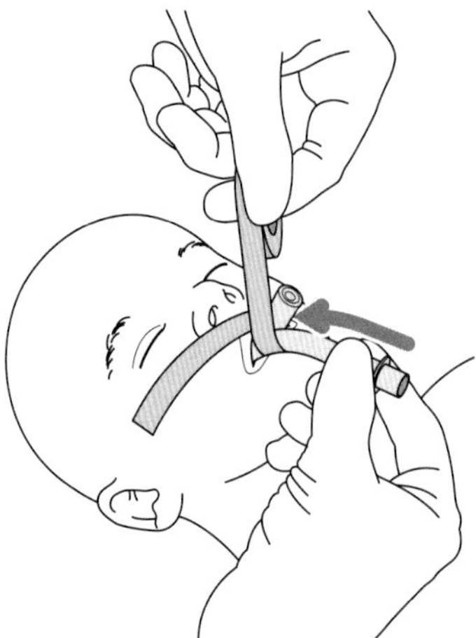

6 Insert bite-block of rolled gauze swabs into patient's mouth. While pushing airway inwards, with adhesive tape looped around airway and bite-block, fix against cheeks on either side

Figure 1.11 Insertion procedure for the Laryngeal Mask Airway (LMA). A size 1½ should be used for an infant approximately 5–10 kg. The cuff should be inserted with the smooth, portion opposed to the roof of the mouth. After correct insertion, the tip of the LMA is positioned in the esophagus. The LMA opening is at the glottis. Inflation of the cuff helps to secure the tube in the proper position so that air passes through the tube into the trachea. (Courtesy of LMA North America, Inc.)

Table 1.3. Laryngeal Mask Airway (LMA) selection guidelines based on patient size with correlating mask and endotracheal tule internal diameter

Selection guidelines			
Mask size	Patient size	Maximum cuff inflation volume (air) (mL)	Maximum endotracheal internal diameter (mm)
1	Neonates/ infants up to 5 kg	4	3.5
1½	Infants 5–10 kg	7	4.0
2	Infants/ children 10–20 kg	10	4.5
2½	Children 20–30 kg	14	5.0
3	Children 30–50 kg	20	6.0, cuffed
4	Adults 50–70 kg	30	6.0, cuffed
5	Adults 70–100 kg	40	7.0, cuffed
6	Large adults <100 kg	50	7.0, cuffed

Source: courtesy of LMA North America.

While the LMA may prevent gastric distention, it will not prevent aspiration and is not a definitive airway. There is increasing literature reporting success with LMA in children where endotracheal intubation was difficult or impossible. Table 1.3 lists the LMA size based on the child's weight. Intubating LMAs, which allow for insertion of an ETT through the LMA, are not available in children's sizes.

Needle cricothyroidotomy with jet insufflation is another temporizing procedure available when airway access and control cannot be accomplished by BVM, LMA, or orotracheal intubation in children under the age of 8 years (Ch. 2).

Emergency cricothyroidotomy is the airway of last resort in an adult with difficult airway. However, cricothyroidotomy is difficult in children and contraindicated in the infant or small child. It can only be performed in the older child in whom the cricothyroid membrane is easily palpable, usually by 8–10 years of age. Other alternative airways used in adults, such as retrograde intubation, lighted stylet, endotracheal tube introducer, and fiberoptic laryngoscope, can also be used in the child with a difficult airway.

Airway considerations in special circumstances

Trisomy 21

Children with Down syndrome have a complicated airway as they have a large tongue, relative hypotonia, and atlantoaxial instability, which makes them more prone to cervical spine injury.

In cases of trauma, cervical spine immobilization is particularly important to stabilize a possible injury and avoid further injury. A curved laryngoscope blade may be necessary to lift the large tongue out of the way. An ETT 1–2 sizes smaller than calculated may be needed since the trachea is usually smaller than in other children of the same age.

Children with cleft palate or congenital syndromes such as Pierre Robin, Treacher-Collins, or Goldenhaar syndromes, recognized by their microagnathia and asymmetric facies, who have respiratory distress may have a predictably difficult airway. Intubation should be undertaken with caution by the emergency physician (EP) with the greatest experience level, as well as with anesthesia backup if possible. Fiberoptic intubation or LMA may be the best option in these children. As stated in the section on RSI, children with known or suspected neuromuscular diseases should be intubated with a non-depolarizing neuromuscular blocker.

Pearls and pitfalls

Pearls

1. Signs of respiratory distress in a pediatric patient may be subtle
2. Use length-based resuscitation tapes to determine equipment sizes and drug dosages
3. The tongue is the most common cause of airway obstruction in the child
4. Use of airway adjuncts (oropharyngeal and nasopharyngeal) can facilitate bag-valve mask ventilation
5. Consider the Laryngeal Mask Airway as a bridge to definitive airway management of patients with microagnathia.

Pitfalls

1. Premedications in rapid sequence intubation can decrease the rapidity of the procedure
2. Beware of atlantoaxial instability in patients with Down syndrome
3. Try to avoid succinylcholine in patients with neuromuscular disease.

Selected references

American Heart Association. 2005 American Heart Association (AHA) guidelines for cardiopulmonary resuscitation (CPR) and emergency cardiovascular care (ECC) of pediatric and neonatal patients: pediatric advanced life support. *Pediatrics* 2006; **117**: 1005–1028.

Gerardi MJ, Sacchetti AD, Cantor RM, *et al.* Rapid-sequence intubation of the pediatric patient. Pediatric Emergency Medicine Committee of the American College of Emergency Physicians. *Ann Emerg Med* 1996;**28**:55–74.

Walls RM, Murphy, MF, Luten RC (eds.). *Manual of Emergency Airway Management*, 3rd edn. Philadelphia, PA: Lippincott Williams & Wilkins, 2008, pp. 263–302.

Chapter 2 Tutorial: Needle cricothyroidotomy and percutaneous transtracheal ventilation

Edward Klofas

Introduction

The management of a patient who is difficult to ventilate is frightening and challenging to the ED provider. Pediatric patients who have failed basic airway maneuvers (suction, head positioning, chin/jaw lift, use of an oropharyngeal or nasopharyngeal airway, and bag-valve mask ventilation) and advanced airway attempts (endotracheal intubation) are candidates for either a needle cricothyroidotomy or percutaneous transtracheal ventilation (PTTV). Cricothyroidotomy is contraindicated in children <8 years of age because of the size of the cricothyroid membrane. Needle cricothyroidotomy or PTTV should be considered in patients with significant orofacial trauma, upper airway bleeding, copious secretions, anatomic anomalies precluding orotracheal intubation, or with partial or complete airway obstruction. Patients in the field requiring prolonged extrication or who are in cramped quarters may be ideal candidates for PTTV if their airway cannot be maintained by less-invasive means.

Complete expiratory airway obstruction is rare as the upper airway is larger during expiration than in inspiration. However, complete expiratory airway obstruction does not allow for the venting off of airway pressure through the glottis and requires considerable modification of the recommended technique described below.

The flow characteristics of the particular device to be used should be verified prior to use and the table of ventilation parameters (Table 2.1, below) may have to be modified accordingly.

Table 2.1. Suggested ventilatory parameters for children and and adults

Weight (kg)	Pressure (psi)	Tidal volume (mL)
12	5	234
20	15	390
30	25	585
40	35	790
>50	50	975

Catheter contraindicted in child <2 years; 16-gauge for children aged 2–5 years (~12–20 kg); 14-gauge for those >5 years.

Equipment

(Figure 2.1 outlines the equipment needed.)

- transtracheal catheter: while a large-bore IV catheter can be used, these catheters kink easily. Commercially available catheters such as the wire-coiled Cook catheter (Cook Critical care, IN) are helpful
- syringe (3 ml) can be fluid filled
- jet ventilation system:
  - high pressure oxygen source (50 psi)
  - high pressure oxygen tubing
  - on/off valve for inspiration
  - Luer Lock.

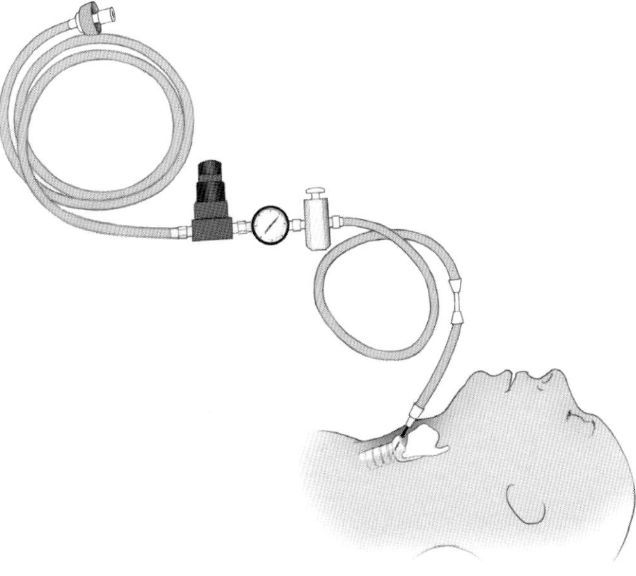

Figure 2.1 Transtracheal jet ventilation equipment and set-up. (Copyright Chris Gralapp; reproduced with permission from Mahadevan SV, Garmel GM. *An Introduction to Clinical Emergency Medicine.* Cambridge, UK: Cambridge University Press, 2005.)

A Practical Guide to Pediatric Emergency Medicine: Caring for Children in the Emergency Department, ed. N. Ewen Amieva-Wang (associate eds. Jamie Shandro, Aparajita Sohoni, and Bernhard Fassl). Published by Cambridge University Press.

The standard percutaneous transtracheal ventilation procedure

The standard PTTV procedure is suitable for adults and children >2 years of age (Fig. 2.2).

1. Expose the neck (may increase exposure by placing a small roll under the patient's neck if not contraindicated by suspected cervical spine injury).
2. Locate the cricothyroid membrane
   a. identify the trachea, palpate the prominent thyroid cartilage anteriorly; the criothyroid membrane is found 1.5–2 cm below the thyroid notch
   b. move finger inferiorly to encounter the depression that is the cricothyroid membrane; leave finger there to serve as a guide
   c. stabilize the larynx by holding the thyroid cartilage between the thumb and middle finger of the non-dominant hand.
3. Prepare skin with an alcohol swab using aseptic technique if possible.
4. Using the index finger of the non-dominant hand on the cricoid membrane as a guide: Puncture the superior aspect of the cricothyroid membrane in the midline, aiming approximately 30 degrees towards the feet.
5. Stabilize the catheter/needle to prevent entering too far and puncturing through the posterior wall of the trachea. This is particularly important with children who have smaller and more compressible tracheas.
6. Confirm intratracheal placement of the needle by freely aspirating air into the syringe. (If fluid-filled syringe is used, bubbles will be seen in the syringe.)
7. **Saftey note:** high-pressure PTTV can have devastating complications if the utmost care is not taken to insure that the PTTV needle is in the trachea and not in the peritracheal soft tissue of the neck.
8. Remove the needle and advance the catheter into the trachea to the hub.
9. Reconfirm intratracheal placement by aspiration air.
10. Remove the syringe holding the catheter firmly in place and tightly against the puncture wound. This will help to prevent localized subcutaneous emphysema at the puncture site.
11. Attach the high-pressure hose with high-pressure regulator device to the high-pressure port of the "e" oxygen cylinder, and the Luer-lock end firmly to the intratracheal catheter.

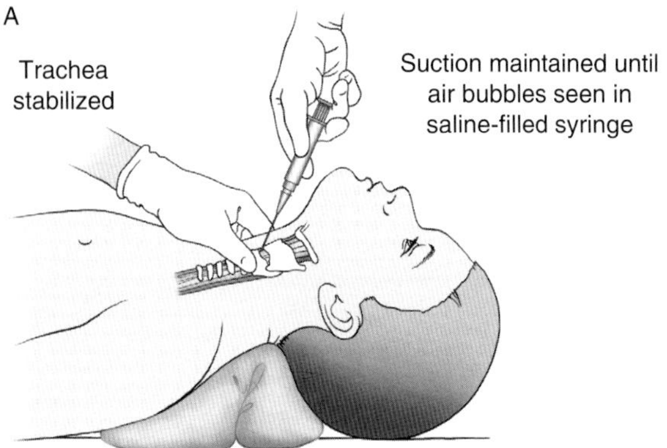

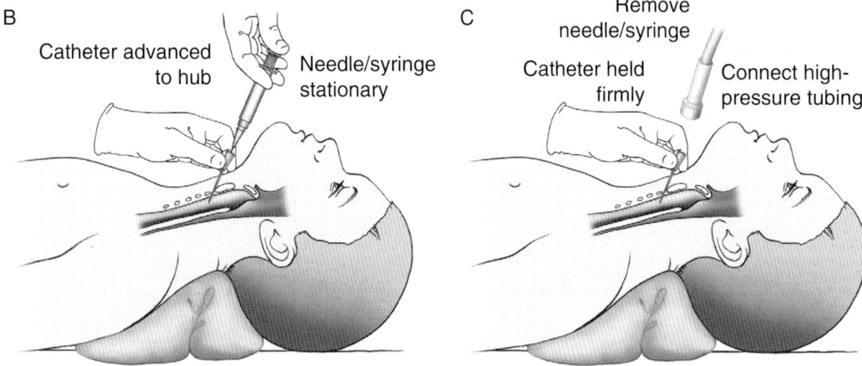

Figure 2.2 Percutaneous transtracheal ventilation. (A) A needle attached to a fluid-filled syringe is inserted through the cricothyroid membrane at a 30 to 45 degree angle from vertical. (B) After the catheter is advanced and placement is assured, the needle and syringe are removed. (C) The catheter is connected to the oxygen delivery system and secured. (Copyright N. Ewen Wang.)

12. While holding the catheter firmly in place, begin ventilation using several short bursts of oxygen to insure correct functioning of the ventilating device and reconfirm correct placement of the catheter. Oxygen should escape freely through the mouth and nose. Be sure to stand clear of the patient's face to avoid being sprayed by secretions.

    It is essential that oxygen escape through the mouth occurs. If not, complete expiratory obstruction might be present, and high pressure ventilation should be stopped (see below).
13. Beginning at this point and continuing throughout the PTTV procedure, observe for signs of complications such as subcutaneous emphysema, cyanosis, or airway obstruction. PTTV should be stopped immediately if these signs appear and the catheter should be removed.
14. Patients should be ventilated using an inspiration/expiration time of 1 s/3 s for a respiratory rate of 15 b/min after the first 5 min. For the first 5 min, the ventilation rate can be increased to 20 b/min (1 s inspiration/2 s expiration) if it is judged that the patient may have been apneic or inadequately ventilating for more than a very brief time.

Modified percutaneous transtracheal ventilation procedure for use in a completely obstructed airway

The modified PTTV procedure should be employed if there is high suspicion of a complete expiratory obstruction, if there is no air expired from the mouth after the first few low-pressure ventilations, or if there are signs of progressive air-trapping or progressive chest expansion.

1. Tracheal cannulization is performed in the standard manner.
2. Standard oxygen tubing connecting the low-pressure regulator to the catheter via a Y-connector should be used. Suggested guidelines:
    - >20 kg body weight: 15 l/min flow, 1 s inspiration/4 s expiration
    - <20 kg body weight: 10 l/min flow, 1 s inspiration/2 s expiration.
3. Inspiration occurs during thumb occlusion of the Y-connector for 1 s. Expiration occurs passively through the catheter and the Y-connector during the 4 s expiratory time.
4. Check placement of catheter by:
    - listening for air exchange through the cannula, nose and mouth
    - observing patient for color and respiratory improvement
    - observing for signs of complications such as subcutaneous emphysema, cyanosis, air-trapping and progressive chest expansion in complete airway obstruction.

Percutaneous transtracheal ventilation should be stopped immediately if these signs appear and the catheter should be removed.

5. The catheter is taped securely in place.

Suggested ventilatory parameters

Table 2.1 lists suggested ventilatory parameters. Suggested ventilatory rates are:

20/min first 5 min, I/E: 1 s on /2 s off
15/min after first 5 min, I/E: 1 s on/3 s off
Adjust based on arterial blood gases as soon as possible.

Complications

The following possible complications must be held in mind:

- subcutaneous emphysema
- barotrauma
- kinked catheter
- obstruction
- esophageal puncture
- pneumothorax
- air embolism
- death.

Selected references

Yealy DM, Stewart RD, Kaplan RM. Myths and Pitfalls in emergency translaryngeal ventilation: correcting misimpressions. *Ann Emerg Med* 1988;**17**: 690–693.

Yealy DM, Plewa MC, Stewart RD. An evaluation of cannulae and oxygen sources for pediatric jet ventilation. *Am J Emerg Med* 1991;**9**:20–23.

Chapter 3

Pediatric shock

Matthew Strehlow

Introduction

Presentation of shock in children differs significantly from that in adults. In children, as opposed to adults, hypotension is a very late finding of cardiovascular dysfunction or shock. Rather, shock is defined as a life-threatening condition characterized by inadequate delivery of oxygen and nutrients to vital organs relative to their metabolic demand. This most frequently results from poor tissue perfusion, but occasionally may be caused by an increase in metabolic demand. The imbalance between oxygen demand and delivery leads to cell ischemia and death, followed by multiple organ dysfunction syndrome. Contrary to adults, where shock is frequently the progression of a chronic, end-stage condition, children in shock frequently have a reversible condition in which full recovery can be achieved if shock is recognized early and treated aggressively.

The overall epidemiology of shock in children, both in the USA and worldwide, is not well delineated. Sepsis accounts for 7% of pediatric deaths in the USA. Pediatric patients with severe sepsis are estimated to have a 10% mortality rate, significantly lower than their adult counterparts. Mortality is heavily weighted towards younger children. Worldwide, hypovolemia secondary to diarrheal illness is the leading cause of shock in children.

Physiology

Adequate oxygen delivery to the tissues is dependent on two components:

- oxygen content in the blood
- cardiac output that matches the metabolic demand of the tissues.

The relationships between the different factors influencing oxygen delivery are shown in Fig. 3.1. In children, a low cardiac output is most commonly caused by a decrease in stroke volume rather than a low heart rate. A decrease in stroke volume frequently results from a decrease in preload or occasionally from decreased contractility. Unlike adults, who may experience hypertensive crises, an increased afterload is a rare primary cause of inadequate cardiac output in children.

Through endogenous vasomediators, the body can increase heart rate, systemic vascular resistance (afterload), cardiac contractility, and venous tone (preload). These compensatory mechanisms function in older children similarly to adults; however, infants have a relatively fixed stroke volume and are dependent on increases in heart rate to increase their cardiac output. When these compensatory mechanisms fail to maintain a blood pressure within the normal range, the patient moves from compensated shock (a normal blood pressure) to hypotensive shock (age-adjusted blood pressure below the 5th percentile). In children, standard practice is to use systolic blood pressure (SBP) to diagnose hypotension (as normative data do not exist for mean arterial pressure (MAP). As automated blood pressure machines indirectly calculate SBP from the measured MAP, falsely elevated blood pressure readings in pediatric shock can occur.

It is important to remember that, despite a normal blood pressure, patients in compensated shock experience hypoperfusion of organ tissues. Compensated shock may last for several hours, during which lactic acid and other metabolites build up in ischemic tissues and accelerate organ dysfunction. Children in compensated shock for an extended period of time may progress rapidly to hypotensive shock and to cardiac arrest.

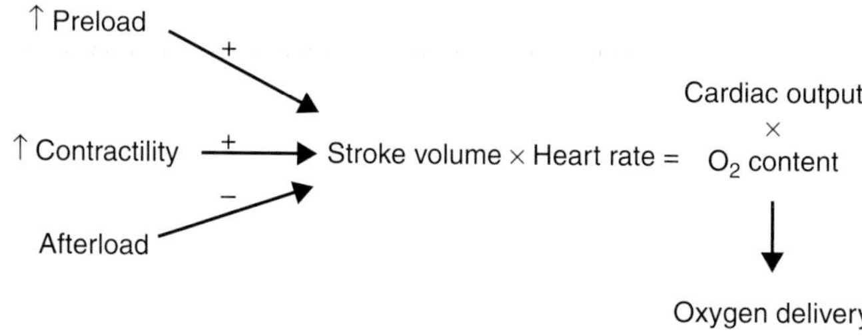

Figure 3.1 Factors influencing oxygen delivery.

A Practical Guide to Pediatric Emergency Medicine: Caring for Children in the Emergency Department, ed. N. Ewen Amieva-Wang (associate eds. Jamie Shandro, Aparajita Sohoni, and Bernhard Fassl). Published by Cambridge University Press.

Clinical presentation

Shock is not a distinct medical illness but a physiologic state that results from a variety of medical conditions that lead to one or more of the following:

- insufficient circulating blood volume (decreased preload) → hypovolemic shock
- changes in vascular resistance (decreased afterload) → distributive shock
- impairment of cardiac function (decreased contractility) → cardiogenic shock
- obstruction of blood flow (decreased preload/increased afterload) → obstructive shock.

Inadequacies of oxygen delivery are compounded by associated conditions that elevate metabolic demand, such as fever and difficulty breathing.

Because of the critical nature of patients in shock, assessment and management of the patient should proceed simultaneously. Most frequently, a child will present with a non-specific illness such as altered mental status or respiratory distress. In potentially critically ill patients, assessment of the airways, breathing, and circulation (ABC) using the pediatric assessment triangle should be performed immediately. Following emergency stabilization measures, a focused history and thorough physical examination help to determine the etiology of the patient's condition (Boxes 3.1 and 3.2).

Box 3.1. Signs of shock

Early signs of shock are frequently seen in later stages and late signs such as altered mental status may present early on depending on the etiology and patient

Early signs

Tachypnea
Tachycardia
Difference between central and peripheral pulses
Weak or bounding peripheral pulses
Delayed capillary refill (>2 s)
Pale or cool skin
Narrowed pulse pressure
Oliguria
Lactic acidosis
Elevated base deficit.

Late signs

Decreased mental status
Weak or absent central pulses
Central cyanosis
Hypotension
Bradycardia.

Differential diagnosis

Shock is commonly divided into four broad categories based on the underlying physiologic derangement (Table 3.1). In order of relative frequency, they are hypovolemic, distributive,

Box 3.2. Historical features helpful in determining the etiology of shock

- Trauma
- Fluid loss
- Signs of infection
- Fever
- Immunocompromised
- Hypothermia
- Allergic reactions and exposures
- Rash
- Congenital heart disease
- Arrhythmia
- Adrenal crisis.

Table 3.1. Categorization and differential diagnosis of shock

Category	Differential diagnosis	Key signs and symptoms
Hypovolemic	Trauma, gastroenteritis, osmotic diuresis (e.g., diabetic ketoacidosis), third space losses (e.g., burns), inadequate fluid intake, non-traumatic hemorrhage	Tachypnea without increased work of breathing, excess fluid loss or inadequate intake (e.g., bleeding, vomiting)
Distributive	Sepsis (frequently presenting with cold shock), anaphylaxis, spinal cord injury	Wide pulse pressure, warm flushed skin, bounding peripheral pulses
Cardiogenic	Congenital heart disease, arrhythmia, myocarditis, cardiomyopathy, ingestion (e.g., beta-blockers, calcium channel blockers)	Tachypnea with increased respiratory effort secondary to pulmonary edema, jugular venous distention, hepatomegaly, cyanosis
Obstructive	Cardiac tamponade, tension pneumothorax, pulmonary embolus, ductal-dependent congenital heart lesions	Distended neck veins, unilateral decreased or absent breath sounds (tension pneumothorax) in first few weeks of life and/or rapidly progressive cyanosis or heart failure (ductal-dependent lesions)

cardiogenic, and obstructive shock. Although these categories often overlap, proper classification of the patient narrows the differential diagnosis and guides evaluation and therapy.

Hypovolemic shock

Hypovolemic shock is characterized by decreased intravascular volume and decreased preload. Decreased volume results from excessive loss or inadequate fluid intake. Sources of volume loss in children include:

- vomiting and/or diarrhea
- osmotic diuresis (e.g., hyperglycemia)
- capillary leak (e.g., burns, sepsis)
- hemorrhage
- inadequate fluid intake, typically in infants and young children.

Pediatric patients are at an increased risk of hypovolemia compared with adults for several reasons. First, children more commonly suffer from gastroenteritis. They may also be unable to communicate their need for hydration or independently access fluids. Additionally, children have a high surface area to volume ratio, which increases insensible losses.

Pediatric patients with non-hemorrhagic volume loss are characterized by a reduction in percentage body weight from baseline: mild (infants 5%, children 3%), moderate (infants 10%, children 5–6%), and severe (infants >15%, children >7%). Many patients with moderate volume loss and all patients with severe volume loss are in a state of hypoperfusion and shock. Hypotensive shock is consistently observed when non-hemorrhagic volume losses exceed 100 ml/kg. When the child's baseline weight is unavailable, clinical signs of shock paired with the history of volume loss are used to estimate the severity of hypovolemia.

Children with hemorrhagic volume loss can lose a significant portion of blood volume prior to displaying obvious signs of shock. Therefore, it is imperative to identify early indicators of blood loss in pediatric patients.

Distributive shock

Distributive shock stems from inappropriate distribution of blood flow, leading to hypoperfusion of many vital tissues and organ systems. Commonly, the skin and skeletal muscle tissue are perfused well beyond their metabolic needs while the splanchnic circulation is hypoperfused. The most frequent causes of distributive shock are sepsis and anaphylaxis; a small number of children will have neurogenic (spinal) shock.

Cardiac output is typically normal or increased as systemic vascular resistance (SVR) is low and the heart rate is elevated. These physiologic changes lead to a wide pulse pressure (diastolic less than one half the systolic), bounding peripheral pulses, and warm, well-perfused skin (warm shock).

Box 3.3. Definitions of systemic inflammatory response syndrome, sepsis, severe sepsis, and septic shock

Systemic inflammatory response syndrome (SIRS)

The presence of at least two of the following four criteria, one of which must be an abnormal temperature or leukocyte count:

- core temperature >38.5°C or <36°C
- tachycardia >2 sd above normal for age *or* persistent bradycardia in a child <1 year old
- respiratory rate >2 sd above normal for age or need for mechanical ventilation
- leukocyte count elevated or depressed, or >10% immature neutrophils.

See also age-specific vital signs (front cover).

Sepsis

SIRS in the setting of a suspected or proven infection.

Severe sepsis

Sepsis plus one of the following organ dysfunctions:

- cardiovascular organ dysfunction
- acute respiratory distress syndrome (ARDS)
- ≥2 other organ dysfunctions.

See criteria of organ dysfunction (Box 3.4).

Septic shock

Sepsis plus cardiovascular organ dysfunction.

Alternatively, patients, particularly those with septic shock, may present with a high SVR and increased afterload. Narrowed pulse pressure, weak pulses, and cool skin (cold shock) are typical findings in these patients. While cold shock is a late finding in adult patients with sepsis, it is frequently observed early in the pediatric population.

Regardless of whether the patient is suffering from warm or cold shock, continued hypoperfusion leads to the build up of lactic acid, inflammatory mediators, and vasoactive substances. These cellular metabolites decrease cardiac output by diminishing contractility and increasing capillary leak.

Sepsis is the most common cause of distributive shock and one of the leading causes of mortality in children. Current definitions of sepsis and organ dysfunction are shown in Boxes 3.3 and 3.4. Of note, in pediatric patients one of the two systemic inflammatory response syndrome (SIRS) criteria necessary for diagnosis must be either an abnormal temperature or an abnormal leukocyte count. Additionally, a low blood pressure is not required to diagnose septic shock if other signs of cardiovascular dysfunction are present, contrary to the diagnosis in adults.

Anaphylactic shock is a multisystem allergic response following exposure to an antigen (Ch. 10). The onset time typically varies from seconds to a few minutes after exposure. The body's response is characterized by systemic vasodilation, capillary leak, and pulmonary constriction. Common signs

Box 3.4. Organ dysfunction criteria

Cardiovascular system

One of the following despite administration of isotonic IV fluids ≥40 ml/kg in 1 h

- hypotension for age (see age-specific vital signs; Table 1 in prelims)
- need for vasoactive drug to maintain blood pressure in normal range
- any two of the following:
  - unexplained metabolic acidosis: base deficit >5.0 mEq/l
  - increased arterial lactate >2× upper limit of normal (ULN)
  - oliguria: urine output <0.5 ml/kg/h
  - prolonged capillary refill >5 s
  - core to peripheral temperature gap >3°C

Respiratory system

Acute respiratory distress syndrome (ARDS) must include PaO_2/FIO_2 <200, bilateral infiltrates, acute onset, no evidence of left heart failure.

- Arterial partial pressure O_2 (PaO_2)/ fraction of inspired oxygen(FIO_2) <300
- PCO_2 >65 torr or >20 mmHg over baseline
- Need for >50% FIO_2 to maintain O_2 saturation ≥92%
- Need for invasive or non-invasive mechanical ventilation.

Neurologic system

- Glasgow Coma Scale ≤11.

Hematologic system

- Platelet count ≤80 000 cells/μl
- International normalized ratio (INR) >2.

Renal system

- Serum creatinine ≥2× ULN for age.

Hepatic sytem

- Total bilirubin ≥4 mg/dl (not applicable to newborns)
- Alanine transaminase (ALT) ≥2× ULN for age.

and symptoms consistent with anaphylactic shock, compared with other etiologies, include urticaria, angioedema, and respiratory distress with wheezing or stridor.

Neurogenic shock, also known as spinal shock, results from injury to the spinal cord above the sixth thoracic spine (T6) or rarely from a head injury. The injury results in the sudden loss of sympathetic innervation of the vasculature leading to uncontrolled vasodilation. Hypotension with a wide pulse pressure and relative bradycardia in patients with possible acute spinal cord injury are the hallmark findings.

Cardiogenic shock

Cardiogenic shock is characterized by decreased cardiac output secondary to myocardial dysfunction. As cardiac output falls, the body responds by increasing heart rate and systemic vascular resistance to maintain perfusion of the heart and brain at the expense of peripheral and splanchnic tissues. With the increased demand on already compromised myocardium, further myocardial dysfunction ensues, and stroke volume and cardiac output fall even further. Urine output decreases as the kidneys retain fluid in an effort to increase preload. Unfortunately, much of this extra blood volume redistributes into the extravascular spaces of the lungs, liver, and peripheral tissues.

Patients most often present with respiratory distress and cyanosis from pulmonary edema. Other signs include hepatic congestion, dependent edema, jugular venous distention, and cool, pale skin. Infants, however, may present with poor feeding and lethargy. Patients in shock who receive IV fluid boluses and develop worsening respiratory distress should be evaluated for cardiogenic shock.

In contrast to adults where ischemic heart disease and long-standing hypertension lead to heart failure and cardiogenic shock, in children primary cardiogenic shock is rare. Causes of cardiogenic shock include:

- congenital heart disease
- myocarditis
- cardiomyopathy: dilated, infiltrative (mucopolysaccharidosis, glycogen storage diseases)
- arrythmias
- metabolic derangements: acidosis, hyperkalemia, hypercalcemia, congenital organic acidemias
- hypothermia
- ischemic heart disease: Kawasaki disease, anomalous coronary artery, myocardial infarction
- poisoning or drug toxicity: beta-blockers, calcium channel blockers, barbiturates, chemotherapeutic agents
- radiation
- traumatic myocardial injury
- thyrotoxicosis
- pheochromocytoma
- phosphodiesterase inhibitors (inodilators).

Obstructive disorders, such as ductal-dependent congenital heart disease and cardiac tamponade, are discussed under obstructive shock.

Obstructive shock

Obstructive shock is characterized by a low cardiac output secondary to a physical impediment to blood flow. Systemic vascular resistance is elevated, resulting in patients whose physical findings parallel those in hypovolemic shock. Immediate identification of the etiology of the obstruction and targeted intervention is critical. There are four primary categories of obstructive shock

- ductal-dependent cardiac lesions
- tension pneumothorax
- cardiac tamponade
- pulmonary embolus.

Ductal-dependent lesions typically present within the first weeks of life and are divided into cyanotic and left ventricular outflow tract obstructive lesions. Cyanotic lesions such as Tetralogy of Fallot are dependent on a patent ductus arteriosus for pulmonary blood flow. Obstructive lesions of the left ventricular outflow tract are ductal dependent for systemic blood flow. Specific signs and symptoms vary with the specific cause of obstruction, but findings of central cyanosis or rapidly progressive congestive heart failure in a newborn should raise suspicion for an obstructive etiology (Chs. 14 and 15).

Tension pneumothorax is caused by the accumulation of air in the pleural space, leading to an increase in intrathoracic pressure, collapse of the lung on the affected side, and deviation of mediastinal structures to the opposite side of the chest cavity. Penetrating traumatic injury and positive pressure ventilation are the common precipitating events. Key findings are rapidly progressive shock and unilateral absent or diminished breath sounds in the appropriate clinical setting.

Cardiac tamponade is characterized by the collection of fluid, blood, or air in the pericardial space. As the pressure within the pericardium rises, cardiac filling is reduced and cardiac output falls. In children, penetrating trauma and cardiac surgery are the most common causes. In a patient with risk factors for cardiac tamponade, a high level of suspicion must be maintained as the classic findings of muffled heart sounds, distended neck veins, and pulsus paradoxus are difficult to discern in the critically ill child.

Pulmonary embolism is blockage of the pulmonary artery or its branches by a clot, air, fat, or other substance. Although rare in children, it may be seen in those with predisposing risk factors such as malignancy, central venous catheters, sickle cell disease, connective tissue disorders, and inherited disorders of coagulation. A rapid onset of respiratory distress, hypoxia, and signs of right heart failure suggest a massive pulmonary embolus; however, the diagnosis is challenging and presentations vary significantly.

Diagnostic studies

Initial diagnostic studies evaluating pediatric shock are employed to determine the etiology of illness, evaluate the severity of hypoperfusion and organ dysfunction, and identify metabolic derangements. Emergency department testing is often broad based and the results non-specific, as it is difficult in the emergency setting to determine the underlying cause of shock.

General laboratory studies include complete blood count (CBC), electrolyte panel, ionized calcium, liver function tests (LFTs), blood urea nitrogen (BUN), creatinine, and glucose level.

Up to 18% of children in shock are hypoglycemic.

Consequently, special attention should be given to rapid determination of their glucose level ($\leq$45 mg/dl for neonates and $\leq$60 mg/dl for older children). Additionally, hypocalcemia is common and should be corrected, as it is associated with significant myocardial dysfunction. Liver and renal function assessment assists in identifying dehydration and determining the severity of organ injury.

Depending on the etiology of shock, other laboratory studies of utility for evaluation and treatment include lactate, urinalysis, blood and urine cultures, cerebrospinal fluid (CSF) evaluation, coagulation studies, ammonia, type and cross-match, arterial or venous blood gas analysis, thyroid stimulating hormone, and cortisol level. Lactate levels and base deficits calculated from blood gases are markers of systemic perfusion. Lacate levels $\geq$4 mmol/l and base deficits $\geq$6 mEq/l suggest significant tissue hypoxia and have been shown to be independent predictors of mortality in shock patients. Elevated ammonia levels in the newborn are suggestive of an inborn error of metabolism.

Initial radiographic evaluation of unstable patients is limited to studies that can be carried out at the bedside. Chest radiographs looking for pneumonia, tension pneumothorax, heart failure, and other causes or complications of shock should be performed. Electrocardiography (ECG) evaluates for arrhythmia, ischemia, drug toxicity, and congenital heart disease.

The role of bedside ultrasound in the evaluation of patients in shock is rapidly expanding. Emergency practitioners are increasingly comfortable with the use of ultrasound for the evaluation of traumatic bleeding, tension pneumothoraces, pericardial tamponade, hypovolemia, cardiac contractility, among others. Multiple ultrasound protocols exist that assist the physician in systematically evaluating undifferentiated shock patients. In one study, the use of early, protocol-based, bedside ultrasonography performed by EPs improved identification of the correct etiology of shock from 50% to 75%.

Management

Life-saving management in pediatric shock centers on rapid recognition and aggressive resuscitation. Guidelines on caring for the critically ill child in emergency medicine, pediatric, and critical care settings focus on the time-dependent nature of management to improve outcomes. Effective implementation of these guidelines has a significant impact on mortality. A retrospective study in children with septic shock demonstrated that patients receiving initial resuscitation in accordance with the American College of Critical Care Medicine pediatric advanced life support (ACCM-PALS) guidelines prior to transfer to a tertiary care facility had a significantly lower mortality (8%) than patients who did not receive appropriate resuscitation (38%).

The goals of resuscitation are the restoration of perfusion and organ function by:

- optimizing oxygen content of blood
- improving cardiac output and the distribution of blood flow
- reducing oxygen demand
- correcting metabolic derangements.

Initial therapy to optimize the oxygen content of blood is through the administration of high-flow oxygen and airway positioning. If the hemoglobin level is <7 mg/dl, transfusion is indicated. In certain conditions such as sepsis and trauma, higher transfusion thresholds may be appropriate (neonates are transfused at higher pressures). Positive pressure ventilation can be added to improve ventilation perfusion mismatching.

Cardiac output is augmented by adjusting preload, contractility, and afterload through the use of IV fluids and vasoactive agents. Peripheral IV access must be established rapidly. If early attempts at peripheral IV access are unsuccessful, intraosseous or central venous access should be obtained without delay.

Fluid resuscitation is initiated with normal saline or lactated Ringer's solution beginning with a bolus administration of 20 ml/kg over 5–20 min depending on patient severity. It is often necessary to repeat boluses to totals of 40–80 ml/kg. Fluid administration through a single IV line by gravity is insufficient to achieve an appropriate flow rate; consequently, a second IV line, pressure bag, rapid infusion device, or syringe push–pull system is required. Despite these measures, it can be difficult to achieve the recommended fluid administration rates in children <40 kg.

Colloids can be considered in patients that are unresponsive to 40–60 ml/kg of crystalloid or in patients with decreased plasma oncotic pressure (malnutrition, hypoproteinemia, nephrotic syndrome). Colloid solutions are advantageous in that a greater proportion of fluid remains in the intravascular space; however, studies have not consistently demonstrated improved outcomes using these fluids. Side effects of colloids include hypersensitivity reactions and coagulopathies, depending on the particular agent administered.

Frequent reassessment during fluid administration for signs of volume overload such as pulmonary congestion and liver engorgement is essential. In addition to cardiogenic shock with pulmonary congestion, other contraindications to aggressive fluid resuscitation include diabetic ketoacidosis and drug overdose by calcium channel blockers or beta-blockers. For cardiogenic shock and cardiovascular drug overdoses, consider a trial of a normal saline bolus of 5–10 ml/kg delivered over 10–20 min. Repeat the fluid bolus if the patient shows signs of clinical improvement.

Decreasing the work of breathing, fever, pain, and anxiety reduces oxygen demand. These problems are reduced by assisting respiration, making the patient comfortable, and administering antipyretics and analgesics as indicated.

Metabolic derangement can potentiate poor perfusion and organ dysfunction. Abnormalities such as hypoglycemia and hypocalcemia should be corrected; however, a metabolic acidosis is common in shock patients and should be addressed by increasing perfusion and ventilation. When the metabolic acidosis is profound or refractory, buffers such as bicarbonate and tromethamine (Tris) are temporizing options that may improve the patient's responsiveness to endogenous and exogenous catecholamines.

Vasoactive agents are used to improve cardiac output and the distribution of blood flow. In general, vasoactive therapies have a limited role in primary hypovolemic and obstructive forms of shock. Table 3.2 lists commonly used vasoactive agents in pediatric patients with shock. The choice of a particular agent depends on the type of shock and the physiology of the patient at a particular time (high SVR/low cardiac output, low SVR/low cardiac output, low SVR/high cardiac output). Children, in contrast to adults, have a greater frequency of high SVR/low cardiac output states. Correspondingly, combined inotrope–vasodilators such as dobutamine and phosphodiesterase inhibitors are more commonly administered in children. Vasoactive agents can be initiated in conjunction with aggressive fluid resuscitation. Patients must be reassessed frequently and treatments modified as their conditions change over time.

Monitoring and end points of resuscitation

Care providers must closely monitor vital signs including oxygen saturation, clinical signs of shock, and urine output. Initially, less-invasive therapeutic end points of resuscitation guide therapy:

- normalization of heart rate and blood pressure
- capillary refill <2 s
- no difference between the strength of central and peripheral pulses
- warm extremities
- urine output ≥1 ml/kg per h
- normal mental status
- decreasing lactate and base deficit.

If patients fail to respond to initial resuscitation measures, more invasive monitoring is indicated; this, if possible, should be performed in conjunction with pediatric critical care specialists. Continuous blood pressure assessment via an arterial line in conjunction with central venous pressure and mixed venous or central venous oxygen saturation (SvO_2, $ScvO_2$) are frequently implemented. These are indirect markers of cardiac output. In the emergency setting, $ScvO_2$ is preferable because it can be measured from any central line; however, an upper extremity central line positioned in the superior vena cava with the tip at the junction with the right atrium is optimal. A typical goal is an $ScvO_2$ ≥70%, as values <70% suggest that the tissue demand for oxygen is exceeding the supply and cardiac output is inadequate. In cases where the cardiac output is elevated, but the distribution of blood flow inappropriate, the $ScvO_2$ may be high but the patient's lactate level will be elevated.

Managing hypovolemic shock

Halting ongoing fluid losses and aggressive fluid resuscitation as outlined above are the mainstays of treatment. Large

Table 3.2. Pharmacologic agents used in the treatment of shock

Drug	Effects	Dose (per kg body weight)	Indications
Dobutamine	Inotrope, vasodilator	2–20 μg/min IV	Cardiogenic and septic shock with high SVR
Dopamine	Vasopressor, inotrope	2–20 μg/min IV	Cardiogenic and distributive shock
Epinephrine	Vasopressor, inotrope	0.1–1 μg/min IV	Cardiogenic and distributive shock
Inamrinone[a]	Inotrope, vasodilator	Loading dose, 0.75–1 mg IV over 5 min (longer if unstable); may repeat twice Infusion, 5–10 μg/min IV	Cardiogenic and unresponsive septic shock with high SVR
Milrinone[a]	Inotrope, vasodilator	Loading dose, 50–75 μg IV over 10–60 min Infusion, 0.5–0.75 μg/min IV	Cardiogenic and unresponsive septic shock with high SVR
Nitroglycerin (glyceryl trinitrate)	Vasodilator	0.25–10 μg/min IV	Cardiogenic shock with high SVR
Norepinephrine	Vasopressor, inotrope	0.1–2 μg/min IV	Distributive shock

SVR, systemic vascular resistance.
[a] Phosphodiesterase inhibitors (inodilators), use of loading dose is optional.

volumes of crystalloid are often necessary (40–80 ml/kg), as only 25% of isotonic crystalloid will remain in the vascular space. Patients with significant or ongoing hemorrhage should receive a 20 ml/kg crystalloid bolus followed by packed red blood cells in 10 ml/kg increments if further fluid resuscitation is necessary. Fresh frozen plasma and platelets should also be considered in patients receiving packed red blood cell transfusion. Vasoactive medications are rarely required in hypovolemic shock unless a concomitant cause of shock is present.

Managing distributive shock

In general, distributive shock is managed with volume expansion, and if hypoperfusion persists, the appropriate vasoactive agents for the patient's physiology are added.

Management of severe sepsis and septic shock centers on controlling infection and rapid restoration of perfusion. Studies in both adults and pediatrics have demonstrated significant mortality reductions in severe sepsis and septic shock patients treated with early, aggressive, goal-directed therapy. Figure 3.2 is a management algorithm for patients with presumed septic shock.

Early administration of antibiotics after the onset of septic shock is associated with improved outcomes. Guidelines recommend that broad-spectrum antibiotics be administered within the first hour after recognition of shock. Attempts should be made to obtain appropriate cultures prior to antibiotic administration but should not delay therapy.

Large volumes of fluid are often necessary during resuscitation of patients with septic shock. The general principles and volumes noted above apply. If respiratory distress develops during fluid resuscitation, early intubation is warranted.

The use of corticosteroids in septic shock patients is debated. Risk factors suggestive of absolute adrenal insufficiency include:

- long-term corticosteroid use
- pituitary or adrenal abnormalities
- severe, unresponsive septic shock and purpura
- catecholamine-resistant shock and an absolute cortisol level <18 μg/dl (496 nmol/l).

Patients with absolute adrenal insufficiency should receive hydrocortisone 50–75 mg/m^2 every 24 h divided every 6 h. Other therapies are not well established. No definitive recommendations exist regarding blood transfusion aimed at improving oxygenation. Intravenous immunoglobulin and extracorporeal membranous oxygenation may have roles in the future. Activated protein C and tight glycemic control therapy are not recommended in children.

Critical to the management of neurogenic shock is the recognition that patients typically have multisystem trauma. Ongoing evaluation during the management of these patients for other causes of shock is vital. In neurogenic shock, blood vessels are dilated and relative hypovolemia exists. Aggressive fluid resuscitation with judicious use of vasoconstrictors, norepinephrine and epinephrine, is best. For the management of anaphylactic shock, see Ch. 10.

Managing cardiogenic shock

Care of pediatric patients in cardiogenic shock focuses on identification of specific etiologies and optimization of cardiac output to decrease pulmonary edema and hypoperfusion.

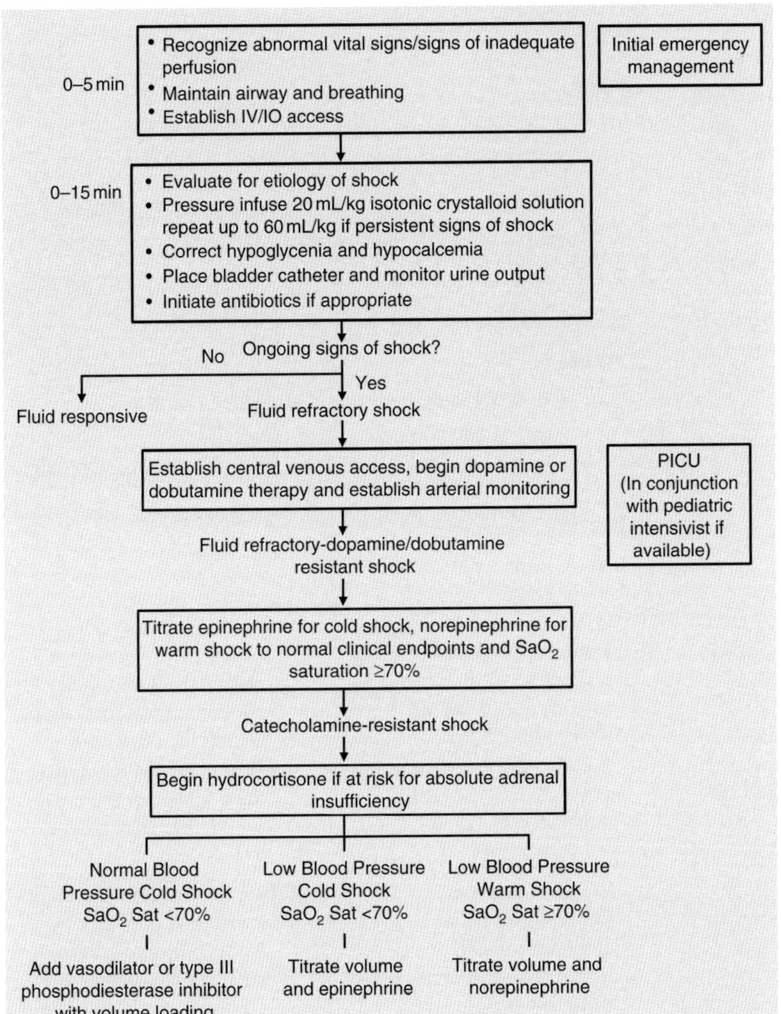

Figure 3.2 Approach to pediatric shock. PICU, pediatirc intensive care unit.

Patients should be placed in a position of comfort and high-flow oxygen administered. If respiratory distress and hypoxia are severe, positive pressure ventilation by continuous or bi-level positive airway pressure or endotracheal intubation and mechanical ventilation is warranted. Small boluses of fluid may be trialed if systemic circulation is compromised and pulmonary congestion is mild.

In the majority of cases, however, pulmonary congestion with an elevated preload and systemic vasoconstriction predominates. Pharmacologic therapy focuses on reducing preload and afterload to decrease pulmonary vascular congestion and improve cardiac output. Vasodilators such as nitrates are first-line treatment options, but in patients with borderline hypotension dobutamine is recommended. Dopamine is the medication of choice for patients who are hypotensive. A vasodilator may be added to dopamine if tolerated. Phosphodiesterase inhibitors have inotropic and vasodilator properties and are an alternative to dobutamine. Once vasodilators have been administered and if blood pressure remains adequate, patients who have increased intravascular volume can be given diuretics. Urine output should be monitored closely.

Managing obstructive shock

Management of obstructive shock is diagnosis dependent and early identification of the specific etiology and intervention to prevent cardiovascular collapse is paramount. Patients may temporarily respond to increasing preload by aggressive fluid resuscitation. Immediate care is decompression for tension pneumothorax, pericardial drainage for pericardial tamponade, prostaglandin E_1 for ductal-dependent cardiac lesions, and removal or dissolution of clot in massive pulmonary embolus. These specific treatments are discussed elsewhere.

Conclusions

Acutely critically ill children are challenging to the most experienced of medical providers. Effective evaluation and management of patients with shock depends on early recognition and intervention prior to cardiovascular collapse. A brief history and thorough physical examination focused on markers of tissue perfusion and signs of specific causes of shock must be performed. Rapid restoration of tissue oxygenation and perfusion typically through aggressive fluid resuscitation, prior to the onset of hypotension, are paramount. If patients are treated early and appropriately, mortality in children with shock can be greatly reduced.

Pearls and pitfalls

Pearls

1. Early recognition and intervention in patients with shock is critical to improve outcomes.
2. Determination of the type of shock guides therapy and an organized approach to evaluation is imperative.
3. Diagnosis of severe sepsis and septic shock in pediatric patients requires the use of age-appropriate definitions.

Pitfalls

1. Failure to recognize pediatric shock because of lack of hypotension.
2. Failure to adequately volume resuscitate the patient in shock.
3. Failure to check a rapid bedside sugar in a patient with shock.

Selected references

Brierley J, Peters MJ. Distinct hemodynamic patterns of septic shock at presentation to pediatric intensive care. *Pediatrics* 2008;**122**: 752–529.

Carcillo JA, Fields AI, for the American College of Critical Care Medicine Task Force Committee Members. Clinical practice parameters for hemodynamic support of pediatric and neonatal patients in septic shock. *Crit Care Med* 2002;**30**: 1365–1378.

Dellinger RP, Levy MM, Carlet JM, *et al.* Surviving Sepsis Campaign: international guidelines for the management of severe sepsis and septic shock. *Crit Care Med* 2008;**36**:296–327 [erratum in *Crit Care Med* 2008;**36**:1394–1396].

Han YY, Carcillo JA, Dragotta MA, *et al.* Early reversal of pediatric–neonatal septic shock by community physicians is associated with improved outcomes. *Pediatrics* 2003;**112**:793–799.

Jones AE, Tayal VS, Sullivan DM, Kline JA. Randomized, controlled trial of immediate versus delayed goal-directed ultrasound to identify the cause of nontraumatic hypotension in emergency department patients. *Crit Care Med* 2004;**32**:1703–1708.

Kumar A, Roberts D, Wood KE, *et al.* Duration of hypotension before initiation of effective antimicrobial therapy is the critical determinant of survival in human septic shock. *Crit Care Med* 2006;**34**: 1589–1596.

Stoner MJ, Goodman DG, Cohen DM, Fernandez SA, Hall MW. Rapid fluid resuscitation in pediatrics: testing the American College of Critical Care Medicine guidelines. *Ann Emerg Med* 2007;**50**: 601–607.

Watson RS, Carcillo JA, Linde-Zwirble WT, *et al.* The epidemiology of severe sepsis in children in the United States. *Am J Respir Crit Care Med* 2003;**167**: 695–701.

Chapter 4

Tutorial: Intraosseous line placement and umbilical venous access

Gregory H. Gilbert and Betsy Encarnacion

Intraosseous line

Intraosseous (IO) infusions establish rapid vascular access in critical situations, particularly if one is unable to secure a peripheral line. This approach may be more feasible and easier for neonates in extremis than a classic umbilical venous catheter. Historically IOs used bone marrow biopsy needles and were not recommended in older children or adults because of the difficulty in penetrating bone. However, the introduction of mechanical devices such as the EZ-IO or the bone injection gun (BIG) (Table 4.1) has rendered IO line placement a viable method of vascular access in all ages (Fig. 4.1). These IO devices have a high success rate in establishing vascular access to draw blood, give medications, and give blood or fluids; the last enables vessels to become more prominent so that an IV or central line can later be placed. The most common site for IO access is the proximal tibia, but the distal tibia, humeral head, and distal femur can also be used (Fig. 4.2).

Placement of IO access should be considered in situations where conventional methods of obtaining venous access are not possible, such as cardiopulmonary arrest, shock, burns, or status epilepticus. Access is like IV access in that it allows for administration of fluids, blood products, and medications. Samples obtained from IO aspirates can also be cultured, analyzed for blood gases, used for blood chemistry, and typed and crossed. Insertion of IO lines is contraindicated at sites with suspected fractures, overlying cellulitis or burns, and when the landmarks cannot be identified. In addition, areas where IO access has been previously attempted unsuccessfully should lead the practitioner to attempt a different site. Instructions for IO catheterization are provided in Box 4.1.

It is also important to know that the most painful part of the procedure, unlike IV access, is infusion. This can be mitigated by first infusing a small amount of lidocaine prior to

Table 4.1. Comparison of the bone injection gun (BIG) and the intraosseous infusion device for pediatric patients (EZ-IO PD)

	Bone injection gun	EZ-IO PD
Design	Spring-loaded device	Battery-powered drill
Pediatric specifics	For children younger than 12 years use an 18-gauge needle	For children lighter than 39 kg use a 15-gauge needle, 15 mm long
Sites used	Promixal tibia	Proximal tibia, distal tibia, distal femur, and the humeral head
Technique	1. Position the gun 90 degrees to the surface of the bone with one hand 2. With the other hand, remove the safety pin and release the trigger 3. Remove the gun and stylet trocar; then attach IO cannula to an IV system	1. Place the needle tip at a 90 degree angle at the insertion site 2. Hold the driver lightly and press the trigger; do not push the driver 3. Guide the needle, feeling for a decrease in resistance indicating penetration into the marrow space 4. Unscrew the stylet and connect the needle to a Luer-Lok set 5. Remove the IO catheter by rotating it clockwise and gently pulling back on the needle

IO, intraosseous infusion.

A Practical Guide to Pediatric Emergency Medicine: Caring for Children in the Emergency Department, ed. N. Ewen Amieva-Wang (associate eds. Jamie Shandro, Aparajita Sohoni, and Bernhard Fassl). Published by Cambridge University Press.

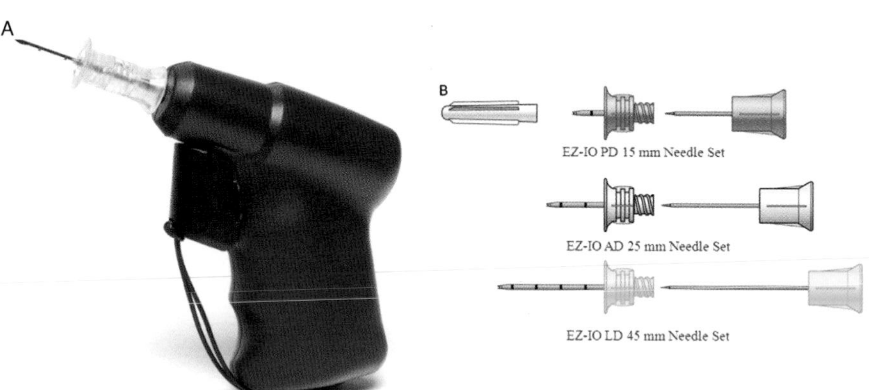

Figure 4.1 Intraosseous access. The EZ IO device and needle sets. (Courtesy of Vidacare Corp.)

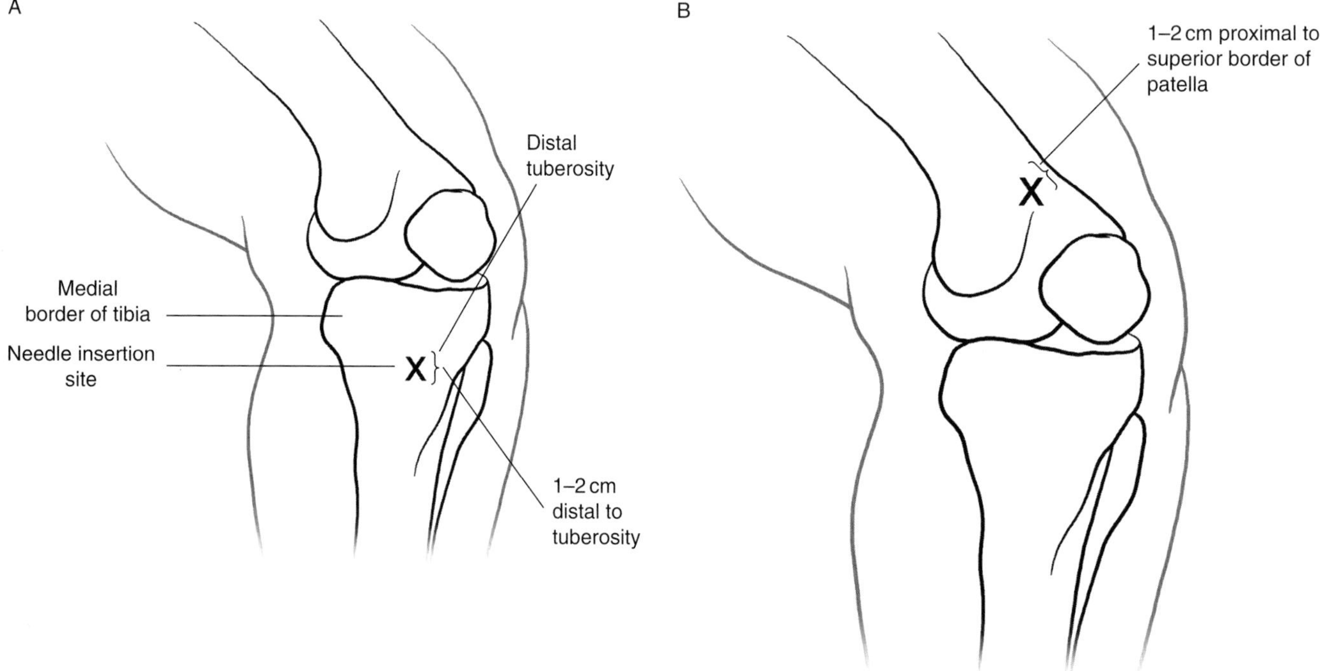

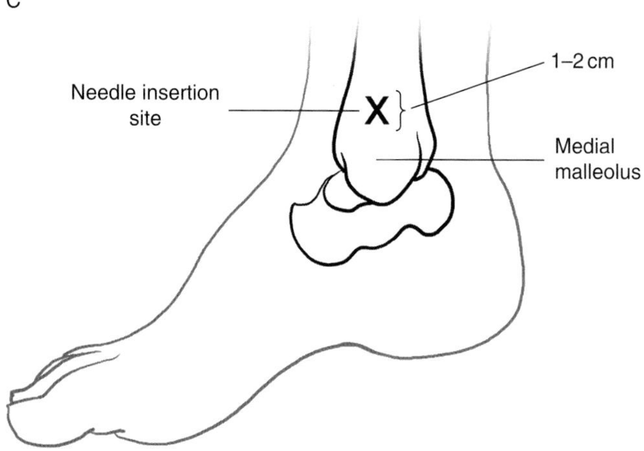

Figure 4.2 Location of intraosseous access sites: (A) proximal tibia; (B) distal femur; (C) distal tibia. (Courtesy of N. Ewen Wang)

Box 4.1. Procedure for placement for an intraosseous (IO) infusion device

1. Identify area to be used; the proximal tibia is most common. Other sites include distal femur, distal tibia, or anterior superior iliac spine.
2. Provide support to popliteal fossa with towels.
3. Cleanse skin.
4. Identify site to be used:
   - anterior tibia: find the medial flat surface 1–3 cm below tibial tuberosity; in infants use tibial tuberosity itself to avoid fracture associated with mid-shaft insertion; insert at an angle of 60–90 degrees
   - distal femur: insert needle midline, 2–3 cm proximal to epicondyle. Use a 75–80 degree angle
   - distal tibia: insert needle perpendicularly posterior to saphenous vein, proximal to medial malleolus.
5. Use firm pressure and screwing motion to advance needle.
6. A sudden decrease in resistance is expected; this is the penetration through the cortex and into the marrow.
7. Attach a syringe to the needle after removing the stylet.
8. Confirm placement with either aspiration of marrow or easy infusion of saline. The IO should be stable in the bone.
9. Secure IO well
10. The IO can be used for code medications and IV fluids. When time allows, it should be flushed with heparinized saline to prevent clot formation.
11. Monitor distal pulses; observe site for signs of extravasation of fluids.
12. Aim to remove needle as soon as possible but within 48 h of placement and replace with conventional vascular access methods.

Box 4.2. Placement of umbilical vein catheter

1. Place infant supine.
2. Cleanse skin.
3. Tie umbilical tape or place a purse-string suture at base of umbilical cord.
4. Cut umbilical cord parallel to skin approximately 2 cm from abdominal wall.
5. Clear clot from umbilical vein (one thin-walled vessel, versus two thick-walled arteries).
6. Holding the umbilical cord with a hemostat, insert catheter (5.0 French) into the umbilical vein with gentle pressure. Continue putting traction on umbilical cord.
7. Blood should flow back with insertion 1–2 cm below the skin. (While umbilical vein catheters are inserted 7–12 cm for resuscitation in the neonatal ICU, in the ED setting they should be used with the catheter placed superficially (3–5 cm) to avoid the need to confirm placement and infusion of inotropes into the liver.)
8. Secure catheter in place.

infusion. Obviously, this is not an important step in the unconscious patient.

Possible complications from the procedure are also important to know, the most common one being failed infusion. This can lead to compartment syndrome if not recognized. In addition, bony fracture or growth plate injury can occur if inserted into the incorrect location; if there is concern for this, a radiograph can be obtained. Lastly, a later complication is infection involving the bone or the skin. Sites should be monitored for signs of infection after IO insertion.

Umbilical vein catheterization

Umbilical venous catheterization is possible for neonates within the first 2 weeks of life in certain instances, such as resuscitation for severely ill patients and for short-term central venous access when peripheral access is not possible. However, preliminary studies suggest that IO placement may be easier and quicker for those who do not frequently perform newborn resuscitation. Instructions for placement of umbilical vein catheter are given in Box 4.2 and Fig. 4.3.

Complications range from uncontrolled bleeding secondary to a loose umbilical tape, creation of a false track while inserting the catheter, and securing an arterial line with mistaken catheterization of one of the two umbilical arteries.

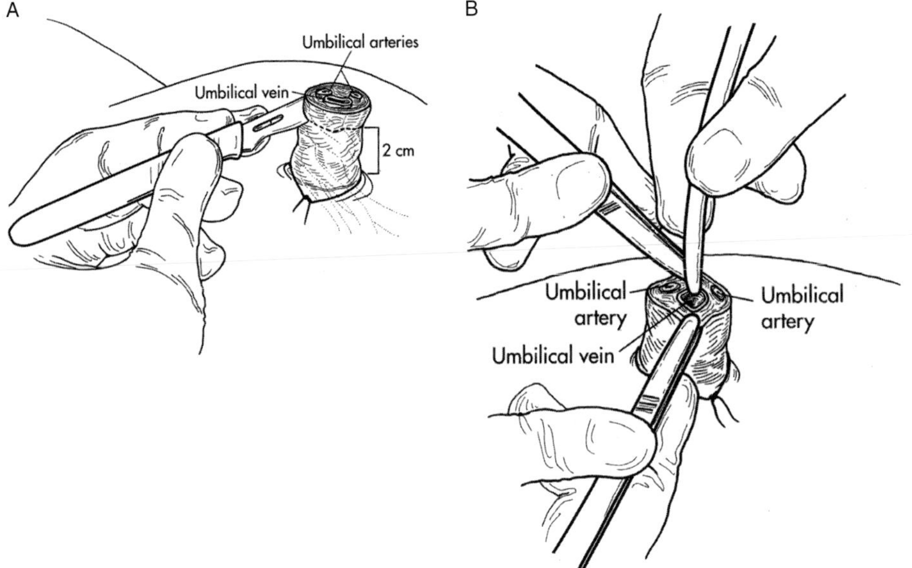

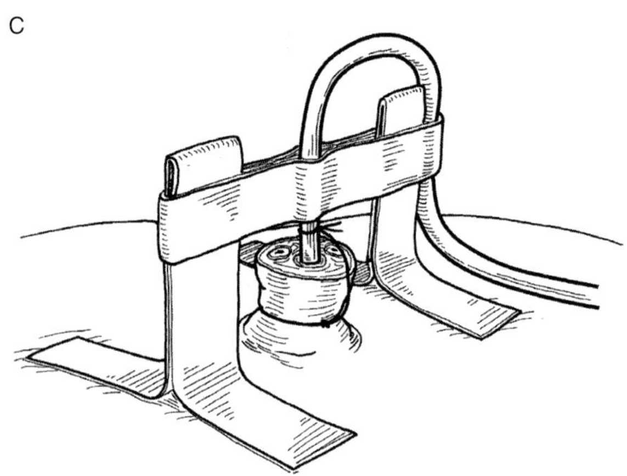

Figure 4.3 Placement of umbilical vein catheter. (A) Cut the umbilical cord for line placement. (B) Insert umbilical catheter in vein. (C) Tape catheter to umbilical wall. (Reproduced with permission from Dieckmann RA, Fiser DH, Selbst SM (eds) *Illustrated Textbook of Pediatric Emergency and Critical Care Procedures*. St. Louis, MO: Mosby, 1997. © 1997 Mosby Inc.)

Selected references

Abe KK, Blum GT, Yamamoto LG. Intraosseous is faster and easier than umbilical venous catheterization in newborn emergency vascular access models. *Am J Emerg Med* 2000; **18**:126–129.

Fiser DH. Intraosseous infusion. *N Engl J Med* 1990. **32**:1579–1581.

McAneney C. Umbilical vessel catheterization. In Dieckmann RA, Fiser DH, Selbst SM (eds) *Illustrated Textbook of Pediatric Emergency and Critical Care Procedures*. St. Louis, MO: Mosby, 1997, pp. 503–505.

Tutorial: Ultrasound-guided vascular access

Teresa S. Wu

Introduction

Indications for vascular access include volume repletion, medication administration, blood product delivery, hemodynamic monitoring, and parenteral nutrition. Vascular access can be particularly difficult to obtain in pediatric patients, and can be complicated by body habitus, volume depletion, scar tissue from previous cannulations, congenital deformities, and patient movement. Peripheral venous access is routinely utilized first, while central venous access is reserved for situations where peripheral access cannot be obtained. If a peripheral vein cannot be readily visualized or palpated, ultrasound can be used to help to localize the vein.

To perform an ultrasound-guided peripheral vein cannulation

The following steps are used for the cannulation.

1. Use a higher frequency probe. Superficial vessels are seen best with higher-frequency transducers. In general, peripheral vein visualization should be performed with a 7.5 to 10 MHz linear array transducer (Fig. 5.1).

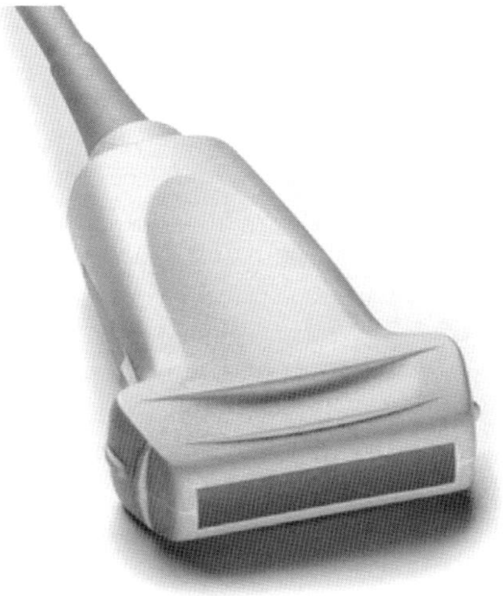

Figure 5.1 Linear array transducer. (Image courtesy of SonoSite, Inc.)

2. Apply a large amount of ultrasound gel to improve the acoustic interface. If the patient is thin and devoid of much subcutaneous fat, use an acoustic standoff pad to improve the sonographic window.
3. If acoustic standoff pads are not available, an acoustic window can be easily created with a small bag of normal saline or a fluid-filled glove sandwiched between two layers of ultrasound gel (Fig. 5.2).

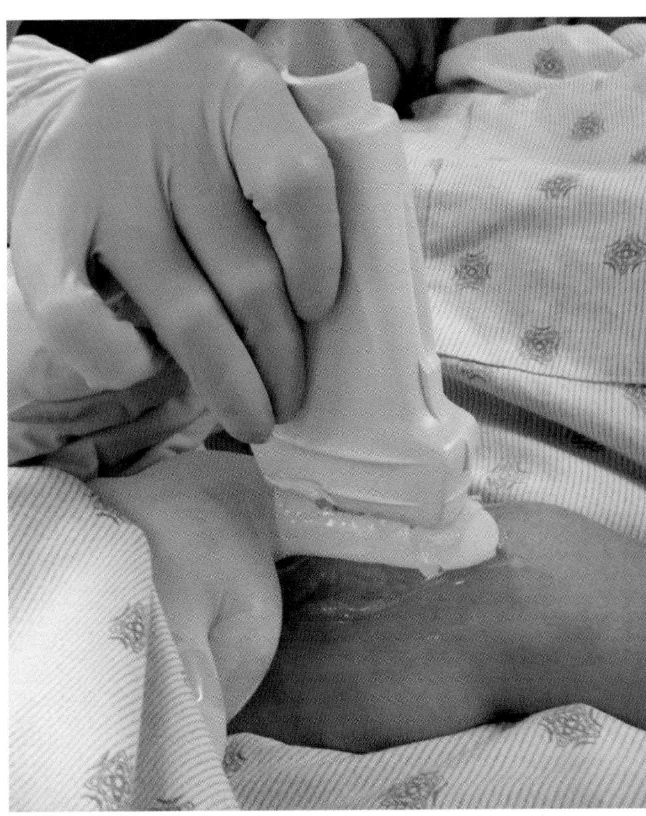

Figure 5.2 Enhancing the acoustic window with a water-filled glove. Scanning through a water-filled glove sandwiched between two layers of gel will provide an excellent acoustic window and allow better visualization of superficial structures.

A Practical Guide to Pediatric Emergency Medicine: Caring for Children in the Emergency Department, ed. N. Ewen Amieva-Wang (associate eds. Jamie Shandro, Aparajita Sohoni, and Bernhard Fassl). Published by Cambridge University Press.

A

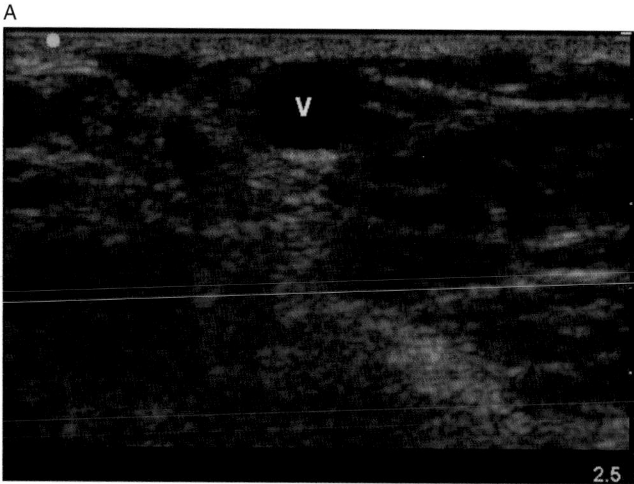

B

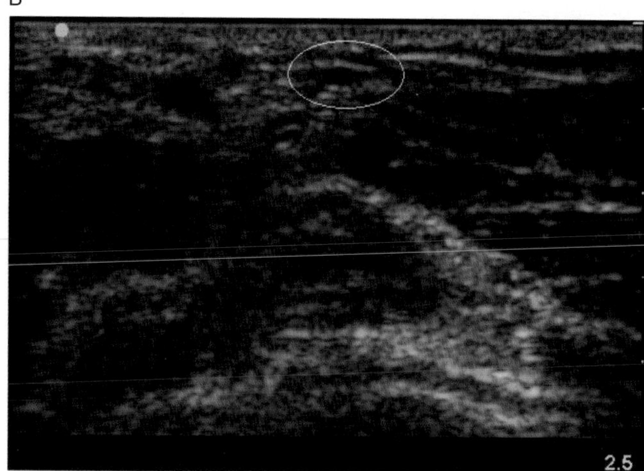

Figure 5.3 (A) Transverse (axial) view of a thin-walled vein (V). (B) Gentle pressure with the ultrasound transducer causes the vein to partially collapse (circled) or "wink".

4. Cleanse and sterilize the area of interest in a standard manner and apply a tourniquet proximally to enhance venous fill.
5. Veins have thinner walls than arteries. On ultrasound, veins will collapse easily under pressure, while arteries will remain patent and pulsatile during the scan (Fig. 5.3).
6. Because veins collapse readily under pressure, care must be taken to prevent inadvertent collapse of superficial veins by minimizing the amount of force applied to the transducer.
7. Application of color Doppler over the vessel of interest can help to distinguish an artery from a vein:
   - flow within an arterial lumen will appear pulsatile; in contrast, a vein will demonstrate a more constant rumble of color flow
   - the color corresponds to the direction of flow (towards or away from the transducer) so blue does not indicate venous and red arterial; the color scale is on the left of the screen and the top color corresponds to flow towards the probe; the bottom color indicates flow away from the probe.
8. Visualize the target vein in both longitudinal and transverse orientations to look for bifurcations and to map out the vessel's anatomical course (Fig. 5.4).
9. Once a peripheral vein has been localized, cannulation can be attempted in a static or dynamic fashion.
10. If the procedure is performed in a dynamic manner, remember to use sterile ultrasound gel and prepare the ultrasound probe in a sterile fashion.
11. When the vessel is being cannulated under dynamic ultrasound guidance, remember that direct visualization of the needle will only be noted when the ultrasound beam is angled directly at the needle. Because the field visualized by ultrasound is so narrow, needle position may need to be inferred by visualizing ring-down artifact, soft tissue changes, and tenting of the wall of the target structure (Figs. 5.5 and 5.6).

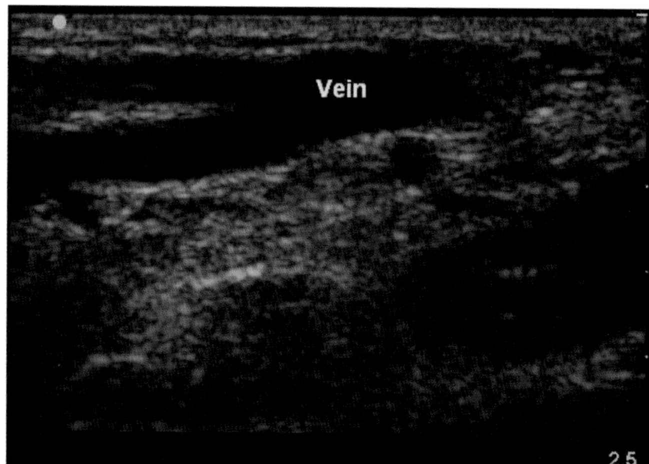

Figure 5.4 Longitudinal (sagittal) view of a peripheral vein.

The three most common sites for central venous catheter placement in children are the femoral, subclavian, and internal jugular veins. Although all three sites provide access to the central circulatory system, in emergency situations where the patient's head and neck region is often difficult to access given simultaneous airway management or cervical spine stabilization, the femoral site is often the most accessible. In adults, central lines in the femoral vein have a higher risk of infection and deep venous thrombosis over the subclavian or internal jugular veins. In children, however, there has been no difference in complications and infection rates based on insertion site. The size of the catheter used during central venous access also differs between children and adults. In children, the catheter used depends on the age and weight of the child.

Central venous access can be obtained using either the landmark-guided approach or under ultrasound guidance. Studies have shown that central lines placed using the

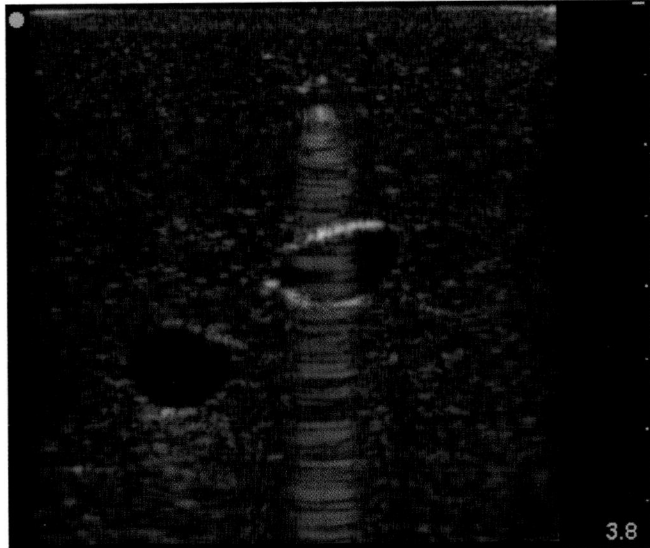

Figure 5.5 Hyperchoic ring-down artifact from the needle advancing towards the vein in a vascular model.

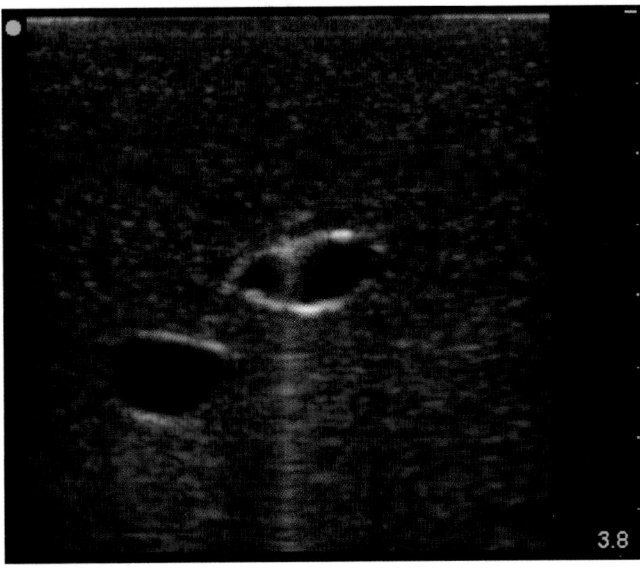

Figure 5.6 Tenting of the vessel wall as the needle is about to enter the lumen of the vein in a vascular model. Note the bright white ring-down artifact coming off the needle.

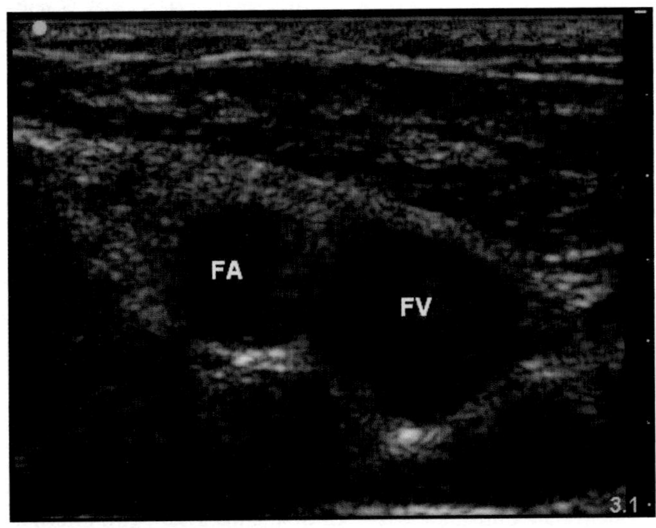

Figure 5.7 Ultrasound image of the right femoral vein (FV) and femoral artery (FA).

landmark technique alone can lead to complications such as inadvertent arterial puncture, multiple punctures through the target vessel, extensive bleeding, or accidental puncture of adjacent structures such as the lung, lymphatic channels, or urinary bladder. The ultrasound-guided approach to central line placement has been described by various specialties, and the consensus remains that ultrasound guidance can improve time to successful cannulation while minimizing complications.

The location of the femoral vein in relationship to the femoral artery is important to establish when attempting femoral vein catheterization to avoid complications such as arterial puncture. In a recent study, children were found to have up to a 12% incidence of femoral vein and artery partial or complete overlap in contrast to the traditionally taught relationship (lateral to medial: nerve–artery–vein–empty space–lymphatics).

Femoral vein access

The following steps are used to access the femoral vein under ultrasound guidance.

1. Apply a large amount of ultrasound gel to improve the acoustic interface.
2. Gently place the 7.5 or 10 MHz linear transducer in a transverse orientation inferior to the middle segment of the inguinal ligament.
3. Under ultrasound, the femoral vein appears as an oval, thin-walled, anechoic structure that collapses easily under pressure. The adjacent femoral artery will be the round, anechoic, thicker-walled, pulsatile structure lying just lateral to the femoral vein. The femoral artery should not collapse under pressure unless the patient is profoundly hypovolemic (Fig. 5.7).
4. Application of color Doppler over the vessel of interest can help to distinguish an artery from a vein:
   - flow within an arterial lumen will appear pulsatile; in contrast, a vein will demonstrate a more constant rumble of color flow
   - the color corresponds to the direction of flow (towards or away from the transducer) so blue does not indicate venous and red arterial; the color scale is on the left of the screen and the top color corresponds to flow towards the probe; the bottom color indicates flow away from the probe.

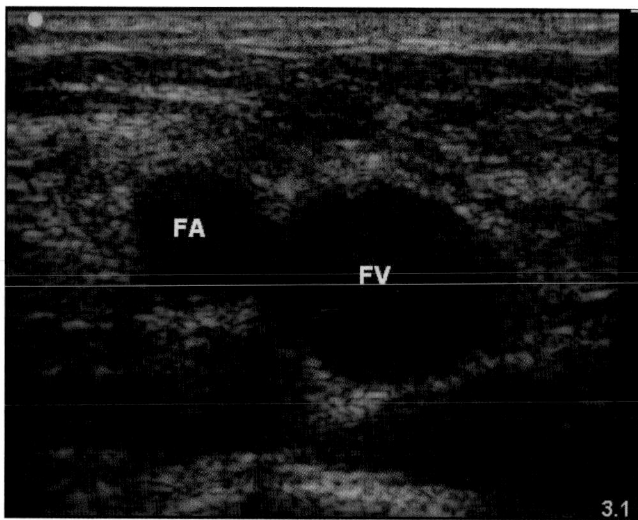

Figure 5.8 Changing the spatial relationship of the femoral vein (FV) and femoral artery (FA) with hip rotation. External rotation and abduction of the right hip increases the distance between the femoral artery and femoral vein.

5. Assess for anatomical variations or abnormal bifurcations by scanning in both a transverse and a longitudinal fashion along the femoral vein. In approximately 25% of patients, the femoral vein may course directly posterior to the femoral artery just below the inguinal ligament.
6. Scan caudally until the femoral vein can be visualized coursing distinctly away from the femoral artery. Patient positioning may alter the relationship of the femoral vein to the femoral artery. Attempt to rotate the femur in different angles to achieve the ideal spatial relationship between the femoral vein and femoral artery (Fig. 5.8).
7. Access the femoral vein in a sterile fashion, utilizing either the static or dynamic ultrasound-guided approach.
8. If the procedure is performed in a dynamic manner, remember to use sterile ultrasound gel and prepare the ultrasound probe in a sterile fashion.
9. When the vessel is being cannulated under dynamic ultrasound guidance, remember that direct visualization of the needle will only be noted when the ultrasound beam is angled directly at the needle. Because the field visualized by ultrasound is so narrow, needle position may need to be inferred by visualizing ring-down artifact, soft tissue changes, and tenting of the wall of the target structure (Fig. 5.5 and Fig. 5.6).

Internal jugular vein access

The following steps are used to access the internal jugular vein under ultrasound guidance.

1. Place the patient in the Trendelenburg position and turn the patient's head gently towards the contralateral side. Turning the patient's head more than 30 degrees past midline may cause compression of the internal jugular vein by the sternocleidomastoid muscle.

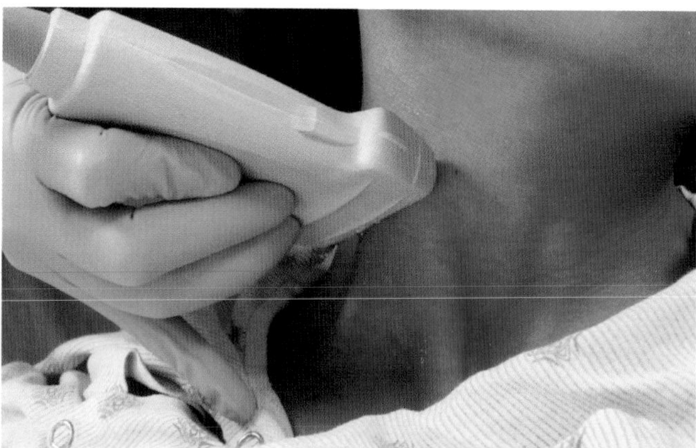

Figure 5.9 Transducer position for visualization of the right internal jugular vein.

2. If the patient is alert and cooperative, have the patient use their sternocleidomastoid muscle to elevate their head momentarily to help to visualize anatomic landmarks. The internal jugular vein lies deep to the sternocleidomastoid muscle, lateral and superficial to the carotid artery.
3. Apply a large amount of ultrasound gel to improve the acoustic interface.
4. Gently place the 7.5 or 10 MHz linear transducer at the bifurcation of the sternal and clavicular heads of the sternocleidomastoid muscle for the standard central approach (Fig. 5.9).
5. Under ultrasound, the internal jugular vein appears as an oval, thin-walled, anechoic structure that collapses easily under pressure. The adjacent carotid artery will be the round, anechoic, thicker-walled, pulsatile structure lying just medial to the internal jugular vein. The carotid artery should not collapse under pressure unless the patient is profoundly hypovolemic (Fig. 5.10).
6. Application of color Doppler over the vessel of interest can help distinguish an artery from a vein:
   - flow within an arterial lumen will appear pulsatile; in contrast, a vein will demonstrate a more constant rumble of color flow
   - the color corresponds to the direction of flow (towards or away from the transducer) so blue does not indicate venous and red arterial; the color scale is on the left of the screen and the top color corresponds to flow towards the probe; the bottom color indicates flow away from the probe.
7. Scan along the internal jugular vein in a transverse and longitudinal fashion to assess for any anatomic or pathologic variations.
8. Access the internal jugular vein in a sterile fashion, utilizing either the static or dynamic ultrasound-guided approach.

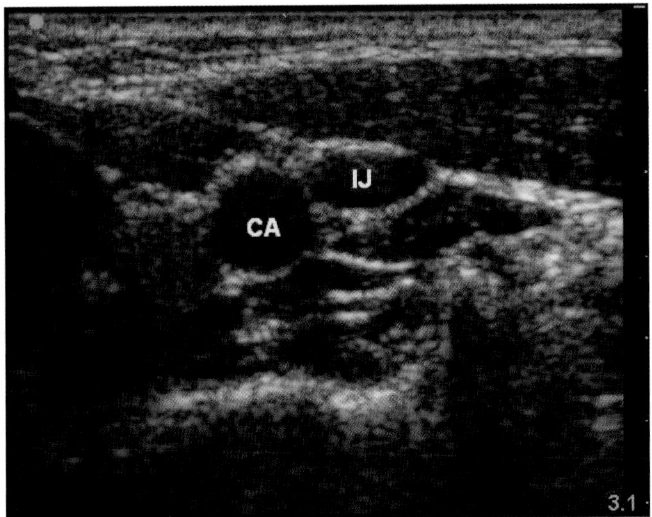

Figure 5.10 Transverse (axial) view of the right internal jugular vein (IJ) and right carotid artery (CA).

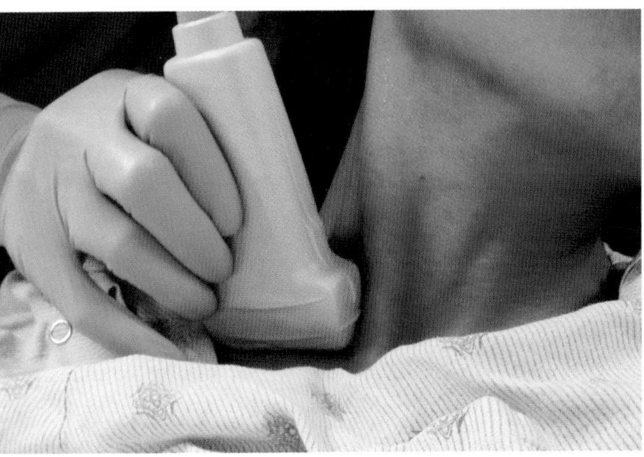

Figure 5.11 Transducer position to visualize the subclavian vein using a supraclavicular approach.

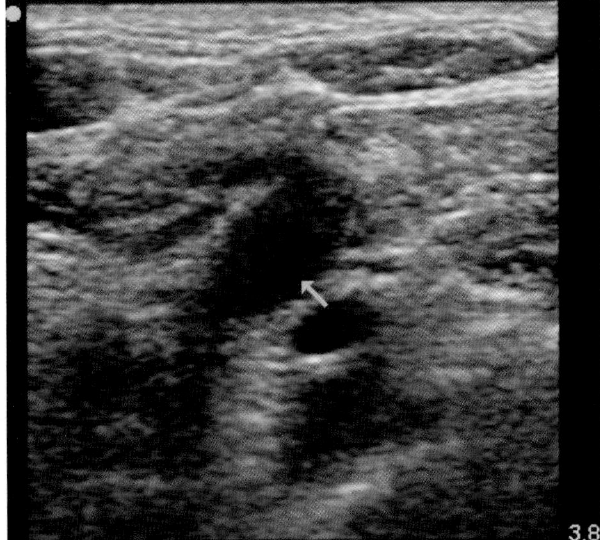

Figure 5.12 Ultrasound image of the subclavian vein (arrow) from a supraclavicular approach.

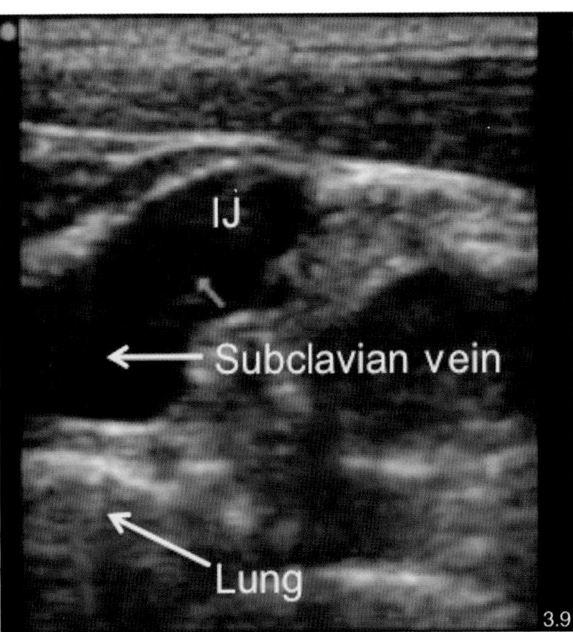

Figure 5.13 Ultrasound image of the internal jugular vein (IJ) joining the subclavian vein from a supraclavicular approach.

9. If the procedure is performed in a dynamic manner, remember to use sterile ultrasound gel and prepare the ultrasound probe in a sterile fashion.
10. When the vessel is being cannulated under dynamic ultrasound guidance, remember that direct visualization of the needle will only be noted when the ultrasound beam is angled directly at the needle. Because the field visualized by ultrasound is so narrow, needle position may need to be inferred by visualizing ring-down artifact, soft tissue changes, and tenting of the wall of the target structure (Fig. 5.5 and Fig. 5.6).

Subclavian vein access

The use of ultrasound guidance via a supraclavicular approach enables the subclavian vein to be visualized as it connects to the caudal portion of the internal jugular vein. The subclavian vein is difficult to visualize with ultrasound if an infraclavicular approach is utilized because the window can be obscured by the clavicle. To circumvent this limitation, the following steps of the supraclavicular approach are used.

1. Apply a large amount of ultrasound gel to improve the acoustic interface.
2. Place the 7.5 to 10 MHz linear transducer in a transverse orientation 1 cm lateral to the sternal notch and just superior to the clavicle (Fig. 5.11).
3. Angle the probe caudally to visualize the subclavian vein lying just lateral to the internal jugular vein. In this plane, the subclavian vein appears as a long, anechoic, thin-walled structure lying just below the hyperechoic clavicle.
4. The thicker-walled, pulsatile subclavian artery may be seen coursing just below the subclavian vein (Fig. 5.12).
5. Fanning the probe in a cranial fashion may provide an image of the internal jugular vein joining the subclavian vein (Fig. 5.13).
6. Scan along the subclavian vein in a transverse fashion to assess for any anatomic or pathologic variations.
7. Access the subclavian vein in a sterile fashion, utilizing either the static or dynamic ultrasound-guided approach.
8. If the procedure is performed in a dynamic manner, remember to use sterile ultrasound gel and prepare the ultrasound probe in a sterile fashion.
9. When the vessel is being cannulated under dynamic ultrasound guidance, remember that direct visualization of the needle will only be noted when the ultrasound beam is angled directly at the needle. Because the field visualized by ultrasound is so narrow, needle position may need to be inferred by visualizing ring-down artifact, soft tissue changes, and tenting of the wall of the target structure (Fig. 5.5 and Fig. 5.6).

Selected references

Chiang VW, Baskin MN. Uses and complications of central venous catheters inserted in a pediatric emergency department. *Pediatr Emerg Care* 2000;**16**:230–232.

McGee DC, Gould MK. Preventing complications of central venous catheterization. *N Engl J Med* 2003;**348**:1123–1133.

Merrer J, De Jonghe B, Golliot F, *et al.* Complications of femoral and subclavian venous catheterization in critically ill patients: a randomized controlled trial. *JAMA* 2001;**286**: 700–707.

O'Grady NP, Alexander M, Dellinger EP, *et al.* Guidelines for the prevention of intravascular catheter-related infections. *Pediatrics* 2002;**110**:e51.

Sheridan RL, Weber JM. Mechanical and infectious complications of central venous cannulation in children: lessons learned from a 10-year experience placing more than 1000 catheters. *J Burn Care Res* 2006;**27**:713–718.

Warkentine FH, Clyde Pierce M, Lorenz D, Kim IK. The anatomic relationship of femoral vein to femoral artery in euvolemic pediatric patients by ultrasonography: implications for pediatric femoral central venous access. *Acad Emerg Med* 2008;**15**:426–430.

Chapter 6

Pediatric resuscitation: the updated American Heart Association guidelines

Stephanie J. Doniger

Introduction

The 2005 recent 2010 revised Pediatric Advanced Life Support (PALS) guidelines from the American Heart Association (AHA) simplified resuscitation for prehospital as well as for advanced providers. Overall, the emphasis is on effective basic life support (BLS) including effective chest compressions, with recommendations for different ages. For the lay rescuer, pediatric guidelines are now applied to children between 1 and 8 years of age. While the 2010 AHA guidelines have changed the order of performance of ABCs in an effort to simplify resuscitation algorithms for the lay provider, they remain the same for health care providers. For the advanced provider, PALS guidelines can be applied to children 1 year of age through to the onset of puberty, determined by the presence of secondary sexual characteristics.

Once it is recognized that a child needs resuscitation, it is important to approach the evaluation and management in a step-wise manner following the mnemonic ABC (airway, breathing, circulation). If there is an abnormality at any step of this ABC assessment, intervention must be initiated at that point to stabilize the patient. In 2010, the AHA published new guidelines for pediatric BLS and PALS. Key updates to BLS for pediatric patients include:

- initiation of CPR: begin with compressions, followed by breathing, and lastly by airway (CBA); for a lone provider, begin with 30 compressions, while for two healthcare providers, 15 compressions is appropriate (instead of the two rescue breaths recommended in the 2005 guidelines)
- depth of chest compressions: compress the chest at least one-third of the anterior–posterior chest diameter, which is approximately 4 cm in infants and 5 cm in children (the 2005 guidelines recommended compression with enough force to depress the chest wall one-third to half the anterior–posterior diameter).

Airway

Evaluation for airway patency

The first priority in life support is evaluating the airway. The provider should look, listen, and feel to determine the status of the airway. Looking for chest rise, listening for breath sounds and air movement, and feeling air movement at the nose and mouth should indicate the patency and efficacy of the airway. Clinical signs of an airway obstruction include breathing difficulty, the inability to speak or breathe, a silent cough, or poor air exchange. It is crucial to determine whether the airway is maintainable by simple maneuvers, or if advanced interventions are required.

Management: opening the airway

Simple measures to restore airway patency include positioning, suctioning, and relieving airway obstruction by a foreign-body. Airway adjuncts such as oropharyngeal and nasopharyngeal airways may assist in opening the airway, and facilitating in delivering oxygen by Bag-Valve Mask. The preferred method of opening the airway for the lay rescuer and the healthcare provider in non-trauma settings is the head tilt–chin lift maneuver for both injured and non-injured victims. In trauma situations in which a cervical spine injury is suspected, a jaw thrust maneuver without a head tilt by healthcare professionals is recommended.

Foreign bodies

In the situation of airway foreign bodies, if the individual is unresponsive, it is recommended to activate the emergency medical services and perform cardiopulmonary resuscitation (CPR). It is unadvisable to perform blind finger sweeps. The recommendation is to perform five back blows and five chest thrusts for infants, and to perform the Heimlich maneuver in older children (Fig. 6.1).

A Practical Guide to Pediatric Emergency Medicine: Caring for Children in the Emergency Department, ed. N. Ewen Amieva-Wang (associate eds. Jamie Shandro, Aparajita Sohoni, and Bernhard Fassl). Published by Cambridge University Press.

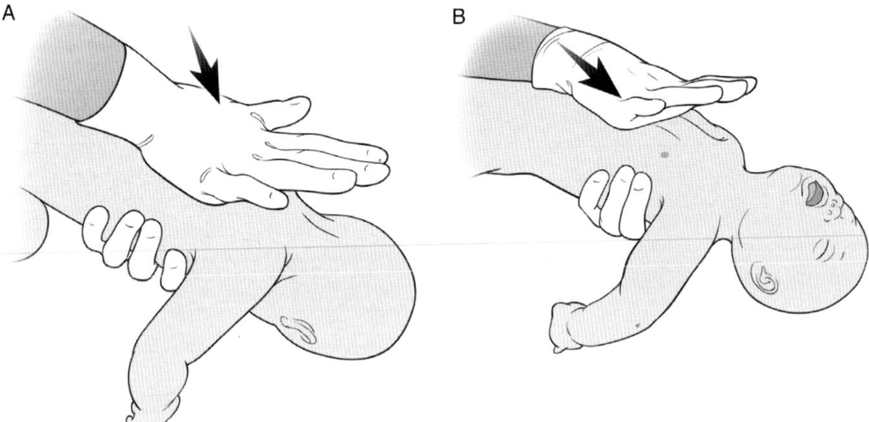

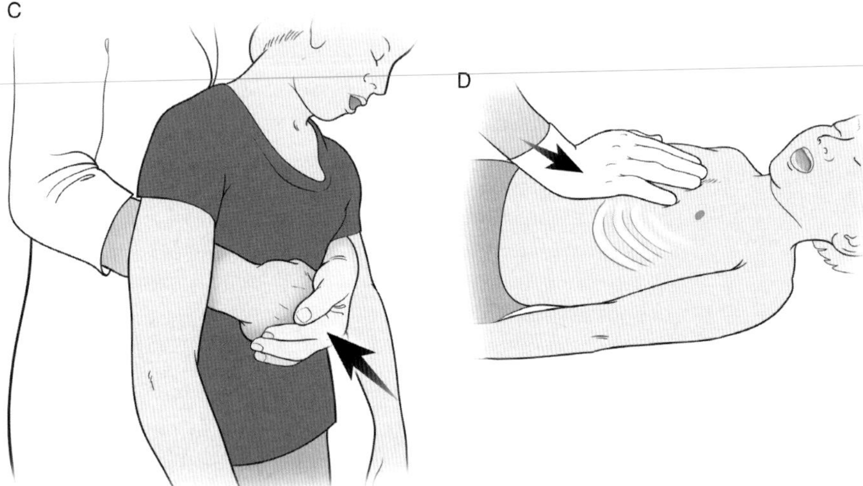

Figure 6.1 Technique for foreign body removal in a child unable to move air. In infants A), alternate five back blows and B) five chest thrusts until the object is expelled. In older children, the rescuer can kneel or stand behind responsive child and C) perform abdominal thrusts. If the child becomes unresponsive, D) abdominal thrusts should be performed on the supine child. (Copyright Chris Gralapp.)

Breathing

Evaluation of adequate breathing

The assessment of breathing includes an evaluation of the respiratory rate and effort, lung sounds, and pulse oximetry. Normal respiratory rates depend on the age of the patient (Table x; inside book cover). Tachypnea is a rate that is more rapid than normal for age, whereas bradypnea is slower than normal for age. Apnea is defined as a complete cessation of breathing for 20 s or more, often with associated change in color or tone. A child may exhibit nasal flaring, retractions or accessory muscle use, or irregular respirations indicating increased respiratory effort. Further factors to assess are adequate and equal chest wall excursion, and the auscultation of air movement. Abnormal lung sounds include stridor, grunting, gurgling, wheezing, and crackles.

Management: respiratory support

Rather than waiting for respiratory arrest, patients who do not exhibit adequate breathing should receive rescue breaths. It is recommended to try "a couple of times" to deliver two effective rescue breaths. In those who are not breathing but have a pulse, only respirations should be delivered, without compressions. The healthcare provider should administer 12–20 breaths/min (1 breath every 3–5 s) for infants and children, and 10–12 breaths/min (1 breath every 5–6 s) for adults. Rescue breaths should be given over 1 s, with enough volume to create visible chest rise. There are no indications stating specific tidal volumes, since it is difficult to estimate tidal volumes delivered during rescue breaths. In fact, much less tidal volume is required during resuscitation than in normal healthy individuals, given that during CPR there is 24–33% less blood flow to the lungs. Therefore, fewer breaths with smaller volumes are needed for oxygenation and ventilation.

The method of maintaining a proper airway depends on the skill level of the provider. For all providers, adequate BVM technique is crucial to sustaining a patient's airway. While intubation provides a definitive airway, intubation must not cause a prolonged interruption in compressions. New PALS guidelines state that a cuffed endotracheal tube may be used in all ages, except in neonates. A cuffed endotracheal tube is particularly useful for those with poor lung compliance, increased airway resistance, or in those with a large glottic air leak. Attention must be paid to tube size, position, and

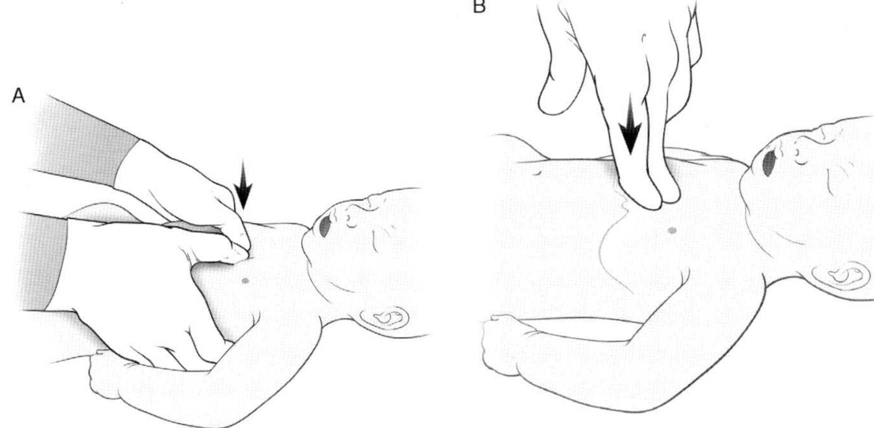

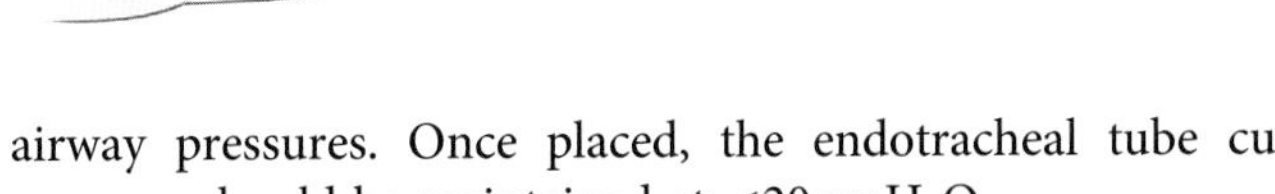

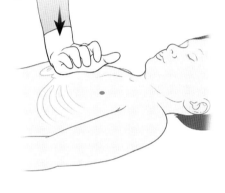

Figure 6.2 The proper positioning in order to perform effective chest compressions in infants and children. (A) In infants, the use of two hands with a thumb-encircling technique is preferred. The thumbs are placed side by side over the lower half of the sternum just below the nipple line, avoiding compression of the xyphoid process. (B) For an infant if there is a lone rescuer, or the provider has small hands, a two finger compression technique is preferred. Two fingers of one hand are placed over the lower half of the sternum just below the nipple line, avoiding compression of the xyphoid process. (C) For older children, the heel of the hand is placed over the lower half of the sternum between the nipple line and bottom of the sternum, avoiding compression of the xyphoid process. The fingers are lifted to avoid compressing the ribs. (Copyright Chris Gralapp.)

airway pressures. Once placed, the endotracheal tube cuff pressure should be maintained at $<20\,\mathrm{cmH_2O}$.

Confirmation of tube placement should include clinical assessment and auscultation of breath sounds. In addition, it is recommended that exhaled carbon dioxide is measured by a calorimetric detector or by capnography. However, their use is limited to those patients exhibiting a perfusing rhythm. In those patients weighing >20 kg, one may consider esophageal detector devices for confirmation of tube placement. It is important to verify endotracheal tube placement after the tube is inserted, during transport, and after the movement of the patient.

Circulation

Evaluation of circulation

The assessment of cardiovascular function primarily includes heart rate and rhythm, and blood pressure. Heart rate and blood pressure vary according to the child's age (Table x; inside book cover). Hypotension is defined as <5th percentile of expected blood pressure for age. In children between 1 and 10 years of age, the 5th percentile systolic blood pressure can be estimated by the formula:

$$\text{5th percentile blood pressure} = 70 + 2(\text{age in years})$$

Other indicators of adequate perfusion include peripheral and central pulses, capillary refill time, skin color, and temperature. A delayed capillary refill time of greater than 2 s represents poor peripheral perfusion and may be a result of dehydration, shock, or hypothermia.

The advanced cardiac evaluation includes the recognition and management of arrhythmias (Ch. 17) with the goal of restoring a perfusing heart rhythm. The resuscitation algorithms begin with differentiating between bradycardia and tachycardia. Upon recognition of a tacycardia, step-wise questioning can help to evaluate the ECG tracing. Is the rhythm regular or irregular? Is the QRS narrow or wide? Does every P wave result in a single QRS? Once this is established, treatment options are considered according to whether or not the patient has a pulse and the presenting rhythm on ECG.

Circulation management

Recommendations for stabilizing the patient's cardiovascular function include performing chest compressions and establishing IV access. The advanced provider must be able to treat arrhythmias.

Effective chest compressions are crucial in improving survival. The AHA now recommends, "push hard and push fast." Interruptions in compressions should be limited to <10 s for interventions such as placing an advanced airway or defibrillation. Rhythm checks should be performed every 2 min, or five cycles of CPR.

Since bradycardia is often a terminal rhythm in children, it is not appropriate to wait for a pulseless arrest to initiate compressions. Compressions should be initiated in newborns with a heart rate <60 beats/min, in children with a heart rate <60 beats/min and poor perfusion, and in patients without a pulse. Compressions should be performed at a rate of 100/min for all ages, except newborns, in whom compressions should occur at a rate of 120/min. The compression to ventilation ratio is 30:2 for single rescuers, while the ratio is 15:2 when there are two providers present. Once an advanced airway is in place, compressions and breaths should be performed continuously without interruption. These universal rates simplify guidelines for providers and, furthermore, allow for sufficient time for adequate chest recoil and to allow for adequate cardiac filling and venous return.

In order to perform adequate compressions for children, the heel of one or two hands should be used to compress the lower half of the sternum to a depth of one-half to one-third of the chest diameter (Fig. 6.2). For infants, the AHA now recommends that two thumbs press on the sternum, with the hands encircling the chest (Fig. 6.2). In addition to compressing the sternum, the hands should squeeze the thorax. This improves coronary artery perfusion pressure and may generate higher systolic and diastolic blood pressures. When performing chest compressions, rescuers should alternate after five cycles of CPR, or 2 min, in order to decrease rescuer fatigue. This switch should be performed in <5 s, in order to minimize interruptions in CPR.

Intravenous or intraosseous (IO) routes are preferred for vascular access and for the administration of all drugs. Drug administration via the endotracheal tube is not recommended, since drug delivery is unpredictable. In addition to lower drug concentrations in the blood, some drugs can cause detrimental β-adrenergic effects. However, if vascular access is unavailable, lipophilic drugs may be administered at higher doses through the endotracheal tube.

Lipophilic drugs that can be given via an endotracheal tube: lidocaine, epinephrine, atropine, and narcan (mnemonic: LEAN).

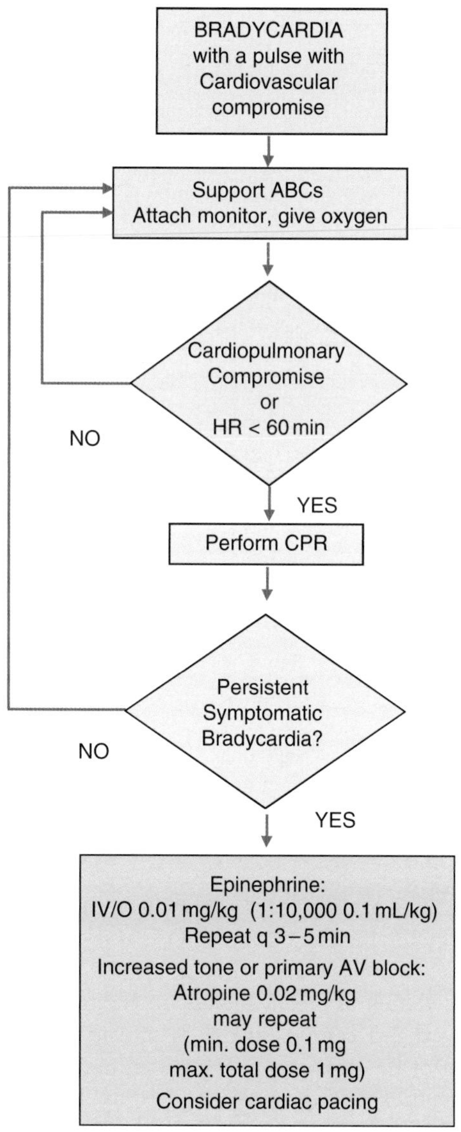

Figure 6.3 Pediatric bradycardia algorithm with pulse and poor perfusion. CPR, cardiopulmonary resuscitation; HR, heart rate; AV, atrioventricular. (Courtesy Dr. Stephanie J. Doniger.)

Defibrillation

In situations of sudden witnessed collapse with ventricular tachycardia or fibrillation, defibrillation is warranted, followed by CPR, and then by drug administration. Use of CPR will provide some blood flow to deliver oxygen and substrate to the heart muscle, thereby making it more likely to abort ventricular fibrillation. A single shock should be administered at a dose of 2 J/kg, followed by immediate CPR. If there is any delay in delivering the shock, CPR should be initiated immediately. In at least 90% of these cases, ventricular fibrillation is eliminated by the first shock. In those cases in which the first shock does not terminate ventricular fibrillation, CPR is of greater value. CPR "primes" the heart for the next defibrillation attempt. In cases of prolonged ventricular fibrillation, it has been shown that giving CPR prior to defibrillation increased survival rates from 4% to 22%.

The updated PALS guidelines emphasize the superiority and greater safety of biphasic over monophasic shocks. Based on adult and animal model studies, biphasic shocks are at least as effective as monophasic shocks but are less harmful. Regardless of the type of defibrillator (monophasic or biphasic), the dosages of defibrillation are now 2 J/kg followed by 4 J/kg for subsequent dosages. It is important to note that stacked shocks are no longer recommended. A single shock is recommended followed by CPR

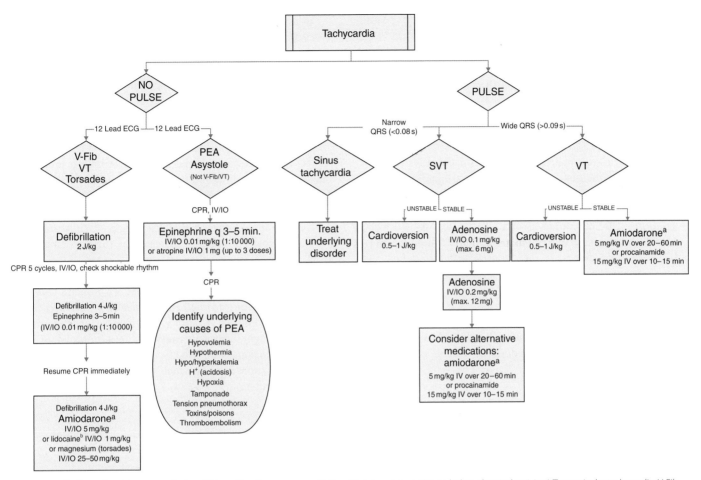

Figure 6.4 Tachycardia with poor perfusion. CPR, cardiopulmonary resuscitation; IO, intraosseous; PEA, pulseless electrical activity; VT, ventricular tachycardia; V-Fib, ventricular fibrillation. [a]Amiodarone: repeat doses of 1–5 mg/kg may be required (max. 15 mg/kg per day). [b]Lidocaine: repeat every 5–10 min after the initial bolus (max. 3 mg/kg) then infuse 20–50 μg/kg per min. (Courtesy Dr. Stephanie J. Doniger.)

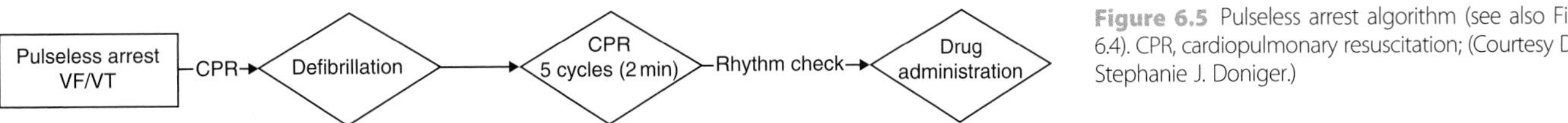

Figure 6.5 Pulseless arrest algorithm (see also Fig. 6.4). CPR, cardiopulmonary resuscitation; (Courtesy Dr. Stephanie J. Doniger.)

largely because of the prolonged period of time required to administer three shocks. Do not interrupt CPR until five cycles or 2 min for a pulse/rhythm check.

Automatic external defibrillators

In the community, automatic external defibrillators (AEDs) have been shown to increase survival rates. There has been sufficient evidence to show that AEDs can safely be used for those >1 year of age. In a sudden witnessed collapse, CPR should be initiated while the AED is being retrieved and attached. If the collapse is unwitnessed, CPR should be performed for five cycles or 2 min prior to the use of the AED. Pediatric AED pads and energy levels should be used in those 1–8 years of age. If the pediatric dose is unavailable, the adult dose is a reasonable alternative.

Rhythm management

The treatment of arrhythmias follows the AHA bradycardia (Fig. 6.3) and tachycardia (Fig. 6.4) algorithms. The presence or absence of a pulse determines which arm of the algorithm to initiate (Fig. 6.5). Of note, sinus tachycardia with adequate perfusion is not in the algorithm; the underlying cause should be treated.

Management

Pharmacologic therapy

For the most part, the algorithm drug dosages are unchanged in the updated 2005 AHA Recommendations. The new recommendations emphasize that drug delivery should not interrupt CPR. The timing of drug delivery is less important than maintaining chest compressions. Amiodarone is the preferred drug for treatment for pulseless arrest. Lidocaine is only recommended when amiodarone is unavailable. Additionally, lidocaine has been replaced by amiodarone and procainamide in the stable ventricular tachycardia algorithm (Fig. 6.4). It is important to note that amiodarone and procainamide should not be administered together as they can lead to severe hypotension and prolongation of the QT interval.

High-dose epinephrine (1:1000 concentration via IV) is not recommended in any age group and is actually associated with a worse outcome. Therefore, the standard recommended dose is (0.01 mg/kg IV/IO of the 1:10 000 solution) for all doses, which correlates to 0.1 ml/kg. Although the preferred routes of administration are IV or IO, it may be given via the endotracheal tube when such access is unable to be obtained (0.1 mg/kg). In exceptional cases, such as beta-blocker overdose, high-dose epinephrine may be considered.

In cases of asystole or pulseless electrical activity (PEA), CPR should be initiated immediately while attempting to identify and treat the underlying causes or the 6 Hs and 5 Ts:

hypovolemia
hypoxia
hydrogen ion (acidosis)
hypo/hyperkalemia
hypoglycemia
hypothermia
toxins
tamponade (cardiac)
tension pneumothorax
thrombosis (coronary or pulmonary)
trauma (hypovolemia).

Pharmacologic therapy consists of epinephrine (0.01 mg/kg IV/IO). Alternatively, for slow rates, atropine may be administered (1 mg IV/IO) (Fig. 6.5).

Post-resuscitative care

Special circumstances: the 2010 AHA guidelines issue specific recommendations for the resuscitation of infants and children with single ventricle physiology, Fontan, hemi-Fontan/bidirectional physiology, and pulmonary hypertension. Infants with single ventricle physiology may benefit from inducing mild hypercarbia ($PaCO_2$ 50–60 mmHg), as may children with Fontan or hemi-Fontan/bidirectional Glenn physiology. In children with pulmonary hypertension, it may be beneficial to correct the hypercarbia, administer medications to decrease pulmonary artery pressure, and perform a trial of nitrous oxide or aerosolized prostacyclin or analogue to reduce pulmonary vascular resistance. For full recommendations for these special patient populations, please see the AHA 2010 Guidelines for PALS (*Circulation* 2010;**122**(suppl 2)).

In general, it is recommended that a normal body temperature is maintained after resuscitative care of neonates and children. Although there is little evidence from children, the 2010 AHA recommendations based on adult evidence include consideration of therapeutic hypothermia for children who remain comatose after cardiac arrest. However, in all cases, it is important to avoid hyperthermia, particularly in very-low-weight infants.

In addition, new recommendations recognize the probable benefits of vasoactive medications, including inodilators (inamrinone, milrinone) to treat after resuscitation in myocardial depression. Further studies are recommended prior to universal initiation of these agents.

New evidence suggests that the length of resuscitation is not an adequate prognostic indicator of survival. Intact survival has been reported even in those cases of prolonged resuscitation and where two doses of epinephrine have been administered. The 2010 AHA guidelines recommend that in all cases of sudden unexplained cardiac death, permission for an unrestricted complete autopsy with tissue for genetic analysis should be sought. This is because of the importance of diagnosing channelopathies, which may have caused the fatal arrhythmia, knowledge of which may be critically important for living relatives.

Pearls and pitfalls

Pearls

1. The Pediatric Advanced Life Support (PALS) may be applied to children from 1 year of age through to puberty.
2. "Push hard, push fast", at 100 compressions/min.
3. Universal compression rate: ventilation 30:2 (lone rescuer), 15:2 (2 rescuers).
4. Once an advanced airway is in place, simultaneously perform compressions and ventilations at a rate of 8–10 ventilations/min.
5. Preferred route for drug administration is IV/IO.
6. Family presence during a resuscitation should be encouraged.

Pitfalls

1. Failure to maintain cervical spine precautions in trauma situations.
2. Inadequate cardiopulmonary resuscitation (CPR) with too few, too shallow, too weak chest compressions or frequent interruptions in CPR.
3. Inaccurate medication dosing, failure to use length-based resuscitation system.

Selected references

Abella B, Alvarado J, Myklebust H, *et al.* Quality of cardiopulmonary resuscitation during in-hospital cardiac arrest. *JAMA* 2005;**293**:363–365.

Berg MD, Schexnayder SM, Chameides L, *et al.* 2010 American Heart Association guidelines for cardiopulmonary resuscitation and emergency cardiovascular care. Part 13: pediatric basic life support. *Circulation* 2010; **122**:S862–S875.

Donoghue A, Nadkarni V, Berg R, *et al.* Out-of-hospital pediatric cardiac arrest: an epidemiologic review and assessment of current knowledge. *Ann Emerg Med* 2005; **46**:512–522.

ECC Committee SaTFotAHA. Highlights of the 2005 American Heart Association Guidelines for Cardiopulmonary Resuscitation and Emergency Cardiovascular Care. *Currents* 2006;**15**:2–10.

Kattwinkel J, Perlman JM, Aziz A, *et al.* 2010 American Heart Association guidelines for cardiopulmonary resuscitation and emergency cardiovascular care. Part 15: neonatal resuscitation. *Circulation* 2010;**122**: S909–S919.

Kleinman ME, Chameides L, Schexnayder SM, *et al.* 2010 American Heart Association guidelines for cardiopulmonary resuscitation and emergency cardiovascular care. Part 14: pediatric advanced life support. *Circulation* 2010;**122**:S876–S908.

Lopez-Herce J, Garcia C, Dominguez P, *et al.* Characteristics and outcome of cardiorespiratory arrest in children. *Resuscitation* 2004;**63**:311–320.

Ralston M, Hazinski M, Zaritsky A, Schexnayder S, Kleinman M. Pediatric assessment. In *Pediatric Advanced Life Support, Provider Manual.* Dallas, TX: American Heart Association, 2006, pp. 1–32.

Chapter 7

Neonatal resuscitation in the emergency department

Stephanie J. Doniger

Introduction

Neonates in the ED are usually born precipitously either en route to, or in, the ED prior to the opportunity to transport the mother to the labor and delivery ward. As such, neonatal advanced life support (NALS) is a rarely used but vital skill. Classically, guidelines for neonatal resuscitation have been historically separate and different from pediatric advanced resuscitation (PALS), contributing to the complexity of management.

In approaching a precipitous delivery, the EP must be prepared to treat both patients – the mother and the neonate. Additional specialists, such as pediatrics and obstetrics, should be consulted as soon as possible, ideally even before the patients have arrived. Three important questions to answer if possible prior to the delivery are:

- estimated gestational age of the neonate
- presence of rupture of membranes and color of the amniotic fluid
- number of births anticipated.

If time allows, questions of prenatal care or other problems with the pregnancy are informative.

The NALS emphasizes an inverted pyramid of care (Fig. 7.1). The majority of children need to be warmed, dried, and stimulated – basic skills frequently forgotten in the stress and chaos of a precipitous birth. Stimulation alone often improves respiratory and cardiovascular status in the newly born. Only 10% of all births will need some intervention to help the neonate to start breathing; only 1% will need extensive resuscitation.

Routine care

Upon delivery, the EP should determine if the neonate is of term gestation, if the infant is breathing or crying, and if the muscle tone is good. If all of these conditions are satisfied, then the infant should be offered routine care (stimulation, warmth, drying). If not, the infant should be warmed and stimulated by

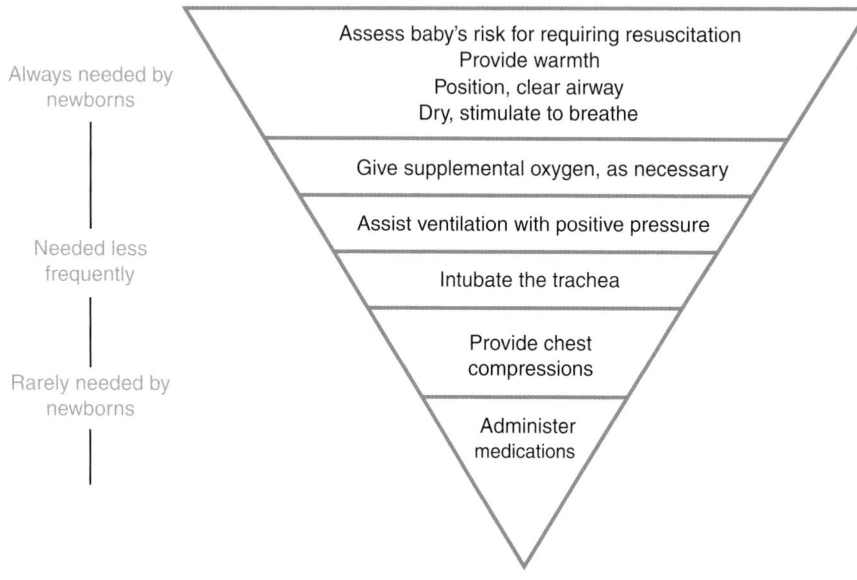

Figure 7.1 Inverted pyramid of neonatal resuscitation. (Reproduced with permission from American Heart Association. *Neonatal Resuscitation Textbook*, 5th edn. Washington, DC: American Heart Association, 2006.)

A Practical Guide to Pediatric Emergency Medicine: Caring for Children in the Emergency Department, ed. N. Ewen Amieva-Wang (associate eds. Jamie Shandro, Aparajita Sohoni, and Bernhard Fassl). Published by Cambridge University Press.

rubbing the back and flicking the heels. The head should be repositioned and the airway should be cleared within the first 30 s after birth. The heart rate should also be determined via palpation of the brachial or umbilical pulse or auscultation.

Airway, breathing

If the neonate does not spontaneously breathe after 30 s of stimulation, has ineffective breathing pattern such as gasping or if the heart rate is <100 beats/min (bpm), positive-pressure ventilation should be started at a rate of 40–60 breaths/min. This can be achieved with the use of a neonatal/pediatric-sized (200–750 ml) self-inflating bag connected to a reservoir, a flow-initiating bag, or a T-piece device. Peak inspiratory pressures as high as 30 cmH_2O are sometimes needed with initial breaths to establish adequate functional residual capacity, although care must be taken to avoid overinflation of the lungs. If a neonate is ventilated with a bag-valve mask for longer than a few minutes, an orogastric tube should be placed to avoid gastric distension. The best indicator of successful ventilation is an increase in the heart rate, tone, color, and spontaneous breathing.

Whenever positive pressure is indicated for resuscitation, supplemental oxygen is recommended, but should not be delayed if oxygen is not available. The standard for term infants is to use fraction of inspired oxygen (FIo_2) of 100%; the oxygen concentration can then be adjusted down according to clinical response. While updated recommendations discuss the possible adverse effects that high oxygen concentrations have on the respiratory physiology and cerebral circulation of newborns, oxygen deprivation and asphyxia also cause tissue damage. Since precipitous births occur rarely in the ED, we believe starting with 100% FIo_2 and adjusting downwards is appropriate.

For those babies who are breathing but have central cyanosis, free-flow oxygen is indicated. It is important to note that a self-inflating bag cannot reliably deliver free-flow oxygen.

In a vigorous infant, it is no longer recommended to perform oropharyngeal and nasopharyngeal suctioning of meconium-stained amniotic fluid at the perineum. Those infants with meconium who are not vigorous, have a heart rate of <100 bpm, or have poor respiratory effort and tone warrant intubation and suctioning of meconium through the endotracheal tube (ETT) at birth.

Circulation

If respirations are assisted, compressions and circulatory support are rarely needed. However compressions should be started if, after 30 s of positive pressure ventilation (Fig. 7.2), the heart rate is not rising or is <60 bpm. Chest compressions should be administered with the thumb technique (Fig. 6.2). If the baby is large, or the EP's hands are small, the two-finger

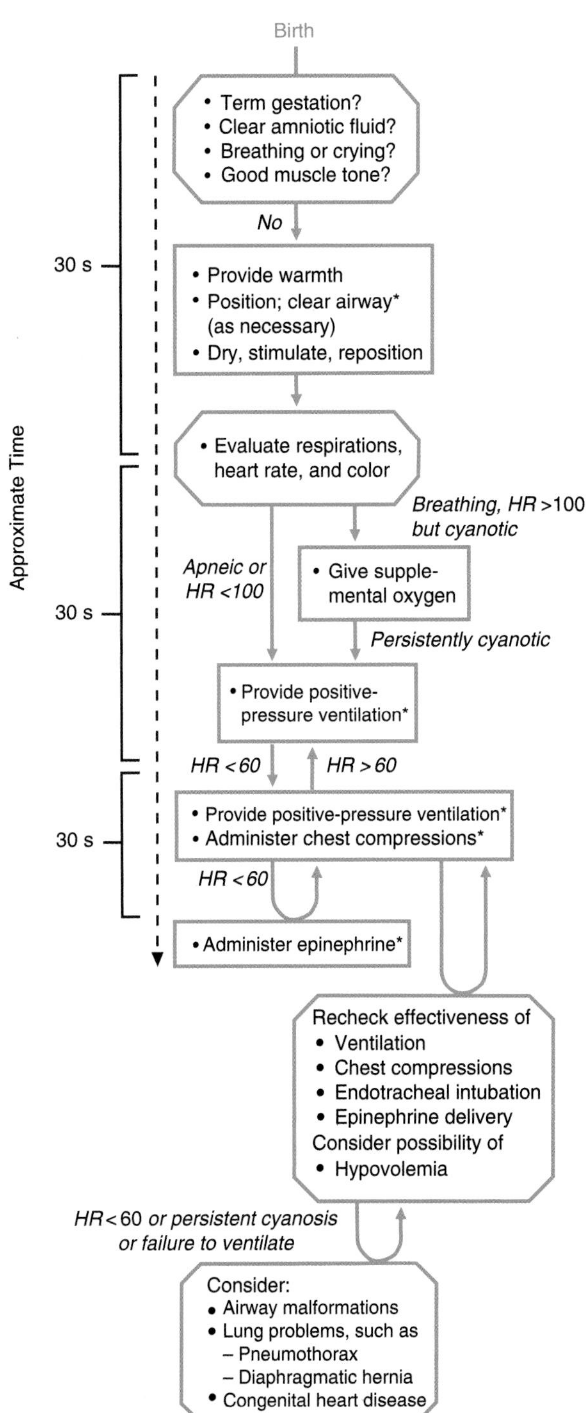

Figure 7.2 Neonatal resuscitation algorithm. HR, heart rate; *Endotracheal intubation may be considered at several steps. (Reproduced with permission from American Heart Association. *Neonatal Resuscitation Textbook*, 5th edn. Washington, DC: American Heart Association, 2006.)

technique using the right middle and second finger to compress while using the other hand to support the newborn's back is indicated (Fig. 6.2).

Compressions and ventilations should be given in a 3:1 ratio of compressions to ventilations with 90 compressions and 30 breaths in 1 min for a total of 120 events/min. When compressions are given continuously after intubation, the rate should be 120 compressions/min. Vascular access can be obtained via peripheral IV, umbilical vein, or an intraosseous line (Ch. 4). Umbilical vein catheterization is an option within the first 5 days of life if there is a length of viable cord to catheterize (Ch. 4). Intubation should also be considered at this time.

In newborn resuscitation, drug therapy is rarely indicated. However, the 2005 American Heart Association recommendations for drug therapy in the newborn focus on the indications for the use of epinephrine and naloxone.

In neonatal resuscitation, as opposed to pediatric resuscitation, epinephrine is always used in the 1:10 000 concentration whether given IV, IO, or through the ETT. Epinephrine should be dosed at 0.1–0.3 ml/kg.

The IV route for epinephrine administration is preferred. Despite the fact that the endotracheal route for drug administration is unpredictable for drug delivery, it is a viable option when there is difficulty obtaining venous access; the dose is 0.3–1 ml/kg. High-dose epinephrine is no longer recommended.

If there is evidence or suspicion of hemorrhage, 10 ml/kg isotonic saline or blood should be administered. Naloxone is no longer recommended in primary resuscitative efforts and should not be given endotracheally. Heart rate and color must first be restored through ventilatory support prior to its administration. It is important to review the mother's history when possible, as naloxone administration with chronic opioid use could result in seizures.

Post-resuscitative care of neonates

Neonates who require all but the minimal intervention should be transferred to a facility where ongoing neonatal care and resuscitation can be provided. Infants who have received prolonged positive-pressure ventilation or chest compressions are at risk for further complications.

Withdrawing resuscitation

Neonatal recommendations include guidelines regarding withholding and withdrawing resuscitative efforts. Such decisions are best made when there are opportunities for parental agreement. It may be reasonable to withhold resuscitation in those conditions associated with an unacceptably high mortality. Such situations include extremely low birth weights (<400 g), young gestational age (<23 weeks), and certain congenital anomalies (anencephaly, trisomy 13). Hospital-specific policies regarding the youngest age at which an infant can be resuscitated in that facility exist, and should be known to the EP. In other situations, the parental desires would dictate resuscitative efforts. This occurs in babies with an uncertain prognosis, borderline survival, a relatively high morbidity rate, and an anticipated high burden to the child. Furthermore, if after 10 min of adequate continuous resuscitation there are still no signs of life (i.e., no heartbeat or respiratory effort), it is reasonable to discontinue resuscitation. This recommendation is based on evidence showing a high mortality rate and likelihood of severe neurodevelopmental disability.

Pearls and pitfalls

Pearls

1. During precipitous ED delivery ask three things: (a) estimated gestational age, (b) whether the membranes have ruptured and if meconium is present, and (c) number of births anticipated.
2. Get additional help.
3. It is no longer recommended to routinely suction at the perineum. If meconium is present but the neonate is vigorous, no suctioning is needed. If the neonate requires suctioning, it should be done via an endotracheal tube.
4. Only 10% of all newborns will require some resuscitation at birth; only 1% will require extensive resuscitation.

Pitfalls

1. Failure to warm, dry and stimulate the newborn.
2. Failure to be aware of interventions for the newborn.

Selected references

Allwood A, Madar R, Baumer J, Readdy L, Wright D. Changes in resuscitation practice at birth. *Arch Dis Child Fetal Neonatal Ed* 2003;**88**:F375–F379.

ECC Committee SaTFotAHA. 2005 American Heart Association Guidelines for Cardiopulmonary Resuscitation and Emergency Cardiovascular Care. Part 13: Neonatal Resuscitation Guidelines. *Circulation* 2005;**112**:188–195.

Haddad B, Mercer B, Livingston J, Talati A, Sibai B. Outcome after successful resuscitation of babies born with apgar scores of 0 at both 1 and 5 minutes. *Am J Obstet Gynecol* 2000;**182**:1210–1214.

Perlman J, Risser R. Cardiopulmonary resuscitation in the delivery room. Associated clinical events. *Arch Pediatr Adolesc Med* 1995;**140**:20–25.

Chapter 8

Tutorial: Pediatric critical care tricks of the trade

James P. Andrus

Airway

1. Following endotracheal intubation, checking the air leak around the endotracheal tube (ETT) indicates that the internal diameter (ID) is the correct size for the patient. The leak should be between 10 and 30 cmH_2O pressure via manometer-assisted auscultation during hand bag ventilation. A leak $<10\,cmH_2O$ indicates the size is too small, and $>30\,cmH_2O$ indicates the ETT is too big.
2. The depth of the ETT should be confirmed by auscultation and chest radiography:
   - neonates (up to 4 kg): Weight(kg)+6
   - <2 years old: approximately 10–12 cm at the gum
   - ≥2 years old: (Age(years)/2) + 12 or (Weight(kg)/5) + 12.
3. For difficult intubations, have an extra set of hands to lift the head while attempting to visualize the airway. Use of a head pillow or donut can be substituted. This realigns the axis of intubation.

Breathing

1. Use a nasal or oropharyngeal airway to utilize the bag-valve mask more effectively.
2. The tongue is the most common cause of airway obstruction. Nasal airways should be avoided in the presence of facial trauma and head trauma with visible fluid leak from the nares. An oral airway may be substituted in unconscious patients.
3. In children, two roles exist for permissive hypercapnea:
   - in respiratory failure caused by acute respiratory distress syndrome (ARDS), pneumonia, asthma, or other parenchymal lung disease: maintenance of pH at 7.25–7.35 can have protective effects on the lungs
   - mild permissive hypercapnea with pH of 7.32–7.40 should be considered in patients with single-ventricle physiology prior to complete correction with the Fontan procedure.

Circulation

1. Always remember that blood vessels in children follow the same anatomic paths as in adults but can be much smaller than in adults.
2. Vessels may be difficult to locate in the presence of shock or edema, in smaller children, and in the "chubby child." Use of ultrasound to guide placement is encouraged. In the presence of severe shock with evidence of end-organ hypoperfusion, rapid progression toward intraosseous access is encouraged.
3. There is variability in the position of the left femoral vein with respect to the artery as they pass under the inguinal ligament. They can switch medial positions and the artery can run anterior to the vein; therefore, ultrasound guidance is encouraged.
4. Calcium-channel blockers should be avoided in children ≤1 year old. The physiology and anatomy of the immature heart of a neonate leads to limited myocardial contractility that is decreased compared with more mature pediatric and adult hearts. The heart develops increased contractility over the first months of life up to approximately 2 years of age. Anatomically, sympathetic nerve fibers within the myocardium increase in total number as does the concentration of norepinephrine. In addition, the immature heart has limited responsiveness to cardiotonic agents because it has a relatively high non-contractile content, decreased availability of releasable norepinephrine, a less-mature sympathetic system, underdeveloped intracellular calcium regulatory mechanisms, and decreased functional reserve capacity. A major component of this relatively decreased cardiac contractility and poor responsiveness to cardiotonic agents is the poorly developed sarcoplasmic reticulum of the neonate and infant. Therefore, children have an extreme dependence on extracellular calcium and increased sensitivity to hypocalcemic states and calcium channel blockade.

A Practical Guide to Pediatric Emergency Medicine: Caring for Children in the Emergency Department, ed. N. Ewen Amieva-Wang (associate eds. Jamie Shandro, Aparajita Sohoni, and Bernhard Fassl). Published by Cambridge University Press.

Selected references

Brodsky JB, Shulman MS, Mark, JBD. Malposition of left-sided double-lumen endobronchial tubes. *Anesthesiology* 1985;**62**: 667–689.

Cote C, Todres ID. The pediatric airway. In Cote C, Ryan J, Todres ID, *et al. A Practice of Anesthesia for Infants and Children*, 2nd edn. Philadelphia, PA: Saunders, 1993, pp. 55–83.

Morgan J, Perreault C, Moran K. The cellular basis of contraction and relaxation in cardiac and vascular smooth muscle. *Am Heart J* 1991;**121**:961–968.

Padman R, Lawless S, van Nessen S. Use of BiPAP by nasal mask in treatment of respiratory insufficiency in pediatric patients. *Pediatr Pulmonol* 1994;**17**:119–123.

Randolph AG, Cook DJ, Gonzales CA, Pribble CG. Ultrasound guidance for placement of central venous catheters: a meta-analysis of the literature. *Cri Care Med* 1996;**24**(12):2053–2058.

Smith GB, Hirsch NP, Ehrenwerth J. Placement of double-lumen endobronchial tubes. *Br J Anaesth* 1986;**58**: 1317–1320.

Chapter 9

Tutorial: Mechanical ventilation in the emergency department

James P. Andrus

Introduction

Initial ventilator management of the pediatric patient is dictated by:

- the underlying illness
- any chronic disease states that may influence the pulmonary pathophysiology
- age
- size of the patient.

These factors help in determining the goals of therapy and the starting point for ventilator settings. However, continued observation of the patient is critical in providing optimal ventilator management to ensure the safety and improvement in the condition of the patient.

Following placement of an endotracheal tube (ETT), confirmation of ideal tube placement should be prioritized. Observation of a capnometer tells if the patient can be ventilated through the ETT as previously placed. Lack of color change indicates inability to ventilate through the ETT and most commonly indicates incorrect placement of the ETT in the esophagus, or tube obstruction. Auscultation of breath sounds gives information as to the depth of placement of the ETT in the trachea. Observation of chest movement for symmetry and degree of excursion provides additional information. Finally a chest radiograph and blood gas should be obtained to confirm placement. At this point, hand ventilation of the patient can assist in determining initial ventilator settings.

Volume control ventilation

The goals of ventilator use can be divided into improved ventilation, improved oxygenation, airway protection, and decreased work of breathing. Although physiologic tidal volumes range from 3 to 6 ml/kg, frequently a slightly higher tidal volume is required because of the underlying poor pulmonary compliance. Therefore, when initiating volume control ventilation (VCV), tidal volumes of 6–10 ml/kg provide a good starting point (Table 9.1). Lower tidal volumes in this range can be employed if the lungs demonstrate essentially normal compliance and the goals of therapy do not require supranormal tidal volumes. Historically, higher tidal volumes in the range 12–15 ml/kg have been used to achieve adequate ventilation; however, this can result in significant ventilator-induced lung injury through shearing forces and should be reserved for only brief periods of time to make rapid physiologic corrections. Whenever excessively high tidal volumes are required to achieve adequate ventilation, special attention should be given to the peak inspiratory pressures (PIP) generated by each breath. Most ventilators are equipped with a monitoring mode. If the PIP that is generated exceeds 35 cmH_2O, then pressure control ventilation (PCV) should be used.

Table 9.1. Initial pediatric ventilator settings by age

Age	Tidal volume (ml/kg)	Peak inspiratory pressure (cmH_2O)	Positive end expiratory pressure (cmH_2O)	Rate (breaths/min)	Fraction of inspired oxygen
Birth to 6 months	6 to 10	12 to 30	5 to 15	30 to 50	1.00
6 months to 2 years	6 to 10	12 to 30	5 to 15	20 to 40	1.00
2–6 years	6 to 10	12 to 30	5 to 15	20 to 30	1.00
≥6 years	6 to 10	12 to 30	5 to 15	12 to 20	1.00

A Practical Guide to Pediatric Emergency Medicine: Caring for Children in the Emergency Department, ed. N. Ewen Amieva-Wang (associate eds. Jamie Shandro, Aparajita Sohoni, and Bernhard Fassl). Published by Cambridge University Press.

Pressure control ventilation

Use of PCV achieves high inspiratory pressures faster than can VCV; therefore, it overcomes airway resistance more efficiently. The initial PIP should be set at 15–30 cmH_2O and the tidal volume should be maintained between 6 and 10 ml/kg. If the ventilator cannot monitor the tidal volumes, observation of chest rise can be used in conjunction with blood gases and chest radiography as indicators of effective tidal volumes.

Use of PCV should be considered over VCV in patients with small airway disease or lower airway obstruction, such as reactive airway disease, brochiolitis, or bronchomalacia, regardless of the patient's primary illness. An ideal initial PIP is 12–30 cmH_2O, but higher pressures in the range 30–50 cmH_2O may be required at the onset of ventilation caused by poor compliance and an elevated arterial partial pressure of carbon dioxide ($PaCO_2$). Whenever initiating PCV, special attention should be given to monitoring serial expired tidal volume and blood gases.

After setting the PIP or tidal volume, consideration should be given to the positive end expiratory pressure (PEEP). The PEEP provides lung recruitment that allows greater surface area for oxygen exchange. PEEP is generally set at 5–15 cmH_2O pressure regardless of age or size, with lower PEEPs reserved for generally healthy lungs, while higher pressures are reserved for lungs with significant atelectasis, poor compliance, or capillary leak. The use of high PEEPs in relatively healthy lungs in hypovolemic or euvolemic individuals may result in decreased venous return and compromised hemodynamics. In general, setting the PEEP to zero, except in patients with extremely high intrinsic PEEP (e.g., in reactive airway disease or bronchiolitis), should be avoided so as to avoid atelectasis when using a low PEEP strategy. Although some advocate the use of no PEEP in patients with single ventricle physiology, there is no evidence to dissuade the use of low levels of PEEP. As a corollary, PEEPs >5 cmH_2O should be avoided in patients with single ventricle physiology to ensure adequate pulmonary blood flow and patency of the systemic to pulmonary conduits.

As mentioned above, PEEP strategies vary with the underlying pulmonary and airway pathophysiology, with high PEEP strategies used for poor pulmonary compliance states associated with parenchymal lung disease. Two different strategies, with evidence to support their use, exist for the treatment of lower airway disease. The easiest to use is the strategy of using low or no PEEP as the patient already has a high intrinsic PEEP to maintain alveolar and airway patency. The second strategy sets the ventilator PEEP to 1–2 cmH_2O above the inflection point on the pressure–volume curve. Manufacturers have equipped many ventilators with monitoring capabilities to allow this strategy. A practitioner experienced in its use should initiate this strategy.

The next step is to set the ventilator rate and inspiratory time (I-time) or I:E ratio. The combination of rate and tidal volume should provide adequate minute ventilation to control $PaCO_2$ in an acceptable range. In general, initial ventilator rates should decrease with patient age and size. For example, neonates and infants should start on rates of 30–50 breaths/min, children 6 months to 2 years of age 20–40 breaths/min, 2–6 years 20–30 breaths/min, and older children 12–20 breaths/min. Use of low tidal volume strategies may necessitate the use of higher rates than considered standard.

In most instances, starting with a fraction of inspired oxygen (FIo_2) of 1.00 is ideal to ensure adequate oxygenation in the presence of pulmonary disease. However, high FIo_2 should be avoided in children with significant mixing lesion at the level of the ventricle or single ventricle physiology prior to the bidirectional Glenn, superior vena cava to pulmonary artery, shunt because this can result in pulmonary overcirculation with a left-to-right shunt with life-threatening systemic hypotension and poor systemic perfusion. Conversely, children at risk of reactive pulmonary hypertension should always be initiated on a FIo_2 of 1.00. Children with reactive pulmonary hypertension frequently benefit from mild hyperventilation initially with later attempts to normalize blood pH.

High-frequency oscillation ventilation

If PCV and VCV fail to improve ventilation at reasonable tidal volumes or PIPs, high-frequency oscillation (HFOV) should be considered in conjunction with a pediatric critical care specialist in a pediatric intensive care unit (PICU) setting. Although HFOV can be a highly efficient method of ventilating patients to achieve

Pearls and pitfalls

Pearls

1. In volume control ventilation (VCV), start with tidal volumes of 6–10 ml/kg.
2. If VCV generates peak inspiratory pressures greater than 35 cmH_2O, then pressure control ventilation should be used.
3. Pressure control ventilation should be considered over VCV in patients with small airway disease or lower airway obstruction, such as reactive airway disease, bronchiolitis, or bronchomalacia, regardless of the patient's primary illness.
4. Whenever there are ventilator problems, the EP should take the patient off the ventilator and hand bag to get a sense of resistance, volumes, and lung compliance.

Pitfalls

1. Failure to realize the use of high positive end expiratory pressures in relatively healthy lungs in hypovolemic or euvolemic individuals may result in decreased venous return and compromised hemodynamics.

carbon dioxide removal, it can have profound hemodynamic effects by impeding venous return. When initiating HFOV, additional fluid boluses and, possibly, the addition of positive inotropic agents, such as dopamine or epinephrine, may be rapidly required. It should be noted that it is very difficult to achieve adequate oxygenation and ventilation with HFOV in children and adults >30 kg and its use may require special pressures and equipment in addition to the oscillatory ventilator.

Hand bagging

Despite an optimal thought process and excellent ventilator planning, there is no substitute for the empiric information gathered with hand ventilation, observation of the chest mechanics, chest radiography, and use of serial blood gases. The optimal method of hand ventilation involves the use of an anesthesia bag and an in-line manometer to provide a sense of the lung compliance and pressure that might be required to achieve the goals of therapy for the individual patient. Even with standard hand ventilation bags and no manometer, hand ventilation can provide a sense of lung compliance and information to assist in guiding initial ventilator settings higher or lower. The most important feature of initial mechanical oxygenation and ventilation of the patient is ongoing monitoring with observation, chest radiography, and serial blood gases to ensure optimal care.

Section 2

Allergy

Chapter 10

Allergic emergencies

Jonathan E. Davis and Robert L. Norris

Introduction

Anaphylaxis is a severe, life-threatening, systemic reaction that can affect all ages. The clinical syndrome is variable and may involve multiple organs, including the skin, CNS and respiratory, GI, and cardiovascular systems (Table 10.1). Respiratory and cardiovascular symptoms cause the greatest concern because they carry the greatest potential for morbidity or mortality. The estimated lifetime prevalence of anaphylaxis is up to 2%, with the incidence peaking in early childhood. In the USA, food allergies are the most common culprit in children, accounting for an estimated 100 total deaths each year.

Allergic emergencies present as a clinical spectrum, ranging from urticaria and angioedema to presyncope, bronchospasm, or cardiovascular collapse. Our definition of anaphylaxis involves allergic symptoms with one or both of the following features:

- respiratory difficulty (caused by bronchospasm or local tissue edema in the pharynx or hypopharynx)
- hemodynamic instability (presyncope, syncope, hypotension or arrhythmia).

Pathophysiology

There are three steps of a classic IgE-mediated allergic or anaphylactic response:

1. *Sensitization.* Allergen exposure leads to the production of IgE antibodies
2. *Early phase reaction.* Subsequent allergen exposure causes IgE-mediated release of preformed substances from mast cells and basophils
3. *Late phase reaction.* Other immune cells produce additional inflammatory mediators.

An anaphylactoid (now termed non-allergic anaphylaxis) reaction is an immediate systemic reaction that mimics anaphylaxis with the release of identical mediators from mast cells and basophils, but is not IgE mediated. Adverse reactions may occur on first exposure to the inciting agent, since prior sensitization is not required. However, the clinical presentation and management of non-allergic and allergic anaphylaxis is identical.

Table 10.1. Target systems in anaphylaxis

System	Symptoms
Cardiovascular	Hypotension, lightheadedness (presyncope), syncope, arrhythmias, chest pain
Respiratory	Upper airway (oropharyngeal, hypopharyngeal or laryngeal) edema; lower airway bronchospasm
Gastrointestinal	Nausea, vomiting, diarrhea, cramping
Skin	Flushing, erythema, pruritus, urticaria, angioedema
Central nervous system	Headache, confusion, altered level of consciousness

Etiologies

There are multiple triggers of anaphylaxis, including foods, medications, insect venoms, latex, and exercise. Food-induced anaphylaxis is the most common single cause of anaphylaxis treated in EDs in the USA, as well as the most common cause of anaphylaxis among pediatric ED patients. Although many infants outgrow allergies to eggs, milk, or soy products, some food allergies (commonly to peanuts, tree nuts, fish, and shellfish) may persist into adulthood.

The pathogenesis and true incidence of exercise-induced anaphylaxis remains unknown. Cases are often unpredictable, difficult to diagnose, and occur in relation to a variety of activities. Anaphylaxis may also occur in relation to environmental factors, such as cold weather. Latex allergies encompass various reactions to the proteins found in natural rubber latex or to the additives used in its processing.

Mortality

Factors associated with severe or fatal anaphylaxis include asthma or an allergy to peanuts and tree nuts (which account for the majority of fatal or near-fatal food reactions in the USA). Adolescents seem to be at particular risk for anaphylaxis, possibly because they engage in risky behaviors despite a

A Practical Guide to Pediatric Emergency Medicine: Caring for Children in the Emergency Department, ed. N. Ewen Amieva-Wang (associate eds. Jamie Shandro, Aparajita Sohoni, and Bernhard Fassl). Published by Cambridge University Press.

known allergy. They are also less likely to recognize allergic triggers, may "deny" symptoms, and may not carry or use their epinephrine self-administration device.

Differential diagnoses

Anaphylaxis must be considered in the differential for any acute-onset respiratory distress, bronchospasm, hypotension, or cardiac arrest. However, it is also important to consider other diagnostic possibilities (Table 10.2). Vasovagal episodes share many of the characteristic features of anaphylaxis, including hypotension, pallor, weakness, nausea, and emesis. These episodes also usually occur with a relatively rapid onset. However, typical vasovagal reactions lack the characteristic cutaneous findings of anaphylaxis such as urticaria, angioedema, flushing, or pruritus. Also, vasovagal syndromes will often spontaneously regress after laying the patient in a supine position; anaphylaxis will not. Lastly, vasovagal reactions are typically associated with bradycardia, whereas a reflex tachycardia is frequently seen in cases of anaphylaxis.

Other forms of shock (i.e., hypovolemic, cardiogenic, or endotoxic) may be confused with anaphylaxis. Flush syndromes (e.g., carcinoid), "restaurant syndromes" (e.g., scombroid poisoning or monosodium glutamate [MSG] reaction), or excessive endogenous production of histamine syndromes (e.g., systemic mastocytosis) may mimic anaphylaxis as well. "Restaurant syndromes" are particularly difficult to distinguish from food-induced anaphylaxis given their shared historical (i.e., food ingestion preceding the reaction) and clinical (i.e., skin flushing) features.

Table 10.2. Differential diagnosis of anaphylaxis

Category	Examples
Anaphylactic and anaphylactoid reactions	Reactions to exogenously administered agents (foods, medications, hymenoptera venom, others) Related to physical factors (exercise; cold, heat, sunlight) Idiopathic
Vasodepressor reactions	Neurocardiogenic reaction
Other forms of shock	Hemorrhagic, cardiogenic, endotoxic
Flush syndromes	Carcinoid
"Restaurant syndromes"	Scombroid poisoning, monosodium glutamate reaction
Excess endogenous production of histamine syndromes	Systemic mastocytosis Urticaria pigmentosa Basophilic leukemia Acute promyelocytic leukemia
Non-organic disease	Panic attack Munchausen's stridor Vocal cord dysfunction syndrome Globus hystericus
Miscellaneous	Hereditary angioedema Angiotensin-converting enzyme Inhibitor-induced angioedema Pheochromocytoma

Angioedema can resemble anaphylaxis in its clinical presentation. Angioedema can result from an allergic or IgE-mediated reaction, hereditary or acquired loss of C1 esterase inhibitor, or be triggered by medications such as angiotensin-converting enzyme (ACE) inhibitors. The proposed mechanism of angioedema in these conditions involves increased levels of bradykinin (a potent vasodilator), leading to capillary leakage and tissue edema. Albeit controversial, acute treatment of hereditary angioedema generally involves the administration of fresh frozen plasma, which transiently repletes the C1 esterase inhibitor protein. There is little evidence that standard treatment modalities for type 1 (IgE-mediated) hypersensitivity reactions (including epinephrine) are of any benefit in hereditary angioedema. However, if the etiology of the angioedema is unknown, it is recommended to treat as for any IgE-mediated or allergic reaction.

Management in the emergency department

Evaluation begins with rapid triage and stabilization of the symptomatic patient. Patients with worsening symptoms or abnormal vital signs should be taken immediately to an area with critical care capabilities. Anaphylaxis is a dynamic process and frequent reassessments are crucial. A severe reaction may not require any treatment if improvement occurs prior to ED arrival. Conversely, patients who present with mild allergic symptoms and initially appear stable still have the potential for rapid deterioration.

History and physical examination

Often the most valuable information comes from those who actually observed the allergic reaction evolve. Interview family, emergency medical services personnel, or anyone else who may have witnessed the episode to elicit specific information regarding the initial presenting signs and symptoms. Although timing was variable, one study in children determined the mean latency period between allergen exposure and symptom onset was around 15 min. Obtain the patient's past medical history, focusing on a prior history of allergy, asthma, or any other pre-existing atopic conditions. A personal or family history of atopy may be a predisposing factor for anaphylaxis. Maintain a particularly high level of vigilance in patients with a history of asthma or reactive airway disease, particularly when poorly controlled, as fatal anaphylactic reactions may be more likely to occur in such individuals.

The clinical presentation of anaphylaxis may vary between children and adults, with respiratory symptoms predominating in children and cardiovascular manifestations predominating in adults. While absence of cutaneous findings speaks against the diagnosis of anaphylaxis in general, it by no means excludes this possibility. The most severe episodes can occur without any cutaneous manifestations whatsoever.

Table 10.3. Common medications utilized in the treatment of allergic emergencies

	Anaphylaxis		Milder reactions	
	Route	**Medication/dosage**	**Route**	**Medication/dosage**
Emergency department				
Epinephrine	IM	0.01 mg/kg (0.1 ml/kg of 1:1000)	IM/SC[a]	0.01 mg/kg
	IV	0.1–2 μg/kg per min infusion	–	–
Histamine H_1 antagonist	IV/IM	Diphenhydramine 1 mg/kg (max. 50 mg)	PO	Cetirizine 2.5–10 mg *or* diphenhydramine 1 mg/kg (max. 25–50 mg)
Histamine H_2 antagonist	IV	Ranitidine 1 mg/kg (max. 50 mg)	PO	Ranitidine 1–2 mg/kg (max. 150 mg)
Corticosteroid	IV	Methylprednisolone 1–2 mg/kg (max. 125 mg)	PO	Prednisone 1–2 mg/kg (max. 60 mg)
Bronchodilator	Nebulized	Albuterol 2.5 mg per dose, may repeat as necessary	–	–
Discharge treatments[b]				
Histamine H_1 antagonist	PO	Cetirizine 2.5–10 mg daily *or* diphenhydramine 1 mg/kg (max. 25–50 mg) every 6 h		
Histamine H_2 antagonist	PO	Ranitidine 1–2 mg/kg (max. 150 mg per dose) twice daily		
Corticosteroid	PO	Prednisone 1–2 mg/kg (max. 60 mg) daily		
Epinephrine self-administration device	IM	0–10 kg: no device available; 10–25 kg: 0.15 mg device; >25 kg: 0.3 mg device		

[a] Epinephrine IM or SC may also be considered for use in milder reactions.
[b] Typical duration of treatment following discharge from ED is 3–7 days.

Recurrent (sometimes termed “biphasic” or “multiphasic”) anaphylaxis is defined as the reappearance of allergic phenomena following the complete resolution of the original reaction and without re-exposure to the inciting allergen. Recurrence may involve minor symptoms such as urticaria, or it may involve more ominous physiologic derangements, including respiratory compromise or hemodynamic instability. Recurrence rates have been reported as high as 20% and can occur up to 72 h after the inciting event.

Life support

Initial attention must focus on the ABCs. Definitive airway management is of paramount importance, as the window for effective intervention may rapidly dwindle if decisions are not made swiftly and decisively. The pediatric airway is smaller in diameter than that in adults, therefore, airway edema has a more profound effect. The administration of supplemental oxygen while establishing large-bore vascular access and infusing crystalloid (i.e., initial 20 ml/kg; then titrate to response, with maximum 80–100 ml/kg) is essential in the majority of cases. Maintain vigilance for early clinical signs of shock. Compensated pediatric shock can present with tachycardia alone; hypotension may be a late finding.

Table 10.3 summarizes the common medications utilized in the treatment of allergic emergencies.

Epinephrine

Use of epinephine could be considered as a second “A” (“adrenaline”) in the ABC for anaphylaxis management. Guidelines uniformly recommend epinephrine as the first-line treatment for severe allergic reactions. While current guidelines recommend prompt administration of epinephrine in any case of anaphylaxis, the question of what precisely constitutes anaphylaxis (i.e., where do a particular patient’s symptoms lie along the clinical spectrum of allergic manifestations) repeatedly arises, fueling uncertainty regarding the appropriateness of epinephrine use. In moderate and severe allergic emergencies, the way to reduce poor outcomes is aggressive management with appropriate doses/routes of epinephrine.

Practitioners should err on the side of administering epinephrine sooner rather than waiting too long.

Epinephrine IM or SC may also be safely and effectively utilized in children for control of milder allergic symptoms, which fail to meet threshold criteria for anaphylaxis.

Epinephrine: by what route?

Recent evidence clearly demonstrates that intramuscular (IM) epinephrine is preferred over subcutaneous (SC) administration, regardless of patient age or setting. Studies show comparatively slow and variable absorption with the SC route, as absorption depends on cutaneous blood flow – a factor already compromised by anaphylaxis and worsened by epinephrine’s potent local vasoconstrictor effects. Virtually all reported adverse outcomes of epinephrine result from IV administration, particularly when administered too rapidly, in an inappropriately concentrated form, or in excessive dosage. Therefore, IV epinephrine should be reserved for those patients with severe cardiovascular compromise (i.e., profound decrease in peripheral perfusion) or when repeated IM epinephrine fails to alleviate symptoms. Overall, continuous dilute, low-dose epinephrine infusion may represent the safest and most effective form of IV delivery, as the dose can be titrated to desired effect, while minimizing the potential for accidental administration of large or concentrated bolus doses. Intravenous epinephrine in the pediatric patient should be used cautiously, and it is paramount that the weight-based dosages be carefully checked in order to avoid an iatrogenic catastrophe.

Epinephrine: how much?

The IM epinephrine dose is (1:1000) 0.01 ml/kg up to 0.3 mg for children.

Epinephrine: is it safe?

Data confirm a very favorable safety profile of epinephrine (particularly by routes other than IV). Otherwise-healthy children have a more attractive risk–benefit ratio for epinephrine in general when compared with adults, and tolerate most of the potential complications better than adults.

Antihistamines

Antihistamines are second-line agents and should never be administered as initial or sole treatment for anaphylaxis. The use of histamine H_1 receptor antagonists (such as diphenhydramine: 1 mg/kg IV [up to 50 mg]) in allergic emergencies is common practice. The newer (second-generation) histamine H_1 receptor antagonists such as cetirizine (Zyrtec), fexofenadine (Allegra), and loratidine (Claritin) may substitute for oral diphenhydramine in patients with milder allergic symptoms. Some practitioners opt to use non-sedating formulations during "waking" hours, with adjunctive use of a single nighttime dose of oral diphenhydramine.

While the precise role of H_2 receptor antagonists in the treatment of allergic emergencies remains unclear, their potential benefit, combined with a low propensity for adverse events, makes their adjunctive use advisable. An agent such as ranitidine can be administered IV (1 mg/kg, max. 50 mg per dose) or orally (1–2 mg/kg, max. 150 mg per dose, twice daily).

Corticosteroids

Although corticosteroids have traditionally been used in the management of anaphylaxis, their effects have never been validated in placebo-controlled trials. However, based on their known beneficial effects, their administration is indicated in the vast majority of allergic emergencies.

Methylprednisolone is typically administered as a 2 mg/kg IV loading dose (max. 125 mg), followed by oral corticosteroids 1–2 mg/kg daily (max. 60 mg daily) for 3 to 7 days.

Similarly, oral steroids may be used initially in the ED for patients with less severe allergic symptoms.

Inhaled bronchodilators

Continuous (or intermittent) nebulized inhaled bronchodilators (e.g., albuterol sulfate) may be used for the treatment of anaphylaxis-induced bronchospasm, either as a routine adjunct or a rescue measure in patients with severe symptoms that remain refractory to epinephrine treatment.

Disposition

One of the most difficult decisions in treating patients with allergic emergencies in the ED is appropriate disposition. Patients with severe reactions or a slow response to standard therapies require admission. Patients with mild reactions can be safely discharged home with a responsible adult. Most patients, however, fall somewhere between. In addition, it is important to appreciate the potential for recurrent anaphylaxis. Factors to consider in determining whether to admit a patient to the hospital are presented in Table 10.4.

There is no firmly established ED observation time for patients considered "low-risk." A recent consensus statement recommended 4 to 6 h of post-anaphylactic observation for

Table 10.4. Factors to consider in determining patient disposition

Factor	High-risk features
Presenting symptom severity	Initially severe symptoms are an important consideration even if symptoms have improved or resolved following initiation of treatment
Anaphylaxis history	Maintain a very low threshold for admission if any prior history of severe, protracted or recurrent anaphylaxis
Particular allergen	"Nut" (peanut or tree nut) reactions are associated with particularly high morbidity and mortality among food allergens
Medical co-morbidities	Conditions such as asthma (particularly high morbidity and mortality in the setting of anaphylaxis), congestive heart failure, renal disease (at risk for fluid overload with volume resuscitation)
Baseline medications	Particularly beta-adrenergic blocker use (including ophthalmic)
Access to medical care	Great distance or reduced access to medical care
Age	Patients at extremes of age have reduced compensatory abilities; adolescents may be at risk for fatal anaphylaxis because of "compliance" issues
Unreliable home situation	Including barriers to appropriate discharge instructions and education

most patients, with more prolonged observation (or hospital admission) for those with severe or refractory symptoms, and in patients with reactive airway disease. Practitioners should have a low threshold for prolonged ED observation or hospital admission, particularly when high-risk features are present. Patients who are discharged should be instructed to contact their primary care providers for follow-up promptly for further education on allergic reactions and testing as indicated.

Discharge medications

Epinephrine self-administration devices should be prescribed to individuals who have a prior history of anaphylaxis. A more difficult decision involves patients who experienced only minor symptoms after exposure to an allergic trigger. However, it is estimated that between 44% and 59% of patients with initially mild symptoms may exhibit life-threatening anaphylaxis after a second exposure to the same allergic trigger. We strongly advocate that any child with a previously severe systemic reaction or peanut/tree nut allergy must be given an Epi-pen.

Patients and caretakers should be instructed on the indications for epinephrine administration and on proper device use prior to ED discharge. The device formulations currently available in the USA include EpiPen/ Twinject (0.3 mg epinephrine) and EpiPen Jr/ Twinject (0.15 mg epinephrine). Current guidelines recommend the 0.15 mg device or traditional ampule/needle/syringe dosing for infants <10 kg, the 0.15 mg device for children weighing 10–25 kg, and the 0.3 mg device for children >25 kg.

Other recommended discharge medications include oral histamine H_1 and H_2 receptor antagonists and corticosteroids. Many authors empirically recommend continuation of oral medications for at least 72 h following ED discharge.

Discharge education

Optimal management of allergic emergencies begins prior to symptom onset, with avoidance of the precipitant whenever possible. In addition, MedicAlert bracelets should be recommended for at-risk individuals. Emergency response plans should be worked out in advance with a child's teachers and caregivers outside the home, including precise instructions on allergen avoidance and use of the child's epinephrine kit as prescribed.

Anaphylactic reactions are life threatening and are almost always unanticipated. Any delay in the recognition of initial signs and symptoms may result in a poor outcome (Box 10.1). Even when there are only mild symptoms initially, the potential for disease progression must be appreciated, and treatment

Box 10.1. Key points

1. **When does an *allergic* reaction become an *anaphylactic* reaction?**
   Involvement of the respiratory (upper or lower) or cardiovascular system is necessary to distinguish anaphylaxis from other allergic phenomena.
2. **When to use epinephrine?**
   Undisputed first-line agent and treatment of choice for anaphylaxis. Maintain a very low threshold for use.
3. **By what route to use epinephrine?**
   Regardless of patient age, IM (particularly in the lateral thigh) is superior to SC. The IV route should only be used for patients in extremis and unresponsive to repeated IM dosages, or those with profound shock.
4. **When to avoid epinephrine?**
   There are no absolute contraindications.
5. **Antihistamines**
   Blockage with H_1 plus H_2 antihistamine combination is best. The addition of an H_2 antagonist carries potential benefits and has a low propensity for adverse events.
6. **Corticosteroids**
   Benefit as a secondary treatment in anaphylaxis extrapolated from known benefit in other allergic diseases; corticosteroids may play a role in reducing the incidence of recurrent anaphylaxis.
7. **Disposition**
   Maintain a low threshold for admission or prolonged ED observation. Be particularly cautious in asthmatics or patients with "nut" allergies.

Pearls and pitfalls

Pearls

1. The clinical presentation of anaphylaxis may vary between children and adults, with respiratory symptoms predominating in children and cardiovascular manifestations predominating in adults.
2. Anaphylaxis may lead to significant morbidity or mortality if not treated early and aggressively.
3. Epinephrine is the undisputed first-line agent in the treatment of anaphylaxis. There are no absolute contraindications to epinephrine use.
4. Definitive airway management should occur early if the airway patency is at risk.
5. The self-administration of epinephrine is a potentially life-saving intervention and should be prescribed to at-risk patients.

Pitfalls

1. Epinephrine IV should be reserved for patients unresponsive to IM dosing.
2. The absence of dermatologic findings such as urticaria, angioedema, or flushing does not exclude the possibility of anaphylaxis.
3. Failure to have contingency plans for surgical airway management when intubating.
4. Failure to maintain a low threshold for prolonged ED observation or hospital admission, particularly when the reaction was severe or if other high-risk features are present.

must begin swiftly and aggressively. Epinephrine is the cornerstone of therapy. Second-line therapies include histamine H_1 and H_2 receptor antagonists and corticosteroids. It is prudent to maintain a low threshold for hospital admission (or prolonged ED observation) in significant reactions, or in the presence of other high-risk features, particularly pre-existing asthma or following "nut"-induced food allergy. Ensuring that patients have continuous access to and familiarity with their epinephrine self-administration device is critical to preventing morbidity and mortality.

Selected references

Joint Task Force on Practice Parameters for the American Academy of Allergy, Asthma and Immunology, the American College of Allergy, Asthma and Immunology, and the Joint Council of Allergy, Asthma and Immunology. The diagnosis and management of anaphylaxis: an updated practice parameter. *J Allergy Clin Immunol* 2005;**115**:3: S483–S523.

Lieberman P. Biphasic anaphylaxis. *Ann Allergy Asthma Immunol* 2005;**95**:217–226.

Sampson HA, Munoz-Furlong A, Bock SA, *et al.* Symposium on the definition and management of anaphylaxis: summary report. *J Allergy Clin Immunol* 2005;**115**:3:584–591.

Sampson HA, Munoz-Furlong A, Campbell RL *et al.* Second symposium on the definition and management of anaphylaxis: summary report: second national institute of allergy and infectious disease/food allergy and anaphylaxis network symposium. *J Allergy Clin Immunol* 2006;**117**:391–397.

Sicherer SH, Simons FER. Self-injectable epinephrine for first-aid management of anaphylaxis. *Pediatrics* 2007;**119**:3:638–646.

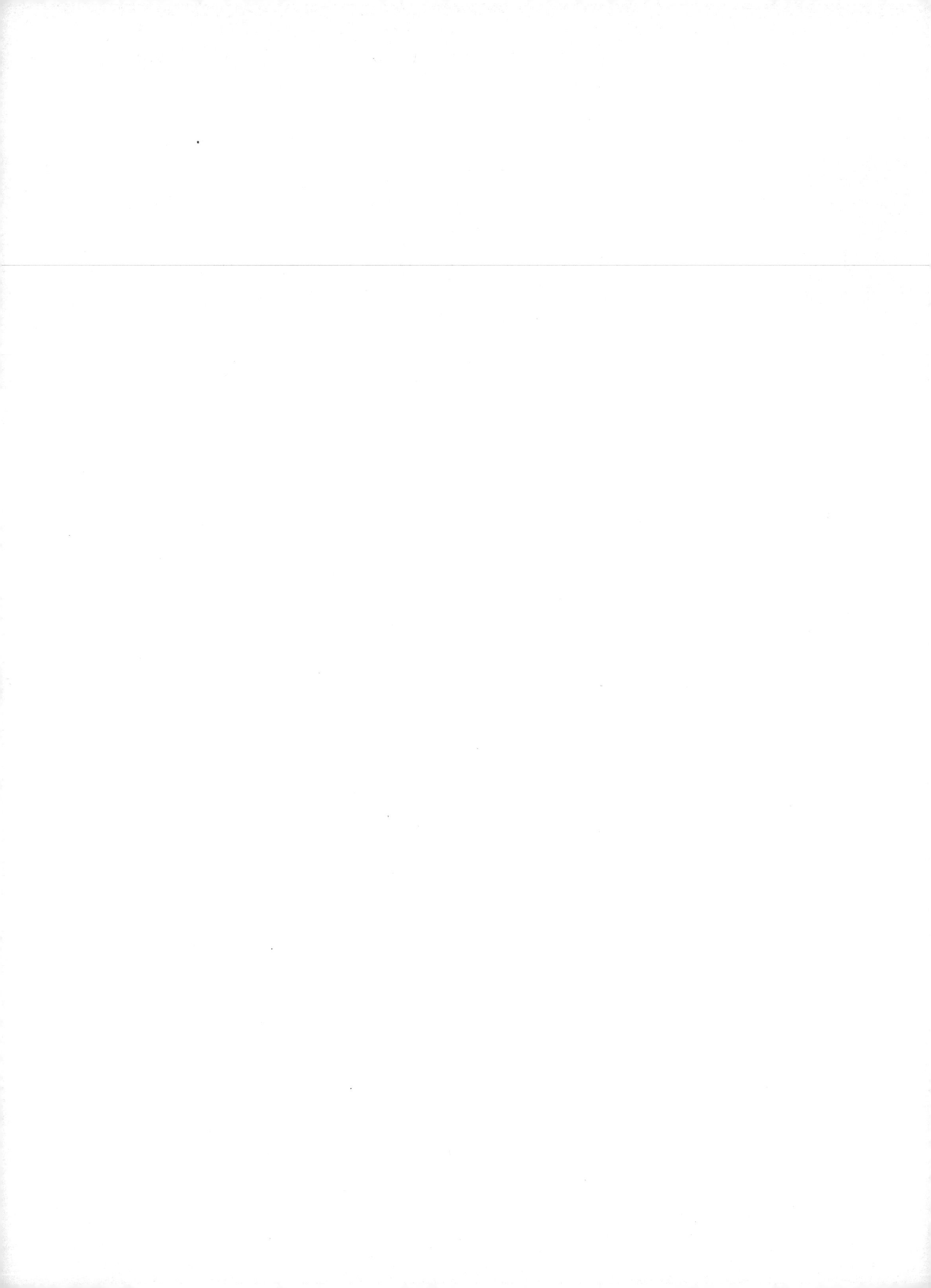

Section 3

Cardiac emergencies

Expert reviewers: Emily Wessler and Anne M. Dubin

Chapter 11

Approach to cardiac examination and murmur evaluation

Daniel Bernstein and Emily Wessler

Introduction

The cardiac history and examination should focus on different features in the child than in the adult. This introduction will discuss a general approach to the pediatric cardiac history and physical examination as well as developmentally based physical findings and diagnoses. Finally, innocent and pathologic heart murmurs in the child will be discussed.

Cardiac history and examination

The birth history is important for infants with possible cardiac problems. It should include a brief review of the pregnancy, infections, and maternal disorders such as diabetes or lupus. Perinatal history includes Apgar scores, presence or absence of respiratory distress or cyanosis, and prior workup performed when the child was discharged from the hospital. The family history should be delineated, including prior family members with congenital heart disease, syndromes associated with congenital heart disease, cardiomyopathies, or sudden death. Heart attack or stroke in any family member under the age of 50 may be an indication of familial hypercholesterolemia.

Auscultation can be difficult in younger children and infants because of their rapid heart rates and lack of cooperation. Attempting to listen to a crying child will rarely yield complete data, and a cardiac diagnosis should not be ruled out until a complete examination is obtained. Ensuring the patient's comfort and cooperation may require the examination to occur in the caretaker's arms or while feeding. Toddlers can usually be distracted with a keychain or toy.

In the immediate newborn period, acrocyanosis (cyanosis of the hands and feet secondary to peripheral vasoconstriction) must be distinguished from central cyanosis (cyanosis of the tongue and mucous membranes); the latter represents true deoxygenation.

In infants, feeding is a significant stressor; therefore, heart failure can manifest as feeding difficulties.

Heart failure can manifest as diaphoresis, tachypnea, falling asleep while feeding, and frequent small feeds. Other symptoms of heart failure in the infant include failure to thrive, nasal flaring, retractions, irritability, and flank or periorbital edema.

In infants and young children, wheezing can be a sign of pulmonary edema.

Older children may have exercise intolerance, pedal edema, anorexia, nausea, vomiting, and abdominal pain. They may also complain of chest pain, palpitations, or syncope.

In adolescents, abdominal complaints are particularly common symptoms of heart failure.

Many adolescents with heart failure have minimal respiratory symptoms.

Knowledge of age-appropriate vital signs is imperative. Careful measurement of the heart rate and respiratory rate are important as tachycardia and tachypnea may represent signs of congestive heart failure. A transcutaneous oxygen saturation is another important and easily obtained component of the vital signs. Neonates and infants with suspected congenital heart disease should always have preductal (right arm) and postductal (right or left leg) saturations measured as well as four extremity blood pressures to rule out coarctation of the aorta. Any significant differential between upper and lower extremity oxygen saturations or blood pressures is a cause for concern.

Height and weight should be plotted against normal growth curves; weight is usually affected by heart disease more than height.

Failure to thrive is an important sign of heart failure in children.

The initial part of the physical examination should be an observation of the child's overall activity level, comfort, and breathing pattern. Signs of respiratory distress include nasal flaring and suprasternal and subcostal retractions. Cyanosis is best noted by the color of nail beds, tongue, or mucous membranes. Clubbing of the distal phalanges is not usually present until the child is 1–2 years of age. The lungs should be auscultated for rales, rhonchi, or wheezing as signs of pulmonary

A Practical Guide to Pediatric Emergency Medicine: Caring for Children in the Emergency Department, ed. N. Ewen Amieva-Wang (associate eds. Jamie Shandro, Aparajita Sohoni, and Bernhard Fassl). Published by Cambridge University Press.

Table 11.1. Common thoracotomy scars

Location	Type of operation
Midline	Any surgery involving cardiopulmonary bypass, i.e., complete repair or palliation of intracardiac lesions
Left lateral	Patent ductus arteriosus ligation, coarctation repair, pulmonary artery band, Blalock–Taussig shunt, some mitral valve repairs, unifocalization of left pulmonary arteries in tetralogy of Fallot with pulmonary atresia
Right lateral	Blalock–Taussig shunt, some atrial septal defect closures, unifocalization of right pulmonary arteries in tetralogy of Fallot with pulmonary atresia, Blalock–Hanlon atrial septectomy

edema. In infants and young children, wheezing can be a sign of congestive heart failure. Hepatomegaly is a common sign in patients with congestive heart failure, and is more easily appreciated in a young child than jugular venous distention.

Edema in young infants will be predominantly facial or flank, whereas pedal edema is more common in older children.

Peripheral perfusion, including presence or absence and quality of upper and lower extremity pulses and capillary refill, should be noted. Radial and femoral pulses should be palpated on each side simultaneously. Normally, the femoral pulse should slightly precede the radial. If this pattern is reversed (radial–femoral delay), it may be a sign of coarctation, particularly in older children and adolescents who have developed collateral vessels around the coarctation.

The cardiac examination should always consist of four components:

- visualization
- palpation
- auscultation for heart sounds
- auscultation for murmurs.

During visual inspection of the chest, a sternotomy or thoracotomy scar may suggest the type of previous cardiac surgery (Table 11.1). Asymmetry of the chest should be noted either as an indication of persistent ventricular enlargement or a paralyzed diaphragm following cardiac surgery. An easily visible point of maximal impulse (PMI) may be a sign of cardiac enlargement, although this can be a normal finding in an individual with a thin chest wall. Next, palpation of the heart for the PMI, heaves, or thrills should be performed. A laterally displaced PMI may indicate left ventricular hypertrophy or enlargement. The PMI may be felt at the lower left sternal border in patients with right ventricular hypertrophy or enlargement, or may be felt in the right chest in patients with dextrocardia. A heave below the sternum may indicate right ventricular hypertrophy or enlargement. Precordial thrills are associated with murmurs of grade IV or greater and are always

Table 11.2. Alterations in the second heart sound and diffential diagnoses

Finding	Differential diagnosis
Widely split	Atrial septal defect, partial anomalous pulmonary venous return, right bundle branch block, pulmonary stenosis, mitral regurgitation, ventricular septal defect
Narrowly split	Pulmonary hypertension, aortic stenosis
Paradoxically split	Left bundle branch block, right ventricle pacing, severe aortic stenosis, patent ductus arteriosus, hypertrophic cardiomyopathy
Single	Dextro-transposition of the great arteries, tetralogy of Fallot, truncus arteriosus, pulmonary hypertension, aortic stenosis, pulmonary stenosis, aortic atresia, pulmonary atresia
Loud P2	Pulmonary hypertension

pathologic. The suprasternal notch is a good place to feel for thrills associated with aortic pathology in younger children, similar to feeling for a carotid thrill in an adult. The presence of a thrill in the suprasternal notch, however, is not necessarily associated with a grade IV murmur.

Auscultation of the heart sounds should be undertaken in a systematic method, noting the quality of the first and second heart sounds, any additional heart sounds, and the regularity of the rate and rhythm. If a murmur is present, it is helpful to try to ignore the murmur and concentrate solely on the heart sounds. The first heart sound (S1) may be decreased in conditions associated with decreased left ventricular compliance, such as moderate to severe aortic stenosis or cardiomyopathy. The second heart sound (S2) is normally physiologically split, widening with inspiration and narrowing or becoming single with expiration.

Changes in S2 are often signs of significant heart disease (Table 11.2). One of the most common congenital heart lesions, the atrial septal defect, is primarily diagnosed by a widely fixed split S2, as the murmur may be relatively nonspecific. The pulmonary component of S2 may be diminished in patients with valvar pulmonary stenosis and increased in patients with pulmonary hypertension. A single S2 may be present in patients with severe stenosis or absence of either aortic or pulmonary valves, preoperatively in patients with dextro-transposition (d-transposition) of the great vessels, and in patients with tetralogy of Fallot who have had a transannular right ventricular outflow tract patch. A systolic ejection click may be heard immediately after the first heart sound, signifying either aortic or pulmonary valve stenosis. The presence of multiple clicks at the lower left sternal border may be a sign of Ebstein anomaly of the tricuspid valve.

A third heart sound (S3), heard during early diastole, may be a normal finding in infants and young children. Pathologically, it may be heard in congestive heart failure or when there is

Table 11.3. Common heart murmurs in patients with acyanotic heart disease

Finding	Differential diagnosis
Systolic ejection murmur at upper left sternal border (± radiating to lungs)	Pulmonary stenosis, peripheral pulmonary stenosis, atrial septal defect (with fixed split second sound), pink tetralogy of Fallot, outlet ventricular septal defect
Systolic ejection murmur at mid left sternal border radiating to upper right sternal border	Aortic stenosis, subaortic stenosis, supravalvar aortic stenosis, hypertrophic cardiomyopathy
Holosystolic murmur lower left sternal border	Ventricular septal defect, atrioventricular septal defect, tricuspid regurgitation, Ebstein's anomaly
Holosystolic murmur apex	Apical ventricular septal defect, mitral regurgitation, dilated cardiomyopathy with mitral regurgitation
Systolic or continuous murmur left sternal border radiating to left subscapular area	Coarctation of the aorta
Mid-diastolic rumble lower left sternal border	Flow murmur across tricuspid valve caused by large atrial septal defect or atrioventricular septal defect, tricuspid stenosis
Mid-diastolic rumble apex	Flow murmur across mitral valve caused by a large ventricular septal defect, atrioventricular septal defect or mitral stenosis
Continuous murmur mid to upper left sternal border and left subclavicular area	Patent ductus arteriosus, aortopulmonary window, collaterals

Table 11.4. Innocent murmurs and their differential diagnosis

Murmur	Characteristics	Differential diagnosis	Distinguishable characteristic
Still's murmur	Medium-pitched ejection type murmur and a characteristic musical or vibratory quality	HCM	HCM murmur increases with Valsalva
		Small VSD	VSD murmur often "squeaky" or harsh
Pulmonary flow murmur	Soft ejection murmur at the mid to left upper sternal border	ASD	ASD also with fixed split S2
		Valvar PS	PS murmur often harsher; mild PS associated with ejection click
Murmur of peripheral pulmonary stenosis	Soft ejection murmur over the left or right chest, often heard in the axillae	Valvar PS	PS murmur often harsher; mild PS associated with ejection click
		Pathologic PPS	Pathologic PPS murmur persists beyond 6 months; often unilateral and harsher
Venous hum	Continuous murmur of low frequency, often with diastolic accentuation, usually heard in infraclavicular area	PDA, AVM	Venous hum disappears with jugular vein compression or movement of head
Mammary soufflé	Continuous murmur over one or both breasts	PDA, AVM	Mammary soufflé disappears with gentle pressure over area of murmur

AS, aortic stenosis; AVM, arteriovenous malformation; HCM, hypertrophic cardiomyopathy; PDA, patent ductus arteriosus; PPS, peripheral pulmonic stenosis; PS, pulmonary stenosis; VSD, ventricular septal defect.

excessive blood return across an atrioventricular valve. A fourth heart sound (S4) is always associated with pathology such as excessive flow across the atrioventricular valves or ventricular dysfunction caused by cardiomyopathy.

Auscultation for murmurs should include description of the murmur's location, radiation, character, intensity, and pitch (Table 11.3). Systolic murmurs are described as either ejection murmurs, which are crescendo–decrescendo murmurs that begin slightly after S1, or holosystolic murmurs if they have the same intensity throughout systole and begin immediately with S1. Diastolic murmurs are almost always associated with pathology and described as early (usually decrescendo) or mid-diastolic (usually rumbling). To-and-fro murmurs are a combination of both systolic and diastolic murmurs, with a quiet interval between. Continuous murmurs are heard throughout both systole and diastole. Although there may be variations in the intensity of the continuous murmur, unlike the to-and-fro murmur, there is never a period of quiet. Murmurs can be classified as innocent (or functional) and organic (Table 11.4).

A complete initial assessment of a child with suspected or known cardiac disease includes obtaining an ECG and a frontal and lateral chest radiograph. In a child on medications such as diuretics or ACE inhibitors, a chemistry panel is essential to evaluate for electrolyte derangements or renal dysfunction, which may be associated with these medications. A CBC may be helpful, as anemia can increase the intensity of most innocent flow murmurs and polycythemia can be a sign of chronic hypoxemia.

Pearls and pitfalls

Pearls

1. Count the heart rate for a full minute.
2. Diastolic murmurs are almost always pathologic.
3. In infants, congestive heart failure often manifests as wheezes rather than rales.
4. In older children and adolescents, heart failure often manifests as abdominal symptoms.
5. Changes in S2 are often associated with significant heart disease.
6. While S3 gallops in infants and young children may be normal, an S4 is always abnormal.

Pitfalls

1. Failure to discuss a consult with the pediatric cardiologist. (Subtle findings may indicate a different level of urgency to the cardiologist than to an emergency room physician.)
2. Failure to refer all patients with murmurs that are not clearly innocent to a pediatric cardiologist.

Selected references

Allen HD, Gutgesell HP, Clark EB, Driscoll DJ. *Moss and Adams' Heart Disease in Infants, Children, and Adolescents Including the Fetus and Young Adult*, 6th edn. Philadelphia, PA: Lippincott Williams & Wilkins, 2001.

Bernstein D. Cardiology. In Bernstein D, Shelov SP (eds.) *Pediatrics for Medical Students*, 2nd edn. Philadelphia, PA: Lippincott Williams & Wilkins, 2003, pp. 261–300.

Bernstein D. The cardiovascular system. In Kliegman RM, Behrman RE, Jenson HB Stanton BF (eds.) *Nelson Textbook of Pediatrics*, 17th edn. Philadelphia, PA: Saunders, 2007, pp. 1851–1997.

Hoffman JIE. Incidence of congenital heart disease: I. Postnatal incidence. *Pediatr Cardiol* 1995;**16**: 103–113.

Jonas RA. *Comprehensive Surgical Management of Congenital Heart Disease*. London: Arnold, 2004.

Keane J, Fyler D, Lock J. *Nadas' Pediatric Cardiology*, 2nd edn. Philadelphia, PA: Hanley & Belfus, 2006.

Mavroudis C, Backer CL. *Pediatric Cardiac Surgery*, 3rd edn. St. Louis, MO: Mosby, 2003.

Rudolph AM, *Congenital Diseases of the Heart: Clinical Physiological Considerations*, 2nd edn. New York: Futura, 2001.

Chapter 12

Tutorial: Basic tools in the evaluation of the pediatric electrocardiograph

Donald H. Schreiber

Introduction

The most common reasons for obtaining an ECG in a child are syncope, chest pain, suspected arrhythmia, seizure, toxic exposure, electrical burns, electrolyte abnormalities, or abnormal physical examination findings such as murmurs. In one large series of 1631 ECGs obtained in 1501 children, the overall accuracy of the ED interpretation of the pediatric ECG was 87%. Clinically significant discordance was present in 212 cases. Of these 212 cases, the discordant findings in descending order were right ventricular hypertrophy, left ventricular hypertrophy, right bundle branch block, and prolonged corrected QT interval (QTc). No cases of myocardial infarction were present in the entire series, reflecting the rarity of this condition in the pediatric patient population.

In contrast to the adult ECG, the interpretation of the pediatric ECG must take into account the normal age-related differences in the heart. By understanding age-related changes in the ECG and utilizing a step-by-step approach, the EP can achieve high rates of accuracy in pediatric ECG interpretation.

This chapter will review the step-wise approach to the pediatric ECG by carefully assessing the rate; rhythm; QRS axis; the presence or absence of hypertrophy; the determination of the PR, QRS, and QTc conduction intervals; and the evaluation of Q waves, ST segments and T waves.

Rate

Cardiac output reflects the product of stroke volume and heart rate. Infants have a fixed stroke volume because of their poorly compliant, stiff ventricular wall, and thus are extremely sensitive to changes in heart rate. The variation in normal heart rate with age must also be appreciated. Table 12.1 highlights the normal ranges in heart rate by age.

Rhythm

While there is little difference in dysrhythmia analysis from adult ECG interpretation, heart rate and interval parameters for arrhythmias are different in children. Intervals that are considered normal for an adult may be wide for a child. For example, the interval parameters seen in ventricular tachycardia differ between adults and children: a QRS complex of >0.08 but <0.12 s can be an indication of ventricular tachycardia in an infant, whereas in an adult, the QRS would be considered normal (Table 12.2).

Table 12.1. Variation in normal heart rate with age

Age	Heart rate (beats/min)
Newborn	145 (90–180)
6 months	145 (105–185)
1 year	132 (105–170)
4 years	108 (72–135)
14 years	85 (60–120)

QRS axis

The determination of the QRS axis takes into account the net deflection of the QRS complex in a particular lead. If the sum of the positive deflection of the R wave and the negative deflection of the S wave in the QRS complex is positive, then the QRS axis is within ±90 degrees of that lead.

The determination of the QRS axis uses a *successive approximation method* utilizing the limb leads.

Step 1. Locate a quadrant, using leads I and aVF (Fig. 12.1). In the top panel of Fig. 12.1, the net QRS deflection of lead I is positive. This means that the QRS axis is in the left hemicircle (i.e., from -90 degrees through 0 to +90 degrees) from the lead I point of view. The net positive QRS deflection in aVF means that the QRS axis is in the lower hemicircle (i.e., from 0 through +90 degrees to +180 degrees) from the aVF point of view. To satisfy the polarity of both leads I and aVF, the QRS axis must be in the lower left quadrant (i.e., 0 to +90 degrees). Utilizing only leads I and aVF, the QRS axis may be determined to

A Practical Guide to Pediatric Emergency Medicine: Caring for Children in the Emergency Department, ed. N. Ewen Amieva-Wang (associate eds. Jamie Shandro, Aparajita Sohoni, and Bernhard Fassl). Published by Cambridge University Press.

Table 12.2. Variation in heart rate and electrocardiograph interval parameters with age

Age	Mean (range) heart rate (beats/min)	Mean (max.) PR interval (s)	Mean (range) QRS axis (degrees)	Mean (max.) QRS interval (s)	Mean (max.) R wave V1 (mm)	Mean (max.) S wave V1 (mm)	Mean R/S ratio V1	Mean (max.) R wave V6 (mm)	Mean (max.) S wave V6 (mm)	Mean R/S ratio V6
0–4 weeks	145 (95–180)	0.10 (0.12)	+110 (30–180)	0.05 (0.07)	13 (24)	7 (18)	1.5	5 (15)	3 (10)	2.0
1–6 months	145 (110–180)	0.11 (0.14)	+70 (10–125)	0.05 (0.075)	10 (19)	5 (15)	1.5	13 (22)	3 (9)	4.0
6–12 months	135 (110–170)	0.11 (0.14)	+60 (10–110)	0.05 (0.075)	10 (20)	7 (18)	1.2	13 (23)	2 (7)	6.0
1–3 years	120 (90–150)	0.11 (0.15)	+60 (10–110)	0.05 (0.075)	9 (18)	8 (21)	0.8	13 (23)	2 (7)	20.0
4–5 years	110 (65–135)	0.13 (0.15)	+60 (0–110)	0.06 (0.075)	8 (16)	11 (23)	0.65	15 (26)	2 (5)	20.0
6–8 years	100 (60–130)	0.14 (0.16)	+60 (−15 to +110)	0.06 (0.075)	6 (13)	12 (25)	0.5	17 (26)	2 (5)	20.0
9–11 years	85 (60–110)	0.14 (0.15)	+60 (−30 to +105)	0.06 (0.085)	5 (12)	12 (25)	0.5	16 (25)	1 (4)	10.0
12–16 years	85 (60–110)	0.15 (0.17)	+60 (−30 to +105)	0.07 (0.085)	4 (10)	11 (22)	0.3	14 (23)	1 (4)	10.0
>16 years	80 (60–100)	0.15 (0.20)	+60 (−30 to +105)	0.08 (0.10)	3 (14)	10 (23)	0.3	10 (21)	1 (13)	9.0

Sources: Davignon *et al.* 1979; Park, 2008.

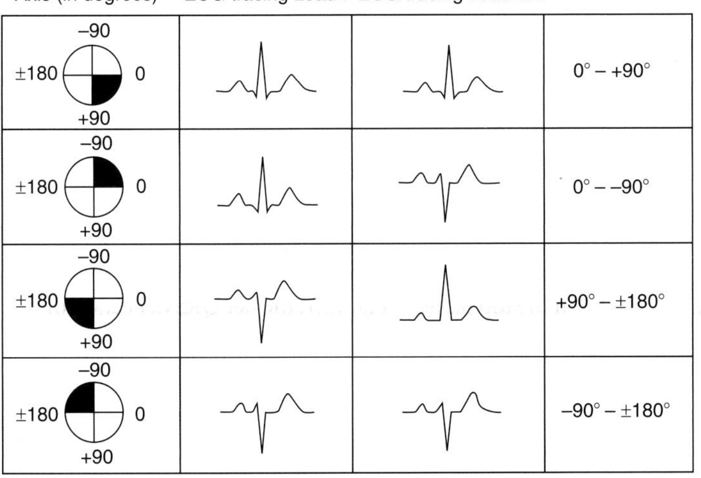

Figure 12.1 Successive approximation method with leads I and avF to determine the QRS axis. (Adapted from Park MK, Guntheroth WG. *How to Read Pediatric ECGs*, 4th edn. Philadelphia, Mosby, 2006. © 2006 Mosby Inc. an affiliate of Elsevier Inc.)

within 90 degrees. The four quadrants can be easily identified based only on the QRS complexes in leads I and aVF.

Step 2. Among the remaining four limb leads, choose the lead with an equiphasic QRS complex (in which the height of the R wave and the depth of the S wave are approximately equal). The QRS axis is perpendicular to the lead with an equiphasic QRS complex in the predetermined quadrant.

Normal QRS axis

The normal ranges of the QRS axis vary with age (Table 12.2). Newborns typically have right axis deviation (RAD) with a mean of +110 degrees compared with adults because of the dominance of the right ventricle. In utero, the heart exhibits right ventricular dominance because pulmonary vascular resistance is higher than systemic vascular resistance. Blood flow bypasses the fetal lungs and is shunted into the systemic circulation through the patent foramen ovale and the patent ductus arteriosus. At birth, even with the physiologic closure of the ductus arteriosus and the foramen ovale, the neonatal ECG still exhibits right ventricular dominance. Over the first 3 years of life, there is a gradual transition to the left ventricular dominant pattern that is characteristic of adulthood.

The RV dominance of infants is expressed on the ECG by RAD and large rightward and/or anterior QRS forces (i.e., tall R waves in lead aVR and the right precordial leads [V1 and V2] and deep S waves in lead I and the left precordial leads [V5 and V6]), compared with the adult ECG. By 3 years of age, the QRS axis has rotated leftward as the left ventricle becomes dominant and approaches the adult mean value of +50 degrees. The mean and ranges of a normal QRS axis according to age are shown in Table 12.2.

An ECG from a 4-day-old child is compared with that of a 5 year old in Fig. 12.2. The infant's ECG demonstrate RAD (+160 degrees) and dominant R waves in the right precordial leads. The T wave in V1 is usually negative. Upright T waves in V1 in this age group would suggest right ventricular hypertrophy (RVH). The 5-year-old child's ECG shows the gradual progression to the adult pattern although evidence of RAD persists. A normal ECG in a young adult is shown in Fig. 12.3.

Adult-type R/S progression in the precordial leads (deep S waves in V1 and V2 and tall R waves in V5 and V6) is rarely seen in the first month or two of life; instead, there may be *complete reversal* of the adult-type R/S progression, with tall R waves in V1 and V2 and deep S waves in V5 and V6. The R wave voltages progressively get larger from V1 through V6 in the normal adult ECG. *Partial reversal* is usually present, with dominant R waves in V1 and V2 as well as in V5 and V6, in children between the ages of 1 month and 3 years.

Abnormal QRS axis

The QRS axis outside of the normal range (Table 12.2) signifies abnormalities in the ventricular depolarization process. Note that hypertrophic changes to the ventricle or bundle branch blocks will produce identical changes in the QRS axis.

Left axis deviation (LAD) is present when the QRS axis is less than the lower limit of normal for the patient's age. It occurs with left ventricular hypertrophy (LVH), left bundle branch block, and left anterior hemiblock.

There is RAD when the QRS axis is greater than the upper limit of normal (ULN) for the patient's age. It occurs with RVH and right bundle branch block.

Hypertrophy

An assessment of atrial and ventricular chamber size is important when analyzing the pediatric ECG for underlying clues to congenital heart abnormalities.

Right atrial enlargement may be diagnosed in the presence of large P waves greater than 3 mV in leads II or V1. Because the right atrium depolarizes before the left atrium, P wave duration greater than 0.08 s in infants and 0.10 s in adolescents indicates left atrial enlargement. Left atrial enlargement is also present when the P wave in VI is notched (P mitrale), biphasic, or deeply inverted. Biatrial hypertrophy is present when the criteria for both left and right atrial enlargement are present.

QRS amplitude, R/S ratio, and abnormal Q waves

The QRS amplitude and R/S ratio are important in the diagnosis of ventricular hypertrophy. With few exceptions, evidence of ventricular hypertrophy with or without associated QRS axis deviation is found on the ECG in patients with congenital heart disease. These values also vary with age. Because of the normal dominance of right ventricular forces in infants and small children, R waves are taller than S waves in the right precordial leads (i.e., V1, V2) and S waves are deeper than R waves in the left precordial leads (i.e., V5, V6) in this age group. Accordingly, the R/S ratio (the ratio of the R wave and S wave voltages) in infants and small children is usually >1 in the right precordial leads and <1 in the left precordial leads.

The criteria for RVH and LVH are listed in Table 12.3. Right ventricular hypertrophy is best seen in leads V1 and V2 with an rSR′, QR (no S), or a pure R (no Q or S) wave. It also may be suggested by the presence of a large S wave in lead V6, upright T waves in leads V1–V3 after the first week of life, or persistence of the right ventricular dominance pattern of the neonate. Similarly, LVH is suggested with the presence of tall R waves in lead V6, large S wave in lead V1, left ventricular "strain" pattern in leads V5 and V6, and an adult-type R wave progression across the precordial leads in the newborn period.

Right ventricular hypertrophy is the most common ventricular abnormality seen on the ECG in congenital heart disease (Fig. 12.4). It may be difficult to distinguish in the early neonatal period because of the normal right ventricular predominance evident on the ECG at this age. Left ventricular hypertophy is found in congenital cardiac syndromes where the right ventricle is small and in those lesions with left ventricular outflow track obstruction. It can also be seen in older children with a patent ductus arteriosus, or larger ventricular septal defect or arterioventricular canal defect.

A

B

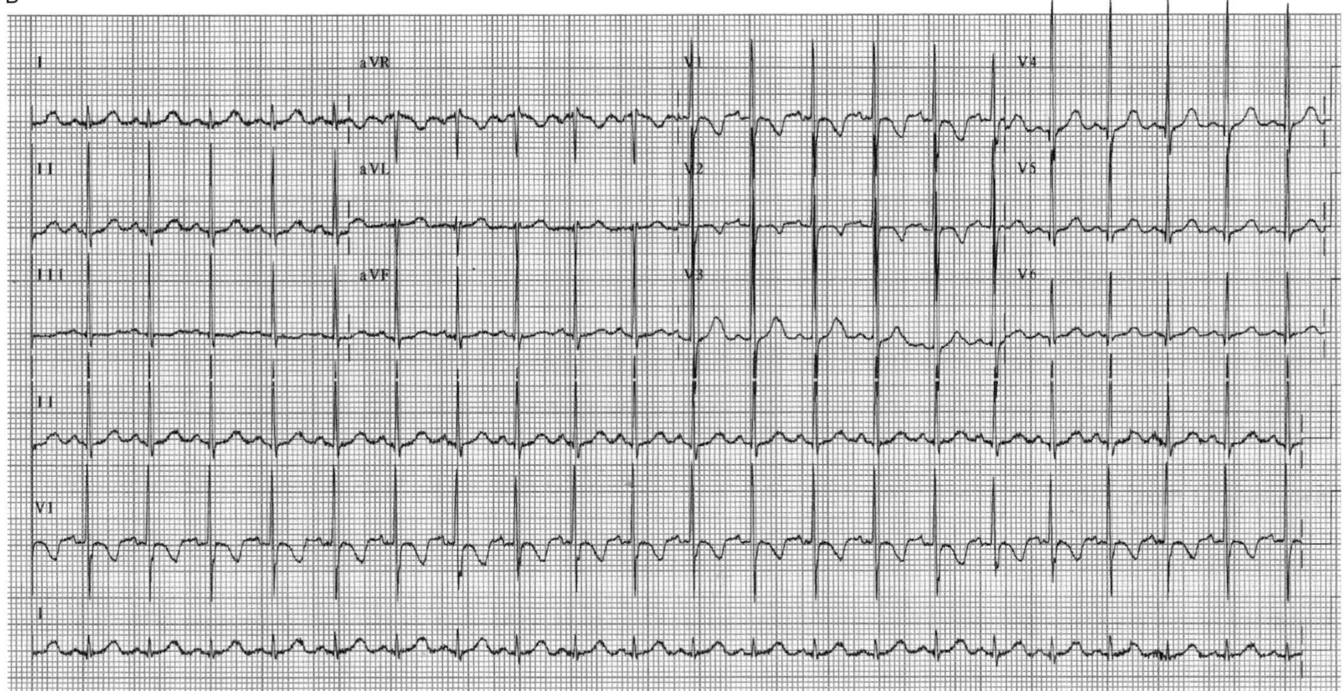

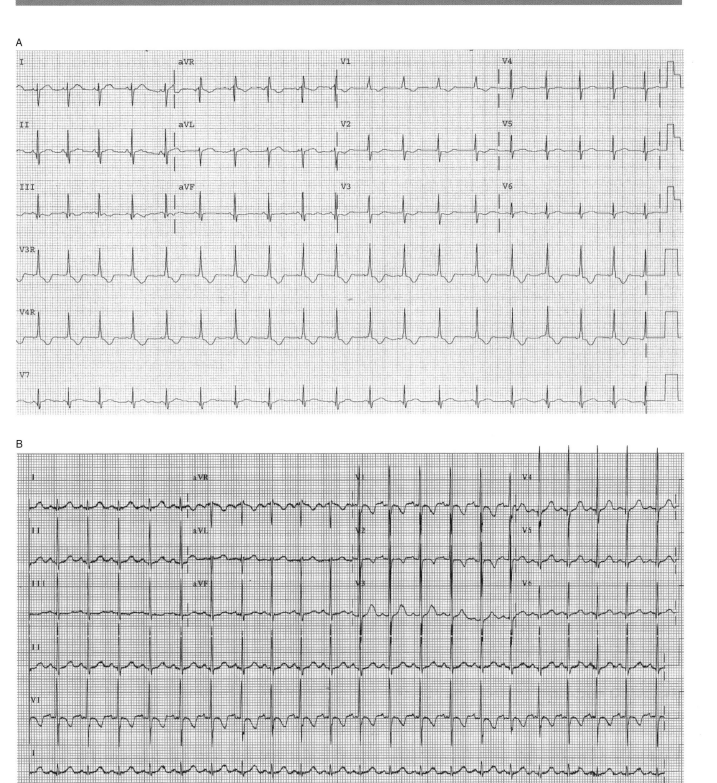

Figure 12.2 Infant and child ECG in right axis deviation (RAD). (A) Normal ECG from a 4-day-old infant, showing RAD (+160 degrees) and dominant R waves in the right precordial leads. The T wave in V1 is usually negative. Upright T waves in V1 in this age group would suggest right ventricular hypertrophy. (B) In this 5-year-old child, the ECG shows the gradual progression to the adult pattern although evidence of RAD persists. (Courtesy Inger Olson.)

Table 12.3. Electrocardiograph criteria for ventricular hypertrophy: the presence of any of these is suspicious for hypertrophy but it is not necessary for all of the criteria to be met

Hypertrophy	Criteria
Right ventricular hypertrophy	R wave greater than the 98th percentile in lead V1 in the absence of ventricular conduction delay
	S wave greater than the 98th percentile in lead V6 in the absence of ventricular conduction delay
	R/S ratio in V1 and V2 greater than the upper limits of normal for age; R/S ratio in V6 <1 after 1 month of age
	Q wave in lead V1 (qR or qRs patterns). A qR pattern may be seen in 10% of newborns
	Right axis deviation for the child's age; positive T wave in V1 >3 days of age
Left ventricular hypertrophy	Left axis deviation for the patient's age
	R wave amplitude greater than 98th percentile in lead V5 or V6
	S wave amplitude greater than 98th percentile in lead V1 or V2
	Abnormal R/S ratio in favor of the LV; R/S ratio in V1 and V2 less than the lower limits of normal for the patient's age (see Table 12.2)
	Q wave amplitude in V5 and V6 greater than 5 mm, as well as tall symmetrical T waves in the same leads
	Inverted T wave in lead V6

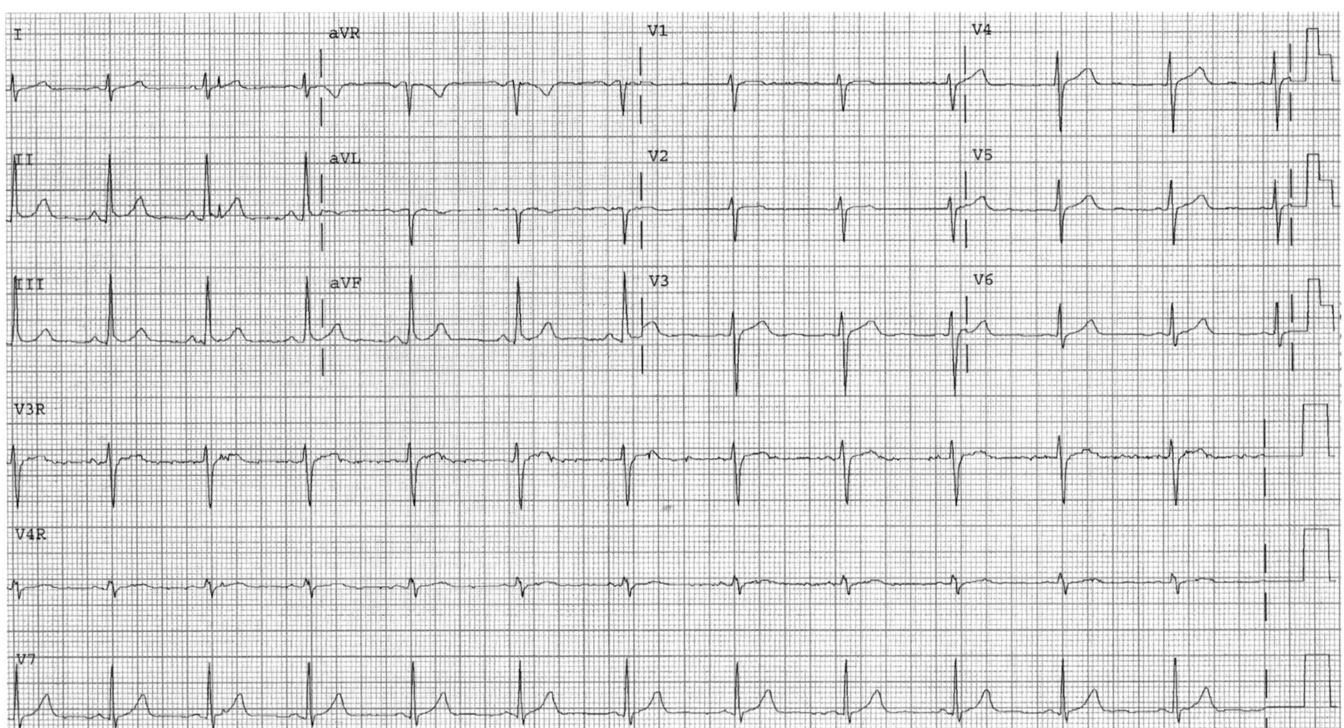

Figure 12.3 Normal ECG in a young adult. (Courtesy Dr. Inger Larson.)

Conduction intervals: PR, QRS and QTc

Conduction intervals are dependent on heart size and myocardial mass. In the neonatal and infant heart, the normal PR, QRS, and QT intervals are, therefore, shorter than their corresponding adult values. The criteria for abnormal prolongation of these intervals overlap normal adult values. For example a PR interval of 0.15 in a 6 month old is abnormal but within normal limits for an adolescent or adult.

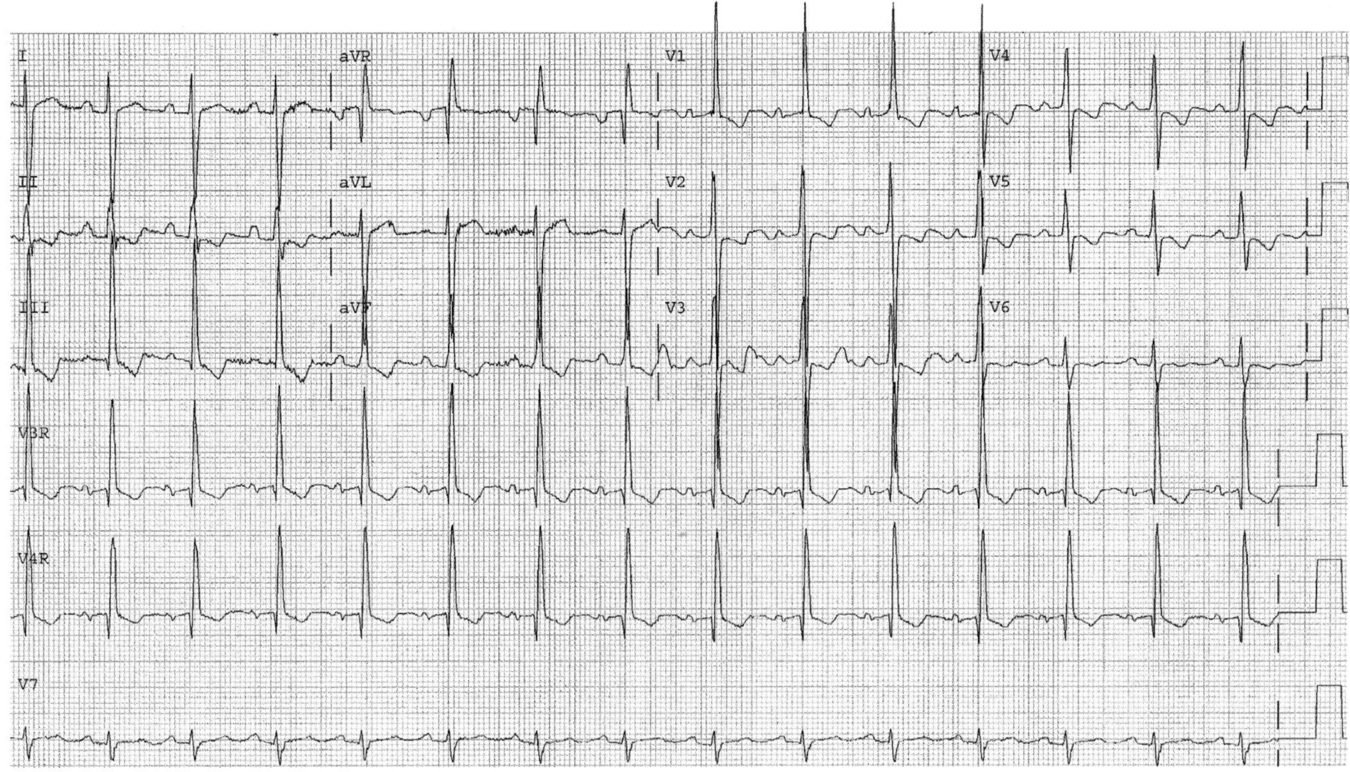

Figure 12.4 This ECG is an example of right ventricular hypertrophy (RVH) in a 10-year-old child with pulmonary hypertension. The QRS duration is normal but at this age persistent evidence of right axis deviation and the pronounced R wave in V1 and V2 indicates RVH and not the normal juvenile pattern. Evidence of tall R waves in leads III and aVR and the S waves in leads I and V6 are beyond the upper limits of normal, indicating an abnormal rightward force. The isolated R wave without S wave in V1 and the R/S ratio greater than 1 in V2 again indicate RVH. (Courtesy Dr. Inger Larson.)

QRS interval

The QRS duration varies with age (Table 12.2). It is shorter in infants and increases with age until adulthood. The QRS duration is abnormally prolonged in a variety of conditions that include right bundle branch block, left bundle branch block, pre-excitation (e.g., Wolff–Parkinson–White syndrome), paced rhythms, and in certain toxic (e.g., tricyclic antidepressant overdose) and metabolic (e.g., hyperkalemia) emergencies. The primary differential diagnosis of wide complex tachyarrhythmias includes ventricular tachycardia and supraventricular tachycardia with aberrancy. There is no clear evidence that Brugada's criteria for ventricular tachycardia in adults applies to the pediatric patient.

QT interval

The QT interval varies primarily with heart rate and is best measured using the heart rate to QTc interval ratio (see also Ch. 19 for the long QT syndrome). The QTc interval is calculated by the use of Bazett's formula:

$$\text{QTc} = \frac{\text{QT measured}}{\sqrt{\text{RR interval}}}$$

According to Bazett's formula, the normal QTc interval (mean ± SD) is 400 ms (±14 ms) with the upper limit of normal 440 ms in children 6 months and older. The QTc interval is slightly longer in the newborn and small infants, with the upper limit of normal being 470 ms in the first week of life and 450 ms in the first 6 months of life.

ST segment and T waves

The normal ST segment is isoelectric. However, in the limb leads, elevation or depression of the ST segment up to 1 mm is not necessarily abnormal in infants and children. An elevation or a depression of the ST segment is judged in relation to the PR segment as the baseline. Some ST segment changes are normal (non-pathologic) and others are abnormal (pathologic).

Tall peaked T waves may be seen in hyperkalemia and LVH. Flat or low T waves may occur in normal newborns or with hypothyroidism, hypokalemia, pericarditis, myocarditis, and myocardial ischemia.

ST segment changes

Slight shift of the ST segment is common in normal children and adolescents. Elevation or depression of up to 1 mm in the limb leads and up to 2 mm in the precordial leads is within normal limits. The most common causes of ST segment changes are normal variants: J-point depression and benign early repolarization.

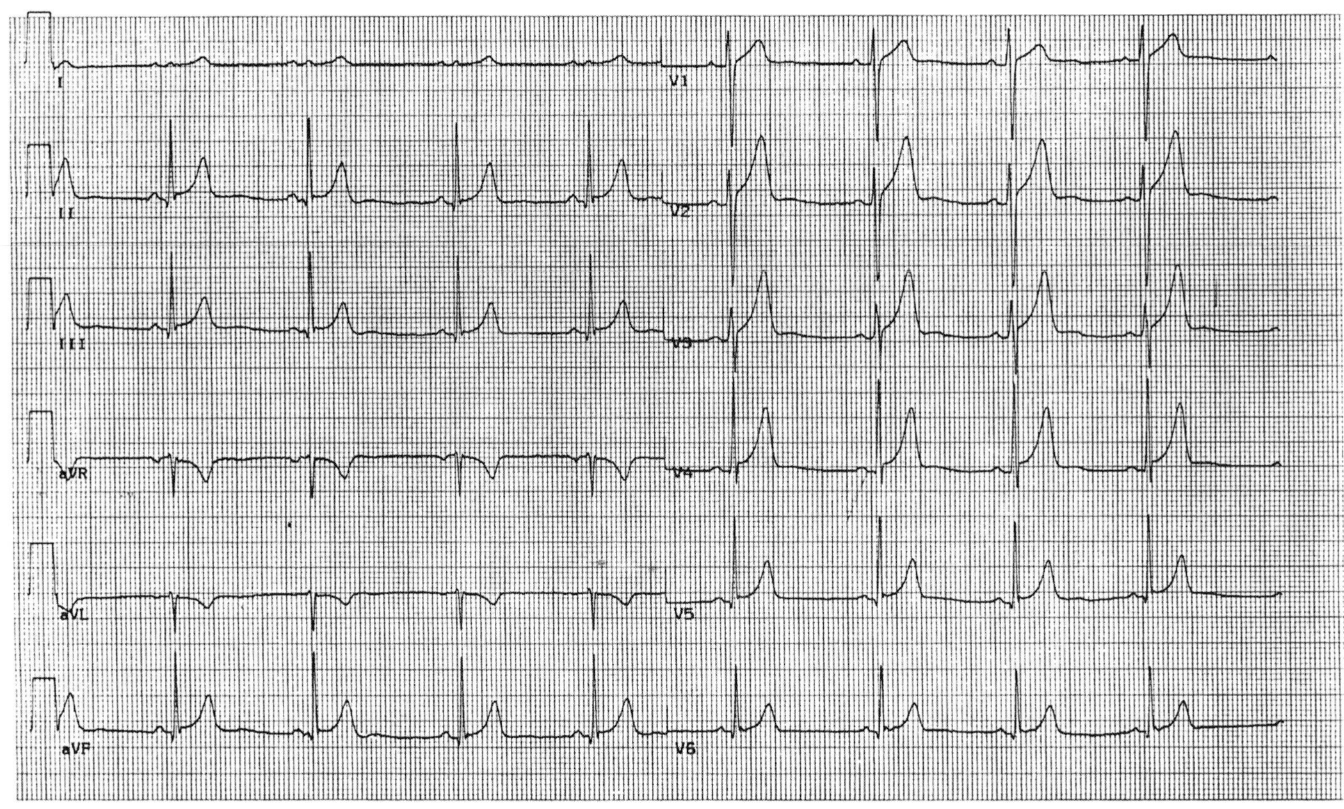

Figure 12.5 This ECG is from a healthy 19-year-old female and shows benign early repolarization and J-point depression. The ST segment elevation is most marked in II, III, aVF, and V2–V6. (Courtesy Donald Schreiber.)

J-point depression

The J-point is the junction point between the QRS complex and the ST segment. It may be depressed below the isolectric line up to 1 mm and is most commonly seen in the precordial leads. The ST segment is usually upsloping and concave and there is no persistent ST segment depression. The J-point depression is seen more often in the precordial leads than in the limb leads.

Benign early repolarization

In benign early repolarization, the ST segments are elevated but are non-pathologic (Fig. 12.5). This condition, seen in healthy adolescents and young adults, resembles the ST segment shift seen in acute pericarditis. However the ST segment is concave up and is usually most prevalent in the precordial leads especially V1–V3. It may be present in the inferior leads as well. It may be easily differentiated from pericarditis because it is not as diffuse and is not associated with PR depression.

Pathologic ST segment changes

Abnormal changes of the ST segment are often accompanied by T wave inversion. Horizontal or downsloping ST segments accompanied by inverted or biphasic T waves or ST segment elevation that is either horizontal or convex are usually all pathologic. During exercise the J-point and ST segment may be depressed but the latter is usually upsloping and the T wave remains upright. This is a normal variant. Pathologic ST segment changes are most commonly seen in LVH (Fig. 12.6) or RVH with strain, pericarditis, myocarditis (Fig. 12.7), and digoxin effect. Compared with the adult patient, myocardial ischemia or infarction is rare in the pediatric patient population but will also show similar abnormal ST segment changes.

Q waves, ventricular hypertrophy and myocardial infarction

Normal mean Q voltages and upper limits are presented in Table 12.2. The average normal Q wave duration is 0.02 s and does not exceed 0.03 s. Abnormal Q waves may manifest themselves as deep and/or wide Q waves in the leads in which they appear. Deep Q waves may be present in ventricular hypertrophy. Deep and wide Q waves are also seen in myocardial infarction but this condition is rare in children. The presence of Q waves in the right precordial leads (e.g., severe RVH) or the absence of Q waves in the left precordial leads (e.g., left bundle branch block) is abnormal.

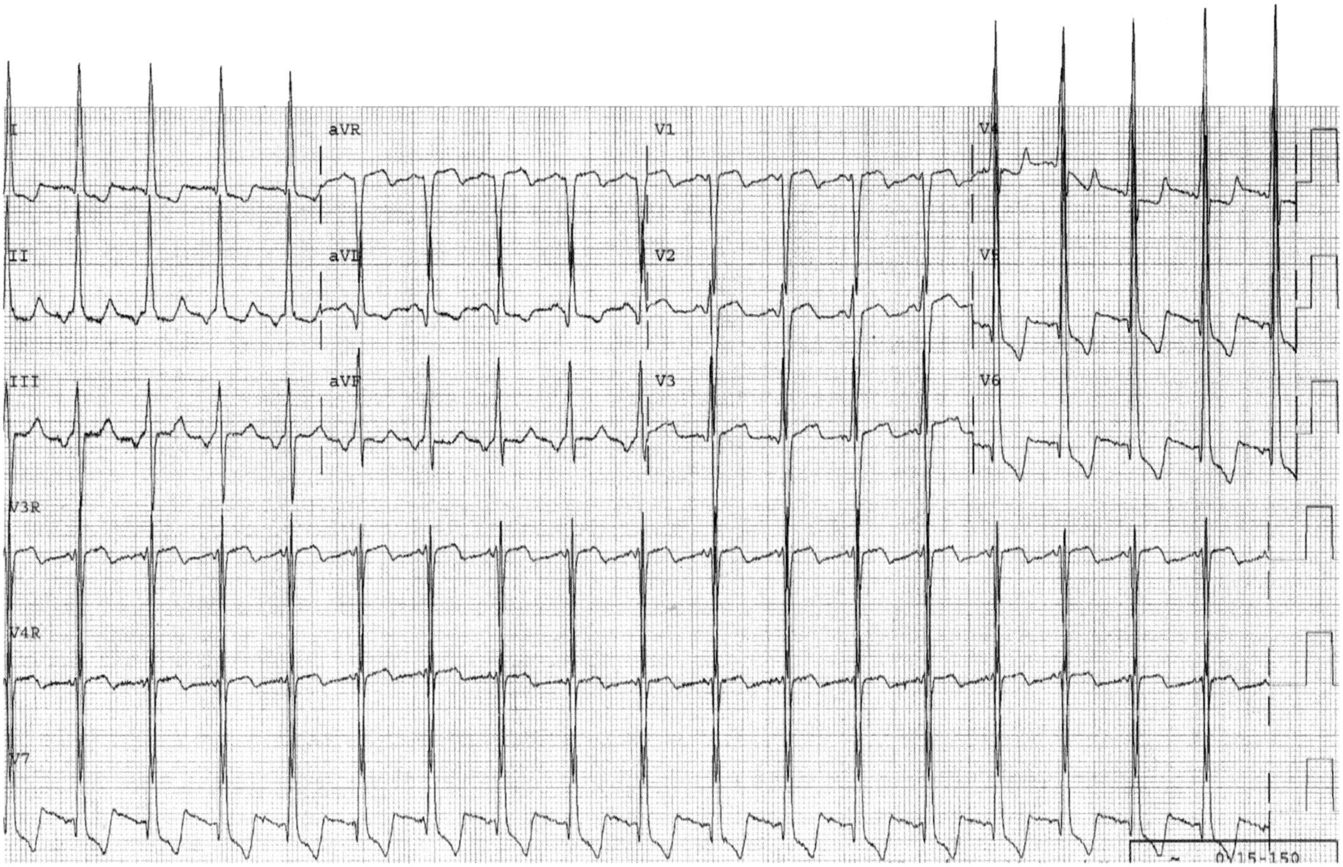

Figure 12.6 This ECG demonstrates left ventricular hypertrophy. The ST segment is downsloping and the T wave is inverted in leads I, aVL, and V4–V6. (Courtesy Dr. Inger Larson.)

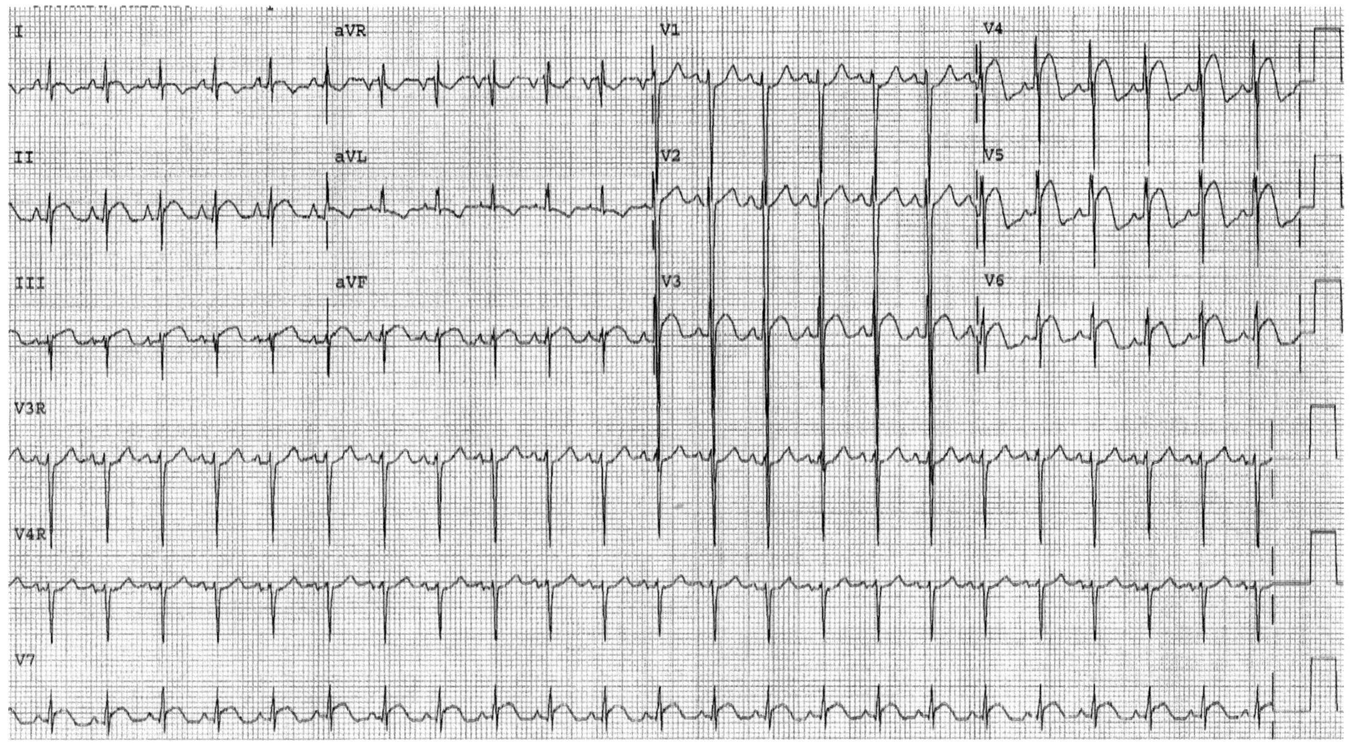

Figure 12.7 This ECG of myocarditis demonstrates diffuse convex ST segment elevation in leads I–III, aVF, and V3–V6. (Courtesy Dr. Inger Larson.)

A simple step by step approach to pediatric ECG interpretation

Step 1. Assess the rate and the rhythm.
Step 2. Check for normal QRS axis.
Step 3. Look at the R and S wave voltages in V1 and V6 and determine if there is any ventricular hypertrophy using the tables provided.
Step 4. Calculate the PR, QRS, and QTc intervals.
Step 5. Evaluate the ST segments, T waves, and, if present, Q waves for possible myocarditis, pericarditis, and, rarely, myocardial infarction.
Step 6. If all are normal, then the ECG is normal!

Conclusions

By combining a logical step-by-step approach with the knowledge of the normal age-related changes in the ECG and a basic understanding of certain important ECG abnormalities, the EP can achieve a high rate of accuracy in pediatric ECG interpretation.

Pearls and pitfalls

Pearls

1. Use of systematic method with special age-specific values for intervals, axes, and voltage criteria will facilitate accurate pediatric ECG interpretation.
2. Right ventricular hypertrophy is the most common ventricular abnormality seen on the ECG in congenital heart disease.

Pitfalls

1. Failure to realize that conduction intervals are dependent on heart size and myocardial mass. In the neonatal and infant heart, the normal PR, QRS, and QT intervals are, therefore, shorter than their corresponding adult values.

Selected references

Davignon A, Rautaharju P, Boisselle E, *et al.* Normal ECG standards for infants and children. *Pediatr Cardiol* 1979;**1**: 123–131.

O'Connor M, McDaniel N, Brady WJ. The pediatric electrocardiogram part I: age related interpretation. *Am J Em Med* 2008;**26**:506–512.

Park MK: *Pediatric Cardiology for Practitioners*, 5th edn. Philadelphia, PA: Mosby Elsevier, 2008.

Sharieff GQ, Rao SO. The pediatric ECG. *Emerg Med Clin North Am* 2006;**24**:195–208.

Wathen JE, Rewens AB, Yetman AT, *et al.* Accuracy of ECG interpretation in the pediatric emergency department. *Ann Emerg Med* 2005;**46**:507–511.

Chapter

13 Chest pain

Aparajita Sohoni

Introduction

While the average adult who presents to an ED with chest pain will undergo a workup to rule out coronary artery disease and ischemic myocardial disease, the average pediatric patient with chest pain should undergo a different workup based on a different list of possible diagnoses. Fortunately, the majority of cases of pediatric chest pain are from a non-life-threatening cause. Still, chest pain in a child engenders considerable fear and anxiety in both parents and medical providers. For the medical provider, approaching the child with chest pain in a systematic fashion will ease this anxiety and help to avoid missing an important diagnosis.

Epidemiology

Chest pain in the pediatric patient is a common phenomenon. The average age at time of presentation is 11–13 years old.

Younger children are more likely to have organic disease, while adolescents are more likely to have psychogenic or idiopathic chest pain.

Overall no sex predilection is seen. The majority of chest pain in pediatric patients is benign in etiology, with <5% of cases of chest pain with a cardiac etiology. Most common category of pediatric chest pain (20–45%) is idiopathic in nature. Table 13.1 lists the major causes of pediatric chest pain with associated frequencies.

Table 13.1. Etiologies of chest pain in pediatric patients

Category	Frequency (%)	Diagnoses
Idiopathic	20–40	
Musculoskeletal	20–30	Muscle strain: history of trauma to the affected muscle Costochondritis: pain at the costochondral junction, usually unilateral, females > males Chest wall contusion: skin changes over site of tenderness, soft tissue swelling Rib fracture: focal pain over affected rib Tietze syndrome: rare, swelling at right sternoclavicular junction or second chondrosternal junction, 70% solitary lesions Slipping rib syndrome: trauma to the 8th, 9th, or 10th costal cartilage, resulting in a slipping movement of the ribs Precordial catch syndrome: benign, sudden onset, localized to periapical region, non-radiating, lasts seconds, pleuritic Zoster: dermatome distribution of pain, followed by vesicle formation
Pulmonary	6–20	Bronchitis, pneumonia, bronchospasm, pleural effusion, pneumothorax, pulmonary embolism
Psychogenic	5–10	Anxiety, emotional stress, depression, hyperventilation
Gastrointestinal	2–10	Esophagitis, esophageal foreign body, referred pain (from peptic ulcer disease, pancreatitis, hepatitis, biliary colic, cholecystitis)
Cardiovascular	<5	Structural abnormalities, coronary arteritis (Kawasaki disease), pericarditis, myocarditis, arrhythmias
Miscellaneous		Cocaine abuse, tobacco use, sickle cell disease

Source: Leung *et al.* 1996.

A Practical Guide to Pediatric Emergency Medicine: Caring for Children in the Emergency Department, ed. N. Ewen Amieva-Wang (associate eds. Jamie Shandro, Aparajita Sohoni, and Bernhard Fassl). Published by Cambridge University Press.

Clinical presentation

Patients with chest pain will present with a range of symptoms or complaints, from isolated chest pain to concomitant shortness of breath or pulmonary symptoms to associated GI symptoms such as nausea and vomiting. While older children may be able to give a succinct history regarding the time course of their chest pain and associated symptoms, younger children may not be able to describe their symptoms or answer specific questions. The key to the evaluation of chest pain, or possible chest pain, is to remember the range of etiologies of chest pain and to ask questions that target individual organ systems. If possible, patients should be questioned about the onset, duration, severity, and frequency of their pain; the location and type of pain (sharp, squeezing, or crushing); the presence of any alleviating and worsening factors; any recent illnesses, trauma, or exercise; as well as about drug use, social stressors, and a thorough family history of cardiac or pulmonary disease.

Diagnosis

In approaching a child with chest pain, careful assessment of age-appropriate vital signs is key. Specifically, the respiratory rate and oxygen saturation will allude to a pulmonary process, while an isolated tachycardia may suggest an arrhythmia. Fever, tachypnea, or tachycardia can be an indication of myocarditis. A careful physical examination should be performed, noting any skin changes (rashes, bruises, or flushing). The entire chest should be palpated to determine any focal tenderness or reproducibility of the chest pain. Careful auscultation of bilateral lung fields should be performed. The heart sounds should also be evaluated for overall quality (as muffled heart sounds or a friction rub may suggest pericarditis), as well as abnormal heart sounds (i.e., murmurs) that could suggest structural heart disease. For every child with chest pain, an assessment of emotional states is a key part of the diagnostic approach – any hyperventilation, overall anxiety, or nervousness should be noted.

The history, physical examination, and subsequent differential diagnosis will guide which test if any is warranted. A chest radiograph, ECG, CBC, erythrocyte sedimentation rate, and urine drug screen represent some of the most common tests obtained in the evaluation of a pediatric patient with chest pain. Sometimes, in the case of pleuritic chest pain, a trial treatment with an inhaler can be therapeutic and diagnostic.

Management/disposition

The treatment of chest pain will vary with the underlying cause. For simple musculoskeletal chest pain, analgesics and rest will usually suffice. For pulmonary symptoms, treatment of the underlying pulmonary disease with inhalers or steroids (in the case of bronchospasm) will usually result in improvement of the chest pain. If structural heart disease or arrhythmias are suspected, consultation with a pediatric cardiologist should be obtained on an emergency or urgent basis. If no underlying cause is found, reassurance should be provided to the patient and their caregivers, along with appropriate return precautions.

What is important to remember in evaluating a pediatric patient with chest pain is that there is significant emotional anxiety on the part of the parents and the patient regarding the presence of chest pain. Chest pain results in a significant change in lifestyle, even if it is ascribed to a benign etiology. In one study, 69% of children had restricted their activities, while approximately 50% of children had missed a day of school because of chest pain. For this reason, caregivers should be counseled in detail regarding the chest pain their child is experiencing, the proposed etiology, plan of care, and what to do if their child does not improve or worsens. Pediatric chest pain, while usually benign, still warrants thorough evaluation and careful disposition planning in order to ensure the best outcome for the patient and family.

Pearls and pitfalls

Pearls

1. Ischemic cardiac disease in an otherwise healthy pediatric patient is rare.
2. The workup of a patient with chest pain should be tailored to the differential diagnosis, in order to avoid excessive testing.
3. Chest pain associated with exercise, dizziness, or syncope is concerning for cardiac disease.

Pitfalls

1. Failure to recognize that younger pediatric patients will be unable to provide a detailed history regarding their chest pain.
2. Failure to recognize that in infants, problems with breathing and eating can indicate underlying structural heart disease.
3. Failure to consult a pediatric cardiologist if there is concern for a patient's chest pain or symptoms being caused by underlying structural heart disease.

Selected references

Cava JR, Sayger PL. Chest pain in children and adolescents. *Pediatr Clin North Am* 2004;**51**:1553–1568, viii.

Leung AK, Robson WL, Cho H. Chest pain in children. *Can Fam Physician* 1996;**42**:1156–1160, 1163–1164.

Massin MM, Bourguignont A, Coremans C, *et al.* Chest pain in pediatric patients presenting to an emergency department or to a cardiac clinic. *Clin Pediatr (Phila)* 2004;**43**:231–238.

Chapter

14 Overview of emergency congenital heart disease: ductal-dependent lesions and acute hypercyanotic "tet" spells

Emily Wessler and Daniel Bernstein

Introduction

The incidence of congenital heart disease (CHD) is approximately 8 per 1000 live births in the western industrialized world. Nearly half of these are significant enough to warrant cardiac catheterization or surgery within the first year of life. Despite major advances in medical and surgical management, CHD is still the leading cause of deaths from congenital malformation. This chapter will first review the fetal and transitional circulation before going on to discuss the differential diagnosis and management of suspected acute presentation of CHD. The CHD tutorial in Ch. 15 will outline a system for classifying CHD based on physiology and present a brief overview of the most common congenital heart conditions. Chapter 16 is a tutorial that reviews the issues of heart transplantation likely to be relevant to the ED physician.

Fetal and transitional circulation

In fetal life, the circulation is arranged in parallel, rather than in series as it is after birth (Fig. 14.1). In the fetus, the placenta, rather than the lungs, serves as the source of oxygen uptake. There are three unique fetal structures that allow mixing of oxygenated and deoxygenated blood in the fetal circulation: the ductus venosus, the foramen ovale, and the ductus arteriosus. Blood that is more highly oxygenated from the placenta travels through the umbilical vein via the ductus venosus to the inferior vena cava and is selectively routed across the foramen ovale into the left atrium. This more-oxygenated blood passes into the left ventricle and then to the ascending aorta to supply the head and neck vessels. Only 10% of the combined fetal cardiac output passes from the ascending aorta across the isthmus of the aortic arch and into the descending aorta. Deoxygenated blood from the superior vena cava enters the right atrium, where it mixes with a portion of the inferior vena cava blood, passes through the right ventricle, and into the main pulmonary artery. Because the lungs are not used for gas exchange in the fetus, the pulmonary vascular bed is vasoconstricted and, therefore, the resistance to flow in the lungs is high. Less than

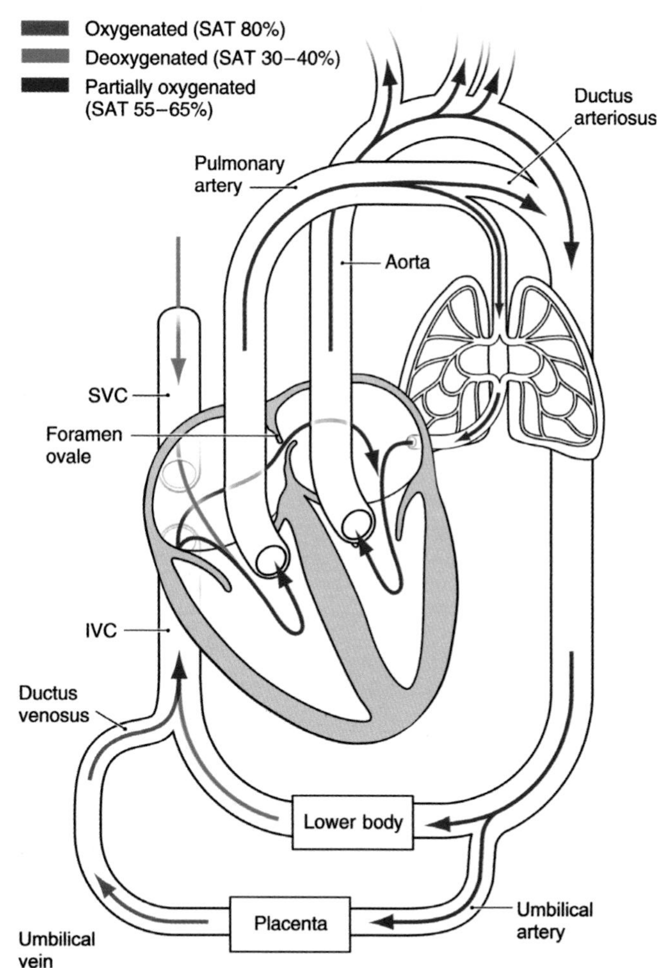

Figure 14.1 The parallel circulation in the late-term fetus showing the three fetal pathways (ductus venosus, foramen ovale, and ductus arteriosus). Oxygenated blood (oxygen saturation [SAT] approximtely 80%) returns from the placenta and mixes with deoxygenated blood returning from the fetal lower body, resulting in an overall oxygen saturation of 60–65% supplying the fetal body. This blood mostly traverses the foramen ovale and enters the left ventricle, which primarily supplies blood to the fetal upper body via the ascending aorta. Venous blood from the fetal upper body preferentially flows through the tricuspid valve and enters the right ventricle which supplies blood to the fetal lower body via the ductus arteriosus and the descending aorta. (Copyright Chris Gralapp.)

A Practical Guide to Pediatric Emergency Medicine: Caring for Children in the Emergency Department, ed. N. Ewen Amieva-Wang (associate eds. Jamie Shandro, Aparajita Sohoni, and Bernhard Fassl). Published by Cambridge University Press.

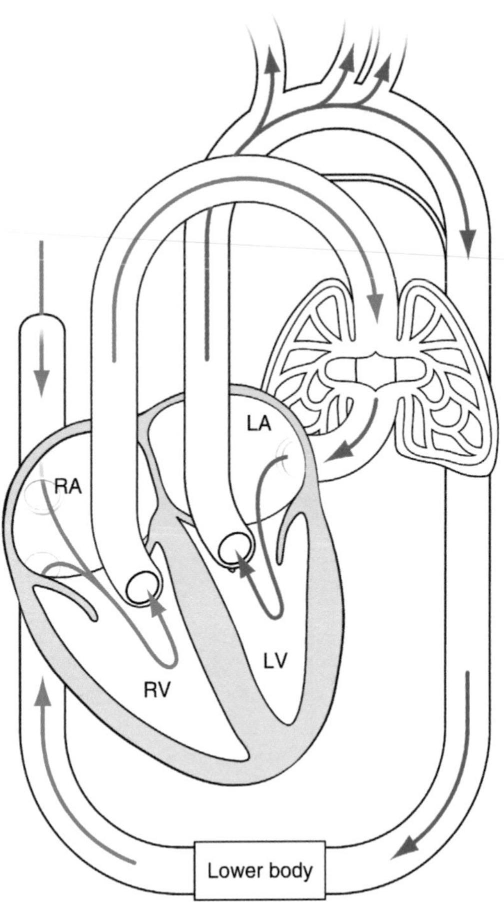

Figure 14.2 The adult circulation demonstrates closure of the three fetal pathways and transition to a series circulation. A, atrium; L, left; R, right; V, ventricle. (Copyright Chris Gralapp.)

7% of fetal cardiac output enters the lungs. The majority of the output from the right ventricle flows right to left across the ductus arteriosus from the pulmonary artery to the descending aorta and eventually into the placental circulation. Consequently, in the fetal circulation, the left ventricle pumps blood primarily to the head and upper body via the ascending aorta and the right ventricle pumps blood primarily to the lower body via the descending aorta. There is mixing of oxygenated blood (from the placenta, not the lungs) and deoxygenated blood (from the fetal venous return) at the right atrium, such that the fetal systemic oxygen saturation is only approximately 65%.

At birth, there are two major changes that occur immediately, leading to a "transitional" circulation. First, with the first breath, there is expansion of the lungs and an increase in arterial partial pressure of oxygen (PO_2), which induces a decrease in pulmonary vascular resistance. Second, the umbilical cord is clamped, removing the low resistance placental circulation and immediately increasing the systemic resistance. Because of this reversal in relative resistances between the systemic and pulmonary systems, blood now flows across the ductus arteriosus from left to right (i.e., from the aorta to the pulmonary artery). In response to the higher systemic PO_2, the ductus arteriosus closes over the first week of life. The entire cardiac output of the right ventricle now flows through the lungs and returns to the left atrium, increasing left atrial volume and pressure, thereby effectively closing the flap of the foramen ovale and preventing the right-to-left shunting of blood across the atrial septum. The foramen ovale may remain "probe patent" until later childhood and can persist in up to 15% of adults. Therefore, within several days of birth, the heart makes a dramatic transition: from the parallel fetal to the series adult circulation (Fig. 14.2). Although the pulmonary vascular resistance falls dramatically at birth, it initially remains elevated compared with "adult" levels, dropping to normal adult levels at approximately 6 weeks of life. This increased resistance to flow into the lungs in the first month of life may delay the onset of symptoms related to those heart lesions with left-to-right shunts, such as ventricular septal defect (see below).

Fetuses with even the most severe CHD can grow and develop normally because of this parallel circulation. However, following birth and the removal of the placenta and fetal pathways, the circulation may be unable to compensate for severe malformations. Since the ductus does not close immediately at birth, it is not unusual for there to be a delay in presentation of neonates with ductal-dependent congenital heart lesions (e.g., coarctation of the aorta or severe tetralogy of Fallot).

Patients with ductal-dependent congenital heart lesions are often diagnosed in the first week or two of life when they present in extemis when the ductus arteriosus finally closes.

Efforts to reopen the fetal pathways with prostaglandin (for the ductus arteriosus) or balloon atrial septostomy (for the foramen ovale) may be life saving in these situations. In general, CHD presents in one of three ways: cyanosis, congestive heart failure, or without symptoms.

Acute presentation

A differential diagnosis of the specific type of CHD can be developed based on the age at presentation and associated signs and symptoms (Table 14.1). Newborns presenting with cyanosis at delivery are most likely to have a CHD that allows minimal or no *effective* pulmonary blood flow such as de-transposition of the great arteries without a large atrial septal defect, or infradiaphragmatic obstructed total anomalous pulmonary venous return. Ductal-dependent right-sided obstructive lesions (e.g., tetralogy of Fallot, pulmonary atresia, tricuspid atresia) may present with cyanosis at several hours of life but often not until later in the first week of life when the ductus begins to constrict. Ductal-dependent left-sided obstructive lesions (critical coarctation, hypoplastic left heart syndrome, or interrupted aortic arch) are most likely to present within the first week of life, either with decreased peripheral perfusion or with cardiogenic shock. Acyanotic left-to-right shunt lesions (e.g., ventricular septal defect) may present with a murmur in the first few days to weeks of life but these patients usually do not develop symptoms of heart failure until after the pulmonary vascular resistance falls, 4–6 weeks after birth.

Table 14.1. Differential diagnosis of congenital and acquired heart disease by age of symptomatic presentation

Age[a]	Lesions
Birth	Lesions with little or no effective pulmonary flow (cyanosis): obstructed total anomalous venous return, transposition of the great vessels with poor mixing
	Lesions causing heart failure in utero: Ebstein's anomaly, arrhythmia, cardiomyopathies
Birth to first week (usually ductal-dependent lesions)	Ductal-dependent right-sided obstructive lesions (cyanosis): tricuspid atresia, critical pulmonic stenosis, tetralogy of Fallot
	Ductal-dependent left-sided obstructive lesions (shock): coarctation, critical aortic stenosis, hypoplastic left heart
	Shunt and mixing lesions (heart failure, ± cyanosis): truncus arteriosus, left-to-right shunts associated with coarctation, PDA in premature infants
4–6 weeks (when pulmonary vascular resistance falls)	Left-to-right shunt lesions (heart failure): VSD, atrioventricular septal defect
	Anomalous left coronary artery from the pulmonary artery
	Arrhythmia, cardiomyopathies
First 3 months to 1 year	Acyanotic lesions (heart failure): VSD, PDA (non-premature infants), non-critical coarctation of the aorta, anomalous left coronary artery from the pulmonary artery, arrhythmia, cardiomyopathies
Late infancy to early childhood	Acyanotic lesions (heart failure): atrial septal defect, coarctation of the aorta
	Arrhythmia, cardiomyopanthies
Adolescence	Acyanotic lesions: coarctation of the aorta (hypertension, claudication), VSD with pulmonary hypertension (heart failure, syncope), aortic stenosis (syncope)
	Arrhythmia, cardiomyopathies

PDA, patent ductus arteriosus; VSD, ventricular septal defect.
[a]Although these ages represent typical times of presentation, there are many exceptions and a high index of suspicion should always be entertained.

Diagnosis and management

In a previously healthy neonate who presents within the first months of life with cyanosis, congestive heart failure, or shock, CHD should be among the top differential diagnoses considered. Because the ductus arteriosus remains open for several days after birth, many of these patients appear normal on discharge from the nursery, only to present with severe cyanosis and cardiovascular collapse when the ductus arteriosus closes.

While sepsis should remain a primary diagnosis in the differential, it is imperative to have a low index of suspicion for significant ductal-dependent CHD in the neonate less than 1 month of age presenting in shock.

Initial stabilization includes ABC. Antibiotics and prostaglandin E_1 (PGE) should be administered. The emergency dosing of prostaglandin E_1 is at 0.05–0.1 μg/kg per min.

A thorough examination must be undertaken, including pre- and postductal saturations, four extremity blood pressures, assessment of heart sounds, and quality of distal pulses. An ECG and chest radiograph can help to narrow the differential to specific CHD diagnoses. Maneuvers to increase the oxygen delivery (e.g., inotropic support, red blood cell transfusion, or volume resuscitation) in combination with maneuvers to decrease oxygen consumption (e.g., intubation, sedation, and muscle relaxation) may also need to be instituted. Consultation with a pediatric cardiologist is essential. Definitive diagnosis is with echocardiogram.

The hyperoxia test

The hyperoxia test can help to guide the differential between pulmonary and cardiac causes of cyanosis in the neonate. An arterial blood gas should be obtained in the right arm on 21% fraction of inspired oxygen to assess the arterial PO_2. The newborn is then placed on 100% oxygen, either via an oxyhood or an endotracheal tube, for 10 min and a repeat arterial blood gas is obtained. (Note that administration of 100% oxygen by nasal cannula is not sufficient and may lead to a false positive hyperoxia test). If the PO_2 is >200 torr, it is most likely that the desaturation is caused by a pulmonary etiology. If the PO_2 is <100 torr, it is most likely that the desaturation is caused by a cardiac etiology. However, there are many situations where the hyperoxia test may be inaccurate, so it should only be used as one additional piece of information in the gathering of data for the differential diagnosis and should not delay consultation with a cardiologist.

Management of acute cyanotic spells

Hypercyanotic episodes ("tet" spells) in tetrology of Fallot are characterized by paroxysms of hyperpnea, prolonged crying, intense cyanosis, and decreased intensity of the murmur of pulmonic stenosis. There are several proposed mechanisms for these episodes, including infundibular spasm of the right ventricular outflow tract especially during crying episodes, increased oxygen demands coupled with limited ability to increase transit of blood through the pulmonary vascular bed, and venous pooling and decreased systemic vascular resistance caused by prolonged recumbent periods.

Management of the "tet spell" includes
- placing the patient in the knee-to-chest position
- morphine for sedation
- intubation only if necessary.

Other treatment modalities include increasing systemic vascular resistance with phenylephrine and the use of beta-blockers.

Conclusions

While an acute presentation of CHD is relatively rare in the ED, prompt recognition and treatment of a ductal-dependent lesion or an acute cyanotic spell can decrease morbidity and mortality. Early consultation with a pediatric cardiologist is essential for any patient with suspected heart disease.

Pearls and pitfalls

Pearls

1. A newborn <2 weeks old who appears septic has an equal chance of having a left-sided obstructive lesion. Consider starting prostaglandin E_1 at 0.05–0.1 μg/kg per min concomitant with antibiotics.
2. In patients with tetrology of Fallot and hypercyanosis, ketamine is a good alternative for intubation as it does not significantly decrease systemic vascular resistance.

Pitfalls

1. Failure to realize that children can have acyanotic ductal-dependent congenital heart disease.
2. Failure to prepare for intubation after administering prostaglandin E_1.
3. Failure to realize that medications that can decrease systemic vascular resistance such as benzodiazepines or other sedatives should be used with extreme caution during a "tet" spell.

Selected references

Allen HD, Driscoll DJ, Shaddy RE, Feltes TF. *Moss and Adams' Heart Disease in Infants, Children, and Adolescents: Including the Fetus and Young Adult*, 7th edn. Philadelphia, PA: Lippincott Williams & Wilkins, 2007.

Bacha EA, Almodovar M, Wessel DL, *et al.* Surgery for coarctation of the aorta in infants weighing <2 kg. *Ann Thorac Surg* 2001;**71**:1260–1264.

Bernstein D. Cardiology. In Bernstein D, Shelov SP (eds.) *Pediatrics for Medical Students*, 2nd edn. Philadelphia, PA: Lippincott Williams & Wilkins, 2003, pp. 261–300.

Bernstein D. The cardiovascular system. In Kliegman RM, Behrman RE, Jenson HB Stanton BF (eds.) *Nelson Textbook of Pediatrics*, 17th edn. Philadelphia, PA: Saunders, 2007, pp. 1851–1997.

Boucek MM, Waltz DA, Edwards LB, *et al.* Registry of the International Society for Heart and Lung Transplantation: Ninth Official Pediatric Heart Transplantation Report, 2006. *J Heart Lung Transplant* 2006;**25**: 893–903.

Bradley SM, Simsic JM, Mulvihill DM. Hypoventilation improves oxygenation after bidirectional superior cavopulmonary connection. *J Thorac Cardiovasc Surg* 2003;**126**:1033–1039.

Gewillig M. The Fontan circulation. *Heart* 2005:**91**;839–846.

Ghanayem NS, Hoffman GM, Mussatto KA, *et al.* Home surveillance program prevents interstage mortality after the Norwood procedure. *J Thorac Cardiovasc Surg* 2003;**126**: 1367–1375.

Hoffman JIE. Incidence of congenital heart disease: I. postnatal incidence. *Pediatr Cardiol* 1995;**16**:103–113.

Jonas RA. *Comprehensive Surgical Management of Congenital Heart Disease.* London: Arnold, 2004.

Keane J, Fyler D, Lock J. *Nadas' Pediatric Cardiology*, 2nd edn. Philadelphia, PA: Hanley & Belfus, 2006.

Mahle WT, Spray TL, Gaynor JW, Clark III BJ. Unexpected death after reconstructive surgery for hypoplastic left heart syndrome. *Ann Thorac Surg* 2001;**71**:61–65.

Mavroudis C, Backer CL. *Pediatric Cardiac Surgery*, 3rd edn. St. Louis, MO: Mosby, 2003.

Park MK, Guntheroth WG. *How to Read Pediatric ECGs*, 4th edn. St. Louis, MO: Mosby, 2006.

Razzouk AJ, Chinnock RE, Gundry SR, *et al.* Transplantation as primary treatment for hypoplastic left heart syndrome: Intermediate term results. *Ann Thorac Surg* 1996;**62**:1–7.

Rudolph AM, *Congenital Diseases of the Heart: Clinical Physiological Considerations*, 2nd edn. New York: Futura, 2001.

Rychik J, Levy H, Gaynor JW, DeCampli WM, Spray TL. Outcome after operations for pulmonary atresia with intact ventricular septum. *J Thorac Cardiovasc Surg* 1998;**116**:924–931.

Chapter 15

Tutorial: Congenital heart disease: specific lesions and operative repair

Emily Wessler and Daniel Bernstein

Classification of congenital heart disease

Defects of congenital heart disease (CHD) can be classified into cyanotic or acyanotic based on physical examination and pulse oximetry, and then further categorized by chest radiograph based on their physiology into those with increased or those with decreased pulmonary blood flow (Table 15.1). This chapter will discuss in more detail the more common specific CHD lesions, their surgical repair (Table 15.2), complications, and prognosis.

Determining the etiology of congestive heart failure (CHF) in a pediatric patient is critically important. Measures that are effective in some situations (e.g., oxygen administration in a patient with cardiomyopathy) may be deleterious in others (oxygen administration in a shunt-dependent patient or a patient with a mixing lesion).

Acyanotic congenital heart lesions

Increased pulmonary blood flow (left-to-right shunt)

Acyanotic patients with increased pulmonary blood flow generally have a left-to-right shunt. The amount of shunting and timing of presentation will depend on the location of the defect and the balance between the systemic and pulmonary resistances. These patients often become symptomatic sometime during the first 2 months of age when the pulmonary vascular resistance finally decreases to adult levels. They present with tachypnea, tachycardia, poor feeding, failure to thrive, and respiratory distress. As the amount of pulmonary blood flow increases, sympathetic activity increases to maintain a normal systemic cardiac output, with resultant tachycardia, diaphoresis,

Table 15.1. Classification of congenital heart disease based on physiology

	Acyanotic heart disease		Cyanotic heart disease	
Pulmonary blood flow (on chest radiograph)	**Increased**	**Normal**	**Decreased**	**Increased**
Physiology	Left-to-right shunt lesions	Obstructive lesions	Right heart obstructive lesions	Transposition or total mixing lesions
Congenital heart lesions	Atrial septal defect, ventricular septal defect, atrioventricular septal defect, patent ductus arteriosus, partial anomalous pulmonary venous return, aortopulmonary window, arteriovenous malformation	Pulmonic stenosis, aortic stenosis, mitral stenosis, coarctation of the aorta	Tetralogy of Fallot, critical pulmonary stenosis (newborns), pulmonary atresia, transposition of the great arteries with pulmonary stenosis, Ebstein's anomaly, tricuspid atresia	D-transposition of the great arteries, truncus arteriosus, hypoplastic left heart, total anomalous pulmonary venous return, single ventricle, tricuspid atresia with transposed great arteries

A Practical Guide to Pediatric Emergency Medicine: Caring for Children in the Emergency Department, ed. N. Ewen Amieva-Wang (associate eds. Jamie Shandro, Aparajita Sohoni, and Bernhard Fassl). Published by Cambridge University Press.

Table 15.2. Eponyms of common surgeries for correction and palliation of congenital heart disease

Name	Synonyms	Congenital heart disease	Operation	Residual defects/major complications	Palliative or complete correction
Stage I palliation	Norwood, Sano, Kishimoto	HLHS, HLHS variants, critical AS	Anastomose PA to diminutive aorta to reconstruct aortic arch, atrial septectomy, BT shunt (Norwood) or RV-to-PA conduit (Sano or Kishimoto)	Cyanosis; volume overload of single right ventricle; in BT shunt may have low diastolic pressures; *try to avoid supplemental oxygen*	Palliation
Bidirectional Glenn	Hemi-Fontan	Single ventricle variants including HLHS, HRHS, unbalanced AVSD, PA/IVS, heterotaxy syndromes, tricuspid atresia	Connect SVC directly to PA; remove or tightly band other sources of pulmonary blood flow	Cyanosis; SVC syndrome; pulmonary AV malformations	Palliation
Fontan	Total cavopulmonary connection, total cavopulmonary isolation	Same as bi-directional Glenn	Connect IVC directly to PA either with external conduit or via the atrium through a lateral tunnel	Mild or no cyanosis, mild exercise intolerance; PLE; arrhythmias; ventricular failure	Palliation
Kawashima		Patients with single ventricle who also have an interrupted IVC (usually with polysplenia syndrome)	Connect SVC to PAs (similar to Glenn shunt); since the IVC drains via the azygous vein, this is nearly a complete Fontan (hepatic veins still enter the RA)	Mild to moderate cyanosis; SVC syndrome; pulmonary AV malformations	Palliation
Blalock–Taussig shunt	BT shunt, modified BT shunt, Great Ormond Street shunt, central shunt	Any lesion with minimal or no pulmonary blood flow directly from the heart, e.g., right-sided obstructive lesions	PTFE tube from subclavian artery to PA (BT shunt) or aorta to PA (central shunt); original BT shunts divided the subclavian artery	Cyanosis; volume overload of heart; risk of shunt clotting; risk of poor coronary perfusion from low diastolic BP	Palliation
Waterston or Potts shunt	Waterston–Cooley, Cooley shunt	Any lesion with minimal or no pulmonary blood flow directly from the heart (e.g., right-sided obstructive lesions)	Waterston is a connection between AscAo and right PA; Potts shunt is a connection between descending aorta and left PA	Cyanosis, volume overload of heart; pulmonary hypertension; risk of poor coronary perfusion from low diastolic BP	Palliation
Damus–Kaye–Stansel	D-K-S	Forms of complex single ventricle, TGA/VSD/PS, Triatresia with TGA	Anastomose PA end to side with aorta, BT shunt or RV-to-PA conduit	Cyanosis (these patients usually undergo subsequent Glenn and Fontan repairs)	Palliation
Ross	Pulmonary autograft	Aortic stenosis	Transpose PV to aortic position; RV-to-PA conduit	Aortic insufficiency, RV-PA conduit stenosis or insufficiency	Complete
Konno, Ross-Konno		Subaortic and aortic annular stenosis	Resection of subaortic stenosis by creation of new VSD encroaching on RV outflow tract, which is then patch closed; may be combined with a Ross procedure	Recurrent sub-AS, sub-PS; if combined with a Ross, then aortic insufficiency and RV-PA conduit stenosis or insufficiency	Complete

Table 15.2. *(cont.)*

Name	Synonyms	Congenital heart disease	Operation	Residual defects/major complications	Palliative or complete correction
Mustard, Senning	Atrial switch	d-TGA	Redirect systemic venous flow to the LV and pulmonary venous flow to the RV via an intra-atrial baffle	Atrial rhythm disturbances; cyanosis if baffle leak, IVC or SVC obstruction, PV obstruction, failure of systemic RV	Complete
Rastelli		d-TGA/VSD/PS	Closure of VSD with a baffle tunneling LV flow to aorta; placement of RV-to-PA conduit	Stenosis or insufficiency of RV-PA conduit; sub-AS caused by stenosis of LV–aorta baffle	Complete
Arterial switch with LeCompte maneuver	Jatene	d-TGA	The great vessels are switched using coronary artery buttons to transfer the coronaries to the new aorta; The PAs are brought anterior to the aorta during the arterial switch operation	Supravalvar PS; rarely supravalvar AS; coronary artery stenosis and ischemia	Complete
Takeuchi		Anomalous left coronary artery from pulmonary artery	Baffle flow of anomalous left coronary artery from the PA to the aorta	Pulmonary stenosis, coronary ischemia	Complete

AVSD, atrioventricular septal defect; BP, blood pressure; BT shunt, Blalock–Taussig shunt; DBP, diastolic blood pressure; DILV, double inlet left ventricle; EDP, end diastolic pressure; HLHS, hypoplastic left heart syndrome; IVC, inferior vena cava; LV, left ventricle; PA, pulmonary artery; PA/IVS, pulmonary atresia/intact ventricular septum; PLE, protein losing enteropathy; PS, pulmonary stenosis; PTFE, polytetrafluoroethylene; PV, pulmonary valve; RV, right ventricle; RV-to-PA, right ventricle to pulmonary artery; SVC, superior vena cava; d-TGA/VSD/PS, d-transposition of the great arteries with ventricular septal defect and pulmonary stenosis; TA, tricuspid atresia; VSD, ventricular septal defect.

and eventual decreased peripheral perfusion, poor urine output, and, rarely, progression to shock. Some of the measures used for emergency treatment of children with congestive heart failure are outlined in Table 15.3.

Septal defects

Isolated **atrial septal defects** (ASDs) rarely demonstrate sufficient left-to-right shunting to manifest overt symptoms of heart failure, although many children may exhibit more subtle signs of slow growth or mild exercise intolerance. **Ventricular septal defects** (VSDs) will vary in their clinical presentation depending on the size of the defect and the location. A small muscular VSD causes a loud, high-pitched, apical systolic murmur but rarely any symptoms. Many of these will close spontaneously within the first few years of life. Larger defects will have a more blowing holosystolic murmur and, if large enough, can lead to pulmonary vascular disease as early as the first year or two of life. Patients with an **atrioventricular septal defect** (atrioventricular canal, or endocardial cushion defect), commonly associated with trisomy 21, will present at various ages, depending on whether the atrial (later presentation) or ventricular (earlier presentation) component is predominant. Non-premature infants or children with a patent ductus arteriosus (PDA) will usually present with a prominent machinery-like continuous heart murmur and may or may not have signs of congestive heart failure depending on the size of the PDA. The timing of surgical correction varies among the defects, with earlier closure of defects recommended in those likely to cause symptoms or pulmonary vascular disease (aortopulmonary window, large PDA, and large VSD) and later closure of defects in those that are less likely to cause symptoms or pulmonary vascular disease, such as an ASD.

Left-to-right shunt lesions after repair

Once the above defects are successfully closed, either surgically or by catheter-based device, there should not be a significant residual murmur. Small residual VSDs may result in a loud, high-pitched murmur for the first few months after surgery until they close spontaneously. If a new murmur is auscultated, particularly in the context of fever, suspicion of endocarditis and/or dehiscence of a patch should be entertained. The long-term outlook for patients with a corrected ASD, VSD, or PDA is excellent, provided that the defect was closed early enough to prevent pulmonary vascular disease. Rare long-term complications include the development of late complete heart block (which may require the emergency institution of temporary pacing) or late post-bypass cardiomyopathy. In contrast,

Table 15.3. Measures used for emergency treatment of children with congestive heart failure

Therapy	Mechanism	Advantages	Disadvantages
General measures			
Oxygen	Improved pulmonary venous saturation	Improves oxygen delivery to tissues	May cause pulmonary vasodilation and increase left-to-right shunting in some patients, potentially decreasing cardiac output
Transfusion of packed red blood cells	Increases oxygen-carrying capacity	Improves oxygen delivery to tissues	Small risk of infection, transfusion reaction
Diuretics			
Furosemide	Inhibits sodium and chloride resorption in loop of Henle and proximal and distal convoluted tubule	Improves pulmonary congestion	Hypokalemia, hyponatremia, hypocalcemia
Hydrochlorothiazide	Inhibits distal convoluted tubule sodium and chloride resorption	Improves pulmonary congestion; calcium sparing	Hypokalemia; hyponatremia; relatively weak diuretic as a single agent
Aldactone	Aldosterone antagonist	Potassium sparing	Very weak diuretic
Positive inotropic agents			
Digitalis	Inhibits Na^{+}-K^{+} ATPase and increases intracellular calcium	Improved inotropy; antiarrhythmic qualities	Increases myocardial oxygen consumption; narrow therapeutic window; may be pro-arrhythmic, toxicity increased by hypokalemia
Dopamine	Beta-adrenergic receptor agonist; increases contractility and heart rate; at low doses may increase renal blood flow	Improved inotropy; may increase renal perfusion	Tachycardia; increases oxygen consumption; arrhythmia; increases afterload at high doses through α-adrenergic effect
Dobutamine	Beta-adrenergic receptor agonist; increases contractility and heart rate; acts peripherally to reduce afterload	Improve inotropy	Hypotension; increases oxygen consumption; tachycardia; arrhythmia
Milrinone	Cyclic-AMP-specific phosphodiesterase inhibitor	Inotropy synergistic with β-agonists	Hypotension
Epinephrine	Agonist for α- and β-adrenoceptors; increases blood pressure, contractility, heart rate; bronchodilator	Improve inotropy	Tachycardia; arrhythmia; increases oxygen consumption; increases afterload
Afterload-reducing agents[a]			
Hydralazine	Direct arteriolar vasodilator	Decreases peripheral vascular resistance, increases heart rate, stroke volume, cardiac output	Hypotension
Prazosine	Peripheral α-adrenoceptor blocker	Isolated reduction in peripheral resistance	Hypotension, reduced preload
Captopril/enalapril	Angiotensin-converting enzyme inhibitors	Decreased peripheral vascular resistance with unchanged or slightly increased cardiac output	Hypotension, may exacerbate renal insufficiency
Nitroprusside	Arterial and venous vasodilator	Easy to titrate, very rapid onset and dissipation	Releases cyanide so must follow levels

[a] Do not use in fixed left ventricular outflow tract obstruction.

patients with atrioventricular septal defects often have residual regurgitation of the mitral or tricuspid valve, occasionally severe enough to cause heart failure symptoms. Some of these patients may require valve replacements during their lifetime.

Normal pulmonary blood flow (obstructive lesions)

Acyanotic patients with normal pulmonary blood flow generally have an obstructive heart lesion. The most common obstructive lesions are valvar pulmonary stenosis, valvular aortic stenosis, and coarctation of the aorta. If there is only mild or moderate obstruction, a normal cardiac output is maintained and patients are usually asymptomatic.

Pulmonary and aortic stenosis

Patients with **pulmonary stenosis** usually present with a murmur but without significant symptoms. The exception is the neonatal period, when patients with severe, or "critical," pulmonary stenosis may present with cyanosis as a result of right-to-left shunting across the foramen ovale. Pulmonary balloon valvuloplasty is usually the treatment of choice and is usually the only procedure these patients will require.

Patients with valvar **aortic stenosis** present with varying signs and symptoms depending on the degree of severity. Mild to moderate stenosis usually presents with a murmur and no symptoms. Severe stenosis in the neonatal period presents as poor peripheral pulses and perfusion and eventual cardiovascular collapse. Older children with moderate to severe aortic stenosis can present with fatigue, exercise intolerance, syncope, or chest pain with exertion. Aortic balloon valvuloplasty is often the first treatment of choice for patients with aortic stenosis; however, unlike pulmonary stenosis, many of these patients require further procedures, repeat valvuloplasties, surgical repair, or valve replacement with a homograft, a bioprosthesis, or a mechanical prosthetic valve. The Ross procedure involves using the patient's own pulmonary valve (pulmonary autograft) to replace the abnormal aortic valve, and placing a right ventricle to pulmonary artery (RV–PA) conduit. If the left ventricular outflow tract is hypoplastic, it can be enlarged through a procedure known as the Konno repair, which literally borrows part of the right ventricular outflow to enhance the size of the left ventricular outflow.

Aortic or pulmonary stenosis after repair

Patients with previously palliated aortic stenosis may develop a severe enough degree of aortic insufficiency to result in symptoms of left heart failure. If valve replacement is necessary and a mechanical valve is utilized, then anticoagulation will be required.

Coarctation of the aorta

Patients with coarctation of the aorta (CoA) may present at any age. Neonates with critical CoA (i.e., where cardiac output is dependent on maintaining a PDA) may present with diminished pulses, diminished peripheral perfusion, or shock, depending on the status of the ductus. When the PDA is open, there may be differential cyanosis in CoA: the hands will be pink and the feet will be blue. Pre- and postductal oxygen saturations will reflect this difference, with ascending aortic blood flow coming from the left ventricle, and descending aortic blood flow from the right ventricle through the ductus.

In older childen and adolescents, CoA may present with hypertension, although some children will complain of claudication and examination may show hypoplasia of the lower extremity muscles. Any child or adolescent who presents to the emergency room with hypertension, regardless of the chief complaint or age, should have pulses in the upper and lower extremities palpated for both discrepancy and radial–femoral delay and have four extremity blood pressures measured. If the lower extremity blood pressure is less than the upper extremity blood pressure, a CoA is likely. The CoA is repaired by resection of the coarctation site with primary anastomosis of the proximal and distal aorta with ligation and division of the PDA, if present.

Coarctation of the aorta after repair

Long-term outcomes are usually quite good, with residual coarctation as the most common long-term complication, more frequently seen when the repair is performed in premature infants. Balloon angioplasty is the treatment of choice for recurrent coarctation, with or without placement of a stent. These patients, particularly those in whom the diagnosis has been delayed until adolescence or young adulthood, are at risk for chronic hypertension. Cardiomyopathy is a rare complication of late repair of CoA.

Cyanotic congenital heart lesions

The major cyanotic congenital heart lesions can be remembered as the 5 Ts:

- truncus arteriosus
- transposition of the great arteries
- tricuspid valvular problems including tricuspid atresia and Ebstein's anomaly
- tetralogy of Fallot (ToF; most common cyanotic heart defect)
- total anomalous pulmonary venous return (TAPVR).

Left-sided obstructive lesions such as hypoplastic left heart syndrome (HLHS) and other single-ventricle variants are also causes of cyanosis.

Increased pulmonary blood flow (mixing lesion)

Patients with cyanotic CHD and increased pulmonary vascular markings on chest radiograph have one of the mixing lesions:

their oxygenation is low because they have inappropriate routing or mixing of systemic venous and pulmonary venous blood flows at the atrial, ventricular or great vessel level, or a combination of these (Table 15.3). They also have a high ratio of pulmonary to systemic blood flow ($\dot{Q}_p$:$\dot{Q}_s$) resulting in increased pulmonary markings on chest radiograph and often clinical signs of pulmonary overcirculation.

d-Transposition of the great arteries

d-Transposition of the great arteries (d-TGA) may present immediately after birth or, if there is an associated VSD, at up to a few months of age. The aorta arises from the right ventricle and the pulmonary artery from the left ventricle, resulting in two parallel circulations. This physiology would be immediately fatal after birth if not for the persistence of one or more of the "fetal" pathways or a VSD, with mixing of desaturated and saturated blood at the atrial, ventricular, and/or ductal level. Because the ductus can remain open for several days after birth, some of these patients present with severe cyanosis and cardiovascular collapse outside the immediate newborn period, a few days after hospital discharge. The combination of low PaO_2, elevated $PaCO_2$, and metabolic acidosis indicates severely compromised circulatory gas exchange and requires emergency initiation of prostaglandin E_1 (PGE) at 0.05–0.1 μg/kg per min to open the ductus. Intubation is often necessary, either secondary to the fragility of the patient's condition or the apnea induced by PGE. If PGE is not effective, these patients require an emergency balloon atrial septostomy by a pediatric cardiologist to provide adequate mixing. In the interim, maneuvers to increase oxygen delivery (e.g., inotropic support, red blood cell transfusion, or volume resuscitation) in combination with maneuvers to decrease oxygen consumption (e.g., intubation, sedation, and muscle relaxation) should be undertaken. Note that these maneuvers will ultimately be ineffective until an adequate site for mixing is established.

d-Transposition of the great arteries after repair

Once surgically corrected by the arterial switch operation, patients with d-TGA should have normal oxygen saturations with minimal, if any, residual lesions. Chest pain in a patient with a history of an arterial switch operation should be aggressively investigated to rule out coronary involvement. An ECG plus creatine phosphokinase-MB (CPK-MB) and troponin levels (markers of heart cell damage) should be obtained to rule out coronary ischemia. Patients who had their repairs before the mid to late 1980s may have had an atrial switch operation (Mustard or Senning). These patients have a much higher incidence of long-term complications, including systemic right ventricular dysfunction, valvar regurgitation, atrial arrhythmias, or obstruction of the superior vena cava, inferior vena cava, or pulmonary veins.

Aortic atresia and hypoplastic left heart syndrome

Severe left-sided obstructive lesions such as aortic atresia and HLHS usually present in the neonatal period or shortly thereafter with decreased peripheral perfusion and cyanosis, and can progress quite rapidly to cardiogenic shock. Some of these complex defects will remain relatively silent until the PDA closes. Initial stabilization of these patients is with PGE, as maintaining patency of the ductus will allow the right ventricle to support the systemic circulation. Secondary treatment may include volume resuscitation, red blood cell transfusion, and inotropic support; however, none of these will be effective without initiation of PGE to open the ductus. Surgical interventions for these patients vary widely depending on the intracardiac anatomy. Both short- and long-term outcomes for patients with HLHS have improved dramatically over the last decade, with many centers reporting 85%–90% first-stage survival. However, because these patients are surviving with one functional ventricle, they should be considered "palliated" rather than "repaired" and are subject to many long-term sequelae (see below).

Hypoplastic left heart syndrome is a complex of heart lesions that include a small or absent left ventricle with hypoplastic or atretic mitral and aortic valves. Prenatal diagnosis is becoming increasingly common, and ideally these patients are managed safely in the hospital immediately after birth through their initial repair. Some patients without prenatal diagnosis are discharged from the hospital and present to the ED with circulatory collapse and multiorgan failure. These patients may present with profound metabolic acidosis and may have only a minimal to moderate decrease in PO_2 and are often misdiagnosed as having sepsis rather than congenital heart disease. Initial management includes PGE to reopen the ductus arteriosus; volume expansion; red blood cell transfusion; IV inotropes, particularly afterload reduction with milrinone to promote systemic cardiac output; and calcium supplementation to improve contractility. In general, over aggressive oxygen administration should be avoided as it can lower the pulmonary vascular resistance and increase blood flow to the lungs ($\dot{Q}_p$) at the expense of the systemic circulation ($\dot{Q}_s$). Intubation, sedation, and muscle relaxation may aid in the control of excessive pulmonary blood flow and shift the $\dot{Q}_p$:$\dot{Q}_s$ in favor of increasing systemic blood flow. At any stage in the palliation of HLHS, signs and symptoms of heart failure secondary to either ventricular failure or severe tricuspid valve regurgitation may be present and anticongestive therapy or inotropic support may be required.

Patients with HLHS undergo at least three palliative operations for separation of their pulmonary and systemic circulations. The stage I palliation reconstructs a "neo-aorta" from a combination of the main pulmonary artery, which has been detached from the branch pulmonary arteries, and the hypoplastic aorta. Pulmonary blood flow is achieved with either a modified Blalock–Taussig shunt (Norwood operation) or with an RV–PA conduit (Sano or Kishimoto operation). These children are very dependent on an appropriate balance of their pulmonary and systemic blood flow ratio. Typical oxygen saturations vary between 70 and 85%. Administration of oxygen can be very detrimental to this balance and should generally be avoided unless the saturation is below 65%. Interstage mortality, that is the time between the stage I palliation and the Glenn operation (see below), has been reported to be as high as 5–10%. However, with the introduction of home monitoring of saturations and daily weight checks, interstage mortality can be almost totally eliminated.

Worsening hypoxia after stage I palliation for HLHS requires careful evaluation. The differential includes: (1) a pulmonary etiology such as atalectasis, pneumonia or pulmonary edema; (2) stenosis of the RV–PA conduit or Blalock–Taussig shunt; (3) decreased cardiac output; or (4) worsening tricuspid valve regurgitation. Appropriate therapy is dependent on the cause of desaturation. Workup should include a chest radiograph, arterial blood gases, lactate, hemoglobin, and echocardiogram to determine the cause of desaturation and direct further treatment.

The second stage operation for HLHS is the bidirectional Glenn operation, which is usually performed between 2 and 6 months of age. The superior vena cava is detached from the right atrium and anastomosed directly to the pulmonary arteries. A previous Blalock–Taussig shunt or RV–PA conduit may be either removed or banded down at this time. These patients are more stable as they are no longer reliant on the delicate balance between systemic and pulmonary vascular resistances for adequate perfusion and oxygenation. Pulmonary blood flow in Glenn shunt physiology is dependent on venous return from the head and neck vessels, and typical oxygen saturations remain in the range 70–85%. For patients with a Glenn shunt who present with hypoxia, oxygen administration is not detrimental. Strategies to improve blood flow through the carotid and subclavian vessels, including hypoventilation, increase cerebral and, therefore, pulmonary blood flow and may improve oxygenation.

The final stage III palliation for HLHS and other single-ventricle disorders is the modified Fontan operation in which the inferior vena cava is anastomosed to the pulmonary arteries. The Fontan operation is now performed either with a lateral tunnel created inside the right atrium or with an external homograft or PTFE conduit. Some centers perform this operation with a small fenestration, allowing a "pop-off" between the pulmonary and systemic circulation, with resultant mild residual hypoxia; others do not routinely fenestrate and those patients have saturations of >90%. Intermediate-term outcomes are generally good, with more than 90% of patients in class I or II of the New York Heart Association classification.

Hypoplastic left heart syndrome after repair

Long-term complications following the Fontan operation include ventricular dysfunction; arrhythmias (particularly intra-atrial re-entrant tachycardia); hypoxemia caused by a fenestration, residual shunts, veno-venous collaterals, or pulmonary arteriovenous malformations; lymphatic dysfunction, with resultant protein-losing enteropathy or plastic bronchitis; and thromboembolic events. Patients with a failed Fontan circuit eventually may require a cardiac transplant (Ch. 16).

Truncus arteriosus

In truncus arteriosus, the primitive truncus fails to divide into an aorta and pulmonary artery. The pulmonary arteries arise from the truncus, either in a main pulmonary trunk or as two separate arteries. There is a large VSD beneath a single truncal valve. The truncal valve itself may be very abnormal with two to five leaflets. Systemic and pulmonary blood flows are mixed at the ventricular level, resulting in mild to moderate cyanosis and increased pulmonary blood flow, which may result in congestive heart failure symptoms after the first few weeks of life when pulmonary vascular resistance falls. These patients are repaired by closing the VSD, allowing the truncal valve to become the aortic valve, separating the pulmonary arteries from the truncus and placing an RV–PA conduit to the pulmonary arteries.

Truncus arteriosus after repair

Results for patients with a repaired truncus arteriosus are usually excellent unless the truncal valve is very deformed, which may result in residual stenosis or insufficiency and eventually may require truncal valve replacement. Even those patients with normal truncal valve function will require replacement of the RV–PA conduit during childhood and adolescence as they grow.

Total anomalous pulmonary venous return

Total anomalous pulmonary venous return is categorized in the group of patients with cyanotic heart disease and increased pulmonary blood flow based on the appearance of pulmonary overcirculation on chest radiograph. However, in this group of patients, the increased pulmonary vascular markings are caused by either pulmonary venous hypertension from obstruction or increased pulmonary blood flow if the veins are unobstructed. There are four types of TAPVR based on where the anomalous pulmonary veins drain: infracardiac (25%), supracardiac (45%), cardiac (25%), and mixed (5%). Both infracardiac and supracardiac types are likely to develop obstruction, although infracardiac veins are always obstructed when the ductus venosus closes. Neonates with obstructed TAPVR present with severe hypoxemia, metabolic acidosis, and severe pulmonary venous congestion. Obstructed TAPVR is one of the few remaining surgical emergencies that requires immediate surgical intervention upon diagnosis as PGE will not relieve the obstruction.

Total anomalous pulmonary venous return after repair

Operative survival is greater than 95%; however, long-term prognosis is more guarded and is dependent on residual or progressive pulmonary vein stenosis. Asymmetrical pulmonary blood flow patterns on chest radiograph increase suspicion for isolated pulmonary vein stenosis. Tachypnea, failure to thrive, diaphoresis, or other signs or symptoms of congestive heart failure may represent pulmonary venous obstruction either at the site of the surgical anastomosis or of individual veins and should be aggressively evaluated.

Decreased pulmonary blood flow (obstructive right heart lesion)

Cyanotic patients with decreased pulmonary blood flow on chest radiograph usually have an obstructive right heart lesion. For cyanosis to occur, there must be two components to their congenital defect: (1) obstruction to pulmonary blood flow at the tricuspid valve, subpulmonary or pulmonary valve, and/or main or branch pulmonary arteries; and (2) a means by which deoxygenated blood can enter the systemic circulation (ASD, patent foramen ovale, or VSD).

Tetralogy of Fallot

Tetralogy of Fallot is an association of four anatomic findings leading to varying degrees of pulmonary outflow tract obstruction. It is thought to be caused by a single major developmental abnormality – anterior deviation of the conal septum – which leads to (1) a malalignment VSD; (2) an overriding aorta; (3) subvalvar, valvar, and/or supravalvar pulmonary stenosis; and (4) right ventricular hypertrophy. In its mildest form, ToF resembles a large non-restrictive VSD and may present with congestive heart failure, the so-called "pink tet." Other patients with moderate pulmonary obstruction have mild to moderate but stable levels of desaturation. If obstruction to pulmonary blood flow is severe or complete (ToF with pulmonary atresia), pulmonary blood flow is dependent on a PDA. These patients usually present with severe cyanosis and circulatory collapse when the ductus closes. Still other patients with ToF and pulmonary atresia may have major aortopulmonary collateral arteries and no PDA; these patients usually have a persistent level of moderate cyanosis during early infancy and are not dependent on PGE for survival.

Patients with any degree of obstruction may develop hypercyanotic spells ("tet" spells).

Repair of ToF involves closure of the ventricular septal defect (usually accomplished through the tricuspid valve avoiding a large ventriculotomy scar); pulmonary valvuloplasty; removal of obstructive infundibular muscle; and a trans-annular patch if the pulmonary valve annulus is hypoplastic or an RV–PA conduit if the pulmonary valve is absent.

Tetralogy of Fallot after repair

Because this disease is variable in its anatomic presentation, long-term results of ToF repair are also varied. The most common postoperative complications result from residual pulmonary stenosis or more commonly from pulmonary insufficiency (more common in those patients with a trans-annular patch), characterized by right heart failure with hepatomegaly, exercise intolerance, failure to thrive, or arrhythmias. Almost all patients who have been repaired will have an abnormal ECG with either an incomplete (rsR′) or complete right bundle branch block pattern. Because ventricular tachycardia is not uncommon in previously repaired ToF, previous ECGs should be reviewed for the "normal" baseline QRS duration and morphology of the individual patient. "Pink tets" and mild "tets" generally have an excellent outcome, similar to simple VSD closures. Patients with severe stenosis or atresia of the pulmonary valve may require life-long surgical reinterventions, including valve replacement or conduit revisions.

Tricuspid atresia

Tricuspid atresia (Triatresia) encompasses a heterogeneous group wherein the primary defect is complete lack of development of the tricuspid valve, resulting in absence of any connection between the right atrium and right ventricle. Tricuspid atresia may present in any of three physiologic states. (1) Associated with significant pulmonary stenosis, in which cyanosis is dominant; these patients usually require a Blalock–Taussig shunt in the neonatal period. (2) With unobstructed pulmonary blood flow with a VSD, in which cyanosis is minimal and congestive heart failure is dominant. These patients may require a pulmonary artery band for initial palliation. (3) With perfectly balanced circulations with just enough pulmonary stenosis to prevent pulmonary overcirculation but not enough to result in significant cyanosis. These patients may be discharged from the neonatal nursery without surgical intervention but need to be monitored closely as outpatients as their VSDs may begin to close or their pulmonary obstruction worsen during the first several months of life, resulting in worsening cyanosis. Patients with tricuspid atresia in combination with transposition of the great vessels usually present with pulmonary overcirculation and heart failure.

Tricuspid atresia after repair

Regardless of initial intervention, these patients will all eventually undergo palliation with a Glenn shunt and Fontan procedure (see above under HLHS for details of these operations and their long-term complications). In general, patients with tricuspid atresia have improved outcomes compared with those with HLHS as their "single ventricle" is an anatomic left rather than anatomic right ventricle.

Other lesions

Two other cyanotic heart lesions with decreased pulmonary blood flow worth mentioning are the tricuspid valvular disorders pulmonary atresia with intact ventricular septum and Ebstein's anomaly. In newborns with the former, pulmonary blood flow is totally dependent on a PDA. Some of these patients may have coronary sinusoids – residual primitive connections between the right ventricle and the coronary arterial bed. In a subset of these patients, the proximal coronary arteries may be stenotic and, therefore, distal coronary perfusion is dependent on blood flowing from the high pressure right ventricle through the sinusoid, known as right ventricular-dependent coronary circulation. These patients are at high risk of sudden cardiac death. Overall survival is less than for those patients without coronary stenoses. Abnormalities on an ECG at any point of life may represent myocardial ischemia or infarction. Cardiac enzymes (CPK-MB or troponin) may be elevated during episodes of cardiac ischemia.

Temporary measures in infancy

In some patients with acyanotic congenital heart disease (e.g., those with atrioventricular septal defect) and in others with cyanotic heart disease with pulmonary overcirculation (e.g., tricuspid atresia with transposed great vessels), repair may not be performed during infancy and instead a temporary pulmonary artery band is placed to reduce pulmonary blood flow, attenuate symptoms, and allow time for the patient to grow.

Problems can occur after this temporary measure. Initially acyanotic patients may develop mild cyanosis if the band is tight or as they grow and the band becomes relatively tighter. They may continue to have some degree of congestive heart failure if the band is loose. Excessive cyanosis is a sign that the patient has "outgrown" the PA band and is ready for the next stage of surgery.

Associated abnormalities

Some patients with congenital heart disease also have abnormalities of left–right patterning of their lungs and abdominal organs. Patients may have complete **situs inversus**, or one of the **heterotaxy** syndromes: asplenia syndrome (right atrial isomerism) or polysplenia syndrome (left atrial isomerism). Most of these patients have complex congenital heart lesions. Although the details are beyond the scope of this chapter, there are several important emergency management principles to remember. First, because of abnormal splenic function, patients with either syndrome are at risk for infection. Second, there is an increased risk of intestinal malrotation, and these patients are at increased risk of volvulus and may present with an acute abdomen.

Pearls and pitfalls

Pearls

1. Hold diuretics and ACE inhibitors and start *slow* volume resuscitation in a child taking anticongestive heart medications who presents with hypotension and dehydration.
2. Patients with fixed left ventricular outflow lesions, such as aortic stenosis and coarctation, should not be given afterload reducing agents.
3. Patients with situs inversus, or one of the heterotaxy syndromes, are at risk for infection secondary to decreased splenic function. They are also at risk for malrotation and volvulus.
4. After complete surgical correction of patent ductus arteriosus, ventricular septal defects, or atrial septal defects, there should be no murmurs. If a new murmur is auscultated, endocarditis or patch dehiscence should be suspected.

Pitfalls

1. Failure to notify and discuss care and follow-up of a cardiac patient with their cardiologist when these patients are seen in the ED.
2. Failure to compare old with new ECG while analyzing potential ventricular arrhythmias in patients with repaired heart defects.

Selected references

Allen HD, Driscoll DJ, Shaddy RE, Feltes TF. *Moss and Adams' Heart Disease in Infants, Children, and Adolescents: Including the Fetus and Young Adult*, 7th edn. Philadelphia, PA: Lippincott Williams & Wilkins, 2007.

Bacha EA, Almodovar M, Wessel DL, Zurakowski D, Mayer Jr. JE Jonas RA, del Nido PJ. Surgery for coarctation of the aorta in infants weighing less than 2 kg. *Ann Thorac Surg* 2001; **71**:1260–1264.

Bernstein D. Cardiology. In Bernstein D, Shelov SP (eds.) *Pediatrics for Medical Students*, 2nd edn. Philadelphia, PA: Lippincott Williams & Wilkins, 2003, pp. 261–300.

Bernstein D. The cardiovascular system. In Kliegman RM, Behrman RE, Jenson HB, Stanton BF. (eds.) *Nelson Textbook of Pediatrics*, 17th edn. Philadelphia, PA: Saunders, 2007, pp. 1851–1997.

Boucek MM, Waltz DA, Edwards LB, *et al.* Registry of the International Society for Heart and Lung Transplantation: Ninth Official Pediatric Heart Transplantation Report,

2006. *J Heart Lung Transplant* 2006;**25**: 893–903.

Bradley SM, Simsic JM, Mulvihill DM. Hypoventilation improves oxygenation after bidirectional superior cavopulmonary connection. *J Thorac Cardiovasc Surg* 2003;**126**:1033–1039.

Gewillig M. The Fontan circulation. *Heart* 2005;**91**:839–846.

Ghanayem NS, Hoffman GM, Mussatto KA, *et al.* Home surveillance program prevents interstage mortality after the Norwood procedure. *J Thorac Cardiovasc Surg* 2003;**126**:1367–1375.

Hoffman JIE. Incidence of congenital heart disease: I. Postnatal incidence. *Pediatr Cardiol* 1995;**16**:103–113.

Jonas RA. *Comprehensive Surgical Management of Congenital Heart Disease*. London: Arnold, 2004.

Keane J, Fyler D, Lock J. *Nadas' Pediatric Cardiology*, 2nd edn. Philadelphia, PA: Hanley & Belfus, 2006.

Mahle WT, Spray TL, Gaynor JW, Clark III BJ. Unexpected death after reconstructive surgery for hypoplastic left heart syndrome. *Ann Thorac Surg* 2001; **71**:61–65.

Mavroudis C, Backer CL. *Pediatric Cardiac Surgery*, 3rd edn. St. Louis, MO: Mosby, 2003.

Park MK, Guntheroth WG. *How to Read Pediatric ECGs*, 4th edn. St. Louis, MO: Mosby, 2006.

Razzouk AJ, Chinnock RE, Gundry SR, *et al.* Transplantation as primary treatment for hypoplastic left heart syndrome: intermediate term results. *Ann Thorac Surg* 1996; **62**:1–7.

Rudolph AM, *Congenital Diseases of the Heart: Clinical Physiological Considerations*, 2nd edn. New York: Futura, 2001.

Rychik J, Levy H, Gaynor JW, DeCampli WM, Spray TL. Outcome after operations for pulmonary atresia with intact ventricular septum. *J Thorac Cardiovasc Surg* 1998;**116**:924–931.

Chapter 16

Tutorial: Heart transplant

Emily Wessler and Daniel Bernstein

Emergency department management

Heart transplantation is performed on approximately 350 infants, children, and adolescents in the USA each year. Historically 1- and 5-year survival rates have been 80% and 68%, respectively, although survival in the most recent era has improved to >90% at 1 year. Immunosuppressants used following heart transplantation can cause significant side effects, including risk of life-threatening infection, renal insufficiency, diabetes, hypertension, malignancy, and hyperlipidemia (Table 16.1). The causes of death early after transplant include rejection, infection, and primary graft failure. The causes of death late after transplant are usually related to graft coronary artery disease (a form of chronic rejection), infection, malignancy, or rejection related to non-compliance. Signs and symptoms of acute rejection may mimic just about any routine childhood illness, including fever, decreased appetite, nausea and vomiting, abdominal pain, tachycardia, tachypnea, abnormal weight gain, irritability, and decreased urine output.

Rejection can present with abdominal symptoms such as pain, nausea, and vomiting.

As these symptoms are non-specific, any symptom whatsoever must be considered as a sign of possible rejection in any patient following heart transplantation. An echocardiogram can evaluate whether rejection is associated with ventricular dysfunction, although echocardiography is insensitive as a screening tool for rejection. It is imperative that any treatment of a patient following heart transplantation be coordinated

Table 16.1. Common maintenance immunosuppressive medications used following heart transplantation

Class	Name	Mechanism of action	Side effects
Antimetabolite	Azathioprine	Suppresses proliferating T lymphocytes	Bone marrow suppression, LFT abnormalities
	Mycophenolate mofetil	Suppresses proliferating T lymphocytes	Bone marrow suppression (although less than with azathioprine), nausea
Calcineurin inhibitors	Cyclosporine	Suppresses proliferating T lymphocytes by blocking interleukin-2 production	Renal insufficiency, hypertension, tremors, seizures, PRESS syndrome (cerebral edema) photosensitivity, gingival hyperplasia, hirsutism
	Tacrolimus	Suppresses proliferating T lymphocytes by blocking interleukin-2 production	Renal insufficiency, hyperkalemia, seizures, tremors, PRESS syndrome (cerebral edema) hypertension, diabetes
Steroids	Prednisone	General immunosuppressant	Cushingoid effects, diabetes, osteoporosis, avascular necrosis, obesity, increased cholesterol, muscle weakness, cataracts, mood swings
Cell cycle inhibitor	Sirolimus	Blocks T cells from entering cell cycle progression	Hypertension, renal insufficiency, tremors, headache, increased cholesterol

A Practical Guide to Pediatric Emergency Medicine: Caring for Children in the Emergency Department, ed. N. Ewen Amieva-Wang (associate eds. Jamie Shandro, Aparajita Sohoni, and Bernhard Fassl). Published by Cambridge University Press.

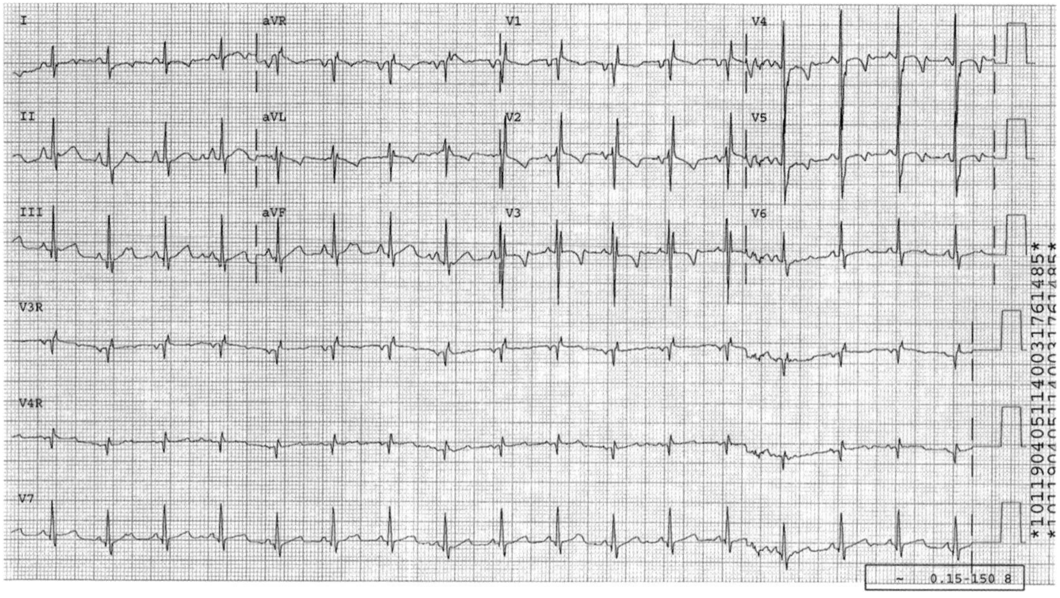

Figure 16.1 The ECG for a 1-year-old cardiac transplant recipient. Note the additional P wave from the native sinus node. (Courtesy Inger Olson.)

with the pediatric heart transplant center that routinely follows that patient. Besides the concern for rejection, many routine medications affect metabolism or clearance of immunosuppressive medications. Consequently, if a heart transplant recipient presents to ED for any reason, the patient's transplant cardiologist must be called, no matter how routine or minor the problem.

If a patient presents with signs of decreased cardiac output or overt cardiogenic shock, IV solumedrol (15 mg/kg IV, max. 1 g) should be administered while awaiting response from the transplant cardiologist.

The ECG of a transplant recipient should look typical for age. In patients who underwent operations in prior decades where the recipient right atrium was anastomosed to the donor right atrium (more recently the anastomosis is carried out at the superior and inferior vena cavae), a second P wave may be present but will be unrelated to the donor rhythm (Fig. 16.1). Arrhythmias are uncommon and both atrial and ventricular arrhythmias may represent rejection.

Pearls and pitfalls

Pearls

1. Signs and symptoms of acute rejection may mimic just about any routine childhood illness.
2. If a patient presents with signs of decreased cardiac output or overt cardiogenic shock, IV solumedrol (15 mg/kg IV, max. 1 g) should be administered.

Pitfalls

1. Failure to notify and discuss care and follow-up of cardiac transplant patient with transplant cardiologist when a heart transplant patient is seen in the ED for any reason, no matter how minor or apparently unrelated to cardiology.

Selected references

Boucek MM, Waltz DA, Edwards LB, *et al.* Registry of the International Society for Heart and Lung Transplantation: Ninth Official Pediatric Heart Transplantation Report, 2006. *J Heart Lung Transplant* 2006;**25**: 893–903.

Razzouk AJ, Chinnock RE, Gundry SR, *et al.* Transplantation as primary treatment for hypoplastic left heart syndrome: Intermediate term results. *Ann Thorac Surg* 1996; **62**:1–7.

Chapter 17

Arrhythmias

Jennifer R. Reid and Alison K. Meadows

Introduction

Arrhythmias in children are rare. For those with arrhythmias, 50% have sinus tachycardia, 13% have supraventricular tachycardia (SVT), 6% have bradycardia, and 5% have atrial fibrillation. The clinical presentation of infants and children with arrhythmias can be challenging. Infants usually present with non-specific symptoms such as vomiting, irritability, and poor perfusion. Children can also present with non-specific symptoms: shortness of breath, syncope, chest or abdominal pain, or palpitations. Children may not be aware of, or able to express, their symptoms: "not feeling right" or "feeling funny" may be their only complaint.

Evaluation of arrhythmias begins with assessing the pulse (fast, slow, or irregular), blood pressure, and oxygen saturation. If there is concern for arrhythmias, a 12-lead ECG is the next step. The first step is recognizing the range of normal pediatric heart rates (Table 12.1). When reviewing pediatric ECG intervals, remember that intervals vary by age (Table 12.2). Most tachyarrhythmias can be differentiated based on the presence of a P wave, and the width of the QRS complex. The most common tachyarrhythmia in children is SVT. Most bradyarrhythmias (sinus bradycardia; first-, second-, or third-degree atrioventricular [AV] block) can be differentiated based on the PR interval and pattern on rhythm strip. Remember to look for a prolonged QT interval; corrected QT interval (QTc) >440 ms in any age is prolonged. These children are at risk for arrhythmias and should be referred to a pediatric cardiologist.

After stabilizing the airway, provide necessary ventilatory support (i.e., oxygen, bag-valve mask ventilation, intubation), and establish IV access. If the patient becomes unstable, cardioversion takes precedence over establishing IV access. The key to managing pediatric arrhythmias is to treat any and all reversible causes. The American Heart Association's mnemonic on the reversible causes of arrhythmias and shock, the 6 Hs and 5 Ts, provides an excellent checklist:

- 6 Hs
  - hypoxia
  - hypovolemia
  - hydrogen ion (acidosis)
  - hypoglycemia
  - hypo/hyperkalemia
  - hypothermia
- 5 Ts
  - trauma
  - toxins
  - tension pneumothorax
  - thrombosis
  - tamponade.

Once a heart rate is recognized as abnormal, it can be classified into one of three broad categories: tachyarrhythmias, bradyarrhythmias, or pulseless arrhythmias. (See also Ch. 6).

Tachyarrhythmias

Tachycardia is defined as a heart rate beyond the upper limit for age. In adults, this is greater than 100 bpm; in infants <3 months, this is greater than 180 bpm. Tachycardia is not necessarily an arrhythmia. Tachycardia can have its origin in the atria, as in sinus tachycardia, SVT, ectopic atrial tachycardia, atrial flutter, or atrial fibrillation; or originate in the ventricles, as in ventricular tachycardia or ventricular fibrillation. The clinical presentation, diagnosis, ED management, and disposition for each of these rhythms is discussed below. Box 17.1 gives the basic treatment guidelines for tachycardia.

Sinus tachycardia

Clinical presentation

Sinus tachycardia can be a normal response to stress, fever, dehydration, or pain. Patients may exhibit symptoms that reflect these causes.

Diagnosis

Sinus tachycardia can be differentiated by the presence of a P wave (with a normal axis) preceding every QRS complex and a narrow QRS complex (Fig. 17.1).

A Practical Guide to Pediatric Emergency Medicine: Caring for Children in the Emergency Department, ed. N. Ewen Amieva-Wang (associate eds. Jamie Shandro, Aparajita Sohoni, and Bernhard Fassl). Published by Cambridge University Press.

Management

Identify and treat the underlying cause: antipyretics, hydration, calming measures.

Disposition/when to admit

Disposition usually depends on the underlying cause. Once causes are addressed, sinus tachycardia should resolve. Unresolved and unexplained sinus tachycardia should warrant further workup and admission.

Supraventricular tachycardia

Clinical presentation

The most common tachyarrhythmia in children is SVT. The onset is usually abrupt, without an antecedent history of illness. Infants may appear "unwell;" they are often mottled, fussy, or feeding poorly. Older children may report palpitations or "feeling unwell." They may or may not have poor perfusion.

Box 17.1. Tachycardia treatment guidelines

1. Support ABCs, give 100% oxygen, attach monitor/defibrillator.
2. Evaluate QRS.
3. Narrow QRS ($\leq$0.08 s): sinus tachycardia or supraventricular tachycardia:
   - sinus tachycardia: treat underlying cause
   - supraventricular tachycardia: treat with (a) vagal maneuvers; (b) adenosine (0.1 mg/kg, max. first dose 6 mg; may double for second dose, max. 12 mg), (c) synchronized cardioversion (0.5 to 1 J/kg; may increase to 2 J/kg); sedate if possible, but do not delay.
4. Wide QRS (>0.08 s): ventricular tachycardia with a pulse (else treat as ventricular fibrillation): synchronized cardioversion (0.5 to 1 J/kg, may increase to 2 J/kg); sedate if possible but do not delay; consider amiodarone (5 mg/kg IV over 20–60 min) *or* procainamide (15 mg/kg IV over 30–60 min), *not* both.

Diagnosis

A re-entrant mechanism is the usual cause of SVT, either from an accessory pathway (Wolff–Parkinson–White syndrome or concealed accessory pathway) or a pathway within the atrioventricular node. It can result in cardiovascular compromise. Sometimes it can be difficult to differentiate sinus tachycardia from SVT (Table 17.1).

In infants, the heart rate during SVT can range between 220 and 320 bpm. In children, the SVT rate usually ranges from 150 to 250 bpm.

Usually, the QRS complex is narrow (<0.08 s), but with aberrant conduction, can appear wide and resemble VT (Fig. 17.2).

Table 17.1. Differential diagnosis: distinguishing sinus tachycardia from supraventricular tachycardia

Feature	Sinus tachycardia	Supraventricular tachycardia
Heart rate: infant (bpm)	<220	>220
Heart rate: child (bpm)	<180	>180
Onset	Gradual: history of illness, fever, dehydration, pain, or injury	Abrupt
P waves	Present	Absent

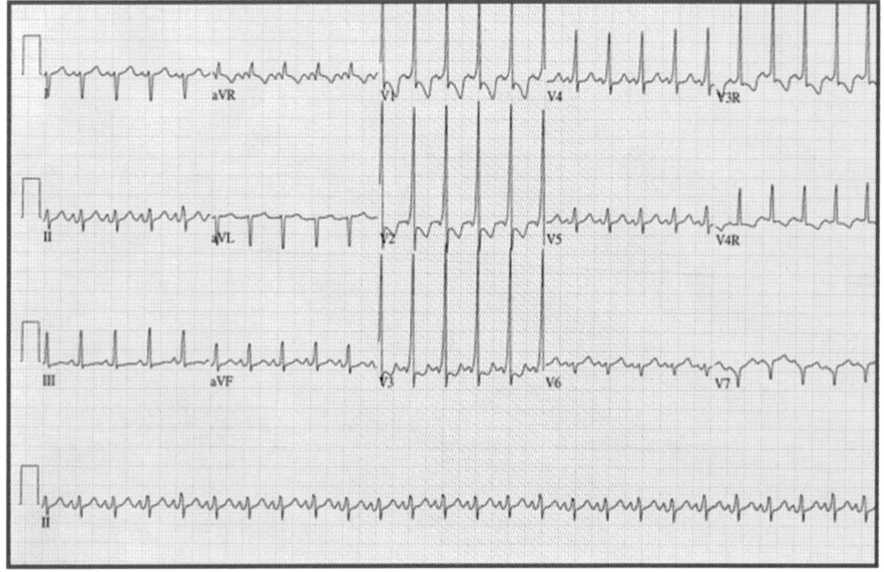

Figure 17.1 Sinus tachycardia. (Courtesy A. Meadows.)

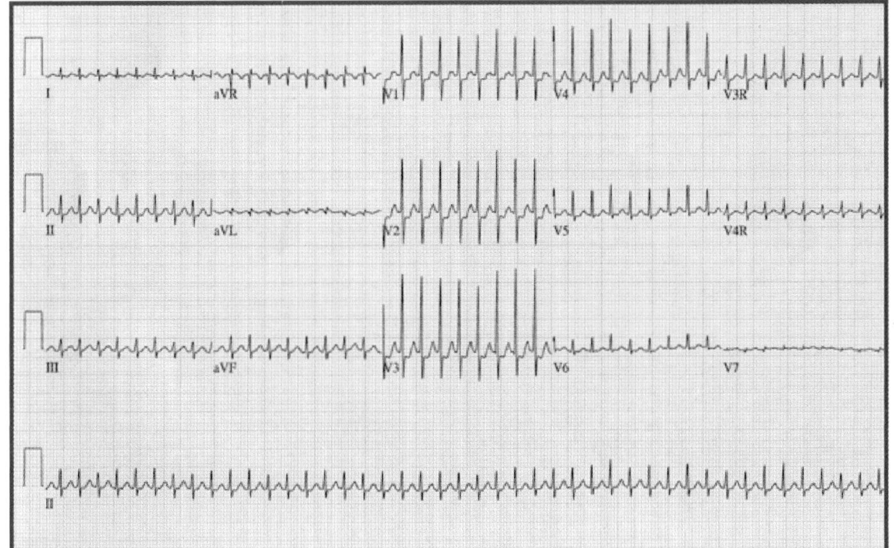

Figure 17.2 Supraventricular tachycardia. (Courtesy A. Meadows.)

Management

If the child is stable with good perfusion, treatment can begin with vagal maneuvers. These include applying an ice-and-water slurry in a bag to the face (leaving the mouth uncovered and not applying pressure to the eyes) for 10–20 s and blowing into an occluded straw or bearing down for 10–20 s. Carotid massage and eyeball pressure are no longer recommended because of their potential for harm.

If vagal maneuvers are unsuccessful, adenosine can be administered. An initial adenosine dose of 0.1 mg/kg should be given as a rapid IV bolus (max. initial dose 6 mg). This dose can be doubled for the second attempt to 0.2 mg/kg and increased to 0.4 mg/kg for a third dose (max. 12 mg dose) if initial doses are unsuccessful in converting the rhythm. Adenosine should be administered as centrally as possible (antecubital vein preferable to hand vein), and followed by an immediate flush. If SVT persists, and the patient remains stable, cardiology consultation is advised. Recall that adenosine will not effectively correct atrial flutter or atrial fibrillation, and may cause bronchoconstriction in asthmatics.

If the child is unstable, synchronized cardioversion should not be delayed. The cardioversion dose is 0.5–1 J/kg, which can be increased to 2 J/kg if lower doses are unsuccessful. A baseline ECG, with a repeat ECG following medical or electrical intervention may help to determine etiology and efficacy. Ideally, a rhythm strip should run continuously throughout attempts at conversion.

Disposition/when to admit

Patients who have an established history of SVT and who respond to one or two doses of adenosine may be discharged after discussion with a pediatric cardiologist. Patients presenting with their first episode of SVT, with SVT unresponsive to adenosine or requiring cardioversion, and patients with cardiovascular instability should be admitted to a pediatric cardiologist.

Atrial flutter

Clinical presentation

Patients may range from asymptomatic to hemodynamically unstable.

Diagnosis

Atrial flutter is extremely uncommon in children. It occurs almost exclusively as a postoperative complication of congenital heart disease repair, or secondary to a stretched or dilated atrium from other causes (cardiomyopathy, myocarditis). The hallmark ECG pattern is a "saw-toothed" baseline, with an atrial rate of approximately 300 bpm. Since the AV node cannot conduct this quickly, the ventricular rate is usually blocked 2:1, 3:1, or 4:1, with a narrow QRS (Fig. 17.3).

Management

Begin with assessment of the ABCs. An unstable patient may need cardioversion, starting at 0.5–1 J/kg and if ineffective, increased to 2 J/kg. A stable patient should be discussed with cardiology prior to intervention. Patients taking digoxin are at risk for ventricular arrhythmias with electrical cardioversion. In a stable patient, the initiation of heparin for prevention of intracardiac thrombus, digoxin and/or beta-blockade for rate control, or more aggressive antiarrhythmic agents (i.e., calcium channel blockers, sotolol, amiodarone) will likely be initiated once admitted. If spontaneous or medical cardioversion does not occur, synchronized cardioversion is usually required.

Disposition/when to admit

A pediatric patient experiencing atrial flutter may be started on digoxin, heparin, beta-blockers, other antiarrhythmics and/or

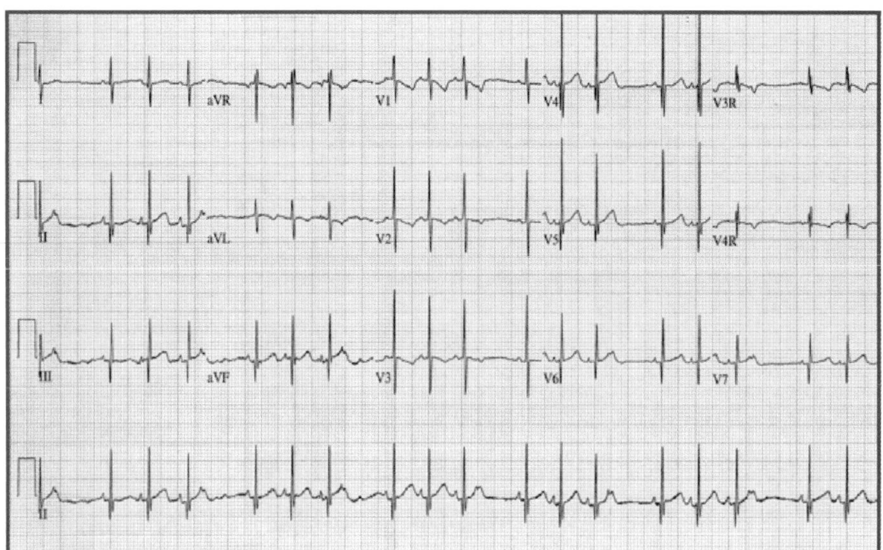

Figure 17.3 Atrial flutter. (Courtesy A. Meadows.)

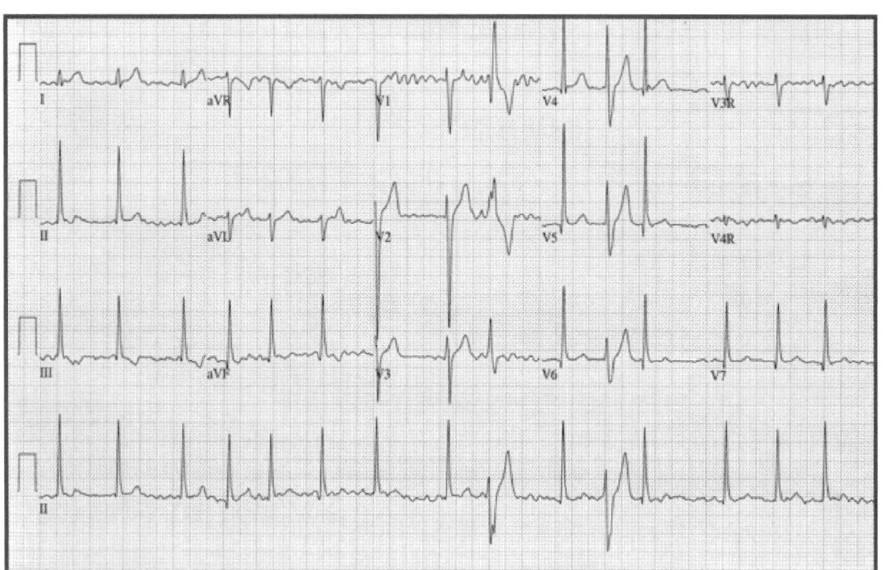

Figure 17.4 Atrial fibrillation. (Courtesy A. Meadows.)

cardioversion. A cardiology consultation and admission are recommended.

Atrial fibrillation

Clinical presentation

Patients may range from asymptomatic to hemodynamically unstable.

Diagnosis

Atrial fibrillation is extremely uncommon in children. It occurs almost exclusively as a postoperative complication of congenital heart disease repair or more rarely from other causes (hyperthyroidism, left atrial dilatation associated with mitral valve disease or cardiomyopathy). The pathophysiology is the random discharge of atrial cells, leading to disorganized atrial contraction with the appearance of "a bag of worms." On ECG, the baseline is "irregularly irregular" with atrial rates ranging from 350 to 600 bpm. QRS complexes are normal (Fig. 17.4).

Management

Begin with assessment of the ABCs. An unstable patient may need cardioversion, starting at 0.5–1 J/kg and if ineffective, increased to 2 J/kg. A stable patient should be discussed with cardiology prior to intervention. If it is unknown how long the child has been in atrial fibrillation, immediate cardioversion runs the risk of thromboembolic sequelae. Ideal management includes rate control with beta-blockers and anticoagulation while evaluating for possible thrombi if the child can tolerate the atrial arrhythmia.

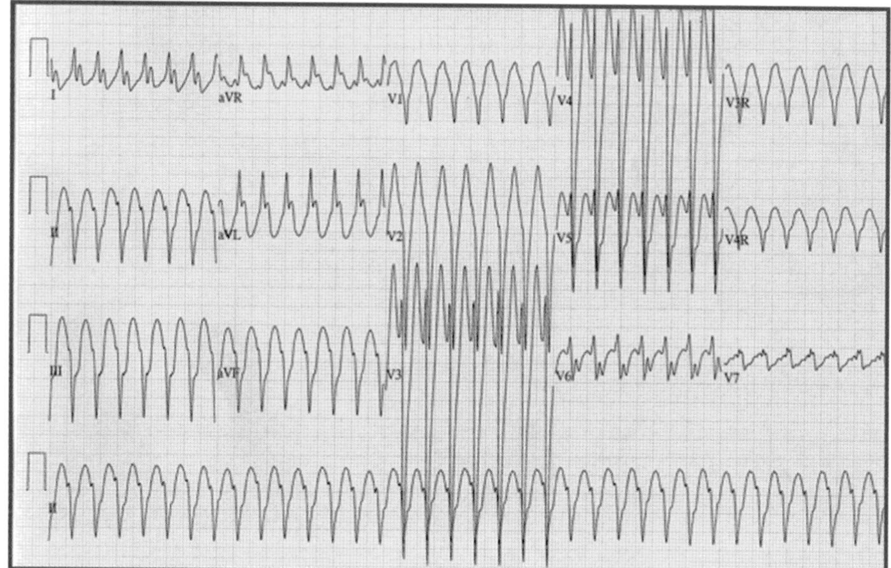

Figure 17.5 Ventricular tachycardia. (Courtesy A. Meadows.)

Disposition/when to admit

A pediatric patient experiencing atrial fibrillation may be started on digoxin, heparin, beta-blockers, other antiarrhythmics and/or cardioversion. A cardiology consultation and admission are recommended.

Ventricular tachycardia

Clinical presentation

Patients may be asymptomatic and cardiovascularly stable, or complaining of dizziness, palpitations, or "feeling unwell." Often, however, patients present with cardiovascular collapse.

Diagnosis

Ventricular tachycardia is rare in pediatrics, but potentially life threatening. The heart rate may vary from normal to as high as 200 bpm, and the QRS complex is usually wider than 0.08 ms. P waves may not be identifiable, or may not be related to the QRS complex (Fig. 17.5).

Most children with ventricular tachycardia have an underlying congenital (prolonged QT) or acquired disorder.

Such acquired disorders include cardiac surgical scars, electrolyte disorder, metabolic abnormality, myocarditis, or drug toxicity.

Management

Urgency depends on clinical status. Assure the ABCs are maintained and determine the presence of a pulse and hemodynamic stability. Ventricular tachycardia in a patient with a pulse should be treated promptly. The child can be treated pharmacologically with amiodarone 5 mg/kg IV over 20–60 min or with procainamide 15 mg/kg IV over 30–60 min. *Do not* administer both amiodarone and procainamide. A patient who remains with ventricular tachycardia and continues to have a pulse can also be treated with synchronized cardioversion, starting at 0.5–1 J/kg and if ineffective, increased to 2 J/kg. Sedation is recommended but should not delay cardioversion. Any patient without a pulse should be treated as a patient in pulseless arrest, see ventricular fibrillation below.

Disposition/when to admit

All patients with ventricular tachycardia warrant cardiology consultation and admission.

Bradyarrhythmias

Determining a slow heart rate requires knowledge of the normal variation in pediatric heart rates by age (Table 12.1). A clinically significant bradycardia is a heart rate less than normal for age, with poor systemic perfusion. Primary bradycardias are the result of congenital and acquired cardiac conditions that affect impulse formation or conduction (congenital abnormality, postsurgical injury, cardiomyopathy, etc.). Secondary bradycardias affect the normal function of the heart and are more common (hypoxia, acidosis, hypotension, drug effects, etc.). The most common cause of bradyarrhythmias in pediatric patients is hypoxia. Box 17.2 outlines the treatment guidelines.

Sinus bradycardia

Clinical presentation

Sinus bradycardia can be asymptomatic (common in competitive athletes or during sleep) or can have non-specific symptoms (altered mental status, dizziness, syncope, fatigue, and shock).

Diagnosis

Evaluation with ECG should show an abnormally slow heart rate for age. P waves should be visible. The QRS complex should be narrow.

Box 17.2. Bradycardia with poor perfusion: treatment guidelines

1. Support ABCs; give 100% oxygen, attach monitor/defibrillator.
2. CPR if heart rate <60 bpm with poor perfusion.
3. Epinephrine IV/IO (0.01 mg/kg 1:10 000; 0.1 ml/kg) or by endotracheal tube (0.1 mg/kg 1:1000; 0.1 ml/kg); can be repeated every 3–5 min.
4. If caused by increased vagal tone or heart block: atropine (0.02 mg/kg, may repeat; min. dose 0.1 mg, max. total dose for child 1 mg).
5. If ongoing bradycardia, consider pacing.

Management

First and foremost, ensure the ABCs. Most pediatric bradycardia will improve or resolve with airway and ventilation support. A heart rate of <60 bpm, with poor perfusion, is an indication for chest compressions. If the patient is still symptomatic, the drug of choice is epinephrine. It can be administered IV/IO at 0.01 mg/kg (0.1 ml/kg of 1:10 000 solution) or by endotracheal tube (ETT) at a dose of 0.1 mg/kg (0.1 ml/kg of 1:1000 solution). It can be dosed every 3 to 5 min. If the response is transient, consider an epinephrine infusion. If increased vagal tone, primary AV block, or cholinergic drug toxicity is suspected, atropine can be given. Cholinergic drug toxicity should be suspected with these clinical symptoms: miosis, bronchorrhea, salivation, emesis, diarrhea, diaphoresis, and muscle weakness. Atropine can be administered IV/IO or by ETT at a dose of 0.02 mg/kg. The minimum dose is 0.1 mg; the maximum total dose for a child is 1 mg and for an adolescent is 2 mg.

Consider cardiac pacing with pads or paddles for patients whose bradyarrhythmias are unresponsive or the result of congenital or acquired heart disease resulting in complete heart block or abnormal sinus node function.

For children <1 year or 10 kg, small or infant size pads or paddles are recommended. For those older than 1 year or >10 kg, large or adult size pads or paddles are recommended.

Pads or paddles should be placed with the heart between them. One pad can be located on the upper right side of the chest, below the clavicle, and the other to the left of the anterior axillary line. Alternatively, one pad can be placed on the anterior chest wall, to the left of the sternum, and the second can be placed over the back. Select the pacer mode on the defibrillator, synchronize, and use the minimal amount of electricity to achieve "capture." Consider sedation and analgesia, as pacing can be painful.

Carefully consider and treat reversible causes. Hypoxia should be treated with supplemental oxygen. Hyperkalemia, resulting in ECG changes, should be treated as an emergency with calcium chloride 10% (20 mg/kg IV, preferably by central line) or calcium gluconate 10% (100 mg/kg/IV). In addition, insulin, glucose, and sodium bicarbonate (1 mEq/kg IV) should be considered. Hypothermia should be addressed with rewarming techniques, avoiding hyperthermia in cardiac arrest patients. Head trauma and impending herniation should be considered and treated. Toxins should be treated with specific antidotes, if available, and supportive care. Toxins that can induce bradyarrhythmias include calcium channel blockers, β-adrenergic blockers, digoxin, clonidine, α_2-adrenergic blockers, opioids, succinylcholine, and cholinesterase inhibitors (organophosphates, nerve agents). Recall that following cardiac transplantation, the heart is "denervated." Its response to sympathomimetic or anticholinergic medications may be unreliable or ineffective, and consider early cardiac pacing in transplant recipients.

Disposition/when to admit

A pediatric patient with symptomatic bradycardia should be admitted. Asymptomatic bradycardia that cannot be attributed to physiologic reasons (athletic conditioning, sleep) warrants follow-up with a primary care provider.

Heart block

Heart block is divided into first degree, second degree (Mobitz I and II), and third degree (Fig. 17.6).

Clinical presentation

Patients may be asymptomatic (particularly with first-degree block), may present with syncope (particularly with heart rates <45 bpm), or with symptoms of congestive heart failure (more likely in third-degree block).

Diagnosis

Evaluation with ECG should distinguish between the types of AV block. First-degree AV block is usually secondary to a delay in conduction through the AV node. The PR interval will be prolonged equally from beat to beat, without any dropped beats. The QRS complex is normal. Compare the measured PR interval with age-specific norms. In second-degree heart block, Mobitz type I (Wenckebach), the PR interval lengthens progressively until a QRS complex is dropped. The QRS complex is normal. This type of block is usually asymptomatic and resolves with activity. Second-degree heart block Mobitz II is "all or none;" there is normal conduction through the AV node until there is block, then normal conduction returns. The result is normal and constant PR interval with an occasional dropped beat or QRS complex. Third-degree heart block shows no relationship (dissociation) between P waves and the QRS complex.

Management

No treatment is indicated for first-degree block, but it may require evaluation for underlying causes, such as Lyme disease or rheumatic fever. Second-degree heart block may require a pacemaker, and third-degree heart block in most cases will require a pacemaker. Atropine may be recommended to temporarily increase the heart rate. Second- or third-degree heart block warrants a pediatric cardiology consultation.

A

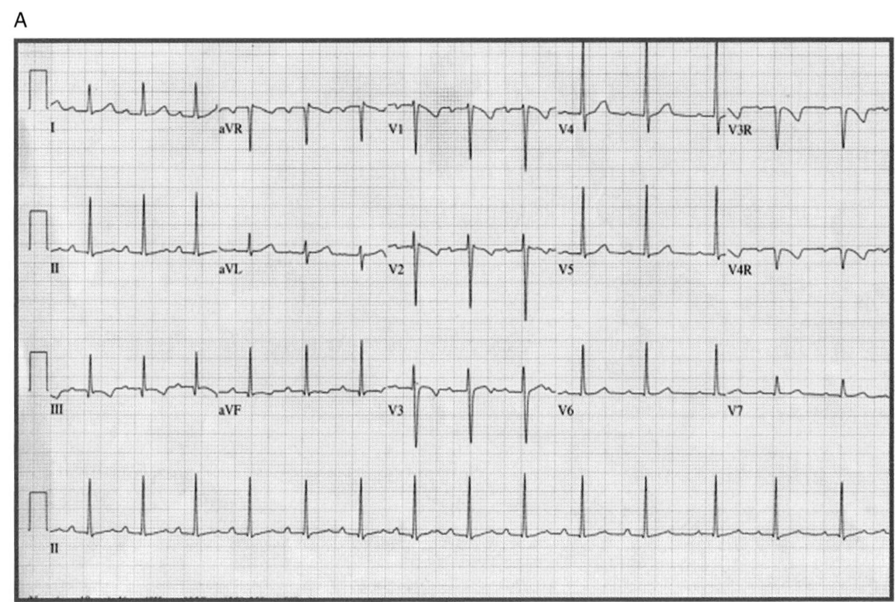

B

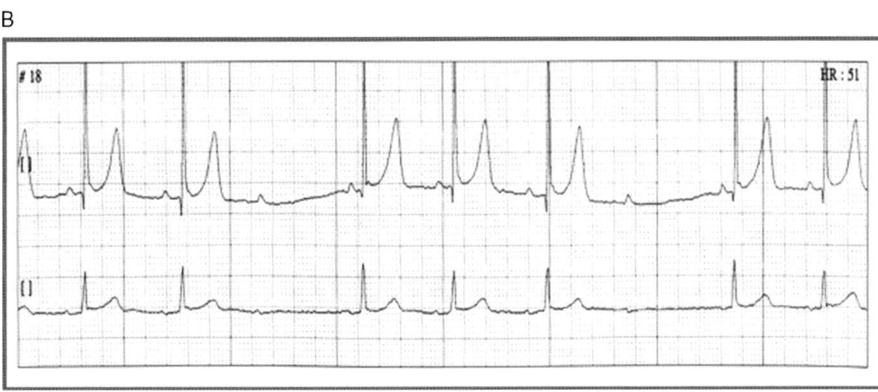

C

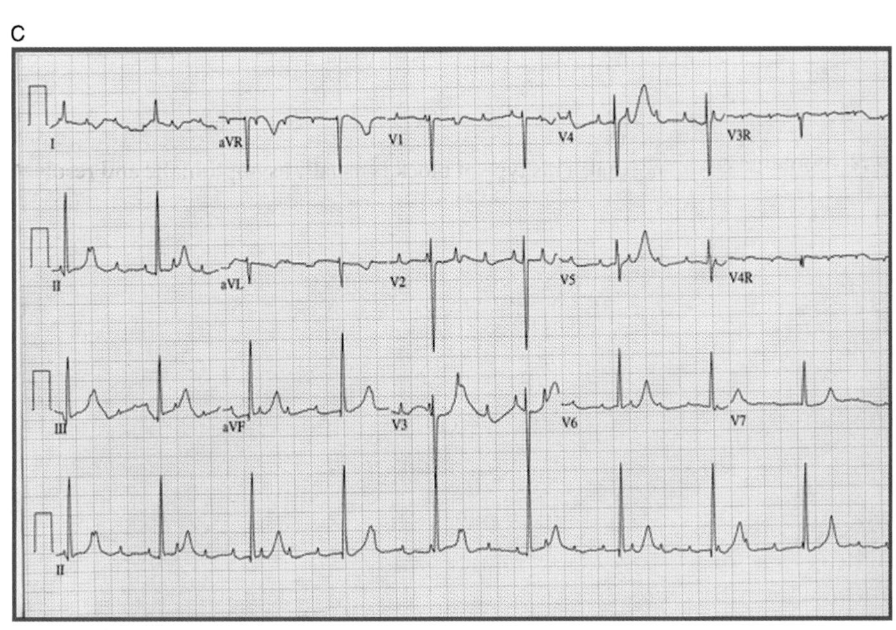

Figure 17.6 Heart block: (A) first degree; (B) second degree; (C) third degree. (Courtesy A. Meadows.)

Disposition/when to admit

A pediatric patient with symptomatic heart block should be admitted. Any patient with third-degree heart block should be admitted. Asymptomatic first- or second-degree heart block should be discussed with, and referred to, a pediatric cardiologist for follow-up.

Pulseless arrhythmias

Pulseless arrest rhythms include ventricular fibrillation, pulseless electrical activity (PEA), and asystole. In pediatrics, this is usually a terminal rhythm secondary to respiratory or cardiac failure when the body is no longer able to compensate. Clinically, the patient's extremities are cool, the skin is cyanotic, respiratory effort has ceased, and a pulse is no longer palpable.

Evaluation should include cardiorespiratory assessment and monitoring, temperature, arterial blood gas, bedside glucose, electrolytes, and ECG. Consider reversible causes: hypoxia, hypovolemia, hydrogen ions (acidosis), hypothermia, hyper/hypokalemia, hypoglycemia, tamponade, toxins, thromboembolism, trauma or tension pneumothorax.

Management of pulseless arrhythmias always begins with the ABCs (Box 17.3). Establish an airway, ventilate with 100% oxygen via bag mask, and begin chest compressions. Continue monitoring cardiac activity and the efficacy of the interventions with heart rate, blood pressure, perfusion, and oxygen saturation. Prepare for IV/IO access and endotracheal intubation. Chest compressions should be administered at a rate of >100/min and ventilations at a rate of 8–10/min. Resuscitation medications should be administered as reviewed in Ch. 6.

Deciding when to terminate resuscitation is complex. Previous studies have shown little to no meaningful survival if spontaneous circulation has not resumed after either two doses of epinephrine have been delivered or 30 min total of resuscitation. This decision should be made on a case-by-case basis, with family involvement if possible. Studies have shown that parents prefer to be present during their child's resuscitation and that being present can assist in the grieving process if death ensues.

Ventricular fibrillation

Clinical presentation

Ventricular fibrillation is a pulseless, non-perfusing rhythm. Patients are in a state of caridorespiratory arrest needing ABC support. It may present as a terminal rhythm secondary to respiratory or cardiac failure, or acutely (after chest trauma).

Diagnosis

This is an uncommon pediatric rhythm. The ECG typically shows wide QRS complexes of varying widths and amplitudes without P waves (Fig. 17.7). There is no pulse.

Box 17.3. Treatment guidelines for pulseless arrhythmias

1. Start CPR, give 100% oxygen, attach monitor/defibrillator.
2. Evaluate rhythm.
3. Treat ventricular fibrillation/tachycardia with
   (a) defibrillation, continued CPR: use an automatic external defibrillator if >1 year of age with pediatric pads for 1–8 years olds *or* use a manual defibrillator with 2 J/kg initial dose and 4 J/kg subsequent defibrillations
   (b) epinephrine IV/IO (0.01 mg/kg 1:10 000; 0.1 ml/kg) or by endotracheal tube (0.1 mg/kg 1:1,000; 0.1 ml/kg); may be repeated every 3–5 min
   (c) consider antiarrhythmic drugs: amiodarone (5 mg/kg IV/IO) or lidocaine (1 mg/kg IV/IO)
   (d) for torsades de pointes: magnesium 25–50 mg/kg IV/IO, max. 2 g.
4. Asystole/PEA: treatment with epinephrine IV/IO (0.01 mg/kg 1:10 000; 0.1 ml/kg) or by endotracheal tube (0.1 mg/kg 1:1,000; 0.1 ml/kg); may repeat every 3–5 min.

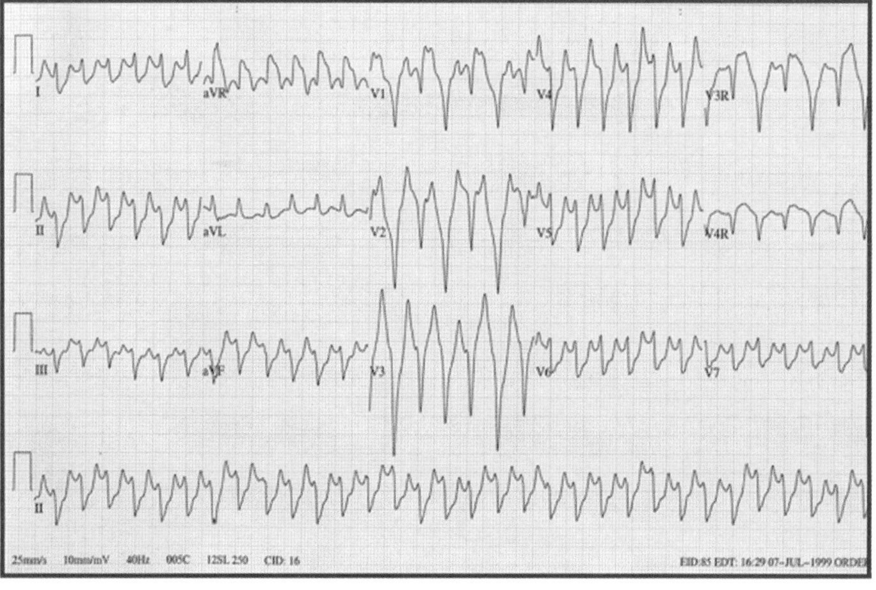

Figure 17.7 Ventricular fibrillation. (Courtesy A. Meadows.)

Management

Management of pulseless arrhythmias always begins with the ABCs. Establish an airway, ventilate with 100% oxygen via bag mask, and begin chest compressions. Defibrillation is the necessary treatment and needs to be instituted without delay. Defibrillation should begin with 2 J/kg for the first shock, increased to 4 J/kg for the second and subsequent attempts. An automated external defibrillator can be used, either in the field or in ED for children >1 year, with pediatric attachments for children between 1–8 years.

If ventricular fibrillation/tachycardia continues, CPR should continue, and the patient should be given epinephrine (0.01 mg/kg [0.1 ml/kg 1:10 000] IV/IO or 0.1 mg/kg [0.1 ml/kg 1:1000] ETT), which can be repeated every 3 to 5 min. Consider antiarrhythmics (e.g., amiodarone 5 mg/kg IV/IO or lidocaine 1 mg/kg IV/IO). If torsades de pointes is present, consider magnesium (25 to 50 mg/kg IV/IO, max. 2 g). After five cycles of CPR, check rhythm, and repeat defibrillation attempts at 4 J/kg if ventricular fibrillation or ventricular tachycardia persists.

Disposition/when to admit

A pediatric patient who has experienced ventricular fibrillation should be admitted.

Pulseless electrical activity

Clinical presentation

Pulseless electrical activity is a pulseless, non-perfusing rhythm. Patients are in a state of cardiorespiratory arrest needing ABC support. It is usually a degenerative, terminal rhythm, or it may present after ventricular tachycardia/fibrillation is treated during resuscitation.

Diagnosis

Pulseless electrical activity is an uncommon pediatric rhythm. The ECG can show any organized electrical activity (T waves, normal or wide QRS complexes, etc.) but there is no pulse.

Management

Management of pulseless arrhythmias always begins with the ABCs. Establish an airway, ventilate with 100% oxygen via bag mask, and begin chest compressions. Treat with epinephrine (0.01 mg/kg [0.1 ml/kg 1:10 000] IV/IO or 0.1 mg/kg [0.1 ml/kg 1:1000] ETT), which can be repeated every 3 to 5 min.

Disposition/when to admit

A pediatric patient who has experienced PEA should be admitted.

Asystole

Clinical presentation

Asystole is a pulseless, non-perfusing rhythm. Patients are in a state of cardiorespiratory arrest needing ABC support. It is usually a terminal rhythm.

Diagnosis

The ECG shows no electrical activity and there is no pulse.

Management

Management of pulseless arrhythmias always begins with the ABCs. Establish an airway, ventilate with 100% oxygen via bag mask, and begin chest compressions. Asystole can be treated with epinephrine (0.01 mg/kg [0.1 ml/kg 1:10 000] IV/IO or 0.1 mg/kg [0.1 ml/kg 1:1000] ETT), which can be repeated every 3 to 5 min.

Postsurgical cardiac arrhythmias

Children who have undergone cardiac surgery can suffer from a variety of complications, including arrhythmias and myocardial failure. Many of these complications occur in the early postoperative course. However, new arrhythmias, such as atrial flutter or atrial fibrillation, heart block, or re-entrant rhythms may develop as the tissue heals. Clinical indicators of postsurgical complications include deterioration in appearance (sweating, failure to thrive, irritability, or shock), increased work of breathing, and poor perfusion.

Management should begin with the ABCs, appropriate monitoring, and the administration of 100% oxygen. Obtain IV access. Obtain an ECG and compare with previous ECGs if possible. Obtain a chest radiograph. An echocardiogram may be needed to evaluate cardiac function and the pericardium. It is essential to consult the cardiac surgeon or cardiologist to

Pearls and pitfalls

Pearls

1. The primary cause of cardiac arrhythmias in children is usually hypoxia.
2. Treatment priorities are determined by adequacy of perfusion.
3. Fast rhythm (>220 bpm in infants and >180 bpm in children) is usually supraventricular tachycardia.
4. Supraventricular tachycardia is the most common pediatric arrhythmia in children with a structurally normal heart.
5. A corrected QT interval (Qtc) >440 ms in any age is pathologic and warrants referral to a cardiologist.
6. First-degree heart block is all right; second-degree heart block is probably all right but third-degree heart block is definitely bad.

Pitfalls

1. Failure to first assess and secure the ABCs in any pediatric patient with an arrhythmia.
2. Failure to treat the underlying cause of the arrhythmia.
3. Use of diltiazem in a child <6 months of age (more sensitive to calcium channel blockers).

discuss the patient's operative history and postoperative course. Each patient with a congenital heart disease is unique and has had a unique course (see Ch. 15). The nuances will help to guide management. Information on the type of repair, potential complications, and therapy can be found on an emergency information form (EIF) that patients should carry.

Selected references

Doniger SJ, and Shariff GQ. Pediatric Dysrhythmias. *Ped Clin North Amer.* 2006;**53**:85–105.

ECC Committee, Subcommittees and Task Forces of the American Heart Association. 2005 American Heart Association guidelines for cardiopulmonary resuscitation and emergency cardiovascular care. *Circulation* 2005;**112**(Suppl. I):IV–156–IV-195.

Sirbaugh PE, Pepe PE, Shook JE, *et al.* A prospective, population-based study of the demographics, epidemiology, management and outcome of out-of-hospital pediatric cardiopulmonary arrest. *Ann of Emergency Med* 1999;**33**: 174–184.

Chapter

18 Endocarditis, myocarditis, and pericardial disease

Cynthia Galvan and Michael A. Gisondi

Introduction

The incidence of pediatric endocarditis and myocarditis is difficult to define, and both entities are categorized by the US National Institutes of Health as rare diseases (prevalence <200 000 in the general population). In the past, both in the USA and globally, infective endocarditis (IE) may have been related to rheumatic heart disease.

Structural heart disease (e.g., a bicuspid aortic valve) exists in 90% of patients with infective endocarditis.

Researchers have found that up to one-third of pediatric patients with myocardial disease who present with heart failure may require a heart transplant as definitive treatment. Meanwhile, pericardial disease is usually associated with an underlying co-morbidity. This chapter will review endocarditis, myocarditis, and pericardial disease and their management in the ED.

Endocarditis

Endocarditis involves the inner layer of the heart, including the valvular structures, and is classified as either infectious or non-infectious. The former occurs in the setting of a damaged cardiac endothelium and simultaneous bacteremia. Gram-positive cocci, which have a predilection for fibronectin in the subendocardial connective tissue, are the most common cause of IE. A vegetation – consisting of bacteria, platelets, and fibrin encased in calcium – then forms. These vegetations can cause valvular regurgitation and heart failure. Pieces of the vegetation can embolize systemically, while bacterial infection can also spread into the cardiac tissue. Infective endocarditis can be acute or subacute. Neonatal endocarditis occurs in hospitalized neonates, commonly in the right heart, and is usually associated with disruption of the endocardium by IV catheters in association with transient bacteremia from trauma to skin or mucous membranes, vigorous endotracheal suctioning, or parenteral hyperalimentation. Right heart IE may be associated with pulmonary septic emboli while left heart IE may be associated with peripheral emboli and vascular phenomena. Mortality varies for IE but can be as high as 40% in some groups, for example high-risk patients with *Staphylococcal aureus* infection.

Clinical presentation and management history

Endocarditis in children typically presents subacutely in the setting of a low-grade fever and somatic complaints.

The infant can present to ED with signs and symptoms of congestive heart failure and septicemia, history of fever, poor feeding, spitting up, irregular breathing patterns, lethargy, and poor tone or skin color. In the older more verbal children, arthralgias, myalgias, weakness, decreased energy, weight loss, rigors, and diaphoresis may be presenting symptoms. Patients who are chronically ill, are hospitalized in long-term care, or who have indwelling lines or catheters are more at risk for bacteremia and right heart endocarditis.

History of prolonged illness or fever with positive blood cultures for *S. aureus* may be suggestive of endocarditis. Any recent instrumentation, central venous catheters, or cardiac surgery should heighten the suspicion for endocarditis. Although rare, in the older teenager or adolescent, a history of intravenous drug use in the setting of fever and illness with a new murmur is suspicious for endocarditis. Lack of endocarditis prophylaxis in the setting of dental procedures in a high-risk population may also heighten the suspicion for endocarditis.

Differential diagnosis

The differential diagnosis for endocarditis includes myocarditis, pericarditis, congestive heart failure from other causes, septicemia, congenital heart disease, and collagen vascular diseases.

Physical examination

Physical examination may identify a new murmur and signs of heart failure. Signs of endocarditis result from associated bacteremia or fungemia, valvulitis, immunologic responses, and embolic phenomena. Embolization to abdominal viscera, brain, extremities, kidneys, and spleen may occur from left

A Practical Guide to Pediatric Emergency Medicine: Caring for Children in the Emergency Department, ed. N. Ewen Amieva-Wang (associate eds. Jamie Shandro, Aparajita Sohoni, and Bernhard Fassl). Published by Cambridge University Press.

Table 18.1. Complications of infective endocarditis by system

System	Complications
Brain	Mycotic aneurysms, abscesses, ischemic and/or hemorrhagic emboli, meningitis
Lungs	Infarcts, abscesses, pneumonia
Heart	Valvulitis, abscesses, ruptured chordae tendonae
Liver	Hepatomegaly
Kidneys	Glomerulonephritis, infarct
Abdominal viscera	Ischemic and/or hemorrhagic emboli
Spleen	Abscesses, infarct, rupture
Bone	Osteomyelitis
Vascular	Non-tender Janeway lesions, tender Osler's nodes, Roth spots (not seen in neonates)
Eyes	Conjunctival and/or retinal lesions

heart IE and to the lungs from right heart IE. Vasculitic stigmata, which include non-tender Janeway lesions, conjunctival hemorrhages, and pulmonary infarcts, as well as Osler's nodes and Roth spots, are less common in children than adults and have not been described in neonates (Table 18.1).

The Modified Duke criteria form the current standard of diagnosing endocarditis via clinical and laboratory results in adults, and have been shown to be useful in the pediatric population (Box 18.1).

Diagnostic studies

Blood cultures are imperative to the diagnosis of IE. While yield is directly related to amount of blood obtained, one set of pediatric blood cultures is considered sufficient. If the patient has no underlying structural heart disease or recent operation, and is not acutely ill, it is reasonable to wait for more thorough workup in-house prior to antibiotic administration. The laboratory should be notified that IE is on the differential and that the blood cultures should be incubated for 2 weeks.

Other laboratory tests may support the diagnosis of IE. They include a CBC, basic metabolic panel, urine analysis, rheumatoid factor, ESR, and C-reactive protein (CRP). If congestive heart failure or myocarditis is suspected, cardiac enzymes and possibly brain natriuretic peptide (BNP) may be checked. Complications involving extracardiac systems should guide further testing. Chest radiography can aid in the diagnosis of related cardiomyopathy, pulmonary infarction/abscesses/emboli, or heart failure.

While the echocardiogram is essential in the diagnosis of endocarditis in the adult, echocardiographic findings of IE are rare in children.

Box 18.1. Modified Duke criteria for diagnosis of infective endocarditis

Major criteria

- *Bacteremia*: two positive blood cultures drawn together or persistently positive blood cultures of organisms typical of infective endocarditis (IE) (*S. viridans, S. bovis, S. aureus*, HACEK group, enterococci).
- *Endocardial involvement*: echocardiogram showing vegetation, abscess, new partial dehiscence of prosthetic valve, new valvular regurgitation (worsening or changing of pre-existing murmur not sufficient).

Minor criteria

- *Predisposition*: predisposing heart condition or IV drug use.
- *Fever*: temperature 38.0°C.
- *Vascular phenomena*: major arterial emboli, septic pulmonary infarcts, mycotic aneurysm, intracranial hemorrhage, conjunctival hemorrhages, Janeway lesions.
- *Immunologic phenomena*: glomerulonephritis, Osler's nodes, Roth spots, rheumatoid factor.
- *Microbiological evidence*

Diagnosis

Definite IEs

- 2 major criteria
- 1 major and 3 minor criteria
- 5 minor criteria.

Possible IE

- 1 major and 1 minor criteria
- 3 minor criteria

Rejected as IE

- firm alternative diagnosis explaining evidence of IE
- resolution of IE syndrome with antibiotic therapy for 4 days
- no pathologic evidence of IE at surgery or autopsy with antibiotic therapy for 4 days
- does not meet criteria for possible IE, as described.

HACEK, *Haemophilus, Actinobacillus, Cardiobacterium, Eikenella, Kingella* spp., and Gram-negative coccillobacilli.

Transesophageal echocardiography is usually not warranted in children but may be performed in the presence of prosthetic valves obscuring adequate view with transthoracic echocardiography or if there is high suspicion for IE but poor echo windows on transthoracic echocardiography.

Management

The diagnosis of endocarditis will not usually be made in the ED. If endocarditis is suspected in the ED, then diagnostic tests, treatment, and disposition should be guided by clinical status, presence of native or prosthetic material, and medication allergies. If the clinical process is subacute, the patient has not had recent cardiac surgery, and the patient is clinically stable, it is reasonable to wait for in-hospital workup with a probable or definite IE diagnosis prior to starting antibiotics. If the patient's clinical status is rapidly deteriorating or the patient has had recent cardiac surgery with foreign material, immediate broad-spectrum antibiotics should be started.

Initial antibiotic treatment ideally should be guided by culture results. In the ED in the setting of acute disease with high suspicion of endocarditis, antibiotic treatment should be initiated only after cultures are obtained. Treatment should cover *Streptococcus viridans*, enterococci, and *S. aureus*, including methicillin-resistant *S. aureus* (MRSA). Broad-spectrum antibiotics should be initiated with coverage modified as the organism and susceptibilities are known. For IE of unknown etiology, vancomycin 40 mg/kg IV in 24 h divided q. 6–12 h *plus* gentamicin 3 mg/kg IM/IV in 24 h divided q. 8 h (max. 240 mg) is suggested. On appropriate therapy, bacteremia may last up to 10 days from start of therapy. In general, antibiotic treatment may range from 2 to 8 weeks and is guided by clinical status and blood culture results.

Disposition

All patients with possible or definite IE must be admitted to the hospital. Patients with a subacute presentation warrant admission to the hospital for further workup. Emergency echocardiogram, evaluation of cardiac function and complications, and admission to the ICU are necessary in the acutely ill. Patients with IE should be in a hospital facility that has access to pediatric cardiac surgery, cardiology, and infectious disease departments.

Myocarditis

Myocarditis involves the thick muscle layer of the heart and may occur in conjunction with endo- or pericarditis.

In the USA, myocarditis is most commonly caused by cardiotropic viruses including adenovirus and enterovirus.

Myocarditis may also be caused by other infections, including protozoans, or immune-mediated processes such as lupus, rheumatic fever, drug hypersensitivity, and transplant rejection. Complications include dilated cardiomyopathy, congestive heart failure, arrhythmias, and heart block. Up to 20–40% of all cases of sudden infant death syndrome have been linked to myocarditis at autopsy.

Risk factors

Risk factors for myocarditis include possible genetic predisposition, pericarditis, opportunistic infections in immunocompromised patients, HIV, and rheumatologic disease.

Clinical presentation and management history

The history usually includes a recent viral illness, flu and cold symptoms, and fatigue, plus chest pain in the older pediatric patient. Increased fatigue, lethargy, poor feeding, sweating with feeds, and poor skin color may be signs of dyspnea on exertion and shortness of breath in the preverbal child. Congestive heart failure or a history of multiple respiratory or GI illnesses should elevate myocarditis in the differential.

Physical examination

Myocarditis comprises a spectrum of presentations ranging from asymptomatic to sudden death. Of patients presenting with acute myocarditis, one-third recover, one-third develop dilated cardiomyopathy, and one-third will die or require cardiac transplantation. Initial diagnosis of myocarditis is commonly missed.

The patient with myocarditis will appear uncomfortable. Vital signs may include hyperthermia, tachycardia, tachypnea, hypoxia, and hypotension. Respiratory distress, including tachypnea, nasal flaring, and intercostal retractions, may be signs of impending cardiovascular collapse. The most common initial complaint in older patients is vague abdominal pain or vomiting. Mid-epigastric tenderness or hepatomegaly secondary to congestive heart failure may be seen on examination. Signs of poor perfusion, including cool or clammy extremities, delayed capillary refill, poor skin tone, and lethargy, may be present. Cardiac examination may reveal tachycardia, a gallop, or murmur, or it may be normal.

Diagnostic testing

The diagnosis of myocarditis in the ED is based on ECG changes, leukocytosis, elevated cardiac markers, abnormal chest radiograph, and echocardiographic evidence.

The ECG changes include sinus tachycardia with low-voltage QRS complexes (<5 mm in all limb leads), ST–T wave changes, PR prolongation, prolongation of the QTc interval, and arrhythmias. Sinus tachycardia is the most common arrhythmia. A tachycardia greater than expected for the degree of fever (10 bpm for each degree of temperature elevation) may indicate myocarditis. Other arrhythmias may be associated with myocarditis, including junctional tachycardias, second- and third-degree atrioventricular (AV) blocks, ventricular ectopy, and ventricular tachycardia. Chest radiography may reveal cardiomegaly, pulmonary edema from congestive heart failure, or support an alternative diagnosis. Urgent echocardiogram should be performed on unstable patients. Myocardial dysfunction, chamber dilation, wall motion abnormalities and AV valve regurgitation may be present on echocardiogram.

Increased inflammatory markers showing leukocytosis with lymphocyte predominance, elevated ESR, and elevated CRP may support a diagnosis of myocarditis. Additional laboratory testing may include a complete metabolic panel including LFTs, BNP, and blood cultures. Aspartate transaminase (AST) has been found to be elevated and may be indicative of end-organ damage, but it is not specific for myocarditis. In-hospital workup may include cardiac catheterization, magnetic resonance imaging (MRI), or endomyocardial biopsy.

Management

Management of myocarditis in the ED should be guided by clinical status and signs of cardiac complications at presentation. Treatment in the ED is mainly supportive. All patients with suspected myocarditis should be admitted for full workup and cardiac evaluation.

Prompt recognition and stabilization of patients with fulminant myocarditis before circulatory collapse is key. Goals of treatment include reducing high ventricular filling pressures, reducing afterload, improving oxygen delivery, and decreasing oxygen demand of myocardial tissue. Institute inotropic support, afterload reducers, and diuretics for heart failure and consider intubation (Box 18.2). The myocardium is irritable, and patients may present with different arrhythmias. If possible, treatment of arrhythmias should be delayed until the patient is in a tertiary care center.

Patients with myocarditis who are acutely ill require hospitalization in a pediatric tertiary care hospital with access to cardiology, cardiothoracic surgery, and ICU. Life-saving cardiopulmonary-sustaining therapies including extracorporeal membrane oxygenation, ventricular assist device, or intra-aortic balloon pump may be necessary.

Box 18.2. Medications commonly used in fulminant myocarditis and congestive heart failure

Inotropic support

Dopamine 5–10 μg/kg per min
Epinephrine 0.03–0.1 μg/kg per min
Milrinone 0.25–1 μg/kg per min
Dobutamine 5–20 μg/kg per min.

Afterload reduction

Milrinone 0.25–1 μg/kg per min
Nitroprusside 0.5–3 μg/kg per min.

Diuresis

Furosemide 1–2 mg/kg IV q. 6–12 h
Chlorthiazide 5–10 mg/kg IV q. 6–24 h.

Antiarrhythmia

Amiodarone 2.5–5 mg/kg IV over 20–60 min (do not exceed 15 mg/kg in 24 h and ensure normal ionized calcium level prior to initiation)
Lidocaine 20–50 μg/kg per min.

Pericardial disease

The pericardium comprises parietal and visceral layers. Pericardial fluid is contained between the two layers and serves to cushion the heart and aid in heart pump function. In pericarditis, or infection and inflammation of the pericardium, an acute increase in the pericardial fluid will limit contraction. Systemic hemodynamics are altered by a change in the consistency and elasticity of the pericardium and in the amount and viscosity of pericardial fluid. Based on the proximity and adherence of the visceral layer to the myocardium, overwhelming inflammation may involve both layers in perimyocarditis.

Pericarditis is caused by infectious, rheumatologic, inflammatory or neoplastic processes, or it may be idiopathic in nature. Viral pericarditis is commonly caused by adenovirus or coxsackievirus.

Cardiac tamponade is a serious complication of pericarditis. When the pericardial sac fills acutely with fluid or purulent (bacterial) material, tamponade physiology ensues. In emergency cardiac tamponade, pressures within the atria and ventricles approach similar values, causing hypotension, cardiovascular collapse, and sudden death if not recognized and treated.

The patient presents with chest pain. Complaints of shortness of breath, dyspnea, anxiety, altered mental status, exercise intolerance, and malaise may also be included in the history. Past medical history often includes recent viral illness. Signs and symptoms include poor feeding, irritability, lethargy, respiratory distress, grunting, and cyanosis; fever may be present in the infant.

Physical examination

Classic findings include a friction rub and chest pain that is relieved when leaning forward. The friction rub is usually heard best anywhere between the apex and the left sternal border with the patient in a forward-sitting position during end-expiration. In the absence of these findings, pericarditis cannot be excluded. Fever, hypotension, tachycardia, tachypnea, hypoxia, and signs of congestive heart failure may be seen in the acutely ill. A gallop rhythm, hepatomegaly, pulmonary crackles, and respiratory distress may be signs of congestive heart failure and may be seen with concurrent myocarditis. Poor skin turgor, poor perfusion, cyanosis, and lethargy are signs of impending cardiac demise. Muffled heart tones, jugular venous distension, hypotension, and pulsus paradoxus (10 mmHg drop in systolic blood pressure with inspiration) are indicative of cardiac tamponade. To measure pulsus paradoxus, if the patient is able to cooperate, he or she should breath normally. The sphygmomanometer cuff is inflated above the systolic blood pressure then deflated slowly until the Korotkoff sounds are heard only during expiration. Then the cuff is deflated again slowly until the Korotkoff sounds are heard during inspiration and expiration. If the difference between these two systolic blood pressures is >10 mmHg, pulsus paradoxus is present.

Diagnostic testing

Diagnosis of acute pericarditis depends on a history of chest pain, clinical signs including a friction rub, and adjunctive testing including echocardiography. An ECG and chest radiograph should be organized and blood drawn for CBC. Additional testing may include a chemistry panel, cardiac markers, BNP, blood cultures, urinalysis, and urine culture. Elevated cardiac markers may indicate myopericarditis.

Classically there are four phases of pericarditis on the ECG (Fig. 18.1): (1) ST elevation (J point pattern) and PR depression in all leads with the reverse in lead aVR and usually

V1 (Fig. 18.2), (2) normalization of the ST segment, (3) T wave inversion, and (4) baseline ECG pattern. Timeline includes days to 2 weeks for phase one, 1–3 weeks for phase two, 3 weeks to several weeks for phase three, and several weeks for phase four. The chest radiograph may reveal a bottle-shaped, globular or enlarged heart.

Emergency echocardiography is necessary in the acutely ill patient. In cases of slow accumulation of pericardial effusions or chronic pericardial effusions, echocardiography may be used to identify tamponade physiology. Tamponade physiology seen on echocardiography includes collapse of the free wall of the right atrium in diastole or pulsus paradoxus of tricuspid valve inflow.

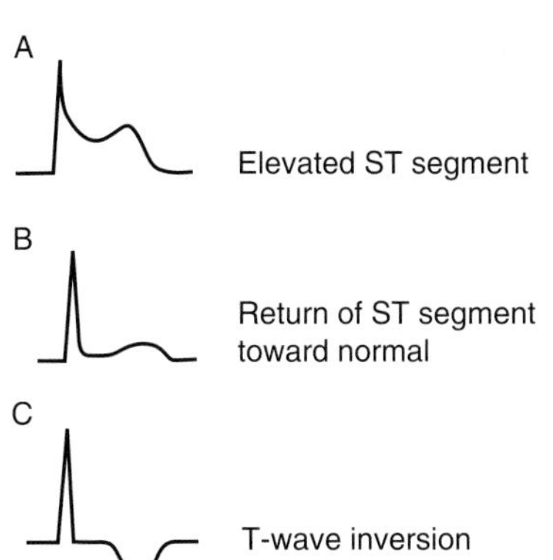

Figure 18.1 Classically, there are four phases of pericarditis on the ECG. (A) ST elevation (J point pattern) and PR depression in all leads with the reverse in lead aVR and usually V1. (B) Normalization of the ST segment. (C) T wave inversion and return to baseline.

Management

The mainstay of treatment of pericardial disease in the ED is aimed at decreasing chest pain and inflammation, managing cardiac tamponade if present, and appropriate consultation of specialists for further management of pericardial effusions. In the acutely ill patient, evaluate the ABCs, establish IV access, and monitor the cardiovascular and respiratory systems. Treatment of acute and recurrent pericarditis includes non-steroidal anti-inflammatory drugs (NSAIDs). Steroids are added to aid in quick decrease of pain and associated inflammation and when systemic lupus erythematosus, juvenile rheumatoid arthritis, or other rheumatologic disorders are suspected. In bacterial pericarditis with purulent pericardial effusion, IV antibiotics should be started and the fluid drained. Malignant effusions from neoplastic disease are treated with drainage and chemotherapy.

Cardiac tamponade is relieved with drainage of pericardial fluid via pericardiocentesis. Bedside pericardiocentesis and/or thoracotomy are needed when the patient presents in cardiac arrest or pulseless electrical activity from cardiac tamponade. In mild or chronic tamponade, non-emergency drains can be placed to drain fluid over time and monitor for reaccumulation. Treatment of constrictive pericarditis includes surgical pericardiotomy and drain placement. It is important not to sedate patients who have tamponade physiology, even for pericardiocentesis, as cardiovascular collapse may ensue.

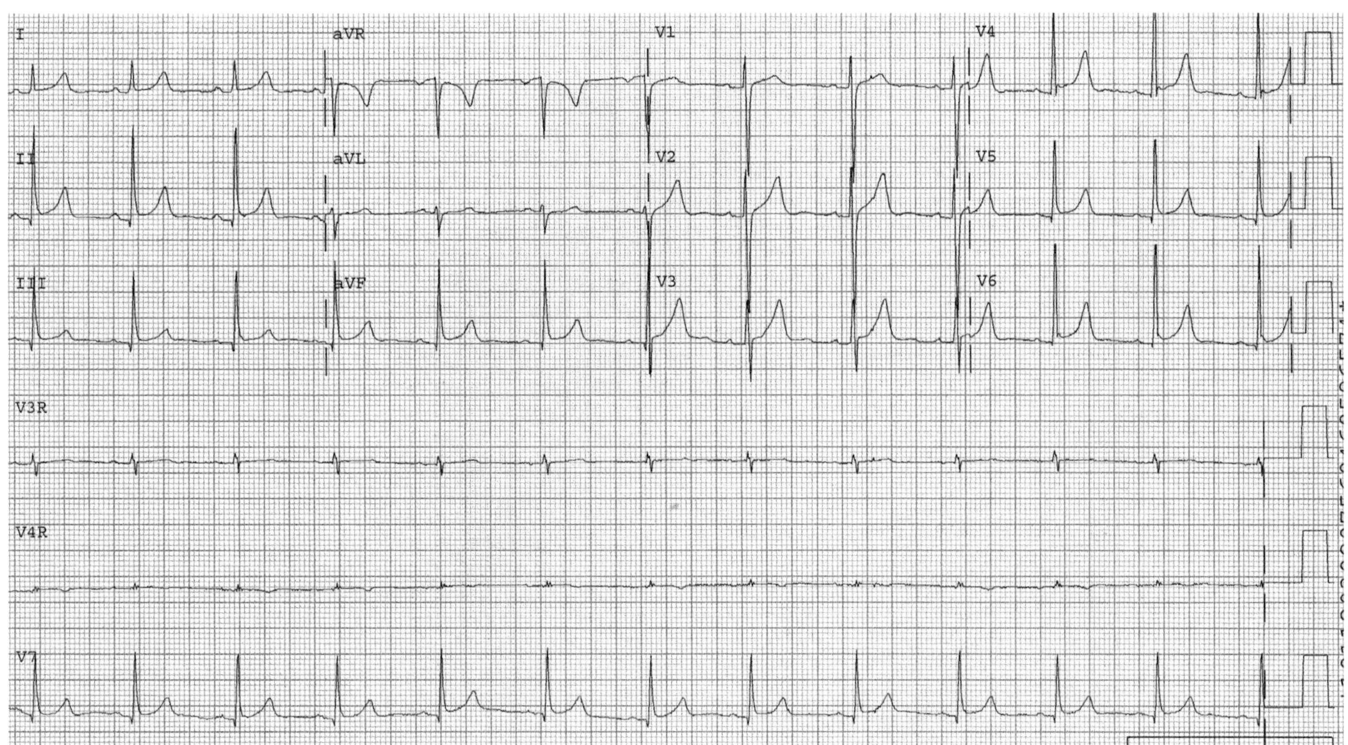

Figure 18.2 Pericarditis. Note the early signs of pericarditis in the ECG: ST elevation (J point pattern) and PR depression in all leads with the reverse in lead aVR and usually in V1. (Courtesy Inger Olson).

Pearls and pitfalls

Pearls

1. Children usually present with the subacute form of bacterial endocarditis.
2. Classic stigmata of endocarditis such as Roth spots, Osler's nodes, and Janeway lesions are rare in children.
3. Endocarditis is rare in children without structural heart disease.
4. Myocarditis, commonly caused by viruses, is usually self-limited but may present as fulminant myocarditis with severe heart failure.

Pitfalls

1. Failure to consider endocarditis in a patient with non-specific symptoms and a new murmur.
2. Failure to recognize myocarditis in a patient with respiratory and gastrointestinal symptoms.

Disposition

All patients with suspected or confirmed new-onset pericarditis should be admitted to the hospital for full workup. Mitigation of chest pain and management of cardiac tamponade should begin in the ED. When fever is present, blood cultures should be obtained prior to institution of antibiotics when possible. All other treatments and workup can be completed as an inpatient. Early consultation with cardiology, cardiac surgery, and the ICU is warranted. In patients with recurrent pericarditis, discharge to home may be considered in consultation with pediatric cardiology if appropriate primary and specialty care follow-up is arranged.

Selected references

Baddour LM, Wilson WR, Bayer AS, *et al.* Infective endocarditis. Diagnosis, antimicrobial therapy, and management of complications. *Circulation* 2005;**111**:e394–e434.

Feldman AM, McNamara D. Myocarditis. *N Engl J Med* 2000;**343**:1388–1398.

Ferrieri P, Gewitz MH, Gerber MA, *et al.* Unique features of infective endocarditis in childhood. *Circulation* 2002;**105**:2115–2126.

Freedman SB, Haladyn JK, Floh A, *et al.* Pediatric myocarditis: emergency department clinical findings and diagnostic evaluation. *Pediatrics* 2007;**120**:1278–1285.

Li J, Sexton DJ, Mick N, *et al.* Proposed modifications to the Duke criteria for the diagnosis of infective endocarditis. *Clin Infect Dis* 2000;**30**:633–638.

Liu PP, Mason JW. Advances in the understanding of myocarditis. *Circulation* 2001;**104**:1076–1082.

Maisch B, Seferović PM, Ristić AD, *et al.* Guidelines on the diagnosis and management of pericardial diseases executive summary. *Eur Heart J* 2004;**25**:587–610.

Spodick DH. Acute pericarditis. *JAMA* 2003;**289**:1150–1153.

Valente AM, Jain R, Scheurer M, *et al.* Frequency of infective endocarditis among infants and children with *Staphylococcus aureus* bacteremia. *Pediatrics* 2005;**115**(1): e15–e19.

Wheeler DS, Kooy NW. A formidable challenge: the diagnosis and treatment of viral myocarditis in children. *Crit Care Clin* 2003;**19**:365–391.

Wilson W, Taubert KA, Gewitz M, *et al.* Prevention of infective endocarditis: guidelines from the AHA. *Circulation* 2007;**116**:1736–1754.

Chapter 19

Syncope

Donald H. Schreiber and Chioma Agbo Boukai

Introduction

Syncope is a loss of consciousness caused by decreased cerebral perfusion to the areas of the brain necessary for consciousness. Up to 15% of children experience a syncopal episode. The prevalence of syncope is higher in females than in males, and peaks during adolescence. The decreased cerebral perfusion resulting in syncope can occur for a myriad of reasons. In vasovagal syncope, autonomic dysfunction occurs, with excessive vagal tone causing bradycardia and decreased cardiac output. Syncope caused by hypovolemia or a dysrhthmia results from a decrease in stroke volume. Syncope may be difficult to distinguish from other entities such as seizures or breath-holding spells (Table 19.1). This chapter will review the different etiologies of syncope and the ED approach to the pediatric patient with syncope. A review of common arrhythmias and structural heart lesions that may present with syncope is also included.

Causes of syncope

Vasovagal syncope is non life-threatening and the most common cause of syncope in children. It is caused by an increased vagal tone that slows the heart rate in conjunction with decreased intravascular volume from pooling of blood in in the venous system. It can be precipitated by a stressful event or pain (particularly GI) and is not uncommon in adolescents and young adults. Vasovagal syncope usually has a presyncopal component as cerebral perfusion decreases. Patients become diaphoretic and dizzy, and often experience visual changes such as tunnel vision. They can also experience headache, palpitations, and shortness of breath. These symptoms resolve if the patient lies down, or in the case of syncope, when the patient regains consciousness. During the event, the patient is usually bradycardic and hypotensive. Recovery is usually rapid once the patient is prone. Patients may also demonstrate brief myoclonic jerking that can be misinterpreted as a seizure.

Cardiogenic syncope is caused by cardiac conditions such as arrhythmias or structural heart disease; it can also result from a precipitous fall in cardiac output. Arrhythmias causing syncope are rare in children without structural heart disease. However, arrhythmias may occur as a result of metabolic derangements, toxic ingestions, or acquired or congenital conduction disorders such as the long QT syndrome, the Brugada syndrome, the Wolff–Parkinson–White (WPW) syndrome, or the congenital short QT syndrome. Heart block can be acquired with Lyme disease, as well as in certain autoimmune disorders such as systemic lupus erythematosus or sarcoidosis. Important clues to the diagnosis are a history of medication ingestion or sudden cardiac death in the family. Of note, children with repaired congenital heart defects such as tetrology of Fallot, or transposition of the great arteries are at risk for arrhythmias that are associated with sudden death. Structural heart lesions such as hypertrophic cardiomyopathy, coronary artery anomalies, valvular aortic stenosis, dilated cardiomyopathy, and pulmonary hypertension can also cause syncope. With these disorders, syncope is usually acute without any prodromal or presyncopal symptoms. Syncope with exercise is also an important clue to a cardiac etiology. The history and physical examination usually point to a cardiac etiology and the ECG is often abnormal.

Other causes of syncope include breath-holding spells, hyperventilation, or hypoglycemia. Seizures may also be mistaken for syncope.

Clinical presentation

A careful history and physical examination are key to the evaluation of a patient with syncope. The history of present illness should include time of last meal, activities prior to the event, patient position at onset of symptoms, and the duration of episode. Particular attention should be paid to the cardiovascular and neurologic symptoms after a syncopal episode. Key aspects of the history that identify those patients with a cardiac abnormality include a previous cardiac history, lack of prodrome, exertional syncope, or a familial history of cardiac arrest or ventricular arrhythmia.

The physical examination of a child after a syncopal episode can often be normal. However, the examination

A Practical Guide to Pediatric Emergency Medicine: Caring for Children in the Emergency Department, ed. N. Ewen Amieva-Wang (associate eds. Jamie Shandro, Aparajita Sohoni, and Bernhard Fassl). Published by Cambridge University Press.

Table 19.1. Causes of syncope in children

Etiology	Causes
Conduction abnormalities	Long QT syndrome, short QT syndrome
	Brugada syndrome
	Familial catecholaminergic polymorphic ventricular tachycardia
	Pre-excitation syndromes (such as Wolff–Parkinson–White)
	Bradyarrhythmias (complete atrioventricular block, sinus node dysfunction)
Structural abnormalities	Hypertrophic cardiomyopathy
	Coronary artery anomalies
	Arrhythmogenic right ventriclular dysplasia/cardiomyopathy
	Aortic stenosis
	Dilated cardiomyopathy
	Pulmonary hypertension
	Acute myocarditis
	Congenital heart disease
Other non-cardiac etiologies	Vasovagal (neurocardiogenic) syndrome, including situational syncope (cough, micturition, hair combing)
	Breath-holding spell
	Orthostatic hypotension (hemorrhage, dehydration, pregnancy)
	Toxic exposure
	Hypoglycemia
	Conditions that mimic syncope: seizure, migraine syndromes, hysterical faint
	Hyperventilation

may reveal a heart murmur suggestive of structural heart disease. Orthostatic changes in blood pressure and pulse associated with dizziness may suggest significant hypovolemia. An abnormal neurological examination suggests a non-cardiac etiology.

Diagnostic studies

The diagnostic workup is guided by the history and physical examination.

Box 19.1. Electrocardiograph features of life-threatening causes of syncope

Prolonged corrected QT interval (QTc)
Brugada pattern
Wolff–Parkinson–White syndrome
Epsilon waves (arrhythmogenic right ventricular dysplasia)
Short corrected QT interval (QTc $\leq$0.30 s)
Conduction delay or atrioventricular block
Signs of myocardial ischemia or infarction
Ventricular hypertrophy or strain patterns
Other arrhythmia (see Ch. 17).

An ECG is considered the standard of care for the evaluation of syncope unless there is a clear vasovagal etiology or clinical evidence of hypovolemia.

A hematocrit, fingerstick glucose, and urine pregnancy test may be useful. Use of non-contrast computed tomography (CT) is not indicated for the evaluation of syncope in the absence of any head injury or neurological abnormalities on physical examination.

Accurate pediatric ECG interpretation can identify serious causes of syncope in children, as well as eliminate the need for admission in a significant number of cases. The key components of the ECG that need to be carefully reviewed in children with syncope are listed in Box 19.1.

Syndromes

Long QT syndrome

Increased QT interval is an important cause of syncope in children. The corrected QT interval (QTc) is calculated by Bazett's formula:

$$\text{QTc} = \frac{\text{QT measured}}{\sqrt{\text{RR interval}}}$$

A prolonged QT interval is defined roughly as greater than 50% of the RR interval and places the patient at higher risk for life-threatening ventricular arrhythmias, particularly torsades de pointes. Long QT intervals may be attributable to one of the long QT syndromes, which may be congenital or acquired. The long QT syndromes are disorders of myocardial repolarization. Congenital long QT syndromes are caused by mutations affecting ion channels of the myocardium. The congenital syndromes include the Jervell and Lange–Nielsen syndrome and the Romano–Ward syndrome. Acquired long QT syndrome is often caused by electrolyte disturbances such as hypocalcemia, hypokalemia, or hypomagnesemia. The acquired syndromes may also occur with myocarditis, hypertrophic and dilated cardiomyopathies, severe malnutrition or anorexia. A number of drugs are also known to precipitate the acquired long QT syndrome by prolonging the QTc interval, such as class IA, IC, and III antiarrhythmic agents, phenothiazines (e.g., thioridazine, chlorpromazine), tricyclic antidepressants, organophosphates toxicity, antibiotics (e.g., ampicillin, erythromycin, levofloxacin, trimethoprim-sulfamethoxazole, amantadine), and antihistamines (e.g., terfenadine).

Patients with the congenital long QT syndrome have significantly higher rates of sudden cardiac death. Prompt referral to a pediatric cardiologist is recommended. The management of congenital long QT syndrome focuses on the reduction of sympathetic input to the myocardium. Initial treatment is with beta-blockers to limit the maximal heart rate during exercise. Beta-blocker therapy has been shown to reduce the incidence of syncope and sudden cardiac death. Dual chamber cardiac pacing is an option for patients with long QT syndrome who remain symptomatic while on beta-blocker therapy. The 2008 American College of Cardiology/American Heart Association/Heart Rhythm Society (ACC/AHA/HRS) guidelines recommend placement of an implantable cardioverter-defibrillator (ICD) for patients with long QT syndrome who have a syncopal event while on beta-blocker therapy.

Wolff–Parkinson–White syndrome

Wolff–Parkinson–White syndrome is an important cause of syncope in children. Its prevalence is approximately 0.25% of the general pediatric population. It arises from abnormal electrical conduction between the atria and the ventricles. In the WPW syndrome, an accessory pathway exists that directly connects the atria and ventricles bypassing the atrioventricular node. This results in an earlier activation of the ventricles with a shortened PR interval. The classic ECG pattern of WPW syndrome shows several characteristic features (Fig. 19.1). The PR interval is shortened (<0.12 s). The shape of the QRS complex with a delta wave represents the abnormal and slower conduction through the ventricle that does not completely follow the His–Purkinje conduction pathways. The delta wave is the abnormal initial upstroke of the QRS complex. The abnormal QRS complex is usually slightly prolonged to more than 0.12 s.

Patients with WPW syndrome require risk stratification, often with electrophysiological studies. Electrophysiology studies should be considered in children <10 years old or who are competitive athletes. Radiofrequency catheter ablation is recommended as first-line therapy for symptomatic patients with WPW syndrome.

Vagal maneuvers can be attempted to manage supraventricular tachycardia associated with WPW syndrome. Patients with a regular orthodromic (narrow complex) supraventricular tachycardia associated with WPW syndrome may be treated with any of the following: adenosine, calcium channel blockers, beta-blockers, or procainamide. The last has the potential advantage because of its safety profile that is independent of the conduction pathway. Amiodarone is reserved as a second-line drug in refractory cases. However patients with symptomatic supraventricular tachycardia associated with WPW syndrome with

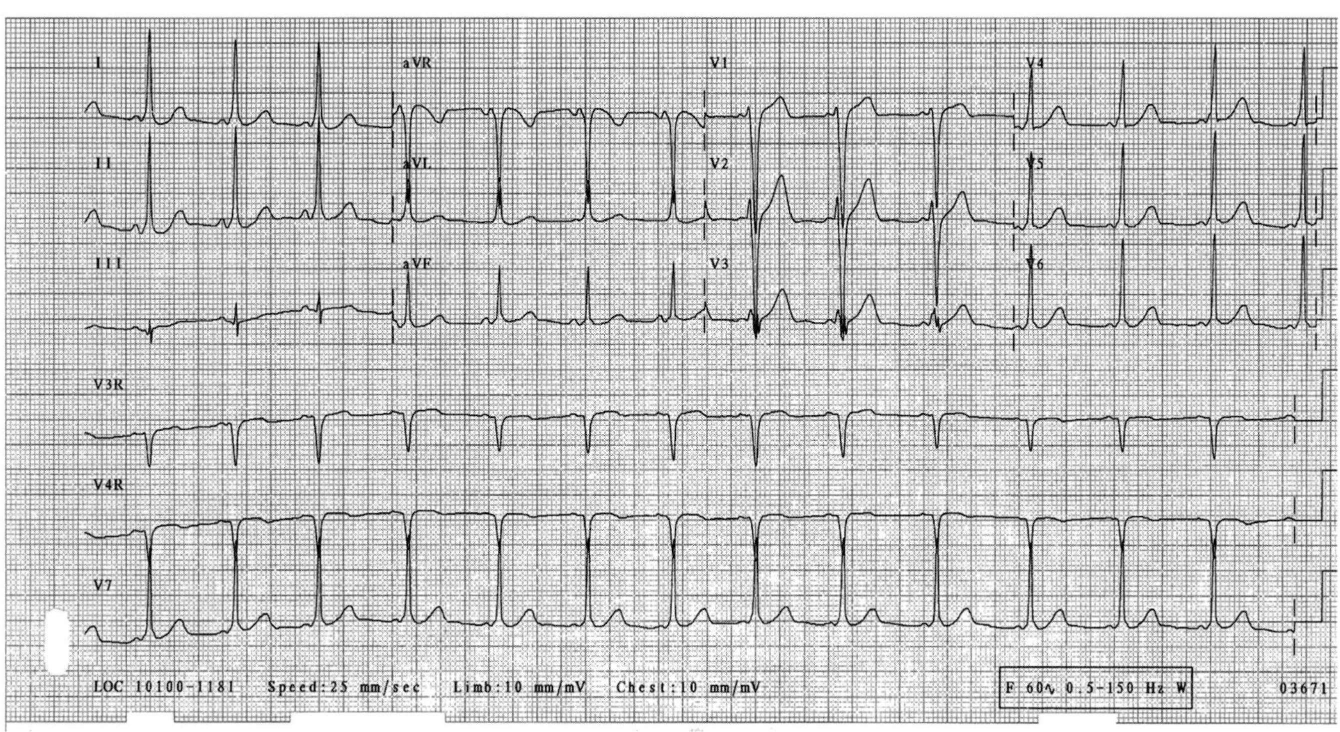

Figure 19.1 This is the ECG of a 15-year-old boy with Wolff–Parkinson–White syndrome. The two main features, shortened PR interval (<0.12 s) and delta wave widening syndrome at the base of the QRS interval, are evident. (Courtesy Inger Olson.)

antidromic conduction (wide complex tachycardia) must never be treated with atrioventricular nodal-blocking agents such as adenosine, calcium channel blockers, or beta-blockers because of the risk of inducing ventricular fibrillation via unopposed rapid conduction down the accessory pathway. Procainamide is, therefore, the drug of choice in a wide complex supraventricular tachycardia.

Patients with WPW syndrome presenting with atrial fibrillation must also not be treated with drugs that slow or block conduction through the atrioventricular node. This may cause an acceleration of the ventricular rate via rapid conduction through the accessory pathway. Procainamide is recommended. For hemodynamically unstable patients with WPW syndrome and atrial fibrillation (Fig. 19.2), prompt cardioversion is recommended in the PALS algorithm.

Brugada syndrome

The Brugada syndrome, first reported by the Brugada brothers in 1992, is a common cause of sudden cardiac death in the minority of patients who suffer a cardiac arrest without structural or atherosclerotic heart disease. It is a genetic disorder thought to be responsible for 4–5% of all sudden cardiac deaths in adults and children. The incidence varies considerably in different populations. The clinical characteristics are similar to the nocturnal sudden death syndrome initially reported from Asia. Patients typically present with syncope or sudden cardiac arrest from ventricular tachycardia.

The syndrome is associated with a specific set of abnormalities seen on the baseline ECG. Not all patients with the Brugada pattern have the Brugada syndrome, but further testing is required. For example, in children, a febrile episode may cause the Brugada pattern seen on the ECG. There are different types of Brugada patterns characterized by varying ECG abnormalities in the precordial leads (V1–V3), such as right bundle branch block (complete or incomplete) and ST segment elevations (Fig. 19.3). A number of drugs can also induce the Brugada-like ECG patterns and occasionally ventricular tachycardia in affected patients (Table 19.2). Patients with the Brugada pattern on the ECG should be promptly referred to a pediatric cardiologist. In the presence of syncope with a family history of sudden cardiac death or documented arrhythmias such as ventricular tachycardia, the Brugada syndrome is more likely. Antiarrhythmic therapy is usually ineffective. While placement of an ICD is the classic treatment, quinidine has been used in children. Urgent referral for electrophysiologic testing is recommended.

Short QT syndrome

A short QT interval is a sign of a digitalis effect, hyperkalemia, hypercalcemia, or hypermagnesemia. It is also seen with hyperthermia and in the short QT syndrome. The

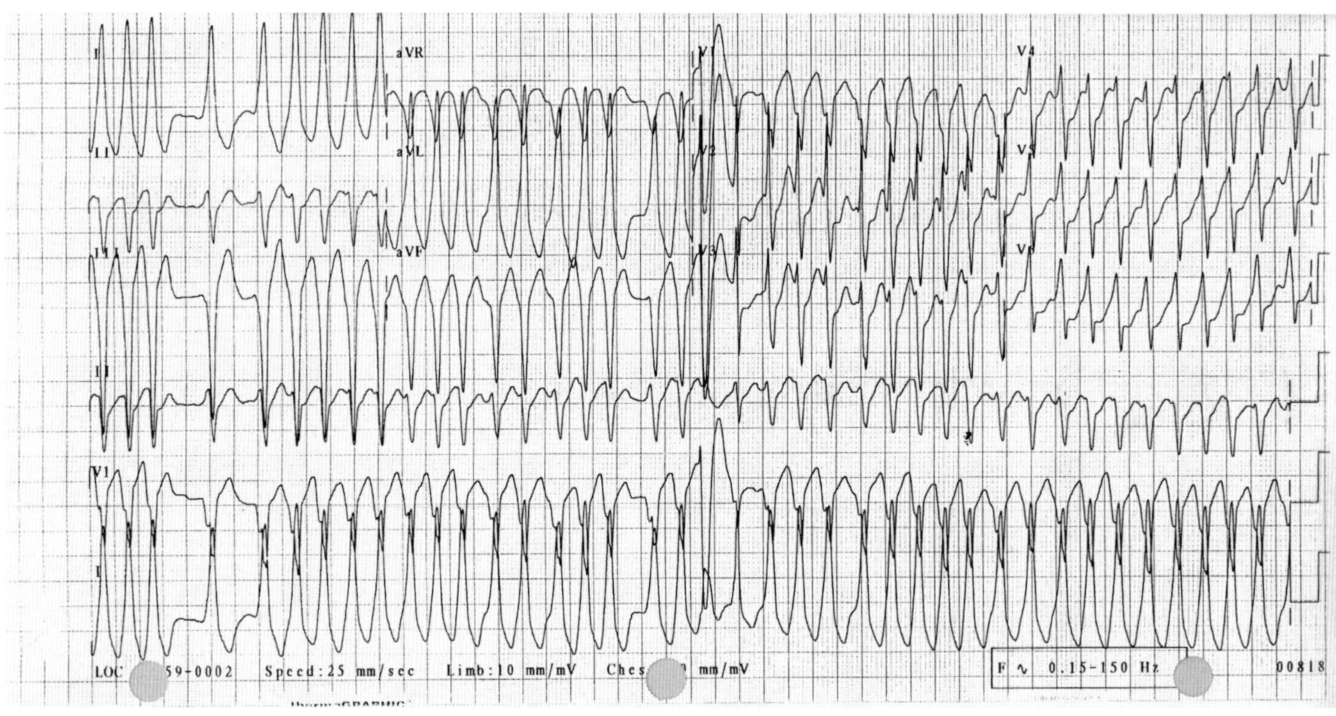

Figure 19.2 Wolff–Parkinson–White (WPW) syndrome with atrial fibrillation (AF). The clinician should consider WPW with AF in patients with an irregular, wide QRS complex tachycardia. Clues that suggest the diagnosis of WPW AF are the irregularity of the rhythm, the rapid ventricular response (much too rapid for conduction down the atrioventricular node), and the wide, bizarre QRS complex, signifying conduction down the aberrant pathway. A careful review of the ECG in Fig. 19.1 reveals that a delta wave is seen in numerous complexes, particularly in the precordial leads. (Reproduced with permission from emed home, http://www.emedhome.com/docs/case012508a.jpg; accessed 11 August 2009.)

last is a familial cause of sudden death associated with a short QTc $\leq$0.30 s.

Arrhythmogenic right ventricular dysplasia

Arrhythmogenic right ventricular dysplasia (ARVD) is a cardiomyopathy that primarily involves the right ventricle but eventually progresses to affect the left ventricle. The cardiomyocytes are replaced by adipose and fibrous tissues, resulting in slowed conduction that forms an arrhythmogenic substrate for re-entry and ventricular tachycardia with a left bundle branch block morphology. Several ECG features have been used as the diagnostic criteria for ARVD including (1) T wave inversion in leads V1 through V3, (2) QRS duration of > 110 ms in leads V1 through V3, and (3) the presence of an epsilon wave. The epsilon wave is the most specific hallmark for the diagnosis of ARVD (Fig. 19.4). Placement of an ICD is the only reliable treatment to prevent sudden cardiac death. For suspected cases, a pediatric cardiology referral is recommended.

Table 19.2. Drugs that can induce Brugada-like electrocardiograph patterns

Drug class	Examples
Antiarrhythmic or antianginal drugs	Sodium channel blockers (some have been used for drug challenge in patients with Brugada type 2 or 3 ECG pattern): class IC drugs (flecainide, pilsicainide, propafenone), class IA drugs (quinidine, ajmaline, procainamide, disopyramide, cibenzoline), lithium
	Calcium channel blockers
	Beta-blockers
	Nitrates
Psychotropic drugs	Tricyclic antidepressants, phenothiazines, selective serotonin reuptake inhibitors (SSRI)
Other	Alcohol intoxication, cocaine, dimenhydrinate

Hypertrophic cardiomyopathy

In the USA, a high school, college, or professional athlete dies on average every 2 weeks from cardiac arrest associated with hypertrophic cardiomyopathy (HCM). Although most cases are diagnosed at 30–40 years of age, 2% of cases are found in children younger than 5 years of age and 7% occur in children younger than 10 years of age. The overall incidence of HCM is approximately 1 in 500. The clinical presentation varies, with patients experiencing chest pain, palpitations, shortness of breath, syncope/near syncopal episodes particularly with exertion, or sudden death. The hallmark anatomic finding in patients with HCM is an asymmetric, hypertrophied septum associated with left ventricle outflow tract obstruction.

Findings on ECG include left atrial enlargement and left ventricular hypertrophy, ST segment abnormalities, T wave inversions, Q waves, and diminished or absent R waves in the lateral leads (Fig. 19.5). Premature atrial and ventricular contractions, supraventricular tachycardia, multifocal ventricular arrhythmias, or atrial fibrillation are common arrhythmias.

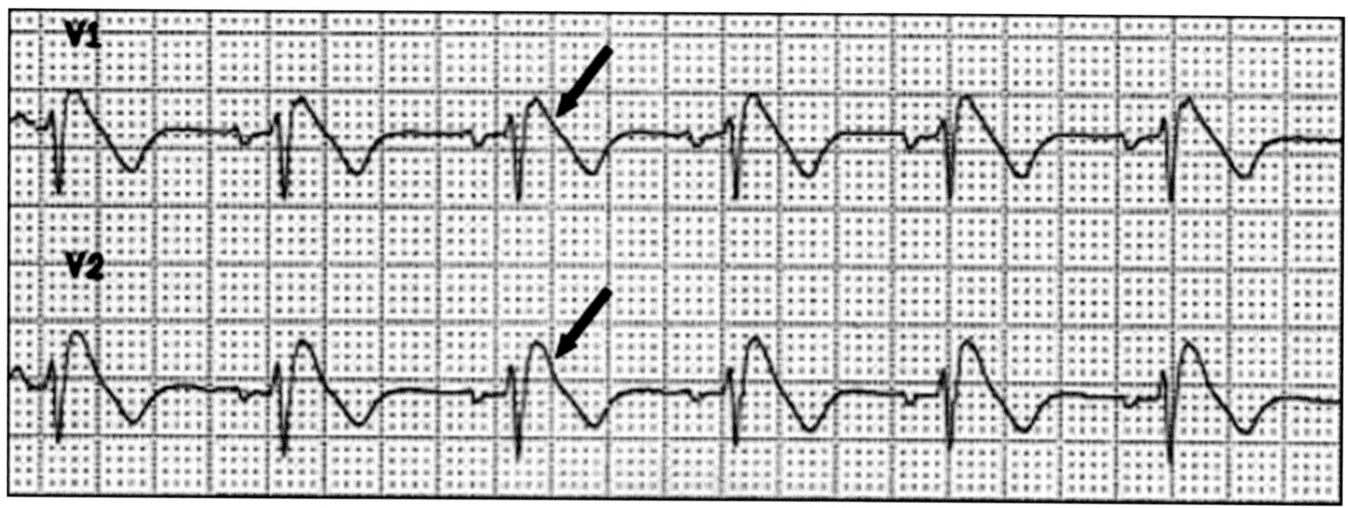

Figure 19.3 Brugada syndrome in a 13-year-old child. The V1 and V2 precordial leads show the typical "coved-type" ST segment elevation (arrowed) with a negative T wave in the type 1 ECG pattern. Also note the incomplete right bundle branch block pattern and that the R′ prime component of the QRS complex is greater than the R component of the R wave (R′ > R) in V1. (With permission from Mivelaz Y, Bernardo SD, Pruvot E, *et al.* Brugada syndrome in childhood: a potential fatal arrhythmia not always recognised by paediatricians. A case report and review of the literature. *Eur J Pediatr* 2006;165:507–511.)

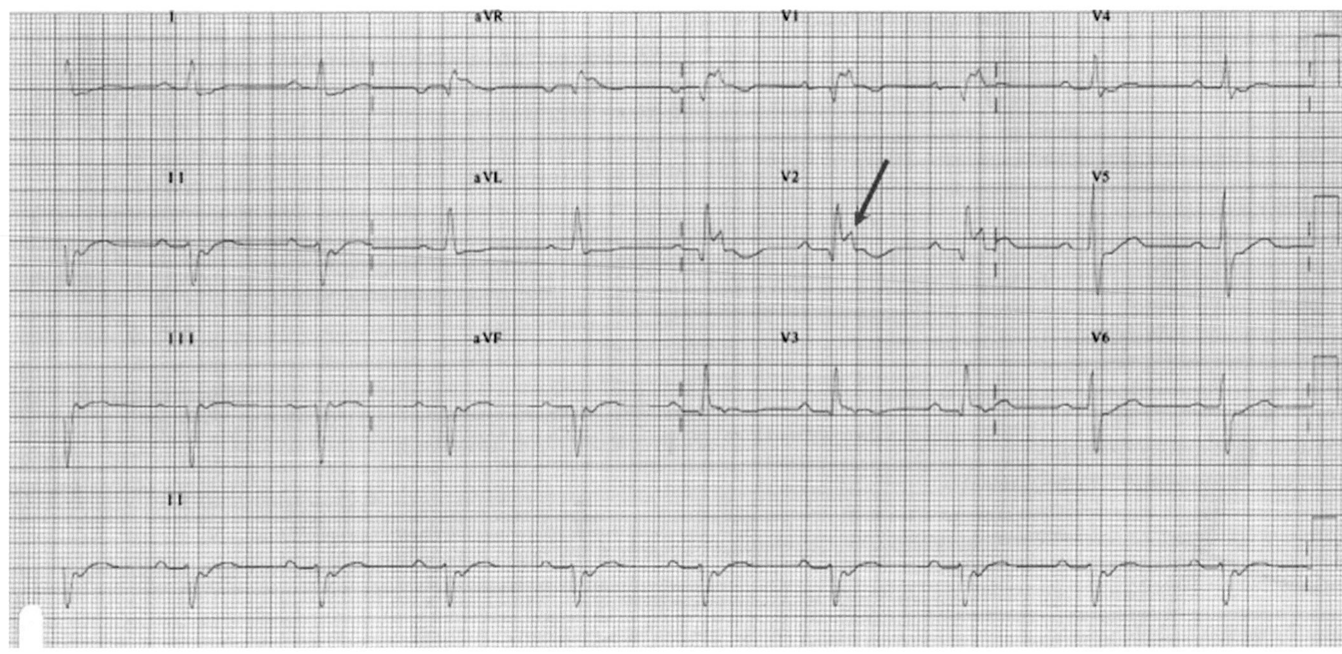

Figure 19.4 Arrhythmogenic right ventricular dysplasia (ARVD). An ECG shows the typical features of prolonged QRS interval in V1–V3, T wave inversion in V1–V3, and an epsilon wave (arrow) in the anterior precordial leads V1 or V2. Left axis deviation is also present, indicating an incomplete left bundle branch block pattern. (Reproduced with permission from You CC, Tseng YT, Hsieh MH. An epsilon wave in arrhythmogenic right ventricular cardiomyopathy/dysplasia. *Int J Cardiol* 2007;119: e63–e64.)

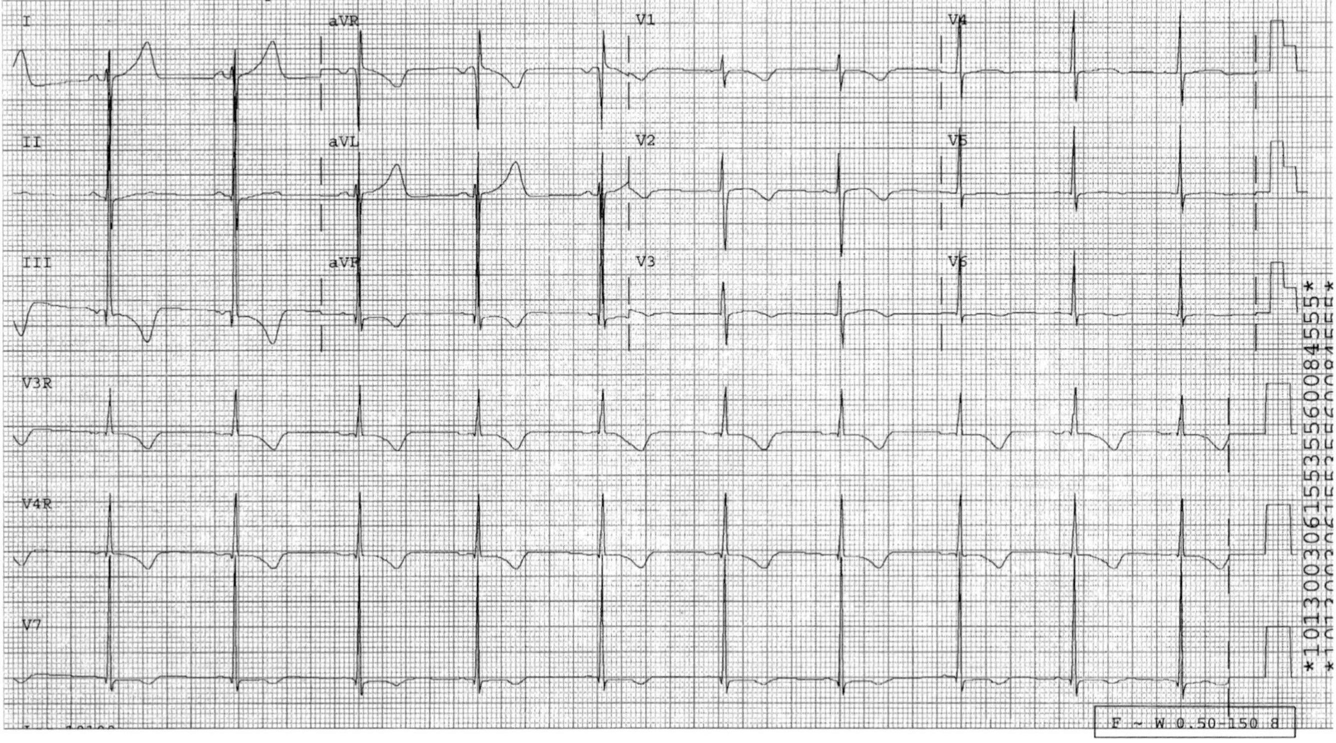

Figure 19.5 Hypertrophic cardiomyopathy. The ECG shows left ventricular hypertrophy with strain pattern. (Courtesy Inger Olson.)

Disposition of patients with syncope

The majority of children who present following a syncopal episode can be safely discharged from the ED after appropriate evaluation. Children with concerning cardiac findings or ECG abnormalities associated with syncope warrant referral to pediatric cardiology and occasionally admission is warranted. Children with a family history of syncope or sudden death, evidence of cardiovascular disease, or syncope with exercise should be referred to cardiology for further evaluation. Children with orthostatic hypotension resistant to rehydration therapy should be considered for prolonged observation or admission.

In WPW syndrome, patients with rapid atrial fibrillation should be admitted. In syncope caused by supraventricular tachycardia and WPW syndrome, a pediatric cardiologist should be consulted to determine further therapy, disposition, and follow-up. Patients with the long QT syndrome should be admitted if they develop syncope while on therapy (with beta-blockers) or if the QTc is >550 ms.

Pearls and pitfalls

Pearls

1. Vasovagal syncope is the most common cause of syncope in children.
2. Syncope during exercise associated with a systolic ejection murmur may be caused by aortic stenosis or hypertrophic cardiomyopathy and requires emergency cardiology consultation.

Pitfalls

1. Failure to ask about family history of sudden death or cardiac disease.
2. Failure to obtain an ECG after a syncopal event.
3. Failure to consult a pediatric cardiologist for review of a questionable or borderline ECG or for a concerning clinical presentation, such as syncope during exercise.

Selected references

Corrado D, Basso C, Thiene G. Arrhythmogenic right ventricular cardiomyopathy: diagnosis, prognosis and treatment. *Heart* 2000;**83**:588–595.

Epstein D. Following the trail of broken hearts. *Sports Illustrated* 2007, Dec 4.

Epstein, AE, DiMarco, JP, Ellenbogen, KA, *et al.* ACC/AHA/HRS 2008 guidelines for device-based therapy of cardiac rhythm abnormalities. A report of the American College of Cardiology/American Heart Association Task Force on Practice Guidelines (Writing Committee to Revise the ACC/AHA/NASPE 2002 Guideline Update for Implantation of Cardiac Pacemakers and Antiarrhythmia Devices): developed in collaboration with the American Association for Thoracic Surgery and Society of Thoracic Surgeons. *Circulation* 2008;**117**: e350–408 [erratum in Circulation 2009;**120**: e34–e35].

Hulot JS, Jouven X, Empana JP *et al.* Natural history and risk stratification of arrhythmogenic right ventricular dysplasia/cardiomyopathy. *Circulation* 2004;**110**: 1879–1874.

Lewis DA, Dhala A. Syncope in the pediatric patient. The cardiologist's perspective. *Pediatr Clin North Am* 1999;**46**:205–219.

McKenna WJ, Thiene G, Nava A *et al.* Diagnosis of arrhythmogenic right ventricular dysplasia/cardiomyopathy. Task Force of the Working Group Myocardial and Pericardial Disease of the European Society of Cardiology and of the Scientific Council of Cardiomyopathies of the International Society and Federation of Cardiology. *Br Heart J* 1994;**71**:215–218.

Peters S. Advances in the diagnostic management of arrhythmogenic right ventricular dysplasia–cardiomyopathy. *Int J Cardiol* 2006;**113**:4–11.

Section

4

Dental emergencies

Expert reviewer: Brian Su-Chieh Liu

Chapter 20

Dental emergencies

Ketan H. Patel

Introduction

While children have similar mechanisms of dental disease and trauma to adults, children present the added complexity and advantage of having both primary (deciduous) and permanent teeth. Children may also be less cooperative than adults with the dental examination, procedures, and treatments. This chapter discusses pediatric dental development, dental trauma, and then oral and dental infections.

Pediatric dental anatomy and development

The individual anatomy of each tooth varies little from primary to permanent dentition (Fig. 20.1). The central pulp containing the neurovascular supply of the tooth is covered by a layer of dentin (microtubules that hydrate and cushion the tooth) and overlaid by enamel. The primary teeth are generally smaller than

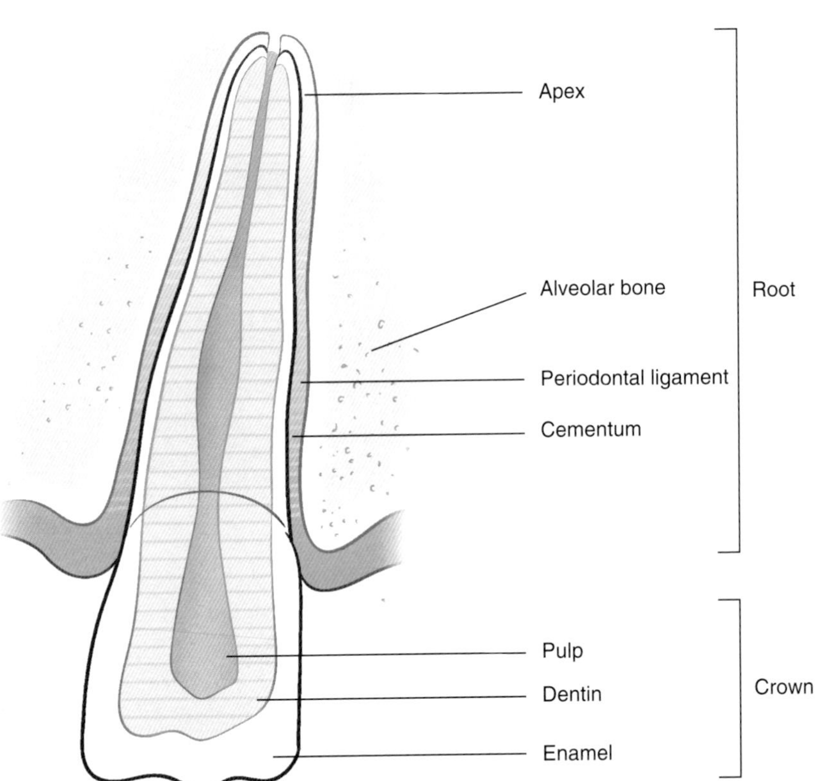

Figure 20.1 Dental anatomy. (Copyright Chris Gralapp.)

A Practical Guide to Pediatric Emergency Medicine: Caring for Children in the Emergency Department, ed. N. Ewen Amieva-Wang (associate eds. Jamie Shandro, Aparajita Sohoni, and Bernhard Fassl). Published by Cambridge University Press.

permanent teeth. Children's teeth have, proportionally, more pulp and less dentin and enamel than adult teeth. This ratio evolves as children get older and is a significant complicating factor in treating children for common dental complaints.

Children have 20 primary teeth, which are eventually replaced by 32 permanent teeth. Eruption of permanent dentition is generally complete except for the third molars, by the time the child is 13 years of age (Fig. 20.2). Identification of a tooth as primary or permanent is very important in most pediatric dental emergencies as management varies greatly based on this determination. Primary teeth are whiter and smaller than permanent teeth; the patient's age and parent's information can also help to identify a tooth.

Communication with dental specialists and other healthcare providers often requires specifically identifying the involved tooth/teeth. An accurate description of the location of the involved tooth is often more useful as lettering and numbering systems are not universally accepted. Description of individual tooth abnormalities may proceed using several descriptive terms including *buccal* (adjacent to the buccal/cheek or lip mucosa) versus *lingual* (adjacent to the tongue) or *palatal* (adjacent to the palate), as well as *apical* (toward the tooth root) versus *coronal* (toward the crown, or visible portion of a tooth). The *incisors* are cutting teeth, which are anterior; *canines* are tearing and cutting teeth lateral to the incisors. *Molars* are wide and flat chewing teeth posteriorly. Normally a tooth is described by using upper or lower first, then left or right, then central or lateral or first or second or third. Figure 20.2 is a guide to common dental terms (i.e., molar, incisor, canine).

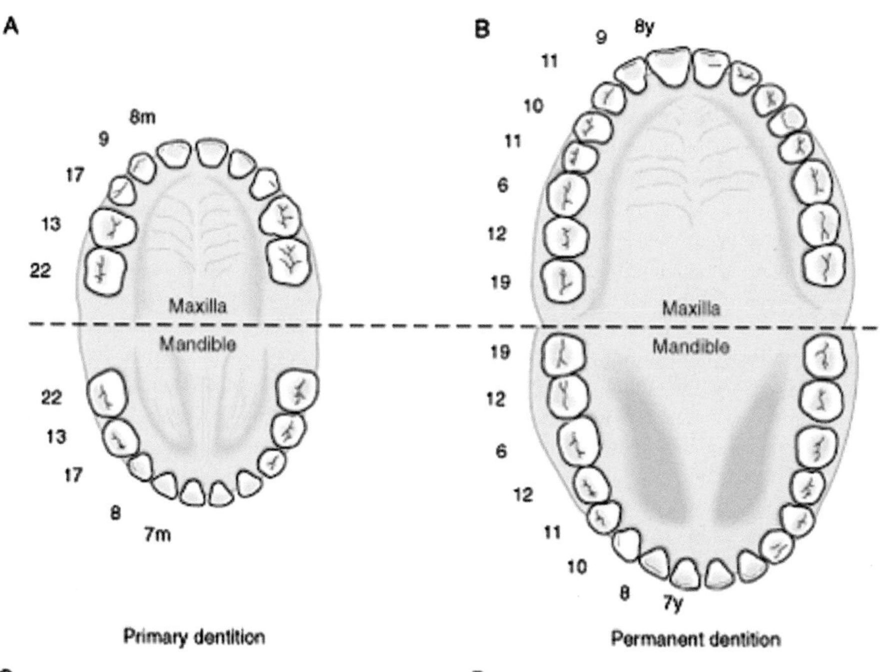

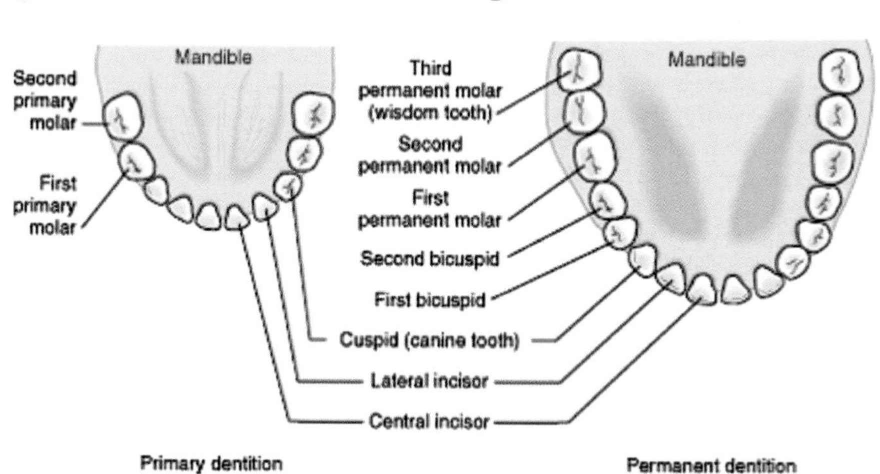

Figure 20.2 Primary and permanent dentition. The numbers represent the average age of eruption for the teeth, indicated in months for the primary teeth and years for the permanent dentition. The names of specific teeth in the primary and permanent dentition are shown. (Reproduced with permission from Zitelli BJ, Davis HW. *Atlas of Pediatric Physical Diagnosis*, 5th edn. Philadelphia, PA: Mosby Elsevier, 2007. © 2007 Mosby Inc., an affiliate of Elsevier Inc.)

Pediatric dental trauma

Dental trauma is the most common pediatric dental emergency. These injuries have functional and cosmetic ramifications. The management differences between child and adult dental trauma revolve around whether the injured tooth is a primary or permanent tooth.

Cracked or split teeth

A cracked or split tooth commonly occurs after direct trauma to the tooth. A subtly cracked tooth may be difficult to see; however, the history of trauma can help in the diagnosis. Pain typically occurs with chewing, and biting down on a tongue blade can reproduce the symptoms. Treatment is the same as for caries: systemic analgesia and referral to a dentist for definitive management as soon as possible. Treatment with antibiotics is not helpful.

Dental fractures

The Ellis classification system is commonly used by non-dentists to describe tooth fractures, but simply describing the anatomy involved in the dental injury is also acceptable (Fig. 20.3). The physical findings and necessary treatment considerations involved with each type of fracture are described below.

Enamel or Ellis I fractures

The enamel or Ellis I fractures are superficial and involve only the enamel. They present mostly a cosmetic issue, with little long-term risk to the tooth. The fracture is white with a chalky texture. These fractures may cause soft tissue lacerations because of their sharp edges. Rough edges can be smoothed with an emery board. Patients should be referred for routine dental evaluation and repair.

Dentin or Ellis II fractures

Fractures involving the dentin are more concerning in children than in adults, as children's teeth contain a greater proportional amount of pulp than dentin. Bacterial contamination of the pulp via the fractured dentin is more likely to occur, with resultant pulpitis and possible need for a partial or full root canal in pediatric patients.

The Ellis II fractures involve the enamel and the dentin and are ivory-yellow in appearance. Because of exposure of the dentin, teeth are most sensitive to cold air or water or direct contact.

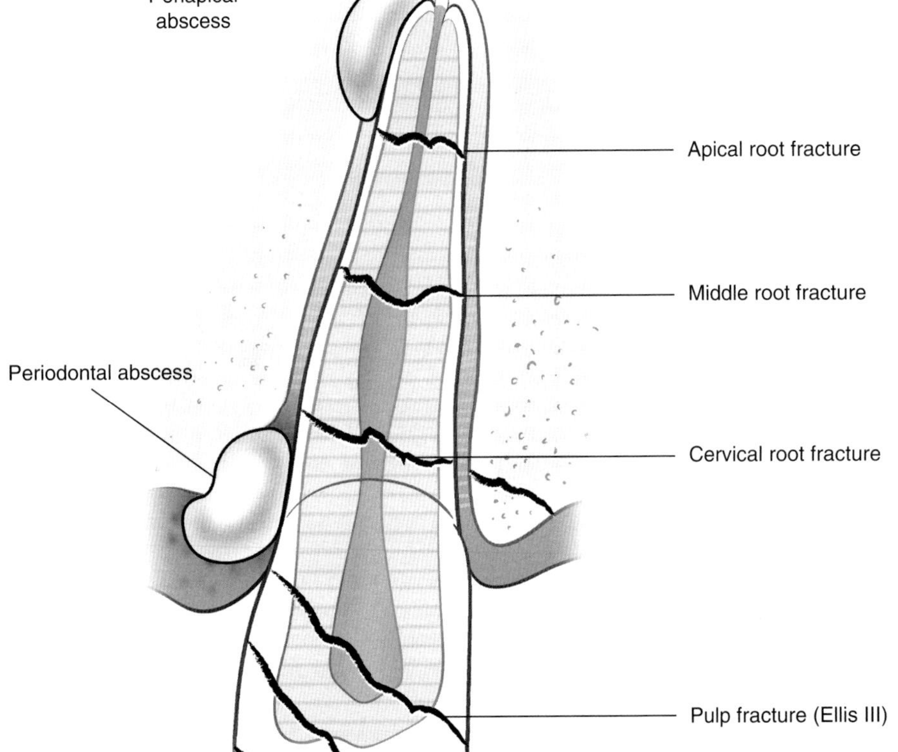

Figure 20.3 Dental fractures and infections. (Copyright Chris Gralapp.)

If a bonding material is available, the exposed dentin should be covered (Ch. 21). Otherwise, urgent follow-up with a dentist should be arranged Pulp or Antibiotics are not indicated for Ellis II tooth fractures.

Pulpor Ellis III fractures

The exposure of the dental pulp makes Ellis III fractures the most serious type of dental fracture. Ellis III fractures are also the most likely to lead to permanent loss of the tooth.

These fractures have a pink blush from formation of drops of blood in the center of the fracture plane. They are usually severely painful unless the neurovascular supply of the tooth has also been disrupted at the tooth apex. Ellis III fractures are true dental emergencies and require emergency dental evaluation and treatment, particularly in children when a primary tooth is involved. A dentist may perform a pulpotomy with additional procedures to preserve the damaged tooth until it is naturally exfoliated and replaced with a permanent tooth. It is preferable to preserve the tooth because the primary teeth have a role in the positioning and development of permanent teeth. If the fracture involves a permanent tooth, pulpotomy may still be successful.

Tooth subluxation

Dental subluxation is characterized by a tooth that is perceptibly loose but still within the socket. The tooth may be mildly or markedly mobile.

Treatment and evaluation is the same in children as with adults. Mildly subluxed teeth (teeth that are mildly mobile in their sockets, sometimes with a ring of blood around the gingival crevice) can be treated with a soft diet for several days.

Extraction may be needed for highly unstable primary teeth. Markedly unstable permanent teeth can be splinted in the ED for 24–48 h or until dental follow-up can be arranged. Antibiotics should also be considered.

Tooth avulsion

A tooth avulsion refers to a tooth that is completely torn from its socket. If the tooth is missing, consider and evaluate for tooth aspiration. If the tooth is available, further management is dictated by whether the tooth is primary or permanent.

In the case of a primary tooth, the tooth is not replaced. Replacement of the tooth will lead to growth abnormalities when eruption of the permanent teeth occurs, although some growth abnormalities can be expected whether or not the tooth is replaced. Referral to a pediatric dentist for placement of a spacer is warranted but is not an emergency requirement.

Permanent teeth are somewhat more complicated from the emergency management perspective. Time is of the essence in tooth reimplantation. Most teeth can be successfully reimplanted if this is done within the first 30 min.

For every minute beyond the 30 min threshold, reimplantation success rates drop by 1%.

Consequently, early reimplantation, preferably in the field, is ideal. Permanent tooth reimplantation is similar in children and adults. The tooth should be handled only by its crown. The root should be cleansed gently with normal saline (or water). The tooth should not be scrubbed to remove debris, as this will damage or remove any remaining periodontal ligament fragments that may still be adherent to the root of the tooth. After suctioning and/or anesthetizing the socket (if needed), the tooth can be gently reinserted. For avulsed incisors, the convex surface of the tooth is buccal, and the concave part lingual. The tooth should be stabilized (Ch. 21).

Disposition after avulsion

Immediate dental follow-up is required. The patient should be started on penicillin, clindamycin, or erythromycin. Most teeth require 2 weeks of stabilization. One week of liquid diet followed by introduction of a soft diet is appropriate.

If a tooth is unable to be reimplanted, emergency dental follow-up is recommended. The tooth should be transported in an appropriate medium to prevent dying of the periodontal ligament. Teeth should never be transported in a dry medium. The options, in order of preference, for dental solutions are as follows.

1. In the socket
2. Hank's Save A Tooth system
3. Patient's mouth (if age appropriate); under the tongue or in the buccal pouch
4. Parent's mouth
5. Milk
6. Saline
7. Water.

Hanks Save A Tooth is available in most EDs and is ideal as a temporary storage medium, particularly for dried teeth or teeth that have been avulsed for greater than 30 min. This solution can restore dried periodontal ligament cells. For this reason, any tooth that has been avulsed and in a dry medium for more than 30 min should be placed in this solution prior to reinsertion. The Hanks Save A Tooth system consists of a container with a basket and solution. The tooth is dropped into the basket and submerged in the solution. For removal, the basket is tipped onto its side to allow the tooth to fall out without manipulation of the root.

Special situations: braces

In facial or dental trauma sustained with the presence of braces, the wire connecting the individual brackets can be cut with any pair of wire-cutters. The actual brackets can be chipped off the affected tooth with the wire-cutters, if needed.

Emergency dental consultations

Emergency dental consultations are rarely available in most emergency practice settings. For this reason, a list of interested dental care providers who are trained in dealing with emergency dental injuries/problems should be compiled before it becomes necessary to call them. This will greatly enhance patient/parent satisfaction and improve dental outcomes.

Pediatric dental infections

Pediatric dental infections can be classified by the affected part of the tooth, ranging from the crown to the apex. The most common dental infections include dental caries, pericoronitis, pulpitis, and periapical abscesses (Fig. 20.3). Dental infections commonly involve several aspects of the tooth and periodontal structures simultaneously.

Teething gingivitis

A child's first tooth appears around 6 months of age. Although not technically a dental infection, the localized inflammation surrounding the erupting tooth can cause gingivitis of the gums, low-grade fevers, irritability, and drooling. A thorough dental examination is warranted before assigning these symptoms to teething. Treatment for a teething infant is generally supportive care using ice rings and systemic analgesics such as ibuprofen. Serious complications have been associated with the use of benzocaine gels.

Topical anesthetics such as benzocaine gels should be avoided in infants.

Erupting cysts or hematomas overlying the emerging tooth usually resolve when the tooth emerges.

Caries

Caries lesions are common in childhood and are the most common cause of odontogenic pain in all patients. Their prevalence varies with socioeconomic status and can be as high as 70% in some low-income groups. Host factors, such as diet and fluoride intake, play an important role in their development. Children can develop early childhood caries from sleeping with a bottle. Pain may be acute or more gradual in onset and often radiates to the temporomandibular joint. The quality of caries-induced pain is variable and may be sharp or dull and achy.

Physical findings for carious teeth are variable and depend on the depth of tooth involved. While an outwardly decayed tooth is obvious, at times the only clue to an underlying caries in a seemingly unblemished tooth is sensitivity to percussion, heat, or cold. Sensitivity to percussion with increased pressure is classic for a periapical abscess, a complication of dental caries.

Management

Analgesia and referral to a general dentist for definitive management is usually sufficient. Use of NSAIDs is indicated and safe in most patients. Narcotic pain medication may be necessary in some acute odontogenic pain. Antibiotic therapy, usually with penicillin, is appropriate in the setting of gingival inflammation or any cellulitis. Clindamycin or erythromycin may be used in children with an allergy to penicillin. Given the importance of primary teeth in the subsequent growth and alignment of the permanent teeth, primary teeth should not be extracted by non-dentists.

Pericoronitis

Pericoronitis is a localized inflammation of the gingival tissue overlying an incompletely erupted tooth. The most common teeth affected are lower third molars. The bacterial plaque accumulation under the gum flap causes infection and severe pain. Pain in the area of the third molars in an older adolescent should prompt consideration of this diagnosis even with no external findings. On examination, the patient usually presents with swelling and reddish gingiva. Dental radiographs may show evidence of tooth impaction.

Management

Antibiotics, saline rinses with or without hydrogen peroxide, and pain management are the mainstays of management. Definitive management by a dentist or oral maxillofacial surgeon should be arranged.

Pulpitis

Pulpitis is a frequent complication in pediatric patients. Pulpitis occurs when the pulp of a tooth becomes infected. This can result from extension of caries into the pulp or from a dental fracture. Pulpitis initially presents as tooth sensitivity to cold or with lying down. Late pulpitis manifests as severe, often excruciating, pain that can be constant or intermittent and triggered by the most innocuous of stimuli, such as air. Pulp infection may extend deeper into the root of the tooth and result in a dental abscess. Pulpitis is diagnosed clinically, with exquisite tenderness to palpation over the affected tooth, while pain on percussion of the surrounding soft tissues may indicate even more severe damage to the pulp.

Management

Treatment of pulpitis is with oral analgesics, systemic antibiotics (penicillin, clindamycin, or erythromycin) and emergency referral to a dentist. The dentist will most likely do a partial or full root canal treatment after carefully examining the tooth.

Dental abscesses

Dental abscesses are a late complication of dental caries or trauma. The infection travels into the root and can extend past the apex of the root. There, the infection can localize within an abscess, spread into the bone (subperiosteal infection), and, in extreme circumstances, spread into the fascial planes of the head and neck. While apical abscesses cannot be observed on oral examination, increased pain with percussion with a tongue blade on the crown of the affected tooth is suggestive. Asking the patient to bite with each individual tooth on a cotton swab is another way to identify an infected tooth. A periapical abscess, or parulis, is a small indurated and tender area at the apex of a tooth. Localized distention of tissues by the abscess causes pain. These abscesses are often visible on the gingival mucosa. Deeper dental abscesses also occur and can cause an overlying cellulitis.

Management

Treatment of dental abscesses is with systemic analgesics and oral antibiotics (usually erythromycin, clindamycin, or penicillin). Ideally a dentist should manage these abscesses. However, if an abscess is fluctuant and the patient has no prompt access to a dentist, incision and drainage of the abscess in the ED may alleviate pain and prevent spontaneous rupture, potentially causing a chronic sinus tract. In the case of a *parulis*, the EP should make a horizontal stab incision into the most fluctuant area of the abscess, extending to the bone, and irrigating with normal saline. Deeper abscesses and those without a clear periapical lesion should be referred to a specialist for treatment. Patients with systemic symptoms, toxic appearance, trismus, immunosuppressed state, and/or evidence of spread into the fascial planes of the face or neck require admission for broad-spectrum parenteral antibiotics and, if indicated, emergency surgical incision and drainage. These complications are rare, but correct diagnosis and appropriate therapy are of the utmost importance in patients who have systemic signs of infection and an odontogenic source.

Periodontal disease: gingivitis and periodontitis

Periodontal disease is a spectrum of disease that extends from minor gingival inflammation (gingivitis) to deeper space infections (periodontitis). Gingivitis is often caused by irritation of the superficial gingival tissues by bacterial plaque. Periodontitis is gingivitis that has penetrated into, and caused loss of, alveolar bone. Gum sensitivity is the primary symptom of gingivitis and, therefore, it rarely leads to ED visits. Gingival bleeding in gingivitis and the perception of mildly mobile teeth in periodontitis may lead to visits.

While gingivitis may be seen in children as a result of poor dental hygiene, for unclear reasons it rarely progresses to periodontitis in prepubertal children. The finding of gingivitis unresponsive to improved oral hygiene measures or periodontitis in a child should trigger an evaluation for underlying systemic illnesses.

A variation on this disease spectrum is acute necrotizing ulcerative gingivitis. Rather than localized inflammation of gingival tissues secondary to irritation from plaque, this involves the invasion of non-necrotic tissue by bacteria. Systemic symptoms such as fever may also be present. This diagnosis in children is rare and should cause concern of more widespread social or medical problems, such as neglect or immunocompromised states.

Management

Enlarged gingival spaces can trap food material and cause acute pain. Loculated areas of pus, or abscesses, should be drained with a stab incision. The patient should be prescribed appropriate antibiotics and instructed in oral saline rinses. Tetracycline is the best initial choice for patients >8 years old with periodontal disease/abscesses. Alternatively, any antibiotic with good Gram-negative and anaerobic coverage should suffice. These measures are only the initial treatment, and referral to a dentist should be arranged.

Postextraction pain

Periosteitis

Immediate pain after extraction is often caused by immediate periosteitis (inflammation of the socket). This pain is often well controlled with NSAIDs and is otherwise self-limited.

Dry socket syndrome

Dry socket syndrome results from premature loss of the post-extraction clot, which normally covers the extracted tooth's socket. Patients usually describe an initial painless period followed by acute onset of severe pain and a foul odor 3–4 days later. This condition represents a localized infection of the bone surrounding the socket and generally occurs after a molar extraction.

Management

Treatment consists of anesthesia using a nerve block, gentle irrigation of the socket, and packing (if age appropriate) of the socket with iodoform gauze saturated with a medicated dental paste. These medicated dental pastes often include eugenol, a common dental topical anesthetic. Patients with dry socket syndrome should be referred back to their dentist for daily packing changes until their condition heals. Patients should be prescribed oral antibiotics (typically penicillin or erythromycin), and systemic analgesics such as narcotics and/or NSAIDs. Initiation of rebleeding in the dry socket by any method is not recommended as it may increase the risk of osteomyelitis.

Pearls and pitfalls

Pearls

1. The likelihood of pulpitis after dentin (Ellis II) fractures is increased in primary teeth because of a greater percentage by volume of pulp.
2. Reimplantation of avulsed permanent teeth should take place as soon as possible, preferably within the first 30 min of the injury.

Pitfalls

1. Primary teeth should not be reimplanted after avulsion because of risk for ankylosis.

Selected references

James T. Oral medicine. In Marx J, Hockberger R, Walls R (eds.) *Rosen's Emergency Medicine: Concepts and Clinical Practice,* 6th edn, Ch. 69. St. Louis, MO: Mosby Elsevier, 2006.

Tinanoff N. Dental caries. In Behrman RE, Kliegman RM, Jenson H (eds.) *Nelson Textbook of Pediatrics*, 17th edn, Ch. 293. Philadelphia, PA: Saunders, 2007.

Chapter 21

Dental procedures

N. Ewen Amieva-Wang and Brian Su-Chieh Liu

Introduction

While dental procedures are best performed by a dentist, there are times when a dentist will not be available for emergency consultation. This chapter will discuss the treatment of a fractured tooth and reimplantation and splinting of an avulsed tooth. Although the actual procedures are similar for adults and children, the indications can differ based on whether the child has primary or permanent dentition. Since dental emergencies require timely action, we recommend the creation of an ED dental box. The dental box should contain:

- different materials used to cap and splint teeth, as well as instructions for the use of these materials
- Frasier suction
- 15 ml syringe with an IV catheter (to irrigate)
- dental cotton rolls
- 2 × 2 and 4 × 4 cotton gauze
- supplies to perform a local or regional block.

Materials

There are many protective materials to cap exposed dentin and pulp secondary to tooth fracture. Calcium hydroxide has been traditionally used. It is inexpensive and easily accessible; however, it can be difficult to adhere to the tooth and may not create an adequate seal on the tooth. Glass ionomer restorative cement or light/heat-cured dental composites are reasonable alternatives to calcium hydroxide. These materials may be easier to use, leading to more successful results. Light-curing calcium hydroxide and calcium hydroxyapatite in a urethane dimethacrylate (UDMA) base is dentin adhering and particularly easy to handle.

Light-curing composite systems work well to splint avulsed teeth. These systems require a hand-held light, wire cutters, and orthodontic wire (0.6–0.7 mm) or even 50 lb nylon fishing wire. While sutures are always available, they are painful and may be difficult to place if the gingival tissue is macerated. The Coe-Pak is a ready-made system designed to adhere to tooth enamel and gingiva; this method is designed to hold a tooth in place for 24 h.

Treatment of tooth fractures

Primary teeth commonly sustain fractures through the enamel of a tooth (Ellis I). These fractures affect cosmesis and not tooth viability. A dentist can file down or repair these cracks in a non-emergency setting. Fractures through the dentin (Ellis II) should be covered within 24–48 h to prevent damage to the dentin and pulp. Fractures through the pulp (Ellis III)

Box 21.1. Covering a tooth fracture

Procedure (Fig. 21.1)

1. Inspect tooth, account for missing fragments, and assess all oral injuries.
2. Anesthetize the wound (local anesthetic, regional block, or procedural sedation).
3. Irrigate and clean the tooth fracture (suction and gauze).
4. Insert dental cotton rolls between the gums and lips to avoid contamination of the fracture.
5. Dry the fracture with gauze and suction (do not over dry).
6. Prepare covering mixture: composite, calcium hydroxide, glass ionomer.
7. Apply the protective covering.
8. Arrange prompt dental follow-up.
9. Recommend a soft diet.

Complications

- Decreased adhesion of tooth covering to tooth.

Tricks of the trade

- Insert dental cotton rolls between the gums and lips
- Take time to prepare work area
- Dry (do not dessicate) the tooth.

A Practical Guide to Pediatric Emergency Medicine: Caring for Children in the Emergency Department, ed. N. Ewen Amieva-Wang (associate eds. Jamie Shandro, Aparajita Sohoni, and Bernhard Fassl). Published by Cambridge University Press.

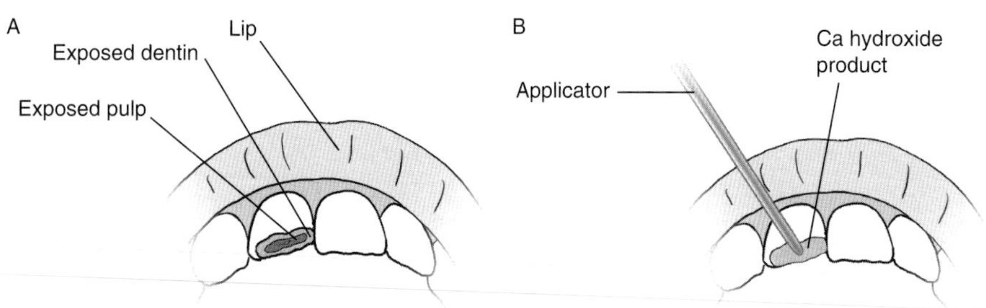

Figure 21.1 Applying a protective covering to a cracked tooth. (A) Upper incisor with a fracture through enamel, dentin, and pulp. (B) After cleaning and drying, a protective coating is then applied. (Copyright N. Ewen Wang.)

Box 21.2. Reimplantation and splinting of tooth

Procedure for reimplantation (Fig. 21.2)

1. Make sure tooth is not a primary tooth.
2. Clean the tooth: hold by crown, swish in Hank's solution, milk, or saline.
3. Inspect the tooth (reimplantation is contraindicated if there is extensive fracture or root fracture).
4. Inspect the tooth socket: gently swab with gauze or suction lightly.
5. Firmly insert the tooth into the socket.
6. Hold the implanted tooth in position: (patient bites on gauze, parent holds it in place).

Procedure for splinting a tooth (light curing method) (Fig. 21.3)

1. Cut orthodontic or fishing wire to a length that covers the injured tooth and the adjacent tooth to either side.
2. Bend the wire to the shape of the tooth arch.
3. Clean the labial surface of the reimplanted tooth and the tooth on either side.
4. Check the patient's occlusion and position the tooth firmly in the socket.
5. Insert dental cotton rolls between the gums and lips to provide a larger area on which to work.
6. Apply etching material to the center of the labial side of each tooth.
7. Wait 15 s and then wash the etching material off the teeth.
8. Apply bonding material; gently dry, then light cure.
9. Apply composite to the center of each tooth.
10. Position the wire on top of the composite.
11. Apply another layer of composite on top of the wire on each tooth.
12. Smooth the composite over the wire, covering the ends with composite.
13. Light cure the composite immediately after application.
14. Check the patient's occlusion.
15. Prescribe antibiotics.
16. Arrange dentist follow-up.

Problems

- Reimplanted tooth not stable
- Tooth splint does not adhere.

Tricks of the trade

- Take time to rinse off tooth, position correctly do not reimplant and then change position
- Splint the tooth
- Take time to prepare work area.

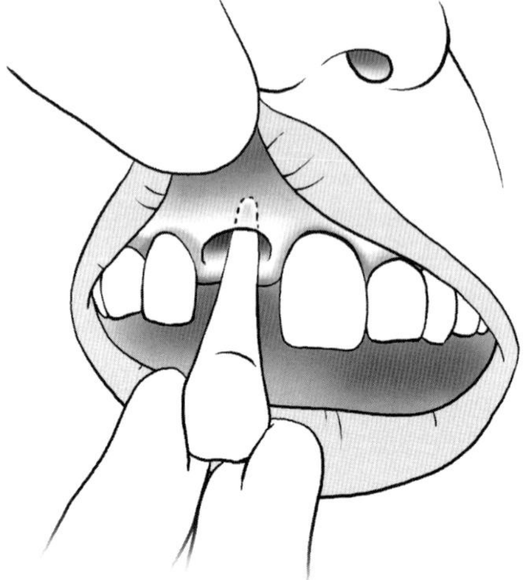

Figure 21.2 Reimplantation of an avulsed tooth. After tooth and area of avulsion are gently rinsed and cleared of debris, the tooth is firmly reimplanted. (Copyright N. Ewen Wang.)

should be promptly covered to avoid destruction and infection of the pulp. In general, the more time the dentin or pulp is exposed to the oral cavity, the higher the chances of permanent damage and the lower the chance of tooth salvage. Although a primary tooth will ultimately be replaced by a permanent tooth, salvaging the primary tooth is important because it can serve as a place-holder or spacer while the permanent dentition grows in. Teeth with large pulp-exposed fractures have a low rate of survival, but covering these fractures can decrease pain and perhaps infection (Box 21.1 and Fig. 21.1).

Reimplantation and splinting of an avulsed tooth

Primary teeth should not be reimplanted. Inappropriately reimplanted teeth can ankylose to the alveolar bone or to the permanent teeth. The successful reimplantation of a permanent tooth, however, can greatly affect appearance and function (Box 21.2 and Figs. 21.2 and 21.3).

Avulsed teeth should be stored and transported in appropriate media. The EP should be careful to leave the

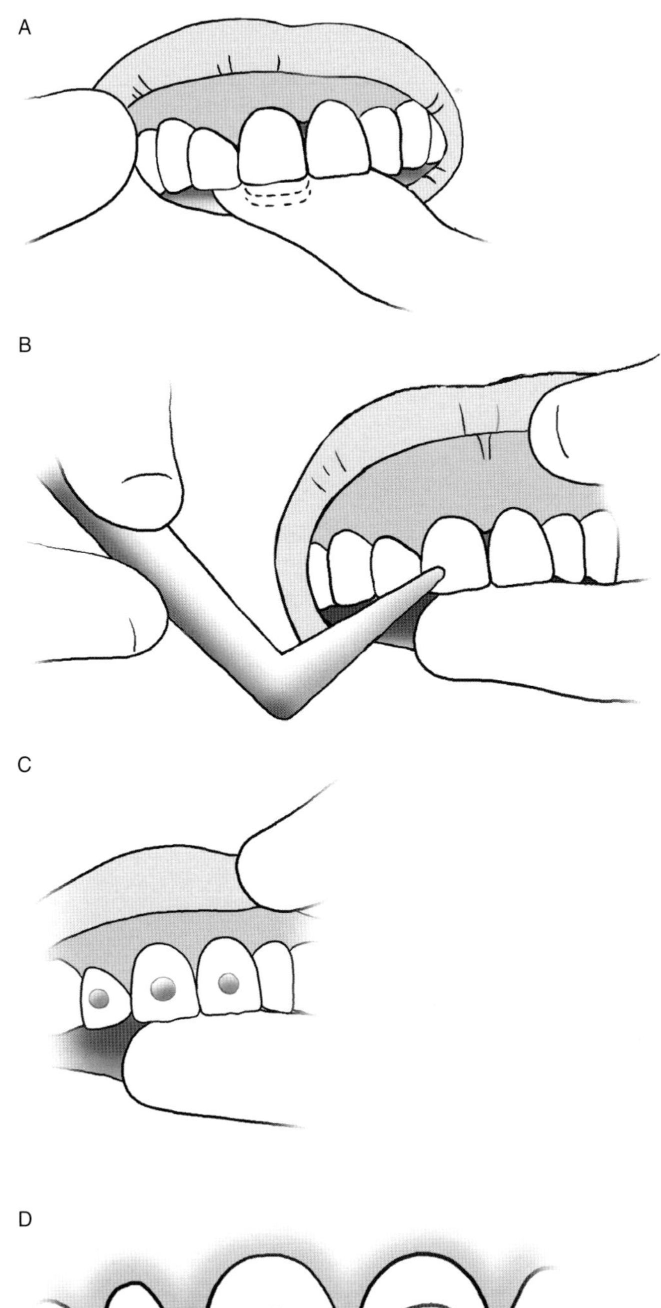

Figure 21.3 Splinting of teeth. (A) The tooth is repositioned or reimplanted firmly. (B) Etchant is placed on the surface of the tooth. (C) After etchant is washed off, bonding material and composite are applied to the avulsed tooth and the teeth on either side. (D) Wire is placed on the top of the composite and a second layer of composite is placed on top of the wire. (Copyright N. Ewen Wang.)

periodontal ligament fibers of the root intact. Handling the tooth by its crown will minimize periodontal ligament trauma. A number of complications can occur with tooth reimplantation:

- ankylosis of implanted tooth to the underlying bone
- infection
- malocclusion (increases ankylosis).

Pearls and pitfalls

Pearls

1. Prompt management of pulp and dentin fractures can increase tooth viability.
2. Covering a primary tooth fracture is indicated.
3. Give antibiotics after tooth reimplantation to minimize inflammation.
4. Organize a "dental box" in the ED to facilitate prompt treatment of dental emergencies.

Pitfalls

1. Failure to promptly reimplant permanent teeth.
2. Failure to provide good discharge instructions including soft diet after tooth reimplantation and capping.
3. Failure to communicate prognosis in a tooth reimplanted after a delay, or in a pulp fracture.
4. Failure to arrange prompt dental follow-up.

Selected references

James T. Oral medicine. In Marx J, Hockberger R, Walls R (eds.) *Rosen's Emergency Medicine: Concepts and Clinical Practice,* 6th edn, Ch. 69. St. Louis, MO: Mosby Elsevier, 2006.

Tinanoff N. Dental caries. In Behrman RE, Kliegman RM, Jenson H (eds.) *Nelson Textbook of Pediatrics*, 17th edn, Ch. 293. Philadelphia, PA: Saunders, 2007.

Section

5

Dermatology

Chapter 22

Approach to pediatric dermatology: introduction and terminology

Theresa M. van der Vlugt

Introduction

The main responsibility of the acute care provider in evaluating a pediatric rash is to identify and treat the rashes that represent serious or life-threatening disease. It is also important to identify contagious viral exanthems, particularly those that can be dangerous to immunosuppressed persons or non-immune pregnant women, such as varicella, rubella, or parvovirus B19. While most other rashes do not require emergency identification, a definitive diagnosis and appropriate treatment can alleviate discomfort and reassure worried families. This introductory chapter defines essential terminology and important dermatology history and then presents a rubric that we will use subsequently in discussing pediatric dermatology.

Understanding dermatologic terminology is essential, as often the diagnosis lies in the description. In order to describe a rash one must remember the basic anatomy of the skin and then describe primary lesions, secondary lesions, color, and configuration or distribution.

Background

The skin consists of the epidermis and dermis, separated by the dermal basement membrane. The epidermis is the most superficial layer of skin, in which keratinocytes on the basement membrane proliferate, become apoptotic, and flatten out into the horny stratum corneum layer, which is continuously shed. It takes 28 days for a newly formed keratinocyte to go through this cycle; this fact can help patients and parents to understand why most rashes do not have a rapid resolution. Melanocytes, the pigment producing cells, are in the epidermis. The dermis, below the basement membrane, is composed of collagen and elastin in a muccopolysaccharide gel, providing strength and elasticity. Finally blood vessels travel in the subcutaneous fat layer and terminate in vascular plexi in the dermis.

Terminology

Primary lesions are the earliest lesions to appear, before any changes from excoriation, super-infection, or treatment. They can be described by answering four basic questions:

Is the lesion colored?
Is the lesion raised?
Is it fluid filled?
Is there scale?

Table 22.1 lists the basic terms and definitions used to describe primary lesions.

Secondary lesions are changes that occur to primary lesions and the surrounding skin with time and treatment. Table 22.2 lists common terms used to describe secondary lesions and Table 22.3 lists important history features.

Color

Rashes can be skin color, brown, red, white, yellow, tan, and blue. Blanching of rash with pressure can be an important sign, indicating whether red blood cells remain within vascular channels (blanching) or have leaked out into the surrounding skin (non-blanching). This section will focus mostly on rashes that are red.

Rashes other than red in color are usually not acute or urgent.

Distribution and configuration

Rashes can be *generalized* or *localized*. Note whether a generalized rash spares or involves the palms, soles, face, or scalp. Often, the distribution on the body can be a clue as to the etiology of the rash (Fig. 22.1).

A generalized *guttate* rash has a raindrop-like distribution, and a *reticulated* rash is in a net-like pattern. A *morbilliform* rash is a diffuse, generalized eruption of erythematous macules and papules (resembling measles); this type of rash is also often called *maculopapular*. When a rash is localized, note whether it

A Practical Guide to Pediatric Emergency Medicine: Caring for Children in the Emergency Department, ed. N. Ewen Amieva-Wang (associate eds. Jamie Shandro, Aparajita Sohoni, and Bernhard Fassl). Published by Cambridge University Press.

Table 22.1. Primary lesion terms and definitions

Term	Definition
Macule/ patch	Circumscribed flat non-palpable area of color change; macules are <1 cm, patches >1 cm
Papule/ plaque	Solid, raised, palpable lesion; papules are 1 cm or less, plaques are >1 cm and often formed of a confluence of papules
Nodule/ tumor	Raised, circumscribed but less distinct solid lesions, with the greatest mass being below the surface of the skin; the skin moves *over* a subcutaneous nodule and *with* an intradermal nodule; nodules are ≤2 cm and larger nodules are called tumors
Wheal	Flat-topped, raised lesions caused by edema in the upper dermis; often pink, blanching, shifting or short lived
Vesicle/ bulla	Circumscribed, raised, clear fluid-filled lesion; vesicles are <1 cm and bullae >1 cm
Pustule	Circumscribed, raised, yellow or white exudate-filled lesion; pustules are <1 cm and often sharply demarcated
Burrows	Linear tracks of erythema or epidermal change, sometimes seemingly wandering; caused by tunneling of animal parasites in the skin
Petechiae/ purpura	Extravasated red blood cells into the dermis; ptechiae are tiny flat red macules, and purpura are larger red or purple macules or plaques; these lesions are non-blanching with pressure

Table 22.2. Secondary lesion terms and definitions

Term	Definition
Excoriation	Abrasion or trauma that causes loss of epidermis, often in linear grooves when self-induced
Crust	Dried exudate of serum, blood, or pus, often combined with collapsed blister roof that results from full-thickness epidermal disruption
Scale	Flaky whitish or skin-colored plates that can be large or miniscule on the surface of the skin; caused by compacted, desquamating layers of the upper epidermis
Fissures	Linear cleavages in the epidermis that can extend to the dermis and are often painful
Erosions/ ulcers	Erosion is loss or necrosis of part or all of the epidermis; ulcer is loss of all of the epidermis and part or all of the dermis; erosions are often the base of a blister where the roof has been lost; erosions heal without scarring, whereas ulcers have scarring
Atrophy	Thinning or loss of the dermis or epidermis in a circumscribed area; skin can be translucent and depressed, and develops fine wrinkles with lateral pressure
Lichenification	Thickened epidermis with exaggerated skin markings, resulting often from chronic trauma, scratching, or rubbing

Table 22.3. Important features of a dermatology history

	History
Appearance	What did the rash first look like? Did the appearance change?
Location	Where did the rash first start on the body? Did it spread, and how (centripetal, centrifugal)?
Timing	When did it start? How long has it lasted?
Symptoms	Itchy or painful? Interfering with sleep?
Constitutional/ associated symptoms	Is there fever, sore throat, cough, headaches, joint pains?
Exposure	Has there been exposure to sun, plants, skin or hair soaps, lotions, cosmetics, pets or animals? Has there been a tick or insect bite?
Travel	Within or outside the USA? Camping or hiking in areas with endemic diseases such as Lyme disease?
Medications	Any recently added (antibiotics, antipyretics) or chronic (antiseizure) medications? Timing of medication changes or additions?
Foods/allergens	Any ingestion of typical allergens (milk, nuts/peanuts, seafood, soy, egg)? Any recent exposure to radiographic contrast?

is in a *dermatomal* distribution, following the skin distribution supplied by a dorsal ganglia. If a localized rash has an unusual shape or borders with straight lines it is more likely to be facticious, abuse-related, or a contact dermatitis. Note whether a rash has any mucosal surface involvement. Individual lesions may be *discrete* (single), *confluent* (single lesions merging together), or *grouped* (single lesions in groups). Groups of lesions may be *linear* (in straight lines), *annular* (in a circular

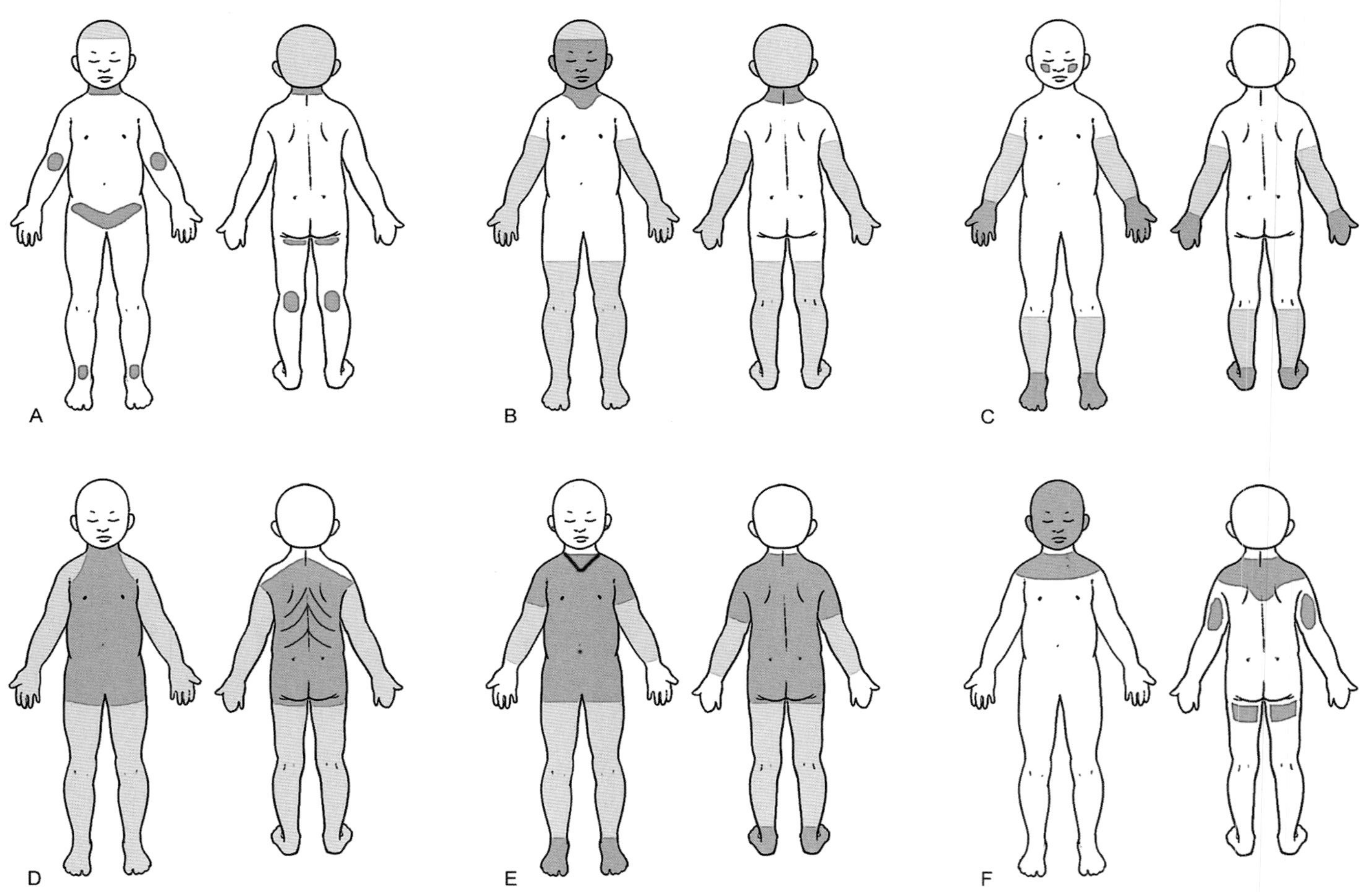

Figure 22.1 Body distribution of different rashes. Darker shading indicates more likely/more intense rash, and lighter shading indicates less likely or less intense rash. (A) Flexural rashes: childhood atopic dermatitis, infantile sebaceous dermatitis, intertrigio/tinea cruris, candida. (B) Sun-exposed sites: sunburn, phototoxic or photoallergic dermatitis, some viral exanthems(centripetal). (C) Acrodermatitis: Papular acrodermatitis, infantile atopic dermatitis, Tinea with or without "id" reaction, dyshidrotic eczema, desquamation following toxic shock or streptococcal infection. (D) Pityriasis rosea distribution: Pityriasis rosea, secondary syphilis, drug reactions, viral exanthems, guttate psoriasis, atopic dermatititis. (E) Clothing-covered sites: Milaria, contact dermatitis (note jewelry/pants-snap markings for nickel allergy), summertime psoriasis. (F) Acneiform rashes Courtesy of T van der Vlugt.

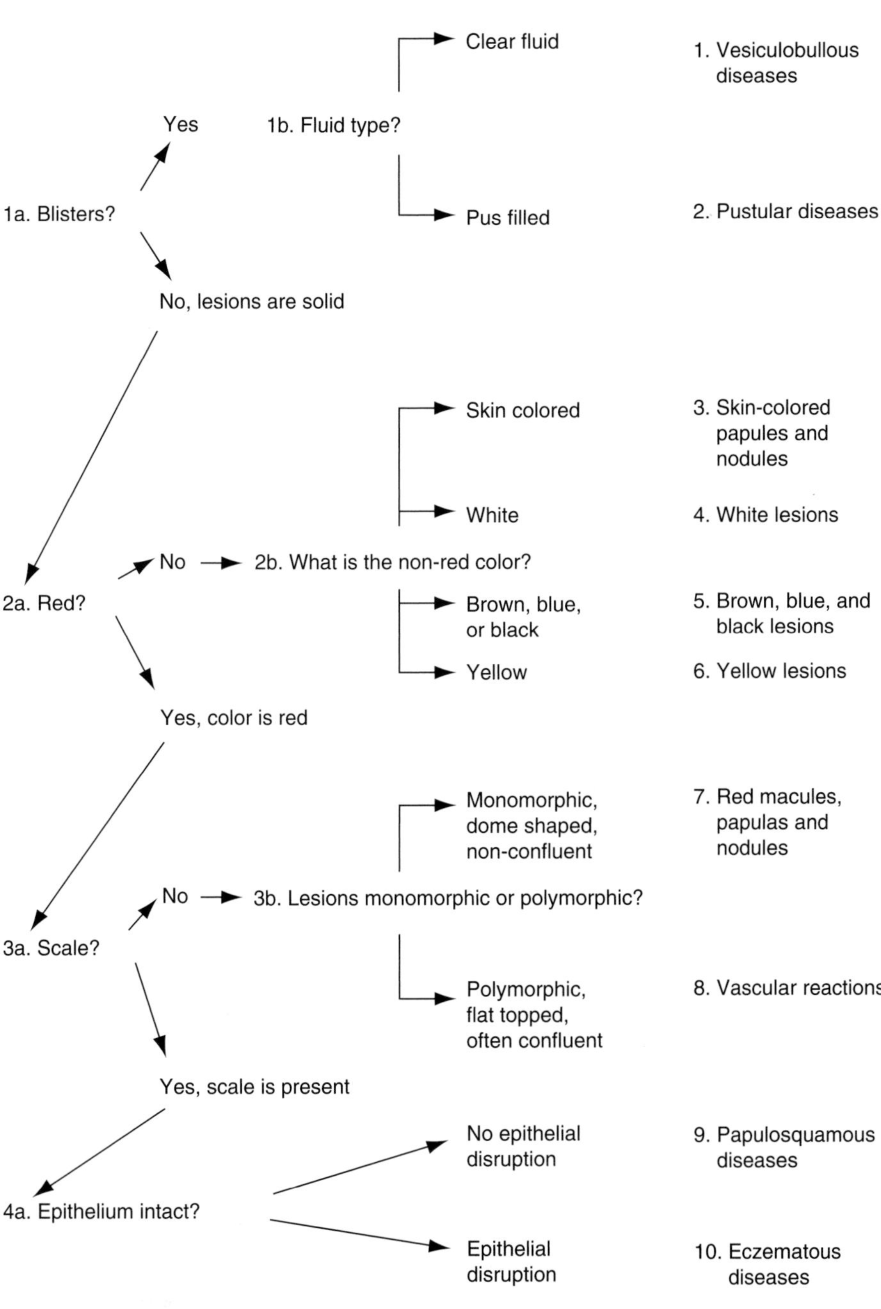

Figure 22.2 Stepwise algorithm for evaluating rash. (Adapted from Lynch PJ *Dermatology* 3rd edn. Baltimore, MD: Williams & Wilkins. 1994.)

arrangement), or *curvilinear, arctuate*, or *whorled* (in curved lines). The borders of a lesion may be *serpiginous* (snake-like, curved, and recurved). Individual coin-like lesions may be described as *nummular* or *discoid*.

History and physical examination

Diagnosis in the vast majority of common skin conditions is made based on the history and physical examination, so a careful, dermatology-focused history is essential. Very few skin problems have confirmatory laboratory or radiographic tests that are available in a timely manner. Important history points are included in Table 22.3. Figure 22.2 shows the step-wise algorithm for evaluating a rash in a child, using a clinical and morphological rubric.

While there are many dermatologic lesions, this section will focus on those relevant for pediatric emergency medicine.

Chapter 23

Dermatologic emergencies: quick reference tables

N. Ewen Amieva-Wang

Three disease entities that cause rash, fever, and hypotension are:

- toxic shock syndrome (Ch. 89)
- Rocky Mountain spotted fever (Ch. 90)
- meningococci infection (Chs. 89 and 92).

The characteristics of these are compared in Table 23.1. Table 23.2 compares staphylococcal scalded skin syndrome and Stevens–Johnson syndrome/toxic epidermal necrolysis.

Table 23.1. Comparison of three diseases that cause rash, fever and hypotension

Characteristic	Toxic shock syndrome (staphylococcal variant)	Rocky Mountain spotted fever	Meningococcal infection
Host	Humans; caused by superantigenic exotoxins	Tick	Humans
History	Associated with foreign bodies (e.g., superabsorbent tampons) and skin wounds	Endemic state, tick	Sporadic, college dormitory outbreaks
Season	–	Spring/summer	Winter/spring
Age	Menstrual-related form occurs in women 15–35 years of age; 50% of cases are not associated with menstruation; occurs in children <2 years with cutaneous lesions	66% in those <15 years of	6–12 months and teenagers/ young adults
Clinical features	May have prodrome of fever, malaise; multisystem failure with hypotension and rash	Headache/fever/rash	Malaise, fever, headache, appears ill
Meningitis	Uncommon	Uncommon	Common
Rash	Starts with erythroderma; desquamation especially of palms and soles at 1–2 weeks after onset of illness	Centripetal spread is hallmark: ankle then soles then trunk Macule/ papule then petechial but 15% spotless	Scattered petechial eruption, angular, often extremities but spares palms and soles Petechial then purpuric
Treatment	Broad-spectrum antibiotic that covers methicillin-resistant *Staphylococcus aureus* (MRSA): vancomycin	Doxycycline (since ED diagnosis is not definitive, cover for meningococcal disease also)	Gram-negative coverage (ceftriazone, cefotaxime)
Mortality	3%	5–25%	10–20%

A Practical Guide to Pediatric Emergency Medicine: Caring for Children in the Emergency Department, ed. N. Ewen Amieva-Wang (associate eds. Jamie Shandro, Aparajita Sohoni, and Bernhard Fassl). Published by Cambridge University Press.

Table 23.2. Comparison of staphylococcal scalded skin syndrome, and Stevens–Johnson syndrome/toxic epidermal necrolysis[a]

Features	Staphylococcal scalded skin syndrome	Stevens–Johnson syndrome	Toxic epidermal necrolysis
Age	Infants	Children	Teenagers/adults
Etiology	*Staphylococcus aureus*	Drugs (anticonvulsants, antibiotics, NSAIDs); also infections: Mycoplasma pneumonia, herpes simplex virus, Epstein–Barr virus	Drugs (anticonvulsants, antibiotics, NSAIDs)
Exfoliating skin	White	Necrotic	Necrotic
Skin biopsy/level of split	Granular layer within epidermis	Full-thickness epidermis	Full-thickness epidermis
Inflammatory cells	Scarce	Prominent	Prominent
Extent		<10% body surface area; also by definition involvement of at least two other mucous membranes	>30% body surface area
Mortality	1–10%	<5%	30%

NSAID, non-steroidal anti-inflammatory drug.
[a] Stevens–Johnson syndrome and toxic epidermal necrolysis are part of a spectrum of disease.

Chapter 24

Cutaneous drug reactions

Theresa M. van der Vlugt

Introduction

Drugs can cause almost any type of skin pathology, by way of allergy, toxicity, or metabolic or environmental interactions. Maculopapular, urticarial, and fixed drug eruptions are common. Depending on the mechanism, reactions can occur within minutes or within weeks or months of starting a medication (Table 24.1). Infants and children have a lower incidence of adverse drug reactions than adults. Definitive treatment for all drug reactions is prompt discontinuation of the suspected drug.

Table 24.1. Onset of drug eruption after ingestion of medication

Time scale	Cause
Hours to 2 days	Acute generalized exanthematous pustulosis
Hours to 7 days	Urticaria, angioedema, phototoxic reactions
1–7 days	Fixed drug eruption, photoallergic reactions
1–21 days	Generalized pustular eruptions
7–14 days	Morbilliform, scarlatiniform, or bullous drug eruptions
7–21 days	Serum sickness-like eruption, vasculitis, serum sickness
14–56 days	Erythema nodosum, Stevens–Johnson syndrome, toxic epidermal necrolysis
30–100 days	Hypersensitivity syndrome, Lichenoid eruptions

Source: Adapted from Weston *et al.* 2007.

Clinical presentation

In evaluating a possible drug reaction, the clinician should (1) exclude alternative causes, particularly infectious; (2) note the interval between introduction of the drug and onset of reaction (Table 24.1); (3) note the morphology of the rash and look for danger signs (Table 24.2); (4) know the "reputation" of the drug for causing a particular reaction in the population; (5) review the patient's history of reactions to other drugs, foods, or the current drug; and (6) elicit any response to withdrawal of drug or rechallenge. Rechallenge should *not* be performed after any serious reaction.

Urticarial or angioedemic drug reaction

See Ch. 10 for an outline of the approach to allergic emergencies.

Table 24.2. Danger signs in drug-induced rashes

Type	Features
Cutaneous	Confluent erythema or erythroderma, facial edema or oropharyngeal/tongue involvement, skin pain, palpable purpura, skin necrosis, blistering or epidermal detachment, positive Nikolsky sign, mucous membrane erosions, urticaria
General	High fever (>40°C), enlarged lymph nodes, arthralgia or arthritis, shortness of breath or wheezing, hypotension
Laboratory findings	Eosinophil count >1000 cells/ml, lymphocytosis with atypical lymphocytes, abnormal results on LFTs

Source: Adapted from Roujeau *et al.* 1994.

A Practical Guide to Pediatric Emergency Medicine: Caring for Children in the Emergency Department, ed. N. Ewen Amieva-Wang (associate eds. Jamie Shandro, Aparajita Sohoni, and Bernhard Fassl). Published by Cambridge University Press.

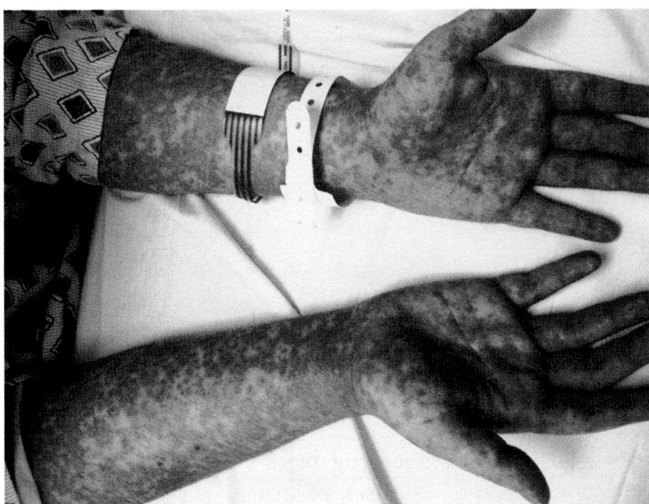

Figure 24.1 Morbilliform drug reaction secondary to sulfa exposure. Rash is symmetrical, discrete, and erythematous with blanching macules. Palms and soles are involved. Rash is pruritic. (Courtesy of T. M. van der Vlugt.)

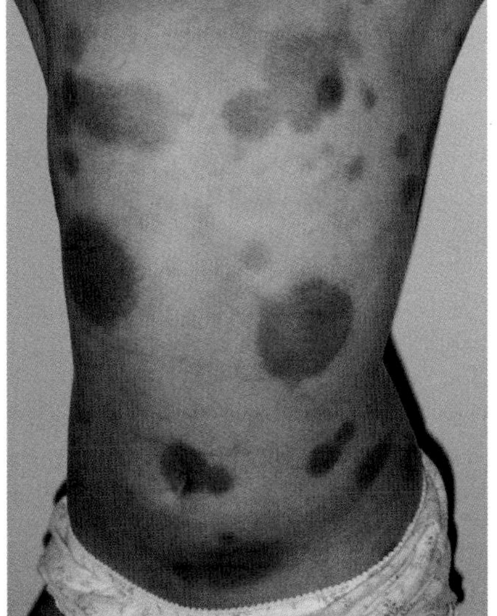

Figure 24.2 Fixed drug eruption. Trimethoprim–sulfamethoxazole-induced oval, erythematous macules with diffuse hyperpigmentation within several lesions. (Courtesy of Logical Images, Inc.)

Morbilliform drug eruptions

Of drug-induced eruptions, 40–75% are a "morbilliform" eruption, usually starting 7–14 days after first ingestion of causative medication. These rashes are symmetrical, discrete, erythematous, partly blanching macules that originate on the trunk and head before spreading to the rest of the body (Fig. 24.1). Palms and soles are frequently involved. Macules can become papules and coalesce into plaques and are variably pruritic. There can be mucous membrane erythema, but mucous membrane lesions are uncommon. Often, there can be associated low-grade fever, malaise, and arthralgia. The rash begins to resolve in 7–14 days, often with superficial desquamation. Morbilliform drug eruption occurs mainly with antibiotics and antiseizure medications. Treatment consists of removing the offending drug and using systemic and topical antipruritics or topical steroids. Oral steroids are sometimes recommended early in the reaction and can help with more severe pruritus.

Fixed drug eruption

Fixed drug eruptions are the second most common type of drug eruption (Fig. 24.2).

In fixed drug eruptions, a sharply demarcated circular or oval red–brown plaque of dermatitis with occasional bullous areas occurs and reoccurs in the same spot with administration or readministration of the causative drug.

Initial lesions are usually solitary, but multiple lesions can occur with rechallenge. Lesions gradually subside but leave post-inflammatory hyperpigmentation that can last months. Common sites include the face, trunk, genitals, hands, and feet.

The most common cause of fixed drug eruptions in children is sulfa drugs.

Misdiagnosis as an insect bite, contact allergy, or post-traumatic change is common, but skin biopsy or rechallenge (unintentional or intentional) will usually differentiate. There is no treatment for the hyperpigmentation, but severely pruritic lesions can be helped by moderate-potency topical steroids (Ch. 34).

Phototoxic and photoallergic reactions

Many drugs can produce adverse cutaneous reactions when the individual taking them is exposed to ultraviolet light. Reactions are generally either phototoxic (very common) or photoallergic (uncommon), and many drugs or substances can cause both types of reaction.

Phototoxic reactions occur when a drug or compound absorbs ultraviolet light, moves to an excited state, then returns to ground state and releases the energy, forming free radicals that directly damage nearby cells. Phototoxic reactions often present as an exaggerated sunburn, often with blistering, followed by desquamation and hyperpigmentation. Hyperpigmentation can also occur without prior erythema or blistering. Bizarre patterning is not uncommon, relating to splashing of a phototoxic compound on skin. Phototoxic reactions occur on first exposure, within minutes to hours of sun exposure, and severity is related both to dose of medication or compound and sun exposure. Phytophotodermatoses are phototoxic reactions to plant compounds (psoralens). Phototoxicity usually occurs from plant substance on the surface of the skin (classically lemons and limes) but sometimes can be from ingested plants (particularly celery). Treatment is only supportive, with cool compresses and analgesics, and avoidance of future exposures.

Photoallergic drug reactions are type 3 hypersensitivity reactions and require prior exposure and sensitization in order to occur. They are not dose related. They occur when ultraviolet light changes a drug molecule present in the skin, creating a sensitizing hapten. Photoallergic drug reactions have an intense painful and/or pruritic, eczemoid dermatitis with erythema, edema, papules, and vesicles; there is crusting and oozing. The rash is most prominent on sun-exposed areas such as the face, upper trunk, and extensor forearms, usually starting approximately 24 h after sun exposure in a sensitized individual. Only minimal sun exposure can be required for a significant reaction. The eruption is very similar to allergic contact dermatitis, as the pathogenesis is identical. Alternatively, sensitized individuals can develop immediate urticaria in response to sunlight as a manifestation of photoallergic reaction (type 1 hypersensitivity). Both topical and systemic medications can cause photoallergy, the most common cause being topical sunscreens containing para-aminobenzoic acid (PABA). Sulfa antibiotics, NSAIDs, and acyclovir can cause photoallergic reactions. Many drugs or plants causing phototoxicity are also able to cause photoallergy. Treatment includes systemic antipruritics, topical corticosteroids, skin-soothing lotions or cold compresses, and avoidance of the sensitizing drug or chemical.

Drug reaction with eosinophilia and systemic symptoms

Drug-induced hypersensitivity syndrome (DIHS), also called drug reaction with eosinophilia and systemic symptoms (DRESS) or the exfoliative dermatitis/fever/hepatitis/lymphadenopathy syndrome, is an uncommon drug reaction starting later (2–8 weeks) after initiating a medication. It can be fatal in 10% of patients.

Aromatic anticonvulsants (phenytoin, carbamezepine, and phenobarbital) are the most common causes of DRESS; sulfonamides are also common culprits.

The rash (Fig. 24.3) begins as facial edema and erythema, becoming diffuse erythroderma with scaling and exfoliative dermatitis. Follicular papules and pustules are often present, and bullae and purpura can be seen. Fever, hepatitis with elevated liver enzymes, and diffuse lymphadenopathy are common, and inflammation of kidney, lung, heart, thyroid, and CNS, plus eosinophilia and atypical lymphocytosis, can occur. Hypersensitivity syndrome can be difficult to distinguish clinically from acute lymphoma or vasculitis/serum sickness, and when severe can resemble Stevens–Johnson syndrome or toxic epidermal necrolysis, but laboratory studies usually differentiate. Cessation of the offending medication is associated with a slow resolution of symptoms over weeks and months. Although there are no formal studies, most experts endorse systemic corticosteroids (1–2 mg/kg daily) for which there is significant anectodal evidence. Steroids should be continued for a few weeks, early cessation of steroids may

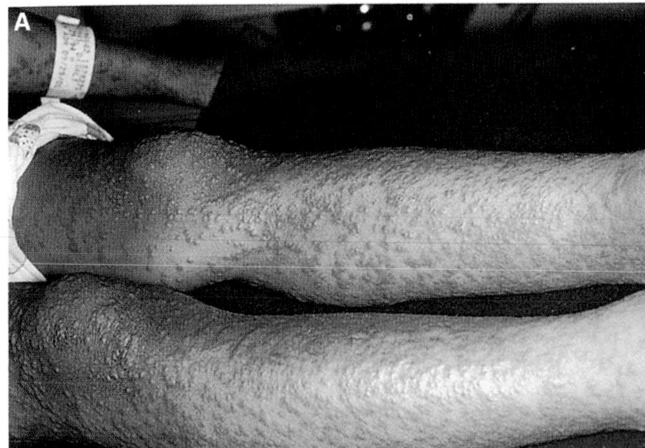

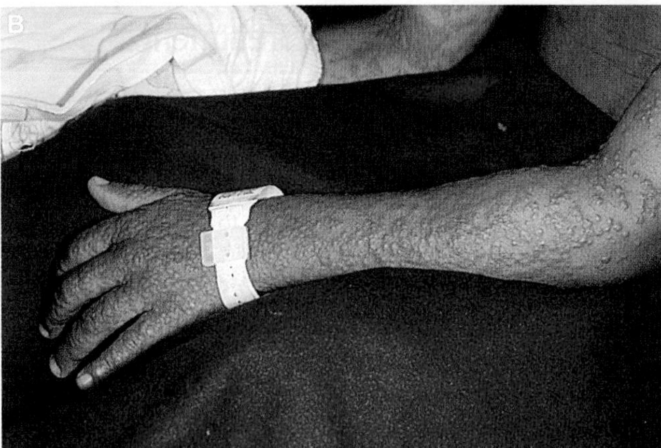

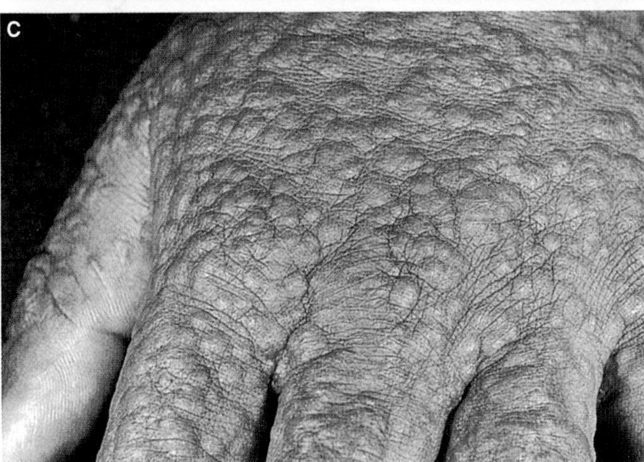

Figure 24.3 Drug-induced hypersensitivity syndrome (DIHS) or drug rash with eosinophilia and systemic symptoms (DRESS). A 7-year-old child presented with an extensive papular rash over his entire body 35 days after he was started on phenytoin. Papular lesions are seen on both legs (A), and arms (B); a close up shows the indurated nature of the rash (C). Mucous membrane involvement is minimal or absent (D). (Reprinted with permission from Shah BR, Lucchesi M (eds). *Atlas of Pediatric Emergency Medicine*. New York: McGraw Hill, 2006.)

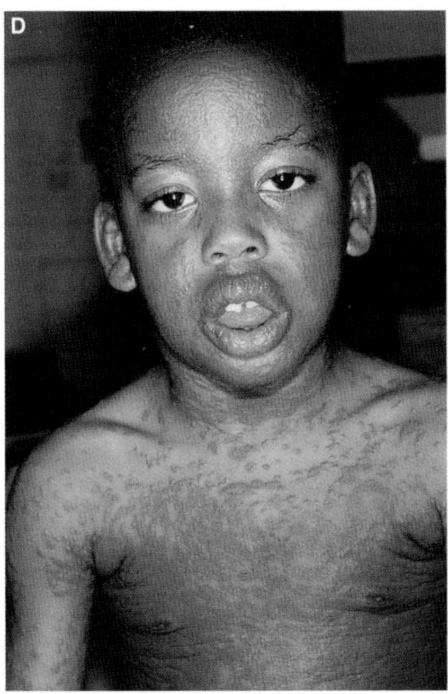

Figure 24.3 *(cont.)*

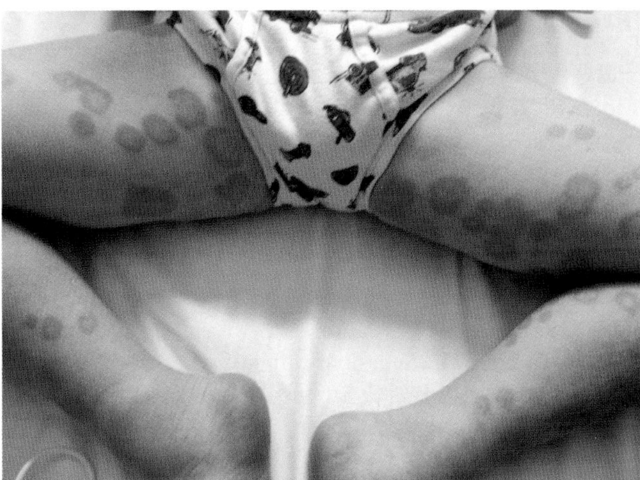

Figure 24.4 Serum-sickness-like drug reaction. Urticarial, erythema multiforme-like rash with characteristic lilac/purplish discoloration as well as arthralgia and periarticular swelling. Note right ankle periarticular swelling. (Courtesy of T. M. van der Vlugt.)

precipitate relapse of rash and hepatitis. Systemic antipruritics may also be of help.

Acute generalized erythematous pustulosis

The rash of acute generalized erythematous pustulosis (AGEP) is a rapid onset of widespread erythema and thousands of pinpoint (0.1 mm) non-follicular pustules, usually in association with fever and within hours to 1–3 days of starting a medication. The condition resolves spontaneously in 4–10 days, with superficial desquamation. Drugs are the most common cause in adults (penicillins, macrolides, sulfonamides, anticonvulsants, NSAIDs, and, rarely, cephalosporins) but children can develop this in response to vaccines or with no drug precipitants (suspected viral etiology.)

Bullous drug eruptions

Vancomycin and NSAIDs have been associated with eruptions of tense bullae, usually on the extremities but sometimes generalized, within 2–4 weeks of starting the drug. This IgA-mediated eruption resolves with drug discontinuation. If cessation of vancomycin is not an immediate option, a severe bullous eruption can be treated with steroids or dapsone.

Erythema nodosum

Erythema nodosum (see Fig. 30.1, p. 161) is the occurrence of ill-defined red, tender subcutaneous nodules, usually on the lower extremities, starting 2–5 weeks after beginning a causative drug. Oral contraceptives are the most common cause, with sulfonamides and sulfonylureas, NSAIDs, and opiates also being implicated. Erythema nodosum is associated with infection (particularly beta-hemolytic streptococci) or inflammatory bowel disease far more commonly than with drugs, but no underlying cause is found for erythema nodosum in most pediatric patients. Treatment consists of rest, elevation, NSAIDs (for non-NSAID-associated reaction), and discontinuation of the offending drug. For patients with recurrent erythema nodosum, systemic or intralesional steroids can be considered.

Serum sickness-like drug reaction

Serum sickness-like reaction (SSLDR) is a drug reaction that mimics true serum sickness, which is an allergic reaction originally caused by administration of non-human antiserum to humans (Fig. 24.4). In SSLDR, 1–3 weeks after first ingesting the causative drug, children develop an urticarial or erythema multiforme-like rash that commonly has central *lilac/purplish* discoloration, along with arthralgia and periarticular swelling, fever, lymphadenopathy, and eosinophilia. Unlike true serum sickness, SSLDR lacks circulating immune complexes, as well as vasculitis, purpura, hypocomplementemia, and renal insufficiency. Cefaclor is the most notorious causative agent, but penicillins, other cephalosporins, minocycline, griseofulvin, sulfonamide, or beta-blockers have been implicated. The syndrome subsides 2–3 weeks after the drug is stopped. Treatment consists of oral antihistamines; a short course of corticosteroids can be given early for severe cases.

Disposition of patients with cutaneous drug reactions

The management and disposition of patients with a drug reaction will be determined by the overall appearance of the patient, their hemodynamic stability, involvement of the airway, and the extent of the rash. Well-appearing patients who have completed a period of observation in the ED uneventfully can be discharged home with close follow-up. Thorough return precautions should be given to caregivers and the importance of cessation of the offending agent should be stressed. It may be helpful to emphasize that even when the offending agent is promptly stopped, the rash may take weeks to completely resolve (see also Ch. 85).

Pearls and pitfalls

Pearls

1. Cutaneous drug reactions can occur at any point after starting a medication.
2. Definitive treatment is to stop the offending medication.
3. Severe drug reactions are less common in pediatric patients than in adults.
4. Most drug rashes do not resolve quickly, even when the causative agent is stopped.

Pitfalls

1. Failure to stop the offending medication.
2. Failure to provide close follow-up for symptom recheck and initiation of a substitute medication.

Selected references

Morelli JG, Tay YK, Rogers M, *et al.* Fixed drug eruptions in children. *J Pediatr* 1999;**134**:365–367.

Roujeu J-C, Stern RS. Severe adverse cutaneous reactions to drugs. *N Engl J Med* 1994;**331**:1272–1285.

Stein KR, Scheinfeld NS. Drug-induced photoallergic and phototoxic reactions. *Expert Opin Drug Saf* 2007;**6**:431–443.

Weston WL, Land AT, Morelli JG. *Color Textbook of Pediatric Dermatology*, 4th edn. Philadelphia, PA: Mosby Elsevier, 2007.

Chapter 25

Dermatitis

Theresa M. van der Vlugt

Introduction

Dermatitis refers to inflammation of the epidermis and superficial dermis, often with an interrupted "eczematous" skin surface that can be fissuring, weeping and crusting. Disorders in this group discussed here are

- atopic dermatitis
- seborrheic dermatitis
- contact dermatitis
- nummular eczema.

Regional dermatitis (scalp and diaper) are discussed in Ch. 26.

Atopic dermatitis

Atopic dermatitis, commonly called "Eczema", is a skin disorder affecting 15–23% of children in the developed world, with a much decreased incidence in the developing world. Its cardinal features are (1) extreme pruritus; (2) early age of onset, with most cases beginning in the first 2 years of life, and the majority of those within the first 6 months; (3) an erythematous, scaling, cracking eruption, often weeping serous fluid and with characteristic age-dependent distributions (Fig. 25.1); and (4) chronic, relapsing-remitting course. All of these features make atopic dermatitis a not uncommon presenting complaint in the emergency setting.

Unrelenting pruritus is such a hallmark of atopic dermatitis that if the rash is *not* itchy, another diagnosis must be suspected.

Two-thirds of patients have a family history. Two-thirds of infants and children with atopic dermatitis will also develop allergic rhinitis, and half will develop asthma; this is the "atopic march." Current thinking is that atopic dermatitis is not caused by allergies to food or environmental triggers but rather is a co-occurrence in an allergic phenotype. Sufferers do have exacerbations of disease in response to stress and environmental triggers (dust mites, heat/sweating, dry air).

Skin findings

Infants present, often in the first 8 weeks of life, with itchy red plaques that scale, crack, and weep on the cheeks, chin, and scalp (Fig. 25.2). The nose is spared (headlight sign). They also have widespread plaques on the extensor surfaces such as knees and elbows, and on the anterior chest. The diaper area can be involved, but also is commonly spared.

The childhood form starts between 1 and 2 years of age and classically involves flexural surfaces such as antecubital and popliteal fossae, post-auricular and nuchal regions, ankles and wrists, and gluteal folds. Atopic dermatitis in adolescents and adults involves the palmar surfaces of hands and feet (Fig. 25.3), worsening involvement of face, neck, and posterior auricular areas, and in some cases continued flexural involvement. Eyelid involvement is common in all stages, and this can aid in diagnosis. Skin can develop pustules and secondary infection. Significant flares of atopic dermatitis usually stop when children are school aged, and approximately half will experience substantial clearing by puberty.

Differential diagnosis

Differential diagnosis includes:

- seborrheic dermatitis
- psoriasis
- inherited immunodeficiency syndromes
- dietary deficiencies, zinc and biotin
- contact dermatitis
- scabies
- tinea corporis.

Seborrheic dermatitis, has a very similar distribution, onset and appearance to atopic dermatitis in infants. It can be nearly impossible to distinguish the two, although there are two major differences: seborrheic dermatitis more frequently involves the diaper area and is not itchy. Consequently, babies with seborrheic dermatitis are "happy babies" and those with atopic dermatitis are not.

A Practical Guide to Pediatric Emergency Medicine: Caring for Children in the Emergency Department, ed. N. Ewen Amieva-Wang (associate eds. Jamie Shandro, Aparajita Sohoni, and Bernhard Fassl). Published by Cambridge University Press.

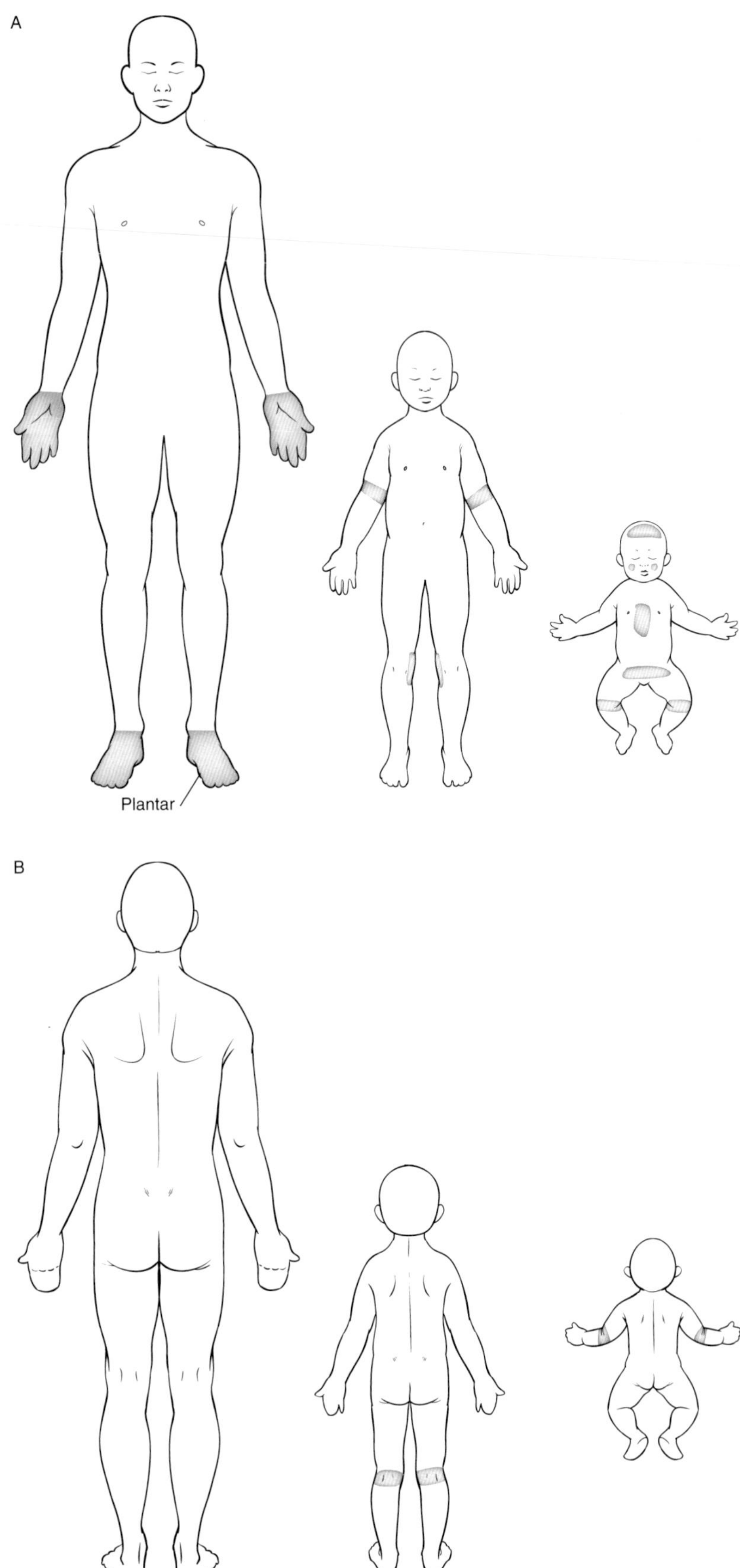

Figure 25.1 Age-dependent distribution of atopic dermatitis. Involvement of the face, scalp, trunk, and extensor surfaces of extremities in infants, flexural skin in toddlers, and hand and feet in preteenagers and adolescents. (Copyright Chris Gralapp.)

A

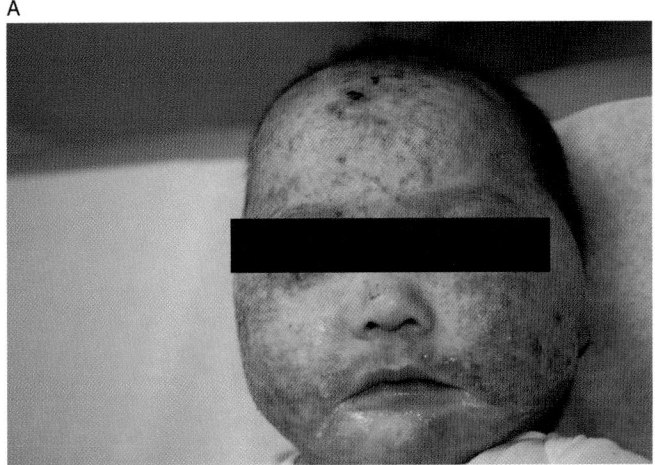

B

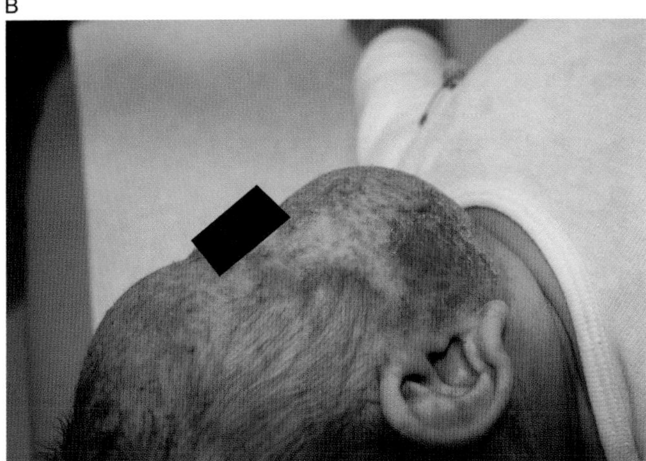

Figure 25.2 Atopic dermatitis in infancy with diffuse dryness, scaling and erythema. (Courtesy Mehran Moseley.)

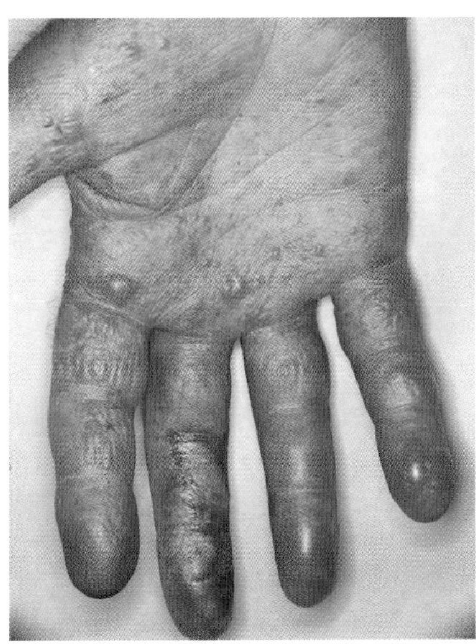

Figure 25.3 Dermatitis of hand and palm in adolescent with atopic dermatitis. (Reproduced with permission from Weston WL, Lane AT, Morelli JG. *Color Textbook of Pediatric Dermatology*, 4th edn. Philadelphia, PA: Mosby Elsevier, 2007. © 2007 Elsevier Inc.)

Psoriasis can mimic atopic dermatitis, and one-third of individuals with psoriasis have an onset in childhood. Again, atopic dermatitis is very pruritic and psoriasis is usually not. The childhood distribution of psoriasis also differs (Fig. 25.4), with psoriasis more common in the diaper area. Psoriatic lesions are well-demarcated patches and plaques with a rim of scale (Fig. 25.5), whereas atopic dermatitis lesions are poorly demarcated. In psoriasis, 25–50% have nail pitting or dimpling, while there is no nail involvement in atopic dermatitis.

Many patients with **inherited immunodeficiency syndromes** (such as Wiscott–Aldritch syndrome, Omenn syndrome, Hyper-IgE syndrome, and severe combined immunodeficiency syndromes) can have an itchy, diffuse, scaling, erythematous dermatitis that starts in infancy even before other symptoms, but they will also have lymphadenopathy, hepatosplenomegaly, recurrent infections, and failure to thrive.

Zinc deficiency and **biotin deficiency** in infancy can both mimic atopic dermatitis, but these patients are irritable, *not* itchy. They also have alopecia, diarrhea, and often marked perineal or perianal lesions with candidal superinfection. These deficiencies should always come to mind with difficult-to-treat diaper dermatitis.

Contact dermatitis is pruritic but very localized. It is uncommon in young children, and in infants is usually caused by nickel allergy from jewelry or snaps.

Scabies in infants and young children can cause a localized allergic reaction and a pruritic generalized dermatitis mimicking atopic dermatitis (Fig. 29.7, p. 158). There are differences in that; scabies mites

- favor flexural creases, interdigital spaces or palms/soles in young infants but usually spare the face (whereas atopic dermatitis usually involves the face)
- cause pustules on hands and feet but spare the soles and palms in young infants
- cause eczematous eruptions on the face and trunk in young infants
- rarely involve the head and neck areas in older children

Children commonly have secondary impetiginous infection. Visible skin burrows are diagnostic, as is demonstration of the eight-legged mite on skin scrapings. Other family members are often involved.

Tinea corporis is not common in infants and is much more common in children and teenagers. It presents as minimally itchy well-demarcated patches or plaques with increased inflammation and scale at the leading edge and often central clearing. Commonly, tinea corporis is treated as atopic dermatitis with topical steroids, which causes spreading and nonclearing of the patches.

Treatment

There is no "cure" for atopic dermatitis. Treatment centers on topical steroids and skin moisturization, with environmental

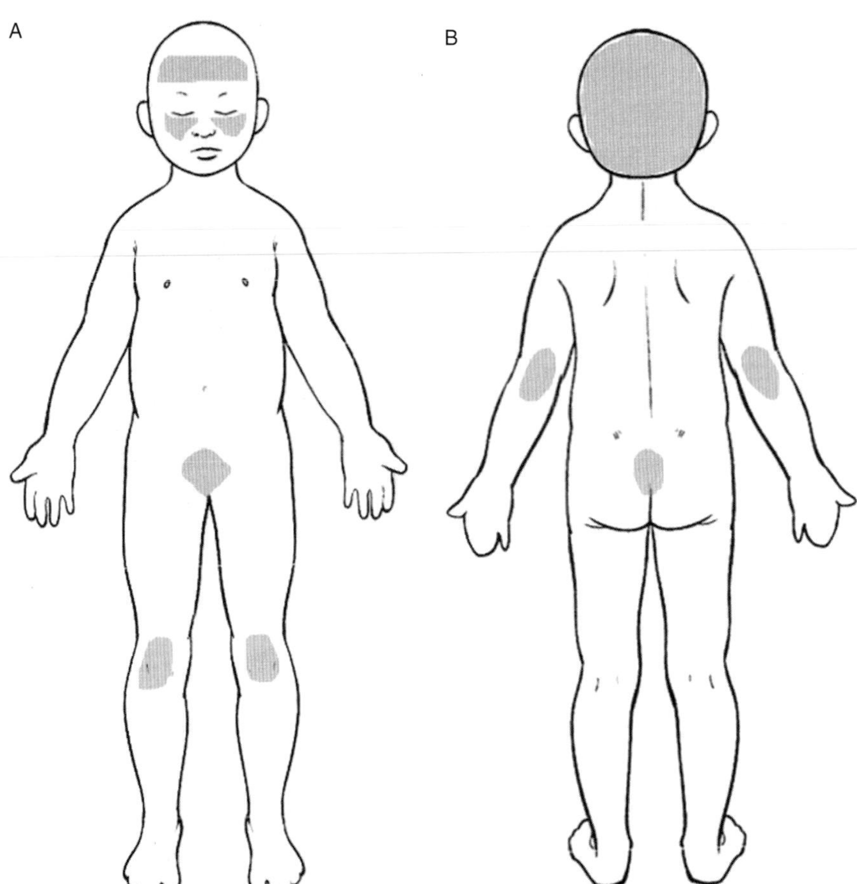

Figure 25.4 Distribution of childhood psoriasis. (Copyright Chris Gralapp.)

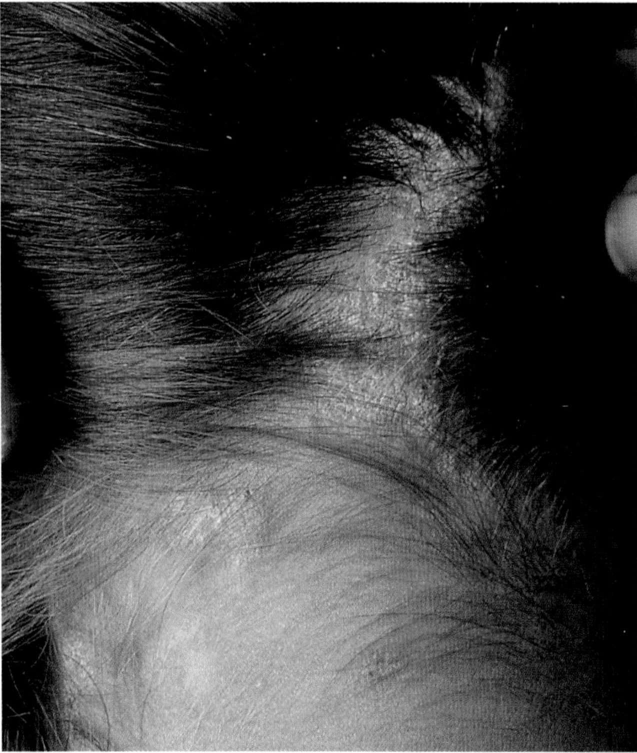

Figure 25.5 Psoriasis with plaques with typical thick silvery scales on the scalp of a child with psoriasis. (Courtesy Hans Kersten.)

modifications. Loose clothing, avoidance of sweating, humidifiers in dry air, and avoidance of fragranced detergents or fabric softeners can all help, as can minimizing skin irritation by scrubbing, washcloths, or brisk toweling. Traditional soaps and detergents should be avoided in favor of synthetic soaps or non-soap cleansers (Dove or Basis, Cetaphil or Aquanil), and baths should be short (5 min). Moisturizers should be applied immediately to skin that has only been patted with a towel to remove water beads. Petrolatum-based moisturizers (Vaseline, Aquaphor) are used for severe disease or in dry skin and dry environments, and water-based moisturizers (Cetaphil, Eucerin) can be used in less severe cases or in the summer. Skin should be moisturized several times a day.

Topical steroids are a mainstay of treatment, and flares of atopic dermatitis in children over age 3–6 months should be first treated with a moderate-potency (class 3–5) steroid cream or ointment twice daily (BID) for 2 weeks, and younger infants with a low-potency steroid BID for 2 weeks (Box 25.1). Studies and experience show that moderate and low-potency steroids can be used for long periods on skin with active dermatitis without significant risk of atrophy or hypothalamic–pituitary–adrenal axis suppression. Steroid penetrance is dramatically increased when steroids are used under an occlusive dressing, so only

Box 25.1. Topical steroids for use in atopic dermatitis

Low-potency topical steroids

Hydrocortisone (0.5%–2.5%): all ages.
Desonide 0.05%: 1 year and older.

Moderate potency

Fluticasone propionate cream 0.05% or ointment. 0.005%: 3 months and older.
Fluocinolone acetonide 0.025%: 1 year and older.
Prednicarbate 0.1%: 1 year and older.
Triamcinolone acetonide 0.1%: widely used for all ages.
Mometasone furoate (cream) 0.1%: 2 years and older.

low-potency steroids should be used in the diaper area or intertriginous zones.

Although the itch is not histamine mediated, many sources advocate the use of a sedating antihistamine 1 h before bedtime (such as diphenhydramine 1.25 mg/kg or hydroxyzine 1 mg/kg) to promote sleep during flares. Certirizine, a non-sedating antihistamine, has been shown to have some steroid-sparing effect in severe atopic dermatitis and can be given as a single dose in the morning.

Children with severe or widespread flares that are interfering with sleep can try "wet dressings." Before bed, steroid cream is applied to the dermatitis, then moisturizer is applied to the whole skin; finally, a pair of close-fitting cotton pajamas that has been soaked in warm water and wrung out until just damp should be put on the child. Then a second set of dry pajamas or a dry sleeper should be put over the damp one. The child's room should be warm enough that the child does not chill but not too warm. Wet dressings can be used for up to seven nights.

Complications

Children with atopic dermatitis have a higher risk of bacterial overgrowth and impetigo in areas of dermatitis, and a risk of more extensive viral infections. *Staphylococcus aureus* can be cultured from the lesions in 93% of the affected children, and 79% carry it in the nares. Patients with chronic atopic dermatitis are susceptible to bacterial superinfection, which can be diagnosed when the condition worsens with pustules, more demarcated or deeper erythema, and the honey-crusts of impetigo. This should be treated for 10–14 days with an oral antibiotic, choice to be determined by local sensitivities, with prior culture when these are complex.

Children with atopic dermatitis exposed to herpes simplex virus (HSV) can develop eczema herpeticum (Ch. 28). There is a widespread outbreak of painful herpetic lesions; patients are irritable and sick, with an increased risk of dehydration and bacterial superinfection. These lesions appear as punched-out erosions or vesicles with umbilication (Fig. 25.6). Eczema herpeticum must always be treated with antibiotics as well as oral or IV acyclovir. Subspecialty consultation should be obtained and hospitalization should be considered.

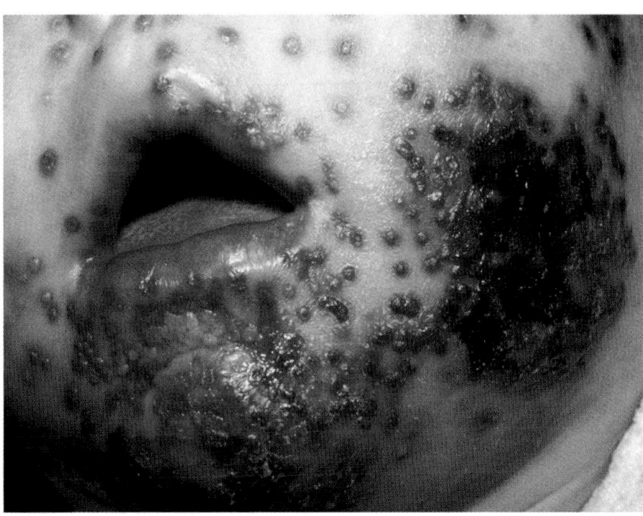

Figure 25.6 Eczema herpeticum: numerous vesicles and erosions from herpes simplex virus infecting atopic dermatitis. (Courtesy of Logical Images Inc.)

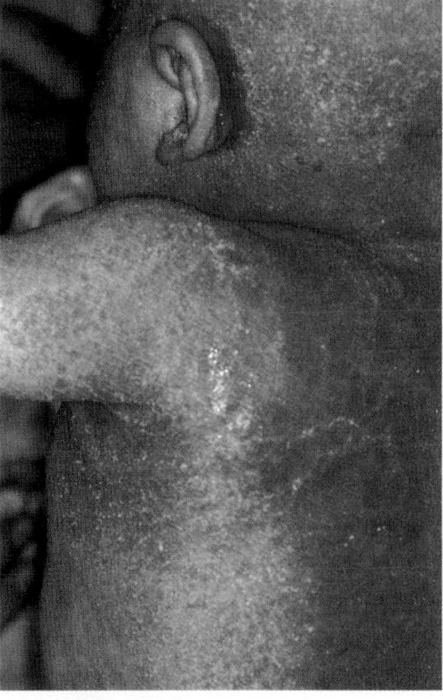

Figure 25.7 Infant seborrheic dermatitis. Greasy scales and erythema on the face, spreading to the neck and trunk. (Reproduced with permission from Weston WL, Lane AT, Morelli JG. *Color Textbook of Pediatric Dermatology*, 4th edn. Philadelphia, PA: Mosby Elsevier, 2007. © 2007 Elsevier Inc.)

Seborrheic dermatitis

Seborrheic dermatitis is characterized by salmon-colored (sometimes only faintly colored) patches with overlying yellowish greasy scale of the scalp, face, flexures, and diaper area in infants (Fig. 25.7). It is common in neonates and young infants, peaking at 8–12 weeks then completely clearing

Table 25.1. Differences between atopic and seborrheic dermatitis

Feature	Atopic dermatitis	Seborrheic dermatitis
Scale	Fine, dry and adherent	Yellowish and slightly greasy
Plaques	Less well defined	Clearly defined
Fissuring and weeping	Common	Rare
Itching	Markedly itchy	Not itchy
Rash in diaper area	Less common	Often involved

by 6–12 months. It is rarely seen in toddlers and children but resurfaces as a common scalp dermatitis ("dandruff") in adolescents, as well as adolescent dermatitis of eyebrows, nasolabial folds, posterior auricular areas, the moustache/beard area, and the hair-bearing chest. Seborrheic dermatitis in adolescents and adults is associated with an overgrowth of *Pityrosporum ovale*, a lipophilic yeast, but it is unclear if this is a problem in the infantile form.

Seborrheic and atopic dermatitis can be indistinguishable in young infants and can even co-occur in the same child. Unlike atopic dermatitis, seborrheic dermatitis is not very itchy even when it is widespread, and it rarely makes infants irritable. Other clues to diagnosis are given in Table 25.1.

Seborrheic dermatitis can be super infected with candida or bacteria, but this usually occurs in the diaper area or neck folds. Candidal superinfection lends to beefy red erythema with satellite papules and pustules, and bacterial superinfection also adds increased erythema and oozing.

Treatment

Treatment of mild cases of infantile seborrheic dermatitis may not be necessary, as spontaneous clearing with age is the rule. Non-clearing or widespread infantile seborrheic dermatitis should prompt consideration of a search for immunodeficiency.

Seborrheic dermatitis on the scalp is best treated with daily hair washing with a simple no-tears shampoo; more adherent or thicker scalp scale can be treated with a thin application of oil (mineral, baby, olive), followed by gentle scalp massage with fingers or a soft toothbrush (de-scaling), then shampooing with either plain or antiseborrheic shampoos (e.g., zinc pyrithionine, selenium sulfide 2.5%, 2% ketoconazole, keratolytic tar + sulfur/salicylic acid/T-gel). Lowest potency (hydrocortisone, desonide) topical steroid creams, lotions, or gels can be used throughout the body and face once or twice a day when there is a significant inflammatory component. Even low-potency steroid creams should not be used for more than a week or two on the face or in the diaper area (under occlusion) in infants. For older patients, consider adding topical azoles (e.g., ketoconazole cream), or sulfur-based lotion (10% sodium sulfacetamide and 5% sulfur).

If candidal superinfection is suspected in the diaper area, nystatin or econazole cream can be added. Topical antibiotics usually suffice for bacterial superinfection. For adolescents, there are a number of useful over-the-counter antiseborrhea shampoos based on tar, ketoconazole, selenium sulfide, salicylic acid, zinc pyrithionine, and 5% tea tree oil. Low-potency topical corticosteroid creams, gels and lotions can be used on the face and in the scalp for itchy or inflammatory cases.

Contact dermatitis

Contact dermatitis is classified as either **irritant** contact dermatitis or **allergic** contact dermatitis. The irritant form arises from direct, prolonged or repeated skin contact with an irritating substance such as harsh detergents or solvents, bubble baths, certain plants (citrus, carrot, spinach), saliva, urine, or feces. It is usually a non-specific inflammation of the epidermis and dermis in a specific but not sharply demarcated region, with or without eczematous (fissuring/weeping) change. It is not immune mediated, and is often *worsened* by application of topical steroids. Treatment involves avoiding the causative irritant and keeping the skin clean and dry but not overdry.

Allergic contact dermatitis is a type 4 hypersensitivity reaction that requires prior sensitization with the offending substance. It is uncommon in children under 1 year of age, and children with atopic dermatitis appear to be somewhat resistant to it. Acute allergic contact dermatitis is typically a sharply demarcated area of erythema, edema, papules, and oozing vesicles and bullae that is extremely pruritic. Forms caused by chronic exposure (such as a habitually worn piece of jewelry) usually lack vesicles and are more lichenified, with fissures and scaling. Nickel in jewelry or metal clothing fasteners is the most common source of allergic contact dermatitis in infants, causing circles of dermatitis where clothing snaps touch the skin (the top snap of jeans classically causes a periumbilical patch), earlobe dermatitis from pierced ears, or a circumferential neck dermatitis from a necklace. Nickel also commonly causes an "id reaction" (dermatophytid reaction), with widespread individual papulovesicles that co-occur or occur shortly after a flare of localized nickel contact dermatitis. Any flare of allergic contact dermatitis, other eczematous dermatitis, or cutaneous fungal infections can precipitate an "id" reaction. If allergic contact dermatitis occurs on the feet, it can be a reaction to chemicals used to treat rubber, to shoe leather, or to dyes, and is often misdiagnosed as tinea pedis. Tinea pedis is uncommon before adolescence and favors the arch and webspaces, which are usually spared in an allergic contact dermatitis related to shoe components.

Urishol-containing plants (poison ivy, oak, and sumac, all *Rhus* family) are a common cause of allergic contact

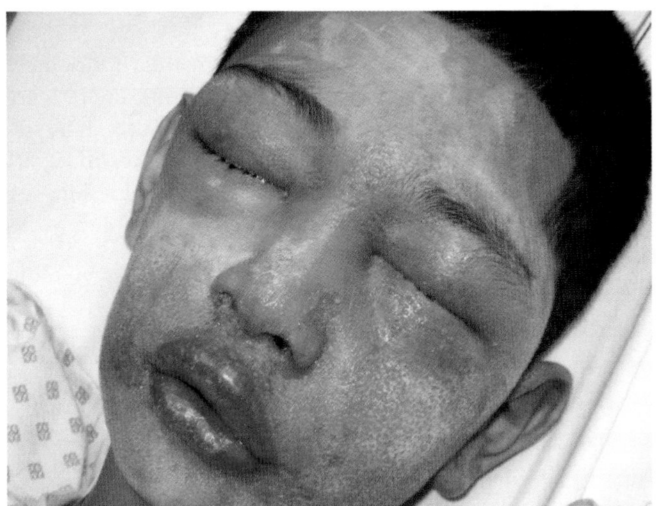

Figure 25.8 Rhus dermatitis of the face. Note facial swelling and fine vesiculation under the eyes with weeping lesions. (Courtesy of T. M. van der Vlugt.)

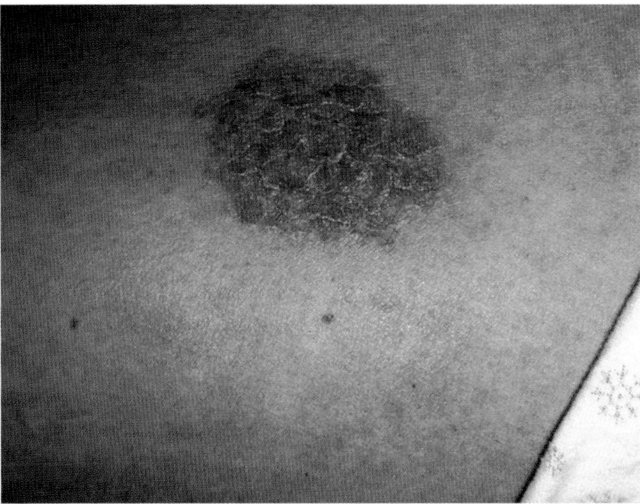

Figure 25.9 Nummular eczema. Coin-shaped lesions on the extremities. (Courtesy Steven Shpall.)

dermatitis, and 70% of the US population is sensitive to them. Contact causes a typical, very itchy, weepy, bullous dermatitis with linear streaks and borders from leaves or branches brushing against skin. Urishol oils bind quickly to skin, and known exposures should be washed with soap and water or a specific solvent (such as Technu) as soon as possible. When not promptly removed, urishol oils can be spread by contact (scratching) to previously uncontaminated skin: this is often the source of facial or genital involvement. Extensive facial exposure can simulate angioedema (Fig. 25.8) but is distinguished from this by fine vesiculation and weeping. Other common sensitizers, with the distribution of the reactions, are:

- *Rhus* plants (poison ivy, oak, sumac; can also cross-react with rind of mango): diverse distribution
- nickel: earlobes, neck, chest, wrist, periumbilical
- neomycin: diverse, often ear canal or from skin application
- potassium dichromate (in shoe leather): foot dermatitis
- rubber additives: foot, waistband or brassiere dermatitis
- lanolin: clothing distribution.

Treatment

Treatment of localized reactions can be accomplished with moderate- or lower-potency topical steroids twice a day, as well as removal of exposure to the offending antigen. Cool wet compresses of water or Burrow's solution can help. Experts disagree on the utility of calamine or other "shake" lotions for itch. Topical anti-itch creams with diphenhydramine or benzocaine can themselves be sensitizers and should be avoided. Severe *Rhus* dermatitis, particularly involving the face or genitals, can benefit from oral antihistamines and oral steroids, such as prednisone 1 mg/kg daily, tapered over 2–3 weeks. Popular steroid "dosepacks" do not provide a long enough course of steroids and can precipitate rebound symptoms when stopped too early. Patients should understand that even with removal of the offending sensitizer and treatment, allergic contact dermatitis does *not* resolve rapidly and can take several weeks to clear.

Pearls and pitfalls

Pearls

1. Atopic dermatitis (eczema) is the "itch that rashes." If the rash is not itchy, suspect another diagnosis.
2. Topical steroids and skin hydration are the cornerstones of eczema care.
3. Seborrheic dermatitis is characterized by salmon-colored patches with overlying yellowish greasy scale of the scalp, face, flexures, and diaper area in infants.

Pitfalls

1. Failure to recognize eczema herpeticum.
2. Failure to distinguish allergic contact dermatitis from tinea pedis.
3. Failure to treat allergic rhus contact dermatitis (such as poison ivy/oak) with a longer, 2–3 week steroid taper (when steroids are required).

Nummular eczema

Nummular eczema or nummular dermatitis is characterized by coin-shaped plaques, usually single or few, on the extensor surfaces of arms of legs, and occasionally on the face and trunk. It starts with tiny pruritic erythematous papules and pustules, which eventually coalesce into an exudative, crusted plaque that is greater than 1 cm and often 2–5 cm in diameter (Fig. 25.9).

It commonly starts around age 5 and is uncommon in younger children. Lesions last for months and will often reoccur, although the condition rarely lasts past puberty. The cause is unknown.

Nummular eczema is frequently confused with impetigo (but does not clear with antibiotics) or tinea corporis (but does not clear with antifungals). It can often look like an allergic contact dermatitis, so careful history is necessary. Nummular eczema can look like psoriasis, but lesions are more solitary, pustular, and oozing than those of psoriasis. It can co-occur in children with atopic dermatitis.

Treatment

Treatment is similar to that of atopic dermatitis. Twice-daily moderate potency steroid creams or ointments (better) are used, as well as oral antihistamines for itching. Topical mupirocin or oral antibiotics are indicated for staphylococcal superinfection. Families should be aware that individual lesions are difficult to resolve, and even with concerted effort 4–6 weeks may pass before improvement is seen.

Selected references

Kiken DA, Silverberg NB. Atopic dermatitis in children, Part 1: epidemiology, clinical features, and complications. *Pediatr Dermatol* 2006;**78**: 241–247.

Kiken DA, Silverberg NB. Atopic dermatitis in children, Part 2: treatment options. *Pediatr Dermatol* 2006;**78**:401–406.

Krol A, Krafchik B. The differential diagnosis of atopic dermatitis in childhood. *Dermatol Ther* 2006;**19**:73–82.

Chapter 26

Regional dermatitis

Theresa M. van der Vlugt

Introduction

Two common sites of dermatitis are the scalp and the diaper area. This chapter will review each of these disease entities. Scalp dermatitis refers to scaling and erythema of the scalp, with or without pruritus or alopecia. This condition may vary by age in a pronounced way (in order of likelihood):

- newborn to 3 months:
  - seborrheic dermatitis
  - atopic dermatitis
  - psoriasis
  - tinea capitis
  - Langerhan cell histiocytosis
  - zinc and biotin deficiencies
- 3 months to 12 years:
  - tinea capitis
  - atopic dermatitis
  - psoriasis
  - seborrheic dermatitis
- 12 years and older:
  - seborrheic dermatitis
  - atopic dermatitis
  - psoriasis
  - tinea capitis
  - contact dermatitis (hair products and dyes).

Alopecia areata has no erythema or scale but will be included here as a common scalp condition in childhood.

Diaper dermatitis affects up to 20% of children under 2 years of age. Persistent diaper dermatitis can be a manifestation of systemic diseases such as psoriasis, Langerhan cell histiocytosis, or zinc or biotin deficiency.

Scalp dermatitis

Clinical presentation and differential diagnosis

Scalp dermatitis may be caused by a number of different conditions that may be differentiated based on patient age and the clinical presentation. Scaling of the scalp in neonates ("cradle cap") is often simply physiologic retention of keratin and not necessarily a sign of pathology.

Tinea capitis and kerion (Fig. 26.1). Tinea capitis presents with scalp scaling and minimal to moderate scalp erythema, as well as patchy alopecia with the "black dot sign" (hairs broken off at skin surface). Severe tinea capitis can have pustules, cervical lymphadenopathy, and id reactions. "Kerion" is a severe infection of tinea capitis with a local, inflamed, boggy swelling of the scalp, often with overlying alopecia and purulent drainage. School-age children, particularly between 3 and 7 years old, are susceptible to tinea scalp infections (tinea capitis), and comparatively resistant to seborrheic dermatitis. Tinea capitis is usually caused by infection with *Trychophyton tonsurans* (>90% in the USA). Dermatophyte scalp infections are often spread from family member to family member, by hair care implements or in crowded conditions.

Seborrheic dermatitis. Infantile seborrheic dermatitis has asymptomatic mild erythema and greasy yellow scale, particularly with eyebrow, nasolabial, and posterior auricular involvement (Fig. 25.7, p. 140). Adolescents are also susceptible to seborrheic dermatitis (dandruff) and additionally get contact dermatitis from hair dyes and shampoos.

Atopic dermatitis. This often first occurs on the scalp and forehead but is very itchy and excoriated (Fig. 25.2, p. 137); plaques are poorly defined and can have patches of alopecia. Lesions are often present elsewhere on the body in typical age-related distributions.

Psoriasis. These lesions are well-defined erythematous plaques, with adherent fine silvery scale (Fig. 25.5, p. 139). The scalp is a common site of involvement in children, as well as the diaper area and flexor knees and elbows.

Langerhans cell histiocytosis. This uncommon dermatitis often presents before 3 months of age, with scalp and flexural "seborrheic" dermatitis overlying reddish-brown or purpuric papules. No response to usual seborrheic treatment is a diagnostic clue.

A Practical Guide to Pediatric Emergency Medicine: Caring for Children in the Emergency Department, ed. N. Ewen Amieva-Wang (associate eds. Jamie Shandro, Aparajita Sohoni, and Bernhard Fassl). Published by Cambridge University Press.

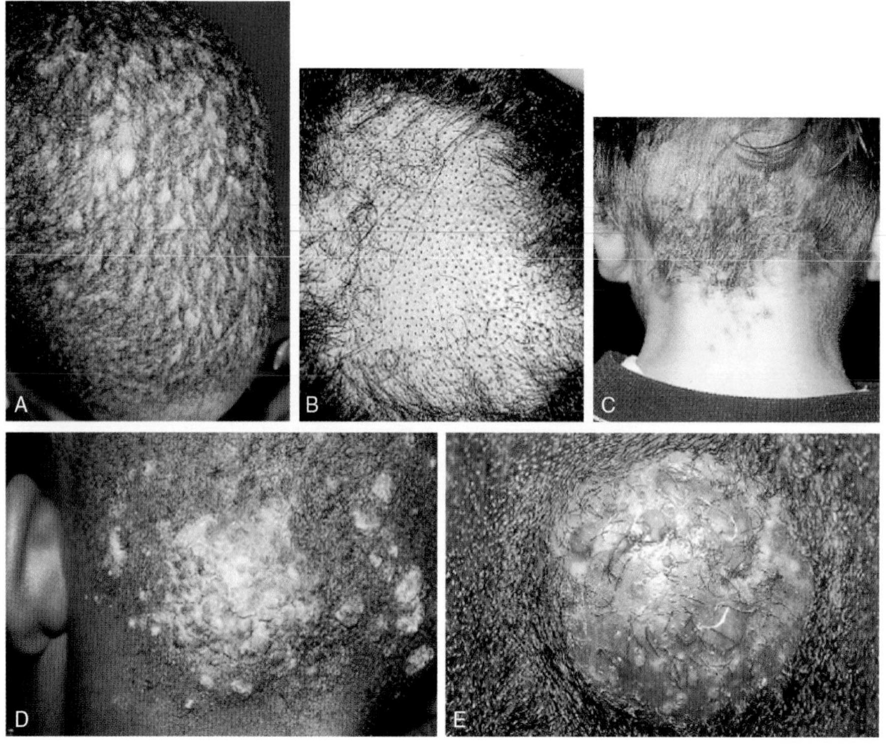

Figure 26.1 Tinea capitis can present in many guises. (A) in this child, mild erythema and scaling of the scalp are associated with spotty alopecia. (B) Infiltration of hair shafts by endothrix has resulted in widespread breakage at the scalp, producing a "salt and pepper" appearance. (C) Superficial papules and pustules have ruptured, producing weeping and crusting lesions, simulating impetigo. (D) This variant of tinea is characterized by thick heaped-up scale. (E) Kerion. A boggy mass has formed as a result of an intense inflammatory response. The lesion is studded with pustules. (Reproduced with permission from Zitelli BJ, Davis HW. *Atlas of Pediatric Physical Diagnosis*, 5th edn. Philadelphia, PA: Mosby Elsevier, 2007. © 2007 Mosby Inc., an affiliate of Elsevier Inc.)

Alopecia areata. Well-circumscribed areas of hair loss appear in otherwise well-appearing children. These areas have no signs of trauma or hair growth, nor do they have erythema or scale. Other parts of the body (eyelashes, eyebrows, sexual hair) may be involved. Alopecia areata is thought to be an autoimmune process. The alopecia in this condition differs from that in tinea capitis in that the latter has scale, erythema, and the "black dot" sign. It differs from that in atopic dermatitis in that atopic dermatitis has severe pruritus and an age-related lesional distribution. Zinc and biotin deficiency have alopecia, but also many other clinical signs.

Diagnostic studies

When tinea capitis is suspected, potassium hydroxide (KOH) microscope evaluation of "black dot" hair scrapings or scrapings of the leading, active edge of a plaque will show septated fungal hyphae. Fungal culture is diagnostic. Clinical diagnosis is usually sufficient for seborrheic dermatitis, atopic dermatitis, and alopecia areata, while psoriasis and Langerhans cell histiocytosis require biopsy for definitive diagnosis.

Treatment

Treatment of tinea capitis must always be systemic; the gold standard is still griseofulvin 20–25 mg/kg daily for 6–8 weeks. Griseofulvin should be taken with milk or fatty food to increase absorption. Consider adjunctive therapy with sporicidal shampoo (selenium sulfide 2.5%). Fluconazole 3–6 mg/kg daily for 2–4 weeks is also effective, as is terbinafine (same dosing as fluconazole, up to 250 mg daily). Both have fewer side effects than itraconazole and ketoconazole. All of these have drug–drug and drug–disease interactions that must be checked before use.

Kerion, in particular, has high risk of permanent scarring alopecia and should also be cultured and treated with antibiotics in addition to systemic antifungals, and also with steroids 0.5–1 mg/kg daily for 2–4 weeks. Children with large, purulent kerion and extensive associated id reactions can appear quite ill and are frequently hospitalized.

For seborrheic dermatitis in infants, daily hair washing with a no-tears shampoo and gentle de-scaling with mineral or olive oil and a soft toothbrush usually suffices. Adolescents or younger children with severe seborrheic dermatitis can use antiseborrheic shampoos (e.g., zinc pyrithionine, selenium sulfide 2.5%, 2% ketoconazole, keratolytic tar + sulfur/salicylic acid/T-gel).

Atopic dermatitis is treated with low- or moderate-potency steroids and skin moisturization, as well as avoidance of triggers (see Ch. 25 for details).

In alopecia areata, topical treatments including steroids may induce short-term hair growth, but in 90% of cases spontaneous hair-growth will eventually recur.

Diaper dermatitis

Diaper dermatitis affects up to 20% of children under 2 years of age. The major causes of diaper dermatitis are:

- irritant contact dermatitis
- allergic contact dermatitis

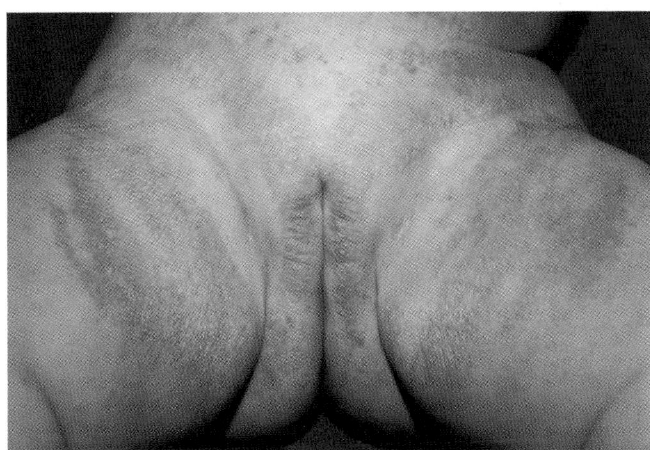

Figure 26.2 Chafing diaper dermatitis with involvement of the convex surface of the thighs, buttocks, and waist area. (Reproduced with permission from Weston WL, Lane AT, Morelli JG. *Color Textbook of Pediatric Dermatology*, 4th edn. Philadelphia, PA: Mosby Elsevier, 2007. © 2007 Elsevier Inc.)

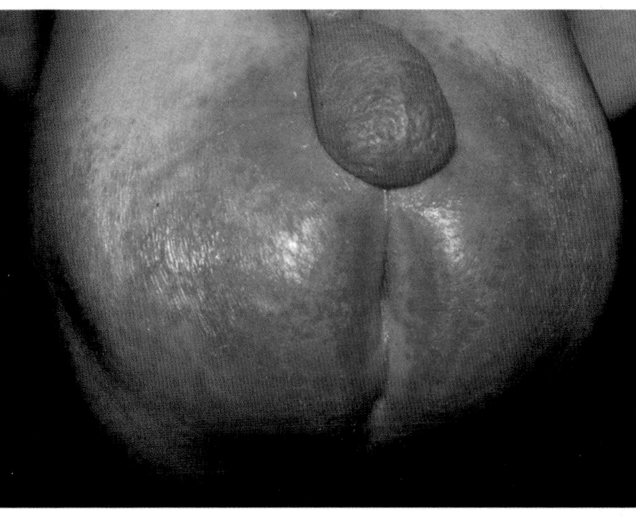

Figure 26.3 Irritant contact diaper dermatitis. Erythema and scaling involve the convex surfaces and intertriginous creases. (Courtesy of Logical Images Inc.)

- candidal infection
- streptococcal and staphylococcal superinfected contact dermatitis
- seborrheic dermatitis
- atopic dermatitis
- psoriasis
- streptococcal perianal or perivaginal cellulitis
- zinc or biotin deficiency
- Langerhans cell histiocytosis.

Persistent diaper dermatitis can be a manifestation of systemic disease, such as psoriasis, Langerhan cell histiocytosis, or zinc or biotin deficiency.

Irritant contact dermatitis. This is the most common diaper dermatitis. It occurs secondary to irritation of urine and feces in the diaper area. It can be "chafing" with mild, shiny, sometimes faintly striated erythema on the convex surfaces of the buttocks, lower abdomen, and thighs (Fig. 26.2).

Wet irritant contact dermatitis. This form can cause erythema and maceration, sometimes with shallow ulcers in the intertriginal folds and on the genitalia (Fig. 26.3). Treatment consists of keeping the skin dry with frequent diaper changes. Urine and feces should be removed promptly from the skin with *water only* if possible. Care should be taken not to overclean, overrub, or otherwise irritate already irritated skin. The clean, dry, diaper-area skin can then be covered with a greasy ointment before the diaper is reapplied. Occlusive plastic or rubber diaper covers should be avoided. Topical steroids should be avoided for this (and most) types of diaper dermatitis.

Candidal diaper dermatitis. In already active diaper dermatitis, the skin can be colonized by *Candida albicans*, often within 72 h. Candidal diaper dermatitis is uncommon after age 1. Candidal dermatitis will often start in the perianal area and can spread to involve the genitals, inguinal creases, buttocks, thighs, and upper abdomen. It is characteristically a beefy-red well-demarcated plaque, with oval-shaped satellite pustules and papules around the periphery (Fig. 26.4). Treatment initiates with local skin care as described above, as well as with topical antifungals (econazole or nystatin cream) twice a day until clear. This can be applied under the barrier ointment used to keep the skin dry. Again, steroid creams should be avoided if possible.

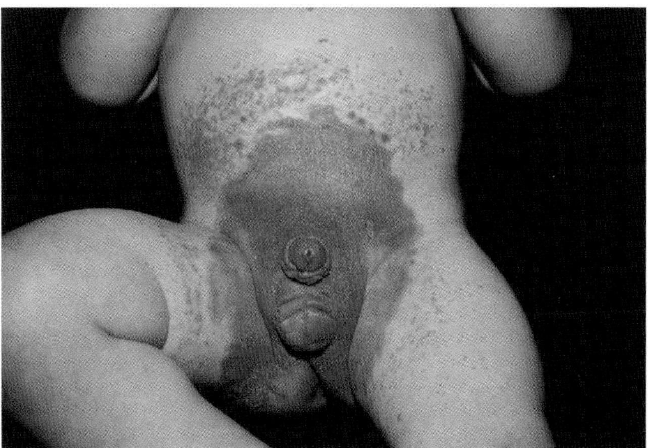

Figure 26.4 Candidal diaper dermatitis with bright red confluent erythema involving the inguinal creases and genitalia. Satellite oval lesions can be seen. (Reproduced with permission from Weston WL, Lane AT, Morelli JG. *Color Textbook of Pediatric Dermatology*, 4th edn. Philadelphia, PA: Mosby Elsevier, 2007. © 2007 Elsevier Inc.)

Atopic dermatitis. This diaper dermatitis is difficult to distinguish from wet irritant contact dermatitis, although

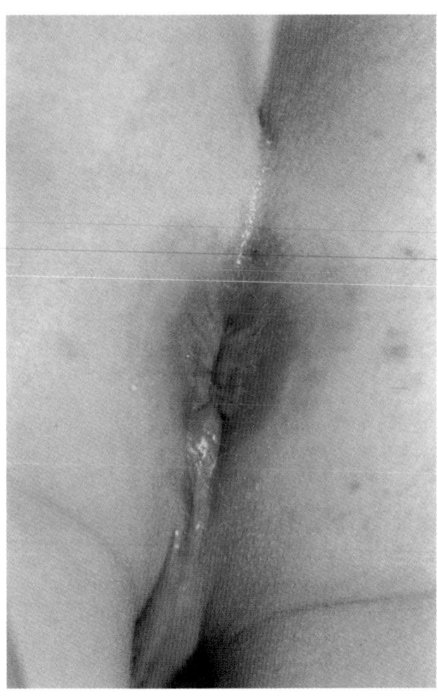

Figure 26.5 Perianal streptococcal infection with acutely red and painful perianal skin. (Reproduced with permission from Weston WL, Lane AT, Morelli JG. *Color Textbook of Pediatric Dermatology*, 4th edn. Philadelphia, PA: Mosby Elsevier, 2007. © 2007 Elsevier Inc.)

Pearls and pitfalls

Pearls

1. Consider seborrheic dermatitis, psoriasis, and candidiasis when the intertriginous areas are involved, and also when there are lesions in other areas of the body.
2. The most common cause of diaper dermatitis is irritant contact dermatitis, which should be treated with non-irritating cleansing, frequent diaper changes and a barrier cream.

Pitfalls

1. Steroids should be avoided in all diaper dermatitis except for atopic dermatitis.
2. Failure to identify a kerion.
3. Failure to consider perianal or perivaginal streptococcal infections.

the diaper area is often spared in atopic dermatitis. Children with diaper atopic dermatitis have stigma of the condition elsewhere in the age-appropriate distributions, and all affected skin is very itchy. In this case steroids are indicated. For most diaper dermatitis, particularly irritant diaper dermatitis, avoid anything stronger than hydrocortisone 1% (and use this only for <1 week).

Seborrheic dermatitis. This is common in the diaper area, but affected children would be expected to have seborrheic dermatitis elsewhere in the appropriate distributions, such as the scalp. A greasy yellow scale is pathognomonic. Spontaneous clearing is the rule.

Perianal or perivaginal streptococcal cellulitis. The usual cause is group A beta-hemolytic streptococci. Streptococcal cellulitis presents as a well-defined circumanal or circumvaginal erythema that is markedly tender and can have fissures, superficial erosions, or purulent discharge (Fig. 26.5). Children often become constipated secondary to retention of painful bowel movements. Diagnosis can be confirmed by bacterial culture or rapid strep testing; if rapid strep testing is negative, *S. aureus* or coliform bacteria may be found on culture. Presumptive treatment with oral penicillin or erythromycin is indicated.

Difficult to treat or persistent diaper dermatitis should prompt a search for zinc or biotin deficiency, Langerhan cell histiocytosis, or severe inherited immunodeficiencies (AIDS, complement deficiencies, hyper-IgE syndrome, Omenn syndrome, X-linked agammaglobulinemia, Wiskott–Aldritch syndrome).

Selected references

Krol A, Krafchik B. The differential diagnosis of atopic dermatitis in childhood. *Dermatol Ther* 2006;**19**:73–82.

Paller AS, Mancini AJ. *Hurwitz Clinical Pediatric Dermatology, a Textbook of Skin Disorders in Childhood and Adolescence.* Philadelphia, PA: Elsevier Saunders, 2006.

Weston WL, Land AT, Morelli JG. *Color Textbook of Pediatric Dermatology*, 4th edn. Philadelphia, PA: Mosby Elsevier, 2007.

Chapter 27 General dermatology

Theresa M. van der Vlugt

Pyogenic granuloma

Pyogenic granuloma is a small acquired vascular tumor, common in children and pregnant women. Pyogenic granulomas are thought to be an abnormal healing response.

Clinical presentation

Pyogenic granuloma presents as a rapidly growing bright red sessile or slightly pedunculated nodule, often at the sites of minor trauma (hands, face, oral mucosa, forearms) (Fig. 27.1). It can have a small collarette of scale at the base, and is usually under 1 cm in diameter. The nodule is usually not painful or itchy. The surface is fragile, often crusted or ulcerated, and it will bleed briskly with even minor trauma, which is the hallmark of this lesion and a common cause of ED presentation.

Treatment

Usually 5–10 min of firm direct pressure is required to stop bleeding. Pyogenic granulomas must be completely excised, preferably by a dermatologist. Some are amenable to laser treatment.

Pityriasis rosea

Pityriasis rosea has long been thought to have a viral etiology caused by seasonal local epidemics, and occasional prodromes, but the cause is still unknown.

Clinical presentation

Classically older children and young adults develop a "herald patch," a pink scaly oval patch of dermatitis with raised borders and central clearing on the trunk, upper arm, neck, or thigh (Fig. 27.2). Incidence of the herald patch is reported variably at 20–80%. A few days or weeks after the herald patch, an eruption of small salmon-pink ovoid macules and faintly raised papules with fine central scale appears on the trunk, scalp, and extremities, sparing the face in 85%. Smaller lesions can have a "collarette" of scale. Lesions follow skin lines of cleavage and can appear in the pathognomonic symmetric "Christmas tree" pattern on the back. Oral and palm or sole lesions are uncommon. The "inverse pattern" of pityriasis rosea, more common in younger children and African-American individuals, has relative truncal sparing and lesions on the face, neck, groin, and axilla.

A

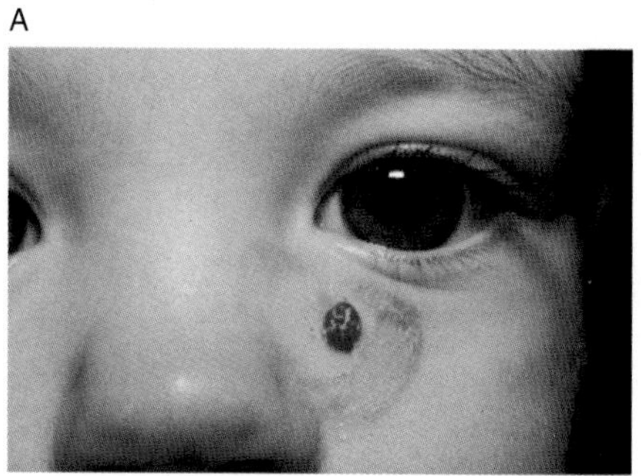

B

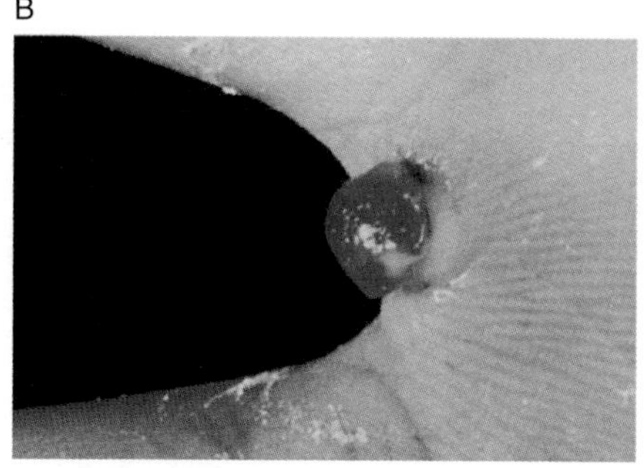

C

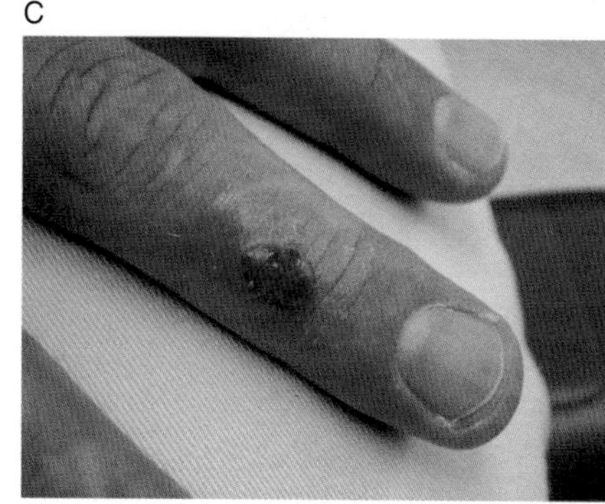

Figure 27.1 Pyogenic granuloma. (A–C) An acquired, vascular papule that is erythematous and friable. The friability of the lesion on the hand (C) is particularly evident. (A,B reprinted with permission from Paller, AS, Manicini AJ (eds.) *Hurwitz Clinical Pediatric Dermatology: A Textbook of Skin Disorders of Childhood and Adolescence* 3rd edn. Philadelphia, PA: Elsevier Saunders, 2006. © 2006 Saunders Inc., an affiliate of Elsevier Inc. C, courtesy Steven Shpall.)

A Practical Guide to Pediatric Emergency Medicine: Caring for Children in the Emergency Department, ed. N. Ewen Amieva-Wang (associate eds. Jamie Shandro, Aparajita Sohoni, and Bernhard Fassl). Published by Cambridge University Press.

A

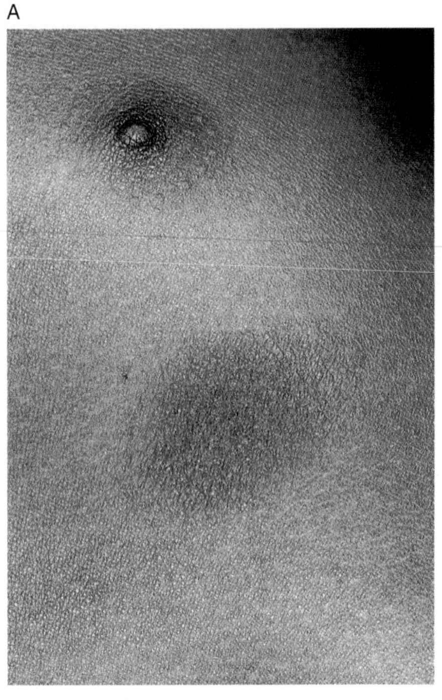

B

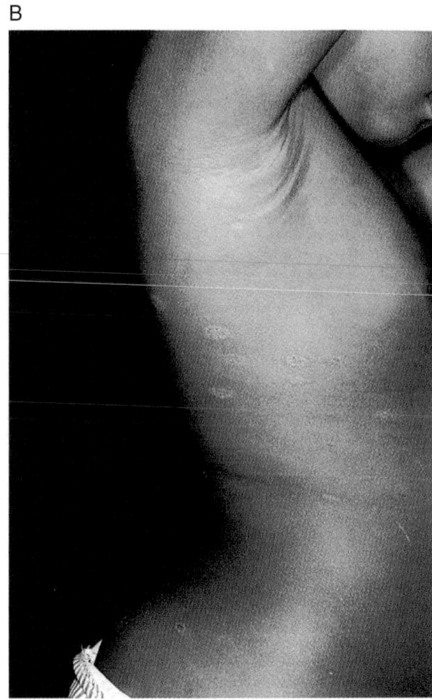

C

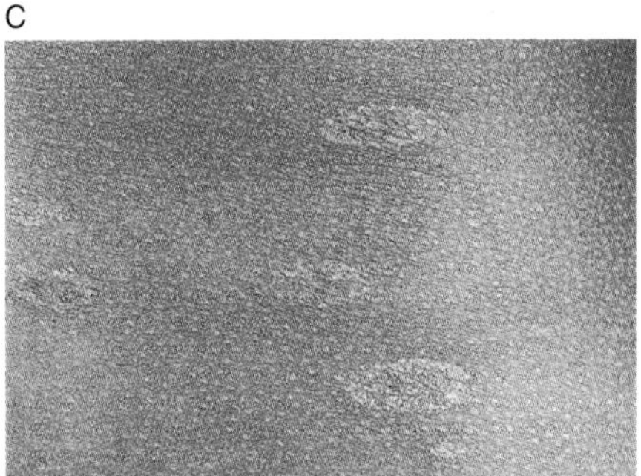

Figure 27.2 Pityriasis rosea (PR). (A) The herald patch preceded the PR eruption by about 10 days in this child. (B,C) Oval-shaped papulosquamous PR eruption; most of the eruptions are truncal in distribution (B). Conformation to skin lines is often more discernible in the anterior and posterior axillary folds and supraclavicular areas. A fine wrinkled tissue-like scale remains attached within the border of the plaque, giving the characteristic ring of "collarette" scale. This can be seen in the close up of the papulosquamous oval-shaped lesions (C). The axes of the oval plaques are distributed along the skin lines. Numerous lesions on the back, oriented along the skin lines (parallel to the ribs) give the appearance of drooping pine-tree branches (Christmas tree distribution). (Reprinted with permission from Shah BR, Lucchesi M (eds). *Atlas of Pediatric Emergency Medicine*. New York: McGraw Hill, 2006.)

Differential diagnosis

Differential diagnosis of the herald patch includes tinea corporis or nummular eczema (Fig. 25.9, p. 142). If the herald patch is mistakenly treated with systemic antifungals, the ensuing widespread eruption can be mistaken for an id reaction or drug reaction. When the herald patch is missed or not present, the generalized eruption can be confused with viral exanthems. Differential diagnosis in sexually active individuals must include syphilis, particularly with palm or sole lesions. Testing samples with KOH will always differentiate tinea; the scale of guttate psoriasis is thicker, silvery, and adherent; secondary syphilis usually has no scale and has concurrent constitutional symptoms. Inverse pityriasis rosea can mimic seborrheic dermatitis but lacks the typical greasy yellow scale of seborrheic dermatitis.

Treatment

Patients are usually asymptomatic and can be reassured that lesions will clear over weeks to months and leave normal skin. Judicious sunlight or mild sunlamp exposure hastens resolution and helps with itching. Oral antihistamines can alleviate pruritus. Steroids can also be considered for dark-skinned individuals with significant neck or face lesions, which are at risk for post-inflammatory hyper- or hypopigmentation.

Cold panniculitis

Cold panniculitis occurs primarily in younger children and toddlers, on the cheeks and other fat-layered areas, in response to popsicles, cold compresses, or cold weather. The fatty tissue of younger children is thought to solidify more readily in the cold because it contains a higher percentage of saturated fat.

Clinical presentation

Lesions are tender, erythematous indurated plaques or nodules on cold-exposed skin, usually on the cheeks or in the perioral area, which are noted a few hours to a few days after cold exposure. They blanch little or not at all, lack the warmth of cellulitis or erysipelas, and there are no constitutional symptoms.

Treatment

Lesions take weeks and sometimes months to completely resolve, leaving a slightly hyperpigmented area that fades with time. There is no treatment other than symptomatic pain relief.

Pearls and pitfalls

Pearls

1. Pyogenic granuloma must be removed by excision. Most bleeding can be controlled with 5–10 min of firm direct pressure.

Pitfalls

1. Failure to recognize pityriasis rosea as a self-resolving rash.
2. Treating cold panniculitis with antibiotics.

Selected references

Bjorje Nelson JS, Stone MS. Update on selected viral exanthems. *Curr Opin Pediatr* 2000;**12**:359–264.

Paller AS, Mancini AJ. *Hurwitz Clinical Pediatric Dermatology, a Textbook of Skin Disorders in Childhood and Adolescence*. Philadelphia, PA: Elsevier Saunders, 2006.

Wagner AM. An 8-year-old girl with an enlarging papule on the eyelid. *Pediatr Ann* 2006;**35**:429–430.

Weston WL, Land AT, Morelli JG. *Color Textbook of Pediatric Dermatology*, 4th edn. Philadelphia, PA: Mosby Elsevier; 2007.

Chapter 28

Herpes simplex infections

Theresa M. van der Vlugt

Introduction

Infections with herpes simplex virus (HSV) types 1 and 2 are common in all age groups worldwide. One-third of the world's population has recurrent HSV-1 infection; 20% have recurrent HSV-2. While more than 80% of primary HSV-1 and HSV-2 infections are asymptomatic, once infection has occurred, the virus is always latent in nerve ganglia and can reactivate. Infected children and adults shed virus during reactivation as well as when they are asymptomatic. There are different presentations of HSV infection in neonates, infants, children, and adolescents.

Neonates, the immunosuppressed, and children with atopic dermatitis are at risk for significant and severe disease.

Clinical presentation

The clinical presentation will vary with the site of infection.

Herpetic gingivostomatitis accounts for 60% of all herpes infections in children 6 months to 5 years (Fig. 28.1), with the possibility of later herpes labialis "cold sore" reactivations. Most are caused by HSV-1. During primary infection, the patient can have high fever, tender cervical adenopathy, poor oral intake because of pain, and bad breath. All forms of recurrent HSV often have a 6–48 h prodrome of tingling, itching, burning, or pain in the distribution where vesicles will appear.

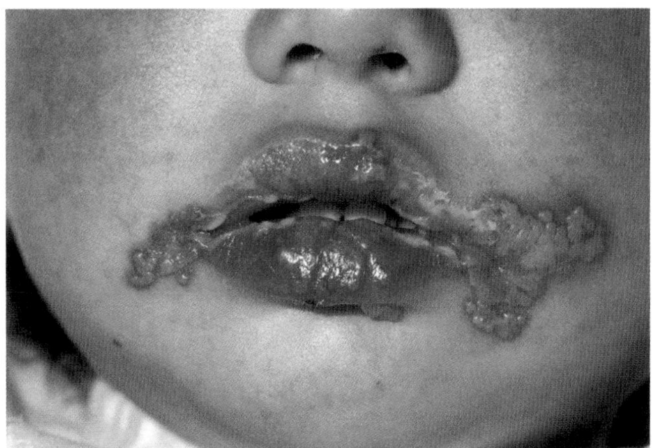

Figure 28.1 Infant with primary herpes gingivostomatitis. (Reproduced with permission from Weston WL, Lane AT, Morelli JG *Color Textbook of Pediatric Dermatology*, 4th edn. Philadelphia, PA: Mosby Elsevier, 2007. © 2007 Elsevier Inc.)

The lesions of herpes are often a continuum between exanthem and enanthem. Herpetic gingivostomatitis starts with small vesicles on an erythematous base on the tongue, gingival mucosa, and anterior palate, and it progresses to painful erosions and ulcerations with a gray or white base. Perioral skin is often involved. It persists for 7–14 days, although the fever persists only 2–6 days.

Herpes labialis ("cold sores" or "fever blisters") is recurrent HSV infection of the lip and occurs in 20–50% of children who have had a previous HSV infection. The lesions of herpes labialis appear as painful grouped vesicles that rupture and crust on the top or bottom lip following sun exposure, stress, an acute febrile illness, or menstruation. These lesions generally last 5–10 days.

Herpes facialis is recurrent outbreaks of clustered vesicles on an erythematous base on the cheek, forehead, or around the eye. Similar crops of lesions occur in and are spread between participants in contact sports such as wrestling or rugby (herpes gladiatorum or herpes rugbeiorum), typically on the head and neck, sometimes on the extremities and trunk. It is important to remember that HSV infection on the face near the eye has the potential for affecting the eye (HSV keratitis). Recurrent herpes facialis or gladiatorum is often confused with impetigo or herpes zoster and can be difficult to distinguish without culture or PCR.

Herpetic keratoconjunctivitis is an ocular emergency and can occur as primary, autoinnoculated, or recurrent infection (Ch. 119).

Herpetic whitlow can develop in thumb-sucking children with herpetic gingivostomatitis or herpes labialis. This is a fingertip infection with deep-seated painful white clustered vesicles on an erythematous base. Herpetic whitlow is often confused with common paronychia but often has no or scant pus on incision and drainage.

A Practical Guide to Pediatric Emergency Medicine: Caring for Children in the Emergency Department, ed. N. Ewen Amieva-Wang (associate eds. Jamie Shandro, Aparajita Sohoni, and Bernhard Fassl). Published by Cambridge University Press.

Genital herpes occurs primarily in adolescents (majority HSV-2, increasingly HSV-1) and its presence in prepubertal children should raise a strong suspicion of sexual abuse. Patients complain of severe pain, itching, dysuria, discharge, and tender inguinal adenopathy. Primary infections may have fever, headache, myalgia, and malaise. There is tremendous variation in severity and presentation of genital herpes. Primary infections tend to be more severe, with the typical vesicles becoming ulcers on vulvar, penile, scrotal, or perianal mucosa. Lesions will last 2–3 weeks before resolution.

Neonatal herpes presents as either disseminated herpes (25%) (Ch. 28), CNS disease with or without skin lesions (30%), or limited skin, eyes, and mouth involvement (Ch. 156). Involvement of the skin, eyes, and mouth usually presents in the first week of life with typical HSV lesions in these areas. Before the availability of antviral drugs, neonatal herpes on the skin, eyes, or mouth previously progressed 60–70% of the time to more severe involvement, but recent use of these drugs has reduced this progression significantly.

Eczema herpeticum/Kaposi's varicelliform eruption (Fig. 25.6, p. 140) occurs in children with atopic dermatitis or other skin disorders that disrupt the epithelial barrier (i.e., seborrheic dermatitis, bullous pemphigoid, or even with severe burns). These skin lesions result in exposure of underlying dermis, which then becomes super infected with HSV-1 or HSV-2. Other viruses have also been implicated in eczema herpeticum. Diagnosis is confirmed with Tzanck smear of a lesion showing multinucleated giant cells, and by other serological testing and skin biopsies.

Diagnosis

Diagnosis is based on pattern recognition for the rash, as well as confirmatory viral culture or polymerase chain reaction (PCR) of lesions, or typical Tzank smear (now rarely performed). Herpetic gingivostomatitis can be confused with herpangina, but the latter is usually strictly posterior pharyngeal and rarely if ever has lip lesions. Hand, foot, and mouth disease and apthous ulcers can be similar, but have many fewer lesions than HSV and no fever.

Management/disposition

The majority of herpes infections seen in the ED are benign in well-appearing children and will require oral antiviral treatment and close outpatient follow-up. Neonates, patients who are immunocompromised, with concern for diffuse, CNS, or multiorgan system involvement, or who appear ill, warrant admission for further evaluation and treatment. Otherwise, the following guidelines should be reviewed for management of outpatient herpes infections:

Primary gingivostomatitis benefits from treatment with oral acyclovir 15 mg/kg per dose (up to 200 mg/dose) five times a day for 7–10 days, when started within the first 72 h, with decreased duration of lesions and significantly decreased time of viral shedding. Famcyclovir and valacyclovir are not FDA approved for children but are used off-label because of easier dosing schedules. Antiviral and over-the-counter creams are minimally effective and not recommended. Topical or systemic analgesics can be necessary. Viscous lidocaine should be used with care because gingival numbness can lead to further buccal trauma from chewing. Dehydration is a common complication of herpetic gingivostomatitis in infants and young children and can require IV rehydration.

Primary genital herpes is treated similarly to gingivostomatitis, but treatment can be started within 6 days of onset of disease. Recurrent labial or genital disease benefits modestly from episodic acyclovir therapy, and treatment may not be necessary for mild occurrences. Continuous suppressive therapy (acyclovir 80 mg/kg daily divided into three doses for 6–12 months) can be used for children with very frequent recurrences.

Herpetic whitlow should also be treated with oral acyclovir. Herpes facialis often does not require treatment, but herpes gladiatorum is often treated with acyclovir to minimize viral shedding or spread to other competitors.

Recurrent herpetic lesions are common throughout life with all forms of HSV infection. Children with HSV reactivation can develop erythema multiforme and even recurrent erythema multiforme, now understood to be an immune-mediated response to HSV antigens in the skin. Bacterial secondary infection of HSV skin lesions can occur. In addition, HSV has been implicated in Bell's palsy, trigeminal neuralgia, ascending myelitis, and post-infectious encephalomyelitis.

Pearls and pitfalls

Pearls

1. Neonatal herpes (Ch. 88) can present as fulminant sepsis within the first week of life (with or without lesions), isolated vesicles on the skin and mucous membranes, or encephalitis with or without skin lesions.
2. All presentations of possible neonatal herpes are an emergency and should prompt immediate evaluation and initiation of therapy with systemic acyclovir.

Pitfalls

1. Failure to treat for herpes simplex virus in a neonate with a seizure or fulminant sepsis.
2. Failure to recognize eczema herpeticum in children with an underlying skin disease.
3. Failure to consider and treat dehydration in children with herpes gingivostomatitis.

In eczema herpeticum, treatment with IV acyclovir should be initiated as soon as possible. Systemic antibiotics to cover possible bacterial superinfection should also be started. The major complications include multisystem involvement (brain, liver, lung, ocular), with significant hemodynamic instability from this generalized infection. Specialty consultation should be obtained and these children should strongly be considered for admission.

Selected references

Amir J, Harel L, Smetana Z, Varsano I. Treatment of herpes simplex gingivostomatitis with acyclovir in children: a randomized double-blind placebo controlled study. *Br Med J* 1997;**314**:1800.

Feigin RD, Cherry JD, Demmler GJ, *et al. Textbook of Pediatric Infectious Diseases*, 5th edn. Philadelphia, PA: Saunders, 2004.

Kimberlin DW. Herpes simplex virus infections in neonates and early childhood. *Pediatr Infect Dis* 2005;**16**:271–281.

Chapter 29

Non-bacterial infections and infestations

Theresa M. van der Vlugt

Introduction

This chapter covers tinea, candida, warts, molluscum, scabies, and lice.

Fungal infections: tinea and candida

Dermatophyte fungi (mainly *Trycophyton* species) digest keratin and can invade the skin, hair, and nails causing tinea corporis/cruris/manum/pedis or "ringworm", tinea capitis (Ch. 26), or tinea unguium (onychomycosis). A small lipophilic yeast (*Malassezia furfur*) causes tinea versicolor. *Candida albicans* causes thrush, intertrigio diaper dermatitis (Ch. 26) and complicated intertrigo.

Clinical presentation

Tinea corporis or "ringworm" is very common in childhood. The classic lesion of tinea corporis is an annular red scaly patch or plaque, often with central clearing, and an active border with scale and sometimes small pustules (Fig. 29.1). The trunk is a common site, and multiple patches can coalesce forming polycyclic or serpiginous borders. When tinea corporis occurs on the face, it is called tinea faciei and when it occurs in the inguinal area or on the inner thighs (usually in adolescents, bilaterally) it is called tinea cruris.

Tinea pedis and unguium occur primarily in adolescents.

Tinea pedis classically causes vesicles and erosions on an erythematous scaly base in the instep of one or both feet, with or without fissuring erythema between the toes. Tinea unguium causes thickened, irregular, discolored toe or fingernails that often detach from the nail bed.

Tinea versicolor is common, and causes multiple (often confluent) ovoid plaques with a fine scale on the trunk, upper arms, and sometimes neck and face. On darkly pigmented skin, plaques appear hypopigmented, and on light skin they appear tan colored (Fig. 29.2).

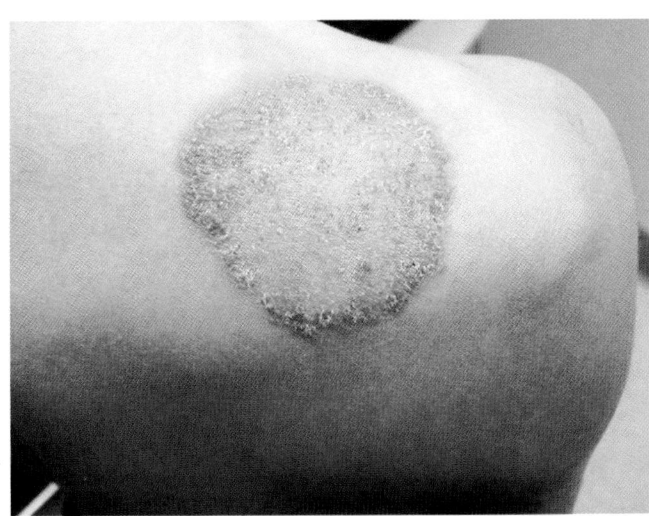

Figure 29.1 Tinea corporis: red scaly plaque with partial clearing in center. (Courtesy of Hans Kersten.)

Differential diagosis

The "herald patch" of pityriasis rosea can mimic tinea corporis, but usually has central scale and not peripheral scale, and an ensuing widespread rash. Granuloma annulare has erythematous annular lesions with central clearing, but the borders are more raised and there is no scale (Fig. 29.3). All forms of atopic dermatitis, particularly nummular eczema (Fig. 25.9, p. 142), can have similar lesions, but patients should have lesions in other body areas; atopic dermatitis lesions are markedly more pruritic and often have weeping fissures, which are uncommon in tinea corporis. Tinea lacks the greasy yellow scale of seborrheic dermatitis. Sarcoidosis and lupus erythematosus can have similar skin lesions to tinea corporis. Erythema chronicum migrans has annular erythema that can expand rapidly (1 cm daily) and has no scale. Of all of these skin lesions, only tinea will have a positive fungal culture or KOH wet-mount microscopy. Differential diagnosis of tinea versicolor includes vitiligo, pityriasis alba, tinea

A Practical Guide to Pediatric Emergency Medicine: Caring for Children in the Emergency Department, ed. N. Ewen Amieva-Wang (associate eds. Jamie Shandro, Aparajita Sohoni, and Bernhard Fassl). Published by Cambridge University Press.

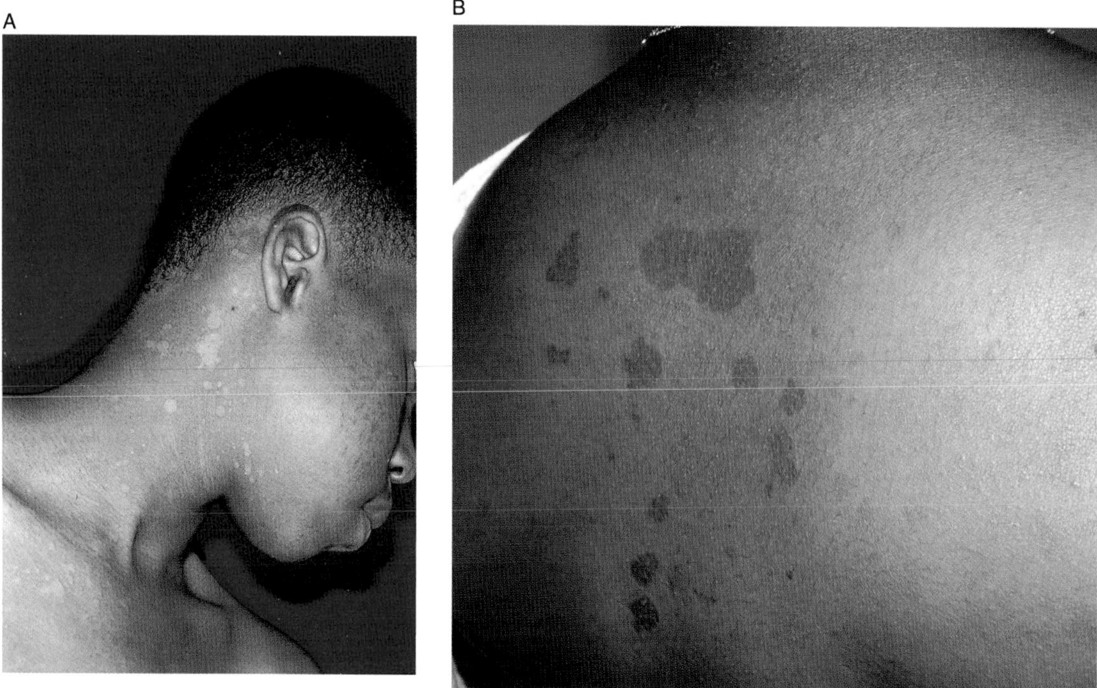

Figure 29.2 Tinea versicolor. (A) Numerous circular, scaly lesions on the neck and anterior chest. The lesions are slightly hypopigmented, confluent macules. Lesions in tinea versicolor can be a variety of colors, including tan, pink, or hypopigmented, as in this case. (B) Here the lesions are hyperpigmented. (A, reprinted with permission from Shah BR, Lucchesi M (eds). *Atlas of Pediatric Emergency Medicine*. New York: McGraw Hill, 2006. B, courtesy Paul Matz.)

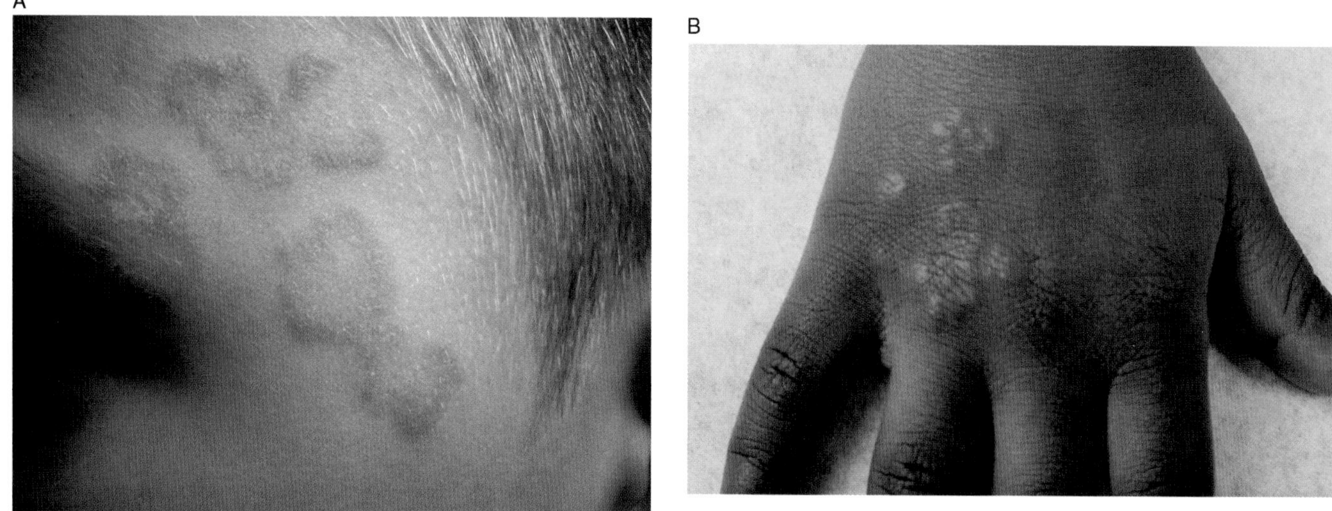

Figure 29.3 Granuloma annulare. Raised ring of subcutaneous nodules with intact overlying skin. These can occur in groups (A) and sometimes nodules can be apparent (B). (Courtesy of Hans Kersten.)

corporis, and prityriasis rosea, but positive fungal scrapings will differentiate.

Diagnostic studies

Skin scrapings for diagnosis should be obtained particularly in cases of prolonged disease unresponsive to prior therapies.

Management

Choice of antifungal drug is important. Nystatin cream is *not* effective against dermatophytes. Conversely, terbinafine and tolnaftate have very little efficacy against *Candida* but are good for dermatophytes. Combination steroid/antifungal creams are aggressively promoted but have been shown to prolong infections and cause skin atrophy and systemic absorption with

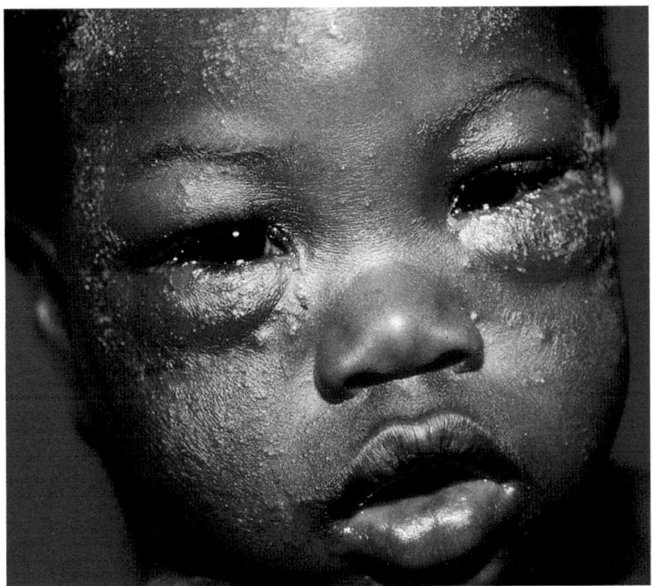

Figure 29.4 Tinea and id reaction. Diffuse vesicular rash in a child being treated for tinea capitis. (Reproduced with permission from Kane KS, Lio PA, Stratigos AJ, Johnson RA (eds). *Color Atlas and Synopsis of Pediatric Dermatology*, 2nd edn. New York: McGraw Hill Medical 2009.)

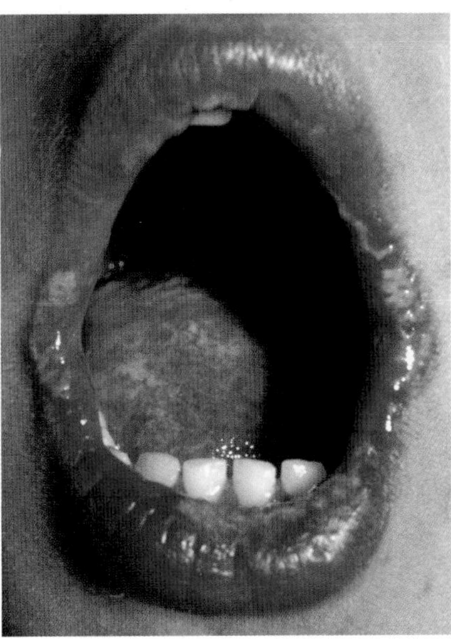

Figure 29.5 White patches on tongue (thrush) with involvement of the corners of the mouth (perleche) caused by *Candida albicans*. (Courtesy of Logical Images Inc.)

prolonged use; therefore, they are not recommended for use outside of specialty consultation.

Systemic (non-topical) therapy can sometimes prompt an id reaction, a widespread papulovesicular dermatitis with small oval lichenified papules on the extremities, trunk, scalp, and face, which are often pruritic (Fig. 29.4). Since this often occurs soon after systemic antifungals are started, it is often mistaken for a drug reaction – it is not! Drug reactions are more erythematous, morbilliform, and widespread. Antifungal drugs should be continued in an id reaction; a short course of topical or oral steroids can be added for the itching of the id reaction itself.

Other fungal infections

Tinea versicolor

Mild infections are treated with selenium sulfide or ketoconazole 2% shampoos applied to skin or with ketoconazole cream.

In *severe* infections, oral agents should be considered.

1. Ketoconazole (Nizoral) 200 mg oral dose (PO) daily for 5 days or 400 mg PO single dose 1–2 h before exercise. Let sweat dry, leave on as long as possible. Repeat in 1 week.
2. Itraconazole (Sporanox) 200–400 mg PO once, repeat in 1 week. Maintain improvement with ketoconazole shampoo and/or cream.

Tinea corporis/pedis/manus/cruris

Topical imidazole creams BID for 2–4 weeks or terbinafine cream. Immunocompromised individuals or those with widespread infections often require systemic therapy with terbinafine (3–6 mg/kg daily), itraconazole (3–5 mg/kg daily) or fluconazole for 2–4 weeks. Systemic therapy is commonly used in tinea faceii.

Tinea capitis

Oral griseofulvin 20 mg/kg daily divided BID for 6–12 weeks until samples are culture negative. Griseofulvin should be taken with milk or fatty food to increase absorption. Consider adjunctive therapy with sporicidal shampoo (selenium sulfide 2.5%). Use prednisone + griseofulvin if kerion is present. Alternative systemic agents are terbinafine or azoles (e.g., itraconazole 3–5 mg/kg daily for 4–6 weeks).

Onychomycosis

Topical terbinafine, azoles, ciclopirox (Penlac) daily, or 4% thymol solution BID for superficial disease. Systemic terbinafine (3–6 mg/kg daily for 1 month) may be curative for severe/symptomatic cases.

Candida albicans

Skin infection by *C. albicans* is seen commonly in infants under 1 year of age and in immunocompromised individuals, but it can occur anywhere skin is persistently warm, moist, or macerated, such as the diaper area or intertriginal body folds (intertrigo). Oral candidiasis or thrush is a common infection of otherwise healthy neonates and infants. *Candida* spp. can cause chronic paronychia in thumb- or finger-sucking infants.

Clinical presentation

Candidal skin infections in the *diaper area* or *intertriginal* body folds present with deeply erythematous plaques with elevated margins and typical satellite papules and pustules (Ch. 26).

Thrush is characterized by white or gray pseudomembranous patches of the tongue, soft and hard palates, and buccal mucosae (Fig. 29.5). It may be painful or painless. Unlike milk or formula curds, the patches are adherent to the underlying tissue; when they are gently scraped off with a tongue depressor or swab, they reveal an erythematous, friable erosion at the base. *Perleche* is a painful fissure at the angle of the mouth, often complicated by candidal infection.

Candidal *paronychia* have nail plate involvement and are less purulent or painful than bacterial paronychia.

Treatment

Candidal skin infections. Treatment always centers on trying to maintain a relatively dry skin environment (frequent diaper changes in infants) to minimize maceration, and antifungal creams (nystatin, oxiconazole, miconazole, ketoconazole, clotrimazole) used two to four times a day for 3–5 days. Nystatin is commonly used in neonates. Miconazole and Zeasorb AF powder can be used for prophlaxis after candidal intertrigio has resolved.

Oral candidiasis (thrush) in infants. Nystatin oral suspension applied to lesions with a swab or fingertip (or a dropperful instilled into each cheek) twice a day for 7–14 days. In infants with recurrent infections, discard pacifiers and bottle nipples (reservoirs) and evaluate mothers for asymptomatic vaginal or nipple infection.

Oral candidiasis (thrush) in older children and adults. Nystatin or clotrimazole troches, sucked five times a day for 7–14 days, or fluconazole 6 mg/kg on day 1, then 3 mg/kg a day for 2 weeks. Immunosuppressed children may need systemic therapy with fluconazole or itraconazole, both 5 mg/kg a day for 21 days.

Perleche. Ketoconazole or miconazole cream BID.

Paronychia. Thymol solution 4% BID, nystatin or imidazole creams BID, or nystatin cream under occlusion nightly for 3–4 nights. Nail plate irregularities will take months to grow out.

Warts

Warts (verruca) are discrete, benign, flesh-colored papules caused by local infection by one of many types of human papillomavirus (HPV). Prevalence in children is estimated at 10%, increasing through childhood and peaking in adolescence. Warts are uncommon in infants and toddlers but more common in children than adults. Warts are most common on knees and hands but can occur anywhere. Warts on the soles of feet are called plantar warts, and are often smooth topped and deep seated. Genital warts are called condyloma, are rarely solitary, and are considered a sexually transmitted disease. Common warts are harmless and frequently self-involuting over years, but have some social stigma and can occasionally be painful.

Clinical presentation

Common warts (verruca vulgaris) are often solitary and have a rough, sometimes "cauliflowered" surface; they disrupt normal skin lines and can have multiple black dots (thrombosed capillaries) within the wart itself.

Treatment

Common warts. Half to two-thirds of cases resolve spontaneously within 2 years. Treatment of warts is not within the purvue of emergency medicine, but common treatments include occluding the wart around-the-clock with duct tape, which is as effective as cryotherapy. Over-the-counter salicylic acid solutions or plasters are effective and can readily be combined with duct tape occlusion.

Facial warts. Further treatment should be deferred to a specialist.

Anogenital condyloma. In children, this should always prompt consideration of sexual abuse, and a careful history and physical examination should be performed.

Molluscum contagiosum

Molluscum contagiosum is a very common skin infection in children caused by infection with a human poxvirus. It is uncommon before the age of 1 year, and most common in ages 2–5. It is spread by contact, fomites, and possibly swimming pool water, and it is more common in wrestlers and swimmers. Children with atopic dermatitis can be disproportionately affected.

Clinical presentation

Molluscum lesions are smooth, pearly papules, often grouped but not coalescent, and can be flesh colored or mildly pink (Fig. 29.6). Papules have a white or yellow center and older papules will have characteristic umbilication. Lesions are usually 2–8 mm, but "giant" molluscum can occur. They occur commonly in the groin, axillae, and popliteal and antecubital

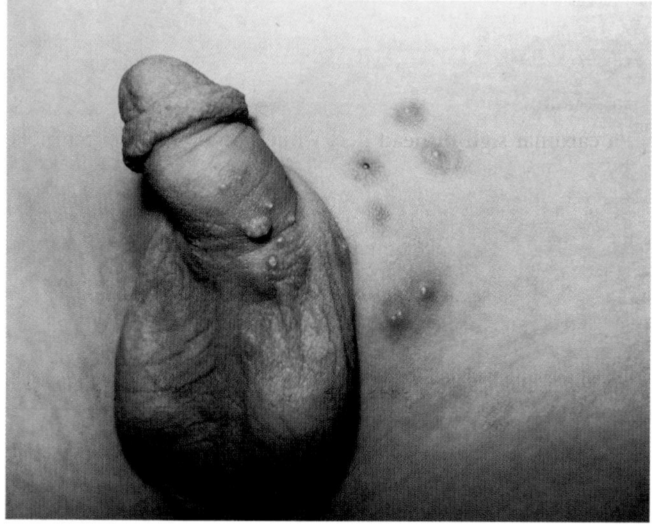

Figure 29.6 Molluscum contagiosum. A centrally umbilicated dome-shaped lesion. These often appear in crops. The lesions can easily become excoriated. (Courtesy S. Shpall.)

fossae, but they can occur anywhere and can be very numerous in immunosuppressed individuals. They can cause a surrounding erythematous mildly scaly dermatitis. They can be mildly itchy, causing koebnerization and autoinoculation. Close inspection revealing the central core will reliably identify molluscum lesions. Rarely does molluscum truly become infected – the inflammatory response that may come with involution can be mistaken for infection.

Treatment

Usually, no treatment is needed since spontaneous resolution is seen in immunocompetent children, often within 6–9 months, but full resolution can take years. Facial or large lesions can be referred to dermatology for more specific treatment.

While molluscum is not contagious to adults, siblings of affected child should not bathe together.

If accompanied by a symptomatic, reactive "molluscum dermatitis," treat with low-potency topical steroids.

If a child has concomitant atopic dermatitis, this should be appropriately treated to avoid facilitating spread of molluscum.

Lice

Humans are the only host for three species of lice: the head louse (*Pediculus humanus capitis*), which is very common in ages 3–12; the body louse (*Pediculus humanus corporis*); and the pubic louse (*Phthirus pubis*). The body louse is the only louse that can transmit other diseases (such as epidemic typhus). Lice infections are spread through close contact and fomites (bedding, headgear, clothing, hairbrushes.)

Clinical presentation

Lice are tiny 1–4 mm wingless six-legged insects with grayish translucent bodies that feed on human blood by direct skin puncture. Female lice lay eggs every 2 weeks, and egg cases called "nits" are tightly attached to the hair shaft close to the scalp. In approximately a week, nits hatch into young lice. Lice bites are very pruritic. Nocturnal scalp itchiness and scratching are a cardinal sign of head lice, while body or pubic itchiness and excoriation are a sign of body or pubic lice. With head lice infestations, cervical lymphadenopathy can be found. Bacterial superinfection of excoriated bites is not uncommon. Body or pubic lice bites can cause bluish crusted macules, maculae ceruleae, on the trunk or in the pubic area.

Diagnosis

Diagnosis is based on finding live lice or finding viable nits on hair shafts.

Nits more than 7 mm out from the scalp are likely to be non-viable.

Nits can persist after therapy. Viable nits may be confirmed by low-power microscopy showing a developing louse in the egg. Care should be taken not to confuse dandruff or retained external hair root sheaths with nits; these can be easily moved along or off a hair shaft, and nits cannot.

Management

Head lice. There are many options: permethrin 1% cream rinse, pyrethrin + piperonyl butoxide, malathion 0.5% lotion, ivermectin, or manual removal. Close contacts should be evaluated for signs/symptoms of infection but are not necessarily treated.

Nit removal. This is often mandated by schools and can be accomplished by combing wet hair with a fine-toothed nit comb (usually packaged with over-the-counter treatments) after nits are softened with a warm wet towel or with vinegar rinses. Cutting hair short is not necessary or helpful.

Body lice. Improve hygiene, launder clothing/bedding, consider permethrin 5% cream or lindane 1% lotion.

Pubic lice. Treat as for head lice plus launder all clothing/bedding.

Eyelash lice. Use petrolatum on eyelashes and lid margins BID for 8 days.

Topical treatments are repeated in 1 week. Most importantly, bedding, headgear, and clothing should be laundered in hot soapy water then dried on hot in a drier; non-washable items can be dry cleaned, sealed in plastic bags for 2–4 weeks, or soaked in rubbing alcohol for an hour. Play areas and furniture should be vacuumed. Failure to clear the home environment is a common cause of apparent "treatment failures."

Scabies

Scabies is a common infestation caused by the eight-legged *Sarcoptes scabiei* mite, an obligate human parasite. Tiny mites burrow into the stratum corneum of the epidermis and tunnel through it at 0.5–5 mm daily. Female mites live 30–40 days and lay eggs as they tunnel, which hatch in 3–4 days. Scabies is spread by casual contact and fomites, and human infections can be asymptomatic for the first 3 weeks.

Clinical presentation

The cardinal symptom of scabies is itching, classically worse at night. Scabies lesions are pruritic erythematous papules, commonly in interdigital webs, dorsal hands, genital areas, flexural areas, and on the abdomen. Face and scalp are usually spared in older children and adults. Older family members often have few lesions, whereas younger children and infants can have dozens (Fig. 29.7). Infants, in particular, can develop a generalized eczematous eruption involving the face, scalp, and trunk, with vesicles (particularly on palmar surfaces). Lesions are almost always excoriated at presentation and can have honey-colored crusts and serous weeping. Finding an S-shaped burrow or track is pathognomonic. Bacterial superinfection can occur from excoriation. Immunosuppressed individuals can have hundreds of mites and scaly widespread dermatitic papules and plaques, known as "Norwegian" scabies.

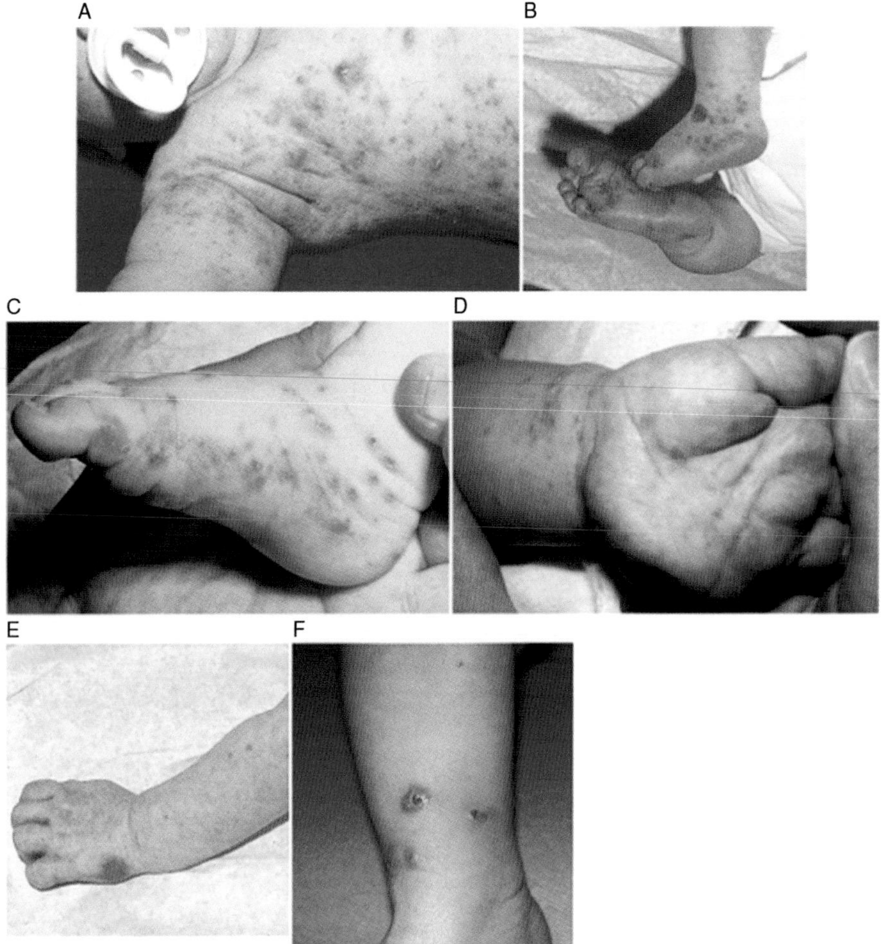

Figure 29.7 Infantile scabies. Widespread pruritic papules, pustules, and vesicles occur over the trunk and axilla (A); the soles, dorsal, lateral, and instep portions of the feet (B,C), where burrows are also evident; the palm of the hand (D); and lateral aspect of the wrist (E). (F) Infants are also more likely to develop an intense nodular reaction to the mite. (Reproduced with permission from Zitelli BJ, Davis HW *Atlas of Pediatric Physical Diagnosis*, 5th edn. Philadelphia, PA: Mosby Elsevier, 2007. © 2007 Mosby Inc., an affiliate of Elsevier Inc.)

Differential diagnosis

In scabies, the differential includes any severely itchy dermatitis, including atopic dermatitis, contact dermatitis, seborrheic dermatitis, or papular urticaria. Scabies must be suspected in any young infant with sudden onset of a severely pruritic dermatitis. Other family members will almost always have a few lesions and should be questioned about itchy lesions and examined. Diagnosis is confirmed by scraping a burrow and viewing the mite in the skin scrapings in immersion oil under 10× microscopy.

Management

Permethrin 5% cream applied overnight everywhere below the head; consider oral ivermectin (one dose 0.2 mg/kg) if immunocompromised. Repeat whole treatment in 1 week.

Infants under 2 months and pregnant women. Permethrin is not recommended and they are treated with sulfur 6% ointment, applied from the neck down for three consecutive nights, then washed off 24 h after the last application.

Close contacts and family members. They should be empirically treated.

Clothing/bedding. All used during the past 3 days should be washed in hot water and dried in a hot dryer.

Itching may persist for several weeks despite curative treatment.

Papular urticaria

Papular urticaria deserves a brief mention as it is a common cause of emergency visits. It is a chronic eruption of grouped multiple itchy pink urticarial papules, often each with a central punctum (Fig. 29.8), that begins in the spring or summer and can re-occur yearly in children ages 18 months to 7 years. It lasts for 3–6 months then resolves. Lesions may be single but are often grouped on the shoulders, upper arms and chest, buttocks, and calves. Lesions may be crusted and weeping from excoriation. Each lesion is the site of a type 4 hypersensitivity reaction to an arthropod bite, usually bedbugs or mites, dog or cat fleas or mites, or even mosquito bites. Lesions last weeks to months, and new crops will occur usually over a 3–6 month

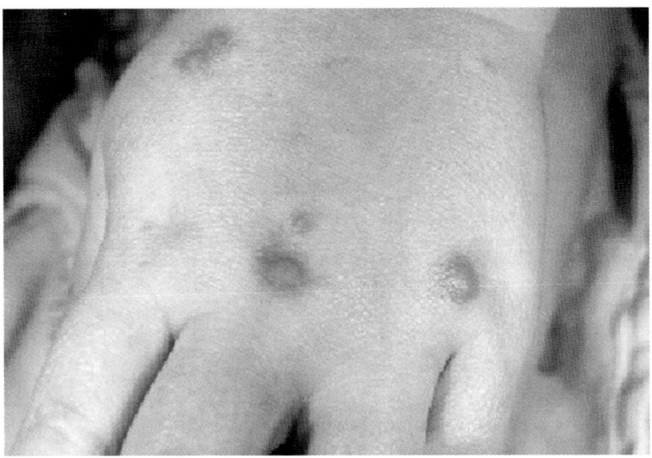

Figure 29.8 Papular urticaria. Edematous, red papules that swell intermittently and become itchy. Excoriated red papules continue to enlarge intermittently for many months. (Reprinted with permission from Paller, AS, Manicini AJ (eds.) *Hurwitz Clinical Pediatric Dermatology: A Textbook of Skin Disorders of Childhood and Adolescence* 3rd edn. Philadelphia, PA: Elsevier Saunders, 2006. © 2006 Saunders Inc., an affiliate of Elsevier Inc.)

period prior to resolution. Often the toddler is the only one in the family with the reaction, so it can be hard to convince parents that insect bites are the culprit; explaining that the child has a hypersensitivity or particular allergy to the bite can help. Children may develop the syndrome only when visiting a particular relative's house, if a pet is present there.

Treatment

Treatment centers on minimizing exposure to the suspected allergenic biting insect, home environment cleaning as per scabies or lice, and having pets treated by a veterinarian for fleas or mites. Oral antihistamines such as cetirizine and topical low- to mid-potency steroid creams or ointments two or three times a day can improve symptoms. Parents must be reminded of the long-lasting nature of type 4 hypersensitivity reactions, and the recurrent nature of this condition, but also reassurred that children usually outgrow the reaction.

Pearls and pitfalls

Pearls

1. Scabies must be suspected in any young infant with sudden onset of a diffuse severely pruritic dermatitis.
2. Nystatin cream is useful for treating superficial candidal infections, but it is *not* effective against dermatophytes.
3. Do not stop systemic antifungal drugs because of a widespread rash on day 2 or 3 of treatment. This is usually an "id" (dematophytid) reaction, not an allergy, and antifungals should be continued.
4. While tinea corporis is common in childhood, tinea pedis and unguum occur primarily in adolescents.
5. Nits more than 7 mm out from the scalp are likely to be non-viable.

Pitfalls

1. Treating tinea with topical steroids; this prolongs and spreads the infection: "tinea incognito."
2. Failure to distinguish pityriasis rosea and granuloma annulare from tinea corporis.

Selected references

Paller AS, Mancini AJ. *Hurwitz Clinical Pediatric Dermatology, a Textbook of Skin Disorders in Childhood and Adolescence.* Philadelphia, PA: Elsevier Saunders, 2006.

Sladden MJ, Johnson GA. Common skin infections in children. *Br Med J.* 2004;**329**:95–99.

Theos, A. Superficial cutaneous fungal infections in children. *Pediatr Ann* 2007;**36**:47–54.

Weston WL, Land AT, Morelli JG. *Color Textbook of Pediatric Dermatology*, 4th edn. Philadelphia, PA: Mosby Elsevier, 2007.

Reactive erythemas

Theresa M. van der Vlugt

Introduction

The "reactive erythemas" involve a somewhat disparate group of skin diseases that are characterized by red rashes without wheals that manifest in different disease states. While erythema nodosum is an erythematous panniculitis, it is also discussed here for comparison with other erythematous lesions. Table 30.1 compares these rashes and Figs. 30.1 to 30.4 illustrate them.

Erythema nodosum

Erythema nodosum is more common in spring and fall, more common in females than males, and can been seen in all ages. It is more common in older children and adolescent girls. The inflammation of the septal fat that causes the lesions of erythema nodosum is considered a reaction to an infectious, autoimmune, malignant, or unknown inflammatory process.

Table 30.1. Reactive erythemas

Diagnosis	Erythema nodosum	Erythema chronicum migrans	Erythema marginatum	Erythema multiforme (EM minor)
Illustration	**Fig. 30.1**	**Fig. 30.2**	**Fig. 30.3**	**Fig. 30.4**
Age	Rare under 2 years; most common in adolescent girls	Typically school age but all ages possible	4–9 years	Young adult, although can occur in younger children and infants
Etiology	Varied; may be infectious (streptococci most common), autoimmune, malignant, or idiopathic	Lyme disease	Acute rheumatic fever (ARF); group A streptococcal infections not causing ARF	Hypersensitivity reaction to HSV type 1, rarely to type 2; not drug related
Distribution	Extensor surfaces, particularly pretibial legs	At site of tick bite	Diffuse	Palms and soles; 25–50% with mild oral mucosal involvement
Lesions	Painful, tender nodules; often symmetric	Pruritic annular lesion; may have central clearing or be uniformly erythematous	Curvilinear semicircular rash, appearing and disappearing diffusely over the body	Target lesion; may become bullous; occasionally will have petechiae in some lesions
Treatment	Workup of underlying disease; NSAIDs, antihistamines	Doxycycline	Treat underlying disease (initiate workup for streptococcal infection)	Supportive care; oral antihistamines, emollients; oral antivirals for recurrent episodes
Resolution	2–6 weeks	Resolves with treatment of underlying disease	May persist after treatment of underlying disease	On average 21 days

NSAID, non-steroidal anti-inflammatory drug.

A
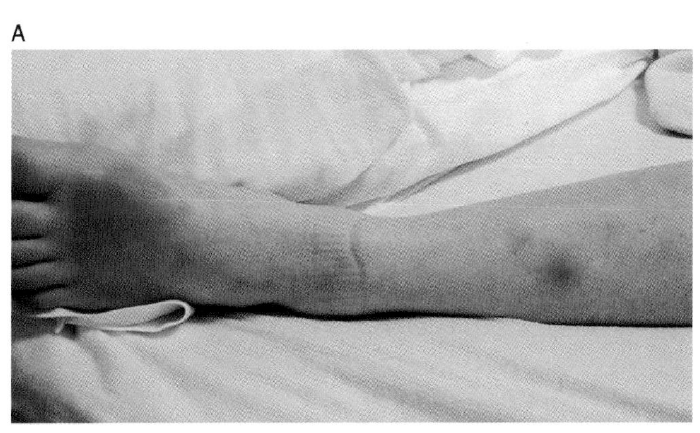

B
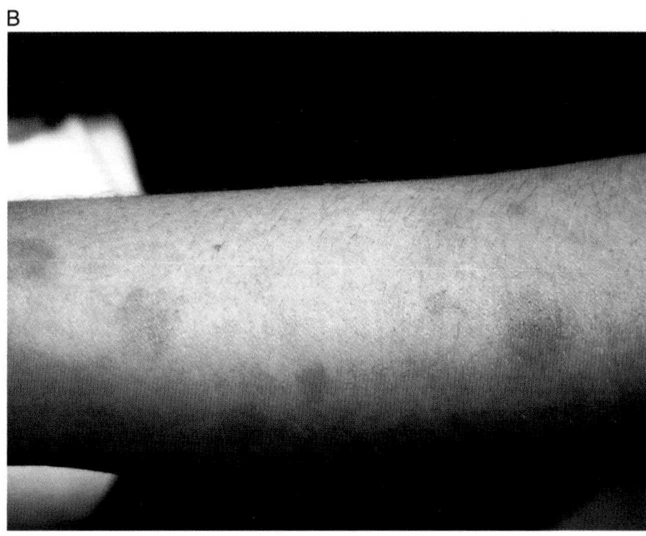

Figure 30.1 Erythema nodosum. Tender red nodules with indistinct borders often simulating bruises. (Courtesy Dr. Paul Matz.).

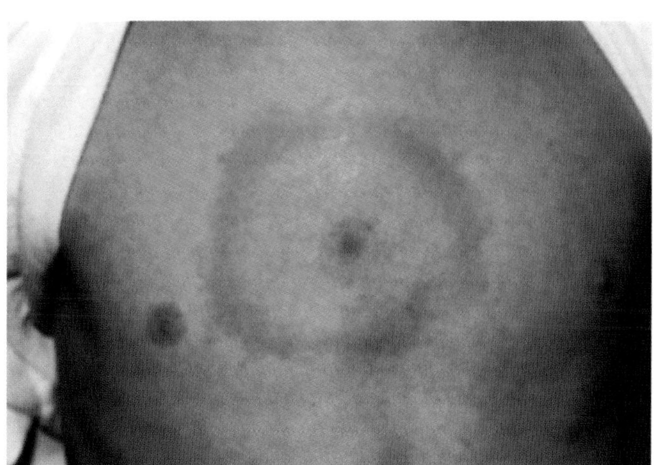

Figure 30.2 Erythema migrans of Lyme disease. Expanding, erythematous, annular patch of early localized Lyme disease. A small red papule is seen centrally at the site of the tick bite. (Reproduced with permission from Paller, AS, Manicini AJ (eds.) *Hurwitz Clinical Pediatric Dermatology: A Textbook of Skin Disorders of Childhood and Adolescence* 3rd edn. Philadelphia, PA: Elsevier Saunders, 2006. © 2006 Saunders Inc., an affiliate of Elsevier Inc.).

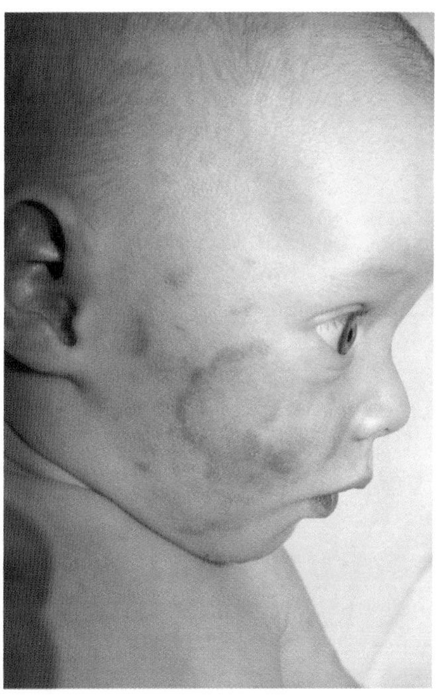

Figure 30.3 Erythema marginatum. Fleeting semi-annular erythema on the face of an infant with acute rheumatic fever. (Reproduced with permission from Weston WL, Lane AT, Morelli JG. *Color Textbook of Pediatric Dermatology*, 4th edn. Philadelphia, PA: Mosby Elsevier, 2007. © 2007 Elsevier Inc).

A non-specific prodrome with low-grade fever, malaise, and occasionally upper respiratory tract infection symptoms may occur in 25% of children and 50% of adults. Up to 90% of children will have associated arthralgias before, during, or after an attack.

Streptococcal infection is usually the most common etiology in children, although many other infections have been reported associated with erythema nodosum.

Drugs (particularly sulfa and oral contraceptives) have also been associated. In 15–35% of cases, no etiology can be found.

Clinical presentation

Lesions are very tender, painful, erythematous, or violaceous subcutaneous nodules or plaques that suddenly appear on extensor surfaces, characteristically the pretibial lower legs. It is often symmetric. Widespread involvement can occur in infants, but it is generally uncommon before age 2.

Diagnostic studies

Workup for erythema nodosum in children usually includes a search for streptococcal disease (rapid strep test, anti-

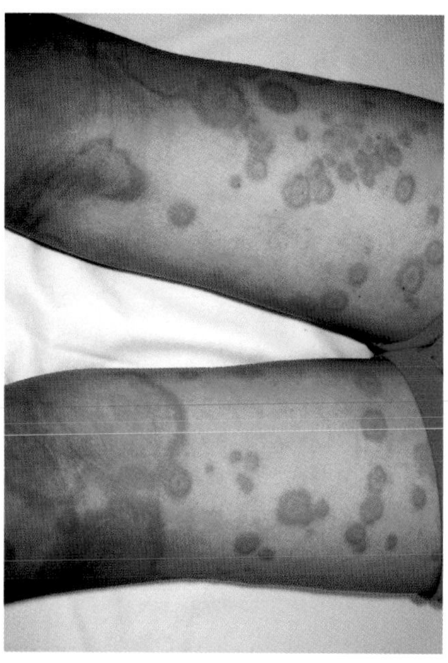

Figure 30.4 Erythema multiforme: Fixed papules with central clearing and duskiness; characteristic "target lesions". (Courtesy of T.M.vanderVlugt.)

streptolysin (ASO) antibody titer, DNase B titer), a chest radiograph to look for tuberculosis or other granulomatous disease, and a PPD test (purified protein derivative test or Mantoux test). More extensive workup is not necessary unless specifically indicated by other symptomatology.

Management

Associated conditions should be treated accordingly, but erythema nodosum itself requires no treatment other than NSAIDs for pain and antihistamines for itch. Oral steroids are *not* routinely recommended. Leg elevation can help. Lesions usually resolve in 2–6 weeks. Recrudescence can occur when associated with ongoing underlying disease, but after resolution is uncommon. Recurrent cases are often associated with recurrent streptococcal infection.

Erythema chronicum migrans

Erythema chronicum migrans is associated with Lyme disease (Ch. 90). The rash occurs at the site of the original tick bite. Multiple concurrent rashes are a marker of early disseminated disease.

Clinical presentation

Erythema chronicum migrans begins as a red papule at the site of the bite, which over 4–20 days develops a surrounding red patch that spreads peripherally. Central clearing can cause it to become annular. It is commonly asymptomatic but can manifest with burning or itching. Systemic symptoms include fever, headache, myalgias and LAN. Without treatment, the rash will resolve in 3 weeks, but systemic sequelae of disseminated or advanced Lyme disease can occur 4 weeks to 1 year after the rash.

Diagnosis

History of a tick bite with characteristic rash is sufficient to make a presumptive diagnosis. Even without a history of bite, erythema chronicum migrans with typical associated symptoms should prompt consideration of treatment in endemic areas.

Management

Early antibiotic therapy with doxycycline can prevent long-term complications of Lyme disease. The erythema chronicum migrans should disappear within 3 days with successful treatment.

Erythema marginatum

Erythema marginatum is part of the Jones criteria for rheumatic fever (Ch. 82). Although it is associated with fever and carditis, it is manifest in only <5% of children with acute rheumatic fever. Erythema marginatum is also associated with streptococcal infections not causing acute rheumatic fever.

Clinical presentation

This is a curvilinear eruption of erythematous semicircles that appears, moves over the skin, and then disappears over a period of hours.

Diagnosis and management

The rash will resolve, however a thorough workup for acute rheumatic fever is warranted.

Erythema multiforme (minor)

Erythema multiforme is now almost universally understood to be distinct from Stevens–Johnson syndrome (erythema multiforme major) and to be in most cases a hypersensitivity reaction to HSV-1 and, rarely, HSV 2 reactivation. Up to 50% of children with erythema multiforme minor can have had an antecedent herpes labialis outbreak, but since primary herpes infections can be asymptomatic it can occur with no prior clinical history of HSV. There are also reports of erythema multiforme associated with Epstein–Barr virus, cytomegalovirus (CMV), coccidiomycosis, and other atypical infections; Mycoplasma, however, is associated with Stevens–Johnson syndrome, not erythema multiforme minor.

Clinical presentation

Erythema multiforme is a diffuse eruption often involving palms and soles, the hallmark lesion of which is the target lesion, also called an iris lesion. Target lesions start without prodrome as round erythematous macules or wheals, which progress with concentric zones of color change, in which the center becomes dusky, sunken, blistered or crusted. Lesions may be bullous, and then are termed bullous erythema multiforme. Close inspection can reveal fine petechiae in some lesions. Lesions develop over 72 h, are fixed, and persist for at least 7 and on average 21 days. There is some mild mucosal involvement in 25–50%, almost always oral, with bullae on the buccal mucosa that break rapidly to form ulcerations with some edema or crusting. Systemic symptoms are rare, but they are more common in patients with oral involvement and consist of low-grade fever, malaise, or occasionally myalgia or arthralgia.

Differential diagnosis

Differential diagnosis of erythema multiforme with oral lesions includes Stevens–Johnson syndrome (Ch. 32), HSV infection, urticaria, and serum sickness-like drug reaction or hypersensitivity vasculitis.

Treatment

Treatment is supportive, with oral antihistamines and emollients. Most lesions resolve without scarring in approximately 3 weeks. Systemic corticosteroids have not been demonstrated to be helpful and can prolong episodes and promote reoccurrences. Although episodic treatment with antiherpetic drugs has not been helpful, those patients with multiple re-occurrences may benefit from suppressive daily acyclovir for a period of 6–12 months.

Pearls and pitfalls

Pearls

1. Erythema multiforme minor is most commonly caused by herpes simplex virus but can occur with no prior clinical history of this infection.
2. Consider treatment for recurrent cases, or referral for skin biopsy.

Pitfalls

1. Failure to arrange close follow-up and strict return precautions for all patients with potentially serious rash.
2. Failure to recognize possible erythema chronicum migrans of Lyme disease.

Selected references

Moraes A, Soares P, Zapata A *et al.* Panniculitis in childhood and adolescence. *Pediatr Int* 2006; **48**:48–35.

Paller AS, Mancini AJ. *Hurwitz Clinical Pediatric Dermatology, A Textbook of Skin Disorders of Childhood and Adolescence.* Philadelphia, PA: Elsevier Saunders, 2006.

Paquet P, Pierard GE. Erythema multiforme and toxic epidermal necrolysis: a comparative study. *Am J Dermatopathol* 1997;**19**:127.

Weston WL, Lane AT, Morelli JG. *Color Textbook of Pediatric Dermatology*, 4th edn. Philadelphia, PA: Mosby Elsevier, 2007.

Chapter 31 Staphylococcal scalded skin syndrome

Theresa M. van der Vlugt

Introduction

Staphylococcal scalded skin syndrome (SSSS) is a severe form of infection caused by an exfoliative exotoxin produced by *Staphylococcus aureus* that is then hematogenously spread. It is most common in children under 5 years of age; older children and adults have usually developed antibodies to the exotoxin. It is often limited to the upper body and face of infants or preschool children, but in neonates can cause diffuse desquamation, once called Ritter's disease or neonatal pemphigus.

Clinical presentation

After a 24-hour prodrome of malaise, irritability, and sometimes skin tenderness, children develop fever and a tender fissuring erythema beginning on the central face, neck, axillae, and groin, which progresses to a diffuse erythroderma. Perioral crusted fissuring around the mouth gives a "sunburst" appearance, but there is no oral mucosal (inside the mouth) erosion or involvement (Fig. 31.1). This can sometimes progress to a more scarlatiniform rash in mild forms, or to large areas of erythema with large superficial blisters that rupture

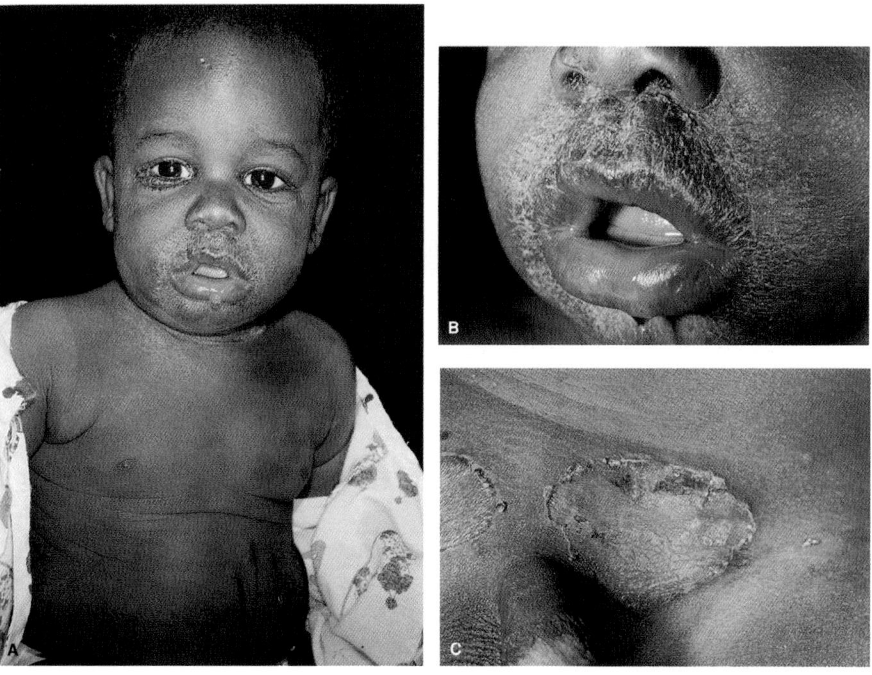

Figure 31.1 Staphylococcal scalded skin syndrome (SSSS). (A,B) Radial sunburst crusting and fissuring around the orifices (mouth, eyes, nose) are hallmarks of SSSS (first day of rash in this patient). Note the absence of any mucous membrane involvement of the mouth or eyes (unlike the prominent mucous membrane involvement seen in toxic epidermal necrolysis or Steven–Johnson syndrome. Within 24 h after these photographs were taken, the skin over the trunk and perineum (C) started wrinkling and flaccid bullae developed, followed by exfoliation in sheets revealing a red scalded-looking surface. In SSSS, *Staphylococcus aureus* is not cultured from the areas of desquamation. (Reprinted with permission from Shah BR, Lucchesi M (eds). *Atlas of Pediatric Emergency Medicine*. New York: McGraw Hill, 2006.)

A Practical Guide to Pediatric Emergency Medicine: Caring for Children in the Emergency Department, ed. N. Ewen Amieva-Wang (associate eds. Jamie Shandro, Aparajita Sohoni, and Bernhard Fassl). Published by Cambridge University Press.

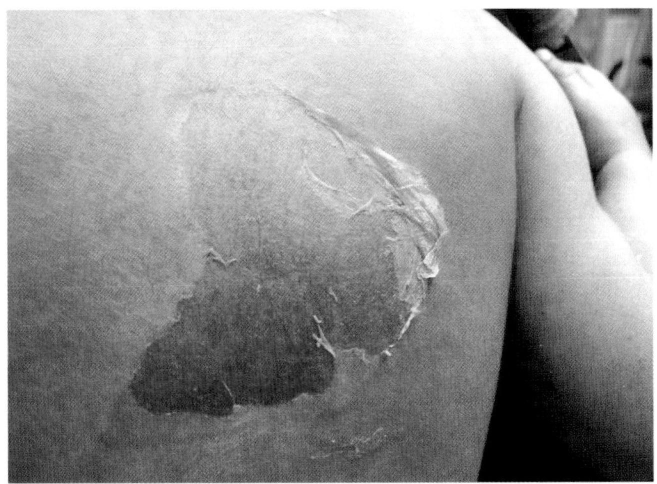

Figure 31.2 Nikolsky sign in child with staphylococcal scalded skin syndrome. Note that just the superficial epidermis is involved. (Courtesy of T. M. van der Vlugt.)

and leave shiny, erythematous tender skin. Nikolsky's sign (Fig. 31.2) is present. Neonates and infants with extensive desquamation can have fluid and electrolyte imbalances and thermal dysregulation. Sepsis or bacteremia, endocarditis, pneumonia, and local cellulitis can also be complications.

Diagnosis

The differential diagnosis involves Stevens–Johnson syndrome/toxic epidermal necrolysis (Ch. 32), Kawasaki disease, scarlet fever, and toxic shock syndrome. Skin biopsy will differentiate all of these, but a careful history and examination with cultures will often suffice. Purely local skin infection from exfoliative exotoxin-producing *S. aureus* is possible (bullous impetigo) but these children are often not particularly ill-appearing.

Usually, diagnosis of SSSS can be made by culture of initial site of infection/skin purulence (such as umbilical stump or circumcision site) or nares and nasopharynx. Blister fluid and desquamating skin are usually sterile except in the case of secondary infection.

Management/disposition

Treatment for SSSS is prompt institution of a semisynthetic penicillinase-resistant penicillin (IV nafcillin or oxacillin, oral dicloxacillin), a first- or second-generation cephalosporin, clindamycin, or erythromycin in penicillin-allergic patients. Clindamycin has the advantage of blocking toxin production. In patients with systemic illness, common treatment choices are IV nafcillin and clindamycin. If methicillin-resistant *S. aureus* (MRSA) is a possibility, vancomycin should be added to initial empiric treatment. Attention should be paid to pain control, including analgesics, gentle handling, white petrolatum dressing for denuded skin, pressure-relieving mattresses, and sterile sheets. In general, admission is usually the rule. Uncomplicated, treated SSSS has a good prognosis and heals without scarring in approximately 14 days. The 4% mortality rate of SSSS is usually associated with the most severe cases.

Pearls and pitfalls

Pearls

1. Staphylococcal scalded skin syndrome (SSSS) occurs more commonly in children <5 years of age.
2. There is *no* mucosal involvement in SSSS.
3. Early and aggressive antibiotic use is key in the management of these patients.

Pitfalls

1. Failure to recognize SSSS and failure to start antibiotic therapy.

Selected references

Aber C, Connelly EA, Schachner LA. Fever and rash in a child: when to worry. *Pediat Ann* 2007;**36**:30–38.

Weston WL, Lane AT, Morelli JG. *Color Textbook of Pediatric Dermatology*, 4th edn. Philadelphia, PA: Mosby Elsevier, 2007.

Chapter

32 Stevens–Johnson syndrome and toxic epidermal necrolysis

Theresa M. van der Vlugt

Introduction

Erythema multiforme (EM), Stevens–Johnson syndrome (SJS), and toxic epidermal necrolysis (TEN) are forms of hypersensitivity reaction in predisposed individuals, and can have similar early characteristics and skin lesions. There is controversy over whether erythema multiforme (previously erythema multiforme minor) and SJS/TEN (previously erythema multiforme major) are distinct entities or different ends of one spectrum. Erythema multiforme does not evolve into SJS or TEN and has no reported mortality. However, SJS and TEN have mortalities of 5% and 30%, respectively. While erythema multiforme and SJS can share similar cutaneous lesions, in erythema multiforme there is no only minor mucous membrane involvement. In SJS, mucosal lesions predominate and are the more severe aspect of SJS. It falls to the clinician, however, to differentiate an essentially benign process like erythema multiforme from the early stages of a potentially life-threatening illness such as SJS/TEN.

Epidemiology

SJS and TEN are uncommon in children, with respective incidences of 1/30 000 and 1/100 000. Both are now widely believed to be two ends of a spectrum of hypersensitivity reaction. In SJS, skin necrosis is primarily in the mucosal membranes and involves <10% of body surface area, while in TEN, necrosis involves mostly the skin and affects >30% of body surface area. There is considerable overlap and we will consider the two entities together.

The major etiology of SJS/TEN is drugs, specifically NSAIDs, sulfonamides, and anticonvulsants, although SJS sometimes occurs secondary to infectious causes, particularly *Mycoplasma* and HSV. Patients with HIV infection, systemic lupus erythematosus, or *HLA-B12* are at higher risk for SJS and TEN. Pathogenesis is thought to be by a genetic inability to detoxify certain drug metabolites, which deposit in the skin and induce epidermal necrolysis.

Clinical presentation

In SJS, there is a characteristic 1–14 day prodrome of fever, malaise, headache, cough, coryza, sore throat, and sometimes vomiting and diarrhea, with at least two mucous membranes involved with swelling, erythema, blistering, erosions, and hemorrhagic crusting. The oral mucosa is always involved in SJS (Fig. 32.1); eye involvement occurs in 80–85% of cases. Painful oral mucosal erosions often interfere with oral intake, and patients must be hospitalized for parenteral hydration or nutrition. Genital, urethral, and rectal involvement can cause constipation and dysuria, and GI and respiratory epithelial involvement can be an overlooked source of morbidity. The

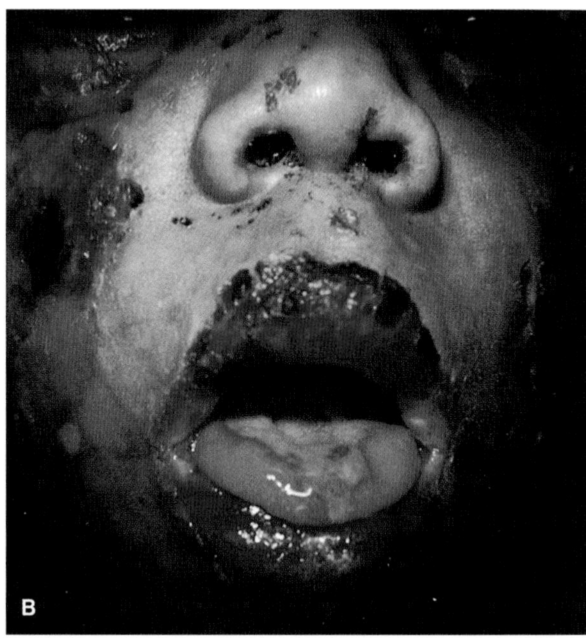

Figure 32.1 Severe Steven–Johnson syndrome, with extensive mucous membrane involvement, hemorrhagic crusting of lips, and mucosal involvement. (Reprinted with permission from Shah BR, Lucchesi M (eds). *Atlas of Pediatric Emergency Medicine*. New York: McGraw Hill, 2006.)

A Practical Guide to Pediatric Emergency Medicine: Caring for Children in the Emergency Department, ed. N. Ewen Amieva-Wang (associate eds. Jamie Shandro, Aparajita Sohoni, and Bernhard Fassl). Published by Cambridge University Press.

Table 32.1. Differential diagnosis of Stevens–Johnson syndrome/toxic epidermal necrolysis

Characteristic	Stevens–Johnson syndrome (SJS)/toxic epidermal necrolysis (TEN)	Toxic shock syndrome	Staphylococcal scalded skin syndrome	Kawasaki disease
Age at presentation	SJS younger; TEN older	Staphylococcal: 15–35 years Streptococcal: 20–50 years	<5 years	<5 years
History	Rash 7–21 days after initiation of drug (antibiotics, anticonvulsants, NSAIDs); and have several day prodrome with fever, upper respiratory tract infection symptoms, vomiting and diarrhea	Pain, flu-like illness, fever, confusion; evidence of soft tissue infection or foreign body	24 h prodrome of malaise, irritability and skin pain, then fever, diffuse erythema	Fever, rash, mucositis
Clinical signs	SJS: involvement of two or more mucous membranes; TEN: red, tender skin, Nikolsky's sign, desquamation deep to epidermis (bloody blister base)	Painful, macular-erythrodermic skin with fever, hypotension, other systemic involvement	Fever, tender skin, plus Nikolsky's sign with desquamation at epidermis (red blister base); no mucosal involvement	Fever, erythematous cracked lips, strawberry tongue, non-purulent conjunctivitis, lymphadenopathy, extremity erythema and edema
Treatment	Supportive care; discontinue drug	Antibiotics	Antibiotics	IV immunoglobulin, high-dose aspirin
Mortality	SJS 5%, TEN 30%	<3% if staphylococcal, 30–70% if streptococcal	1–10%	Low; varies with severity of coronary artery involvement

NSAID, non-steroidal anti-inflammatory drug.

skin rash of SJS usually develops later than the mucosal manifestations and has erythematous dusky-red macules and atypical two-zone targets, predominantly on the trunk and limbs, including palms, soles, face, and ears. Older lesions can have bullae, erosions, or purpura.

The rash of TEN often begins after a similar prodrome to SJS with diffuse burning erythroderma. Lesions evolve over days to form purpuric macules, atypical targets with bullae, and erosions. The hair-bearing scalp is always spared in both SJS and TEN. A hallmark of TEN is Nikolsky's sign (Fig. 31.2), when light mechanical pressure applied to the skin causes the epidermis to wrinkle up like wet tissue paper and peel off. Confluent purpuric macules or erythrodermic areas produce large areas of blistering and sheet-like epidermal detachment. The rash progresses over approximately 4 days, and risk of death arises from sepsis and fluid and electrolyte imbalance. The skin re-epithelializes over weeks, and patients often have scarring and strictures, as well as post-inflammatory depigmentation.

Diagnosis

The differential diagnosis of SJS/TEN includes Kawasaki disease, staphylococcal scalded skin syndrome, and toxic shock syndrome. Diagnosis can always be clarified by skin biopsy and subtle differences in clinical findings and history (Table 32.1).

Management/disposition

There is widespread consensus that patients with significant epidermal loss should be treated in a burn center (or at least ICU) setting. Although mild SJS can show significant improvement

Pearls and pitfalls

Pearls

1. Stevens–Johnson syndrome/toxic epidermal necrolysis are dermatologic emergencies with significant mortality risks.
2. Dermatology should be consulted as an emergency for definitive diagnosis and to guide further treatment.
3. Supportive care may evolve to include aggressive fluid resuscitation, antibiotics, and even pressors.

Pitfalls

1. Failure to recognize the extent of skin involvement.
2. Failure to arrange for appropriate level of care.
3. Failure to search for and stop the offending drug or agent.
4. Failure to recognize potential for death from these dermatologic conditions.

within 1–2 weeks, SJS and TEN can take over a month to resolve. Treatment for SJS and TEN is mainly supportive, with IV fluids, parenteral nutrition when necessary, maintaining a sterile environment in the presence of extensive desquamation, pain control, and treating secondary infections as they arise. Early opthalmological consultation is important. Prompt withdrawal of causative medications is associated with a substantial decrease in mortality. Pediatric dermatology and intensivists should be consulted early regarding the management of patients with suspected SJS or TEN in order to minimize risks of morbidity or mortality.

Selected references

Forman R, Koren G, Shear NH. Erythema multiforme, Stevens–Johnson syndrome and toxic epidermal necrolysis in children, a review of 10 years' experience. *Drug Saf* 2002;**25**:965–972.

Paller AS, Mancini AJ. *Hurwitz Clinical Pediatric Dermatology* 3rd edn. Philadelphia, PA: Elsevier Saunders, 2006, pp. 535–541.

Prendiville, J. Stevens–Johnson syndrome and toxic epidermal necrolysis. In James W (ed.) *Advances in Dermatology*, Vol. **18**. St. Louis, MO: Mosby, 2002, pp. 151–173.

Chapter 33

Urticaria and angioedema

Theresa M. van der Vlugt

Introduction

Urticaria or hives are caused by IgE-mediated leakage of extracellular fluid into the skin structures. Up to a quarter of the population has experienced urticaria. This IgE-mediated reaction is usually triggered by viral infections, foods, medications, or insect stings (Table 33.1). Urticaria can also occur secondary to physical stimuli such as cold or exercise. While the EP must assure that urticaria is not one symptom of a systemic allergic reaction, or anaphylaxis (Ch. 10) many patients have isolated urticaria. In children, the majority of cases are acute; chronic urticaria is associated with autoimmune disease in greater than 50% of cases.

Angioedema is non-pitting edema of deeper layers of skin and mucous membranes, often causing swelling of the lips, face, hands, feet, genitals, or bowel wall. While angioedema can also be IgE mediated, angioedema can also occur through activation of the kinin pathway and build up of the potent vasodilator bradykinin. (This is the mechanism of ACE inhibitor-induced angioedema.) In hereditary angioedema, lack or poor function of C1 esterase inhibitor causes increased levels of bradykinin. While hereditary angioedema is a rare cause of angioedema, it can have a high mortality rate through laryngeal swelling and airway compromise. The majority of patients develop symptoms before age 5, which worsen during adolescence. Presenting symptoms are usually cutaneous angioedema of an extremity, with dysphagia or recurrent colicky abdominal pain.

Table 33.1. Some causes of urticaria/angioedema

Type	Causes
Foods	Peanuts, tree nuts, milk, wheat, soy, eggs, fish/shellfish, strawberries, tomatoes, others (particularly foods that cross-react with latex, such as avocado, banana, chestnut)
Medications	Penicillin, sulfas, cephalosporins, vancomycin, antiepileptics, aspirin, non-steroidal anti-inflammatory drugs, opiates, amphetamines
Chemicals	Radiocontrast dye, latex, formaldehyde, monosodium glutamate, food dyes, preservatives, alcohol
Physical:	Delayed pressure, cold, cholinergic/exercise-induced, solar
Environmental	Dust mites, molds, pollens
Infection	Streptococcal, Mycoplasma, Epstein–Barr virus, viral upper respiratory tract or gastroesophageal infection
Systemic disease	Systemic lupus erythematosus, juvenile rheumatoid arthritis, polyarteritis nodosa, rheumatic fever, inflammatory bowel disease/Crohn's/ulcerative colitis, hereditary angioedema
Venoms	*Hymenoptera*, fire ant, jellyfish

History and presentation

The EP should try to identify the causative agent (Table 33.1). Important components of the history include family history; past similar episodes; recent exposures, including medications, bites, and other illness; time of onset; duration; location; and associated symptoms.

Lesions of urticaria, called wheals or hives, are flat topped, edematous, erythematous plaques that blanch with pressure; they have oval or irregular raised borders (Fig. 33.1). They can be 0.5 to 15 cm in diameter, appear quickly, and typically last 30 min to 3 h. Individual wheals coalesce and fade, and new ones appear during an attack. Skin edema in the wheals can accentuate central pallor or clearing, causing the appearance of an erythematous border. Hives are often very itchy.

Angioedema usually manifests as swelling with indistinct borders, usually in the face, lips, and extremities. It is associated with more pain than pruritus.

Table 33.2. Common medications utilized in the treatment of urticaria

Medication	Route	Dosage	Indications
Epinephrine	IM	(1:1000) 0.01 ml/kg up to 0.3 mg	Severe reaction or widespread urticaria causing discomfort
	Nebulized	0.25–0.5 ml of 2.25% racemic epinephrine diluted 1:8, or 1 ml 1:1000 standard epinephrine	Upper airway angioedema or stridor
Histamine H_1 antagonist	IV/IM	Diphenhydramine 1 mg/kg (max. 50 mg)	First-line treatment of urticaria and angioedema
	PO	Cetirizine 2.5–10 mg *or* diphenhydramine 1 mg/kg (max. 25–50 mg)	First-line treatment of urticaria and angioedema
Corticosteroid	PO	Prednisone 1–2 mg/kg (max. 60 mg)	Routine use not recommended; indications include persistent urticaria, severe angioedema

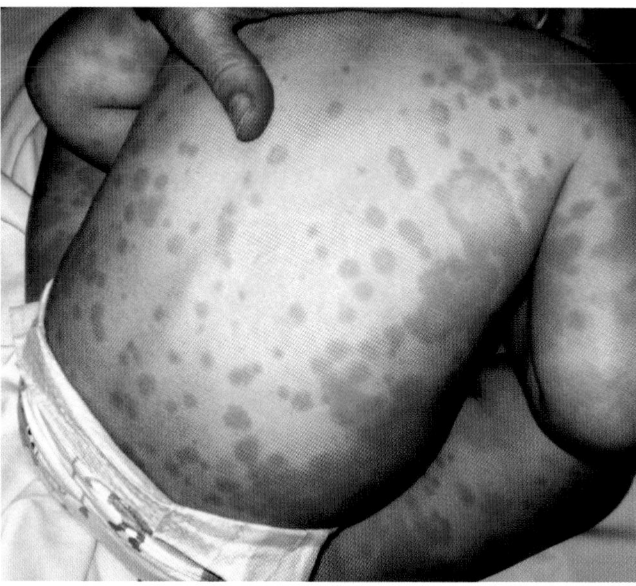

Figure 33.1 Raised migratory and blanching wheals of urticaria. (Courtesy of T. M. van der Vlugt.)

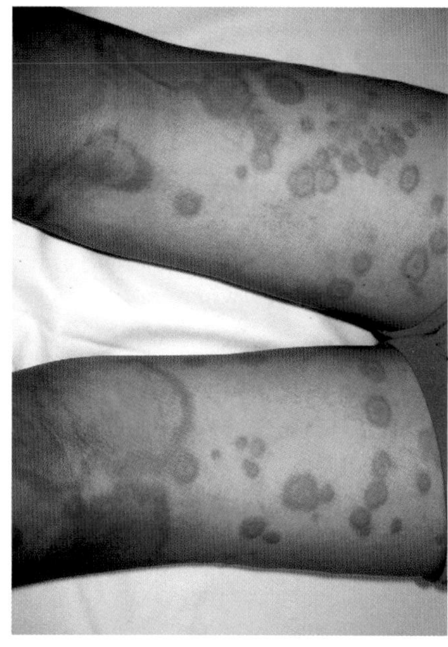

Figure 33.2 Erythema multiforme: Fixed papules with central clearing and duskiness; characteristic "target lesions". (Courtesy of T. M. van der Vlugt.)

Box 33.1. Differential diagnosis of urticaria and angioedema

Urticaria

Erythema multiforme: lesions are fixed, present for >7 days and often dusky color. It does not respond to epinephrine.

Reactive erythemas: erythema chronicum migrans, erythema marginatum, erythema annulare, erythema multiforme, erythema nodosum: see Ch. 30.

Gustatory flushing: occurs in infancy with introduction of solid foods. There is fixed erythema of the cheek, with possible associated sweating or tearing of the eye caused by cross-linking of parasympathetic nerve fibers of parotid gland to sympathetic fibers of sweat glands. It occurs with all salivation not with certain foods.

Angioedema

Cellulitis

Erysipelas

Lymphedema

Facial contact dermatitis: particularly from *Rhus* spp.

The diagnosis of acute urticaria and angioedema is clinical. Urticaria is most often confused with erythema multiforme (Fig. 33.2). Angioedema must be differentiated from infection (Box 33.1).

Treatment and management

The assessment of complete ABCs is vital to ensure that urticaria or angioedema are not a manifestation of anaphylaxis or causing respiratory compromise. For all histamine-related urticaria and angioedema, antihistamines, corticosteroids, and epinephrine are the primary treatments (Table 33.2).

Kinin-mediated angioedema (hereditary, acquired, ACE inhibitor related) respond poorly if at all to epinephrine, antihistamines, and steroids. Early definitive airway management (endotracheal intubation or surgical airway) should be pursued if laryngeal edema is suspected or worsening in these conditions. Hereditary and acquired angioedema have specific treatments because of their pathophysiology. Acute attacks are managed with IV fluids, early definitive airway management, and IV fresh frozen plasma (FFP) (which contains C1 esterase inhibitor [C1-INH]). Purified C1 esterase inhibitor replacement protein is the only proven effective therapy and was approved in 2008 for use in the USA but is not yet routinely available.

Disposition

The EP should counsel the patient to avoid suspected causative agents and refer the patient to an allergist. All patients presenting to the ED with any form of suspected IgE-mediated allergy causing urticaria or angioedema *must* be discharged with a prescription for injectable epinephrine, instructions for allergen avoidance or medication discontinuance, and a follow-up plan.

The inciting agent for patients with angioedema should be identified and discontinued. Keep these patients for observation or admit until the edema is significantly improving.

Pearls and pitfalls

Pearls

1. Urticaria is transient. The lesions move through the course of the day and usually last $<$24 h.
2. Urticaria will resolve with epinephrine treatment, erythema multiforme will not.
3. More than 50% of cases of urticaria in children are caused by viral infection.
4. Hereditary angioedema is unresponsive to antihistamines and epinephrine; it is treated with early airway management and fresh frozen plasma.
5. Rheumatologic disease should be high in the differential diagnosis of chronic urticaria, particularly in conjunction with other symptoms.

Pitfalls

1. Failure to differentiate isolated urticaria from anaphylaxis.
2. Failure to insure that angioedema is improving prior to discharge and the inciting agent has been identified and stopped.
3. Failure to prescribe Epi-pen, as well as follow-up instructions for patients presenting with angioedema.

Selected references

Bailey E, Shaker M. An update of childhood urticaria and angioedema. *Curr Opin Pediatr* 2008;**20**:425–430.

Baxi S, Dinakar C. Urticaria and angioedema. *Immunol Allergy Clin North Am* 2005;**25**:353–367.

Krishnamurthy A, Naguwa SM, Gershwin ME. Pediatric angioedema. *Clinic Rev Allerg Immunol* 2008;**34**:250–259.

Sackesen C, Sekerel BE, Orhan F, *et al.* The etiology of different forms of urticaria in childhood. *Pediatr Dermatol* 2004;**21**:102–108.

Chapter 34

Tutorial: Dermatologic medications and dermatologic diagnostics

David R. Berk

Dermatologic medications

Topical medications: general principles

Topical medicines contain active ingredient(s) and a vehicle.

- Amount
  - pay attention to quantity prescribed; avoid prescribing too little or too much topical medication (Table 34.1).
  - 1 fingertip unit (FTU) is 2 cm of cream on fingertip = 0.5 g.
  - 1 g cream (or ~0.95 g ointment) = 2 FTU. This covers approximately 100 cm^2, or the surface area of four adult hands.
- Application: show the patient how to apply the medication, location, quantity, and frequency.
- Penetration of topical medicines varies:
  - increases with occlusion (e.g., diapers), hydration, inflammation, skin breakage (e.g., atopic dermatitis), heat
  - varies with anatomic site: scrotum > cheeks > abdomen and chest > scalp and axillae > back > forearms > palms > ankles > soles.

Table 34.1. Amount for dispense by age and location

Age group and location	Amount required for 2 weeks of twice daily application (g)
1–2 years[a]	
Head/neck	20
Upper extremity	20
Lower extremity	30
Chest/abdomen	30
Back/buttocks	45
6–10 years	
Head/neck	30
Upper extremity	35
Lower extremity	65
Chest/abdomen	50
Back/buttocks	70

[a] For 3–6 month of age, 15–20 g are required for each of the following sites: head/neck, upper extremity, lower extremity, chest/abdomen, and back/buttocks. For 3–5 years, amounts to dispense are approximately between those for 1–2 years and 6–10 years.

Source: adapted from Weston WL, Land AT, Morelli JG. *Color Textbook of Pediatric Dermatology*, 3rd edn. Philadelphia, PA: Mosby, 2002. © 2002 Mosby Inc.

Vehicles

Ointments. Greases ± small amount of water, messy and may cause heat retention but have fewer allergens. Excellent for atopic dermatitis, psoriasis, emolliation. Avoid for moist areas.

Creams. Emulsions of water and oil, generally containing more fragrances and preservatives and more cosmetically acceptable/elegant. Good for face; best applied to wet skin.

Lotions. Mostly water.

Solutions. Include alcohol and propylene glycol and have minimal residue. Good for scalp and moist areas (e.g., webspaces); may sting if skin breakage.

Gels. Good penetration and minimal residue but very drying and may sting/burn if skin breakage; good for application on the scalp and for acne products.

Plasters/tapes. Easy to direct medicine where desired; good for lichen simplex chronicus (Cordran tape) and warts (salicylic acid products).

Pastes. Creams/ointments + powder; good barrier products for diaper area (e.g., zinc oxide paste).

Powders. Include fine talc particles; good for moist areas (drying effect) but poor drug delivery.

Moisturizers

- In general, the thicker the better: ointments, thick creams, and oils are preferred.

A Practical Guide to Pediatric Emergency Medicine: Caring for Children in the Emergency Department, ed. N. Ewen Amieva-Wang (associate eds. Jamie Shandro, Aparajita Sohoni, and Bernhard Fassl). Published by Cambridge University Press.

- Petroleum jelly avoids potential allergens and may work the best. Next best option is a thick cream. Lotions are mainly water and least effective as moisturizers. Avoid products with fragrances.
- Apply to damp skin as this retains hydration and avoids drying the skin after washing or bathing.
- Moisturizers with keratolytic effect contain urea, lactic acid, and glycolic acid. Helpful for keratosis pilaris, psoriasis, and palmoplantar hyperkeratosis.

Steroids

Topical drugs

Be familiar with standard topical steroid potency chart (Table 34.2).

Low potency. Used for infants or the face/groin/axillae of older patients. Examples include hydrocortisone 2.5%, desonide. For most diaper dermatitis, particularly irritant diaper dermatitis, avoid anything stronger than hydrocortisone 1% (and only use it for <1 week).

Mid potency. Used for psoriasis, atopic dermatitis. Examples include triamcinolone 0.1%, mometasone.

High potency. Use in younger children should usually be limited to short courses (e.g., several weeks; it can be continued for longer periods but patient should be followed monthly). It is good for lichen simplex chronicus, thick psoriatic plaques, and acute poison ivy/oak; palms/soles. Examples include fluocinonide ointment, clobetasol.

When a dermatitis improves after initiating a treatment, topical steroids are tapered off and the improvement maintained with moisturizers. Avoid oral steroids (see indications below).

Moderate and high potency topical steroids may demonstrate tachyphylaxis, or decreasing responsiveness to medicine after several days of application.

Side effects include local irritation, striae, atrophy, steroid acne, tinea incognito, perioral dermatitis, hypopigmentation, glaucoma, facial erythema and telangiectasia, granuloma gluteal infantum (severe nodular diaper dermatitis), hypertrichosis, purpura, and delayed wound healing.

Occlusion enhances potency/penetration, whether artificial/intended (under tape or Saran Wrap) or unavoidable/unintended (diaper area, intertriginous areas).

Oral drugs

Indications include inflammatory dermatoses (e.g., severe allergic contact dermatitis) and bullous dermatoses. Oral steroids are rarely truly indicated for atopic dermatitis or urticaria and should be avoided in psoriasis. Generic prednisolone may not be palatable to children. If so, prescribe Orapred 15 mg/5 ml.

Table 34.2. Potency by class for common topical corticosteroids

Class and generic name	Brand name
Class 1: superpotent	
Clobetasol propionate ointment/cream, 0.05%	Temovate
Betamethasone dipropionate ointment/cream, 0.05%	Diprolene, Diprosone
Halobetasol propionate ointment/cream, 0.05%	Ultravate
Class 2: potent	
Desoximetasone ointment/cream, 0.25%; gel, 0.05%	Topicort
Fluocinonide ointment/cream/gel, 0.05%	Lidex
Mometasone furoate ointment 0.1%	Elocon
Triamcinolone acetonide ointment, 0.5%	Kenalog
Class 3: upper mid-strength	
Betamethasone valerate ointment, 0.01%	Valisone
Fluticasone propionate ointment, 0.005%	Cutivate
Fluocinonide cream, 0.05%	Lidex E cream
Triamcinolone acetonide cream, 0.5%	Aristocort HP
Class 4: mid-strength	
Betamethasone valerate lotion, 0.01%	Valisone, Luxiq
Desoximetasone cream/gel 0.05%	Topicort LP
Hydrocortisone valerate ointment, 0.2%	Westcort
Mometasone furoate cream, 0.1%	Elocon
Triamcinolone acetonide ointment, 0.1%	Kenalog
Class 5: lower mid-strength	
Betamethasone valerate cream, 0.01%	Valisone
Fluocinolone acetonide oil, 0.01%	Dermasmoothe FS
Fluticasone propionate cream, 0.05%	Cutivate
Hydrocortisone butyrate cream, 0.1%	Locoid
Hydrocortisone valerate cream, 0.2%	Westcort
Triamcinolone acetonide lotion, 0.1%	Kenalog
Class 6: mild	
Desonide cream, 0.05%	Desowen
Fluocinolone acetonide cream, solution, 0.01%	Synalar
Prednicarbate 0.1% cream	Dermatop
Class 7: least potent	
Hydrocortisone cream/ointment/lotion, 0.5%, 1%; cream/lotion, 2.5%	Hytone

Side effects include irritability, GI upset (give with ranitidine 2–4 mg/kg daily PO, divided BID if treating infants), hypertension, growth retardation, vaccine ineffectiveness, insomnia, hypothalamic–pituitary–adrenal axis suppression.

Antifungal drugs

Topical drugs

There are several classes of antifungal drugs (Table 34.3):

- polyenes bind ergosterol
- azoles inhibit 14-alpha demethylase
- allylamines inhibit squalene epoxidase.

Dry areas are best treated with creams, intertriginous areas with solutions, and moist areas with powders (but more helpful for prophylaxis than treatment).

Avoid combination products with steroid and antifungal drug: the combination can be counterproductive and contain inappropriately potent steroid.

Oral drugs

In general, tinea capitis requires oral therapy, whereas most tinea corporis/pedis/versicolor (superficial infections) can be treated with topical drugs.

Onychomycosis often responds slowly if at all to either topical or oral antifungal drugs, but topical drugs should usually be tried first.

For most dermatophyte infections in children, griseofulvin is the treatment of choice (except onychomycosis).

Check pretreatment LFTs if prescribing terbinafine or azoles.

Griseofulvin

Dose: 125 mg/5 ml. Give with food as fats increase absorption.
Mechanism: inhibits microtubules.
Pediatric patients: give 20 mg/kg/d divided BID (max. 1 g/day) for 1.5–2 months (do not give only 10 mg/kg per day!).
Contraindications: hepatic failure, lupus, porphyria.
Side effects: agranulocytosis, lupus, photosensitivity, disulfiram-like reaction, oral contraceptive failure.
Interactions: CYP3A4 inducer, so lowers levels of cyclosporin A, oral contraceptives, warfarin.

Fluconazole

Dose: 50, 100, 150 mg, or 40 mg/ml.
Mechanism: inhibits lanosterol 14-α demethylase.
Pediatric patients: 3–6 mg/kg daily.
Contraindication: cisapride, causes arrhythmia.
Interactions: CYP2C9 and CYP3A4 inhibitor so enhances warfarin, oral contraceptives, phenytoin, zidovudine, theophylline, terfenadine. Rifampin decreases fluconazole levels, while cimetidine and hydrochlorothiazide increase fluconazole levels.

Table 34.3. Common topical antifungal drugs

Class and generic name	Brand name	Over the counter/ prescription
Imidazole		
Clotrimazole	Lotrimin	Both
Miconazole	Desenex, Micatin, Monistat, Zeasorb AF	OTC
Ketoconazole	Nizoral	Both
Econazole	Spectazole	Rx
Oxiconazole	Oxistat	Rx
Allylamine		
Terbinafine	Lamisil	OTC
Naftifine	Naftin	Rx
Butenafine	Mentax	Rx
Polyene		
Nystatin[a]	Mycostatin	Rx
Thiocarbamate		
Tolnaftate[b]	Tinactin, Zeasorb AF	OTC
Hydroxypyridone		
Ciclopirox	Loprox	Rx

OTC, over the counter; Rx, prescription.
[a] Nystatin should not be used for dermatophytes
[b] Tolnaftate should not be used for candida.

Itraconazole

Dose: 100 mg, 10 mg/ml. Take with orange juice/carbonated beverage.
Mechanism: inhibits lanosterol 14-α demethylase.
Pediatric patients: For onychomycosis, give a pulse dose 1 week/month

- 10–20 kg: 50 mg daily
- 20–30 kg: 100 mg daily
- 30–40 kg: 100/200 mg alternating daily
- 40–50 kg: 200 mg daily
- >50 kg: 200 mg BID.

Treatment duration: fingernails, 1.5 months; toenails, 3 months. Check LFTs after 1 month.
Tinea versicolor: adult-size: 200 mg once, repeat in 1 week.
Tinea capitis: 3–5 mg/kg day divided BID for 1 month.
Contraindication: ventricular dysfunction; cisapride (arrhythmia).
Interactions: CYP3A4 inhibitor so affects metabolism, and hence blood levels, of multiple compounds including seizure medications, felodipine, oral contraceptives, digoxin, warfarin, statins, and oral hypoglycemic drugs.

Terbinafine

Dose: (Lamisil) 250 mg tablets. Only available in tablet form.

Mechanism: inhibits squalene epoxidase.

Onychomycosis: adult-size: 250 mg PO daily for 12 weeks, or pulse dose 250 mg BID for 1 week/month for 3 months.

Tinea capitis: 3–6 mg/kg daily for 1 month

- <20 kg: ¼ tablet PO daily
- 20–40 kg: ½ tablet PO daily
- >40 kg – 1 tablet PO daily.

Side effects: subacute cutaneous lupus erythematosus, taste/visual disturbance, headache, diarrhea.

Interactions: lowers oral contraceptive; CYP2D6 inhibitor so increases theophylline, TCA, narcotics levels. Rifampin decreases and cimetidine/terfinadine increases terbinafine levels.

Caution: with renal or hepatic insufficiency.

Treatment of specific fungal infections

Tinea versicolor

Mild: selenium sulfide or ketoconazole 2% shampoos, ketoconazole cream.

Severe: Consider oral agents:

- ketoconazole 200 mg PO daily for 5 days or 400 mg PO 1–2 h before exercise. Let sweat dry, leave on as long as possible. Repeat in 1 week.
- Itraconazole 200 mg PO once, repeat in 1 week. Maintain improvement with ketoconazole shampoo and/or cream.

Tinea corporis/pedis/manus/cruris

Topical imidazole or terbinafine cream.

Tinea capitis

Oral griseofulvin 20 mg/kg daily divided BID for 6–12 weeks until culture negative. Griseofulvin should be taken with milk or fatty food to increase absorption. Consider adjunctive therapy with sporicidal shampoo (selenium sulfide 2.5%). Use prednisone + griseofulvin if kerion present. Alternative systemic agents are terbinafine or azoles (e.g., itraconazole 3–5 mg/kg daily for 4–6 weeks).

Onychomycosis

Topical terbinafine, azoles, ciclopirox daily, or 4% thymol solution BID for mild disease. Systemic terbinafine (3–6 mg/kg daily for 1 month) may be curative for severe/symptomatic cases.

Candidal infections

Neonatal candidiasis: nystatin or imidazole creams.

Diaper dermatitis: avoid irritants; ensure frequent diaper changes; use absorptive diapers, barrier creams, topical antifungal (e.g., nystatin or azole cream) for secondary infection.

Perleche: ketoconazole cream, Miconazole cream BID.

Intertrigo: miconazole cream BID or clotrimazole cream BID until resolves, then use miconazole or Zeasorb AF powder for prophylaxis.

Thrush: nystatin swish and swallow four times a day (QID); clotrimazole troche five times daily; fluconazole 6 mg/kg on day 1, then 3 mg/kg a day for 2 weeks.

Eczema treatment

Generous emolliation: large quantities, around-the-clock (every diaper change in infants), particularly after bathing; consider humidifier.

Irritants: avoid irritants (e.g., wool, very hot water, drying soaps, medicated antidandruff shampoos – tend to be drying).

Topical steriods: low- to moderate-potency topical corticosteroids BID. A frequent combination is desonide ointment for face/skin folds/mild areas and mometasone ointment for more severe areas on the body. Alternatively, hydrocortisone 2.5% ointment and triamcinolone 0.1% ointment are cheap alternatives, which may be dispensed in large (one pound) quantities.

Antihistamines: for itching (e.g., hydroxyzine 10 mg/5 ml, 2 mg/kg per day divided QID)

Calcineurin inhibitors: tacrolimus 0.03% ointment, pimecrolimus cream; good option for facial eczema, particularly eyelids and perioral; patient may experience burning feeling as a side effect.

Severe disease: phototherapy or cyclosporine are preferred.

Bacterial superinfection: consider short course of mupirocin ointment BID and dilute bleach baths (one-half cup of regular Clorox bleach in standard 50-gallon bathtub that is one-quarter filled with lukewarm water) several times per week.

Pityriasis alba: use moisturizers, photoprotection, and only low-potency topical corticosteroids (e.g., desonide lotion). Repigmentation often takes many months.

Do not miss eczema herpeticum.

Allergic contact dermatitis treatment

- Avoid allergen; thorough washing after exposed.
- Patch testing if allergen is unknown.
- Use cool compresses.
- Calamine lotion (disadvantage is that it is drying, but that can be helpful for acutely oozing dermatitis) and oral antihistamines.
- Avoid topical antihistamines; high rate of causing contact dermatitis.

- Can use high-potency steroids for short periods or mid-potency steroids for involvement of large body surface areas.
- Recommend use of a topical barrier cream before expected *Rhus* exposure (IvyBlock, others).
- Following *Rhus* exposure, specific solvent washes (Technu, others) can avert or minimize rash.
- If rash is severe (widespread, acutely oozing and weeping in an uncomfortable patient, facial involvement), consider systemic corticosteroids with taper (total ~2–3 weeks).

Seborrheic dermatitis treatment

Cradle cap. Antiseborrheic shampoos (e.g., zinc pyrithionine, selenium sulfide 2.5%, 2% ketoconazole, keratolytic tar + sulfur/salicylic acid/T-gel); de-scale with mineral oil and soft brush.

Pruritic or persistent lesions. Topical corticosteroids. On face, try low-potency topical steroids (e.g., hydrocortisone 2.5% cream). For older patients, consider adding topical azoles (e.g., ketoconazole cream), or sulfur-based lotion (10% sodium sulfacetamide and 5% sulfur).

Infantile seborrheic dermatitis carries a good prognosis, with resolution often by 8–12 months, but may recur at puberty.

Pityriasis rosea treatment

Often, no treatment is needed.

Symptomatic (pruritus). Consider antihistamines or mid-potency topical steroid (e.g., triamcinolone 0.1% cream); little evidence that antibiotics/antivirals offer any benefit.

Resolution. Modest sunlight or sunlamp exposure is well known to hasten resolution of the rash, which occurs over 2–4 months; if has lasted longer, consider psoriasis or pityriasis lichenoides chronica.

Test for syphilis if patient is sexually active.

Common wart treatment

Half to two-thirds of warts resolve spontaneously within 2 years.

Common treatment options include salicylic acid (17% gel, 40% pad), cryotherapy (q month), duct tape occlusion, and imiquimod cream (daily).

Molluscum contagiosum treatment

Molluscum contagiosum is common in the genital area and is not a sign of abuse. Usually, no treatment is needed since spontaneous resolution is seen in immunocompetent children, often within 6–9 months, but full resolution can take years.

Rarely does molluscum truly become infected; the inflammatory response that may come with involution can be mistaken for infection.

Antiparasitic therapies

Pediculosis

Head lice. There are many options: permethrin 1% cream rinse, pyrethrin + piperonyl butoxide, malathion 0.5% lotion, ivermectin, manual removal. Close contacts should be evaluated for signs/symptoms of infection but do not necessarily require treatment.

Body lice. Improve hygiene, launder clothing/bedding, consider permethrin 5% cream.

Pubic lice. Treat as for head lice treatment plus launder all clothing/bedding; use petroleum for eyelashes.

Treatments are repeated after 1 week. Nits far from the scalp are non-viable.

Scabies

- Apply 5% permethrin cream *everywhere* below the head at night; consider oral ivermectin (one dose 0.2 mg/kg) if immunocompromised.
- The whole treatment is repeated in 1 week.
- Close contacts and family members should be empirically treated.
- Clothing/bedding used during the past 3 days should be washed (hot water).

Itching may persist for several weeks despite curative treatment.

Dermatologic diagnostics

Potassium hydroxide preparations

Useful in the evaluation of fungal infections.

- Using a 15-blade, scrape superficial scale onto a glass slide; should not cause pain or bleeding.
- Add several drops of 10–20% KOH.
- Add cover slip.
- Yield improves if the slide is left to sit for 5–20 min so that cell walls dissolve. Alternatively, slide can be gently heated with a match underneath.
- 20% KOH in dimethyl sulfoxide (DMSO) does not require heating.
- Look for hyphae or spores.
- Oral lesions (candidiasis) and onychomycosis can be evaluated similarly.
- Yield may improve if scale from leading edge of lesion is scraped.

- Yield may be low if patient has recently applied topical antifungal.
- Examination with KOH (or with immersion oil) of hair shafts can be helpful to identify nits in suspected pediculosis.

Chlorazole is an ink-containing alternative to KOH.

Scabies preparation

- Choose a high-yield location: wrists, webspaces, feet of infants.
- Choose a high-yield lesion: burrow, unexcoriated papule.
- Apply mineral oil to slide.
- Dip 15-blade in mineral oil, then scrape the lesion.
- Scraping should be more vigorous/deeper than with KOH examination for tinea; it is not uncommon for slight bleeding to occur.
- Look at low power for scabies organism, scybala (stool), or eggs.
- If the patient is an infant or toddler, it may be easier to scrape an affected adult family member if present.

This examination can be performed with KOH instead of mineral oil.

Tzanck smear

Useful in the evaluation of HSV and varicella zoster virus. In a child who is systemically ill, do not wait for the test result before initiating aciclovir treatment.

- Unroof vesicle with 15-blade.
- Scrape base of lesion and apply to glass slide.
- Stain with Giema or Wright stains.
- Look for multinucleate giant epithelial cells on high power.
- This is rapid and inexpensive but it cannot distinguish HSV from varicella zoster virus.
- The effectiveness depends on the lesion stage (good for vesicular stage) and experience of investigator.
- Sensitivity reported as 50–80% or higher, and specificity reported as 90–100%.
- The sample for direct fluorescent antibody testing for definitive diagnosis must also be taken from the base of an unroofed vesicle.

Wood's lamp examination

A Wood's lamp is used for a number of pigmentary disorders, erythrasma, and tinea capitis.

- Depigmented lesions enhance, helping to define the clinical borders of the lesions and distinguish depigmented processes from hypopigmented processes.
- Erythrasma demonstrates coral red fluorescence.
- Tinea capitis caused by *Microsporum* sp. demonstrates green fluorescence. (Woods lamp examination is no longer of much utility in the USA as *T. tonsurans* does not fluoresce.) Tinea versicolor fluoresces faint orange if unwashed for a >24 h.

Diascopy

- Apply glass slide with pressure over lesion.
- Vascular lesions demonstrate characteristic blanching.

Section

6

Ear, nose, and throat

Expert reviewer: Anna Messner

Chapter 35

Allergic rhinitis and sinusitis

Aparajita Sohoni

Allergic rhinitis

Up to 30% of children are affected by allergic rhinitis. Allergic rhinitis can occur seasonally secondary to tree, grass, and weed pollens while perennial allergic rhinitis is often caused by more ubiquitous environmental antigens such as pet dander, mold spores, and dust mites. Allergic rhinitis is an IgE-mediated hypersensitivity reaction. Repeated exposure to an antigen results in vasodilation, stimulation of itch receptors, mucosal edema and secretions, and sneezing.

Clinical presentation and diagnosis

A child with allergic rhinitis presents with pruritus of the nose and eyes, watery and profuse rhinorrhea, nasal congestion, and sneezing. Additional symptoms include redness and tearing of the eyes, cough, snoring, noisy breathing and "popping" of the ears. Differential diagnosis of nasal discharge includes nasal foreign body; however, examination and history are usually sufficient to confirm or disprove this diagnosis.

The examination can reveal a mouth breather, who may have a darkened area over the infraorbital ridge secondary to venous congestion ("allergic shiners"), a transverse wrinkle over the nose caused by constant rubbing of the nose ("allergic salute"), and pale and edematous nasal mucosa with secretions.

Management

Although allergic rhinitis is usually a chronic problem and is ideally followed by a pediatrician or otolaryngologist, children without primary care will present to the ED. Patients should be educated about allergen recognition and avoidance. Inhaled nasal steroids are the recommended first-line treatment of allergic rhinitis. Children can also be prescribed a second-generation antihistamine. Two are available in liquid form, loratidine (2 years and older) and cetirizine (6 months and older). First-generation antihistamines can be used but they have increased sedating effects as well as paradoxical agitation. While antihistamine/decongestant combinations have been shown to work more effectively than antihistamines alone, their use is contraindicated in young children. Nasal decongestant sprays are not recommended in the treatment of allergic rhinitis because of potential for tachyphylaxis with resultant rebound congestion.

Pearls and pitfalls: allergic rhinitis

Pearls

1. Always exclude the diagnosis of nasal foreign body.
2. Treatment includes education about allergen avoidance, inhaled nasal corticosteroids, and second-generation antihistamines.

Pitfalls

1. Prescription of intranasal decongestant sprays as regular use can cause rebound congestion.
2. Failure to warn parents of sedating effects of first generation antihistamines.

Sinusitis

Children are thought to contract six to eight viral upper respiratory tract infections (URIs) annually. Anywhere from 5% to 13% of these may evolve into a case of bacterial sinusitis. Sinusitis refers to an inflammatory process of either infectious or non-infectious etiology that involves one or both of the paranasal sinuses. Pediatric sinus cavities develop at different ages. The ethmoid and maxillary sinuses are present at birth and are the most commonly infected in the infant population. The sphenoid sinus does not fully develop until 3 years of age, while the frontal sinuses are not formed until 7 years of age. These sinuses do not pneumatize until mid or late adolescence, at which point they become the most common site of sinusitis in the late adolescent (Fig. 35.1).

Sinusitis is classified by the duration of symptoms:

- *acute bacterial sinusitis*: bacterial infection of paranasal sinuses lasting <30 days
- *chronic sinusitis*: paranasal sinus inflammation longer than 90 days

A Practical Guide to Pediatric Emergency Medicine: Caring for Children in the Emergency Department, ed. N. Ewen Amieva-Wang (associate eds. Jamie Shandro, Aparajita Sohoni, and Bernhard Fassl). Published by Cambridge University Press.

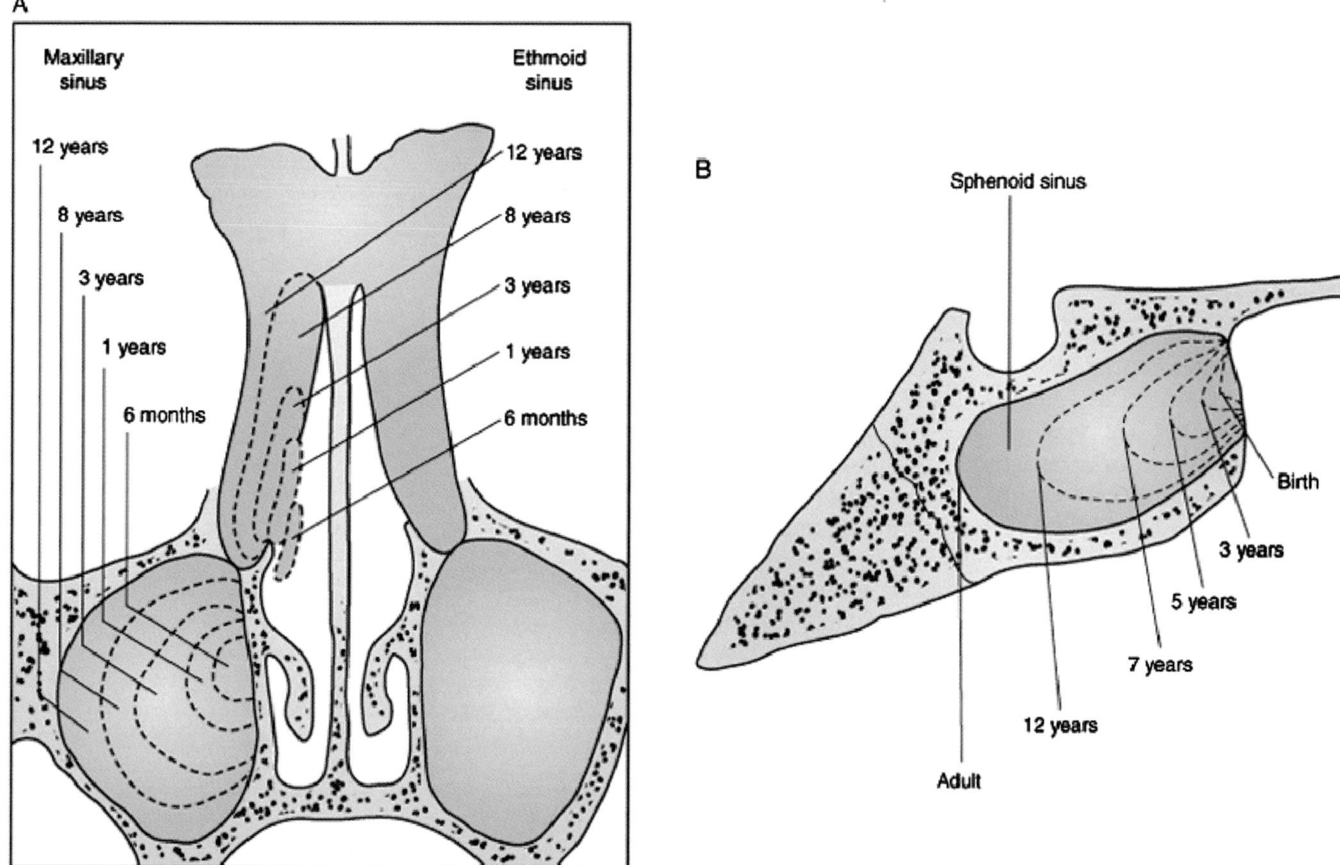

Figure 35.1 Development of paranasal, maxillary and ethmoid sinuses. (A) Note that development occurs throughout childhood and may not be complete until 12 years of age. (B) The sphenoid sinus, which sits under the pitutitary fossa, develops very slowly and may not even be well aerated for the first 5 to 6 years of life. (Reproduced with permission from Zitelli BJ, Davis HW *Atlas of Pediatric Physical Diagnosis* 5th edn. Philadelphia, PA: Mosby Elsevier, 2007. © 2007 Mosby Inc., an affiliate of Elsevier Inc.)

- *subacute bacterial sinusitis*: paranasal sinus infection lasting 30–90 days
- *recurrent acute bacterial sinusitis*: discrete episodes of paranasal sinus infection lasting <30 days, with intervening 10 day periods without symptoms.

Pathophysiology

Sinus cavities are air-filled spaces lined with a ciliated columnar epithelium. Mucosal inflammation and resultant blockage of the osteomeatal complex can obstruct drainage and create an environment favorable for bacterial growth. Specifically, the low pH of the occluded mucus and the decreased oxygen concentration encourage bacterial proliferation. Other systemic conditions, such as viral URIs (viral rhinosinusitis), allergic rhinitis, gastroesophageal reflux disease, structural abnormalities (i.e., deviated septum), immunodeficient states (i.e., IgA deficiency, severe combined immunodeficiency), ciliary dysfunction, or cystic fibrosis will predispose a patient to develop sinusitis.

The bacteria most frequently isolated from patients with acute sinusitis are *Streptococcus pneumonia* (30%), *Haemophilus influenzae* (20%), and *Moraxella catarrhalis* (20%). Chronic sinusitis is commonly caused by polymicrobial infection including these bacteria, as well as *Staphylococcus aureus*, and anerobes (i.e., *Bacteroides* and *Fusobacterium* spp.). Fungal infections in pediatric patients are increasingly identified and most commonly include *Bipolaris*, *Curvularia*, and *Aspergillus* spp. *Pseudomonas aeruginosa* is frequently isolated in patients with cystic fibrosis, in immunosuppressed patients, or in those patients who have completed multiple courses of antibiotics without improvement in their symptoms.

Clinical presentation

Viral URIs frequently precede the development of acute or chronic sinusitis. Bacterial sinusitis should be considered when symptoms of the viral URI have continued for more than 7–10 days or when severe clinical symptoms, such as fever and purulent nasal discharge, have progressed rapidly (i.e., within 3 days of onset). Common presenting complaints include nasal congestion, purulent nasal discharge, facial or sinus pressure, and associated symptoms such as tooth pain, headache, or cough. Younger children may present with irritability or emesis from excessive mucus production or coughing.

Rarely, patients with advanced sinusitis may present with periorbital cellulitis, orbital cellulitis, cavernous sinus infection, intracerebral involvement (i.e., intracranial abscess, empyema), or CNS infection (i.e., meningitis or epidural abscess). Associated symptoms include periorbital swelling, proptosis, visual loss, headaches, altered mental status, neck pain, or other evidence of systemic illness.

Diagnosis

Diagnosis of pediatric sinusitis is primarily made by history. Physical examination findings are frequently not helpful for making the diagnosis of acute sinusitis or for distinguishing between bacterial and viral etiologies. In older or more cooperative patients, facial tenderness, or pain with percussion over the sinuses, may be elicited. Transillumination of the maxillary sinuses to detect the presence of fluid is not reliable in children <10 years old.

Imaging studies, such as radiographs, are not recommended in children because radiography cannot fully visualize ethmoid disease. Use of CT can more reliably show mucosal thickening, air–fluid levels, and associated possible orbital or intracranial complications. The disadvantages of CT scans include the radiation dosage and the high incidence of soft tissue findings in asymptomatic patients. A CT scan of the sinuses should be ordered if the patient appears ill or if there is concern for spread of infection beyond the sinuses. Although MRI is better in delineating sinus disease, it is considered too high cost – both monetarily and given the need for pediatric sedation – to make its use routine for this diagnosis.

Management

The decision of when to start antibiotics for the treatment of sinusitis is controversial for several reasons. First, resolution of symptoms without antibiotic therapy is known to occur in 50–60% of cases of acute sinusitis. Increasing resistance of *S. pneumoniae* to macrolides and penicillin, and the beta-lactamase-producing capability of *H. influenzae* and *M. catarrhalis* has already precluded the use of a number of antibiotics. For this reason, a growing number of clinicians will choose not to prescribe antibiotics unless there is failure to improve after an appropriate amount of time, or if the patient presents with particularly severe symptoms. The recommendation from the Joint Council of Allergy, Asthma, and Immunology to treat with antibiotics is based on the finding that antibiotic use results in a more rapid resolution of symptoms.

A second controversy surrounding antibiotic use in sinusitis is how to avoid the unnecessary prescribing of antibiotics for what may be a viral infection. To avoid this, the general recommendation is to observe patients who present with mild symptoms within the first 7–10 days of illness until the 10 days have passed. At that time, if the symptoms are progressing or failing to improve, a course of antibiotics should be prescribed (Table 35.1). However, patients who show dramatic progression of symptoms within the first 3 days of illness, or are otherwise ill-appearing, should be prescribed antibiotics immediately.

Once prescribed antibiotics, the patient should be re-examined in 3–4 days to ensure improvement of symptoms. Failure to improve may suggest bacterial resistance, the

Table 35.1. Antibiotic therapy for bacterial sinusitis

Antibiotic	Dosage	Indications
Amoxicillin	90 mg/kg daily PO in two divided doses	Uncomplicated mild–moderate sinusitis
Azithromycin	10 mg/kg (max. 500 mg) one dose PO on day 1; 5 mg/kg (max. 250 mg) PO once daily on days 2–5	Penicillin allergy, uncomplicated mild–moderate sinusitis
Amoxicillin–clavulanate	80–90 mg/kg amoxicillin with 6.4 mg/kg clavulanate PO daily in two divided doses	Severe sinusitis; daycare attendance; recent antibiotic use
Ceftriaxone	50 mg/kg IM or IV daily	Unable to take oral antibiotics; consider IV use for refractory chronic sinusitis

Pearls and pitfalls: sinusitis

Pearls

1. The majority of pediatric sinus infections are viral and will resolve without antibiotics.
2. For uncomplicated acute sinusitis, nasal steroids do not need to be prescribed.
3. If antibiotics are prescribed, close follow-up (2–4 days) should be arranged.

Pitfalls

1. Any ill-appearing patient, or those with rapidly progressing symptoms, should be prescribed antibiotics.
2. A CT scan is useful for evaluation of intracranial, orbital, or periorbital spread of disease.

Special situation

1. Any immunocompromised patient with suspicion for sinusitis should be placed on antibiotics and have close follow-up with a specialist.

presence of another offending agent (i.e., fungal), or an alternative etiology responsible for the sinusitis (i.e., nasal polyps). While the duration of antibiotic therapy is also controversial, it is generally accepted that treatment of acute sinusitis should be for 10–14 days, while chronic sinusitis warrants at least 4 weeks of antibiotic therapy.

Nasal and systemic steroids have not been shown to speed resolution of symptoms. Intranasal steroids are not recommended for routine treatment of sinusitis, although systemic steroids may be prescribed for patients who have failed to improve with a trial of antibiotics or if there is persistent nasal congestion. Adjunctive treatment aids include nasal saline irrigation, mucolytics, decongestants, and astringents. At this time, there is no evidence supporting the use or non-use of these methods.

In severe sinusitis, or in a patient with a known complicating co-morbidity, consultation with the otorhinolaryngology service can guide further management issues. Surgical drainage of the sinuses is considered only when significant periorbital, orbital, or intracranial complications are suspected.

Disposition

The majority of pediatric patients with acute sinusitis are well enough to be discharged home for follow-up with their pediatrician. Suspicion for systemic illness or concerning co-morbidity should weigh heavily in determining the disposition of the patient. Close follow-up should always be arranged, and return precautions should be explained to the caregivers.

Selected references

American Academy of Pediatrics. Clinical practice guideline: management of sinusitis. *Pediatrics* 2001;**108**:798–808.

Principi N, Esposito S. New insights into pediatric rhinosinusitis. *Pediatr Allergy Immunol* 2007;**18** (Suppl.):7–9.

Slavin RG, Spector SL, Bernstein IL, *et al.* The diagnosis and management of sinusitis: a practice parameter update. *J Allergy Clin Immunol* 2005;**116**(Suppl.):S13–S47.

Tan R, Spector S. Pediatric sinusitis. *Curr Allergy Asthma Rep* 2007;7: 421–426.

Chapter 36

Ear, nose, and throat foreign bodies

Tammy Foster

Introduction

With the development of the pincer grasp as early as 9 months of age, children often maneuver small objects into their ears, mouth, or nose. A wide variety of ear, nose, and throat (ENT) foreign bodies are encountered in pediatric emergency medicine, including food particles, pebbles, plant material, small toys, beads, styrofoam pellets, and pencil erasers. Button batteries must always be considered, as their alkaline contents can cause liquefaction necrosis of the surrounding tissue.

Children most commonly present with ENT foreign bodies between the ages of 2 and 4 years. The symptoms produced will vary with location, composition, and the length of time the item has been present. A history of foreign body insertion may not be obtainable. Organic matter causes more local reaction than inorganic, and moisture facilitates suppuration. Presenting complaints may include unilateral purulent nasal or aural discharge, epistaxis, drooling, halitosis, or ear or throat pain. Inflammation associated with undiagnosed or incompletely removed foreign bodies may be difficult to distinguish from a primary infectious or neoplastic process.

Unless there is developmental delay or psychiatric disease, ear and nasal foreign bodies in older children and adults are usually accidental and may include insects or the tip of a cotton swab in the ear. Oropharyngeal foreign bodies are usually related to eating. During swallowing, the base of the tongue pushes a bolus of food posteriorly. Any sharp object contained within that bolus may become embedded in the tonsil, the tonsillar pillar, the pharyngeal wall, or the tongue base itself. These foreign bodies commonly cause dysphagia and rarely cause respiratory symptoms. An infant who refuses to eat or who has difficulty handling secretions should be evaluated for a foreign body. Airway and esophageal foreign bodies are addressed in Chs. 178 and 72, respectively. It is important to note, however, that while adults can describe what happened and usually present immediately, more than half of children exhibit minimal signs or symptoms of the event. Subtle or delayed presentation is more common in the pediatric population. Pediatric foreign body aspiration may be accompanied by choking, cyanosis, wheezing, or coughing, but many children have minimal signs and symptoms at the time of evaluation.

An abrasion or ulcer of the posterior pharynx or esophagus may produce a foreign body sensation in the throat. An inadequately chewed corn chip or an irritating pill such as tetracycline may be the cause. However, if a patient complains of a foreign body of the throat, a diligent search is indicated. Objects that remain impacted have the potential for mucosal perforation and deep soft tissue infection. Many cases of otolaryngolic disease of undetermined etiology are caused by foreign bodies. Unilateral purulent nasal discharge and halitosis are classic presenting complaints, but retained particles can cause subsequent granuloma formation with the gross appearance of a tumor or inflammatory process.

Evaluation

Evaluation is primarily by physical examination. A complete physical examination is necessary to rule out additional foreign bodies and underlying illness. Discomfort from otitis media, otitis externa, or pharyngitis may have prompted the foreign body insertion. Consider the possibility of coincident aspiration or ingestion.

Laboratory testing is not usually indicated. In the case of possible oropharyngeal foreign body, a soft tissue neck radiography may elucidate a foreign body if it cannot be seen on physical examination. If a patient is unable to manage secretions or swallow liquids or solids, or there is strong suspicion of foreign body based on history, ENT should be consulted.

The ear is best examined with the pinna superiorly and posteriorly retracted to straighten the external auditory canal (EAC). In infants, however, the pinna may have to be gently retracted posteriorly and downward for optimal view.

Nasal foreign bodies are most commonly found on the floor of the nasal cavity below the inferior turbinate or anterior to the middle turbinate.

Oropharyngeal foreign bodies may be seen by direct inspection or laryngoscopy. Older children may accurately

A Practical Guide to Pediatric Emergency Medicine: Caring for Children in the Emergency Department, ed. N. Ewen Amieva-Wang (associate eds. Jamie Shandro, Aparajita Sohoni, and Bernhard Fassl). Published by Cambridge University Press.

indicate the site to be examined. Tonsillar injury refers sensation to the area around the greater cornu of the hyoid bone. Vague localization to the suprasternal notch can imply a foreign body anywhere in the esophagus. Fish bones usually lodge in the soft palate or tonsil, rarely in the hypopharynx or esophagus. Palpation with a finger should be avoided because of the risk of further displacing the object.

To increase the chance of successful visualization and removal of the foreign body, take the time to obtain proper instruments and to position the patient optimally. In facilities with ENT consultant or where next day follow-up is reliable, foreign body removal can be deferred. If there is no pediatric ENT backup, sedation may be necessary for patients unable to cooperate with the procedure.

If button batteries are involved, swallowing is impaired, or there is a possibility of airway compromise, emergency ENT consultation is warranted. Emergency consultation is also warranted if there is impaired swallowing, respiratory symptoms, suspected aspiration, fever, or toxicity.

Button battery ingestion always requires prompt ENT consultation.

Management

Removal of a foreign body from the ear

Equipment. Otoscope with removable lens, nasal speculum, headlamp, bayonet forceps, alligator forceps, 60 ml syringe, 20 g angiocatheter, emesis basin, soft-tipped Frazier suction catheter.

Local anesthesia is rarely used for ear foreign body removal because of the complex innervation of the EAC. Avoid pushing the object deeper into the canal. Edema of the canal wall can trap an object such that surgical removal becomes necessary. Live insects in the ear should be immobilized with mineral oil or viscous lidocaine before removal. Examine the ear before and after each removal attempt. Assess for completeness of removal and check for trauma to the canal. Document the integrity of the tympanic membrane. A perforated membrane should prompt a call to the otolaryngologist for urgent follow-up.

Techniques for removal of ear foreign bodies include mechanical extraction, irrigation, and suction.

Mechanical extraction. Position the patient comfortably and place the otoscope in the ear, stabilized by the examiner's hand against the patient's face. Move the otoscope lens to one side. Introduce the bayonet or alligator forceps through the lens until the object is grasped. Slowly withdraw the forceps and offending item.

Irrigation. A water stream is *contraindicated* if there is any possibility of tympanic membrane perforation, or in the case of button batteries because of the potential to accelerate leakage of corrosive material. Vegetable matter, such as a bean or popcorn kernel, should not be irrigated with water because it may swell and become impacted. Attach a 20 g angiocatheter to a 60 ml syringe. Warmed irrigation fluid greatly enhances patient comfort (water or normal saline). Position the patient comfortably with an emesis basin under the affected ear. Gently place the angiocatheter in the EAC and slowly inject irrigation fluid until the foreign body washes out.

Suction. Connect the soft-tipped suction catheter or Frazier suction to low wall suction and position the patient comfortably. Visualize the object with the otoscope and retract the lens to one side. Introduce the catheter and advance until the foreign body is contacted. Gently withdraw both the item and the catheter.

Other methods. Acetone is reported to safely remove chewing gum, Styrofoam, and cyanoacrylate glue (superglue) from the ear canal. Ethyl chloride also dissolves Styrofoam beads in the ear. Some metallic foreign bodies may be removed by a magnet.

Attempts should be abandoned if the object migrates further, or if significant pain, bleeding, or swelling occurs. Repeated attempts may result in infection, perforation, and prolonged morbidity. If unsuccessful, next day otolaryngology clinic follow-up is usually adequate, but emergency consultation could be pursued if tympanic membrane rupture or infection is suspected. Antibiotics in topical or oral form may be indicated for canal or tympanic membrane trauma or otitis media.

Removal of a foreign body from the nose

Equipment. Nasal speculum, headlamp, bayonet forceps, alligator forceps, soft-tipped suction catheter, hooked probe or sculpted paperclip. (To make a sculpted paperclip, use Kelly forceps to bend the rounded end of the clip into a scoop. Check that the paperclip edges remain smooth after bending.)

The nasal mucosa should be prepared with neosynephrine or oxymetalozine to decrease mucosal edema. Nebulized lidocaine can be used for local anesthesia, although it may not be necessary and it may obscure the view.

Mechanical extraction. Depending on the item's texture and shape, use the preferred instrument to grasp or scoop the object out of the nasal cavity. Smooth, round items such as plastic beads are not easy to grasp with forceps, but the sculpted paperclip can often be eased behind them. If a balloon catheter can be passed behind the object, it can be inflated and the foreign body pulled out, but use care not to push the object further into the nasopharynx. There are reports of the use of cyanoacrylate glue to remove foreign bodies by applying the glue to the end of a wooden or plastic applicator stick, holding it in contact with foreign body for 1 min, then withdrawing both the stick and the foreign object. Some metallic foreign bodies may be removed by a magnet.

Suction. If using suction, turn it to 100–140 mmHg and ideally use a Frazier suction tube topped with a lightly lubricated pressure equalizer (PE) tube for a better seal.

Other methods. Positive pressure ventilation to the mouth has been successfully used to force foreign bodies out of small children's noses. There is a theoretical risk of barotrauma to the tympanic membranes or lower airway, but this has not been reported. Application of vasoconstrictor medication (neosynephrine spray) may facilitate success. Occlude the unobstructed nare with a finger. A cooperative child can then simply blow his nose, or the parent can provide a gentle puff of air directly to the child's mouth. Alternatively, the clinician may use a bag-valve mask to provide the positive pressure.

Examine the nose after removal attempts to evaluate for trauma to the nasal mucosa, epistaxis, or migration of the foreign body posteriorly. If attempts are unsuccessful, next day follow-up in the specialty clinic is an option as long as the patient exhibits no constitutional symptoms such as fever or lethargy. Antibiotics would be indicated only in cases of incomplete or traumatic removal, or unsuccessful removal with signs of sinusitis.

Removal of a foreign body from the oropharynx

Equipment. Tongue blade, headlamp, mirror, direct laryngoscope, cetacaine spray, forceps or tonsil hemostat, suction.

With the patient sitting in a chair, inspect the oropharynx with a tongue depressor, looking for foreign bodies or abrasions. Grasp the tongue with 4 × 4 gauze and pull gently, taking care not to lacerate the frenulum on the lower incisors. Inspect the hypopharynx directly or with a warmed mirror. Cetacaine spray or viscous or nebulized lidocaine may be used for anesthesia but is not necessary in the case of a simple pharyngeal or tonsillar foreign body. Have the patient raise his soft palate by panting "like a dog." Search for abrasions or foreign bodies, paying special attention to the base of the tongue, tonsils, and vallecula. A small fish bone is frequently difficult to see and may look like a strand of mucus. An indirect laryngoscope or fiberoptic nasopharyngoscope may be helpful. When the object is found, carefully grasp and remove it with the forceps or hemostat.

If unsuccessful and symptoms are mild, test the patient's ability to swallow, first with water and then a small piece of bread or crackers. Occasionally, swallowing a food bolus dislodges the item and eliminates the foreign body sensation.

Emergency consultation is warranted in cases of impaired swallowing, suspected respiratory compromise, or evidence of infection. Serious infectious complications of oropharyngeal foreign bodies include retropharyngneal abscess and mediastinitis.

If inspection does not reveal a foreign body and the patient is afebrile, comfortable, and able to swallow, outpatient follow-up in 1–2 days is appropriate. Advise parents that if an abrasion is the cause of the foreign body sensation, symptoms should resolve within 24 h. Antibiotics are generally not necessary.

Disposition

Schedule follow-up with otolaryngology if there is any question of retained foreign body or significant risk of post-procedure complication such as infection.

Discharge instructions must include advice to return if there is fever, progressive discomfort, or inability to tolerate oral fluids.

Pearls and pitfalls

Pearls

1. Gather all supplies and use optimal positioning for a successful first attempt.
2. Conscious sedation may be necessary in younger children. Have topical anesthetic (EMLA or similar) at two IV sites early.
3. Subtle or delayed presentation is more common in the pediatric population.

Pitfalls

1. Failure to realize that otolaryngolic disease of undetermined etiology could be caused by a foreign body.
2. Failure to examine carefully after removal of foreign material to ensure complete removal, and document the presence or absence of complications.

Selected references

Bressler K, Shelton C. Ear foreign-body removal: a review of 98 consecutive cases. *Laryngoscope* 1993;**103**:367–370.

Chan TC, Ufberg J, Harrigan RA, Vilke GM. Nasal foreign body removal. *J Emerg Med* 2004;**26**:441–445.

Chisholm EJ, Barber-Craig H, Farrell R. Chewing gum removal from the ear using acetone. *J Laryngol Otol* 2003;**117**:325.

Davies PH, Benger JR. Foreign bodies in the nose and ear: a review of techniques for removal in the emergency department. *J Accid Emerg Med* 2000;**17**:91–94.

DiMuzio J Jr., Deschler, DG. Emergency department management of foreign bodies of the external ear canal in children. *Otol Neurotol* 2002;**23**:473–475.

Navitsky RC, Beamsley A, McLaughlin S. Nasal positive-pressure technique for nasal foreign body removal in children. *Am J Emerg Med* 2002;**20**:103–104.

Ngan JH, Fok PJ, Lai EC, Branicki FJ, Wong J. A prospective study of fish bone ingestion: experience with 358 patients. *Ann Surg* 1990;**11**:459–462.

Thompson SK, Wein RO, Dutcher PO. External auditory canal foreign body removal: management practices and outcomes. *Laryngoscope* 2003;**113**:1912–1915.

Chapter 37

Epistaxis and nasal fractures

Amy B. Kunihiro and Aparajita Sohoni

Epistaxis

Epistaxis is a common entity in children; 56% of children aged 6–10 years and 30% of children under the age of 5 have had at least one bloody nose. Pediatric epistaxis is rarely severe. Most cases resolve spontaneously or with manual compression. The most common causes of epistaxis are trauma (e.g., nose picking), nasal foreign body, dry mucosa, or rhinitis. The peak incidence of epistaxis occurs in dry environments and in colder weather.

The majority are anterior nosebleeds, arising from Kiesselbach's plexus in the anterior nasal septum. This plexus is about 0.5 cm from the tip of the nose. As the nasal mucosa is closely adherent to the septum, the underlying vessels have little protection. The more rare posterior bleed tends to arise from the branches of the sphenopalatine artery. Even less common in pediatric patients are episodes of epistaxis caused by systemic conditions, such as bleeding disorders or medications.

Evaluation

Before locating the source of the nosebleed, the patient should be evaluated for airway and hemodynamic stability. Sedation and/or analgesia may be needed, as a child with epistaxis can be difficult to examine. Use of a topical vasoconstrictor (0.05% oxymetazoline hydrochloride, or 0.25, 0.5 or 1% phenylephrine) can facilitate the examination. It can be squirted into the nose by spray bottle or applied to a cotton pledget and pushed into the nostril for 5 min. After application, direct pressure should be held for 5 min.

The majority of pediatric nosebleeds are anterior. Examining the vestibule and anterior septum can be accomplished by pushing the tip of the nose upwards with one's thumb. More thorough evaluation can be accomplished using a nasal speculum with a headlight or head mirror. A posterior bleeding site should be pursued if an anterior site cannot be identified. Posterior sites tend to bleed more profusely, present with blood in the oropharynx, and bleed from both nares, although all of these can occur with anterior bleeding as well. Evaluation of a posterior bleeding site should be performed by an otolaryngologist using flexible or rigid endoscopy. Any child that has a history or examination suggestive of a systemic disease or bleeding disorder, or has severe refractory or recurrent epistaxis, warrants laboratory evaluation. This may include CBC, tests for coagulation (partial thromboplastin time [PTT] and prothrombin time [PT]), and bleeding time.

Treatment

Mild epistaxis that resolves quickly requires education in the event of recurrence (i.e., compression), and ways to prevent it (see Disposition, below). Active bleeding usually responds to compression in children. This entails squeezing the nasal alae together for a minimum of 5 min, without letting go, to ensure constant pressure to Kiesselbach's plexus. The child should sit upright and slightly bent forward to minimize the chance of aspiration from blood entering the hypopharynx.

Most anterior bleeds stop within 10 min of compression. If this does not occur, cautery can be tried in a cooperative patient. Topical application of lidocaine or cocaine for anesthesia should be applied first. Either silver nitrate sticks or electric cautery can be used on a relatively dry surface, starting proximally. Cautery will not work if proximal hemostasis has not been achieved. Do not cauterize both sides of the septum as this could cause perforation of the septum.

If compression and cautery are not successful, nasal packing is the next option to control bleeding. If this step is required, consultation with an otolaryngologist is warranted for both packing placement and evaluation of the underlying cause of bleeding. Packing is generally done with Merocel, or can be accomplished with Gelfoam, Surgicel, or Vaseline gauze. Merocel and Vaseline packs are generally left in for several days, usually no more than 5, and then removed by the otolaryngologist. Antibiotics are warranted for underlying sinusitis but are not proven to reliably prevent toxic shock syndrome, although it is standard of care in emergency medicine to place a child with packing on prophylactic antibiotics for a 5-day course.

A Practical Guide to Pediatric Emergency Medicine: Caring for Children in the Emergency Department, ed. N. Ewen Amieva-Wang (associate eds. Jamie Shandro, Aparajita Sohoni, and Bernhard Fassl). Published by Cambridge University Press.

Disposition

Most patients who have had epistaxis can be safely discharged home. Those patients who only required compression can be instructed to perform this technique at home for any rebleeding. It should also be suggested to humidify the mucosa to prevent recurrence. This can be achieved through the use of saline nasal spray (over the counter) three or four times a day, or a humidifier in the child's room (for children without pulmonary or allergy problems). Children who have been cauterized should follow-up with an otolaryngologist or their pediatrician if rebleeding occurs. Children who have had packing placed and are not admitted to the hospital should see the otolaryngologist in 1–5 days to have the packing removed and for re-evaluation. In children who had bleeding secondary to allergic rhinitis, use of nasal corticosteroid spray should be discontinued. An oral anithistamine can be suggested in its place, with caution to avoid dryness of the mucosa.

Pearls and pitfalls: epistaxis

Pearls

1. Evaluation and treatment of epistaxis requires a cooperative patient. Sedation (with a close eye on the airway) may be needed for more difficult or severe cases.
2. Ensure the stability of the patient's respiratory and hemodynamic status before evaluating the site of bleeding.
3. Posterior bleeding requires the evaluation of an otolaryngologist.
4. Nasal packing should be done in consultation with an otolaryngologist and requires follow-up with an otolaryngologist within 1–5 days.

Pitfalls

1. Failure to arrange close follow-up if nasal packing has been inserted.
2. Failure to assess for a posterior bleed if an anterior source has not been found.

Nasal fractures

Nasal fractures are uncommon in children under 5. Because a child's nose has a more prominent soft cartilaginous portion than an adult nose, the force from a blow will be dissipated by the cartilage across the mid-face, resulting in more significant ecchymosis and edema to the mid-face. If a fracture does occur, the nasal bones and septum will deviate and/or depress.

Evaluation

All children presenting with nasal trauma also need to be assessed for associated injuries to the cervical spine, chest, eyes, teeth, and CNS. Signs and symptoms of more extensive injuries than just to the nose include diplopia, change in visual acuity, neck pain, malocclusion, and sensory deficits, to name a few.

Inspection of the nose should include palpation of facial and nasal bones and internal examination of the nose. Application of a vasoconstricting agent to the nasal mucosa may aid in evaluation. Along with obvious nasal deformity and swelling, pertinent findings include malocclusion and instability of the palate (suggests mid-facial LeFort fracture); tenderness to palpation of the tip of the nose (suggests septal hematoma); tenderness and/or instability of the anterior nasal spine, felt from beneath the upper lip (suggests severe septal trauma); the presence of clear fluid in the nasal cavity (suggests CSF leak secondary to a skull fracture); and tenderness over the frontal sinus (suggests sinus fracture). Epistaxis commonly accompanies nasal trauma but has usually resolved by the time of ED evaluation. If epistaxis persists, direct pressure or sometimes nasal packing is required for bleeding cessation.

Septal hematoma is a rare complication of nasal trauma that warrants otolaryngological evaluation. Signs of hematoma include a bluish or reddish asymmetric septum, swelling of the nasal mucosa causing obstruction to airflow, and a mass that does not change in size after vasoconstrictor application.

Radiographs are not recommended in the routine evaluation of nasal fractures. The nasal bones of children are not fused and are primarily cartilaginous, and so are poorly visualized on plain films.

Management

In children, if there is no septal deviation or hematoma, and minimal swelling, the child does not need follow-up. All others should be seen by an otolaryngologist within 1–3 days. This allows resolution of edema to permit thorough evaluation of any nasal structural abnormality. Postponement of evaluation beyond 7 days makes reduction of nasal fractures much more difficult because of the occurrence of fibrous union between the fractured parts.

Pearls and pitfalls: nasal fractures

Pearls

1. Radiographs are unnecessary and notoriously poor at showing nasal fractures in children.
2. Always consider injury to other facial structures and organs in a child with facial trauma.

Pitfalls

1. Failure to arrange close follow-up (2–3 days) with an ENT specialist in patients with a nasal fracture and moderate-severe swelling.

Lymphadenopathy

Heather Ross Ogle

Introduction

Lymph nodes can become enlarged in reaction to a local infection (reactive nodes); they can be inflamed and infected themselves (lymphadenitis), and they can enlarge in response to systemic disease (infection or neoplasm.) The various cervical lymph node chains drain different spaces in the neck (Fig. 38.1):

- submental/submandibular: oral/dental processes
- submandibular: cheeks
- preauricular: scalp, nasopharynx, orbit (conjunctivitis)
- anterior cervical: mid-face, oral cavity, tonsil
- posterior cervical: nasopharynx
- supraclavicular: often not head/neck source, always abnormal.

Lymphadenopathy is the most common cause of pediatric neck masses.

Neck masses are covered in Ch. 39.

Reactive lymph nodes

Palpable cervical nodes under 1 cm in diameter occur in greater than half of well pediatric patients. Typical reactive lymph nodes are usually multiple, smaller than 1–2 cm, discrete, and firm. They are non-tender and mobile with no superficial skin changes. While these nodes often resolve 2–3 weeks after a local infection, such as an upper respiratory tract infection, they can persist. These nodes are benign and require no treatment.

Lymphadenitis

Inflamed and infected lymph nodes are enlarged, tender, and can be fluctuant. The overlying skin can be warm and erythematous. The most common site of adenitis in the neck is the submandibular region. Lymphadenitis is usually caused by

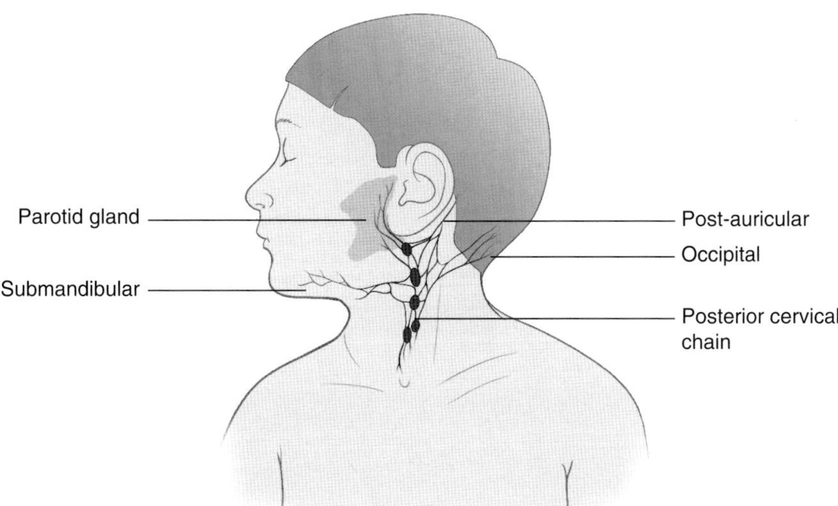

Figure 38.1 Distribution of the superficial cervical lymph nodes. Note also the location of the parotid gland, which can extend slightly posterior to the pinna. (Copyright Chris Gralapp.)

A Practical Guide to Pediatric Emergency Medicine: Caring for Children in the Emergency Department, ed. N. Ewen Amieva-Wang (associate eds. Jamie Shandro, Aparajita Sohoni, and Bernhard Fassl). Published by Cambridge University Press.

Staphylococcus aureus and group A streptococci. Lymphadenitis tends to suppurate and lead to abscess more often in children than adults. Lymph nodes that have grown markedly in size or that are fluctuant should be examined by ultrasound for possible abscess formation.

Management

The majority of patients respond to appropriate outpatient antibiotic therapy for methicillin-resistant *S. aureus* (MRSA). Pediatric ENT follow-up is required to assure resolution or arrange further evaluation. Patients with rapidly enlarged lymph nodes or abscesses must be admitted for IV antibiotics and possible surgical procedures.

Tuberculous and non-tuberculous mycobacteria are other causes of cervical adenitis (scrofula). Patients with mycobacterial infection classically have a single large cervical lymph node. The overlying skin may have a characteristic violaceous color. A PPD test (purified protein derivative test or Mantoux test) is usually strongly reactive. A chest radiograph should be done to rule out active pulmonary disease. Treatment is the same as for pulmonary tuberculosis (Ch. 99). In children, infection with non-tuberculous mycobacteria is more common than with tuberculous mycobacteria and rarely causes fever or systemic symptoms. The chest radiograph is usually normal, and PPD reactions are normal or intermediate in reactivity. The treatment is less definitive, as the non-tuberculous mycobacteria are notoriously resistant to traditional antituberculous drugs.

Cat scratch disease is caused by *Bartonella henselae*, a Gram-negative rod that can be cultured from 30–60% of cats. Classically there is exposure to a young kitten. Clinical symptoms include unilateral, regional lymphadenopathy with or without low-grade fevers, and malaise. The symptoms usually resolve over several weeks with no treatment. Antibiotics should be started in patients with severe systemic symptoms and in the immunocompromised. These patients should also be referred to infectious disease specialists.

Systemic infection

Usually lymph node enlargement secondary to a systemic infection is associated with other signs of infection. Infectious mononucleosis, caused by Epstein–Barr virus causes an exudative tonsillitis with impressive cervical lymphadenopathy in the adolescent population. Cervical lymphadenitis may also accompany infection with CMV or the human immunodeficiency virus (HIV).

Selected reference

Bernius N, Perlin D. Pediatric ear, nose, and throat emergencies. *Pediatr Clin North Am* 2006;**53**: 195–214.

Chapter 39

Neck masses

Heather Ross Ogle

Introduction

The majority of neck masses in children are benign. Pediatric neck masses can be categorized as congenital, inflammatory, and, rarely, neoplastic.

Anatomy

The neck has been traditionally divided into anterior and posterior triangles by the sternocleidomastoid muscle. These landmarks are helpful to precisely locate a mass, possibly diagnose the etiology and to describe the mass to consultants.

Clinical presentation

Typically a child will be brought to the ED with either an incidental mass found by the parent, or a symptomatic infected mass. Emergency management of a neck mass is determined initially by its local effect on the airway and adjacent structures, as well as by the nature of the mass.

Differential diagnosis

The patient's age, the location of the mass, the time course of its development, and the associated symptoms will determine the differential for a pediatric neck mass (Table 39.1).

Table 39.1. Differential of neck masses by age

Age group	Mass
Infant	Sternocleidomastoid tumor of infancy (also known as fibromatosis colli or congenital torticollis), hemangioma, lymphatic malformation (old term cystic hygroma), branchial cleft cyst, rhabdomyosarcoma
Child	Reactive lymphadenopathy, branchial cleft cyst, thyroglossal duct cyst, lymphatic and vascular malformation
Young adult	Reactive lymphadenopathy, mononucleosis, lymphoma, branchial cleft cyst, thyroglossal duct cyst
Adult	Submandibular gland infection, neoplasm, lymphoma, thyroid disorder

Congenital masses

Vascular malformations

Hemangiomas are dense masses of dilated vessels that result from vascular malformation within fetal mesenchymal tissue. They are the most common head and neck tumor of infants and children, with an incidence of 1% at birth and 10% at 1 year of age. Females are three to five times more likely to be affected than males. Hemangiomata generally present within a few months of birth, proliferate over the subsequent 2–12 months and then slowly involute. Approximately 70% of cases resolve by age 7.

An infant with cutaneous vascular lesions and stridor should be suspected of having a subglottic hemangioma.

However, subglottic hemangioma can occur without cutaneous manifestations 50% of the time. The child is usually asymptomatic at birth, but during a phase of rapid growth develops progressive respiratory distress with symptoms of hoarseness, stridor, and cough. The clinical picture may be mistaken for acute infectious croup. However, if the patient has a history of multiple episodes, or is very young, the EP should suspect a non-infectious etiology.

Racemic epinephrine can be used to treat stridor. Infants <2 months with stridor should have a prompt ENT consult. Diagnosis is made by laryngoscopy. Usually management is watchful waiting, as these lesions will regress.

Lymphatic malformations

The majority of lymphatic malformations are soft, compressible masses evident at birth and 80–90% will be identified by age 2 years. They affect both sexes equally, with an incidence of approximately 1/10 000 live births. While lymphatic malformations can occur anywhere in the body, they most commonly form in the posterior triangle of the neck. These lesions

A Practical Guide to Pediatric Emergency Medicine: Caring for Children in the Emergency Department, ed. N. Ewen Amieva-Wang (associate eds. Jamie Shandro, Aparajita Sohoni, and Bernhard Fassl). Published by Cambridge University Press.

transilluminate, and the overlying skin may have a bluish hue. These benign lesions grow in proportion to the child and, unlike hemangiomas, almost never spontaneously involute. They can present after a sudden increase in size secondary to infection or intralesional hemorrhage. Complications include airway obstruction, hemorrhage, and infection.

Morbidity depends primarily on the anatomic location of the malformation, and is related to cosmetic disfigurement and impingement on nerves, vessels, and lymphatics. If the patient has no airway compromise, removal as an outpatient can be arranged. An infected lymphatic malformation should be treated with IV antibiotics, and definitive surgery should be performed once the infection has resolved.

Branchial cleft and thyroglossal duct cysts

Incomplete obliteration of the embryonic branchial apparatus leads to anomalies such as cysts, sinuses or fistulae. Branchial cleft cysts often are not diagnosed until they become infected in late childhood and early adulthood. These infections can manifest as a pit draining mucous along the anterior border of the sternocleidomastoid muscle or as an erythematous, fluctuant mass anterior to the muscle.

Thyroglossal duct cysts occur equally in males and females and are usually detected in the first decade of life, presenting as a mobile, gradually enlarging, non-tender midline mass anywhere from the floor of the mouth to the suprasternal notch. Arrested descent of the thyroid gland through the thyroglossal duct can also result in ectopic thyroid tissue. Infected thyroglossal duct cysts manifest as tender, enlarging masses with or without associated dysphagia, dysphonia, drainage, or fever.

Suspected branchial cleft or thyroglossal duct cysts do not need imaging within the ED. Infections should be treated with appropriate antibiotics, with referral to a pediatric surgery or otolaryngology clinic for elective excision as they tend to get reinfected.

Neoplastic masses

Neck neoplastic lesions have two peaks of incidence in childhood, 2–5 years and 15–19 years. Lymphoma accounts for more than 55% of head and neck tumors in children, and usually presents in adolescent years; 40% of rhabdomyosarcoma tumors occur in the head and neck region.

On physical examination, the lymph nodes are hard, matted and fixed in position.

A swollen supraclavicular node is malignant until proven otherwise.

These nodes grow slowly but over a long period of time. Often lymphadenopathy is accompanied by weight loss, fever and other symptoms.

Patients with suspected malignancy should have screening CBC, and chest radiograph and be admitted to oncology.

Other masses

The sternomastoid tumor of infancy/congenital torticollis, also known as pseudotumor of infancy, is a fibrotic lesion of the distal sternocleidomastoid muscle and usually presents within 1 to 3 weeks of birth. An association with breach delivery and forceps delivery has been reported. The patient may exhibit a head tuck to the ipsilateral side and chin pointed away from the lesion. A hard, non-tender mass can usually be palpated within the body of the sternocleidomastoid muscle.

Usually, aggressive physical therapy and range of motion exercises lead to resolution by the first birthday. Rarely, an untreated case may lead to long-term torticollis.

Pearls and pitfalls

Pearls

1. Sternocleidomastoid tumor of infancy is a common neck mass in the neonate.
2. Branchial cleft cysts can present as a painless, fluctuant anterior triangle mass in infants or a superinfected anterior mass in older children.
3. Thyroglossal duct cysts are usually midline structures that manifest with superinfection.
4. Lymphatic malformations most commonly manifest in the posterior triangle of the neck.

Pitfalls

1. Diagnosis of repeated episodes of stridor in a neonate or young child as croup.
2. Failure to realize that 50% of subglottic hemangiomas present without cutaneous signs.

Selected references

Burezq H, Williams B, Chitte SA. Management of cystic hygromas: 30 year experience. *J Craniofac Surg* 2006;**17**:815–818.

Thomsen JR, Koltai PJ. Sternomastoid tumor of infancy. *Ann Otol Rhinol Laryngol* 1989;**98**:955–959.

Torsiglieri, AJ. Pediatric neck masses: guidelines for evaluation. *Int J Pediatr Otorhinolaryngol* 1988;**16**:199–210.

Triglia JM, Nicollas R. First branchial cleft anomalies. *Arch Otolaryngol Head Neck Surg* 1998;**124**:291–295.

Common ear, nose, and throat complaints: otitis media, mastoiditis, and otitis externa

Amy B. Kunihiro and Aparajita Sohoni

Otitis media

Ear pain is a common presentation to the ED. It often is a true emergency for the parent in the middle of the night, with a child crying inconsolably for unknown reasons. The terminology is important: serous otitis media, also called otitis media with effusion or non-supporative otitis media, refers to the presence of fluid behind the tympanic membrane without associated signs and symptoms of infection. It can sometimes precede or follow an episode of acute otitis media (AOM), which is an infection of middle ear fluid.

The incidence of AOM is bimodal, with a first peak between the ages of 6 and 18 months of age and the second, smaller peak at 5 years. Acute otitis media has occurred in 80–90% of by the age of 3 years, and those children who have not had it by 3 years are unlikely to have severe or recurrent disease. Risk factors for AOM include:

- child aged 6–18 months
- breast-fed for <3 months
- primary or secondary exposure to tobacco smoke
- daycare
- ethnicity: Native American, Alaskan, or Canadian Eskimo
- pacifier use
- family history of AOM.

Clinical presentation

Generally otitis media begins with congestion in the respiratory mucosa (nose, eustachian tube, or nasopharynx) secondary to a viral upper respiratory infection or allergy. This congestion obstructs the eustachian tube at the narrowest part, resulting in negative pressure in the middle ear. Secretions accumulate in the middle ear as a result of this negative pressure. Bacteria and viruses of the upper respiratory tract then colonize these secretions. When this fluid becomes infected, it is referred to as AOM. The most common viruses isolated from the middle ear are respiratory syncytial virus, rhinovirus, adenovirus, and influenza. The three most commonly found bacteria are *Streptococcus pneumoniae*, *Haemophilus influenzae*, and *Moraxella catarrhalis*. An increased number of AOM infections are caused by non-typable *Haemophilus* and *Pneumococcus* strains not covered by current vaccines.

Diagnosis

The differential diagnosis of ear pain includes referred pain from the throat, otitis externa, and middle ear effusion. A red tympanic membrane can be caused by crying and fever. Decreased tympanic membrane mobility can be caused by scarring.

A middle ear effusion is present in both AOM and serous otitis media, an entity which does not require antibiotics. In 2004, the American Academy of Pediatrics (AAP) and American Academy of Family Physicians (AAFP) published guidelines for defining AOM. The diagnosis requires the presence of each of the following:

- a history of recent and abrupt onset of signs and symptoms of middle ear inflammation and effusion
- the presence of a middle ear effusion (bulging of the tympanic membrane, limited or absent mobility of the membrane, tympanic membrane retraction, presence of air fluid level, or otorrhea)
- signs or symptoms of middle ear inflammation (either distinct erythema of the tympanic membrane or distinct otalgia).

AOM can also be diagnosed if the tympanic membrane is perforated, if there is acute purulent discharge, and if otitis externa has been excluded.

AOM in the presence of purulent conjunctivitis has been shown to be predominantly caused by non-typable *H. influenzae*.

Bullous myringitis can cause sudden severe pain. It is caused by bacteria and viruses.

Treatment

In 2004, the AAP/AAFP also published guidelines for treatment of AOM based on certainty of diagnosis and severity of illness (Table 40.1). The guidelines define severe illness as temperature ≥39°C or severe otalgia. In an effort to decrease unnecessary antibiotic use in the treatment of AOM, multiple

A Practical Guide to Pediatric Emergency Medicine: Caring for Children in the Emergency Department, ed. N. Ewen Amieva-Wang (associate eds. Jamie Shandro, Aparajita Sohoni, and Bernhard Fassl). Published by Cambridge University Press.

Table 40.1. American Academy of Pediatrics and American Academy of Family Physicians treatment option recommendations

	Age <6 months	Age 6 months to 2 years	Age >2 years
Uncertain diagnosis	Antibiotics	Antibiotics if severe illness; if illness not severe, consider observation	Observation only option
Certain diagnosis	Antibiotics	Antibiotics	Antibiotics if severe illness; if not severe illness, consider observation

Box 40.1. Antibiotics typically used in treatment of acute otitis media

Amoxicillin: 80–90 mg/kg PO daily, divided BID.
Amoxicillin/clavulanate (dose based on amoxicillin component): 90 mg/kg daily, divided BID.
Azithromycin: (10 mg/kg PO on day 1 (max. 500 mg); then 5 mg/kg PO daily for 4 more days (max. 250 mg/day).
Clarithromycin: 15 mg/kg PO daily, divided BID.
Ceftriaxone: 50 mg/kg IM or IV once daily for 3 days.
Cefuroxime: suspension 30 mg/kg PO daily, divided BID (max. 1 g/day).
Cefpodoxime: 10 mg/kg PO once daily (max. 800 mg/day).

studies have evaluated a "wait and see" approach to its antibiotic treatment. The observation-only approach is contingent on starting antibiotics promptly if symptoms persist or worsen. In published studies, 60–90% of patients did not start antibiotics.

High-dose amoxicillin, which allows for good antibiotic penetration of the middle ear, is the first antibiotic of choice for treatment of AOM (Box 40.1). Children with allergies to penicillin, treated with an antibiotic within the prior 30 days, already on amoxicillin for AOM prophylaxis, or presenting with concurrent purulent conjunctivitis (suggesting *H. influenzae* that can be resistant to amoxicillin) should not be prescribed amoxicillin. Amoxicillin/clavulanate (Augmentin) is an alternative antibiotic choice (in the non-penicillin allergic patient). For children with severe, type 1 allergic reactions to penicillin, appropriate antibiotics include azithromycin, clarithromycin, or erythromycin plus sulfafurazole (sulfisoxazole). Children with a mild allergic reaction to penicillin can be placed on cefuroxime, cefpodoxime, or cefdinir.

Children receiving antibiotics who are 6 years and older and with mild or moderate AOM should receive a 5–7 day course. Children under the age of 6, or any child with severe disease, should receive a 10 day course of antibiotics.

Perhaps one of the most important aspects of treating AOM is the treatment of pain. Acetaminophen and NSAIDs are recommended for systemic analgesia. Antipyrine/benzocaine/glycerin (Auralgan) ear drops can work well in older patients tolerant of ear drops. The use of decongestants or antihistamines is not recommended in the treatment of pediatric AOM.

Failure to improve

Amoxicillin/clavulanate is the recommended drug for patients who fail initial treatment, defined as a lack of improvement within 48–72 h after initiation of antimicrobial therapy. In these cases, alternative antibiotics include cefpodoxime, cefdinir, and cefuroxime. Ceftriaxone IM given every day for 3 days can also be used for treatment failures, and for children who cannot tolerate oral antibiotic.

Disposition and follow-up

Symptoms of AOM should resolve within 24–72 h with appropriate antibiotic therapy. Patients who fail to improve should be reassessed by medical personnel. A middle ear effusion commonly persists after AOM, which can affect speech and cognitive ability. Therefore follow-up is recommended 8–12 weeks after AOM is diagnosed to evaluate for resolution of the effusion. Children who are older than 2 years and who have not had any language or cognitive problems following AOM do not need this follow-up unless there is a concern for hearing loss. Patients with more than three episodes of AOM per year should be evaluated for placement of myringotomy tubes. Suppurative complications of untreated AOM such as mastoiditis are rare in developed countries.

Pearls and pitfalls: otitis media

Pearls

1. A red ear is not necessarily acute otitis media (AOM). There must be evidence of effusion as well as inflammation.
2. High-dose amoxicillin (80–90 mg/kg daily) is the recommended initial dosing for treatment of AOM.
3. The 2004 AAP guidelines have allowed for "wait and see treatment" in subsets of patients.
4. Multiple cases of AOM can affect a child's long-term hearing and thus development.

Pitfalls

1. Failure to refer to pediatric ENT after multiple episodes of AOM (>3).
2. AOM in a neonate is difficult to diagnose; if diagnosed it warrants hospital admission and full workup.

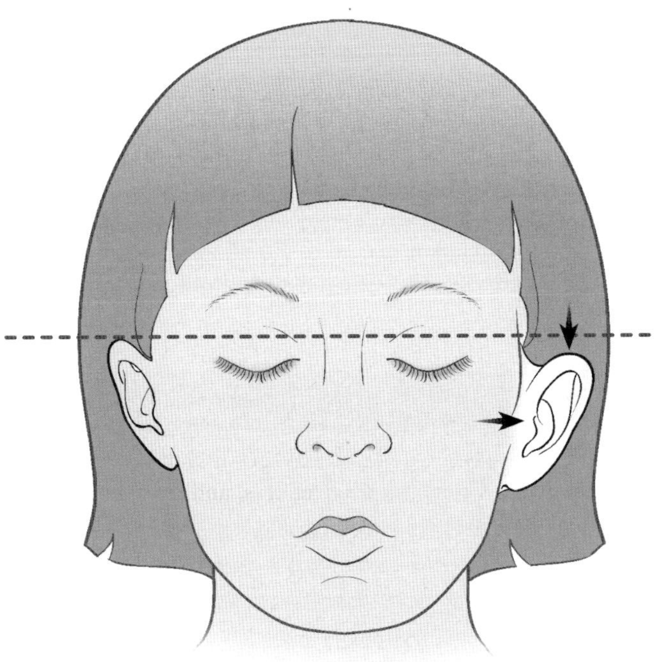

Figure 40.1 Physical findings in mastoiditis. Note the external ear is pushed down and out. (Copyright Chris Gralapp.)

Mastoiditis

Mastoiditis is a rare complication of AOM. The mastoid air cells are connected with the middle ear through a small canal (the aditus ad antrum) at the superior end of the middle ear. Because of this, there may be some inflammation of the mastoid with a routine AOM without there being clinical mastoiditis. However, if the mastoid air cells become filled with fluid they can potentially form an abscess or cause bony destruction. The accumulation of fluid or infected fluid can track back through the antrum, with resultant resolution of the mastoiditis; move laterally to the surface and form a subperiosteal abscess; move anteriorly and form an abscess below the pinna or behind the sterncleidomastoid muscle; move medially into the petrous air cells of the temporal bone (petrositis); or move posteriorly to the occipital bone.

Clinical presentation and diagnosis

Patients present with otalgia and fever, as in AOM, but also present with postauricular tenderness, erythema, and swelling, and sometimes supraauricular tenderness (Fig. 40.1). Imaging with CT or MRI has the most diagnostic utility in mastoiditis. In the ED, CT is generally more available, but MRI should be considered if there is clinical suspicion for intracranial complications.

Management and disposition

Admission for IV antibiotics is necessary if a diagnosis of mastoiditis is made. Cefuroxime (50–150 mg/kg daily IV) is usually the initial antimicrobial of choice. Otolaryngology should be consulted when the diagnosis is made. Surgical procedures that may be warranted include tympanocentesis and myringotomy with tube placement, and mastoidectomy in the case of bony destruction (in as much as 50% of those with mastoiditis).

Otitis externa

Otitis externa, or swimmer's ear, is an inflammation of the external auditory canal (EAC). It is more common in the summer months when water activities are prevalent, as well as in humid regions.

The cerumen in the EAC and the acidic environment of the EAC are natural barriers to growth of bacteria. Breakdown of this natural barrier is the first step in the pathogenesis of otitis externa. Trauma to the EAC by scratching or overzealous "cleaning" of the canal in an attempt to remove cerumen destroys the cerumen barrier. Cerumen itself is acidic, so destruction of this barrier, or constant contact with water (swimming or humid environment), will increase the pH of the EAC. The resulting warm, alkaline, moist canal serves as a breeding ground for bacteria. The most common bacteria in otitis externa infections are *Pseudomonas aeruginosa* and *Staphylococcus aureus*.

Diagnosis

The most common presentation of otitis externa is a painful, pruritic ear, with a tender EAC. The child may have clear or purulent otorrhea, and there may be a component of hearing loss caused by the edema of the EAC. The pain can become intolerable as the otitis externa becomes more severe, and any movement of the preauricular skin, as with mastication, may cause ear pain. On examination, the child will have pain when the pinna is pulled superiorly or tragal pressure is applied. The canal is typically edematous. In severe cases, fever, lymphadenopathy, and periauricular erythema may be present.

Management

Treatment consists of treating the infection, reducing inflammation, pain control, and avoidance of promoting factors.

While cleaning has been recommended in the literature, it is painful and generally not necessary.

If the canal is open, start antibiotic drops; if the canal is closed, quickly place a wick before starting ear antibiotic drops.

The usual medication for treatment of otitis externa is an acidic solution combining an antibiotic, antiseptic, and steroid; however, patients treated with and without antibiotic-containing regimens have similar cure rates. Reasonable options include ciprofloxacin/hydrocortisone, neomycin/polymyxin B/hydrocortisone, gentamicin or ofloxacin, or tobramycin/dexamethasone for a 10-day course. If the EAC is so edematous as to prevent instillation of medication, a wick or piece of gauze should be gently inserted to facilitate medication delivery to the EAC. To place medicine in the ear, the child should be lying on his or her side with the affected ear facing upwards and should remain in this position for 3 min after medication is placed in the ear. Treatment of a patient with a perforated tympanic membrane includes otic drops as well as oral antibiotics, although in true otitis externa, the tympanic membrane is not usually visible. (If the membrane is clearly visualized, the patient probably has AOM with a perforation.) Aminoglycoside- or alchohol-containing drops should not be used in the cases of tympanic membrane perforation, nor neomycin/polymyxin B/hydrocortisone or any acidic/antiseptic agents. A reasonable choice in this situation would be ofloxacin.

The pain in otitis externa will be diminished after initiation of topical therapy, but acetaminophen or ibuprofen, and occasionally narcotic analgesics, may be needed for additional pain control.

Disposition and follow-up

Parents should be counseled to never put "anything smaller than your elbow" into their child's ear; ears do not need to be cleaned by parents. While the child is being treated for otitis externa, the ear should be protected from water. Any water activity should be suspended for the duration of treatment, and a cotton ball coated with petroleum jelly should be placed in the child's ear while bathing. In a child who is a competitive swimmer, consideration can be given to resumption of activity within 2–3 days of starting treatment if their pain has resolved and they have well-fitting ear plugs.

Follow-up is recommended within 1–2 days if symptoms have not improved with appropriate therapy. If symptoms are improving, follow-up is warranted in 1–2 weeks. If a wick is in place, follow-up should occur within 1–3 days.

Prevention of otitis externa in the frequent swimmer is recommended with the use of OTC drops designed to treat swimmers' ear. These drops are usually alcohol/glycerin or alcohol/acetic acid combinations placed in the ear after swimming. The child can also dry the ears on a low setting with a hair dryer.

Pearls and pitfalls: otitis externa

1. Pain with superior movement of the auricle or pressure on the tragus is a reliable sign of otitis externa.
2. A wick placed in the external auditory canal may be necessary to deliver medication to the canal if severe edema is present. Cleansing or irrigation of the ear canal is extremely painful and is not generally necessary in the ED.
3. Malignant otitis externa is rare in the pediatric patient.

Pitfalls

1. Failure to consider a diagnosis of suppurative otitis media if the tympanic membrane is perforated.
2. Failure to teach children and their families how to prevent otitis externa.

Selected references

American Academy of Family Physicians, American Academy of Otolaryngology – Head and Neck Surgery, and American Academy of Pediatrics Subcommittee on Otitis Media With Effusion. Clinical practice guideline: otitis media with effusion. *Pediatrics* 2004;**113**:1412–1429.

American Academy of Pediatrics Subcommittee on Management of Acute Otitis Media and American Academy of Family Physicians. Clinical practice guideline: diagnosis and management of acute otitis media. *Pediatrics* 2004;**113**:1451–1465.

Flynn, C, Griffin, G, Schultz, J. Decongestants and antihistamines for acute otitis media in children. *Cochrane Database Syst Rev* 2004;**3**:CD001727.

Spiro DM, Arnold DH. The concept and practice of a wait-and-see approach to acute otitis media. *Curr Opin Pediatr* 2008;**20**:72–78.

van Balen, FA, Smit, WM, Zuithoff, NP, Verheij, TJ. Clinical efficacy of three common treatments in acute otitis externa in primary care: randomised controlled trial. *BMJ* 2003;**327**:1201.

Chapter 41

Pharyngotonsillitis and deep neck infections

Melissa S. DeFreest

Introduction

Acute pharyngotonsillitis refers to inflammation involving both the pharynx and tonsils and is the second most commonly diagnosed pediatric illness. Deep neck infections usually occur as a complication of pharyngotonsillitis and include peritonsillar abscess, retropharyngeal abscess, parapharyngeal abscess and Lemierre syndrome.

Pharyngotonsillitis

Common conditions causing acute pharyngotonsillitis are respiratory viruses, the group A beta-hemolytic streptococcus *Streptococcus pyogenes* (GABHS; causing "strep throat"), and Epstein–Barr virus (infectious mononucleosis). Other causes of sore throat include gonococcal pharyngitis, epiglottitis (also called supraglottitis), and deep neck infections such as peritonsillar abscess, retropharyngeal abscess, and parapharyngeal abscess. A rare cause of acute pharyngotonsillitis in the USA is diphtheria, which should be considered in the unimmunized child.

Common respiratory viruses that can cause acute pharyngotonsillitis include adenovirus, influenza virus, parainfluenza virus, rhinovirus, and respiratory syncytial virus. Less commonly, acute pharyngotonsillitis can be caused by coxsackievirus (herpangina and hand-foot-mouth disease), echovirus, and HSV (gingivostomatitis). Typical symptoms of acute pharyngotonsillitis that suggest viral etiology include concomitant conjunctivitis, cough, coryza, stomatitis, ulcerative lesions, viral exanthem, and/or diarrhea with absence of fever.

Streptococcus pyogenes infection

Infection with GABHS is responsible for 15–30% of acute pharyngitis in children. These infections are most common in temperate climates during the winter and early spring in children aged 5–15.

Clinical presentation

Signs and symptoms suggestive of GABHS include acute sore throat, fever, dysphagia, pharyngotonsillar erythema with exudates, anterior cervical lymphadenitis, and known exposure to GABHS. Headache, abdominal pain, nausea, vomiting, palatal petechiae, and a scarlatiniform rash may be present.

Streptococcal pharyngitis is unlikely in a child <5 years of age unless there has been a close exposure.

Diagnostic studies

A rapid antigen detection test (RADT or rapid strep test) should be performed when GABHS is suspected. A positive RADT is considered confirmatory and should be treated with antibiotics. Sensitivity of RADTs is 80–90%; therefore, a negative test requires a confirmatory throat culture.

Treatment

Current practice guidelines for treatment of children with acute pharyngotonsillitis recommend withholding antibiotics unless a RADT or throat culture is positive for GABHS. Antibiotic treatment shortens the course of clinical symptoms and prevents both disease transmission and development of complications such as acute rheumatic fever and deep neck infections. Antibiotic treatment does not prevent development of post-streptococcal glomerulonephritis.

In patients with acute GABHS pharyngitis, the recommended first-line therapy remains penicillin V (phenoxymethylpenicillin) (Box 41.1). Alternative antibiotics include amoxicillin, macrolides, oral cephalosporins, and clindamycin. An earlier onset of pain relief can be achieved by using oral dexamethasone (single dose 0.6 mg/kg PO to maximum dose of 10 mg) as an adjuvant therapy for acute GABHS.

Symptomatic treatment with NSAIDs or acetaminophen and throat lozenges or sprays should also be recommended.

Infectious mononucleosis

Epstein–Barr virus infection in younger children often is asymptomatic or non-specific; adolescents develop symptomatic infectious mononucleosis. This should be considered in adolescents with severe pharyngitis.

A Practical Guide to Pediatric Emergency Medicine: Caring for Children in the Emergency Department, ed. N. Ewen Amieva-Wang (associate eds. Jamie Shandro, Aparajita Sohoni, and Bernhard Fassl). Published by Cambridge University Press.

Box 41.1. Treatment of pharyngotonsillitis and abscesses

Acute GABHS pharyngotonsillitis

Commonly age >5 to young adult.

Primary antibiotic therapy: penicillin V PO for 10 days

Alternative antibiotic therapy: benzathine benzylpenicillin G IM single dose

Adjuvant therapy

- second-generation cephalosporin for 4–6 days
- clindamycin or azithromycin PO for 5 days
- clarithromycin or erythromycin PO for 10 days.

Supportive therapy

- hydration IV or PO if needed
- acetaminophen (paracetamol) 15 mg/kg PO q. 4 h
- ibuprofen 10 mg/kg PO q. 6 h
- consider dexamethasone (0.6 mg/kg to max. dose 10 mg).

Acute viral pharyngotonsillitis

Any age, but includes infectious mononucleosis, which is commonly adolescent.

- IV or PO hydration if needed
- acetaminophen 15 mg/kg PO q. 4 h
- ibuprofen 10 mg/kg PO q. 6 h
- consider dexamethasone treatment if significant pharyngeal edema: (0.6 mg/kg to max. dose 10 mg).

Deep space infections of neck

Peritonsillar abscess (PTA; commonly adolescent), retropharyngeal abscess (commonly <4 years), parapharyngeal abscess (commonly >8 years).

- CBC with differential, blood cultures
- culture and sensitivity of abscess aspirate
- IV or PO hydration and analgesia
- imaging studies (may not be needed for PTA)
- broad-spectrum antibiotics IV (PO may be adequate for PTA)
- surgical consult and hospital admission (may not be needed for PTA).

From Gilbert *et al.*, 2008.

Clinical presentation

The typical presentation of infectious mononucleosis includes sore throat, lymphadenopathy, fever, and tonsillar enlargement. Fatigue, palatal petechiae, splenomegaly, and atypical lymphocytosis are also suggestive.

Diagnostic studies

A positive heterophile antibody test (i.e., Monospot) is considered confirmatory although a negative heterophile antibody test cannot reliably exclude infectious mononucleosis in the pediatric age group. A patient with ≥20% atypical lymphocytes or ≥10% atypical lymphocytes with ≥50% lymphocytes and a negative rapid test for GABHS should be treated presumptively as having infectious mononucleosis.

Management

Management is symptomatic and includes hydration, NSAIDs or acetaminophen, and throat lozenges or sprays. Although there is scant evidence, steroids can be used to decrease symptoms. Because of the risk of splenic rupture, contact sports should be avoided for at least 4 weeks and until the patient is completely asymptomatic.

Gonococcal pharyngitis

Gonococcal pharyngitis is rare in children and is caused by infection with *Neisseria gonorrhoeae* (the gonococcus). It should be considered in sexually active patients or in patients in whom sexual abuse is suspected. It may cause an exudative pharyngitis but is more commonly diagnosed only by culture when suspicion is entertained and appropriate culture for *N. gonorrheae* is performed. Evaluation should include a throat culture for *N. gonorrheae* and appropriate screening for other sexually transmitted infections. Gonococcal pharyngotonsillitis should be treated with a one time dose of IM ceftriaxone. Treatment is necessary to prevent both transmission and disseminated disease, and cases of suspected sexual abuse must be reported.

Diphtheria

Diphtheria is a rare cause of life-threatening pharyngotonsillitis; it presents with cervical lymphadenopathy and a thick pharyngeal membrane. Membranes may extend into the airway and cause airway compromise. Removal of the membrane results in bleeding. Disease is caused by infection with *Corynebacterium diphtheriae* in unimmunized individuals. *C. diphtheriae* toxin may cause pharyngeal muscle paralysis, cranial nerve palsies, cardiac toxicity, and polyneuropathy. Treatment consists of antitoxin in addition to antibiotics. Antibiotics decrease the production of toxins and transmission of disease. Recommended initial antibiotic therapy includes 5 days of benzathine penicillin followed by 5 days of oral penicillin V or 7–14 days of IV erythromycin.

Disposition in pharyngotonsillitis

Most children with acute pharyngotonsillitis can be safely discharged home. Admission should be considered for any child with signs of respiratory compromise, dehydration, or who is "toxic" in appearance.

Deep neck infections

Deep neck infections include peritonsillar abscess (PTA; "quinsy"), retropharyngeal abscess (RPA), parapharyngeal abscess (PPA or lateral pharyngeal abscess), and Lemierre's disease (Fig. 41.1). They are often a complication of acute pharyngotonsillitis caused by contiguous spread from local sites. All are potentially life threatening.

Peritonsillar abscess is the most common deep neck infection in pediatric patients and is usually seen in the adolescent years. It is typically in the region of the upper pole of the tonsil and involves the soft palate. Characteristics include unilateral

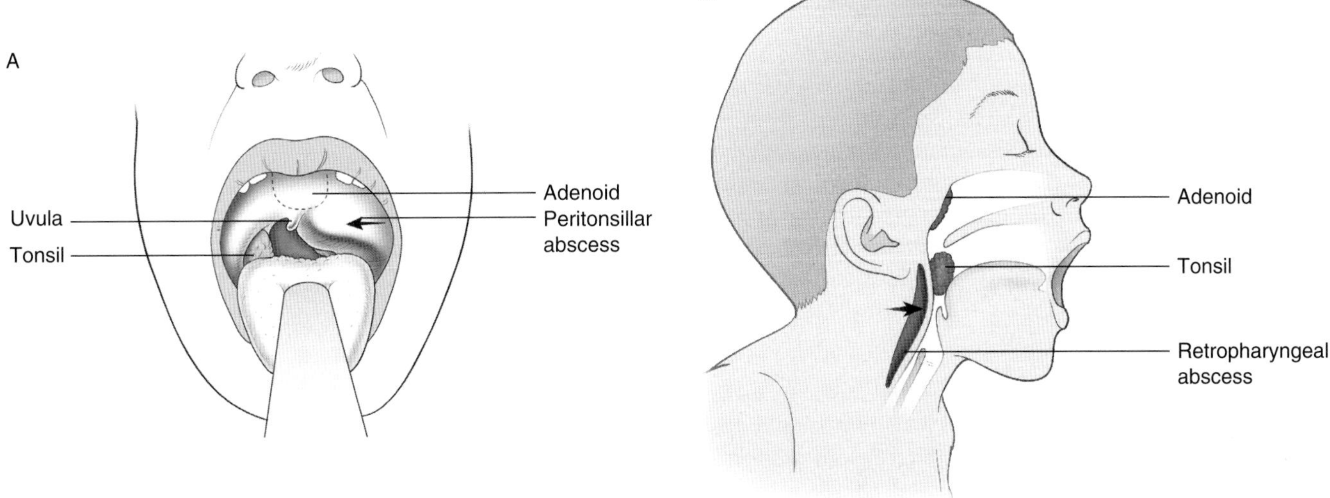

Figure 41.1 Deep neck infections and their location. (A) peritonsillar abcess causes fluctuance and uvular deviation. (B) A retropharyngeal abscess occurs along the retropharyngeal space and swelling is not necessarily visible on oral inspection. Note the location of the adenoid and tonsillar tissue, which can become inflamed in adenoiditis and tonsillitis. (Copyright Chris Gralapp.)

tonsillar/peritonsillar swelling, uvular deviation, trismus, and/or muffled voice. Workup should include CBC with differential and culture/sensitivity of abscess contents. Imaging for PTA is rarely needed unless trismus prevents adequate examination of the oropharynx. If imaging is necessary, CT scan is the preferred modality and should be obtained with IV contrast.

Retropharyngeal abscess usually occurs in early childhood as a result of extension of oropharyngeal infection to the retropharyngeal lymph nodes, with subsequent suppuration. It is most common between the ages 2 and 4 years, and infection is located between the posterior pharynx and prevertebral fascia. A unilateral posterior pharyngeal bulge may be seen on examination, although this is often absent.

Children with RPA present with limitation of neck movement, particularly neck extension, as a result of inflammation of the paraspinous muscles. This may be mistaken as a sign of meningitis.

Other characteristics include neck pain, sore throat, and/or neck mass. Respiratory distress and stridor are rare. If RPA is suspected, imaging should be performed. A widened retropharyngeal space on soft tissue lateral neck radiograph is suggestive of RPA, and RPA should be suspected if the retropharyngeal space is greater than 7 mm at C2 or 14 mm at C6 on a true lateral radiograph performed during inspiration with the neck in extension. A CT scan with IV contrast is the definitive test in suspected RPA. Laboratory evaluation should include CBC with differential and blood cultures.

Parapharyngeal abscesses, in the parapharyngeal area (also called the lateral pharyngeal or pharyngomaxillary area) above the hyoid bone in the upper neck are rare. They usually occur in children older than 8 years. Infection can be in the anterior or posterior pharyngomaxillary space and can cause swelling of the parotid area, trismus, and/or tonsil prolapse.

All deep neck abscesses are typically polymicrobial.

Death from abscess can be the result of infection, rupture with aspiration, airway obstruction, erosion into major blood vessels, and extension into the mediastinum. Careful attention to the airway must be maintained at all times.

Treatment

Treatment of PTA can sometimes be accomplished in the ED. It includes IV or PO hydration, analgesia, antibiotics and either needle aspiration or surgical drainage of the abscess. Consider otolaryngology consult for drainage unless the procedure can be safely performed in the ED setting. Hospital admission for IV hydration, pain control, and antibiotics may be necessary. Steroid use for treatment of PTA is of unproven benefit.

Treatment of RPAs and PPAs require admission, IV antibiotics, and otolaryngology consult for possible drainage (Box 41.1). The classic teaching is that all RPAs and PPAs require surgical drainage. However, hospital admission, observation, and a trial of IV antibiotics without surgical drainage under the auspices of a surgeon can sometimes be effective for very small abscesses.

Lemierre's disease

Lemierre's disease is a very rare entity. It refers to septic thrombophlebitis of the internal jugular vein with metastatic spread. It occurs after acute oropharyngeal infection, most commonly of the palatine tonsils and peritonsillar tissue. The most common etiologic agent is *Fusobacterium necrophorum*. Classical presentation includes pharyngitis, a tender/swollen neck, and pulmonary infiltrates. Additional features may include fever, trismus, cranial nerve palsies, pain/swelling along the sternocleidomastoid, dysphagia, spasm of the sternocleidomastoid, Horner syndrome, and hematogenous spread ("metastasis") to other sites. These patients usually appear toxic with varying degrees of respiratory distress. Evaluation of suspected Lemierre's disease should include laboratory studies, including blood cultures. Imaging of the neck with CT will demonstrate thrombophlebitis of the internal jugular vein. Once a diagnosis has been made, imaging of the brain is necessary to exclude intracerebral thrombosis, particularly if the infection arose from mastoiditis. Untreated Lemierre's disease is usually fatal.

Disposition

A PTA can often be drained and then the child can be treated as an outpatient. Patients with possible RPA or PPA should have appropriate imaging studies to definitively rule out abscess or should be evaluated by an otolaryngologist. Children with RPA or PPA should be admitted for IV antibiotics and/or surgical drainage by otalaryngology. Lemierre's disease requires admission, IV antibiotics, and neurosurgical consultation.

Pearls and pitfalls

Pearls

1. Most acute pharyngotonsillitis is caused by viruses.
2. Antibiotics are not prescribed for pharyngotonsillitis without a positive rapid antigen strep test or throat culture (exception is diphtherial pharyngotonsillitis).
3. Deep neck infection should always be included in the differential diagnosis of sore throat.

Pitfalls

1. Failure to treat group A beta-hemolytic streptococcal infection with antibiotics may result in post-streptococcal sequelae such as acute rheumatic fever.
2. Failure to counsel children with infectious mononucleosis to abstain from contact sports because of the risk of splenic rupture.

Selected references

Brook I. Microbiology and management of peritonsillar, retropharyngeal, and parapharyngeal abscesses. *J Oral Maxillofac Surg* 2004;**62**:1545–1550.

Bulloch B, Kabani A, Tenenbein M. Oral dexamethasone for the treatment of pain in children with acute pharyngitis: a randomized, double-blind, placebo-controlled trial. *Ann Emerg Med* 2003;**41**: 601–608.

Chirinos JA, Lichtenstein DM, Garcia J, Tamariz LJ. The evolution of Lemierre syndrome. *Medicine* 2002;**81**:458–465.

Craig FW, Schunk JE. Retropharyngeal abscess in children: clinical presentation, utility of imaging, and current management. *Pediatrics* 2003;**111**:1394–1398.

Gilbert DN, Moellering Jr, RC, Eliopoulos GM, Sande MA. (eds.) *The Sanford Guide to Antimicrobial Therapy*, 40th edn. Madison, WI: Too Cold for Antimicrobial Therapy, 2010.

Postoperative tonsillectomy

N. Ewen Amieva-Wang and Anna Messner

The tonsils and adenoids are oral pharyngeal lymphoid tissue which can become inflamed (see Fig. 41.1, p. 199). Tonsillectomy and adenoidectomy are common pediatric surgeries. Complications include bleeding, pain, and dehydration. Bleeding is the most serious complication of tonsillectomy/adenoidectomy. Bleeding can occur relatively soon after surgery but is most common on postoperative days 5–7. Significant hemorrhage can occur up to 2 weeks after surgery. Serious bleeding requiring return to the operating room is estimated to occur in 1–2% of cases.

In all cases of postoperative tonsillectomy bleeding, the surgeon should be notified.

The patient should have IV access and be blood typed and cross-matched if necessary.

Pain and dehydration should not be underestimated. Children should have liquid pain medication; if the child cannot take oral fluids, IV hydration should be provided. Occasionally parents will bring children in for halitosis, which is common and normal after tonsillectomy surgery. Parent can be reassured that the halitosis will resolve within 2 weeks. Often children have been given antibiotics postoperatively to help with the halitosis. On physical examination, extensive exudate often covers the tonsillar beds; this is normal. Rarely is there an infection requiring additional antibiotics. Therefore, consult with the surgeon prior to giving antibiotics.

Pain control following tonsillectomy is extremely important. Young children (<7 years of age) typically do well with liquid or rectal acetaminophen every 4 h. The key to pain control is to emphasize that the parent should not wait for the patient to complain of pain but instead use a regular pain medication schedule (including waking the patient up in the night to give the pain medication.) Some otolaryngologists recommend acetaminophen alternating with ibuprofen but others avoid ibuprofen in the postoperative period because of the theoretical increased risk of hemorrhage. In older children, liquid hydrocodone/acetaminophen (Lortab) can be given every 6 h or liquid acetaminophen and codeine. Narcotics should be avoided in young children with a history of obstructive sleep apnea because of the risk of respiratory depression.

Pearls and pitfalls

Pearls

1. Postoperative tonsils always look infected, usually they are not.

Pitfalls

1. Failure to consult the surgeon who did the tonsillectomy if there is postoperative bleeding, no matter how little.

A Practical Guide to Pediatric Emergency Medicine: Caring for Children in the Emergency Department, ed. N. Ewen Amieva-Wang (associate eds. Jamie Shandro, Aparajita Sohoni, and Bernhard Fassl). Published by Cambridge University Press.

Section

7

Endocrine emergencies

Expert reviewers: Darrell M. Wilson and Nikta Forghani

Chapter 43

Diabetic emergencies

Alice Chiao and Aparajita Sohoni

Introduction

Diabetes mellitus (DM) is one of the most common chronic diseases of childhood. Type I DM is caused by autoimmune destruction of the pancreatic insulin-producing islet cells. Three-quarters of these patients will present during childhood, with a bimodal peaks around ages 4–6 and then at ages 10–14 years. Type II DM is caused by insulin resistance. Typically Type II DM is adult onset although there is an increasing incidence in children, presenting in obese, postpubertal adolescents. This chapter will focus on the major emergency of DM, hyperglycemia, and in particular on diabetic ketoacidosis (DKA). We will briefly discuss also hypoglycemia in the face of DM.

The incidence of type I DM is estimated at approximately 2/1000 the population. With the growing epidemic of childhood obesity, an increasing prevalence of pediatric-onset type II DM has been detected. Although studies of the exact incidence and prevalence vary, recent data estimates the prevalence of type II DM in those aged 10–19 years as 0.42/1000 population. Non-Hispanic Whites have the lowest incidence, while American-Indian youth have the highest incidence. Type II DM is thought to develop in the pediatric population in a similar fashion to adults; namely through a combination of insulin resistance and impaired pancreatic beta-cell function. Both factors are modulated by both genetic and acquired factors, such as race/ethnicity, obesity, family history of similar conditions, and lifestyle.

Hyperglycemia in children is most often caused by a form of DM, more commonly type I. The criterion for diagnosing diabetes in pediatric patients does not differ from adults: namely, a random blood glucose of greater than 200 mg/dl (2.0 g/l) with associated symptoms of diabetes (polyuria, polydipsia, polyphagia). While intermediate disease states exist (termed prediabetes or impaired glucose tolerance), this chapter will focus on the management of the two most common causes of hyperglycemia: type I and type II DM.

Diabetic ketoacidosis

Diabetic ketoacidosis is a state of metabolic decompensation caused by a lack of intracellular availability of glucose. This cellular starvation state is induced by either a lack of insulin or a resistance to insulin and results in the utilization of other metabolic substrates for glucose and fatty acid breakdown, inducing a ketotic state. The initial presentation of DM is DKA in approximately 25% of patients with type I DM as well as in 25% of African-American patients with type II DM.

In children, the most frequent cause of DKA in an established diabetic is failure to monitor insulin or failure to take sufficient insulin. In new-onset pediatric DKA, while a viral syndrome may often unmask the diabetes, rarely do children develop DKA as the result of a treatable infection. Other precipitants include non-compliance with insulin regimen, changes of adolescence, and insulin pump failure.

More commonly, patients with type II DM will present with hyperglycemia in the absence of ketosis. This hyperglycemia can be profound (<1000 mg/dl) and may cause severe dehydration and evolve into **hyperglycemic hyperosmolar syndrome** (HHS).

Clinical manifestations

Diabetic ketoacidosis often has an insidious onset, particularly when the child does not carry the diagnosis of diabetes. While some children may have classic signs such polydipsia, polyphagia, and polyuria, non-specific symptoms of hyperglycemia and DKA may include vomiting, abdominal pain, fatigue, and fever.

On physical examination, a child in DKA may present with:

- altered mental status
- signs of shock, dehydration: tachycardia, shock, poor perfusion
- an odor of acetone on the breath, suggesting an underlying metabolic acidosis (lack of "fruity odor" does not rule out DKA, as not everyone can smell ketones)
- respiratory compensation for metabolic acidosis: Kussmaul respirations.

A Practical Guide to Pediatric Emergency Medicine: Caring for Children in the Emergency Department, ed. N. Ewen Amieva-Wang (associate eds. Jamie Shandro, Aparajita Sohoni, and Bernhard Fassl). Published by Cambridge University Press.

Diagnostic studies

Diabetic ketoacidosis is characterized by uncontrolled hyperglycemia (>2.5 g/l), ketosis, and acidemia (pH <7.3 or bicarbonate <15 mEq/l).

In the ED, a patient with suspected DKA or HHS should receive a thorough laboratory evaluation including:

1. Bedside glucose check via fingerstick immediately upon evaluating the patient to confirm hyperglycemia.
2. Venous blood gas to assess acidosis.
3. Basic metabolic panel, calcium, magnesium, and phosphate levels to assess for the presence of an anion gap, the overall level of dehydration, and electrolyte depletion and to officially check the serum glucose level:
   - initial serum potassium levels may be high as acidosis causes efflux of potassium from cells in exchange for hydrogen ion absorption; however, patients with hyperglycemia or DKA are profoundly total body potassium depleted
   - serum potassium concentrations should be monitored closely and replaced once insulin therapy is initiated to prevent the development of potentially malignant arrhythmias
   - serum sodium levels are usually low, because the osmotic effect of hyperglycemia draws water into the intravascular space; the expected decrease in measured serum sodium concentration from hyperglycemia may be calculated using the formula

     1.6 mEq/dl decrease in sodium level for every 100 mg/dl increase in serum glucose above 100 mg/dl
4. Serum ketones are a marker for the degree of ketoacidosis. The standard laboratory ketone assay measures acetoacetate and acetone and not beta-hydroxybutyrate. Point of care blood ketone meters are now available and quite accurate.
5. Urinalysis to evaluate for glucosuria or ketonuria.
6. Blood, urine, vaginal, and throat cultures should also be considered particularly in the ill or febrile child, although treatable infection precipitating DKA in a child is rare.
7. Ancillary laboratory studies where the results will not alter the ED course but will serve in long-term management of the patient: glycosylated hemoglobin levels (HbA1c), C-peptide levels, insulin autoantibodies, and lipid panels.
   - thyroid function tests are not helpful acutely as most patients have sick euthyroid
   - insulin autoantibodies should be drawn prior to treatment if possible.

Management of diabetic ketoacidosis

In the ED, there are several critical goals of management (Box 43.1). These include:

Volume resuscitation. Virtually all children in DKA have intravascular volume depletion and require prompt fluid resuscitation.

Initiation of insulin therapy. Insulin promotes transport of glucose to the intracellular state and ends ketone formation.

Monitoring and assessing. Hourly monitoring of blood glucose levels, identification and treatment of the precipitating event, and prevention of the complications of rapid shifts in serum osmolarity.

Electrolytes. Monitoring of electrolyte levels (particularly potassium and sodium), and of appropriate reversal of metabolic acidosis (serum bicarbonate and ketones).

Box 43.1. Management of diabetic ketoacidosis

Step 1 Volume resuscitation

(a) Isotonic saline should be administered at 20 ml/kg over 1 h or less.

(b) For patients with signs of hypovolemic shock, a second bolus of 10 ml/kg should be given over the second hour.

(c) Once adequate signs of circulation are established, the fluid should be switched to an isotonic solution at 1.5–2× maintenance for the first 4–6 h; after this time, the IV fluids should be switched to one-half normal saline if the sodium concentration is rising appropriately.

Care should be taken to avoid over rapid hydration as it is thought to contribute to cerebral edema.

Step 2 Treating insulin deficiency and hyperglycemia

The degree of hyperglycemia will most rapidly correct during the initial volume expansion phase. This is convenient, as it will allow for laboratory results to be received, and a patient's potassium level will be known prior to administering any insulin.

(a) After initiation of volume replacement, regular insulin infusion is initiated at 0.1 U/kg per h IV (insulin bolus is not recommended).

(b) As the serum glucose level approaches 250–300 mg/dl, 5% dextrose is added to the IV fluids with the goal of maintaining serum glucose at 150–250 mg/dl during the insulin infusion. The insulin infusion rate is adjusted to avoid a rapid fall in blood glucose only if the acidosis is resolving.

(c) The insulin drip should not be discontinued until the patient's ketoacidosis has resolved (bicarbonate >18 mg/dl), as it is required to eliminate ketoacids from the patient's body and reverse the fasting, catabolic state.

Step 3 Monitoring blood glucose and electrolytes

Potassium repletion should begin as soon as the serum potassium level is known and patient has demonstrated ability to urinate; generally, replacement should begin if the potassium level is <5.0–5.5 mEq/l.

(a) Intravenous potassium chloride (20–40 mEq/l) should be administered if the potassium levels are low.

(b) Serum bicarbonate should be monitored every 1–2 h: ideally the metabolic acidosis should resolve within the first 24 h of insulin therapy and is a measure of adequacy

Box 43.1. *(cont.)*

of insulin administration to reverse the catabolic diabetic ketoacidosis state.

(c) Inadequate normalization of bicarbonate levels can indicate a relative lack of insulin. If other causes such as hypovolemia and infection are ruled out, the insulin drip should be increased in conjunction with endocrinology consult.

(d) An increase in insulin dosing requires an increase in the dextrose delivery rate in order to avoid hypoglycemia.

Complications of diabetic ketoacidosis

Rare but serious complications of DKA include cerebral edema, sepsis, acute renal failure, electrolyte disturbances, and resulting cardiac arrhythmias.

Cerebral edema occurs in up to 1% of pediatric patients in DKA, and carries a high mortality rate (>20%).

Of the survivors of cerebral edema, 1–5% have permanent neurological injury. Causative factors are controversial. Recent studies have suggested a correlation between bicarbonate treatment, initial elevated BUN, and cerebral edema; however, the mechanisms remain unknown. Symptoms of cerebral edema include lethargy, altered level of consciousness (ALOC), and occasionally seizures. Treatment is supportive and may require intubation and mannitol administration in consultation with pediatric intensivists.

Management of hyperglycemia

The management of patients with type II DM and hyperglycemia will depend on their clinical presentation. For those patients who present with mild symptomatic hyperglycemia (glucose 126–200 mg/dl) and the absence of ketosis, initiation of glycemic control may be appropriate. However, often presentation in the ED is an opportunity for patient education. Further testing plus initiation of diabetes medication and education should be performed by a pediatric endocrinologist.

For patients who present with moderate–severe hyperglycemia (glucose >200 mg/dl) and ketosis, IV fluids and insulin therapy should be used to provide rapid metabolic control. The degree of dehydration from the osmotic diuresis caused by hyperglycemia should not be underestimated, and the same fluid bolus should be given to these patients. Once the ketosis is reversed and the DM is confirmed, oral antihyperglycemics can be introduced and insulin weaned gradually (Table 43.1). True hyperosmolar non-ketotic coma is very infrequent in pediatric populations, but has a fatality rate of as high as 14% when it occurs.

Table 43.1. Hyperglycemia medications and dosages

Medication	Dosage
Regular insulin	0.1 U/kg per h IV drip (no bolus); 0.05 U/kg per h in children <5 years
Potassium chloride[a]	0.5–1 mEq/kg per h IV infusion (max. 10 mEq/h)
Ondansetron (for severe nausea and vomiting)[b]	0.1 mg/kg IV or PO (frequency varies as there are no specific FDA regulations; it is generally accepted to use three doses in 24 h for non-chemotherapy-associated uses; individual institution protocols may vary)

[a] Frequency of potassium chloride administration will be guided by patient's potassium level.
[b] Antiemetics causing drowsiness such as Phenergan are contraindicated in diabetic ketoacidosis.

Disposition

Any child with a new diagnosis of DM, significant hyperglycemia, or DKA should be hospitalized at a facility with appropriate pediatric specialists including endocrinologists and intensivists, and resources for patient and family education. Critical long-term interventions for these patients include screening for associated cardiovascular risk factors such as hyperlipidemia, hypertension, and obesity and initiating appropriate family interventions such as diet control, education, and close follow-up.

Hypoglycemia in type I diabetes

Hypoglycemia is the most common complication of type I diabetes. Hypoglycemia in DM is managed differently from hypoglycemia without the diagnosis of DM. Hypoglycemia occurs when insulin administered exceeds glucose intake. Risk of hypoglycemia depends on patient age, duration of DM diagnosis, family understanding of the disease, degree of glycemic control, physical activity, oral intake, and concurrent illness.

Clinical presentation

Hypoglycemia in younger children tends to be more severe, because these children are less able to communicate symptoms, and food intake and activity are less controlled. Children maintained with strict glycemic control and children on fixed insulin regimens versus insulin pump and intermittent bolus insulin have increased risk of hypoglycemia. Increased physical activity is also a well known cause of hypoglycemia.

Hypoglycemic symptoms are classified as adrenergic and neuroglycopenic. Adrenergic symptoms include diaphoresis, palpitations, and tremor. Neuroglycopenic symptoms include confusion, ALOC, and seizures. Death can occur with prolonged hypoglycemia. Children with long-standing diabetes tend to have decreased adrenergic responses and, therefore, have a risk of severe or recurrent hypoglycemia with decreased awareness.

Management

Hypoglycemia can be symptomatic or asymptomatic. Diabetic children with hypoglycemia should be given glucose in accordance with the level of hypoglycemia. Mild and moderate hypoglycemia with normal level of consciousness should be treated initially with oral concentrated simple carbohydrates (glucose tablets or juice). In order to maintain glucose levels, initial glucose should be followed by intake of complex carbohydrates.

Severe hypoglycemia (ALOC, seizures) is treated with glucagon.

- ≤20 kg: 0.02 to 0.03 mg/kg or 0.5 mg
- >20 kg: 1 mg and/or IV 25% dextrose (D25; bolus of 0.1 mg/kg).

Fingerstick blood glucose (FSG) should be checked every 15 min until normal blood sugars are obtained. Of note, if a child is on an insulin pump, this can simply be temporarily disconnected.

Also important in the management is to ascertain why the child developed hypoglycemia and to educate and institute measures so this does not recur.

Disposition

Children with a known cause of hypoglycemia, a therapeutic regimen of short-acting insulin, and who have maintained euglycemia after a hypoglycemic episode may be discharged home with reliable family. A child who is unable to tolerate oral intake, continues to have hypoglycemia, or has an unreliable social situation should be admitted to the hospital.

Pearls and pitfalls

Pearls

1. Avoid overaggressive correction of serum blood glucose, dehydration, and acidosis in the patient with diabetic ketoacidosis (DKA).
2. Bicarbonate therapy is not routinely recommended in the treatment of DKA.
3. Patient and family education is key.
4. Insulin bolus is not used in children with DKA.

Pitfalls

1. Failure to monitor for electrolyte shifts after initiating insulin treatment.
2. Insulin bolus and too rapid a fall in blood glucose.
3. Initiating aggressive insulin therapy before correcting potassium level, potentially causing life-threatening hypokalemia.
4. Initiating aggressive potassium therapy before insulin.

Selected references

Dunger DB, Sperling MA, Acerini CL, *et al.* ESPE/LWPES consensus statement on diabetic ketoacidosis in children and adolescents. *Arch Dis Child* 2004;**89**:188–194.

Glaser B. Risk factors for cerebral edema in children with diabetic ketoacidosis. *N Engl J Med* 2001;**344**:264–269.

Levin DL. Cerebral edema in diabetic ketoacidosis. *Pediatr Crit Care Med* 2008;**9**:320–329.

Rosenbloom AL. Hyperglycemic crises and their complications in children. *J Pediatr Endocrinol Metab* 2007;**20**:5–18.

Endocrine disorders

Nikta Forghani and Darrell M. Wilson

Introduction

Endocrine emergencies constitute a small but important percentage of pediatric emergencies. These entities are often difficult to diagnose because they are relatively rare and the signs and symptoms are non-specific. In addition, since the clinical course of many endocrine disorders can be indolent, patients will often not present with the underlying problem as the chief complaint. Prompt recognition of symptoms and early diagnosis can lead to a favorable outcome in most cases. Although the management of endocrine emergencies is often similar in adults and children, their presentations can be quite different, particularly in very young children when endocrine disorders can often be confused with other more common problems such as sepsis, failure to thrive, or feeding intolerance. This chapter will cover the most common pediatric endocrine emergencies: adrenal, thyroid, and parathyroid hormone disease. Diabetes and neonatal endocrine emergencies are discussed elsewhere (Chs. 43 and 157, respectively).

Since endocrinology has such a large scope and often mimics more common disorders, it is difficult to present a general approach to identify all endocrine emergencies. In almost all cases, however, management includes hormone replacement or blocking, resuscitation, and stabilization. The diagnostic workup can be initiated in the emergency room.

It is always prudent to hold 5–10 ml of serum in a red top tube for further analysis.

Table 44.1 lists the most common signs and symptoms, as well as the basic diagnostic and therapeutic approach to the more common emergencies.

Adrenal emergencies

Acute adrenal insufficiency is a life-threatening disorder characterized by hypotension and shock.

Understanding the pathophysiology and diagnostic workup for adrenal insufficiency can clarify the acute management. Although evaluation and management of adrenal insufficiency is similar in neonates and older children, presentation and etiology are often different.

Infants, children and adolescents with suspected adrenal insufficiency should be given hydrocortisone 25, 50, or 100 mg, respectively, as a stress dose.

Congenital adrenal hyperplasia (CAH) is an inherited disorder with 21-hydroxylase deficiency; this enzyme is involved in the production of cortisol and aldosterone (Fig. 44.1). Among other effects, this leads to a salt-wasting syndrome. Build up of the substrates of the enzyme also leads to excess production of androgens in the long term.

Adrenal insufficiency

After the neonatal period, causes other than CAH should be considered if a patient presents with salt-losing adrenal crisis:

- primary adrenal insufficiency
  - autoimmune disorders
  - congenital adrenal hypoplasia
  - adrenocorticotropic hormone (ACTH) resistance syndromes
  - metabolic disorders
  - adrenoleukodystrophy
  - infections:
    - tuberculosis
    - sepsis
    - viral
  - infiltrative/destructive
  - hemorrhage
- secondary adrenal insufficiency
  - hypothalamic tumors, radiation, or surgery
  - hypopituitarism
  - ACTH insufficiency
  - withdrawal from glucocorticoid therapy.

Diseases that cause destruction of bilateral adrenal glands and lead to both glucocorticoid and mineralocorticoid deficiencies include autoimmunity, adrenal hemorrhage, and infection.

A Practical Guide to Pediatric Emergency Medicine: Caring for Children in the Emergency Department, ed. N. Ewen Amieva-Wang (associate eds. Jamie Shandro, Aparajita Sohoni, and Bernhard Fassl). Published by Cambridge University Press.

Table 44.1 Endocrine disease affecting children

Disease	Clinical features	Laboratory findings	ED management	Ancillary tests
Diabetic ketoacidosis (Ch. 43)	Polyphagia, polydipsia, polyuria, nausea, vomiting, weight loss	Serum glucose >200 mg/dl; ketosis (urine or serum); bicarbonate <16 mEq/l	Fluid resuscitation; insulin (0.1 U/kg per h), glucose tolerance test	Insulin antibodies, celiac screen
Primary adrenal insufficiency/ glucocorticoid and mineralocorticoid deficiency	Virilized female, or male neonate; 2 weeks old; nausea, vomiting, shock; increased pigmentation of flexor surfaces and gums	Hyponatremia, hypoglycemia, hyperkalemia	Volume resuscitation with normal saline 20 ml/kg Dextrose bolus, then IV fluid D5-NS Hydrocortisone IV (25 mg infant; 50 mg child; 100 mg adolescent) Treat hyperkalemia as necessary (Ch. 55) Mineralocorticoid replacement often necessary after initial resuscitation (fludrocortisone 0.1–0.2 mg orally once, then BID)	Serum cortisol (5 ml red top tube), ACTH, 17 hydroxyprogesterone
Secondary adrenal insufficiency/isolated glucocorticoid deficiency	Features of chronic steroid use; CNS lesion (headache, growth failure)	Hypoglycemia, hypotension; usually no or mild hyponatremia; no hyperkalemia	Hydrocortisone as above or triple regular dose; no mineralocorticoid needed Treat symptomatic hyponatremia in the ED (Ch. 54)	Stimulated cortisol; free T_4; sodium; serum and urine osmolality
Syndrome of inappropriate secretion of antidiuretic hormone (SIADH) associated with CNS, pulmonary lesions, neoplasm	CNS symptoms	Hyponatremia		Serum sodium
Diabetes insipidus	Polyuria, polydipsia, dehydration	Hypernatremia, hyperosmolality, low urine osmolarity	Replace volume; replace free water deficit over 48 h	Workup for possible central mass
Pheochromocytoma	Headache, palpitations, diaphoresis, episodic hypertension	High urine or serum catecholamines	Decrease blood pressure	Urinary catecholamines, CT/MRI to localize tumor
Neonatal thyrotoxicosis	Child of mother with Graves' disease; microcephaly, tachycardia, congestive heart failure (Ch. 54)	Low TSH, high T_4	Antithyroid medication; high-dose iodine; beta-blocker if severely hypertensive, tachycardic	
Thyroid storm (Table 44.1)	Goiter, hypertension, tachycardia, hyperpyrexia, agitation	Low (undetectable) TSH, high T_4	Antithyroid medication, high-dose iodine, beta-blocker, restore volume, correct electrolyte disturbances, identify precipitating factor, empiric broad-spectrum antibiotics[a]	Thyroid-stimulating antibody

Table 44.1 *(cont.)*

Disease	Clinical features	Laboratory findings	ED management	Ancillary tests
Hypocalcemia (Ch. 57)	Non-specific: fatigue, weakness, abdominal pain, bone pain, seizure	Low calcium (<8 mg/dl in full-term infants or children)	Calcium treatment (Box 44.1)	Phosphate, magnesium, creatinine, alkaline phosphatase, parathormone, 25-hydroxy-vitamin D, 1,25-hydroxy-vitamin D, urine calcium/creatinine
Hypercalcemia: (Ch. 56)	Non-specific: fatigue, weakness, abdominal pain, seizure	High calcium (>10 mg/dl)	Volume resuscitation acutely	Parathormone, PTH-related peptide, 25-hydroxy-vitamin D
Neonatal hypoglycemia (Chs. 157 and 168)	Poor feeding, lethargy, vomiting, seizure	Blood glucose (<50 mg/dl)	Dextrose 10% 2.5–5 ml/kg or dextrose 25% 1–2 ml/kg; an infusion of 10% dextrose should then be initiated at a rate of 8–10 mg/kg per min to maintain the blood sugar >70 mg/dl	Critical sample

ACTH, adrenocorticotropic hormone; D5-NS, 5% Dextrose–Normal Saline; TSH, thyroid-stimulating hormone; T_4, thyroxine.

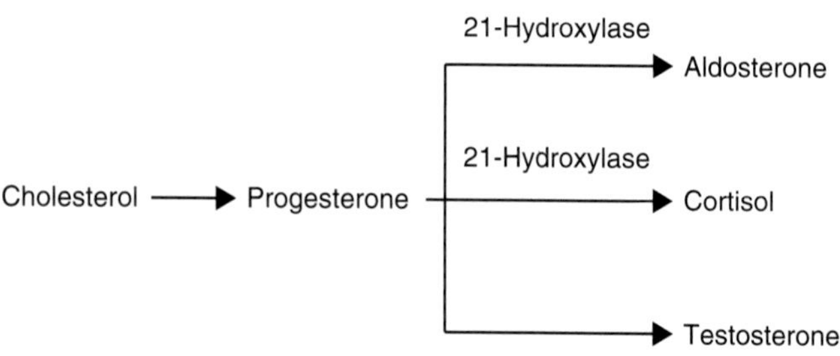

Figure 44.1 Steroid pathway disruption in 21-hydroxylase deficiency. The lack of the enzyme 21-hydroxylase results in an inability of the adrenal gland to synthesize aldosterone or cortisol. Instead steroid precursors are shunted into testosterone synthesis, resulting in increased testosterone and thus masculinization of females with this defect.

Primary adrenal insufficiency, disease within the adrenal gland, should be differentiated from secondary adrenal insufficiency, or the impaired release of ACTH from the pituitary (Table 44.2).

Patients with secondary adrenal insufficiency have isolated cortisol deficiency and do not have mineralocorticoid deficiency or salt loss.

Deficiencies in mineralocorticoids or salt levels do not occur because ACTH does not control the renin–angiotensin–aldosterone axis. A CNS lesion causing impaired production or release of ACTH is the most common etiology. In patients who have used high-dose steroids, endogenous ACTH production will often be suppressed; therefore, withdrawal of steroids without enough recovery time for the ACTH–adrenal axis can lead to profound glucocorticoid deficiency, particularly in the context of an acute illness. Insufficient replacement (failing to increase doses during an acute illness or missed doses) can also result in adrenal crisis.

Table 44.2. Differences between primary and secondary adrenal insufficiency

	Primary adrenal insufficiency	Secondary adrenal insufficiency
History	Fatigue, nausea, salt craving	Fatigue, headache, visual changes
Physical examination	Hyperpigmentation, weight loss	Central incisor, microphallus, signs of other pituitary deficiencies (growth hormone deficiency, thyroid hormone deficiency, diabetes insipidus)
Laboratory findings	High ACTH, low cortisol, low sodium, high potassium	Low ACTH, low cortisol, low or normal sodium, normal potassium

ACTH, adrenocorticotropic hormone.

Glucocorticoid and mineralocorticoid deficiency

In an older child, primary adrenal insufficiency is often characterized by a progressive increase in the pigmentation of the

Table 44.3. Initial stress doses of hydrocortisone (Solucortef IV)

Age	Dose (mg)
Infants	25
Children	50
Adolescents	100

skin at the flexor surfaces, as well as the gum line. Overproduction of propiomelanocortin, an ACTH precursor, leads to increased melanin synthesis, which results in hyperpigmentation. Patients often have GI complaints including nausea and vomiting. Fatigue, weight loss, and salt craving may also be prominent complaints. In patients with autoimmune adrenal insufficiency, alopecia and monilial lesions of the skin or nails may be present.

Isolated glucocorticoid deficiency

Patients with ACTH deficiency can be mildly hyponatremic because cortisol is important in the excretion of free water, but should not be hyperkalemic. In fact, ACTH deficiency can often mask symptoms of diabetes insipidus, a factor that should be considered when cortisol replacement is initiated. Other differences include a lack of hyperpigmentation in patients with secondary adrenal insufficiency because, in fact, ACTH levels are low. Although patients with secondary adrenal insufficiency can be severely hypoglycemic (presenting with seizures), more acute symptoms of dehydration and shock seen in primary adrenal insufficiency are usually not seen because the patients are not mineralocorticoid deficient.

Secondary adrenal insufficiency implies that there is a most likely a problem with the development of the pituitary gland or hypothalamus or the occurrence of a mass in or around that area causing inadequate production or release of ACTH. In infants, associated signs such as a microphallus, a central incisor, or other midline defects may be seen. In older, verbal children there may be accompanying symptoms of headaches or visual changes. Therefore, other pituitary hormones should be evaluated and MRI imaging of the brain (specifically of the hypothalamus and pituitary gland) should be done. Finally, prior steroid use can be an important key in patients with secondary adrenal insufficiency and should be considered.

Diagnosis and management

In terms of the evaluation of these patients, obtaining an ACTH and ideally a stimulated (or random) cortisol level prior to the initiation of glucocorticoid therapy is important. If this is not possible, drawing 5 ml of serum for future analysis prior to starting therapy can be helpful diagnostically. Therapeutically, parenteral hydrocortisone is the mainstay of therapy, using the guidelines outlined in Table 44.3 for the initial dose. Hydrocortisone is the preferred glucocorticoid because of its physiologic resemblance to cortisol and cross-over mineralocorticoid activity.

Table 44.4. Treatments for thyroid storm

Symptom	Treatment	Dosing
Hyperthyroidism	Antithyroid medication	Methimazole 0.5–1 mg/kg daily, divided TID
	High-dose iodine	Lugol's solution 1 drop q. 8 h
	Glucocorticoids	Hydrocortisone 100 mg/m^{2}daily, divided q. 6 h
Tachycardia, hypertension	Beta-blocker (contraindicated in heart failure, asthma)	Propranolol 0.5–1 mg/kg daily, divided BID–QID
Hyperpyrexia	Acetaminophen, cooling blankets	Acetaminophen 15 mg/kg dose q. 4 h

Thyroid emergencies

Thyroid storm

Thyroid storm is a very rare event in pediatrics and is usually precipitated by surgery, infection, trauma, new-onset diabetic ketoacidosis, and, less frequently, by non-compliance with antithyroid treatment and radioiodine therapy. It can also be the presenting symptom of Graves' disease for an undiagnosed neonate (Ch. 157) or child.

The vast majority of children with a thyroid storm will have a goiter; they typically present with hyperpyrexia, diaphoresis, widened pulse pressure, and hypertension.

Tachycardia can be severe and can lead to high-output cardiac failure. Older patients can also have GI complaints, including nausea, vomiting, and diarrhea, as well as altered behavior, seizures, and coma.

Management should focus on correcting the hyperthyroidism, restoring homeostasis, and identifying and treating the precipitating factor (Table 44.4). Methimazole can be used to prevent thyroid hormone synthesis. As oral anti-thyroid medication may take a few days to take effect, oral iodine or IV iodine (given as radiographic contrast dyes) should be used in this situation. Finally, glucocorticoids can be used as they also inhibit thyroid hormone secretion and decrease the conversion of thyroxine (T_4) to triiodothyronine (T_3). Patients with severe hyperthyroidism are also thought to be relatively adrenally insufficient, further making glucocorticoid treatment useful.

It is essential to restore fluid balance to normal and to correct electrolyte disturbances. Some patients may be in shock and will need aggressive fluid replacement, and others will need diuresis because of congestive heart failure. This should take place on a pediatric ICU where invasive monitoring and inotropic support can be utilized, as life-threatening tachyarrhythmias can occur.

Beta-blockers can help to minimize the adrenergic tone; propranolol is preferred as it can also be given IV or as a drip. Hyperthermia should be treated aggressively using cooling blankets and acetaminophen. Aspirin should not be used in pediatrics, as it can also increase serum free T_4 and T_3 by interfering with protein binding. It is also important to identify and treat the factor that led to the decompensation. Broad-spectrum antibiotics should be used once the appropriate investigations have been done.

Hypoparathyroidism and hypocalcemia

Hypocalcemia is a commonly encountered emergency in pediatrics. Children are commonly asymptomatic until levels are very low, which is when patients often present to emergency medical care. While hypocalcemia can be viewed simplistically as an electrolyte deficiency (see also Ch. 56), it is actually usually a manifestation of hypoparathyroidism or vitamin D deficiency.

Hypocalcemia is defined as a serum calcium level <7 mg/dl in premature infants and <8 mg/dl in full-term infants or children.

Pathophysiology

Calcium is the most abundant mineral in the body, most of which is found in bone, leaving <1% in the serum. Calcium levels are under the tight regulatory control of several hormones, including parathyroid hormone (PTH), calcitonin, and vitamin D (Fig. 44.2). Other factors that contribute to calcium homeostasis include hepatic and renal function, phosphate and magnesium levels.

Parathyroid hormone is released in response to decreased levels of ionized calcium. Parathyroid hormone acts directly on the cells of the distal renal tubule to increase calcium and decrease phosphorus reabsorption, mobilize calcium from the bone, and stimulate 1α-hydroxylase activity in the kidney, converting 25-hydroxyvitamin D to 1,25-dihydroxyvitamin D, the active form of vitamin D. 1, 25-Dihydroxyvitamin D promotes calcium and phosphorus absorption from the GI tract and resorption from the renal tubules. Magnesium is essential for the release of PTH from the parathyroid gland and magnesium deficiency alone can cause hypoparathyroidism.

The most common etiologies of hypocalcemia are related to vitamin D or PTH deficiency or resistance. Given the pattern of calcium and phosphorus levels, the etiology of hypocalcemia can often be elucidated. If both calcium and phosphorus are low, it is suggestive of vitamin D deficiency, whereas if the phosphorus level is high, it is more suggestive of PTH deficiency. Finally, dietary intake of calcium is an important consideration, particularly in patients with impaired oral intake (dependent on a gastric tube or total parenteral nutrition).

Neonatal pathophysiology

Calcium is transferred actively from the maternal circulation to the fetus. The majority of fetal calcium accrual occurs in the third trimester. This process results in higher plasma calcium concentrations in the fetus than in the mother and leads to fetal hypercalcemia, with total calcium concentrations of 10–11 mg/dl in umbilical cord blood at term. After the abrupt cessation of placental transfer of calcium at birth, total serum calcium concentration falls temporarily to 8–9 mg/dl at 24 h of life, eventually rising to levels seen in older children and adults by 2 weeks of age. Since the fetus' own PTH production is suppressed during pregnancy by the maternal transfer of calcium, all neonates have a relative hypoparathyroidism at birth. Infants rely on oral calcium from breast milk in the first few days of life until their own parathyroid gland increases PTH secretion.

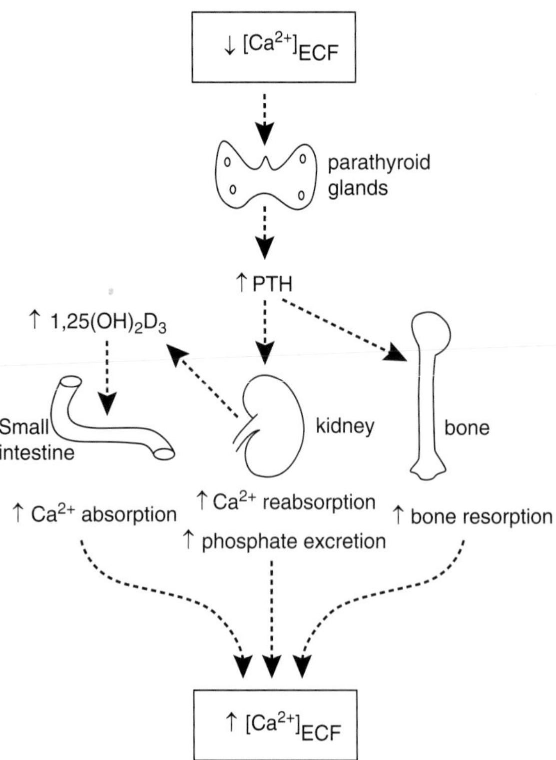

Figure 44.2 Calcium homeostasis. ECF, extracellular fliud; PTH, parathormone; $1,25(OH)_2$-D_3, 1,25-dihydroxyvitamin D_3.

Causes of hypocalcemia

Transient hypocalcemia in neonates

Infants who are sick, premature, or have oral-motor dysfunction can have an exaggerated period of hypocalcemia when feeding is impaired. Premature or other ill infants also may have renal dysfunction, leading to inappropriate calcium excretion or a relative resistance of the immature kidney to PTH. Some infants may have exaggerated PTH suppression or deficiency intrauterine, also leading to early hypocalcemia. Infants of mothers with hyperparathyroidism or infants of diabetic mothers who have magnesium deficiency (magnesuria caused by glucosuria) will have a transient period of hypoparathyroidism as their bodies will need an extended period of time to recover from intrauterine deficiencies. In the above circumstances, infants can have profound symptomatic hypocalcemia in the first few days of their life. They may need initial support to maintain their calcium level but will eventually be able to maintain their calcium once the disease process resolves. Another important etiology of hypocalcemia that generally presents after the first few days of life is the ingestion of cow's milk, which has a high phosphate content; this results in hyperphosphatemia and increased calcium and phosphate deposition, leading to hypocalcemia. These children will also need temporary support with encouragement of breast feeding or a low phosphate formula.

Hypoparathyroidism

Permanent hypoparathyroidism is usually caused by impaired synthesis or secretion of the PTH either from a congenital absence (often associated with 22q11 deletion or DiGeorge syndrome) or from loss of the parathyroid gland surgically or through an autoimmune process.

Hypovitaminosis D

Vitamin D deficiency is still an important etiology of hypocalcemia in children. This can be caused by decreased intake or production of vitamin D. Nutritional vitamin D deficiency is relatively common, and some studies report an incidence of 10–25% in children. Neonates are particularly susceptible as they rely on maternal transfer of vitamin D. If the mother is vitamin D deficient and vitamin D supplementation has not been provided for an exclusively breast-fed infant, symptomatic hypocalcemia can occur. Profound vitamin D deficiency can occur in older infants who are exclusively breast-fed after the first 6 months of life or are malnourished, particularly if dark skinned or without adequate sun exposure. These patients should have physical signs of rickets, including widening of the ends of long bones or prominence of the costochondral junctions of the ribs (rachitic rosary). Young children may have pain at the ends of long bones and may have physical developmental delays to avoid putting pressure on their bones, for example not walking or crawling at age-appropriate times.

Clinical presentation

Profound hypocalcemia manifests as CNS irritability and poor muscular contractility. Low calcium levels decrease the threshold of excitation of neurons, causing them to have repetitive responses to a single stimulus. Because neuronal excitability occurs in both sensory and motor nerves, hypocalcemia produces a wide range of peripheral and CNS effects, including paresthesiae, tetany (i.e., contraction of hands, arms, feet, larynx, bronchioles), seizures, and even psychiatric changes. In severe cases, cardiac function may also be impaired because of poor muscle contractility.

In neonates, parents may first observe myoclonic jerks or hyperresponsiveness, which is often mistaken for normal behavior. Other symptoms reported include poor feeding, vomiting, or lethargy; however, many parents report no symptoms until an actual convulsive episode has occurred. In older children, more common symptoms of cramping or paresthesiae can be present, but children can also be completely asymptomatic until they present to medical attention because of a seizure. On physical examination, hypocalcemic neonates may be difficult to identify as only mild irritability or subtle changes in reflexes may be present. Laryngospasm causing stridor or bronchospasm causing wheezing are very late signs of hypocalcemia and are rarely present. Classically, physical findings in older patients with neuromuscular irritability caused by latent tetany are Trousseau's and Chvostek's signs. Trousseau's sign is the induction of carpal spasm by inflation of a sphygmomanometer above systolic blood pressure for 2–3 min. Trousseau's sign depends upon the effect of ischemia to increase excitability of the nerve trunk under the cuff. Chvostek's sign is contraction of the ipsilateral facial muscles elicited by tapping the facial nerve just anterior to the ear. Contraction of the corner of the mouth alone occurs in approximately 25% of normal adults and even higher rates in children. It is important to remember that although Trousseau's sign is more specific than Chvostek's sign, both may be negative in patients with hypocalcemia, even in those with hypocalcemic seizures.

Laboratory evaluation

The laboratory evaluation for hypocalcemia is reflective of the possible disease etiologies. A complete evaluation for the child includes:

- total calcium, ionized calcium
- phosphorus
- magnesium
- alkaline phosphatase
- bicarbonate
- pH
- renal function: BUN and creatinine
- LFTs
- intact parathormone (iPTH)
- vitamin D: 25-hydroxy- and 1,25-hydroxyvitamin D
- urine calcium/creatinine ratio
- genetic analysis: fluorescent in situ hybridization (FISH) for 22q11.

It is important to remember that hypoalbuminemia can affect serum calcium as most calcium is protein bound. If albumin levels are low, serum calcium levels should be corrected using the simple equation:

$$\text{Corrected calcium} = [0.8 \times (\text{Normal albumin} - \text{Patient albumin})] + \text{Serum calcium}$$

Ionized calcium levels can also be used, but alkalosis can lead to increased protein binding of ionized calcium, falsely lowering these values, so assessing a serum bicarbonate or blood pH is necessary for correlation. Acidosis correspondingly increases ionized calcium levels. Obtaining an intact parathyroid hormone (iPTH) measure in conjunction with calcium is vital as iPTH levels can be variable when calcium is normal but, of

Box 44.1. Treatment of hypocalcemia

1. Either calcium gluconate or chloride can be used; calcium gluconate is less caustic:
   - calcium gluconate: bolus of 100 mg/kg or 1 ml/kg.
   - calcium chloride: 20 mg/kg over 3–4 min.

   Repeated boluses may be given, particularly if a patient continues to actively seize or be symptomatic.
2. After acute recovery, a calcium infusion should be started, delivering 50–100 mg/kg of elemental calcium daily, depending on the severity of hypocalcemia. This can also be accomplished with scheduled doses of IV calcium, although the effects of a dose typically last 4–6 h, so it should be given at minimum every 6 h.
3. If hypomagnesemia is present: 0.5 mEq/kg (6 mg/kg) or 0.125 ml/kg of 50% magnesium sulfate is given.
4. If hypoparathyroidism is suspected,1, 25-dihydroxy-vitamin D or 25-hydroxy-vitamin D (calcitriol) can also be used to boost intestinal absorption of calcium. Onset of action of calcitriol is rapid and its half-life is 4–6 h. Although an IV form is available, oral calcitriol is often used as a single dose of 0.25–0.5 μg acutely and then scheduled twice a day.

course, are expected to be high when calcium levels are low. Vitamin D levels are also important – both 25-hydroxy- and 1,25-hydroxyvitamin D should be obtained. Finally, urine should be sent for a spot calcium to creatinine ratio.

In a neonate, maternal samples can also be helful in the evaluation:

- calcium
- phosphorus
- magnesium
- iPTH
- 25-hydroxyvitamin D.

Finally, if the neonate has any signs of cardiac dysfunction or dysmorphic features, FISH analysis for the 22q11 deletion should be completed.

Treatment

Emergency treatment for hypocalcemia primarily includes IV calcium, regardless of etiology (Box 44.1). Either calcium gluconate or chloride can be used, but unless a central line is used, calcium gluconate is preferred as it is less caustic. However, even calcium gluconate can be caustic so ensuring proper dilution of the solution is important as extravasation of the IV calcium into the tissue can cause serious injury. Patients should be under cardiac monitoring as hypercalcemia, even transiently, can cause clinically significant bradycardia or other rhythmic disturbances.

Any magnesium deficiency should also be treated as hypomagnesemia can often prevent normalization of calcium levels. Patients with profound hypocalcemia should be admitted to an ICU with constant monitoring until the calcium levels are stabilized, and they will need to continue to be monitored closely after the transition to oral calcium. If patients are found to be vitamin D deficient, after initial stabilization and maintenance with calcium, large doses of calciferol (ergocalciferol) or colecalciferol are needed to replenish depleted stores.

Pearls and pitfalls

Pearls

1. Infants, children and adolescents with suspected adrenal insufficiency should be given hydrocortisone 25, 50, or 75 mg, respectively, stress dose.
2. In a child with a suspected endocrinologic condition, hold 5 ml of blood in a red top tube prior to initiating any treatments to aid in the diagnostic workup.
3. A bedside blood sugar and electrolytes are the most critical parts of the laboratory evaluation in a patient with suspected adrenal insufficiency.
4. Any patient with a history of Graves' disease presenting with a high fever, hypertension, and tachycardia should be evaluated for thyroid storm.

Pitfalls

1. Failure to consider hypocalcemia in any child or neonate with seizures.
2. Failure to administer parenteral calcium to a symptomatic hypocalcemic child.

Selected references

Buckingham B. The hyperthyroid fetus and infant. *NeoReviews* 2000;**1**:103–109.

Fleisher G. *Endocrine Emergencies. Textbook of Pediatric Emergency Medicine.* Philadelphia, PA: Lippincott Williams & Wilkins, 2005.

Hsu SC. Perinatal calcium metabolism: physiology and pathophysiology. *Semin Neonatol* 2004;**9**:23–36.

Kahler S. Metabolic disorders associated with neonatal hypoglycemia. *NeoReviews* 2004;**5**:e377–e381.

Levine L. Congenital adrenal hyperplasia. *Pediatr Rev* 2000;**21**:159–171.

Schulman D. Adrenal insufficiency: still a cause of morbidity and death in childhood. *Pediatrics* 2007;**119**:e484–e494.

Singh J. the investigation of hypocalcemia and rickets. *Arch Dis Child* 2003;**88**: 403–407.

Sperling M. *Pediatric Endocrinology.* Philadelphia, PA: Saunders, 2008.

Styne D. *Pediatric Endocrinology.* Philadeplphia, PA: Lippincott Williams & Wilkins, 2004.

Section

8

Environmental emergencies

Chapter 45

Drowning and submersion

David Kammer and Steven H. Mitchell

Introduction

Drowning disproportionately affects children. For each drowning-related death, an estimated 16 child submersion victims are seen in the ED. In a study of 709 unintentional drownings near Seattle, Washington, 29% of those 1–4 years of age, mostly infant, drowned in a bathtub, while 36%, mostly toddlers, drowned in a pool. In older children, alcohol and high-risk behavior plays a significant role in drowning-related deaths.

The term "drowning" was defined by the 2002 World Congress on Drowning as "a process resulting in primary respiratory impairment from submersion/immersion in liquid" regardless of outcome. In the past, the term "drowning" implied mortality within 24 h, while the term "near drowning" was used to imply 24 h of survival after an episode of liquid aspiration owing to immersion. Historically, "dry drowning" has been used to refer to drowning victims found without aspirated water into their lungs, and in the lay press to refer to victims who die of asphyxiation while on dry land shortly after a submersion event. It is now believed that drowning without aspiration is unlikely, and previous reports of "dry drowning" may have been caused by osmotic uptake of fresh water in the lungs, or death that occurred prior to submersion. More commonly "secondary drowning" is used in the medical literature. The phenomenon of suffocating on dry land after an aspiration event is most likely acute respiratory distress syndrome, which is not uncommon after aspiration. The term "secondary drowning" has also been used to describe a drowning event that occurs as a result of some other insult or injury, such as seizure or head trauma. This occurs in roughly 13% of all drownings. Current recommendations urge the avoidance of these terms in favor of less confusing terms such as "death due to drowning", "drowning secondary to seizure", and "fulminant pulmonary edema after drowning".

Pediatric patients differ from adults mostly in terms of survival. They are less likely to develop ventricular fibrillation and are more likely to receive some protective effects from hypothermia. The management of the pediatric drowning patient, however, is very similar to the management of the adult drowning patient; they differ only in terms of which resuscitation algorithms are used.

Pathophysiology

The aspiration of water in a drowning victim is often immediately followed by breath-holding or laryngospasm, although eventually hypoxia leads to termination of these protective mechanisms and water is aspirated. As water enters the lungs it destroys surfactant and causes the development of alveolar edema, which alters alveolar gas exchange and increases intrapulmonary shunting. These effects of aspiration cause hypoxia to occur more quickly in a drowning victim than in an individual who is simply deprived of oxygen, and they may impede gas exchange during resuscitation.

Hypothermia is a common development in victims of drowning (Ch. 47). Primary hypothermia occurs when a victim is submerged in water that is substantially colder than body temperature. Such a submersion can result in decreased muscle coordination and weakness (around 35°C core body temperature) and progress to obtundation and eventual loss of consciousness (at approximately 30°C). A more immediate phenomenon, known as "immersion syndrome," has been described as a sudden syncope upon contact with cold water, possibly as a result of a vagal response. These primary causes of hypothermia are in contrast to secondary hypothermia, which develops from exposure during submersion or resuscitation.

Despite earlier reports from animal models, neither fresh nor saltwater drownings commonly result in clinically significant electrolyte abnormalities. Most significant arrhythmias develop secondary to hypoxia and the resulting metabolic and respiratory acidosis.

Treatment and management

Rescue and recovery

All rescue and recovery attempts should bear in mind the safety of the rescuer. Struggling victims should be approached

A Practical Guide to Pediatric Emergency Medicine: Caring for Children in the Emergency Department, ed. N. Ewen Amieva-Wang (associate eds. Jamie Shandro, Aparajita Sohoni, and Bernhard Fassl). Published by Cambridge University Press.

with an intermediate device, such as a rescue torpedo, as drowning individuals can, in desperation, turn a would-be rescuer into a second victim. If the drowning has not taken place in immediate proximity to a dry surface, such as in a pool or a bathtub, rescue breathing should begin while the victim is still in the water. Effective chest compressions cannot be preformed while the victim is floating. Rescuers should have a high index of suspicion for spinal cord injuries in any situation that may have involved diving or recreational water equipment. In these situations the cervical spine should be immobilized in a neutral position and the patient floated onto a backboard before removal from the water. Wet garments should be removed, and the patient insulated.

Evaluation

Important historical information includes duration of submersion, water temperature, duration and resuscitative efforts at the scene, concern for possible trauma or abuse, history of drug or alcohol use, and past medical history. Patients who are seen in the ED after a significant aspiration event, even if they have spontaneously recovered, should be evaluated with a core temperature, a chest film, and an arterial blood gas.

Resuscitation

Breathing and ventilation are the most important aspects of resuscitation in the drowning victim and the American Heart Association (AHA) Basic Life Support (BLS) and Pediatric Advanced Life Support (PALS) resuscitation should be initiated immediately. Efforts to clear liquid from the airway or lung by positioning, rolling or suctioning are generally unnecessary, and delay ventilation. Most drowning victims aspirate relatively little water and fresh water is often absorbed into systemic circulation. Abdominal thrusts (the Heimlich maneuver) are not an effective method for removing water from the lungs and increase the chances that a victim will vomit. If a foreign body obstructing the airway is suspected, chest compressions may be a more effective mechanism to expel the offending material and are preferred in the unconscious victim.

No modifications are required to the BLS cardiopulmonary resuscitation algorithms for application to drowning victims. In a patient who is very cold, a pulse may be difficult to palpate. In general, breathing, coughing, or movement in response to rescue breaths are good signs of circulation, but if any doubt is present, chest compressions should be initiated and an automated external defibrillator (AED) employed. Drowning victims swallow far more water than they aspirate and up to 86% of victims vomit during resuscitation. When the patient vomits, the victim's head should be turned, or the victim log-rolled, and the mouth should be swept or suctioned to prevent aspiration. Application of cricoid pressure by a second rescuer during resuscitation may reduce the risk of regurgitation. Apneic patients should be intubated at the earliest opportunity. All submersion victims, regardless of level of intervention required at the scene, should receive oxygen and monitoring and be transported to a hospital. En route, CPR should be continued with interruptions in chest compressions minimized. Victims who are breathing spontaneously and not requiring cervical spine immobilization may benefit from being transported in the left lateral decubitus position.

In the pulseless victim, PALS protocols should be initiated. Drug administration by the IV routes is preferred to endotracheal administration because of possible complications in absorption from pulmonary edema. Pulseless cardiac arrest upon arrival in the ED carries a very poor prognosis for the pediatric victim.

Duration of resuscitation and prognosis

The question of how long to continue resuscitation efforts is difficult. One study of pediatric drowning in temperate water found that submersion duration >25 min or resuscitation duration >25 min was associated with 100% mortality. Shorter submersion (<5 min) or resuscitation (<10 min) times are associated with lower mortality or major morbidity, from 9–13%. Patients who have reactive pupils, are in a normal sinus rhythm, or are conscious at the scene of submersion have only 0–1% mortality. These results suggest that patients who were submerged longer than 25 min or who have undergone more

Pearls and pitfalls

Pearls

1. Therapy in ED is directed toward standard basic life support and pediatric advanced life support.
2. Vomiting of water is common and can complicate resuscitation efforts. Early intubation can help to protect the airway from further aspiration.
3. Electrolyte and volume abnormalities are not clinically relevant problems in most victims of fresh or saltwater drowning.
4. Resuscitation lasting longer than 25 min for drowning victims in non-icy water is associated with a dismal prognosis.

Pitfalls

1. Failure to protection spinal cord injury during airway manipulation and transport; drowning victims must be presumed to have a cervical spine injury.
2. Failure to measure a core temperature; drowning victims are often hypothermic.
3. Failure to admit and observe patients who have a significant submersion history, or who are even minimally symptomatic, as delayed pulmonary edema can develop up to 24 h after a submersion event.

than 25 min of active resuscitation would not benefit from prolonged resuscitative efforts.

Extremely cold, or icy, water temperatures may encourage providers to sustain resuscitation for a longer time as case reports in the pediatric literature document incidents of full recovery after 45 min of resuscitation for victims in icy waters. Of victims who survive, approximately 15% have severe neurological deficits.

Disposition

Patients who had minimal submersion time, no episodes of respiratory distress, and a normal physical examination and neurologic status in the ED can be observed for 8 h and discharged with a reliable caregiver if still asymptomatic. All patients who were submerged from more than 1 min, who required rescue breathing, are symptomatic or who were at any point cyanotic or apneic should be held for observation for at least 24 h. Fulminant pulmonary edema can develop hours after aspiration in a seemingly healthy patient. Patients who received CPR, have abnormal chest films, or an abnormal arterial blood gas should be admitted to the ICU.

The use of prophylactic antibiotics and corticosteroids are not substantiated in the literature and may predicate worse outcomes. Despite evidence that some pulmonary edema in drowning victims may result from increased central venous pressure, the use of furosemide is not recommended.

Selected references

Durrer B, Brugger H, Syme D. Advanced challenges in resuscitation: special challenges in EEC-hypothermia. *Resuscitation* 2001;**50**:243–244.

European Resuscitation Council Part 8: advanced challenges in resuscitation. Section 3: special challenges in ECC. 3B: submersion or near-drowning. *Resuscitation* 2000;**46**:273–277.

Fuchs S. Cardiopulmonary resuscitation and pediatric advanced life support update for the emergency physician. *Pediatr Emerg Care* 2008;**24**:561–565; quiz 6–8.

Idris A, Berg R, Bierens J, *et al.* Recommended guidelines for uniform reporting of data from drowning: the "Utstein style." *Resuscitation* 2003;**59**: 45–57.

Moon R, Long R. Drowning and near-drowning. *Emerg Med (Fremantle)* 2002;**14**: 377–386.

Perk L, Borger van de Burg F, Berendsen H, van't Wout J. Full recovery after 45 min accidental submersion. *Intensive Care Med* 2002;**28**:524.

Quan L, Cummings P. Characteristics of drowning by different age groups. *Inj Prev* 2003;**9**:163–168.

Szpilman D, Elmann J, Cruze Filho F. Dry-drowning: fact or fiction. In *World Congress on Drowning*, Amsterdam, 2002, poster 5.2.

Chapter 46

Frostbite and localized cold injury

Medley O'Keefe Gatewood and David A. Townes

Introduction

Localized cold injuries include both freezing and non-freezing syndromes, which may occur independently or in conjunction with systemic hypothermia. Frostbite is a localized freezing injury, while frostnip, chilblains, cold-induced panniculitis, and trenchfoot are non-freezing localized injuries.

Frostbite and frostnip

Frostbite occurs when environmental exposure to cold results in localized tissue damage. It can occur on any skin surface but is usually limited to exposed skin. Frostnip is essentially a less severe form of frostbite where no tissue damage has occurred. It is often painful but resolves completely with rewarming. Similar to burns, frostbite is categorized as first, second, third, and fourth degree, with increasing severity and worsening prognosis. It is also classified as superficial versus deep. Early signs of frostbite include blanching of the skin followed by numbness, pallor, mottling, and development of a hard wooden or waxy texture. Classification of frostbite with associated symptoms is shown in Table 46.1.

Both frostbite and frostnip occur most commonly on the ears, nose, cheeks, fingers, toes, hands, and feet. Children and adolescents are at risk through outdoor recreational activities, inappropriate use of cold compresses, inadequate clothing, dehydration, inactivity, and fatigue. Predisposing factors to frostbite and other localized cold injuries in children are listed in Table 46.2. Most patients sustain frostbite following only 1 to 3 h of exposure to a cold environment. When exposed to cold temperatures, an initial response is vasoconstriction in the skin as a protective measure to maintain core body temperature. Ice crystal formation occurs when tissue temperature drops to −2°C (85.1°F). Upon rewarming, reperfusion of damaged endothelium results in release of inflammatory mediators and further tissue destruction. Assessment of tissue viability in the first hours following injury is often inaccurate.

Management

Management of frostbite begins with removal of wet, cold, and constricting garments. In the prehospital setting, the injured areas should be covered with warm, dry, padded gauze. Affected digits should be dressed separately. It is important

Table 46.1. Classification of frostbite

Classification	Signs	Symptoms
Superficial		
First degree: partial skin freezing	Erythema, edema, no blisters	Numbness, stinging and burning; throbbing and aching possible; may have hyperhidrosis
Second degree: full-thickness skin freezing	Erythema, substantial edema, clear vesicles and blisters	Numbness, followed by aching and throbbing; possible vasomotor disturbance
Deep		
Third degree: full-thickness skin and subcutaneous freezing	Violaceous/hemorrhagic blisters, skin necrosis, blue-gray discoloration of skin	Initially no sensation ("like a block of wood"); later, shooting pains, burning, throbbing, aching
Fourth degree: full-thickness skin, subcutaneous tissue, muscle, tendon, and bone freezing	Little edema; initially mottled, deep red, or cyanotic; eventually dry, black, mummified	Possible joint discomfort

A Practical Guide to Pediatric Emergency Medicine: Caring for Children in the Emergency Department, ed. N. Ewen Amieva-Wang (associate eds. Jamie Shandro, Aparajita Sohoni, and Bernhard Fassl). Published by Cambridge University Press.

Table 46.2. Predisposing factors to localized cold injury

	Factors
Physiologic	Dehydration, overexertion, trauma, physical conditioning, diaphoresis, hypoxia, mental status, fatigue, hunger, starvation, intoxicants
Mechanical	Wet or tight clothing, inadequate insulation, immobility
Environmental	Ambient temperature, humidity, duration of exposure, wind chill factor, altitude, body surface area exposed, heat loss
Cardiovascular	Cold-induced vasoconstriction, hypovolemia, shock, anemia, sickle cell disease, diabetes, arteritis, Raynaud syndrome

Source: adapted from Danzl DF. Frostbite. In Marx JA, Hockberger R, Walls R (eds.) *Rosen's Emergency Medicine: Concepts and Clinical Practice*, 6th edn, Ch. 137. Philadelphia, PA: Mosby 2006.

not to rub or expose areas of frostbite to dry heat. Rewarming should not be initiated if there is any possibility of refreezing (i.e., in the field, during transport) because this will lead to increased tissue damage.

In children presenting to the ED within 24 h of frostbite injury, the frozen areas should be rewarmed rapidly by immersion in water.
If an area has already thawed, it should not be rewarmed.

The water is used at 40–42°C (104–108°F) for 20 to 40 min or until the most distal part is completely thawed; an erythematous flush is visible when this occurs.

Rewarming may be very painful, and judicious analgesia with IV narcotics may be necessary.

The advantage of sterile aspiration of intact clear blisters is unclear and intact blisters are currently thought to be best left intact. Debridement of ruptured blisters is indicated. Hemorrhagic blisters should be left alone as debridement appears to extend the level of injury.

Further treatment includes administration of oral ibuprofen to limit the release of inflammatory mediators and the application of topical aloe vera or antibiotic ointment to the affected areas. Elevation and splinting of the involved area should be done to minimize swelling. It may be covered with a loose, padded dressing.

Areas of frostbite are at increased risk for infection. The need for antibiotics should be based on the clinical evaluation, noting that in severe cases, streptococcal prophylaxis is warranted. Broad-spectrum prophylaxis should be considered if excessive heat was used to thaw tissue, since liquefaction and infection are inevitable. All patients with frostbite should have a tetanus booster immunization if not current. In severe cases of frostbite, a burn specialist and/or plastic surgeon should be consulted. Definitive surgical therapy is usually delayed until a clear level of demarcation is seen.

Non-freezing localized cold injuries

Chilblains

Chilblains (or pernio) consists of painful, inflamed skin lesions caused by repetitive exposure to damp, non-freezing ambient temperatures. The lesions appear <24 h after exposure and usually affect the face, the dorsa of the hands and feet, and the pretibial areas. Skin changes include edema, erythematous or violaceous macules, papules, nodules, or plaques, which may form vesicles or ulcerate. Patients may experience burning, paresthesiae, and pruritus. Blue nodules may develop upon rewarming and may last for several days. Management of chilblains is primarily supportive. Nifedipine, topical corticosteroids, and sometimes oral prednisone have been shown to be helpful in ameliorating the symptoms of chilblains. Affected areas are more prone to reinjury.

Trenchfoot

Trenchfoot, or immersion foot, develops over hours to days from prolonged exposure to damp or wet cold at temperatures above freezing. At first, tingling and numbness develop in the affected area. The area appears pale and mottled and may be anesthetic, pulseless, and immobile. After rewarming, a hyperemic phase occurs characterized by hot, red, painful, dry swollen feet. The pain can be excruciating and is often what incites presentation for medical care. Edema and bullae may develop, and in severe cases gangrene may ensue. Long-term

Pearls and pitfalls

Pearls

1. There is no tissue damage in frostnip and it is completely reversible with rewarming.
2. Chilblains is a non-freezing cold injury with symptomatic dermatologic manifestations.
3. Cold-induced panniculitis results in non-tender skin lesions following focal cold exposure; these resolve over weeks to months.
4. Frostbite involves tissue damage and may result in tissue loss even with proper therapy.
5. Treatment of frostbite involves rewarming the affected area in water heated to 40–42°C (104–108°F).

Pitfalls

1. The initial presentation of frostbite may be deceptively benign.
2. In frostbite, it may take weeks for the demarcation line for tissue viability to become evident.
3. Premature termination of thawing is a common error in the treatment of frostbite.

hyperhidrosis and cold sensitivity are common. Anesthesia of the area may be permanent. With trenchfoot, the best therapy is preventive. Preventive measures include frequent sock changes and never sleeping with wet socks and boots. Once symptoms develop, feet should be kept warm, dry and elevated.

Cold-induced panniculitis

Cold-induced panniculitis is a self-limiting condition characterized by skin plaques or nodules, usually seen around 2 days after local or focal cold exposure and most commonly seen on the face. There is often a history of eating a popsicle or ice cream, using a frozen teething ring, or being exposed to cold weather within the preceding several days. It is more common in infants and younger children because of the higher fat content of their subcutaneous tissue. This fatty tissue solidifies following exposure to cold, resulting in red to violaceous subcutaneous lesions with a firm, rubbery texture. In contrast to frostbite, the lesions are non-tender. There is no specific therapy and lesions usually clear within weeks to months without scarring.

Disposition

Except in very minor cases, all children with frostbite should be hospitalized for 24 to 48 h to determine the extent of injury. Admission to plastic surgical or burn unit should be considered for severe cases.

Children with frostnip, chilblains, trenchfoot, and cold-induced panniculitis may be discharged with specific instructions and good follow-up.

Selected references

Danzl DF. Frostbite. In Marx JA, Hockberger R, Walls R (eds.) *Rosen's Emergency Medicine: Concepts and Clinical Practice,* 6th edn, Ch. 137. Philadelphia, PA: Mosby, 2006.

Ulrich AS, Rathlev NK. Hypothermia and localized cold injuries. *Emerg Med Clin of North Am* 2004;**22**:281–298.

Chapter 47

Hypothermia

Medley O'Keefe Gatewood and David A. Townes

Introduction

Cold injury constitutes a spectrum of injury and illness including hypothermia and localized cold injury. Hypothermia is defined as a core body temperature <35°C (95°F). It is categorized as *mild* (32–35°C/90–95°F), *moderate* (28–32°C/82–90°F) and *severe* (<28°C/<82°F).

Neonates, infants, and children are at greater risk for hypothermia compared with adults for several reasons. They have a larger body surface area (BSA) to mass ratio compared with adults. A 7-lb (3-kg) infant, for example, has 2.5 times more BSA per unit weight than a 140-lb (64-kg) adult. Also, an infant's head takes up a larger proportion of the body than does the head of an adult, further contributing to accelerated heat loss if left exposed. Thermoregulation in children is less efficient than in adults as their thermoregulatory mechanisms are underdeveloped. Infants respond to cold stress by increasing metabolism through an increase in motor activity, or non-shivering thermogenesis. Finally, infants and small children have inadequate subcutaneous fatty tissue to insulate them from exposure in a cold environment.

Shivering, a normal thermoregulatory response in adults, is relatively ineffective in children and completely absent in infants.

In any age group, there are factors that predispose an individual to hypothermia. These include decreased heat production, increased heat loss, and impaired thermoregulation.

Decreased heat production. Hypothermia may result from decreased heat production in the setting of hypoglycemia, hypopituitarism, hypoadrenalism, hypothyroidism, and malnutrition. These etiologies should be considered in patients presenting with unexplained hypothermia who fail to rewarm with standard therapy.

Increased heat loss. This is the most common form of hypothermia encountered in the pediatric population. It may result in hypothermia through both immersion and non-immersion etiologies. Non-immersion etiologies include toxic or pharmacologic ingestions and burns. Of special note is rapid heat loss in a newborn after an emergency delivery.

Impaired thermoregulation. Hypothermia may result if the hypothalamus fails to regulate core body temperature, as in the setting of CNS trauma or mass, toxic and metabolic derangements, sepsis, or chronic disease.

Accidental hypothermia from environmental exposure is common in infants and young children as they are not capable of certain adaptive behavioral responses and must rely on caregivers to provide shelter and appropriate clothing. While most commonly seen in colder climates, accidental hypothermia may develop in young children indoors during the summer in temperate regions. Factors including wind chill and wet or inadequate clothing may cause hypothermia, even in the presence of non-freezing ambient temperatures. Cold-water immersion and near drowning are causes of accidental hypothermia in children.

Pathophysiology

When exposed to a cold environment, the body's thermoregulatory mechanisms attempt to maintain the core temperature through a combination of vasoconstriction, shivering, muscle contraction, and non-shivering thermogenesis. Shivering, for example, increases the rate of heat production two to five times.

There are three main mechanisms by which body heat may be lost to the environment:

Conduction. Heat loss occurs through contact of the individual with material such as wet clothing or cold water.

Convection. Heat loss results when there is airflow around the individual either by movement of the individual or wind. The conversion of liquid on the body surface to gas in the air results in evaporation heat loss.

Radiation. Heat loss occurs whenever there is a temperature gradient between the environment and the individual.

A Practical Guide to Pediatric Emergency Medicine: Caring for Children in the Emergency Department, ed. N. Ewen Amieva-Wang (associate eds. Jamie Shandro, Aparajita Sohoni, and Bernhard Fassl). Published by Cambridge University Press.

Table 47.1. Stages of hypothermia

Degree of hypothermia	Features
Mild (32°C to 35°C)	Reduced cerebral blood flow; confusion and irrational behavior Vasoconstriction: pale, cool skin Increased heart rate and mean arterial pressure, tachypnea Shivering, except in infants and neonates
Moderate (28°C to 32°C)	Further decrease in level of consciousness Shivering absent, muscle rigidity Skin may be cyanotic and edematous Decreased respiratory drive Reduced ventricular compliance leading to hypotension and arrhythmias, particularly bradyarrythmias and atrial fibrillation Pupils become dilated May have mild clotting abnormalities and paralytic ileus
Severe (22°C to 28°C)	Usually comatose, pupils fixed and dilated, reflexes absent, including corneal or oculocephalic reflexes Ventricular arrhythmias, significant hypotension or absent pulse Vasoconstriction elevates venous pressure "Cold diuresis" with profound acidemia and prerenal failure, carbon dioxide retention and respiratory acidosis; respiratory arrest is likely Hematologic changes include hemoconcentration, sludging, thrombocytopenia, leukopenia, and disseminated intravascular coagulation
Profound (<22°C)	Asystole develops, the EEG is flat

Hypothermia occurs when the thermoregulatory mechanisms are overwhelmed causing a drop in core body temperature. Core temperatures below 35°C (95°F) are associated with failure of the thermoregulatory system and can lead to progressive multiorgan dysfunction. Even small deviations in core body temperature may have dramatic effects on body function and physiology (Table 47.1).

In older children and adults, manifestations of hypothermia are consistent with the core temperature.

In neonates and infants, physical findings in hypothermia are often non-specific and may include irritability, lethargy and poor feeding.

In general, as the body's core temperature begins to fall, there is an initial increase in metabolic function and physiology, with elevated heart and respiratory rate and shivering. Maximum shivering thermogenesis occurs at 35°C (95°F). With continued fall in core temperature, this trend is reversed, with decreased heart and respiratory rate, absence of shivering at approximately 31°C (87.8°F), and decreased oxygen demand. Oxygen demand is reduced by 25% at 32°C (89.6°F), by 50% at 28°C (82.4°F) and by 75% at 22°C (68°F). Hypothermia affects all systems of the body including cardiovascular, renal, pulmonary and CNS.

Cardiovascular system

Hypothermia causes decreased depolarization of cardiac pacemaker cells, resulting in bradycardia. Since this bradycardia is not mediated by the vagus nerve, it can be refractory to standard therapies such as atropine. In addition to bradycardia, mean arterial pressure and cardiac output decrease, and the characteristic J or Osborne wave may be seen on ECG. This positive deflection in the height of the terminal portion of the QRS complex near the QRS–ST junction is seen in approximately 80% of individuals with a core temperature below 35°C (95°F), most commonly in the inferior and lateral leads. Both ventricular and, more commonly, atrial arrhythmias may result from hypothermia when the core temperature is below 30°C (86°F). Ventricular fibrillation may occur spontaneously at core temperatures below 25°C (77°F) and aystole at 18°C (64.4°F).

Central nervous system

Hypothermia progressively depresses the CNS. As core temperature drops, there is a linear reduction in CNS metabolism (Table 47.1). Individuals with a core temperature of 34°C (93.2°F) will demonstrate amnesia, dysarthria, and poor judgement. At core temperatures below 33°C (91.4°F), brain electrical activity is abnormal, and when the core temperature drops to approximately 20°C (68°F), an electroencephalogram may appear consistent with brain death.

Hypothermia has a protective cerebral effect if hypothermia precedes hypoxia. This is most likely to occur in cold-water submersion, where rapid development of hypothermia may precede significant hypoxia. This most likely accounts for an observed increased icy water survival (at temperatures below 5–10°C or 41–50°F).

Renal system

Exposure to a cold environment initially induces diuresis regardless of an individual's hydration status. This "cold diuresis" is essentially glomerular infiltrate, which does not clear nitrogen waste.

Pulmonary system

Hypothermia initially stimulates respiration, but this is then followed by a progressive decrease in ventilation in proportion to the overall decrease in metabolism. Carbon dioxide production decreases with decreasing metabolism, but ultimately the decreased respiratory drive associated with severe hypothermia results in carbon dioxide retention and respiratory acidosis. Decreased ciliary motility, viscous bronchorrhea and non-cardiogenic pulmonary edema also contribute to the respiratory compromise witnessed in hypothermia.

Diagnosis

The first step in making the diagnosis of hypothermia is suspecting the diagnosis; it is often recognized late. The diagnosis is confirmed utilizing a proper low-reading thermometer. Oral temperatures are unreliable and standard oral thermometers record only down to 35°C (95°F). Tympanic thermometers closely reflect the hypothalamic temperature although reliability of these devices remains uncertain. When done properly, rectal temperatures are the most reliable and are the method of choice in most settings.

Management

In the majority of situations, treatment of the pediatric patient with hypothermia should begin in the field by removing wet garments and surrounding the child with a source of heat such as warmed blankets, hot water bottles, or the body of a rescuer. In mild hypothermia where the child is awake and alert, this may be supplemented with warm oral fluids. In moderate and severe hypothermia, the child should be placed on an ECG monitor. The child may be hypovolemic secondary to increased losses and decreased intake.

During the initial assessment of the hypothermic child, a rescuer should spend a full minute palpating for a pulse. Cardiopulmonary resuscitation (CPR) should be initiated if no pulse or respirations are present. Although stimulation of the airway may precipitate ventricular arrhythmias in the severely hypothermic patient, the benefits of ventilation and oxygenation far outweigh risks. In severe hypothermia where there is no spontaneous cardiopulmonary activity, it is important to initiate CPR but it may be beneficial to withhold rewarming until extracorporeal rewarming can be initiated. During transport, it is important to take special precautions to minimize transfers, excess movements, or jarring of the litter as this may precipitate an arrhythmia.

On arrival to the ED, the hypothermic child should be evaluated for other injuries or illnesses that may have contributed to the hypothermia, such as trauma, submersion, intoxication, and underlying disease. In patients with moderate to severe hypothermia, a Foley catheter is inserted to enable monitoring of urine output. Nasogastric tube insertion should be avoided until the core temperature is above 30°C, as it may lead to arrhythmia.

Children with severe hypothermia may appear to be dead with fixed and dilated pupils, blue skin, no discernable pulse, no discernable breathing, and rigid muscles. They may be unresponsive to any stimuli. Do not assume that a child is dead until their core temperature is above 32°C (89.6°F). Children with severe bradycardia or asystole can recover without sequelae. Pediatric victims of accidental hypothermia have been successfully resuscitated from temperatures as low as 14.2°C (57.6°F).

If the child is in ventricular fibrillation and their core temperature is below 29.5°C (85.1°F), direct current (DC) cardioversion or standard cardiac medications are unlikely to be helpful. In these situations it is important to continue CPR before and during rapid rewarming measures until the core temperature is above 29.5°C (85.1°F). If ventricular fibrillation occurs at a core temperature of 29.5–32°C (85.1–89.6°F), it is reasonable to make one attempt at DC cardioversion or defibrillation with 2 J/kg. If this fails, continue CPR during rewarming until the temperature is above 32°C (89.6°F). At that temperature, if the arrhythmia has not spontaneously resolved, utilize standard Pediatric Advanced Life Support (PALS). There is some evidence that bretylium tosylate may work in the treatment of hypothermic adults with arrhythmias.

Obtain an ECG, arterial blood gas, urinalysis, and blood for measurements of CBC with platelets, electrolytes, glucose, amylase, renal and liver function, and coagulation studies. Laboratory findings may be inconsistent, depending on the degree of hypothermia. After the initial assessment and resuscitation, the mainstay of treatment for hypothermia is rewarming. This may be accomplished through passive external rewarming, active external rewarming, and active internal or core rewarming (Table 47.2).

Table 47.2. Rewarming methods for hypothermia in children

Rewarming method	Techniques
Passive external	Place in warm environment; insulation (blankets, dry clothes)
Active external	Apply exogenous heat source to patient's skin (radiant heat, forced air, hot packs, electric or plumbed heating blankets); use neonatal incubator
Active internal	Heated humidified oxygen
"Core rewarming"	Warmed IV fluid infusion, heated irrigation (peritoneal, bladder, gastrointestinal, thoracic, and mediastinal lavage), extracorporeal rewarming, heated hemodialysis, cardiopulmonary bypass

Passive external rewarming

Passive external rewarming simply involves placing the patient in a warm environment and insulating them with blankets to minimize heat loss. This method of warming is reserved for generally well patients with mild hypothermia who are awake and alert and have stable cardiovascular function.

Active external rewarming

Active external rewarming should be employed in patients with moderate hypothermia. This technique involves the direct transfer of heat to the patient's skin from an exogenous heat source, such as radiant heat, forced air, hot packs, and electric or plumbed heating blankets. It is important to closely monitor children being warmed with these devices as they may burn the child. Neonates require an incubator for this form of rewarming.

One of the potential complications of active external rewarming is "rewarming shock." The two processes that contribute to rewarming shock are the temperature equilibration between the periphery and the core, and the rewarming-induced peripheral vasodilatation, which shunts cold blood from the periphery to the core. Rewarming shock may be avoided by rewaming the core as well as the periphery through active core rewarming with warmed IV fluid infusion and administration of heated oxygen.

Active internal/core rewarming

Patients with severe hypothermia require active internal or core rewarming. Active core rewarming methods include administration of heated humidified oxygen (40–45°C [104–113°F]) by mask or endotrachial tube and infusion of warmed IV fluid infusion (40–42°C [104–107.6°F]) at maximal flow rates. These interventions should raise the core temperature by approximately 2.5°C/h. Normal saline is the fluid of choice.

Heated irrigation techniques such as peritoneal, bladder, GI, thoracic, and mediastinal lavage are invasive, resource consuming, and of debatable therapeutic effect in practice. Of these, peritoneal irrigation is usually the most feasible. Peritoneal lavage with warmed (40–45°C [104–113°F]) crystalloid at 10–20 ml/kg per h is effective, achieving a rewarming rate of 4°C/h. Lavage of the GI tract and bladder can be done with warmed saline. In refractory cases where there is asystole or ventricular fibrillation, closed thoracic or mediastinal lavage may be considered if extracorporeal rewarming such as hemodialysis or cardiopulmonary bypass (CPB) are not available.

In severe hypothermia, the rewarming method of choice is extracorporeal rewarming including heated dialysis and CPB with a heat exchanger. With CPB, rewarming occurs at approximately 9.5°C/h. Some authors recommend CPB via emergency median sternotomy as femoral–femoral cannulation may prove inadequate in small children. Extracorporeal rewarming should be considered in the severely hypothermic patient in cardiac arrest in whom no contraindications to CPB exist. Use of CPB provides rapid, uniform core rewarming and avoids afterdrop. In patients with less severe hypothermia and preserved circulation, early rewarming and by other techniques may be preferable.

Disposition

Children with hypothermia and an initial core temperature below 35°C should be admitted to the hospital; those with an initial core temperature below 32°C require admission to an ICU.

Pearls and pitfalls

Pearls

1. Children have a larger body surface area to mass ratio than adults.
2. Children, infants, and neonates possess less subcutaneous fatty tissue than adults.
3. Infants do not shiver but rely on non-shivering thermogenesis (the production of heat by metabolism) to generate heat.
4. Thermoregulation is less efficient in children, infants, and neonates.
5. Children are not capable of adaptive behavioral responses to cold stress.

Pitfalls

1. Failure to realize that symptoms of cold injury in neonates and infants are non-specific and include irritability, lethargy, and poor feeding.
2. Do not assume that a hypothermic child is dead until their core temperature is above 32°C (89.6°F).
3. Standard treatment of arrhythmias including cardioversion and standard cardiac medications are unlikely to be effective in children with a core temperature below 29.5°C (85.1°C).

Selected references

APLS Steering Committee. *The Pediatric Emergency Medicine Course*, 4th edn. Sudbury, MA: Jones & Bartlett for the American Academy of Pediatrics and the American College of Emergency Physicians, 2006.

Danzl DF. Frostbite. In Marx JA, Hockberger R, Walls R (eds.) *Rosen's Emergency Medicine: Concepts and Clinical Practice,* 6th edn, Ch. 137. Philadelphia, PA: Mosby 2006.

Danzl DF, Pozos RS. Accidental hypothermia. *N Engl J Med* 1994;**331**:1756–1760.

Danzl DF, Pozos RS, Hamlet MP. Accidental hypothermia. In Auerbach PS (ed.) *Wilderness Medicine*, 4th edn. Philadelphia, PA: Mosby, 2001, pp. 51–103.

Ulrich AS, Rathlev NK. Hypothermia and localized cold injuries. *Emerg Med Clin of North Am* 2004;**22**:281–298.

Chapter 48

Burns

Luigi DiStefano

Introduction

Burns constitute a major cause of injury-related mortality and morbidity in the pediatric population, being the second most common cause of unintentional injury-related death in children aged 5–9 years. They also contribute to significant morbidity in children of all ages and are a frequent cause of non-fatal injury, with severe burns often resulting in lifelong disability. Besides direct contact with a flame, there are multiple sources of thermal injury in children, including scald injury, injuries from fireworks, electrical injuries (see Ch. 50), and chemical burns. Chemical burns are managed very similarly in children and adults and will not be discussed in detail here. Approximately 70% of pediatric burn injuries are caused by direct contact with hot liquids.

Pathophysiology

There are several pathophysiologic factors involved in burn injuries. Direct tissue injury and immediate cell death occurs as a result of the burn itself, usually only to skin, although deeper tissue layers are affected in severe cases. Surrounding tissue develops a state of ischemia as a result of decreased local perfusion, and this causes a subsequent release of cytokines and other inflammatory mediators, which leads to an increase in capillary permeability and local edema. In a minor burn, typically <15% body surface area (BSA), the reaction is confined to the local tissues. In instances in which the burn covers >15%–20% BSA, systemic signs and symptoms manifest, including hypotension, end-organ dysfunction, and, in severe cases, myocardial depression and other physiologic derangements more commonly associated with severe sepsis. These burns also induce a hypermetabolic state, causing increases in catecholamine release and gluconeogenesis, as well as relative increases in insulin resistance and protein catabolism. Pediatric patients are at higher risk of developing dehydration and shock from burns because of their increased BSA to volume ratio.

Classification of burns

Burn thickness

Burn thickness can be classified as superficial, superficial partial-thickness, deep partial-thickness, and full thickness. These refer to the depth of the skin that is involved in the burn. Burns that also involve deeper structures, such as muscle, fascia, or bone, are still considered fourth-degree burns.

First-degree (superficial) burns. These involve the epidermis only. The skin is dry, red, and very *painful* to touch and *blanching* is present.

Second-degree (superficial partial thickness) burns. These involve the epidermis and the superficial portion of the dermis. The skin is weepy, red, and very *painful* to touch. Blisters are often present. *Blanching* is also present.

Second-degree (deep partial thickness) burns. Deeper second-degree burns affecting the epidermis and deep portions of the dermis give rise to skin that is patchy red and white, with blistering being very common. The burn is painful only to direct pressure. These are *non-blanching.*

Third-degree (full-thickness) burns. The entire epidermis and dermis is involved and the area affected appears white and waxy or gray and charred. The skin is dry; wounds are *painless* and *non-blanching.*

Burn surface area

Burn surface area in children can be estimated using the Lund and Browder chart (Fig. 48.1). The palm (not including the fingers) of the patient reflects roughly 1% of the patient's BSA and can also be used to estimate the total burn area. Special care should be taken to note any burns on the *hands, feet, face, genitalia, perineum,* and those across *major joints,* as these may meet stricter criteria for transfer to a burn center.

Clinical presentation

In minor burns, a careful history should be obtained, being careful to note the type of burn, length of exposure to the burn

A Practical Guide to Pediatric Emergency Medicine: Caring for Children in the Emergency Department, ed. N. Ewen Amieva-Wang (associate eds. Jamie Shandro, Aparajita Sohoni, and Bernhard Fassl). Published by Cambridge University Press.

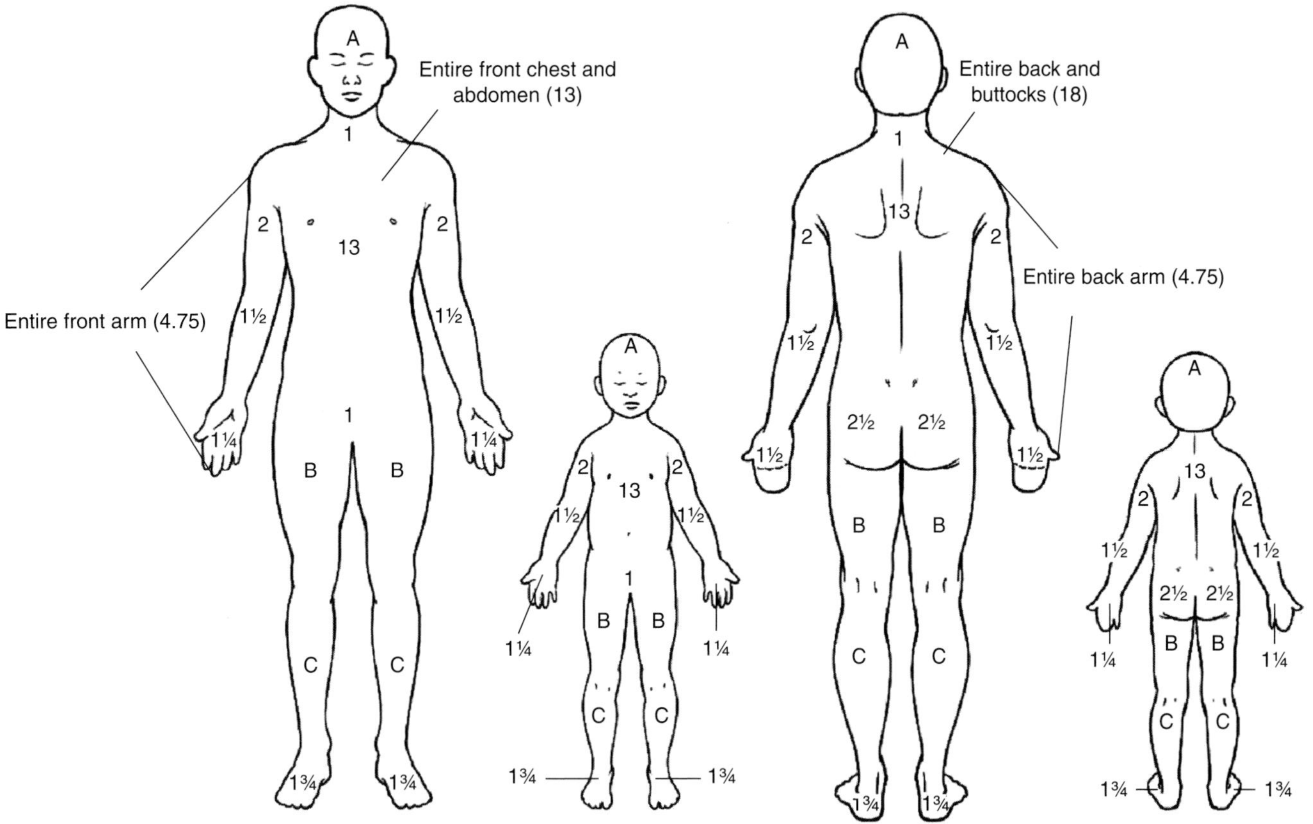

LUND-BROWDER CHART

Relative percentage of body surface area is affected by growth

Age in years	0	1	5	10	15	Adult
A head (back or front)	9½	8½	6½	5½	4½	3½
B one thigh (back or front)	2¾	3¼	4	4¼	4½	4¾
C one leg (back or front)	2½	2½	2¾	3	3¼	3½

Figure 48.1 Estimated percentage of total body surface area. The Lund–Browder chart is the most accurate method for estimating burn extent and must be used in the evaluation of all pediatric patients with burns. Use the numbers written on each body area and substitute the correct figures for age for the areas A–C.

agent, presence of any concomitant trauma, and what, if any, prehospital care has been performed. One should also ask about the possibility of inhalational injuries; facial burns that occurred in a small enclosed space are at higher risk of causing airway edema than facial burns from an outdoors flame. In the case of chemical burns, the type of chemical is of great import. In more severe cases, there may not initially be time to take a full history.

Patients with moderate to severe burns should be approached in a similar fashion to those with trauma. *Airway* security is of paramount importance in the burn victim. An edematous or non-patent airway is an indication for emergency endotracheal intubation. The EP should have a low threshold for calling for help in these situations as burn airways can be very edematous and difficult to secure. Once airway patency/security has been established, special attention should be paid to the oropharynx and nares, looking for evidence of inhalational injury, such as singed nose hairs, carbonaceous sputum, and oropharyngeal burns or edema. Intravenous access should be established promptly in all patients apart from those with the most minor burns.

Once ABC has been established and stabilized, a careful secondary survey of the patient should be performed. The patient's mental status should be examined first, followed by a careful head to toe examination and establishment of the depth and extent of the patient's burns, and any concomitant injuries. With facial burns, perform a corneal fluorescein (Wood's lamp) examination to evaluate for corneal burns.

When to intubate?

Inhalational and airway injuries remain one of the most common causes of death in burn victims, and there is no reliable way to consistently predict which patients will develop airway compromise. Certain clinical features exist that are sometimes correlated with airway edema and/or inhalational injury requiring intubation. These include:

- persistent cough, stridor or wheezing
- carbonaceous sputum or severe blistering in the oropharynx
- severe facial burns (third degree or worse)
- circumferential neck burns
- altered mental status in the setting of moderate to severe burn injury
- respiratory distress or failure
- worsening hypoxia or hypercapnia.

If any of these clinical features are present, and the history is suggestive of a significant inhalational injury, endotracheal intubation should be performed or at least seriously considered, as airway edema in the setting of inhalational injury will only worsen over time. Intubation should also be strongly considered when the patient is being transferred to a burn center and clinical features of inhalation injury are present. If rapid-sequence intubation is being performed, succinylcholine can be safely used within 48 h of a burn injury without significant risk of hyperkalemia.

Management

Fluid resuscitation

Pediatric patients whose burns exceed 15% BSA will be more likely to exhibit systemic signs and symptoms of vasoactive mediator release, and should receive IV fluid resuscitation. The appropriate amount of fluids can be calculated using the Parkland Formula:

Total lactated Ringer's solution $= 4 \times$ weight (kg) $\times$ %BSA.

The first half of this fluid should be administered over the first 8 h post injury. The rest of the volume should be infused over the next 16 h.

Maintenance fluid should be given in addition. The fluid of choice is lactated Ringer's solution. In children <20 kg, Dextrose 5% + lactated Ringer's solution (D5LR) should be used to support metabolic needs. A goal endpoint for fluid resuscitation is a urine output of 1 ml/kg per h.

Treatment of the burns

In the immediate post-burn period, burn wounds can be covered with a clean, dry dressing. Once the patient has been stabilized, dressings soaked in cool saline may be used, which also assist in the reduction of wound pain. There are a number of options for antiseptic membrane dressings that may be used for more definitive coverage. Superficial burns in patients who will be discharged home can be dressed with bacitracin or other simple antibiotic ointment and a dry dressing.

Escharotomy should be performed if there is significant limb ischemia from a circumferential burn (with evidence of neurovascular compromise), or if there is respiratory compromise from significant thoracic or abdominal burns.

Pain control

Pain should be managed aggressively. In major burns, fentanyl is the most appropriate choice of the opiate analgesic family as it causes the least hemodynamic derangement. Morphine is an acceptable substitute. Minor burns in patients who will not be admitted to the hospital can be managed using oral analgesia, such as acetaminophen with codeine, or acetaminophen alone, depending on the severity of pain. Ibuprofen is also effective in pain management because of its anti-inflammatory properties, and is also effective in conjunction with opiates. Tetanus status should be checked and a tetanus booster given if needed.

Diagnostic studies

Diagnostic studies such as a CBC and basic electrolye panel should be performed on any systemically affected patient who will be admitted for burn care. In addition, a urinalysis should be obtained to screen for possible myoglobinuria if any suspected muscle injury is present. A carboxyhemoglobin level should be sent in cases of suspected inhalational injury.

Disposition

Disposition is determined by the severity of the burn. The American Burn Association has established guidelines for transfer to a local burn center. These include:

- age <10 with >10% total BSA affected (second degree or greater)
- age >10 with >20% total BSA affected (second degree or greater)
- full-thickness burns >5% total BSA
- inhalational injury
- burns to the face, hands, feet, genitalia, eyes, or joints (second degree or greater)
- significant major associated trauma (requires that the burn center also be a trauma center).

Patients who do not meet these criteria should be admitted to the presenting institution if any of the following are present:

- age <10 with 5–10% total BSA affected
- age >10 and >10% BSA affected
- inability to take PO fluids
- full-thickness burns >2%
- high-voltage injuries
- circumferential injury
- suspected child abuse.

Non-accidental burns

Burns are one of the most common modalities of abuse (Ch. 135). Some studies estimate that up to 18% of burn injuries in children <24 months may result from abuse or neglect. Specific burn patterns can help to distinguish between accidental and non-accidental burns. Scald burns with hot water are the most common form of this injury.

Children who are the victims of non-accidental burns are more likely to have certain red flags in the history and physical examination. History factors include delay in presentation >24 h, lack of immediate burn or wound care, burn attributed to a sibling, and a history from the parent or caregiver inconsistent with the pattern of injury or the patient's developmental level. Physical findings associated with abuse or neglect include discrete burn margins, also known as tide marks when seen on the extremities, lack of splash burns, unburned areas within the burned area (most commonly seen on the buttocks), a stocking–glove distribution of burns, well-demarcated circular or "point" burns, usually from a cigarette or cigar, and concomitant bruising, fractures, or other trauma.

The EP is often the first caregiver to encounter these injuries, and as such must have a high index of suspicion for non-accidental injury. Such cases should prompt consultation with the ER social worker and child protective services to open an investigation.

Pearls and pitfalls

Pearls

1. The ABC approach is the mainstay of burn resuscitation and the initial assessment of the burn patient.
2. Fluid resusciation is crucial in the critically injured burn patient. Maintenance rate of fluid must be added to the Parkland calculation.
3. A thorough physical examination is essential to identify any burns in areas not immediately visible.

Pitfalls

1. Failure to consider non-accidental burns when evaluating the patient.

Selected references

Botash AS, Fuller PG, Blatt SD, Cunningham A, Weinberger HL. Child abuse, sudden infant death syndrome, and psychosocial development. *Curr Opin Pediatrics* 1996;**8**:195–200.

Sheridan RL. Burns. *Crit Care Med* 2002;**30**(Suppl.): S500–S514.

Sheridan RL. Outpatient burn care in the emergency department. *Pediatr Emerg Care* 2005;**21**:449–459.

Sheridan RL, Ryan CM, Petras LM, *et al.* Burns in children younger than two years of age: an experience with 200 consecutive admissions. *Pediatrics* 1997;**100**:721–723.

Stoddard FJ, Sheridan RL, Saxe GN, *et al.* Treatment of pain in acutely burned children. *J Burn Care Rehabil* 2002;**23**:135–156.

Chapter 49

Heat-related illness

Benjamin Constance and Jamie Shandro

Introduction

Heat-related illnesses can range in severity from irritating heat rash to life-threatening heat stroke. Heat illness arises when the body's homeostatic mechanisms for regulating temperature are no longer able to compensate for an increase in heat production or exposure. Pediatric patients possess unique challenges to thermoregulation and deserve special consideration. Very young children have underdeveloped thermoregulatory controls and depend on others to modify their environment, layer clothing, and provide hydration. Teenage athletes are under tremendous pressure to perform and are at risk of overexerting themselves in hot and humid conditions. Over 1000 cases of heat exhaustion are reported annually among US athletes, and heatstroke is reported as the third leading cause of death among US high school athletes.

Pathophysiology

The human body regulates its temperature to remain at 37°C (±0.6). Endogenous heat, generated from within the body, is produced as a byproduct of metabolism and is increased through muscle activities such as shivering. Exogenous, or external, heat causes a rise in temperature when it exceeds that of the body. Heat loss begins with the transfer of heat from the core to the skin by circulating blood and ends with the transfer of this heat to the environment via conducation, convection, evaporation, or radiation. In warmer climates, when the ambient temperature is equal to or exceeds that of the body, evaporation rather than radiation becomes the dominant mechanism of heat loss. Evaporation becomes increasingly less effective as humidity rises and its effectiveness in cooling the body approaches zero at a humidity of 90–95%.

Thermoregulation in children differs from that in adults in a few key ways. Children make more endogenous heat per kilogram than adults, and they have a higher surface area to body mass ratio, allowing for more efficient transfer of heat from the environment to their bodies. Younger children have lower sweat production than adolescents and adults, which results in less effective evaporative cooling. Young children often do not choose their environment and may not be able to communicate that they are overheating. Older children may be pressured to perform in athletic competitions in hot weather with limited breaks.

Recreational drugs can increase heat production, including cocaine, amphetamines (e.g. 3,4-methylenedioxy-*N*-methylamphetamine, MDMA or ecstasy) and LSD (lysergic acid diethylamide). Several medical conditions can also result in dysfunctional thermoregulation, including anorexia nervosa, spina bifida, quadriplegia, scleroderma, cystic fibrosis, salicylate ingestion, and developmental delay. In contrast to febrile illness where thermoregulatory mechanisms remain intact, core temperatures in heat illness can rise to the level that causes direct cell injury and protein denaturation.

Clinical presentation

Prickly heat (miliaria rubra)

Also known as "heat rash," miliaria rubra is a pruritic, erythematous, maculopapular rash often on the face, upper trunk, and the neck (Fig. 156.3, p. 742). This rash is common in young children and results from tight fitting clothing in hot and humid conditions obstructing epidermal and dermal sweat ducts. This rash can become pustular as the macerated skin becomes secondarily infected with staphylococci.

Heat cramps

Heat cramps often occur as sporadic muscle spasms in voluntary muscle groups after vigorous exercise. They most often occur during rest or while showering after excercise. Involved muscle groups typically include the lower extremities, abdomen, and shoulders. It is believed that heat cramps are primarily caused by electrolyte depletion resulting from hypotonic rehydration solutions such as free water. Cramps may be palpated as tense muscle groups and are sometimes precipitated by passive motion or sudden cold environments. Spasms typically last only a few seconds to minutes but may be painful and prompt emergency care.

A Practical Guide to Pediatric Emergency Medicine: Caring for Children in the Emergency Department, ed. N. Ewen Amieva-Wang (associate eds. Jamie Shandro, Aparajita Sohoni, and Bernhard Fassl). Published by Cambridge University Press.

Table 49.1. Heat exhaustion versus heat stroke

Features	Heat exhaustion	Heat stroke
Core temperature	38°C to 40°C (100.4°F to 104°F)	May be >40°C (>104°F)
Dehydration	Mild to moderate	Usually severe
Sweating	Profuse	Flushed with hot, dry skin (anhidrosis)
Symptoms	Thirst, nausea, vomiting, headache; feels faint or has collapsed	Dizziness, vertigo, syncope, confusion, delirium, vomiting and diarrhea; shock with end-organ damage

Heat exhaustion

Once a thermal insult overcomes homeostatic cooling mechanisms, the core body temperature rises above 38°C and heat exhaustion ensues. Heat exhaustion is defined as an elevation in body temperature to between 38°C and 40°C and is accompanied by mild to moderate dehydration with or without electrolyte disturbances. Without treatment, heat exhaustion can rapidly progress to life-threatening heat stroke. Heat exhaustion is the most common heat illness in athletes. Patients may complain of fatigue, thirst, nausea, and syncope. Clinical signs may include vomiting, diarrhea, hyperventilation, tachycardia, and orthostatic hypotension. Absence of neurological deficits is often used to differentiate heat exhaustion from heat stroke (Table 49.1). Because heat exhaustion presents with a vague clinical syndrome at times, including normothermia, consider a broad differential diagnosis including infection, drug ingestion, neuroleptic malignant and serotonin syndromes, and endocrine emergencies.

Heat stroke

Heat stroke is a medical emergency distinguished from heat exhaustion by the presence of neurological dysfunction and a core body temperature >40.5°C (Table 49.1). At this stage of heat illness, the body's thermoregulatory mechanisms have been overwhelmed. Complications may include permanent end organ damage to the heart, liver, kidneys, or the CNS.

Heat stroke can be thought of as being either classic or exertional in etiology. Classic heat stroke is characterized by a decreased ability to sweat and restricted access to fluids, most commonly developing over days. Children trapped in overheated vehicles, however, may rapidly develop classic heat stroke. In daytime temperatures of 23°C (73°F), vehicle temperatures can exceed 50°C (122°F).

Classic heat stroke presents with the triad of altered mental status, hyperthermia, and hot, dry skin. Exertional heat stroke occurs in otherwise healthy individuals such as adolescent athletes undergoing strenuous activity in warm and humid environments.

In contrast to the anhidrosis of classic heat stroke, patients with exertional heat stroke may present with diffuse sweating.

Heat stroke is a multisystem disease and may present with neurologic abnormalities, cardiogenic shock, respiratory distress, and multiorgan failure. Presenting signs include abnormal mental status (delirium, seizures, hallucinations), vomiting, diarrhea, hyperventilation with respiratory alkalosis, pulmonary edema, oliguria, muscle spasms, and either anhidrosis or profuse sweating. Recognition and treatment of heat stroke must be prompt because of its associated high morbidity and mortality, 17–70%.

Management

Prickly heat (miliaria rubra)

Heat rash can generally be treated with the conservative measures of wearing clean, loose-fitting clothing and avoiding creams, oil-based lubricants, and talc. Parents should monitor children for overheating and the development of skin irritation. Cool baths may be soothing for itching, and antibiotics should only be prescribed if the rash becomes diffuse and pustular.

Heat cramps

Initial treatment of heat cramps includes moving the patient to a cool environment, rest, and massage of affected muscles. Rehydration fluids should contain basic electrolytes, which can be made by adding 1 to 2 teaspoons of table salt to 1 pint of water (10 g to 570 ml). Severe cramps may respond better to IV rehydration with normal saline 20 ml/kg body weight over 30 min. Patients and parents should be educated on heat cramp prevention by encouraging rehydration solutions with electrolytes, stretching before vigorous exercise, and ending activity with a cool-down.

Heat exhaustion

Initial treatment of heat exhaustion consists of removing the patient from hot and humid environments and encouraging them to rest in a cool environment. Rapid cooling is generally not necessary. Laboratory evaluation should include electrolytes, BUN, and hematocrit. Initial fluid replacement should start with IV rehydration (20 ml/kg bolus of normal saline) followed by oral rehydration as tolerated. Oral salt tablet supplements should be avoided as they may precipitate vomiting and airway compromise. Antipyretics play no role in the treatment of heat-related illnesses. If the patient is able to tolerate oral rehydration after IV fluid boluses and correction of electrolyte imbalance, they may be safely discharged home with adequate follow-up and instructions to rest, continue to drink fluids, and avoid heat stress for 1–2 days. If symptoms persist for greater than 2 h, however, observation is warranted to rule-out potential progression to heat stroke or other alternative diagnosis.

Box 49.1. Treatment of heat stroke

1. Rapidly cool the patient until core temperature is <39°C (<102.2°F).
2. Rehydrate with IV normal saline.
3. Consider vasopressor therapy for persistent hypotension or shock despite rehydration.
4. Treat coagulopathy if hemorrhage is present.
5. Treat shivering and seizures with benzodiazepines.
6. Monitor for pulmonary and cerebral edema.
7. Intubate and initiate mechanical ventilation for respiratory failure.

Heat stroke

Management of patients with heat stroke begins with removal of the patient from the offending environment. Vital signs should include an accurate rectal or esophageal temperature. Initial laboratory investigation should include a basic metabolic panel, CBC, LFTs, urinalysis, arterial blood gas, and coagulation panel. Possible abnormalities include hyper- or hyponatremia, hypokalemia, hypoglycemia, renal failure, and metabolic acidosis. Coagulopathies are common in heat stroke, and signs of hemorrhage such as hematuria, hemoptysis, and GI bleeding are poor prognostic indicators.

The patient should be rapidly cooled to <40°C (104°F) as quickly as possible to prevent further tissue damage (Box 49.1). Lower rates of mortality have been observed in patients cooled more rapidly. This can be accomplished by actively cooling the patient with cold-water immersion, or passively by evaporative cooling combined with cold packs applied to groin and axilla. The latter method may be safer for the patient and allow for consistent monitoring while still providing effective cooling. Do this by removing the patient's clothing, moistening the body with water, and exposing them to air currents from mechanical or manual fanning. Antipyretics do not have a role in the treatment of heat stroke and may precipitate further liver damage. Rehydrate with a 20 ml/kg bolus of normal saline and repeat as necessary depending upon vital signs and urinary output. Place a urinary catheter to monitor urine output. In severely affected patients, a nasogastric tube will help to decompress the stomach and prevent aspiration of gastric contents. For patients with a base deficit >6 or persistent hypotension, consider central line placement to monitor central venous pressure.

Once the core temperature is <40°C (104°F), care is mainly supportive. Avoid active cooling below the goal of 39°C (102.2°F) as this may lead to hypothermia. Once the body begins cooling, shivering may commence and increase oxygen consumption and endogenous heat production. For this reason, consider treating shivering with diazepam 0.1–0.3 mg/kg per dose IV. Consider vasopressor therapy (dopamine or dobutamine) for persistent hypotension despite aggressive fluid resuscitation. Treat severe coagulopathy with fresh frozen plasma and platelets if hemorrhage is present. After initial stabilization, monitor the patient with special attention to mental status, perfusion, peripheral pulses, and urine output. Make arrangements to transfer the patient to a pediatric intensive care service for further monitoring and treatment.

Disposition

Most patients with heat-related illnesses can be safely discharged home after cooling, toleration of oral rehydration, and assurance of adequate follow-up. In patients where a concern for dehydration exists, they should be evaluated for electrolyte deficiencies. If symptoms persist for greater than 2 h, or if the presentation is concerning for heat stroke, then continued observation or inpatient admission is warranted. Heat stroke is a medical emergency and warrants ICU admission upon initial evaluation and stabilization in the ED.

Pearls and pitfalls

Pearls

1. Children have several unique risk factors for developing heat-related illnesses, including the inability to control their environment, an increased surface area to body mass ratio, and less effective heat dissipation.
2. Initial management of most heat-related illnesses consists of moving the patient to a cool environment, removal of tight clothing, and rehydration.
3. Heat stroke is a life-threatening condition and warrants aggressive medical management.
4. The classic triad of heat stroke is hyperpyrexia, severe CNS disturbances, and anhidrosis.

Pitfalls

1. Failure to recognize that heat-related illnesses can mimic other medical conditions and patients will not necessarily present with an elevated body temperature.
2. Use of antipyretics, which play no role in the treatment of heat-related illnesses.

Selected references

Committee on Sports Medicine, American Academy of Pediatrics. Climatic heat stress and the exercising child. *Pediatrics* 2000;**106**:158–159.

Grubenhoff MD, Joseph A. Heat-related illness. *Clin Pediatr Emerg Med* 2007;**8**:59–64.

Hoffman JL. Environmental emergencies. Heat-related illness in children. *Clin Pediatr Emerg Med* 2001;**2**:203–210.

Chapter

50 Electrical and lightning injuries

Robert L. Norris

Introduction

Children make up a significant proportion of victims of electrical injuries. There are two age groups of children who most commonly suffer electrical injuries. The first is toddlers, who are often injured in the home as they explore their environment and come in contact with unprotected electrical sources such as exposed outlets or extension cords. The second group is adolescents, particularly young males, who are injured as they engage in risky behaviors such as climbing high-voltage power poles. Lightning, a unique form of electrical injury, causes as many as 300 deaths in the USA each year, while another 1000 to 1500 victims survive with varying disability. This chapter reviews the pathophysiology and management of electrical injuries – both from electrical sources (referred to simply as electrical injuries) and from lightning.

Pathophysiology

Electrical current involves the flow of electrons through a circuit from an area of high concentration to an area of lower concentration. There are four major mechanisms of injury that follow exposure to an electrical source: true electrical injury, flash burns, flame burns, and blunt trauma. True electrical injury, the primary topic of this chapter, occurs as current actually passes through tissues in the body. Cellular damage occurs primarily as electrical energy is converted to heat, but also from protein degradation. The second mechanism of injury, flash burns, occurs when a victim comes into close proximity to the very hot cloud of electrons that surrounds all electrical sources (the "arc"). Flash burns can occur without any actual current flowing through the victim's tissues, although they are often associated with true electrical injury. The temperatures in electrical arcs may exceed 4000°C, and result in simple, although sometimes severe, thermal injuries. Flame burns occur as articles of clothing or jewelry worn by the victim are ignited by the electrical source. Finally, blunt trauma can occur from the massive muscle contractions stimulated by contact with an electrical source, or from the victim being thrown from a source or falling from a height.

There are six major characteristics of electricity that are important in determining the severity of true electrical injuries following any particular exposure:

- voltage: low (<1000 V) versus high (≥1000 V)
- amperage
- resistance
- current type: alternating versus direct
- duration of exposure
- pathway.

Amperage and voltage

The primary mechanism by which electricity causes injury to tissues is through the conversion of electrical energy into heat. The amount of heating that occurs is given by Joule's law: heat $= A^2Rt$, where A is amperage, R is tissue resistance, and t is duration of exposure. The precise amperage involved in an electrical exposure is rarely known; what is generally available in the history, however, is the voltage of the source. Ohm's law, $A = V/R$, gives the relationship between amperage (A), voltage (V), and resistance (R).

Voltage sources are arbitrarily defined as low (<1000 V) and high (≥1000 V). The higher the voltage, generally, the more serious the exposure. Household current in the USA is low voltage, generally either 110 or 220 volts, and is the most common source of electrical injury in children <6 years of age. Older children and adolescents are more commonly injured by high-voltage sources (e.g., power lines).

Resistance

The tissues of the human body have varying degrees of resistance to electrical current flow. In decreasing order of resistance are bone, fat, tendon, skin, muscle, blood vessels, and nerves. The higher the resistance of the tissues traversed, the greater the temperatures generated as the current flows. The resistance of the skin, being the body's first line of defense to electrical exposure, initially determines the amount of current that will enter the victim. Given the generally high resistance of dry skin

A Practical Guide to Pediatric Emergency Medicine: Caring for Children in the Emergency Department, ed. N. Ewen Amieva-Wang (associate eds. Jamie Shandro, Aparajita Sohoni, and Bernhard Fassl). Published by Cambridge University Press.

and the significant heat generated at the points of entrance and exit of the current, cutaneous burns at these sites can be significant. If the resistance of the skin is significantly lowered by being wet with sweat or water, cutaneous burns may be less impressive but internal derangements more severe (e.g., cardiac arrhythmias). Internal effects of electrical burns depend on the pathway taken by the current through the body. The massive heat produced as current flows through long bones, for example, can result in significant thermal injury to overlying muscles and tendons.

Current type

Current types are either alternating (AC) or direct (DC). Alternating current involves the movement of electricity such that the direction of flow of electrons within the circuit changes polarity at a set number of cycles per second (Hertz; Hz). Alternating current tends to be significantly more dangerous than direct current of similar intensities. This is largely because skeletal muscle is prone to tetanic contraction stimulated by current alternating at a rate of 15–150 Hz. For this reason, household current, which alternates at 60 Hz, can be very dangerous. When a victim places a hand on an AC source in this range, tetanic contraction of the strong flexor muscles may effectively "lock" the victim's grip onto the source, prolonging the exposure.

Direct current flows in one direction and tends to cause a single massive muscle contraction, often propelling the victim away from the electrical source, particularly if the voltage is high, thus limiting the duration of exposure. Different types of current induce different arrythmias. Alternating currents increase the risk of current passing through the myocardium during the vulnerable refractory period of the cardiac cycle, resulting in ventricular fibrillation. Direct current (including lightning) tends to act as a massive, single cardioversion stimulus, instantly depolarizing the entire myocardium and resulting in asystole.

Duration of exposure

Time of exposure is important in determining severity of injury, with longer contacts producing more severe injury. With lightning strikes, the exceedingly brief duration of exposure (milliseconds) explains why many victims of such massive electrical exposure actually survive the incident.

Pathway

The pathway that the current takes through the body as it passes from the source to the ground determines which organs are at greatest risk of injury and complications. The most common pathway is a hand-to-foot pattern, where the victim contacts the source with a hand and is grounded through one or both feet. A hand-to-hand pattern allows the current to flow directly across the mediastinum and its structures, placing the victim at risk for acute myocardial injuries and cardiac arrhythmias.

Electrical injuries

The physiologic effects that can be seen following electrical injury are summarized in Table 50.1. It is important to keep in mind that the degree of internal injury may be very poorly estimated based on the extent of cutaneous burns. Severely damaged tissues may underlie apparently normal, unburned skin. For this reason, standard burn formulae for fluid resuscitation are not applied to victims of electrical injury (see Management).

Lightning pathophysiology

Victims struck by lightning are generally struck in one of four ways. The most lethal mechanism is a direct strike, which generally occurs to the head. More commonly, however, a victim is injured while in contact with an object that is struck ("contact strike") or while in close proximity to another object that is struck and some of the current splashes off the object onto the victim ("splash"). Victims may also be injured via ground potential. In this case, lightning strikes the ground in relative close proximity to the victim, who is standing with one foot closer to the site of the strike than the other. An electrical potential is established between the victim's feet and current flows through the victim's lower extremities.

Lighting can be thought of as a massive DC discharge with up to 100 million volts and 200 000 amperes. Devastating effects of such an intense strike are generally offset by the extremely short duration of the exposure, measured in milliseconds. The vast majority of the electrical current flashes over the outside of the victim's body and does not cause massive internal injury. As the current flashes over the victim, it may superheat body sweat or any moisture from accompanying rain and cause superficial cutaneous burns. Likewise, the victim's clothing may explode, and any metal worn may be vaporized (with concomitant underlying serious direct thermal burns). A pathognomonic finding in many lightning strike victims is the presence of Lichtenberg figures: fine, dendritic-appearing erythematous changes in the superficial skin, thought to result from ionization in the cutaneous tissues. These changes, unlike true burns, are ephemeral and disappear within hours.

A relatively small leakage of current into the victim during the strike can short-circuit the CNS, causing loss of consciousness in >70%, along with respiratory and cardiac arrest. The initial arrhythmia in most victims is asystole. In many cases, the inherent automaticity of the young victim's myocardium may restart contractions. The victim will often continue in respiratory arrest because of the simultaneous short-circuiting of the brainstem respiratory center, necessitating prompt respiratory and ventilatory support to prevent secondary anoxic deterioration to ventricular fibrillation. Other physical consequences of lighting strike may be similar to those of electricity, including blunt trauma (Table 50.1). Tympanic membrane rupture occurs in at least 50% of lightning strike victims.

Table 50.1. Adverse effects of electrical exposure

Area/system	Effects
Head	
Skull	Skull fracture or traumatic brain injury
Ears	Tympanic membrane rupture (occurs in >50% of victims struck by lightning)
Eyes	Fixed and dilated pupils (temporary autonomic dysfunction, should not be used as a sign of brain death in such cases); cataracts (often delayed for months following injury; more common with lightning injuries)
Neck/back	Spinal injuries (following massive tetanic contraction of paraspinous muscles or occurring when the victim is thrown from the source or falls from a height)
Trunk	
Heart	Lethal arrhythmias, ventricular fibrillation (with low-voltage AC sources), asystole (high-voltage AC and DC sources), conduction blocks, non-specific ST–T wave abnormalities, myocardial injury (ischemia, infarction, contusion)
Lungs	Pulmonary contusions/burns, pneumothorax
Kidneys	Renal insufficiency (due to direct electrical effects or rhabdomyolysis)
Gastrointestinal tract	Ileus, Gastrointestinal perforations Solid organ injury (often related to blunt trauma)
Musculoskeletal	
Muscle	Rhabdomyolysis
Bones	Fractures, dislocations (classic: posterior shoulder dislocation); less common with lightning injuries
Neurologic	Loss of consciousnes, respiratory arrest, numbness, weakness, paralysis (usually temporary); permanent neurologic injury (often delayed in onset; may be progressive); keraunoparalysis (see text)
Vascular	Hypertension, medial necrosis and thrombosis, delayed arterial aneurysm formation and hemorrhage
Psychiatric	Psychoses, depression, anxiety, phobias, post-traumatic stress disorder
Skin	
General	Cutaneous burns, entrance and exit wounds; burns may be full thickness; surface burns tend to underestimate the degree of deeper tissue trauma; flash burns
Flexor crease	Burns in flexor creases of wrists, antecubital fossae, axillae (pathognomonic for AC injury)
Sweat	Superheating
Lichtenberg figures	Reddish fern-like patterns on the skin (pathognomonic for lightning exposure)
Clothes etc.	Ignition of clothing; vaporization of jewelry or other metal objects on the body

AC, alternating current; DC, direct current.

Keraunoparalysis is a unique neurological finding that may immediately follow lightning strike; it involves temporary paralysis, numbness, and pulselessness of the extremities.

It is usually the lower extremities that are affected by keraunoparalysis. It is thought to be related to autonomic dysfunction and severe vasospasm, and generally resolves within hours without any specific therapy.

Management

Electricity exposure

The ABCs take priority, along with continued Pediatric Advanced Life Support (PALS) and Advanced Trauma Life Support (ATLS) as needed. Victims of electrically induced cardiopulmonary arrest should receive prolonged, aggressive resuscitation efforts, as successful outcomes in such scenarios may occur. Cardiac and pulse oximetry monitoring should be immediately instituted, and IV lines, if not already in place, should be started for infusion of physiologic saline. Unburned access sites are preferred, but placement through burned tissue is done if necessary.

Standard burn formulae are unreliable in guiding fluid resuscitation of electrically injured victims.

In electrical injury, fluid administration aims to achieve a urine output of approximately 0.5–1.0 ml/kg per h if the urine is clear of myoglobin, and at least 1.0 ml/kg per h if myoglobin is present.

The physical examination of the electrically injured child must be careful and complete in order to identify occult injuries. An ECG is obtained to look for any evidence of cardiac injury, and the patient is placed on a cardiac monitor throughout the ED stay. The ECG changes may include non-specific ST–T wave changes, arrhythmias, conduction delays, or evidence of ischemia or frank infarction. Standard laboratory tests are obtained, including a CBC, serum electrolytes, glucose, renal and liver function tests, and a serum creatinine phosphokinase (CPK) and myoglobin. Overall serum CPK elevation tends to correlate with the severity of injury and the need for eventual major surgery, including amputation. Elevated serum CPK-MB fractions are of unclear significance following electrical injury, as this enzyme may be released from electrically traumatized tissues and does not necessarily indicate direct myocardial injury. The role of serum troponins in identifying myocardial injury following electrical exposures is unknown.

An indwelling urinary catheter is placed if the patient appears moderately to severely injured – to monitor urine output as a guide to fluid therapy and to check for development of myoglobinuria. Myoglobin can be detected using a bedside urine dipstick test. A positive test for "blood" in the absence of red blood cells on microscopic examination is consistent with the presence of myoglobin or free hemoglobin in the urine. In addition, urine output and myoglobin excretion can be augmented with urine alkalinization (to a target urine pH of 7.0 without raising the blood pH above 7.5). Aggressive fluid resuscitation and maintenance of urine output may be protective against acute tubular necrosis and acute renal failure. Patients with serious injury should have a nasogastric tube placed to decompress the GI tract, as an ileus commonly occurs following such exposures. If there is evidence of significant extremity trauma, the patient should be admitted to closely monitor the involved limbs for evidence of compartment syndrome. Burns may be severe enough to require escharotomy and/or fasciotomy. Anywhere from 11% to 65% of high-voltage injuries result in significant extremity amputation.

Burn wounds are managed in standard fashion. Consultation with a burn center is prudent, both for recommendations for early management (as these may vary regionally) and for follow-up care or transfer as needed. Tetanus immunization status is updated as necessary.

Specialty consultations are appropriate in injuries that appear significant. Otolaryngology should be consulted for suspected tympanic membrane rupture. Ophthalmology should see the patient to evaluate for evidence of ocular damage (including lens injuries that might result in delayed cataract formation). Children with oral commissure burns from chewing on an electrical cord should be seen by a plastic or maxillofacial surgeon, as they will require splinting of the lips and, likely, multiple surgical procedures to correct the devastating cosmetic effects that can follow. In addition, as a significant percentage of these patients will develop delayed labial artery bleeding following these burns, parents should be educated as to how to tamponade such bleeding and the patient should be followed up closely. Some authorities recommend admitting such patients for monitoring until the burn eschar separates.

Lightning strike

Hospital management of lightning-injured children parallels that of those injured by other electrical sources. The reduced potential for severe muscle trauma dictates a more prudent approach to volume resuscitation, particularly if brain injury or cerebral edema is present. Nevertheless, organ perfusion and urine output should still be carefully monitored. If myoglobinuria is present, similar resuscitation guidelines apply. Keraunoparalysis can generally be managed with expectant observation.

Disposition

After electrical injury

Children exposed to low-voltage household current, without any loss of consciousness, and who are relatively asymptomatic (except possibly for a minor burn at the contact site), can be discharged after 4 h of observation and monitoring in the ED if their ECG is normal. In more serious cases requiring admission, if the patient is cardiovascularly stable in the ED and has a normal ECG, further cardiac monitoring during the hospital stay is probably unnecessary. The risk of delayed arrhythmias, regardless of the source of exposure, is extremely low.

Patients with a history of cardiac arrhythmia or arrest, a loss of consciousness, concern for significant internal injury or compartment syndrome, or an abnormal ECG should be admitted to a monitored setting. The proper time interval for cardiac monitoring has not been firmly established, but 24 to 48 h seems appropriate. Cardiac arrhythmias of consequence, however, usually occur at the time of the electrical exposure and not in a delayed fashion.

The American Burn Association classifies all significant electrical burns as major burn injuries, necessitating transfer to a burn center for further evaluation and management. Such

Pearls and pitfalls

Pearls

1. Perform a careful physical examination in the child with an electrical injury; it is easy to miss occult injuries.
2. Transfer children with significant electrical injuries to a burn center for further evaluation and definitive care.

Pitfalls

1. Failure to suspect deep tissue injury (including compartment syndrome) following high-voltage electrical exposures.
2. Failure to provide cardiac monitoring for children following electric exposure when there is a history of loss of consciousness, arrhythmia or an abnormal ECG.
3. Failure to assess for evidence of myoglobinuria and provide fluid resuscitation; rhabdomyolysis may lead to acute renal failure.
4. Failure to consider the possibility of non-accidental trauma or neglect.

centers have the expertise necessary to determine if and when injured extremities, particularly following high-voltage exposures, require exploration, compartment release, debridement, and further management. When treating a pediatric victim of electrical injury, a high index of suspicion should be maintained for the possibility of non-accidental trauma or child neglect.

After lightning strike

Victims of lightning strike should be admitted for observation, in order to rule out occult injury. Again, transfer to a burn specialty center is prudent. There are no data available on which to base a decision regarding cardiac monitoring of such victims. Twenty-four hours of cardiac monitoring is a reasonable approach at this time.

Selected references

Arnoldo BD, Purdue GF, Kowalske K, *et al.* Electrical injuries: a 20-year review. *J Burn Care Rehabil* 2004:**25**:479–484.

Arnoldo B, Klein M, Gibran NS. Practice guidelines for the management of electrical injuries. *J Burn Care Res* 2006;**27**:439–447.

Maghsoudi Hemmat, Adyani Y, Ahmadian N. Electrical and lightning injuries. *J Burn Care Res* 2007;**28**:255–261.

Spies C, Trohman R. Narrative review: electrocution and life-threatening electrical injuries. *Ann Int Med* 2006;**145**(7):531–537.

Chapter 51

Venomous bites and stings

Robert L. Norris

Introduction

Bites and stings of venomous creatures are common occurrences and most often are little more than painful annoyances. On occasion, however, the effects can be severe, and potentially life threatening. In the 2006 report of calls to the American Association of Poison Control Centers, 82 133 were related to bites and stings, with approximately one-third of these involving victims under the age of 19. This chapter discusses the most significant biting and stinging terrestrial venomous creatures, including hymenoptera, spiders, scorpions, and snakes.

The evaluation of pediatric victims of venomous bites or stings may be hampered by an unclear history of the circumstances and the possible offending organism, particularly with preverbal children. It is possible that the overall effects of some venomous bites and stings may be relatively more severe in children than in adults. Children generally receive a similar venom load as would an adult from the offending animal, yet have less circulating blood volume to dilute venom effects.

Hymenoptera

The stinging insects of the order Hymenoptera, which includes bees, wasps, yellow jackets, hornets, and fire ants, are the most common causes of envenomation in children. There are at least 40–50 deaths following insect stings each year in the USA, with the vast majority caused by anaphylactic reactions.

Venoms

Hymenopteran venoms contain a number of physiologically active components, including vasoactive amines (histamine, serotonin, acetylcholine, epinephrine, norepinephrine, dopamine), peptides (melittin, apamin), and enzymes (phospholipase A, hyaluronidase).

Signs and symptoms

Most hymenopteran stings result in little more than an initially painful, and subsequently pruritic, wheal at the sting site. On occasion, the local reaction is more extensive and exaggerated, with swelling and discomfort progressing over the course of approximately 24 to 48 h and lasting 5 to 10 days. The risk of later, more severe systemic reactions in victims experiencing exaggerated local reactions appears to be only 5–10%.

Fire ant stings tend to be multiple as a disturbed colony of ants swarms up the involved extremity, with each ant stinging multiple times in rapid succession. Over a period of up to 24 h, tiny papules followed by sterile pseudopustules form at the sites of stings. These may remain pruritic for weeks but generally heal well.

In approximately 0.4–0.8% of children, hymenopteran stings can initiate a type 1, IgE-mediated anaphylactic reaction that can manifest with diffuse urticaria, bronchospasm, nausea, vomiting, abdominal pain, and possibly life-threatening laryngeal edema and hypotension. More than 80% of severe allergic reactions begin within 10 min of the sting. Occasionally, children are involved in a massive stinging scenario, when a hive is disturbed. The estimated median lethal venom dose in humans has been estimated at approximately 19 stings per kilogram body weight. Presentation in such scenarios may closely resemble anaphylaxis.

Management

Initial management of most hymenopteran stings includes removing any retained stinger (generally occurs with honeybee stings) and local ice application to control pain and swelling. Care of typical local hymenopteran stings is conservative (ice, analgesics, and antihistamines). Tetanus status should be updated when indicated. Intense pruritus following a sting can be effectively treated with potent topical steroids. If the child develops an exaggerated local reaction, a 5-day course of oral steroids (e.g., prednisolone, 1–2 mg/kg daily) with an antihistamine will give significant relief.

If the victim has a history of systemic reactions to prior stings or demonstrates evidence of a systemic reaction, epinephrine should be administered IM, and the patient should be treated as outlined in Ch. 10.

Laboratory studies are unnecessary following most hymenoptera stings. If the child presents with anaphylaxis or a massive envenomation, standard laboratory studies (CBC, blood

A Practical Guide to Pediatric Emergency Medicine: Caring for Children in the Emergency Department, ed. N. Ewen Amieva-Wang (associate eds. Jamie Shandro, Aparajita Sohoni, and Bernhard Fassl). Published by Cambridge University Press.

A

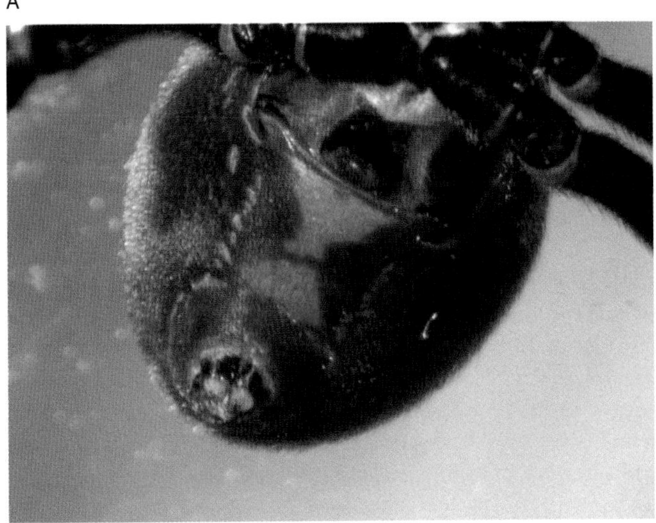

B

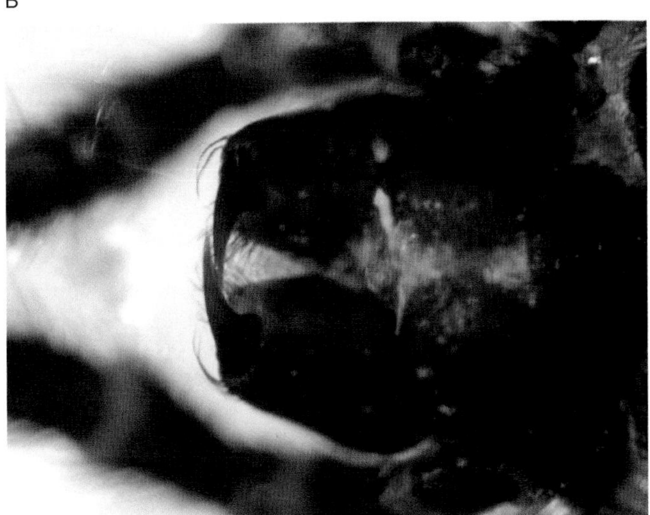

Figure 51.1 Black widow spider. (A) Belly with distinct hourglass pattern. (B) Chelicerae and fangs. (Courtesy of M. Amieva).

sugar, electrolytes) should be obtained, along with studies to rule out rhabdomyolysis (creatinine phosphokinase and myoglobin).

Disposition

Children with typical local reactions can be discharged home after evaluation. Parents should be advised to continue local ice and oral antihistamines as needed and to watch for signs of infection. Children with mild to moderate systemic reactions should be observed in the ED for 4 to 6 h prior to discharge. If the reaction is more severe (e.g., airway compromise, severe bronchospasm, or hypotension), the child should be admitted for 24 h of close observation. Laryngeal edema is the number one cause of death following such reactions.

Children with moderate to severe anaphylaxis related to hymenopteran stings should be referred for allergy testing and possible desensitization therapy, which is very effective at reducing the risk of recurrent anaphylaxis following a future sting. Regardless of the offending insect, children with diffuse hives should receive a prescription for an epinephrine self-administration kit.

Spiders

There are no spiders that can be considered truly deadly. There are, however, some spiders of medical significance throughout much of the world, and these can be broadly divided into two major groups: those that cause a neurotoxic envenoming syndrome and those that cause tissue necrosis.

Neurotoxic spiders

The major neurotoxic spiders are the widow spiders (*Latrodectus* spp.) (Fig. 51.1), the funnel web spiders (*Atrax* and *Hydranyche* spp., found in Australia), and the banana spiders (*Phoneutria* spp., indigenous to Latin America). These neurotoxic spiders all possess venoms that act at neural synapses: neuromuscular junctions and at adrenergic junctions.

Signs and symptoms

Bites by the neurotoxic spiders tend to be very painful, and the offending spider is often seen. Systemic effects may stem from autonomic nervous system stimulation and include hypertension, tachycardia, bradycardia, hypersalivation, diaphoresis, and diffuse muscle spasms.

Management

Management of neurotoxic spider envenomation centers on supportive care. There are several *Latrodectus* antivenoms available, and each appears to be effective regardless of which species of widow spider was responsible for the bite. There also exists an antivenom for the Sydney funnel web spider, the only species of funnel web that has caused documented human fatalities. These antivenoms should be used in significant bites with potentially serious systemic effects. The package insert for the appropriate product is used to guide therapy.

In the USA, *Latrodectus* antivenom is administered to reverse serious systemic effects of widow spider envenomation; one vial is administered either IM or IV. Efficacy is usually noted within 1 h of administration, with reversal of systemic toxicity and relief of pain being noted. Occasionally, a second vial is necessary.

Anytime a heterologous antiserum is administered to an envenomated victim, there is some risk of an acute anaphylactoid reaction.

Administration should be done with the treating physician at the bedside, with the patient closely monitored, and all medications and equipment necessary to reverse an anaphylactoid reaction immediately available. If antivenom is to be withheld or is not available, generous doses of opioid analgesics and benzodiazepines may be used to ease symptoms (though this may require as long as 72 h of therapy). In severe bites that are potentially life threatening, antivenom should be administered. Tetanus immunization is indicated following spider bites.

Disposition

Most victims of neurotoxic spider bite, even those requiring antivenom, can be discharged from the ED if they have a satisfactory response to therapy. Parents should be warned to return if there is any recurrence of venom effects. Those with more severe bites should be admitted for 24 h of monitoring.

Necrotizing spiders

While there are many spiders that may cause a small amount of local tissue damage following their bite, the spiders most notorious for their dermonecrotic potential are the violin spiders of the genus *Loxosceles*. The best known member of this genus is the brown recluse (*Loxosceles reclusa*), found in the mid-western and southern portions of the USA. The venom of *Loxosceles* spiders contains a phospholipase enzyme, sphingomyelinase D, which attacks cell membranes and can lead to local tissue damage that may be severe. The bite of this spider is generally painless and initially goes unnoticed. A few hours following the bite, pain related to focal ischemia begins at the site. Within a day, the site may have a central clear or blood-filled vesicle with surrounding ecchymosis and a rim of pale ischemia. The resulting ulcerative lesion may gradually expand over a period of days to weeks until healing begins.

Rare cases of systemic loxoscelism appear to be more common in young children than in adults. They may present with findings of systemic toxicity, including fever, chills, nausea, malaise, diffuse macular rash, and petechiae, and they may develop hemolysis or coagulopathy.

Management

For necrotizing spider bites, including intermittent local ice therapy for the first 72 h and administration of antibiotics if there is any question of secondary infection. Daily wound cleansings, combined with splinting of the bitten area, should be done until the wound is healed.

Nothing has been proven effective in limiting the degree of necrosis that may occur following a spider bite. There is no role for steroids in managing necrotic arachnidism. Dapsone, although used anecdotally in managing *Loxosceles* bites in adults, is not approved for use in children and should not be prescribed.

Children appearing systemically unwell should be admitted and undergo laboratory evaluation (CBC, coagulation studies, and urinalysis). Systemic loxoscelism is managed with IV hydration, management of renal failure as needed, and a brief course of systemic steroids to stabilize red blood cell membranes. Although there are documented fatalities following bites by the South American violin spider (*Loxosceles laeta*), there has never been a definitively proven fatality following a brown recluse bite in the USA. There is no commercially available antivenom in the USA for management of necrotizing spider bites such as those from *Loxosceles* spp. Tetanus status should be updated as indicated.

Disposition

Victims with potentially necrotic bites should be followed for a few days with daily wound checks. Local, intermittent cooling therapy should be continued for approximately 72 h. Any child with a probable necrotizing spider bite and evidence of systemic involvement should be admitted to watch for the rare complication of hemolysis and coagulopathy.

Scorpions

While most of the >1000 species of scorpions are relatively innocuous – causing nothing more than a painful sting without systemic effects – there are a handful of species that are dangerously toxic to humans. In the USA, the only significantly toxic scorpion is the bark scorpion (*Centruroides sculpturatus*) found in Arizona and just across its borders.

The venoms of the medically significant scorpions all contain low-molecular-weight polypeptide neurotoxins that affect sodium and potassium channels and result in autonomic and cardiovascular dysfunction.

Signs and symptoms

Most scorpion stings result in local pain and swelling that is relatively short lived. The more-toxic scorpions can stimulate an autonomic storm in victims, particularly small children. While adults with these stings may present with pain and little else, some children may present with restlessness, agitation, roving/disconjugate eye movements, hypertension, hypersalivation, respiratory distress, and diaphoresis. In life-threatening cases, the victim may develop hypertensive crisis and acute cardiac failure. Because of the rapid absorption and distribution of venom toxins following scorpion sting, the onset and progression of severe signs and symptoms can be rapid.

Management

Initial hospital management involves managing the ABCs. Analgesic management of these painful stings should be cautious as there is evidence of a synergistic interaction of opioid pain relievers with neurotoxic scorpion venom. Cautious sedation of agitated children, using benzodiazepines, can be beneficial.

There is significant regional variation worldwide related to management of scorpion stings. While antivenoms for many medically important species exist, their use and efficacy are somewhat controversial. In Arizona, after scorpion antivenom availability ceased (through production issues), admissions to

ICU for children stung by bark scorpions increased. Management of bark scorpion stings is limited to airway management, cautious sedation, and other supportive measures, although there are promising studies of anti-*centruroides* anti-venom.

Disposition

Children with significant stings, in the absence of a suitable antivenom or who fail to fully respond to antivenom therapy, should be admitted to the hospital for 24 h for monitoring.

Snakes

Children also make up a substantial proportion of snakebite victims throughout the world. The most important venomous snakes in the world fall into two families: Viperidae and Elapidae. The viperids are further broken down into the Old World vipers (subfamily Viperinae) and the pitvipers of both hemispheres (subfamily Crotalinae). In the USA, the most important venomous snakes are the pitvipers, including the rattlesnakes (*Crotalus* and *Sistrurus* spp.) and the cottonmouth water moccasins and copperheads (*Agkistrodon* spp.). The only USA snakes belonging to the Elapidae family are the coral snakes (*Micrurus* and *Micruroides* spp.). Bites by the secretive coral snakes are relatively uncommon.

Venoms

Snake venoms are complex and contain mixtures of enzymes and low-molecular-weight polypeptides. As a group, viperid snakes tend to cause local tissue changes, coagulation abnormalities, and hemodynamic shock, while elapids tend to cause a neurotoxic clinical picture (in severe cases causing complete paralysis and respiratory failure).

Signs and symptoms

A large proportion of snakebites are inflicted by harmless snakes, many of which are easily mistaken for dangerous venomous snakes because of their color patterns or behavior. Even a venomous snake may bite without injecting any substantial quantity of venom (a "dry bite"). The incidence of dry bites may be somewhere between 25 and 70%.

With envenomation, the bites of most vipers cause significant local pain, swelling, ecchymosis, and variable necrosis of the bitten extremity. Pain and swelling typically begin very quickly following the bite and progress over hours to days, and may be accompanied by serum-filled or hemorrhagic blebs. The victim may develop hypotension and respiratory distress. Seriously envenomed victims of viper bite often develop a consumptive coagulopathy.

Management

Historically recommended first aid techniques are of no proven benefit and may be truly harmful. The following interventions should be avoided: incisions, suction, tourniquets, ice, electric shock, application of herbal remedies, and administration of alcohol. Without doubt, the most important aspect of venomous snakebite management is prompt transportation of the victim to appropriate medical care and immobilization of the affected area.

Box 51.1. Indications for snake antivenom administration

- Evidence of systemic toxicity.
- Hemodynamic or respiratory instability (e.g., hypotension, respiratory distress).
- Hemotoxicity
  - clinically significant bleeding
  - abnormal coagulation studies (PT, activated PTT, fibrinogen, fibrin degradation products, platelet count).
- Neurotoxicity: any evidence of toxicity
  - usually beginning with cranial nerve abnormalities (e.g., ptosis, intraocular muscle weakness)
  - progressing to descending paralysis that may result in terminal respiratory failure if unmanaged.
- Local soft tissue swelling
  - continuing to progress rapidly (after any tourniquet or constriction band that may have erroneously been applied has been removed)
  - involves at least half of the bitten extremity or crosses a joint.

Attention is directed to the ABCs with support given as needed. The bitten extremity should be marked at two or more sites proximal to the bite site for repeated measurements of circumferences to assess for progressive soft tissue swelling. Standard laboratory analyses should be obtained, including a CBC, coagulation studies, fibrinogen, and serum chemistries including creatine phosphokinase.

The wound should be managed with frequent cleansing and immobilization. Serum-filled or hemorrhagic vesicles and blebs should be left intact when possible. Exposed tissue can be treated with wet-to-dry dressings or non-occlusive dressings. Ultimately, reconstructive surgery with skin grafts and muscle/tendon grafts may be necessary for optimal functional outcome. Antibiotics should be reserved for those with suspected secondary infection of the bite site. Prophylactic antibiotics should not be used unless a "rescuer" made incisions into the wound in the field or applied mouth suction to the bite site.

Any child with a significant envenomation should receive an appropriate antivenom as soon as possible (Box 51.1). Antivenom, when given in a timely fashion, is quite effective in managing systemic effects of envenomation, such as coagulopathy or neuropathy. Its benefit in preventing local tissue damage is not established.

Antivenoms are relatively specific for the snake species against which they are designed to protect. There is no benefit to administering an antivenom for an unrelated species, and there is certainly unacceptable risk (anaphylactoid reaction) and expense with such an approach. Therefore, if it is determined that the child requires antivenom, a search for the appropriate product should begin as soon as possible. If the

Box 51.2. Dosing regimen for CroFab

1. Each vial of CroFab should be reconstituted in 10 ml of sterile water.
2. Four to six reconstituted vials are diluted into 250 ml normal saline. The overall amount of dilution can be altered for smaller patients, or for those who are fluid sensitive.
3. The initial CroFab infusion should begin at 25–50 ml/h for 10 min. If no acute allergic reaction occurs, the infusion can be increased to 250 ml/h.
4. The envenomation syndrome should be frequently assessed and improvement should be noted at 1 h following the infusion.
5. If no improvement is noted at 1 h after infusion, a repeated dose should be given.
6. Once the reaction appears to be diminishing (indicated by improvement in coagulation studies, no further progression of swelling, absence of systemic symptoms), maintenance doses of two vials should be given every 6 h for 18 h until control is achieved.

The package insert describes the dosing regimen in detail.

bite involves an unusual snake, such as a captive, exotic species, a regional poison control center may be of assistance in locating the nearest effective antivenom.

The most commonly used antivenom for snakebites sustained in the USA is CroFab (Crotalidae polyvalent immune Fab ovine antivenom). CroFab can be used in the management of any snake bite from the crotaline family (water moccasins, copperheads, or rattlesnakes). CroFab is an antivenom derived from the venom of four snake species, and while the majority of clinical trials were done in adults, its use is also recommended in pediatric patients. CroFab antivenom should be administered to any patient with progression of the envenomation reaction or syndrome (Box 51.1). Relative contraindications to the use of CroFab include a hypersensitivity to papain or papayas. The dosing is the same regardless of weight or age, as the dose of antivenom is targeted towards the amount of venom inoculated, and not to the weight of the patient (Box 51.2).

Anytime AV is administered to an envenomated victim, there is some risk of an acute anaphylactoid reaction. Administration should be done with the treating physician at the bedside, with the patient closely monitored, and all medications and equipment necessary to reverse an anaphylactoid reaction immediately available. CroFab has an overall low rate of acute adverse reactions. However, allergic symptoms such as rash, pruritus, and wheezing have been reported.

At present, there is no commercially available anti-venom in the USA for coral snake bites. Care is supportive with respiratory assistance as needed.

A diagnostic and therapeutic modality that may be useful in victims of neurotoxic snake envenomation is a neostigmine test. This acetycholine esterase inhibitor may reverse objective neurotoxic findings in postsynaptic blockade. The neostigmine test should be tried in any snakebite victim with evidence of cranial nerve dysfunction or skeletal muscle weakness. If objective improvement occurs, further neostigmine (and atropine) is given as needed to maintain neurological function and potentially obviate the need for endotracheal intubation and ventilatory support. If, at 1 h following the test dose, no improvement is seen, further neostigmine will not help.

In the hospital, children with significant soft tissue swelling should have the bitten extremity elevated above heart level and its neurovascular status checked regularly. The risk of compartment syndrome following venomous snakebite is present but low, even in the face of what appears to be severe extremity swelling, because most of the edema is in the subcutaneous tissues rather than the muscle compartment. Compartment pressures should be checked before considering surgical decompression.

Disposition

Any child with a potential venomous snakebite should be admitted to a closely observed setting for at least 24 h, regardless of whether evidence of envenomation exists or antivenom is to be given. At discharge from the hospital, the family should be warned of the signs and symptoms of serum sickness. Serum sickness presents at 1 to 2 weeks following

Pearls and pitfalls

Pearls

1. Perform a careful history and physical examination to ascertain whether a venomous bite or sting may be the cause of signs and symptoms in an agitated, distressed, preverbal child (e.g., possible neurotoxic spider bite or scorpion sting).
2. Administer antivenom when appropriate and available to a child with significant envenomation.
3. Have all medications and equipment necessary to treat an anaphylactoid reaction immediately available when administering antivenom therapy.
4. Warn parents and guardians of the signs and symptoms of delayed serum sickness after the administration of antivenom.

Pitfalls

1. Failure to prescribe an epinephrine self-administration kit to a child being discharged following a possible anaphylactic reaction to a bite or sting (and instruct the family in proper use of the device).
2. Failure to consult an expert in cases of serious envenomation.
3. Failure to evaluate a child with significant limb swelling following a venomous snakebite for possible development of a compartment syndrome.
4. Failure to admit a child with significant envenomation.

antivenom administration and manifests with fever, myalgias, arthralgias, urticaria, and potentially renal and neurological involvement. With CroFab, the rate of serum sickness is low, but may present up to 3 weeks from initial administration. It is easily treated with a course of oral steroids combined with antihistamines and acetaminophen for symptomatic relief. Coagulopathy can recur up to 2 weeks after envenomation; children should be warned to avoid areas of risk during this period.

Conclusions

Bites and stings in children are common occurrences. The vast majority of these result in little more than local discomfort and itching. Occasionally, children suffer more serious bites or stings. A careful approach by the treating physician, with involvement of an envenomation specialist when necessary and available, will generally offer the child the best chances of optimal recovery.

Selected references

Graudins A, Padula M, Broady K, Nicholson GM. Red-back spider (*Latrodectus hasselti*) antivenom prevents the toxicity of widow spider venoms. *Ann Emerg Med* 2001;**37**:154–160.

Moffitt JE, Golden DBK, Reisman RE, *et al.* Stinging insect hypersensitivity: a practice parameter update. *J Allergy Clin Immunol* 2004;**114**:869–886.

Norris RL, Bush SP. Bites by venomous reptiles in the Americas. In Auerbach PS (ed.) *Wilderness Medicine*, 5th edn. St. Louis, MO: Mosby, 2007, pp. 1051–1085.

Pizon AF, Riley BD, LoVecchio F, Gill R. Safety and efficacy of Crotalidae Polyvalent Immune Fab in pediatric crotaline envenomations. *Acad Emerg Med* 2007;**14**:373–376.

Swanson DL, Vetter RS. Bites of brown recluse spiders and suspected necrotic arachnidism. *New Engl J Med* 2005;**352**:700–707.

White ML, Liebelt EL. Update on antidotes for pediatric poisoning. *Pediatr Emerg Care* 2006;**22**:740–746.

Section

9

Fluids and electrolytes

Expert reviewers: Steven Alexander and Nikta Forghani

Chapter 52

Introduction to electrolyte disorders

Erik Shraga

Introduction

The majority of electrolyte abnormalities detected in the ED are often incidental findings on laboratory panels drawn for screening purposes. However, in certain clinical situations, electrolyte imbalances should be anticipated and treated as an emergency (such as hyperkalemia in acute renal failure, hypoglycemia, hyponatremia, or hypocalcemia with seizure). Since EPs rely on laboratory results to confirm clinical decisions, it is also important to understand the shortcomings of these measurements. For example, potassium is mostly intracellular, and measuring serum potassium concentration is, therefore, a poor reflection of total body potassium. Another commonly encountered example is severe hyperglycemia causing an erroneously low sodium concentration. This introductory chapter will discuss electrolyte homeostasis and some general principles. Subsequent chapters in this section will address the diagnosis and management of specific electrolyte disorders.

Background

Water is by far the most abundant constituent of the human body. The percentage of the human body composed of water decreases with age. The term neonate is approximately 75% water by weight, the young child 65%, while the older child and adolescent are 60%. Females tend to have slightly lower total body water content than males. As adipose tissue has relatively little water, obese patients have a lower percentage of their body weight as water.

The majority of total body water is in the intracellular space. This accounts for approximately 40% of body weight. As males tend to have more muscle mass, they also have more intracellular water than females. Approximately 25% of body weight is extracellular fluid, which is composed of interstitial fluid and plasma. The balance between interstitial fluid and plasma fluid is regulated by the hydrostatic and oncotic pressure differences between these two spaces. This may also be affected by the integrity of the capillary membrane.

The equilibrium between intracellular and extracellular fluid is regulated by osmolality, as cell membranes are freely permeable to water. Normal plasma osmolality is 285–295 mOsm/kg. This can be measured directly from a plasma sample in the laboratory. The plasma osmolality can also be estimated using measurements of the most common extracellular constituents of osmolality:

$$2\text{Na}^{+}(\text{mEq/l}) + [\text{BUN}(\text{mg/dl})/2.8] + [\text{Glucose}(\text{mg/dl})/18]$$

where BUN is blood urea nitrogen. As urea freely crosses the cell membrane it is not considered a significant force in contributing to plasma osmolality. Therefore, the equation for osmolality can be simplified to:

$$2\text{Na}^{+}(\text{mEq/l}) + [\text{Glucose}(\text{mg/dl})/18]$$

In periods of hyperglycemia, increased plasma glucose is an effective osmole and draws water out of the intracellular space, thereby diluting the sodium concentration in the plasma, which can lead to lower measured sodium values. A "corrected" sodium value can be calculated:

$$\text{Na}^{+}(\text{mEq/l})\ \text{measured} + 1.6[\text{Glucose}(\text{mg/dl}) - 100]/100$$

Assuming there are no exogenous unmeasured osmoles, such as mannitol, methanol, or ethylene glycol, the estimated osmolality should be within 10 mOsm/kg of the measured value. A difference between the measured and estimated osmolality is suggestive of methanol or ethylene glycol toxicity. This is known as the osmolar gap.

Sodium

As sodium is the main extracellular cation and a significant component of osmolality, it is also an indicator of the free water and hydration status of a child. In general, a low serum sodium reflects an increase in total body free water and high serum sodium reflects a free water deficit (see Ch. 54).

A Practical Guide to Pediatric Emergency Medicine: Caring for Children in the Emergency Department, ed. N. Ewen Amieva-Wang (associate eds. Jamie Shandro, Aparajita Sohoni, and Bernhard Fassl). Published by Cambridge University Press.

Imbalances of blood sodium commonly manifest with CNS disorders.

Hyponatremia

The definition of hyponatremia is a serum sodium of <135 mEq/l. It is important to evaluate for the presence of other osmoles that could cause a pseudohyponatremia. Hyperglycemia, as mentioned, can shift fluid into the extracellular space causing a lower measured serum sodium value. Hyperproteinemia and hyperlipidemia can also cause falsely lowered serum sodium levels.

The greatest clinical concern in the setting of hyponatremia is cerebral edema caused by the osmotic flow of water into cells causing cell swelling. Additionally, hyponatremia can decrease cerebral blood flow. Symptoms of hyponatremia include headache, nausea, emesis, and weakness. Eventually, this can lead to herniation, dilated pupils, seizures, and death. Children tend to develop symptomatic hyponatremia at higher levels of sodium than do adults. This predisposition is presumed to be related to the brain to skull ratio of children.

Hypernatremia

The definition of hypernatremia is a serum sodium greater than 145 mEq/l. The body protects against hypernatremia through secretion of antidiuretic hormone (vasopressin) and stimulation of thirst. Hypernatremia is often seen when a patient has limited access to free water. In pediatrics, this is the situation in infants, who depend on caretakers for all of their oral intake.

Hypernatremia can cause cell shrinkage by shifting water out of the intracellular space. This can cause significant shrinkage of the brain if the serum sodium increases acutely. If the hypernatremia is more chronic in onset, the brain adapts by increasing the content of idiogenic osmoles that help to regulate intracellular fluid. Clinical signs of hypernatremia include irritability, increased tone, and hyperreflexia. These can progress to seizures, lethargy and coma.

Potassium

The vast majority of total volume potassium is in the intracellular space at a concentration of approximately 150 mEq/l (see Ch. 55). Potassium has a myriad of functions. It regulates intracellular osmolality as the major cation and also has a key role in balancing pH, which affects intracellular enzyme function. Potassium is also integral in muscle contraction as well as in generating the neuron action potential.

Imbalances in potassium usually manifest as disorders in cardiac and muscular function.

Hyperkalemia

An excess of potassium can disrupt the functioning of nerves and muscles. Clinical symptoms are usually not evident at serum potassium levels <7 mEq/l. Initial manifestations usually include muscle weakness, starting in the lower extremities. This can progress to paralysis. In addition to skeletal muscle, hyperkalemia can also cause dysfunction of cardiac muscle with classic ECG changes (Ch. 55).

Hypokalemia

Similar to too much potassium, too little potassium can also cause muscle weakness starting in the lower extremities. Hypokalemic weakness can also progress to paralysis. This can, again, affect all types of muscle, including respiratory muscles and the muscles of the GI tract. Cardiac effects include premature beats, bradycardia, heart block, tachycardia, and fibrillation. The ECG changes include a depressed ST segment and a low T wave (the opposite of the peaked T wave seen in hyperkalemia) (Ch. 55). In hypokalemia, always consider hypomagnesemia and in emergency situations treat both.

Calcium

The vast majority of total body calcium is contained as hydroxyapatite in bone. The body works to maintain serum calcium levels at the expense of bone in the context of inadequate calcium intake. Calcium is also important in coagulation, muscle contraction, and neuromuscular activation. As calcium is often bound to albumin and other proteins, the serum calcium level can be measured inaccurately in the setting of hypoalbuminemia. Ionized calcium is the preferred measure of active calcium. Alternatively, the corrected calcium can be estimated using the following equation:

$$\text{Ca}(\text{measured}) + 0.8[\text{Albumin}(\text{normal}) - \text{Albumin}(\text{measured})]$$

Hypercalcemia

Symptomatic hypercalcemia is relatively rare. Children are usually asymptomatic until the serum calcium level is >15 mg/dl. Symptoms include nausea, emesis, disorientation, and polyuria. In infants, hypercalcemia may present as failure to thrive or poor feeding. Serious cardiac sequelae of hypercalcemia include hypertension, shortened QT interval, and ventricular arrythmias.

Hypocalcemia

Hypocalcemia can have significant clinical implications. In school-aged children, paresthesiae are a common manifestation. In infants, hypocalcemia most commonly presents as generalized tonic–clonic seizures. Early hypocalcemia of neonates commonly presents as seizures within the first 72 h of life.

Neonatal hypocalcemia is most commonly caused by a transient hypoparathyroidism. Formula-fed infants or infants incorrectly fed with cow's milk can also present with severe hypocalcemia related to excessive intake of phosphorus in the setting of an immature parathyroid gland. Causes of hypocalcemia in older children include hypoparathyroidism, pseudohypoparathyroidism, vitamin D deficiency, tumor lysis, pancreatitis, and sepsis.

Magnesium

The majority of body magnesium is in the bone and intracellular space; <3% is in the serum. Homeostasis is maintained by dietary intake and GI absorption and kidney excretion. Unlike sodium, potassium, and calcium, there is no immediate hormonal modulation of magnesium excretion from body stores. The most severe manifestations of magnesium disorders are cardiac arrhythmias.

Conclusions

Electrolyte disorders are common and may present in a myriad of fashions. Pediatric patients are more susceptible to manifesting systemic symptoms from an electrolyte abnormality. The remainder Section 9 will detail each of the more common electrolyte abnormalities, their causes, diagnostic approach, and management.

Pearls and pitfalls

Pearls

1. Disorders of sodium balance manifest with CNS disorders.
2. Disorders of potassium balance manifest as cardiac arrhythmias, muscular spasticity and weakness.
3. In situations of potassium deficiency, also consider and treat magnesium deficiency.
4. If a child is not in extremis, consider oral versus IV repletion of potassium.

Pitfalls

1. Failure to consider electrolyte abnormalities in situations of CNS, cardiac dysfunction and weakness.

Selected references

Behrman RE, Kliegman RM, Jenson H. *Nelson Textbook of Pediatrics*, 17th edn. Philadelphia, PA: Saunders, 2007.

Centers for Disease Control and Prevention. Managing acute gastroenteritis among children: oral rehydration, maintenance, and nutritional therapy. *MMWR Morb Mort Wkly Rep* 2003;**52**:RR-16.

Jospe N, Forbes G. Fluid and electrolytes: clinical aspects. *Pediatr Rev*1996;**17**:395–403; quiz 404.

Lin M, Liu S, Lim I. Disorders of water imbalance. *Emerg Med Clin North Am* 2005;**23**:749–770.

Meyers A. Fluid and electrolyte therapy for children. *Curr Opin Pediatr* 1994;**6**: 303–309.

Moritz ML, Ayus JC. Disorders of water metabolism in children: hyponatremia and hypernatremia. *Pediatr Rev* 2002;**23**:371–380.

Ruth JL, Wassner SJ. Body composition: salt and water. *Pediatr Rev* 2006;**27**: 181–188.

Steiner MJ, DeWalt DA, Byerley JS. Is this child dehydrated? *JAMA*. 2004;**291**: 2746–2754.

Chapter 53

Tutorial: Fluids and electrolytes

Nicole Marsico and Rebecca Blankenburg

Introduction

In the ED, IV hydration is often used. While the average adult can usually tolerate a standard one liter bolus of isotonic fluid, children are more difficult to hydrate intravenously. This may be for several reasons: the average child's inability to cooperate with IV placement, difficulty in finding IV access, and the complexity of administering weight-based maintenance fluids. This tutorial will discuss

- signs of dehydration
- oral rehydration
- bolus fluids
- maintenance fluids
- fluids for special patients.

Estimating dehydration

Unfortunately, it is often impossible in the ED setting to obtain past accurate weights from the child's primary care physician, or from past visits to the ED. This is often not possible in the ED. Assessment of dehydration should include a targeted history and physical and vital sign measurements. Key aspects of the history include urine output, duration of illness, presence of diarrhea and emesis, and ability to tolerate oral liquids. Vital sign measurement should include weight, respiratory rate and character of respirations, temperature, pulse, and blood pressure. The physical examination should include assessment of skin turgor on the anterior abdominal wall and measurment of capillary refill time of the palmar surface of a finger at ambient temperature. No one test has demonstrated excellent reliability and accuracy. The presence of normal urine output makes dehydration less likely, but decreased urine output based on caregiver report does not have strong predictive power (Table 53.1).

Fluid resuscitation fluids

Dehydration can be treated with either enteral or IV fluid replacement. Rapid correction of dehydration should be done with isotonic fluids. The two main crystalloid isotonic solutions are normal saline and lactated Ringer's solution.

Treat all moderate to severe hypovolemic dehydration promptly with 20 ml/kg boluses of isotonic fluid until signs of severe hypovolemia resolve. Colloid (red cells, fresh frozen plasma, cryoprecipitate) may be preferred in the setting of acute blood loss, coagulopathy, or hypoalbuminemia. The child should be reassessed during and after the saline boluses, and similar isotonic fluid infusions should be repeated as needed until adequate perfusion is restored

Crystalloid and enteral replacement fluids have different electrolyte compositions (Tables 53.2 and 53.3). Commercially prepared oral replacement fluids are preferred to juices or sports drinks, which have a high concentration of sugar and higher osmolality and, thus, cause an osmotic diuresis or diarrhea.

Route of administration depends on resources and access. Enteral therapy is effective, although often overlooked in the ED and hospital setting. Oral rehydration solution can be given in small 5 ml portions every 5 to 10 min. A nasogastric tube may be placed to more efficiently administer enteral fluids in an uncooperative child. Fluids can be administered through the tube either as boluses or at a continuous rate similar to IV fluids. Several reports suggest that oral rehydration is equivalent to IV fluid administration in the treatment of mild or moderate dehydration. Oral rehydration should not be used in severe hypovolemia. With severe hypovolemia in the setting of actual or evolving circulatory compromise, emergency IV fluid therapy should begin with rapid infusion of 20 ml/kg of isotonic saline.

A Practical Guide to Pediatric Emergency Medicine: Caring for Children in the Emergency Department, ed. N. Ewen Amieva-Wang (associate eds. Jamie Shandro, Aparajita Sohoni, and Bernhard Fassl). Published by Cambridge University Press.

Table 53.1. Evaluation of the degree of dehydration

Symptom	Minimal (<3%)	Dehydration Mild to moderate (3–9%)	Severe (>9%)
Mental status	Alert	Normal or irritable, fatigued	Apathetic, lethargic, non-responsive
Thirst	Drinks normally, may refuse liquids	Normal to increased	Drinks poorly
Heart rate	Normal	Normal to increased	Tachycardia; bradycardia may be present in very severe cases
Pulse quality	Normal	Normal to decreased	Weak, thready, or unable to assess
Respirations	Normal	Normal to fast	Deep or shallow breathing, Kussmaul breathing
Eyes	Normal	Slightly sunken	Deeply sunken
Tears	Present	Decreased	Absent
Oropharynx	Moist	Dry	Parched
Skin turgor	Instant recoil	Recoil <2 s	Recoil >2 s
Capillary refill	Normal	Prolonged	Prolonged
Extremities	Warm	Cool	Cold, mottled
Urine output	Normal to decreased	Decreased	Minimal

Source: Adapted from Centers for Disease Control and Prevention, 2003.

Table 53.2. Electrolyte composition of different fluids used for rehydration

Fluid	Sodium (mEq/l)	Chloride (mEq/l)	Potassium (mEq/l)	Calcium (mEq/l)	Lactate (mEq/l)
LR	130	109	4	3	28
NS	154	154	–	–	–
½NS	77	77	–	–	–
¼NS	38.5	38.5	–	–	–
3% Saline	514	514	–	–	–

LR, lactated Ringer's solution; NS, normal saline.

In children, the most common cause of dehydration is acute gastroenteritis.

The US Centers for Disease Control and Prevention (CDC), World Health Organization (WHO) and American Academy of Pediatrics have joint official recommendations regarding fluid replacement in this scenario, which can also be applicable to children presenting with dehydration from other illnesses (Table 53.4).

Maintenance fluids

What are maintenance fluids?

For a normal (previously healthy) child, the total daily maintenance fluid equals the urine output plus insensible losses plus any other losses. Urine output accounts for two-thirds of total maintenance needs and insensible losses for one-third.

In a child who has diarrhea, vomiting, or other ongoing losses, the maintenance fluids must include the increased needs (Box 53.1). Fever, increased sweating, increased respiratory rate, tracheostomy, or drooling will all increase insensible losses and this must be kept in mind when estimating a child's maintenance fluids. Similarly, if a child has decreased urination, this also must be considered when determining their amount of maintenance fluids (see also the special cases below).

The **Holliday–Segar method** calculates the daily rate of fluid administration assuming that a child has normal urine output and insensible losses, and no extra losses.

Table 53.3. Composition of oral rehydration solution

Oral rehydration solution	Glucose (g/dl)	Sodium (mEq/l)	Chloride (mEq/l)	Potassium (mEq/l)	Base (mEq/l)	Osmolality (mosms/l)
Pedialyte	2.5	45	35	20	30	250
WHO	2	90	80	20	30	310
LiquiLyte	2.2	19.5	44.2	34.6	29.6	
Apple juice	11.9	0.4	–	26	–	700
Gatorade	5.9	21	17	2.5	None	377

Table 53.4. Recommendations for fluid replacement in gastroenteritis

Degree of dehydration	Rehydration therapy	Replacement of losses	Nutrition
Minimal	NA	<10 kg: 60–120 ml ORS for each diarrhea or emesis >10 kg: 120–140 ml ORS for each diarrhea or emesis	Continue age-appropriate diet after hydration; continue breast-feeding
Mild to moderate	50–100 ml/kg ORS over initial 3–4 h	<10 kg: 60–120 ml ORS for each diarrhea or emesis >10 kg: 120–140 ml ORS for each diarrhea or emesis	Continue age-appropriate diet after hydration; continue breast-feeding
Severe	20 ml/kg IV bolus of LR or NS until perfusion improves; *then* 100 ml/kg ORS over 4 h *or* D5½NS IV at twice maintenance	<10 kg: 60–120 ml ORS PO/NG *or* D5½NS + 20 mEq/l KCl IV for each diarrhea or emesis >10 kg: 120–140 ml ORS PO/NG *or* D5½NS + 20 mEq/l KCl IV for each diarrhea or emesis	Continue age-appropriate diet after hydration; continue breast-feeding

D5, dextrose 5%; LR, lactated Ringer's solution; NS, normal saline; NG, nasogastric tube; ORS, oral rehydration solution.
Source: Adapted from Centers for Disease Control and Prevention, 2003.

The **4:2:1 rule** refers to the hourly rate of fluid administration assuming that a child has normal urine output and insensible losses, and no extra losses.

Maintenance fluid composition

Maintenance fluid composition differs from solutions used to replace deficits and ongoing losses; fluid is required to provide sufficient sodium and potassium.

It is inappropriate to replace deficits and ongoing losses solely by increasing the amount or rate of maintenance fluids. Rather, it is preferable to measure the amount of losses and consider the type of loss (i.e., which electrolytes are likely being lost) and replace them accordingly.

Special circumstances

Neonates

Because neonates have difficulty renally clearing electrolytes in the first few days of life, 10% dextrose in water (D10W) is used.

day of life 1: D10W at 80 ml/kg daily
day of life 2: D10W at 100 ml/kg daily
day of life 3: D10W at 120 ml/kg daily.

Usually around day of life 3–4, electrolytes can begin to be added to the IV fluids. Premature neonates have increased insensible losses through their skin because of their immature skin and increased body surface area. It is advisable to consult with a neonatologist on premature infants <40 weeks of adjusted gestational age, and neonates requiring IV fluids in the ED.

Children with cardiac disease

Because children with many congenital cardiac disorders are likely to develop congestive heart failure, it is recommended to proceed with fluid administration more cautiously:

- for resuscitation fluids, give 5–10 ml/kg boluses, and reassess for congestive heart failure after each bolus
- for maintenance fluids, start with half to two-thirds maintenance fluids and adjust according to effect and clinical signs/symptoms of congestive heart failure.

Box 53.1. Maintenance fluids

Normal maintenance fluids

Maintenance fluids = Urine output + Insensible losses

- Daily sodium requirement: 2–5 mEq/kg
- Daily potassium requirement: 2–4 mEq/kg.

Maintenance fluid required depends on the child's weight:

- body weight <20 kg: D5½NS + 10 mEq/l KCl
- body weight ≥20 kg: D5½NS + 20 mEq/l KCl

Holliday–Segar method for daily maintenance fluids

children 0–10 kg: 100 ml/kg

children 11–20 kg: 1000 ml + 50 ml/kg for each 1 kg over 10 kg

children >20 kg: 1500 ml + 20 ml/kg for each 1 kg over 20 kg.

4:2:1 Rule (hourly fluid rate)

Hourly maintenance fluids are given by:

4 ml/kg per h for the first 10 kg of child's weight, plus

2 ml/kg per h for the second 10 kg of child's weight, plus

1 ml/kg per h for each 1 kg in weight after the first 20 kg.

Child with additional losses

Maintenance fluids = Urine output + Insensible losses + Ongoing losses

Children with renal disease

In children with known or potential renal disease, it is important to carefully assess their ability to produce urine. If they have normal urine output, then proceed with regular maintenance fluids, although potassium should not be added to their fluid until the ability to urinate is established.

In children who have anuria or oliguria, one must be careful both in the amount and type of fluids given. They will need less fluid as their "maintenance" needs are significantly decreased since they have less or no urine output.

"Maintenance" fluids for anuric children are one-third of those for a normal child.

This maintenance volume assumes no increased losses from other sources (vomiting, diarrhea, etc.) because insensible losses are usually approximately one-third of the amount calculated by the 4:2:1 rule. In oliguric children, one needs to replace both the insensible losses and the urine output; a good way to do this is to closely measure the urine output every 4–6 h and add the estimated insensible losses and then replace it over the following 4–6 h. In terms of type of fluid chosen, it is advisable to not place any potassium in their fluids, as it will be harder for their kidneys to clear the potassium. Often, people will choose dextrose 5% in half normal saline (D5½NS).

Children with hypoalbuminemia or other low protein states

Because children with hypoalbuminemia and other low protein states have decreased oncotic pressure, they are more likely to develop third-spacing and pulmonary edema with isotonic fluid administration. These patients may benefit from administration of 5% albumin followed by furosemide. If they are severely hypoalbuminemic, they might require 25% albumin 0.5 g/kg, with furosemide 0.5 mg/kg IV (max. 20 mg) halfway through administration and repeated at the end of the infusion. It is advisable to proceed cautiously in these children as it is easy to cause pulmonary edema.

Conclusions

Rehydrating an otherwise healthy child, with no underlying chronic diseases, is relatively simple. Providers should be familiar with special circumstances in which alterations in fluid choice or rate of administration may need to be made.

Pearls and pitfalls

Pearls

1. Give weight-based IV fluid boluses to rehydrate a child.
2. Urine output is one of the most sensitive indications of dehydration.
3. Administer small fluid boluses (5–10 ml/kg) to children with underlying cardiac or renal disease or who are hypoalbuminemic.

Pitfalls

1. Not every dehydrated child needs IV fluids; remember oral or nasogastric routes.
2. Failure to diagnose and treat hypovolemic shock before the onset of hypotension, which is the final sign of severe hypovolemic shock in children, appearing late in the course of events.

Selected references

Centers for Disease Control and Prevention. Managing acute gastroenteritis among children: oral rehydration, maintenance, and nutritional therapy. *MMWR Morb Mort Wkly Rep* 2003;**52**:RR-16.

Jospe N, Forbes G. Fluid and electrolytes: clinical aspects. *Pediatr Rev* 1996;**17**:395–403; quiz 404.

Lin M, Liu S, Lim I. Disorders of water imbalance. *Emerg Med Clin North Am* 2005;**23**:749–770.

Moritz ML, Ayus JC. Disorders of water metabolism in children: hyponatremia and hypernatremia. *Pediatr Rev* 2002;**23**:371–380.

Ruth JL, Wassner SJ. Body composition: salt and water. *Pediatr Rev* 2006;**27**: 181–188.

Steiner MJ, DeWalt DA, Byerley JS. Is this child dehydrated? *JAMA* 2004;**291**:2746–2754.

Chapter 54

Disorders of sodium balance

Barbara Dahl, Bernhard Fassl, and Nikta Forghani

Introduction

Disorders of sodium usually manifest with CNS symptoms. While volume status is reflected by the plasma concentration of sodium, hypo- and hypernatremia can occur in hypo-, hyper-, and euvolemic states depending on the ratio of sodium to plasma. Disorders of sodium balance are discussed by etiology and treatment rather than by this conventional rubric.

Hyponatremia

Hyponatremia is defined as serum sodium (Na) concentration of <135 mEq/l. Hyponatremia is the most common electrolyte abnormality encountered in clinical practice, with an incidence of 1.5% of all pediatric hospital admissions.

Clinical manifestations

Clinical manifestations vary from an asymptomatic state to severe organ dysfunction.

CNS symptoms. Factors that contribute to development of CNS symptoms are

- the rate at which serum sodium levels change
- the serum sodium level itself
- the duration of the abnormal serum sodium level
- the presence of additional risk factors
- the presence of excessive antidiuretic hormone (ADH; vasopressin)
- additional risk factors include age <16 years, male gender, and presence of hypoxia.

CNS signs/symptons of hyponatremia include:

- early signs: anorexia, headache, nausea, emesis
- advanced signs of encephalopathy: dilated pupils, seizures, respiratory arrest, coma.

Cardiovascular symptoms: hypotension, tachycardia.

Musculoskeletal symptoms: weakness, muscle cramps.

Etiology

Hyponatremia is the consequence of one of a number of processes (Table 54.1).

In children, the most common cause of hyponatremia is loss of sodium from the GI tract. Diarrhea is responsible for most incidents of hyponatremia in children. In the absence of a GI illness history the clinician should consider:

- sodium losses by the kidneys (use of diuretics)
- water retention by the kidney:
  - acute or chronic renal insufficiency
  - excessive antidiuretic hormone (ADH) secretion
- chronic illnesses: cirrhosis, cardiac failure, or renal failure
- other excess fluid losses (excessive sweating, GI fistulae or drainage tubes, pancreatitis, burns) that have been replaced primarily by hypotonic fluids
- endocrine causes: cortisol deficiency (central and adrenal), hypothyroidism
- drugs: MDMA (ecstasy), medications.

Box 54.1 outlines a step-by-step method for the workup and diagnosis of hyponatremia etiology. Table 54.2 summarizes potential causes.

Special consideration: severe hyponatremia (<125 mEq/l) in infants

The most common cause of severe hyponatremia in small infants is *incorrect mixing of infant formula* by the caregiver. A detailed history about exact water:formula mixing ratio is mandatory.

The clinician should also consider the following possible etiologies of severe hyponatremia:

- adrenal insufficiency/congenital adrenal hyperplasia: common associated clinical findings are skin hyperpigementation, ambiguous genitalia, hyperkalemia
- cystic fibrosis: hyponatremia is a common *initial* presentation in infancy.

A Practical Guide to Pediatric Emergency Medicine: Caring for Children in the Emergency Department, ed. N. Ewen Amieva-Wang (associate eds. Jamie Shandro, Aparajita Sohoni, and Bernhard Fassl). Published by Cambridge University Press.

Table 54.1. Overview of causes of hyponatremia

Type	Conditions
Hypovolemic hyponatremia	
Extrarenal conditions	GI conditions: vomiting, diarrhea, tubes, fistulae
	Sweat: cystic fibrosis
	Cerebral salt-wasting syndrome
	Drugs
Third-spacing conditions	Pancreatitis, burns, muscle trauma, peritonitis, effusions, ascites
Renal losses	Diuretic excess, osmotic diuresis, renal salt-wasting, adrenal insufficiency, metabolic alkalosis, pseudohypoaldosteronism
Normovolemic hyponatremia	
Extrarenal conditions	Syndrome of inappropriate antidiuretic hormone hypersecretion
	CNS disease: tumor, trauma, infection, cerebrovascular accident
	Pulmonary disease: pneumonia, lung abscess, tuberculosis, cystic fibrosis, positive-pressure ventilation
	Carcinoma: lung, pancreas, thymoma, ovary, lymphoma
	Drugs: exogenous vasopressin, non-steroidal anti-inflammatory drugs, nicotine, diuretics, chlorpropamide, carbamazepine, tricyclic antidepressants, selective serotonin reuptake inhibitors, vincristine, thioridazine, cyclophosphamide, clofibrate
	Surgery: postoperative losses
	Idiopathic (most common)
	Water intoxication from IV therapy, tap-water enema, psychogenic water drinking
	Other: glucocorticoid deficiency, hypothyroidism
Hypervolemic hyponatremia	
Extrarenal	Congestive heart failure, cirrhosis
Renal conditions	Nephrotic syndrome, acute or chronic renal failure
Other	Hyperglycemia, hyperlipidemia, hyperosmolar states

Principles of treatment

The most common and devastating effects of hyponatremia are of CNS origin. Therefore, being aware of the risk factors that lead to hyponatremia and hyponatremic encephalopathy is important. Asymptomatic hyponatremia can be treated with fluid restriction while additional investigation of etiology is being undertaken (if cause is not clear based on history). In asymptomatic children, hypertonic saline can actually be harmful. However, any child with symptomatic hyponatremia (change in mental state or seizures) should be treated immediately and monitored closely.

1 ml/kg of 3% saline will raise serum sodium by 1 mEq/l.

End points of treatment are (a) an alert and seizure-free patient, (b) an increase of 20–25 mEq/l in serum sodium, or (c) 125–130 mEq/l, whichever comes first.

Rate of sodium correction

The rate of sodium correction is different depending on whether the hyponatremia is acute or chronic. Acute evolution of hyponatremia leaves little opportunity for compensatory extrusion of CNS intracellular solutes. The ultimate danger for these patients is brainstem herniation when sodium levels fall below 120 mEq/l. The therapeutic goal is to increase the serum sodium level rapidly by 4–6 mEq/l over the first 1–2 h if a patient is showing clinical signs of increased intracranial pressure and actively seizing.

Chronic hyponatremia must be managed with extreme care. Overly rapid correction of hyponatremia has been associated with the development of the osmotic demyelination syndrome (also known as central pontine myelinolysis), characterized by focal demyelination in the pons and extrapontine areas associated with serious neurologic sequelae.

Regardless of the therapeutic approach, serum sodium must be monitored closely and corrected no faster than 10–12 mEq/l in the first 24 h and 18 mEq/l in the first 48 h. Box 54.2 gives the protocol for calculating sodium replacement.

Disposition

- Transfer patients with symptomatic hyponatremia to a pediatric ICU for appropriate treatment and close monitoring.
- Consult an endocrinologist when patients have suspected hypothyroidism or adrenal insufficiency.
- Consult a nephrologist when patients have salt-losing nephropathy, renal failure, or recalcitrant hyponatremia, or for assistance with fluid and electrolyte therapy in complex clinical situations.

Box 54.1. Diagnosis and workup for severe hyponatremia (serum Na <125 mEq/l)

STEP 1 CONFIRM HYPONATREMIA

1. Exclude measurement error.
2. Look for clues in patient history:
   - feeding with hypotonic formula or free water during infancy
   - conditions causing GI fluid loss, e.g., diarrhea, vomiting, fistulae
   - renal disorders, e.g., salt-losing nephropathy, acute renal failure, chronic renal failure
   - postoperative states
   - psychiatric conditions, coma
   - drug use
   - CNS disease
   - pulmonary diseases
   - hypothyroidism
   - adrenal insufficiency
   - cirrhosis
   - congestive heart failure
   - AIDS.

STEP 2 OBTAIN FURTHER ANALYSES

Obtain potassium, BUN creatinine, bicarbonate, glucose. Consider triglycerides, serum protein. The following results assist diagnosis:

- potassium elevated: adrenal causes
- BUN elevated: hypovolemia
- creatinine elevated: acute/chronic renal failure
- bicarbonate elevated: metabolic acidosis/alkalosis
- glucose, proteins, and triglycerides: excludes pseudohyponatremia
  - each 100 mg/dl increase in the glucose above 100 mg/dl leads to a 1.6 mEq/l decrease in the sodium concentration
  - triglycerides (mg/dl) × 0.002 = decrease in plasma sodium (mEq/l)
  - [plasma protein (g/dl) – 8] × 0.25 = decrease in plasma sodium (mEq/l).

STEP 3 URINE AND SERUM OSMOLALITY

Measurement of urine and serum sodium and creatinine:

- reduction in serum and urine osmolality: excess water load
- urine sodium <20 mEq/l: extrarenal losses
- urine sodium >20 mEq/l: renal losses
- normovolemic hyponatremia (syndrome of inappropriate antidiuretic hormone hypersecretion [SIADH], endocrine causes)
- urine sodium >120 mEq/l: hyponatremia caused by an edemic state (e.g., cardiac, cirrhosis).

STEP 4 SPECIAL STUDIES

- If adrenal insufficiency suspected, measure 17-hydroxyprogesterone, ACTH, cortisol, aldosterone, plasma renin activity.
- If hypothyroidism is suspected, measure free thyroxine and thyroid-stimulating hormone.

Box 54.1. *(cont.)*

- If SIADH is suspected, measure ADH (vasopressin). *Important*: sample for ADH should be taken and sent off *before* correction of sodium.
- Imaging of head with CT for patients with altered mental status.

Table 54.2. Overview of causes of hypernatremia

Type of loss	Causes
Gastrointestinal losses of free water	Diarrhea, emesis, nasogastric suction, ostomy, osmotic cathartic
Renal water losses	Osmotic diuretics, diabetes mellitus, acute tubular necrosis, obstructive uropathy, diabetes insipidus (nephrogenic, central)
Cutaneous water losses	Sweating, burns
Intake	Decreased free water intake: incorrectly mixed infant formula; water restriction in tube-fed children
Endocrine causes	Excessive sodium intake: iatrogenic (hypertonic fluid administration), salt water ingestion Hyperaldosteronism

Box 54.2. Sodium replacement

$$\text{Sodium requirement (mEq)} = 0.6\text{BW(kg)}[\text{Sodium(desired)} - \text{Sodium(serum)}]$$

where BW is body weight (kg).

$$\text{Volume of hypertonic saline} = \text{Sodium(required)(mEq)} \times 1000/\text{Sodium(infusate)(mEq/l)}$$

Hypernatremia

The definition of hypernatremia is a serum sodium concentration greater than 145 mEq/l. The body protects against hypernatremia through secretion of ADH and stimulation of thirst.

Pearls and pitfalls: hyponatremia

Pearls

1. Disorders of sodium balance manifest with CNS disorders.
2. Hyponatremia is a common cause of neonatal seizures.
3. Common causes of hyponatremia in infancy are incorrect mixing of formula, congenital adrenal hyperplasia, and cystic fibrosis.
4. Diarrhea is responsible for most incidents of hyponatremia in children.

Pitfalls

1. Failure to consider the possibility of sampling or analysis error, hyperglycemia, hyperproteinemia, or hyperlipidemia before making the diagnosis of hyponatremia.
2. Failure to quickly recognize and correct severe acute hyponatremia.
3. Correcting serum sodium level too rapidly in patients with chronic hyer- or hyponatremia.

Clinical manifestations

Hypernatremia can cause cell shrinkage by shifting water out of the intracellular space. This can cause significant shrinkage of the brain if serum sodium increases acutely. Symptoms are:

- CNS symptoms: irritability, increased tone, hyperreflexia; these can progress to seizures, lethargy and coma
- other symptoms: physical findings of dehydration or even hypovolemic shock, with tachycardia, orthostasis, and hypotension.

Etiology

Hypernatremia is most commonly seen when a patient has limited access to free water. In pediatrics, this is seen in infants who depend on caretakers for all of their intake. This can also occur in patients with gastroenteritis with excessive diarrhea and vomiting, which can result in severe hypernatremic dehydration. Some diagnostic clues can be derived from the serum sodium levels:

- >190 mEq/l usually associated with excessive long-term salt consumption (exceedingly rare in children)
- >170 mEq/l usually indicates diabetes insipidus
- 150–170 mEq/l usually indicates dehydration.

Table 54.2 gives an overview of causes of hypernatremia and Box 54.3 gives the protocol for diagnosis and workup.

Box 54.3. Diagnosis and workup for hypernatremia

STEP 1 BASIC WORKUP

Confirm hyponatremia; the kidneys' normal response to hypernatremia is excretion of a minimal amount of maximally concentrated urine.

Measure urine and serum osmolality and urine sodium levels:

- if urine osmolarity is high, suspect extrarenal hypotonic fluid losses (e.g., vomiting, diarrhea)
- urine is also concentrated in salt overload states, although the total volume should increase.

Measure serum glucose to ensure that osmotic diuresis has not occurred:

- isotonic urine osmolality can be observed with diuretics, osmotic diuresis
- hypotonic urine and polyuria are characteristic of diabetes insipidus.

STEP 2 FURTHER STUDIES

Measure serum ADH (vasopressin). *Important*: samples for ADH must be taken before serum sodium is corrected.

Carry out an ADH stimulation test.

Box 54.4. Free water replacement

$$\text{Free water deficit (ml)} = 4\,\text{ml} \times \text{lean BW (kg)} \times [\text{Serum sodium(desired change)(mEq/l)}]$$

The free water content of available fluids: ½NS contains 50% free water, ¼NS contains 75% free water.

Principles of treatment

- Patients should be assessed for signs of hypovolemic shock and this should be corrected with boluses of normal saline or colloid.
- Once the patient is hemodynamically stable, a calculation of the free water deficit should be made (Box 54.4).

Pearls and pitfalls: hypernatremia

Pearls

1. Decreased water intake in children dependent on adults for feeding is the most common cause of hypernatremia.
2. Hypernatremia is commonly associated with dehydration and poor perfusion.

Pitfalls

1. Failure to realize that over-rapid hydration can cause CNS deficits in hypernatremic patients.
2. Failure to consider the possibility of neglect/abuse in patients with hypernatremia who are debilitated.

The free water deficit should be corrected to include maintenance fluids and replacement of any ongoing losses. This can be calculated using the equation in Box 54.4 and consideration of the free water content of available fluids. An alternative is to run either ½NS or ¼NS at a rate 20–50% above the maintenance rate. Serum sodium should be monitored initially on an hourly basis.

The rate of correction should not exceed 1 mEq/h or 15 mEq in a 24 h period.

In extreme hypernatremia with serum sodium concentrations >170 mEq/l, serum sodium should be corrected even more slowly, with a goal serum sodium of 150 mEq/l after 48 to 72 h of therapy.

Special situation: diabetes insipidus

In children 3 months to 12 years, desmopressin (DDAVP) 5–30 μg daily is given intranasally in one or two divided doses. An endocrinologist or nephrologist should be consulted before initiation. If DDAVP works and fluids are not appropriately managed during this therapy, a too-rapid correction can occur.

Caution: during correction, serum sodium levels should be closely monitored and fluid therapy switched to oral as soon as possible to prevent too rapid a correction, which can lead to cerebral edema and death.

Selected references

Ichikawa I. A bridge over troubled water: mixed water and electrolyte disorders. *Pediatr Nephrol* 1998;**12**:160–167.

Moritz ML, Ayus JC. Disorders of water metabolism in children: hyponatremia and hypernatermia, *Pediatr Rev* 2002;**23**:371–380.

Moritz ML, Ayus JC. Dysnatremias in the critical care setting. *Contrib Nephrol* 2004;**144**:132–157.

Ranadive SA, Rosenthal SM. Pediatric disorders of water balance. *Endocrinol Metab Clin North Am* 2009;**38**:663–672.

Ruth JL, Wassner SJ. Body composition: salt and water. *Pediatr Rev* 2006;**27**:181–187.

Chapter

55 Disorders of potassium balance

Barbara Dahl and Bernhard Fassl

Introduction

Potassium regulates intracellular osmolality as the major cation and also has a key role in balancing pH, which affects intracellular enzyme function. Potassium is integral in the contraction of all forms of muscle as well as in generating the neuron action potential.

Imbalances in potassium usually manifest as disorders in cardiac and muscular function.

Hyperkalemia

The normal potassium level in the blood is 3.5–5.0 mEq/l. Potassium levels of

- 5.1–6.0 mEq/l : mild hyperkalemia
- 6.1–7.0 mEq/l : moderate hyperkalemia
- >7 mEq/l : severe hyperkalemia.

Clinical manifestations

Clinical changes are not usually evident at serum potassium levels <7 meq/l. Initial manifestations usually include muscle *weakness* starting in the lower extremities. This weakness can progress to paralysis. In addition to skeletal muscle effects, hyperkalemia can also cause dysfunction of cardiac muscle. This is first evident in the ECG as *peaked T waves*, defined as sharp and symmetric T waves that are greater than 10 mm in height in the precordial leads on an ECG and greater than 5 mm in height in the limb leads (Fig. 55.1).

Persistent hyperkalemia can lead to further ECG changes including elongation of the PR interval and widening of the QRS complex until it becomes a sine wave. Eventually hyperkalemia can lead to either asystole or ventricular fibrillation.

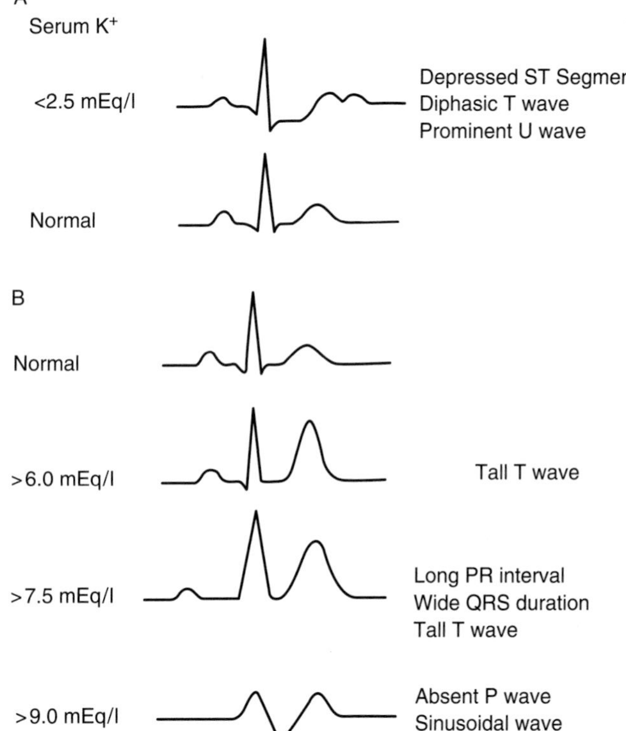

Figure 55.1 Hypo- and hyperkalemia. (A) ECG changes in hypokalemia. As the serum potassium decreases below 2.5 mEq/l, the ST segment becomes depressed, the T wave becomes diphasic, and prominent U waves can occur. (B) In hyperkalemia, at serum potassium levels greater that 6.0 mEq/l, the T waves become tall and peaked; potassium > 7.5mEq/l results in long PR interval, widened QRS; potassium >9.0 mEq/l results in absent P waves and a sinusoidal QRS complex.

Etiology

Acute renal failure, medication effects, and laboratory sampling errors are the most common causes of hyperkalemia (Table 55.1).

Diagnosis

Box 55.1 gives the workup needed for diagnosis of hyperkalemia.

Special consideration: hyperkalemia in small infants

Infants with hyperkalemia should be examined for clinical signs of congenital adrenal hyperplasia (CAH). These include skin hyperpigmentation, ambiguous genitalia (in females), and presence of hyponatremia.

A Practical Guide to Pediatric Emergency Medicine: Caring for Children in the Emergency Department, ed. N. Ewen Amieva-Wang (associate eds. Jamie Shandro, Aparajita Sohoni, and Bernhard Fassl). Published by Cambridge University Press.

Table 55.1. Overview of causes of hyperkalemia

Effects	Causes
Renal causes	Decreased or impaired potassium excretion, acute or chronic renal failure (most common), potassium-sparing diuretics, urinary obstruction
Disease	Sickle cell disease, Addison disease, systemic lupus erythematosus
Potassium overload	Additions of potassium into extracellular space, potassium supplements (e.g., PO/IV potassium, salt substitutes),
Injury	Rhabdomyolysis, hemolysis (e.g., venipuncture, blood transfusions, burns, tumor lysis)
Transmembrane shifts (shift of potassium from the intracellular to extracellular space)	Metabolic acidosis, medication effects, insulin deficiency, acute digitalis toxicity, beta-blockers, succinylcholine
Factitious or pseudohyperkalemia	Improper blood collection (ischemic blood draw from venipuncture technique), laboratory error, leukocytosis, thrombocytosis
Drugs	Succinylcholine, digoxin, fluoride, beta-blockers, ACE inhibitors, angiotensin II receptor blockers, potassium-sparing diuretics, cyclosporine, NSAIDs, trimethoprim

Box 55.1. Diagnosis and workup for hyperkalemia

STEP 1 CONFIRM HYPERKALEMIA

1. Exclude measurement error
   - redraw blood sample to verify potassium level, avoiding "milking" of extremity to obtain blood
   - check for signs of hemolysis.
2. Look for clues in patient history
   - chronic renal illness
   - potassium supplementation
   - muscle injury/trauma
   - metabolic acidosis
   - medications.

STEP 2 OBTAIN FURTHER ANALYSES

Measurements will relate to patient history:

- BUN and creatinine level: evaluation of renal function
- glucose: for patient with diabetes mellitus
- digoxin: for patients taking a digitalis medication
- arterial blood gases: if acidosis is suspected
- urinalysis for proteinuria/hematuria: if signs of renal insufficiency are present (glomerulonephritis, tubular damage).

STEP 3 OTHER STUDIES

1. Continuous cardiac monitoring: indicated in all degrees of hyperkalemia, particularly in moderate–severe hyperkalemia
   - ECG findings: generally correlate with the potassium level, but potentially life-threatening arrhythmias can occur without warning at almost any level of hyperkalemia
   - early ECG changes include peaked T waves, shortened QT interval, ST segment depression
2. Endocrinologic workup in neonates with moderate–severe hyperkalemia or if a clinical suspicion of congenital adrenal hyperplasia (CAH).
   Check 17-hydroxyprogesterone, ACTH, cortisol, aldosterone, plasma renin activity.

Pearls and pitfalls: hyperkalemia

Pearls

1. Sampling errors are the most common causes of hyperkalemia.
2. Disorders of potassium balance manifest as cardiac arrhythmias and muscle weakness.
3. Symptomatic hyperkalemia (presence of muscle weakness, ECG changes) must be treated promptly.
4. Hyperkalemia in small infants can be a sign of congenital adrenal hyperplasia.

Pitfalls

1. Failure to recheck an abnormal potassium blood level.
2. Failure to diagnose hypokalemia in patients with non-specific complaints.

Principles of treatment

Treatment options for hyperkalemia include several methods to attempt to reduce the plasma potassium level. Most importantly, *if there is any evidence of ECG changes, calcium should be administered* to stabilize the cardiac membrane. This stabilization effect is transient, so additional doses may be necessary if the plasma potassium level cannot be lowered through the other treatments.

Treatment of hyperkalemia should be approached in a stepwise fashion (Box 55.2).

Hypokalemia

The reference range for serum potassium is 3.5–5 mEq/l, with total body potassium stores of approximately 50 mEq/kg (i.e., approximately 3500 mEq in a 70 kg person). Serum potassium levels of:

Box 55.2. Treatment of hyperkalemia

STEP 1 STABILIZE CARDIAC MUSCLE
- Calcium chloride 10–20 mg/kg IV, IO *or*
- Calcium gluconate 10% 100 mg/kg (1 ml/kg) IV.

STEP 2 SHIFT POTASSIUM BACK INTO CELLS
- Glucose dextrose 25% with water (D25W) 2 ml/kg IV over 30 min *plus* insulin 0.1 U/kg.
- Albuterol 0.1–0.3 mg/kg nebulized over 20 min.
- Sodium bicarbonate1–2 mEq/kg IV, IO.

STEP 3 REMOVE POTASSIUM
- Sodium polystyrene sulfonate 1–2 g/kg per rectum or PO.
- Furosemide 1–2 mg/kg IV.
- Hemodialysis.

- <3.5 mEq/l: mild hypokalemia
- 2.5–3 mEq/l: moderate hypokalemia
- <2.5 mEq/l: severe hypokalemia.

Clinical manifestations

Skeletal muscle weakness. Hypokalemia affects muscle contractions and can cause muscle weakness starting in the lower extremities. Hypokalemic weakness can also progress to paralysis and can affect respiratory muscle strength.

Smooth muscle dysfunction. Hypokalemia can cause ileus, constipation, nausea, vomiting, abdominal cramping in GI tract; hypotension as a result of vascular effects.

Cardiac effects. Premature beats, bradycardia, heart block, tachycardia and fibrillation can all occur. The ECG changes include a depressed ST segment and a low T wave (the opposite of the peaked T wave seen in hyperkalemia) (Fig. 55.1).

CNS effects. Delirium and coma.

Etiology

The most common cause of hypokalemia in children is GI potassium loss during episodes of gastroenteritis, particularly in rotavirus infections (Table 55.2). Box 55.3 outlines the workup needed for diagnosis of hyperkalemia.

Principles of treatment

Rapid parenteral administration of potassium should be reserved for only severely symptomatic hypokalemia as rapid increase of potassium has been associated with adverse effects.

- For severe hypokalemia, potassium chloride is usually recommended to be given at a dose of 0.5–1 mEq/kg IV given over 30–60 min (max. adult dose 40 mEq).
- If clinical symptoms are not severe, then oral or slower parenteral replacement is recommended.

Table 55.2. Causes of hypokalemia

Effect	Causes
Renal losses	Renal tubular acidosis, hyperaldosteronism, magnesium depletion, leukemia (mechanism uncertain)
Gastrointestinal losses	Vomiting or nasogastric suctioning, diarrhea, enemas or laxative use, ileus
Medication effects	Diuretics (most common cause), beta-adrenergic agonists, steroids, theophylline, aminoglycosides
Transcellular shift	Insulin, alkalosis
Malnutrition or decreased dietary intake	

Source: Greenbaum, 2007.

Box 55.3. Diagnosis and workup for hypokalemia

STEP 1 CONFIRM HYPOKALEMIA
1. Exclude measurement error.
2. Look for clues in patient history:
   - GI illness, diarrhea, laxatives
   - medications
   - renal disorders.

STEP 2 OBTAIN FURTHER ANALYSES
Measure potassium, BUN, creatinine, bicarbonate, glucose, magnesium, calcium, phosphorus. Consider digoxin levels and arterial blood gases (ABG):
- assesses renal function
- excludes other electrolyte disturbances
- hypokalemia can potentiate digitalis-induced arrhythmias if the patient is taking a digitalis preparation
- alkalosis can cause potassium to shift from extracellular to intracellular compartment.

STEP 3 OTHER STUDIES
- Imaging studies: CT scan of the adrenal glands is indicated if mineralocorticoid excess is evident (rarely needed as an emergency).
- ECG:
  - T wave flattening or inverted T waves
  - prominent U wave that appears as QT prolongation
  - ST segment depression
  - ventricular arrhythmias (e.g., premature ventricular contractions, torsade de pointes, ventricular fibrillation)
  - atrial arrhythmias (e.g., premature atrial contractions, atrial fibrillation).

- In considering IV replacement fluids, other electrolyte deficiencies can be considered and combined in the replacement (i.e., if the patient also has low phosphorus, potassium phosphate could be added instead of potassium chloride).

Pearls and pitfalls: hypokalemia

Pearls

1. Severe hypokalemia can result in skeletal, smooth, and heart muscle dysfunction.
2. The most common cause of hypokalemia in children is GI losses during episodes of gastroenteritis.
3. Disorders of potassium balance manifest as cardiac arrhythmias and muscular spasticity and weakness.
4. The safest way to replenish potassium is by mouth.

Pitfalls

1. Failure to monitor rate of potassium replacement; if this is replaced too quick, it can induce symptomatic hyperkalemia even though the total body reserves of potassium might still be less than normal.
2. Failure to monitor and repeat potassium levels during replacement therapy.
3. Failure to recognize and correct other co-existent metabolic disorders (e.g., hypomagnesemia).

- It is important to note that, while adults are often symptomatic with serum potassium levels of 2.5 or lower, children are often more resilient and asymptomatic at this level.

Ongoing monitoring

Cardiac monitoring should be instituted and serum potassium measured every 1–3 h.

Selected references

Chevalier RL. What are normal potassium concentrations in the neonate? What is a reasonable approach to hyperkalemia in the newborn with normal renal function? *Adv Pediatr* 1998;**18**:360–361.

Feld LG, Kaskel FJ, Schoeneman MJ. The approach to fluid and electrolyte therapy in pediatrics. *Adv Pediatr* 1988;**35**:497–535.

Greenbaum LA. Pathophysiology of body fluids and fluid therapy. In Behrman RE, Kliegman RM, Jenson HB (eds.) *Nelson Textbook of Pediatrics*, 17th edn. Philadelphia, PA: Saunders, 2007, pp. 267–319.

Nash PL. Potassium and sodium homeostasis in the neonate. *Neonatal Netw* 2007;**26**:125–128.

Disorders of calcium and magnesium

Barbara Dahl, Bernhard Fassl, and Nikta Forghani

Calcium

The vast majority of total body calcium is contained as hydroxyapatite in bone. The body works to maintain serum calcium levels at the expense of bone in the context of inadequate calcium intake. Calcium is also important in coagulation, muscle contraction, and neuromuscular activation. As calcium is often bound to albumin and other proteins, the reported serum calcium level can be inaccurate in the setting of hypoalbuminemia. Ionized calcium is the preferred measure of active calcium. Alternatively, the corrected calcium (mg/dl) can be estimated using the following equation:

$$\mathrm{Ca(measured\ total)(mg/dl)} + 0.8[4.0 - \mathrm{Albumin(measured)(g/dl)}]$$

where 4.0 g/dl is the average albumin level.

Normal serum calcium is 8.9–10.1 mg/dl, or an ionized calcium of 4.5–5.1 mg/dl. Normal term newborns have slightly lower calcium levels and prematurely born infants may have levels as low as 7 mg/dl.

Calcium homoeostasis is maintained through a complex interaction of vitamin D, parathyroid hormone (PTH), and calcitonin (see Ch. 44).

Hypercalcemia

Symptomatic hypercalcemia is relatively rare. Children are usually asymptomatic until the serum calcium level is >15 mg/dl.

Clinical manifestations

Symptoms can include nausea, emesis, disorientation, and polyuria. In infants, hypercalcemia may present as failure to thrive or poor feeding. Serious cardiac sequelae of hypercalcemia include hypertension, shortened QT interval and ventricular arrythmias.

Etiology

Table 56.1 gives the causes of hypercalcemia.

Diagnosis and suggested workup

Additional studies include a full electrolyte panel, BUN, creatinine, phosphorus, PTH, 25-hydroxyvitamin D level and urine calcium and creatinine.

Principles of management

Box 56.1 describes the management of hypercalcemia.

Table 56.1. Causes of hypercalcemia

Factor	Causes
Parathyroid hormone excess	Primary hyperparathyroidism, transient hyperparathyroidism in neonatal period
Vitamin D excess	Hypervitaminosis, thyrotoxicosis, fat necrosis, granulomatous disease, tuberculosis, fungal infections, lymphoma
Excess calcium intake	Calcium supplements, total parenteral nutrition
Excess calcium reabsorption	Thiazide diuretics, familial hypocalciuria
Increased calcium release from bone	Thyrotoxicosis, hypervitaminosis A, malignancy, immobilization, renal osteodystrophy

Source: adapted from Greenbaum, 2007.

A Practical Guide to Pediatric Emergency Medicine: Caring for Children in the Emergency Department, ed. N. Ewen Amieva-Wang (associate eds. Jamie Shandro, Aparajita Sohoni, and Bernhard Fassl). Published by Cambridge University Press.

Box 56.1. Management of hypercalcemia

Initial therapy

Initial treatment should include hydration with boluses of normal saline, as hypercalcemia often causes polyuria and dehydration. Correcting dehydration will also allow for better renal excretion of calcium.

Once dehydration is corrected

Loop diuretics can also help to increase renal excretion. If hypercalcemia persists, consultation with a pediatric endocrinologist should be made prior to administering medications such as calcitonin or apmidronate to further lower calcium.

All children with symptomatic hypercalcemia should be admitted.

Hypocalcemia

Hypocalcemia is a serum calcium <8.0 mg/dl in children and term infants. Total protein or albumin is necessary to interpret total (but not ionized) calcium levels. Hypocalcemia in children is usually caused by PTH or vitamin D deficiency or pathology.

Clinical manifestations

Signs and symptoms of hypocalcemia depend on age, severity of hypocalcemia, and chronicity of hypocalcemia (acute versus chronic changes). Symptoms are not necessarily tied to a specific calcium blood level:

- *mildly symptomatic acute hypocalcemia*:
  - irritability
  - diarrhea, nausea
  - feeding problems
- *severely symptomatic acute hypocalcemia*:
  - tetany
  - seizures
  - positive Chvostek/Trousseau signs
  - cardiac: prolonged QT, cardiac failure, shock
- *chronic hypocalcemia*:
  - paresthesiae
  - rickets
  - soft tissue calcifications
  - decreased muscle tone, weakness.

Presentation varies with age:

- school-aged children: paresthesiae are a common manifestation
- infants: most commonly generalized tonic–clonic seizures
- neonates: early hypocalcemia commonly presents as seizures within the first 72 h of life.

Etiology

- *Neonatal hypocalcemia*
  - most commonly caused by transient hypoparathyroidism
  - formula-fed infants or infants incorrectly fed with cow's milk can also present with severe hypocalcemia related to excessive intake of phosphorus in the setting of an immature parathyroid gland.
  - exclusively breast-fed infants are at risk of vitamin D deficiency
- *Hypocalcemia in older children*:
  - hypoparathyroidism, pseudohypoparathyroidism (PTH resistance)
  - vitamin D deficiency, calcium, phosphorus, nutritional deficiencies
  - intestinal malabsorption syndromes, e.g., cystic fibrosis or short gut syndrome
  - altered Vitamin D metabolism in genetic disorders, liver disease, renal failure
  - renal calcium losses in renal failure, medications, renal tubular disorder
  - other: tumor lysis, pancreatitis, and sepsis.

Box 56.2 gives the workup for diagnosis of hypocalcemia.

Box 56.2. Diagnosis and suggested workup for hypocalcemia

STEP 1 CONFIRM HYPOCALCEMIA

1. Exclude measurement error.
2. An ionized calcium should always be measured if there is clinical concern for hypocalcemia.

STEP 2 ANALYSES FOR SEVERE HYPOCALCEMIA

- ECG: QT prolongation.
- Serum phosphorus, magnesium.
- Serum alkaline phosphatase.
- Parathyroid hormone, 25-hydroxyvitamin D, 1,25-dihydroxyvitamin D.
- Screen for kidney function: BUN, creatinine.
- Liver function tests, including albumin.
- Urine analysis for urine creatinine:calcium ratio.

Principles of management

Box 56.3 give the principles of management. A number of general principles apply:

- calcium gluconate is preferable when only peripheral IV access is available, as calcium chloride can cause severe chemical burns if it extravasates
- the dose of calcium gluconate can be repeated as frequently as needed while calcium levels are monitored and continue to be low
- consider starting a continuous infusion if multiple boluses are needed
- all children with symptomatic hypocalcemia should be admitted
- patients with severe hypocalcemia should be admitted to the ICU; it takes several days of treatment for serum calcium levels to normalize.

Box 56.3. Principles of management of hypocalcemia

Mildly symptomatic acute hypocalcemia

1. Oral calcium replacement: should not be used for initial management of symptomatic hypocalcemia.
2. Calcium gluconate 10% IV: for a neonate/older child use calcium gluconate to provide 50–100 mg elemental calcium/kg daily in divided doses, q. 4–8 h or as continuous infusion.

Severely symptomatic acute hypocalcemia

1. Calcium gluconate 10% IV: 1–2 ml/kg (100–200 mg/kg). Calcium gluconate is preferable when only peripheral access is available.
2. Continue to use bolus doses if the patient continues to be symptomatic or is still hypocalcemic.
3. Calcium chloride IV (with central access): 20 mg/kg over 3–4 min.
4. Correct hypomagnesemia: 0.5 mEq/kg (6 mg/kg) or 0.125 ml/kg of 50% magnesium sulfate.

Chronic hypocalcemia

Treatment can be deferred to inpatient physician.

Magnesium

Magnesium is another common electrolyte in the body. Its main function is to serve as a cofactor in many enzymatic reactions. It is also necessary for nerve conduction.

Hypermagnesemia

The most common form of hypermagnesemia seen in the pediatric population is in neonates born to mothers who received IV magnesium therapy. Other causes include increased intake with laxative and antacids or decreased excretion by the kidneys.

Clinical manifestations

Symptoms of hypermagnesemia include hypotonia, hyporeflexia, weakness, and even paralysis. Patients are not usually symptomatic until the serum magnesium is >4.5 mg/dl. Severe hypermagnesemia (>15 mg/dl) can cause complete heart block and cardiac arrest, often preceded by prolongation of PR, QRS, and QT intervals on ECG.

Management

Most patients are able to excrete excess magnesium, except in the setting of renal failure, when dialysis may be indicated. Increased fluid hydration and loop diuretics can help to expediate renal excretion of excess magnesium. In the case of ECG changes, calcium gluconate 100 mg/kg IV can have a temporary effect on stabilizing the heart.

Hypomagnesemia

Hypomagnesemia is most often caused by excessive renal or GI losses. It can also be seen in acute pancreatitis. Infants of diabetic mothers can also present with hypomagnesemia as a result of chronic maternal magnesium losses. Symptoms of hypomagnesemia are most often associated with an accompanying hypocalcemia caused by impairment of PTH release. These symptoms can include seizures and/or tetany. This usually occurs at serum magnesium levels <0.7 mg/dl.

Management

Treatment of symptomatic hypomagnesemia is achieved in the acute setting with IV magnesium sulfate at doses of 25 to 50 mg/kg infused slowly over 4 h. This dose can be repeated up to every 6 h. Replacement can also be achieved with oral magnesium supplements.

Pearls and pitfalls

Pearls

1. Any patient presenting with a seizure should be assessed for hypocalcemia.
2. If hypocalcemia is confirmed, intact parathyroid hormone and vitamin D should be measured together with basic electrolytes.
3. Initial therapy should include hydration with boluses of normal saline, as hypercalcemia often causes polyuria and dehydration.

Pitfalls

1. Failure to monitor for electrolyte shifts after initiating treatment for hypercalcemia.
2. Failure to correct hypomagnesemia when trying to treat hypocalcemia.
3. Failure to correct for serum albumin level when considering a diagnosis of hypocalcemia.

Selected references

Feld LG, Kaskel FJ, Schoeneman MJ. The approach to fluid and electrolyte therapy in pediatrics. *Adv Pediatr* 1988;**35**:497–535.

Hsu SC, Levine MA. Perinatal calcium metabolism: physiology and pathophysiology. *Semin Neonatol* 2004;**9**:23–36.

Zhou P, Markowitz M. Hypocalcemia in infants and children. *Pediatr Rev* 2009;**30**:190–192.

Hypoglycemia

Barbara Dahl, Bernhard Fassl, and Nikta Forghani

Introduction

Glucose plays a central role in energy production in the human body and is the preferred energy substrate of the brain. Glucose levels are carefully maintained through complex interactions of the autonomic nervous system and by hormones to enhance glucose production from protein or fat stores (gluconeogenesis) and from breakdown of glycogen (glycogenolysis). Hypoglycemia is defined as:

- in children, a blood glucose of <45 mg/dl
- in neonates, a blood glucose of <30 mg/dl (1.65 mmol/l) in the first 24 h of life and <40 mg/dl (2.5 mmol/l) thereafter; however, there is considerable disagreement about the "normality" of these blood glucose levels in newborns if associated conditions such as hypoxemia and ischemia are present.

Table 57.1 shows the spectrum of hypoglycemia and the numerical ranges associated with each stage.

Table 57.1. Spectrum of hypoglycemia

Severity	Blood glucose (mg/dl)	Symptoms
Mild	40–45	Asymptomatic
Moderate	30–40	Tachycardia, sweating, weakness, irritability
Severe	20–30	Seizures or altered mental status
Very severe	<20	Coma, shock, seizure status

Clinical manifestations

The clinical presentation of hypoglycemia differs significantly according to the patient's age. In newborns and small infants, hypoglycemia can present with:

- hypotonia, poor feeding, lethargy
- respiratory distress, cyanosis
- apnea, hypothermia
- seizures.

In childhood, hypoglycemia usually presents as behavior problems, ravenous appetite, and inattention. In these patients, hypoglycemia may be misdiagnosed as epilepsy or attention-deficit hyperactivity disorder.

The clinical symptoms associated with hypoglycemia can also be categorized by organ system. Specifically, hypoglycemia causes adrenergic activation and a depletion of glucose to the CNS (neuroglycopenia). The adrenergic response produces tachycardia, diaphoresis, trembling, and hunger. The CNS symptoms include altered mental status, lethargy, weakness, headache, irritability, seizures, or coma.

Of note, the younger the child is, the more difficult it may be to make this diagnosis. For example, newborns and infants with hypoglycemia often present with respiratory distress or episodes of ALOC. Hypoglycemia should always be ruled out in the neonatal population, especially given the difficulty with obtaining hard clinical or historical signs in this age group.

Etiology

Causes of hypoglycemia in the immediate newborn period differ significantly from those in later infancy or childhood. Most cases of mild hypoglycemia in childhood are associated with prolonged fasting such as in GI illnesses. In these cases, hypoglycemia is easily reversible and does not recur. This form of hypoglycemia is associated with significant ketosis (ketotic hypoglycemia) secondary to fatty acid breakdown and ketone formation to compensate for low glucose availability. Severe or recurrent hypoglycemia, particularly in small infants, warrants a full workup. Most cases are associated with hyperinsulinemic states during pregnancy or small-for-gestational-age infants or premature infants. **Hypoglycemia of the newborn** is the most common cause of hypoglycemia in children. It is caused by either inadequate substrate availability to allow the newborn to resume adequate glucose production after birth or by a hyperinsulinemic state in the neonate.

A Practical Guide to Pediatric Emergency Medicine: Caring for Children in the Emergency Department, ed. N. Ewen Amieva-Wang (associate eds. Jamie Shandro, Aparajita Sohoni, and Bernhard Fassl). Published by Cambridge University Press.

Hypoglycemia in otherwise normal infants and children (ketotic hypoglycemia)

The most common reason for hypoglycemia in a toddler is ketotic hypoglycemia, which is thought to be caused by insufficient muscle stores of alanine and, therefore, impaired defenses against a fasting state. Children will often present with their first episode at 18–36 months, but cases have been documented as early as 9 months. Commonly, the history will include a prolonged fast (a missed dinner meal or illness causing decreased oral intake) overnight and morning hypoglycemia in an otherwise healthy child. The child may also be underweight, contributing to low muscle stores. The hypoglycemia can be quite severe and may even result in a seizure. The presence of ketones is essential for this diagnosis as fatty acid oxidation defects can also present at this age. Of course, this is a diagnosis of exclusion, and other more severe reasons for ketotic hypoglycemia should also be explored and ruled out. After acute intervention with dextrose, the treatment simply includes avoidance of prolonged periods of fasting. Most children will "grow out" of this condition by 10 years of age.

Persistent/recurrent hypoglycemia at all ages or severe hypoglycemia in the postnatal period

Persistent or recurrent hypoglycemia at any age, or severe hypoglycemia in the postnatal period is associated with a wide variety of conditions:

- inadequate glucose consumption: feeding problems (cleft palate, oropharyngeal malformations, fistulae, etc.)
- impaired glucose production: liver disease/damage, impaired glycogenolysis (e.g., glucose 6-phosphatase deficiency), impaired gluconeogenesis (e.g., hyperglycinemia, pyruvate decarboxylase deficiency)
- inborn errors of metabolism: fatty acid oxidation defects (carnitine deficiencies), enzyme defects (galactosemia, hereditary fructose intolerance), aminoacidopathies (tyrosinemia, maple syrup urine disease, propionic acidemia, glutaric aciduria, methylmalonic acidemia)
- hormone deficiencies: panhypopituitarism, growth hormone deficiency, ACTH deficiency, Addison's disease, glucagon deficiency
- insulin excess: beta-cell hyperplasia, nesidioblastosis, familial leucine sensitivity
- liver disease
- drugs/toxins (ingestions): salicylates, alcohol, propranolol, Vacor rat poison (*N*-3-pyridylmethyl *N*′-*p*-nitrophenyl urea), oral hypoglycemic agents (sulfonylureas), insulin
- systemic illnesses: sepsis, shock
- other: factitious hypoglycemia.

Diagnosis and workup

The workup of hypoglycemia depends on the age of the child, the severity of the hypoglycemic episode, and the frequency of attacks. For example, mild hypoglycemia that is easily reversible in an older child with a history of vomiting/diarrhea and poor intake usually does not require a full workup and is best treated symptomatically until the underlying disease has improved. However, hypoglycemia in infants can be caused by a multitude of conditions and usually requires hospital admission and careful diagnostic workup. Box 57.1 provides a suggested diagnostic approach according to patient age.

Box 57.1. Diagnostic workup for a child with hypoglycemia

STEP 1 INITIAL WORKUP

1. Confirm hypoglycemia.
2. Look for clues as to the etiology in the patient history and physical examination:
   - large for gestational age (LGA) infant, infant of diabetic mother
   - premature infant, small for gestational age (SGA)
   - macroglossia, ear creases: (Beckwith–Wiedeman syndrome)
   - ambiguous genitalia: congenital adrenal hyperplasia
   - hyperkalemia: congenital adrenal hyperplasia (CAH)
   - micropenis: panhypopituitarism
   - darkening of skin: Addison disease
   - recurrent hypoglycemia with minor illnesses: inborn error of metabolism (IEM)
   - presents as shock: IEM, commonly fatty acid oxidation defect
   - lack of metabolic acidosis or urine/serum ketones: fatty acid oxidation defect
   - ingestion in older children: sulfonylureas, salicylate
   - conjugated hyperbilirubinemia: liver disease, common also in IEMs such as galactosemia, tyrosinemia.
3. Check serum electrolytes, bicarbonate, urine and serum ketones; check bilirubin if jaundiced.

STEP 2 FOR SEVERE/RECURRENT HYPOGLYCEMIA

Note: All metabolic studies are best sent before the metabolic state of the child is fully corrected.

1. Check serum insulin level, growth hormone (GH), cortisol, lactate, pyruvate, ammonia, amino acids, carnitine and acylcarnitine; check urine organic acids.
2. Test for IEM if there is known or suspected liver disease, metabolic acidosis, or abnormal odors detected on examination.
3. Consider the following findings to help to narrow the differential (if results are available in the ED):
   - inappropriate insulin:glucose ratio (>0.25): islet cell hyperplasia, exogenous insulin
   - low GH: isolated GH deficiency, hypopituitarism
   - low cortisol: CAH, hypoituitarism, adrenal insufficiency.

Box 57.2. Treatment of hypoglycemia by severity

Mild and moderate hypoglycemia (blood glucose 30–45 mg/dl)

Patients with blood glucose 40–45 mg/dl are usually asymptomatic; as blood glucose reduces to 30–40 mg/dl, patients become tachycardic with sweating, weakness, and irritability.

1. Glucose IV or oral: 0.25 g/kg.
2. Orange juice (oral): 20 ml/kg.
3. Dextrose: an initial IV bolus of 0.25 g/kg (2.5 ml/kg 10% dextrose or 1 ml/kg 25% dextrose).
4. Maintenance dextrose: 6–8 mg/kg per min IV, by giving 10% dextrose at 1.5× maintenance rate.
5. Evaluate for underlying causes: sepsis, infection.
6. Recheck blood glucose every 30 min.

Note: Route of administration depends on child age and associated conditions such as vomiting or ability to drink.

Severe and very severe hypoglycemia (blood glucose <30 mg/dl)

When blood glucose falls to 20–30 mg/dl, there can be seizures or altered mental status; a further reduction to <20 mg/dl leads to coma, shock, and seizures.

1. Glucose IV: 0.25 g/kg.
2. Dextrose: an initial IV bolus of 0.25 g/kg (2.5 ml/kg 10% dextrose or 1 ml/kg 25% dextrose).
3. Maintenance dextrose: 6–8 mg/kg per min IV, by giving 10% dextrose at 1.5× maintenance rate.
4. Recheck glucose every 15 min.
5. Treat seizures: lorazepam 0.1 mg/kg; phenobarbital load 15 mg/kg.
6. Treat shock: fluid boluses.
7. Evaluate for underlying causes: sepsis, infection.
8. If glucose level remains <40 mg/dl or patient remains symptomatic: repeat bolus and increase maintainance to 10–12 mg/kg per min.
9. Hyperinsulinism: treatment-refractory hypoglycemia is often caused by hyperinsulinism. Hyperinsulinism may require extended periods of IV glucose administration and continuous glucose monitoring. The diagnosis of hyperinsulinism depends on documentation of an inappropriately elevated insulin:glucose ratio (>0.25).
   - consult with ICU and endocrinologist.
   - consider glucagon 0.03 mg/kg SC or IM to max. of 1 mg.
   - consider hydrocortisone 75–100 mg/m^2.

Management

Hypoglycemia should be treated as quickly as possible. Rapid correction is essential to prevent further metabolic decompensation and irreversible damage to the brain. Patients of all ages with hypoglycemia require supportive care, IV access, supplemental oxygen, and close monitoring. The treatment goal is to keep blood glucose levels >45 mg/dl. Box 57.2 shows treatment options for the varying levels of hypoglycemia.

Disposition

Any child with hypoglycemia not directly related to insulin therapy should be admitted for careful glucose monitoring and further evaluation. If hyperinsulinism is suspected, a multidisciplinary approach (involving pediatric endocrinologists, surgeons, and pathologists) will be required during hospitalization to determine the underlying cause.

Pearls and pitfalls

Pearls

1. Most cases of mild hypoglycemia in childhood are associated with prolonged fasting such as in GI illnesses. In these cases hypoglycemia is easily reversible and does not recur. This form of hypoglycemia is associated with significant ketosis.
2. Hypoglycemia in infants and children usually requires hospital admission and careful diagnostic workup.
3. Hypoglycemia should be treated expeditiously to avoid neurologic complications.
4. Consider ingestion or poisoning in an older child with new-onset hypoglycemia.

Pitfalls

1. Failure to perform a sepsis workup in a hypoglycemic infant.
2. Failure to consider/make the diagnosis of hypoglycemia in a child who presents with non-specific symptoms (ie vomiting, lethargy, seizure).
3. Failure to expeditiously treat hypoglycemia to avoid neurologic complications.
4. Failure to monitor for and treat recurrent hypoglycemia in the ED.

Selected references

Flood R, Chiang V. Rate and prediction of infection in children with diabetic ketoacidosis. *Am J Emerg Med* 2001;**19**:270–273.

Fourtner SH, Weinzimer SA, Levitt Katz LE. Hyperglycemic hyperosmolar non-ketotic syndrome in children with type 2 diabetes. *Pediatr Diabetes* 2005;**6**:129–135.

Glaser N, Barnett P, McCaslin I, for the Pediatric Emergency Medicine Collaborative Research Committee of the American Academy of Pediatrics. Risk factors for cerebral edema in children with diabetic ketoacidosis. The Pediatric Emergency Medicine Collaborative Research Committee of the American Academy of Pediatrics. *N Engl J Med* 2001;**344**:264–269.

Lawrence SE, Cummings EA, Gaboury I, Daneman D. Population-based study of incidence and risk factors for cerebral edema in pediatric diabetic ketoacidosis. *J Pediatr* 2005;**146**:688–692.

Levin DL. Cerebral edema in diabetic ketoacidosis. *Pediatr Crit Care Med* 2008;**9**:320–329.

Rosenbloom AL. Hyperglycemic crises and their complications in children. *J Pediatr Endocrinol Metab* 2007; **20**:5–18.

Sherry NA, Levitsky LL. Management of diabetic ketoacidosis in children and adolescents. *Paediatr Drugs* 2008;**10**:209–215.

Sperling, M, Dunger, D, Acerini, C, *et al.* ESPE/LWPES consensus statement on diabetic ketoacidosis in children and adolescents. *J Pediatr* 2003;**113**:133–140.

Section

10 Gastrointestinal emergencies

Expert reviewers: Dorsey M. Bass, Janice Lowe, and Claudia Mueller

Chapter 58 Gastrointestinal introduction and abdominal pain

Marcela P. Mendenhall, Ram S. Duriseti, and Teresa S. Wu

Introduction to gastrointestinal disorders

Abdominal complaints represent approximately 10% of ED visits. Emergency conditions are usually secondary to infection, vascular compromise, bleeding, or rapid dehydration (Table 58.1). Abdominal emergencies in neonates are rare, but represent unique clinical entities which must be recognized promptly to avoid life-threatening complications. These are discussed in Ch. 157.

Many different pathologies can manifest with GI complaints. Abdominal pain is caused not only by GI etiologies but also by hemotologic, infectious, respiratory, and toxicological causes. Similarly, vomiting can be caused by systemic illness as well as pathology in almost any organ system. Jaundice can occur from hematologic disorders, resulting in increased circulating bilirubin, as well as from liver dysfunction (Chs. 64 and 67).

This chapter will begin the discussion of GI pathology, addressing the symptoms of undifferentiated abdominal pain. Other chapters will cover specific diagnoses and a special chapter (Ch. 73) will discuss appropriate diagnostic imaging for different suspected causes of GI pathology.

Pediatric abdominal pain

The approach to a child with abdominal pain presents a challenge. The limited expressive capacity of children, the fear and anxiety induced by interacting with strangers, and the child's limited cognitive capacity all complicate a clinical complaint that is notoriously nebulous. The complaint of abdominal pain can indicate an acute surgical or medical GI condition, but it can also be associated with extra-abdominal etiologies such as pharyngitis and lower lobe pneumonia. Children can also have unique GI diagnoses such as intussusception that do not usually occur in adults.

Presentation and clinical evaluation of a child with abdominal pain

Abdominal pain can be considered in three distinct categories: visceral/splanchnic, parietal/somatic, and referred pain. This can potentially aid in diagnosis; however, often a child cannot describe the pain. The complaint of pain should be distinguished from the presence of tenderness on palpation. One of the most important portions of the pediatric examination is observing the child before the clinician enters the room. Observing their level of activity, their willingness to run/jump/move, absence of movement while lying in bed, or bouts of crying suggestive of pain are invaluable to formulating a clinical impression. We prefer distracted abdominal examinations for the anxious child. Either distraction with a light, keys, or other device during the examination or having a trusted parent hold the child over the shoulder with the child's back facing the examiner serves this purpose well. Even in the seemingly calm child, separating them from the parent to place them on a bed for a "proper examination" will be suboptimal in a large number of children because of the induced anxiety, agitation, and crying.

One helpful diagnostic aid in evaluating the cause of abdominal pain is the age of the patient. Different abdominal diagnoses are more common in certain age groups (Table 58.2).

While the PQRST (pain, quality, radiation, severity and timing) of the abdominal pain is always important, it is critical to actively elicit associated symptoms; relationship of pain with meals, urination, defecation and movement; and the effect of the pain on level of activity. Children often are not able or will not offer this history. If a child is school age, the parent will often not know the quality of the stools (constipation) or the number of times a child has urinated or defecated during the day. In the adolescent child, sexual history should be obtained alone without parents or friends in the room.

Surgical conditions presenting with abdominal pain usually have characteristic histories or associated physical findings.

A Practical Guide to Pediatric Emergency Medicine: Caring for Children in the Emergency Department, ed. N. Ewen Amieva-Wang (associate eds. Jamie Shandro, Aparajita Sohoni, and Bernhard Fassl). Published by Cambridge University Press.

Table 58.1. Age-based differential diagnoses of abdominal emergencies

Disease by age group	Clinical presentation
Neonates	
Malrotation with mid-gut volvulus	Bilious or chronic intermittent vomiting, abdominal pain, feeding difficulties or failure to thrive; while malrotation can manifest at any age, 50–75% present at <1 month of age, 90% present at <1 year of age
Necrotizing enterocolitis	Vomiting, abdominal distention, ± fever; often with feeding intolerance, temperature instability
Omphalitis	Erythema of umbilicus, ± fever, ± history of delayed cord separation; usually occurs on day of life 5–9, just prior to cord separation
Hirschsprung's disease	Abdominal distention, diarrhea
Infant	
Pyloric stenosis	Projectile, non-bilious vomiting; 2 to 6 weeks of age
Incarcerated inguinal hernia	Inguinal mass, vomiting; any age
Meckel's diverticulum	Rectal bleeding or bilious vomiting; any age
Intussusception	Vomiting, colicky abdominal pain, listlessness; 3 months to 3 years; most common in those aged 5–9 months
Malrotation with mid-gut volvulus	As in neonate
Child	
Appendicitis	Vomiting, anorexia, abdominal pain ± fever; can present at any age but morbidity and mortality are significantly greater the younger the patient
Meckel's diverticulum	As in infant
Intussusception	As in infant
Adolescent	
Appendicitis	Typically vague periumbilical pain that migrates into the RLQ; fever, anorexia, nausea and vomiting often accompany the pain. Appendicitis is uncommon in infants (<5% of cases)
Ectopic pregnancy	Clinical symptoms usually manifest 4–8 weeks after conception; symptoms of early pregnancy (nausea, breast tenderness) classically associated with amenorrhea, vaginal bleeding, and abdominal pain, ± cervical motion tenderness, ± adnexal mass
Ruptured/hemorrhagic ovarian cysts	Symptoms of severe abdominal pain, which can mimic peritonitis

Physical findings of distention, localized abdominal tenderness, rebound, guarding, or decreased bowel sounds are concerning for a surgical abdomen. Intussusception commonly occurs in children under 1 year of age. It is associated with colicky abdominal pain and listlessness; an abdominal mass can be present (see Ch. 66). Two-thirds of cases of malrotation with volvulus are diagnosed within the first month of life and are associated with bilious vomiting (see Ch. 157). Appendicitis (rare under 3 years of age) classically presents with dull periumbilical pain migrating to the right lower quadrant (RLQ) and associated signs of infection, but it can present atypically. Testicular torsion, inguinal hernia, ovarian cyst, rupture or torsion, tubo-ovarian abscess, and ectopic pregnancy can usually be ruled in or out with careful history and physical examination or ancillary testing in the case of pregnancy. Abdominal pain associated with GI bleeding deserves careful evaluation (see Ch. 63).

Serious medical conditions associated with abdominal pain should also have historical clues as well as physical findings. Gastroenteritis causes discomfort associated with vomiting and diarrhea. Pneumonia and pelvic inflammatory disease may or may not be occult. Urinary tract infection and viral infections, including streptococcal pharyngitis, can also cause vague abdominal pain. The vasculitis Henoch–Schönlein purpura (see Ch. 85), which is a uniquely pediatric diagnosis, can also cause severe abdominal pain. It can be associated with purpuric lesions on the lower extremities (see Fig. 85.3, p. 381) and renal symptoms but often the abdominal pain occurs initially.

Abdominal pain that occurs chronically with no associated symptoms and with a normal growth pattern and physical

Table 58.2. Age-based differential for abdominal pain

Age group	Causes
Infants	Anatomic abnormalities of the GI tract
	Hirschsprung's disease
	Incarcerated hernia
	Infantile colic
	Necrotizing enterocolitis
	Pyloric stenosis
	Intestinal malrotation ± volvulus
	Intussusception
	Gastroesophageal reflux disease (GERD)
	Milk protein allergy
Toddler/ preschooler	Anatomic abnormalities of the GI tract
	Appendicitis
	Foreign body ingestion
	Henoch–Schönlein purpura
	Incarcerated hernia
	Intestinal malrotation ± volvulus
	Intussusception
	Plumbism
School age	Appendicitis
	Diabetes
	Hemolytic uremic syndrome
	Henoch–Schönlein purpura
	Mesenteric lymphadenitis
	Psychogenic abdominal pain
Pre-teen/teenager	Abdominal epilepsy
	Crohn's disease
	Diabetes mellitus
	Mononucleosis
	Ovarian cyst
	Ovarian or testicular torsion
	Pelvic inflammatory disease
	Psychogenic abdominal pain
	Pregnancy (intrauterine or ectopic)
	Ulcerative colitis
Any age	Anatomic abnormalities of the GI tract
	Child abuse
	Cholelithiasis/cholecystitis
	Constipation
	Cystic fibrosis
	Foreign body/bezoar
	Food intolerance
	Gastritis
	Gastroenteritis
	Hepatitis
	Mumps
	Pancreatitis
	Peptic ulcer disease
	Pinworms
	Perforated viscus/peritonitis
	Pharyngitis
	Pneumonia
	Pyelonephritis
	Sickle cell anemia
	Small bowel obstruction
	Trauma
	Tumor
	Urinary tract infection
	Urolithiasis
	Venomous bites or stings

examination is probably benign. Constipation is underdiagnosed and inadequately treated by both primary and emergency clinicians. Lactose intolerance, celiac disease, irritable bowel, and functional abdominal pain are also on the differential.

Diagnostic evaluation and management

Pain control should be offered to all children upon their arrival to the ED. Studies have shown that even narcotics do not impede the diagnosis of a surgical abdomen. Acetaminophen can often provide appropriate relief for vague pain.

Given the number of children that visit the ED for abdominal pain, it is not practical, or probable, to obtain laboratory analyses on all even if they were diagnostic. Laboratory tests and imaging should be based upon the history and physical examination.

Observation and serial examinations

In EDs with pediatric observation units, GI illness is the second most common cause of admission to the unit. In the case of appendicitis, brief periods of observation on the order of 10 to 12 h increased diagnostic accuracy for appendicitis, decreasing both false positives and false negatives. Repeat examination is not precluded by the absence of an observation unit. It is our routine practice to bring patients back for re-examination within 6 to 12 h, or sooner as symptoms dictate, or to keep the patient in the main ED for 6 h of observation when patient flow permits. While not formally studied, in our experience, observation is a safe and effective means to provide a thorough evaluation while decreasing exposure to potentially harmful ionizing radiation.

Disposition

In patients with no final diagnosis or definitive etiology of abdominal pain, close follow-up should be arranged. The patient should understand that no diagnosis is not the same as "not having anything wrong." Patients who are dehydrated or unable to tolerate liquids should be admitted for IV hydration. Children with persistent severe pain or the possibility of a surgical abdomen should be admitted and observed.

Pearls and pitfalls

Pearls

1. In the infant, vomiting with abdominal distention equals a life-threatening process until proven otherwise.
2. Bilious vomiting in a neonate is mechanical intestinal obstruction secondary to malrotation and volvulus until proven otherwise.

Pitfalls

1. Failure to consider an age-based differential diagnosis in cases of abdominal pain.
2. Failure to consider Henoch–Schönlein purpura in a child with abdominal pain and a purpuric rash on the buttocks and lower extremities.

Selected references

McCollough M, Sharieff G. Abdominal pain in children. *Pediatr Clin North Am* 2006;**53**:107–137, vi.

Mace S. Pediatric observation medicine. *Emerg Med Clin North Am* 2001;**19**:239–254.

Chapter 59

Appendicitis

Aparajita Sohoni

Introduction

Appendicitis is a common pediatric disease, with approximately 70 000 cases diagnosed annually in the USA. The natural course of appendicitis occurs over a 24–36 h time period, during which the appendiceal lumen first becomes occluded (either by a fecolith, lymphoid tissue, a foreign body, or rarely malignancies or parasites) and then distended. The distension progresses until arterial insufficiency and subsequent tissue ischemia result. Bacterial translocation into the wall of the appendix produces transmural inflammation, followed by invasion into the parietal peritoneum. The pain pattern described by patients classically involves periumbilical pain migrating to the RLQ as the appendiceal inflammation progresses.

Pediatric patients differ from adults in their ability to provide a history or comply with a physical examination, in the range of diagnostic studies available, and in the likelihood of complications such as perforation or abscess formation. Within the pediatric age group, the risk of appendicitis varies with age. Neonates only rarely develop appendicitis as the appendix has a "less-susceptible" funnel-shape at this age. Neonates are frequently in a recumbent position, do not usually have upper respiratory tract or GI infections causing lymphadenopathy, and consume a soft diet. These factors contribute to the low incidence of appendicitis in this age group.

In older children (1 year of age and older), the shape of the appendix transitions into the typical adult shape. This structure is more susceptible to obstruction, thus increasing the likelihood of developing appendicitis. The maturing appendix is also more susceptible to rupture, making the incidence of appendiceal perforation at time of diagnosis relatively high in the pediatric population. One-third of children will have ruptured prior to operative intervention. This percentage also varies with the age of the child: those younger than 4 years have higher perforation rates (80–100%), while adolescents aged 10–17 years have lower rates (10–20%).

Clinical presentation

The history and physical examination is key to the diagnosis of appendicitis. While older adolescents may be able to give an accurate history, in younger children and infants the parents or caregivers should be questioned regarding the onset of symptoms and change in patterns of behavior, eating, irritability, stooling, urination, and presence or absence of fever.

Pediatric patients with appendicitis almost universally present with abdominal pain. However the validity of the symptoms and signs of appendicitis in pediatric patients is controversial. It is suggested in the literature that absence of RLQ pain or fever decrease, and migration of pain to the RLQ, and the presence of vomiting or diarrhea increase the likelihood of appendicitis.

A thorough physical examination to exclude other causes of abdominal pain is key. The physical examination should be done after positioning the child supine. The examiner should focus on the child's face for evidence of pain or discomfort rather than looking at the abdomen. The examiner should also avoid expecting verbal responses to questions such as "Does this hurt?" given the child's anxiety, suggestibility, and emotional maturity. The presence of guarding, indicating localized peritonitis, and rigidity, suggesting generalized peritonitis, should be assessed. If the patient is not compliant with the physical examination, alternative maneuvers to assess for peritonitis such as having the patient hop from one foot to the other, bumping the bed prior to examining the patient, or examining the patient while he/she is asleep may be useful.

Diagnostic studies

The appropriate way to diagnose appendicitis in a pediatric patient is a controversial topic. If the clinical examination and history are strongly suggestive, imaging may be withheld if the pediatric surgeon is amenable. If imaging is warranted, the main modalities are ultrasound or CT of the abdomen and pelvis. Concern for radiation-induced-malignancy, particularly

A Practical Guide to Pediatric Emergency Medicine: Caring for Children in the Emergency Department, ed. N. Ewen Amieva-Wang (associate eds. Jamie Shandro, Aparajita Sohoni, and Bernhard Fassl). Published by Cambridge University Press.

in the pediatric population, has increased the desire for, and use of, abdominal ultrasound. Ultrasound is an appropriate first-line diagnostic test for appendicitis. If the appendix is not seen on ultrasound, or if the findings are equivocal, a CT should be obtained where there is a high level of suspicion for appendicitis.

Additional studies in the workup of a patient with possible appendicitis include a urinalysis to exclude urinary tract infections or pyelonephritis. White blood cells in the urine can also result from an inflamed appendix overlying the bladder, so care should be taken when interpreting these results. A CBC may also be done.

Management

Initial management of a patient with acute appendicitis consists of prompt antibiotic and IV fluid resuscitation as well as early surgical consultation. Antibiotics should be started once the diagnosis of acute appendicitis is made to prevent wound infection or intra-abdominal abscess formation when perforation has already occurred. Appropriate choices include cefoxitin or piperacillin/tazobactam. In penicillin-allergic patients, gentamicin in combination with either clindamycin or metronidazole is appropriate. Given the higher rates of perforation in pediatric patients, surgeons should be consulted immediately after the diagnosis has been made, or even prior to imaging in strongly suspected cases to avoid diagnostic irradiation. An appendectomy, either laparoscopic or open, is the recommended surgical intervention for acute appendicitis.

If the appendix has already perforated, surgical intervention will not necessarily be performed initially and aggressive antibiotic therapy should be continued. Pain medications, antiemetics, and antipyretics should also be administered as needed.

Disposition

All patients with acute appendicitis should be admitted to a surgical service or transferred to a hospital with a pediatric surgical service.

Pearls and pitfalls

Pearls

1. Pediatric patients have higher rates of perforated appendicitis.
2. Ultrasound is a valid first-line imaging study for the diagnosis of pediatric appendicitis.
3. Antibiotics and fluid resuscitation along with surgery consultation should be initiated as soon as the diagnosis of acute appendicitis is made.

Pitfalls

1. In patients in whom appendicitis is suspected and imaging deemed necessary, ultrasound should be the imaging modality of choice, followed by CT scan if the appendix was not identified.
2. All patients should have appendicitis precautions and close follow-up if discharged.

Selected references

Brennan GD. Pediatric appendicitis: pathophysiology and appropriate use of diagnostic imaging. *CJEM* 2006;**8**:425–432.

Bundy DG, Byerley JS, Liles EA, *et al.* Does this child have appendicitis? *JAMA* 2007;**298**:438–451.

Klein MD. Clinical approach to a child with abdominal pain who might have appendicitis. *Pediatr Radiol* 2007;**37**:11–14.

Chapter 60

Cholelithiasis

Bill Schroeder

Introduction

Although frequent and well studied in adults, gallstones are uncommon in children and the risk factors for their development are still not fully understood (Table 60.1).

Historically, hemolytic diseases such as sickle cell anemia, glucose-6-phosphate dehydrogenase deficiency and spherocytosis have been the most important risk factors for gallstones in children.

Up to 60% of the gallstones in children occur in children 6–12 years of age with documented hemolysis. The prevalence of cholelithiasis in children with hemolytic disease at one children's hospital was 40%. Other risk factors include total parenteral nutrition, GI surgery, and therapy with furosemide or third-generation cephalosporins, particularly in infants being treated for a urinary tract infection. It is becoming more apparent that some common risk factors for adults such as obesity, ileal disease, and family history are also predisposing factors in older children.

One of the biggest differences between gallstones in adults and children is their composition. The vast majority of gallstones in adults are made up of cholesterol (approximately 70–85%). Conversely, more than 70% of gallstones in children are pigmented while only 15%–20% of gallstones are made of cholesterol. This is clinically important because pigmented stones are more likely to be radiopaque since they are commonly composed of calcium salts of unconjugated bilirubin. Plain abdominal radiographs will identify an estimated

Table 60.1. Risk factors for cholelithiasis in children and adolescents

	Infants and children	**Adolescents**
Hemolytic disease	Sickle cell anemia, spherocytosis	Sickle cell anemia, spherocytosis
Gallbladder stasis	Yes	Yes
Prolonged total parenteral nutrition, starvation	Yes	Yes
Starvation	Yes	Rapid weight loss
Medications	Furosemide, third-generation cephalosporins	Oral contraceptives
Illeal resection	Necrotizing enterocolitis, volvulus, trauma	Crohn's disease, trauma
Obesity	–	Yes
Pregnancy	–	Yes
Prematurity	Yes	–
Cystic fibrosis	Yes	Yes
Prolonged hospital stay	Yes	–
Bronchopulmonary dysplasia	Yes	–
Chronic liver disease	Yes	–
Treatment of childhood cancer	–	Yes

A Practical Guide to Pediatric Emergency Medicine: Caring for Children in the Emergency Department, ed. N. Ewen Amieva-Wang (associate eds. Jamie Shandro, Aparajita Sohoni, and Bernhard Fassl). Published by Cambridge University Press.

36–47% of gallstones in children but only 15% in adults. Cholesterol-containing stones are most commonly found in obese adolescent girls who have a strong family history of gallstones. However, they also affect children with ileal disease or bile acid malabsorption, such as in Crohn's disease, ileal resection, and cystic fibrosis.

Clinical presentation

Children with cholelithiasis will often present with the classic symptoms of RUQ pain that radiates to the right scapula accompanied by nausea and vomiting. The most important quality of the pain is that it is recurrent. Also, it is important to keep in mind that younger children are notorious for being unable to localize pain. Children with hemolytic diseases often present with non-specific abdominal pain that is similar to the pain they experience during a hemolytic crisis. Other symptoms that may be helpful are a palpable mass in the RUQ and an intolerance to fatty foods in older children. The infants usually present with non-specific symptoms, the most common of which are fever, vomiting and dehydration.

Management

Management of cholelithiasis in children and adolescents is similar to that of adults and includes pain management, cholecystectomy, or endoscopic retrograde cholangiography. Resolution of the abdominal pain is common after operative management, but not guaranteed. In a recent study, 45% of children had a recurrence of their pain after cholecystectomy or endoscopic retrograde cholangiopancreatography. Attempting to dissolve the gallstones with oral ursodeoxycholic acid is usually not beneficial and generally not recommended. Cholelithiasis diagnosed in infants generally resolves on its own, usually within 1 year, and complications such as cholecystitis are rare.

Disposition

As with management, the disposition is essentially the same in children as in adults. The asymptomatic child can be sent home with follow-up and serial ultrasounds as many stones will resolve on their own, particularly in infants. Children with signs of cholecystitis, choledocholithiasis, or uncontrollable pain secondary to biliary colic should be admitted and treated accordingly.

Pearls and pitfalls

Pearls

1. Gallstones in the pediatric population will continue to increase in prevalence as the average body mass index continues to rise in children and adolescents.
2. Overall the diagnosis and management of cholelithiasis in children is similar to adults.
3. Children with hemolytic disease are at increased risk for cholelithiasis over the general pediatric population.

Pitfalls

1. Failure to consider cholelithiasis in a child with signs, symptoms and risk factors, particularly hemolytic disease.
2. Failure to realize that gallstones in children are more often pigmented and radiopaque than in adults.

Selected references

Kaechele V, Wabtsch M, Thiere D, *et al.* Prevalence of gallbladder stone disease in obese children and adolescents: influence of the degree of obesity, sex and pubertal development. *J Pediatr Gastroenterol Nutr* 2006;**42**:66–70.

Klar A, Branski D, Akerman Y, *et al.* Sludge ball, pseudolithiasis, cholelithiasis, and choledocholithiasis from intrauterine life to 2 years: a 13 year follow-up. *J Pediatr Gastroenterol Nutr* 2005;**40**:477–480.

Rescora F. Cholelithiasis, cholecystitis, and common bile duct stones. *Curr Opin Pediatr* 1997;**9**:276–282.

Wesdorp I, Bosman D, de Graaff A, *et al.* Clinical presentations and predisposing factors of cholelithiasis and sludge in children. *J Pediatr Gastroenterol Nutr* 2000;**31**:411–417.

Chapter 61

Failure to thrive

Marcela P. Mendenhall

Introduction

Failure to thrive (FTT) is classically defined as inadequate weight gain or growth velocity (weight less than the third percentile for age and gender, weight-for-height less than the fifth percentile, or the crossing of two major percentiles on the standard weight curves below a previously established rate of growth). However, it is noteworthy that by definition approximately 3% of normal healthy infants and children will fall below the third percentile. Failure to thrive is classified further into organic or non-organic etiologies, with organic FTT reflecting an underlying medical condition and non-organic FTT mirroring environmental or social problems in the child's life. A mixed etiology may be present when the effects of the organic disease are combined with concurrent psychosocial problems. Non-organic FTT, however, accounts for approximately 70% of total presenting cases.

Failure to thrive is the result of inadequate energy intake, inadequate nutrient absorption or increased losses, increased energy requirements, or ineffective energy utilization (Table 61.1). Inadequate energy intake can be divided into two groups: inadequate nutrient intake or inadequate appetite/inability to eat large amounts. Inadequate nutrient intake may result from inappropriate feeding technique, inappropriate nutrient intake (excess fruit juice or milk intake, incorrect mixing of formula, too little milk letdown), gastroesophageal reflux disease (GERD), mechanical problems (cleft palate, nasal obstruction, adenoid hypertrophy, dental problems, etc.), suck or swallow

Table 61.1. Failure to thrive: age-based differential diagnosis

Feature	Neonatal	3–6 months	7–12 months	>12 months
Inadequate nutrition intake				
Method	Poor suck; breast feeding problems; poor feeding tolerance	Under feeding	Feeding problems, as in younger patients	Coercive feeding
Diet	Poorly mixed formula; inadequate number of feedings	Milk-protein intolerance; improper formula mixing		
Environment	Neglect	Socioeconomic issues		Highly distractable child; distracting environment
Inadequate intake/ability to eat sufficiently				
Digestion and absorption	Metabolic disease, chromosomal anomalies	Celiac disease, cystic fibrosis	Celiac disease, intestinal parasites	Celiac disease, intestinal parasites
Inefficient use of calories	Anatomic defect, chromosomal anomalies	Oral motor dysfunction, congestive heart disease, gastroesophageal reflux		Irritable bowel disease, acquired illness
Psychiatric				New psychosocial stress, eating disorders

A Practical Guide to Pediatric Emergency Medicine: Caring for Children in the Emergency Department, ed. N. Ewen Amieva-Wang (associate eds. Jamie Shandro, Aparajita Sohoni, and Bernhard Fassl). Published by Cambridge University Press.

problems (CNS or neuromuscular problems, esophageal dysmotility), psychosocial problems, or economic deprivation. Inadequate appetite or inability to eat large amounts can result from cardiopulmonary disease, hypo/hypertonia, cerebral palsy, chronic infection or immunodeficiency, anemia, GERD, mechanical digestive problems, chronic constipation, or genetic syndromes. Digestion and absorption of nutrients could be affected by disorders such as cystic fibrosis, celiac disease, short bowel, Crohn's disease, parasites, and chronic cholestasis.

Excessive caloric demand could result from cardiac disease, pulmonary disease, inflammatory bowel disease, acquired immunodeficiency syndrome (AIDS), malignancy, or hyperthyroidism. Inefficient utilization of calories could result from cardiac or pulmonary disease, hyperthyroidism, malignancy, chronic irritable bowel disease, chronic/recurrent infection, renal tubular acidosis, chronic renal or hepatic disease, storage diseases, diabetes mellitus, and inborn errors of metabolism. Lastly, abnormalities of hormonal control of nutrient metabolism can lead to growth retardation. Therefore, a careful history and physical examination must be performed to elicit any clues that could focus the diagnostic approach.

Clinical presentation

Failure to thrive in the infant or child presents in a myriad of ways. Rarely presenting as a primary complaint, clues suggesting FTT can be elicited with a thorough history and examination. Red flags include lack of weight gain, relative decreased weight in comparison to height and head circumference, symmetric weight and height reduction compared with head circumference, and finally stunted weight, height, and head circumference. When presenting as a primary complaint, the patient with FTT is usually referred from their primary care physician who has tried outpatient management without success.

Diagnosis

A thorough history and physical are key to recognizing FTT. The history should include birth history: specifically any medical complications of the pregnancy, known intrauterine growth restriction, toxin or infectious exposures, the mother's emotional response to the pregnancy, gestational age, complications of delivery and problems immediately postpartum. History should also include recurrent infection such as otitis media; pneumonia; and family history, including thyroid disorders, immune disorders, celiac disease, and malignancy.

Social history should elucidate any recent travel, stressors in the infant/child's life, as well as any changes in the family structure. In addition to drug allergies, food allergies should also be elicited as well as diet, specifically how the infant's formula is mixed. Review of systems should look for diarrhea, constipation, snoring or mouth breathing, wheezing or stridor, vomiting or spitting up, gagging, tactile hypersensitivity, prolonged feeding time, polyuria, polydipsia, or polyphagia.

The physical examination starts with key measurements, including height, weight, and head circumference. First and foremost, care must be taken to plot the infant or child on the correct growth chart. Clues in the physical examination include impediments to feeding such as cleft palate, choanal atresia, hypotonia, poor suck, and cardiopulmonary disease.

Initial screening laboratory analyses in the ED may include a CBC, basic or comprehensive metabolic panel (BMP or CMP), urinalysis, lead testing, or inflammatory markers. Anemia often accompanies malnutrition. Electrolyte derangements and acidosis can provide clues as to etiology. Urinalysis is a helpful screening tool for renal and metabolic problems, and ESR and CRP are screening tools for inflammation or infection. Focused testing, usually pursued by the primary care clinician or the inpatient team, may include stool analysis for fat malabsorption and sweat testing to exclude cystic fibrosis, an endocrinologic workup, an immunologic workup, a metabolic workup, a celiac disease workup, inflammatory bowel disease workup, thyroid testing (PPD [Mantoux] test), and even HIV testing. Imaging may be useful including abdominal and chest radiograph, ultrasound, CT or upper GI radiographic series with swallow of dye.

Management

Disposition and subsequent management of FTT depends on the severity. Any failure to gain weight in an infant <2 months of age requires very good follow-up and consideration for admission.

Indications for hospitalization include severe malnutrition, dehydration, serious intercurrent illness, psychosocial issues putting the child at risk for further harm, and failure to respond to months of outpatient management. Management may be enhanced during a hospitalization by providing a controlled environment to assess caloric intake, feeding techniques and parent–child interactions. Overall, in the absence of severe malnutrition or social disarray, FTT evaluation is best done as an outpatient.

Pearls and pitfalls

Pearls

1. Admit a child to the hospital with failure to thrive that is thought to be a result of social causes or neglect, for inpatient evaluation and management.

Pitfalls

1. Failure to recognize failure to thrive by only addressing the presenting complaint or acute illness.
2. Failing to ensure adequate follow-up.
3. Failing to screen for social and physical neglect.

Chapter 62

General gastrointestinal complaints: constipation and gastroesophageal reflux

Marcela P. Mendenhall

Constipation

Introduction

Constipation is a common affliction for infants and children. As infants grow, their intestines continue to mature. Intestinal transit time increases significantly in the first 2 years of life, resulting in decreased stool frequency and increased stool volume. Consequently, infantile and early childhood constipation accounts for nearly 5% of all outpatient visits and more than 25% of referrals to a pediatric gastroenterologist. The etiology is multisystemic and includes diet, psychosocial, and developmental issues as well as possible anatomic, congenital, infectious, inflammatory, metabolic, or endocrinologic derangements.

Constipation is defined by the hard nature of the stool, pain associated with its passage, or the failure to pass three stools in 1 week. Infantile constipation most often results from the inability to coordinate pelvic floor relaxation with the valsalva maneuver. This etiology is most often seen in infants presenting with the isolated complaint of straining with stools and warrants parental reassurance only. Another common etiology of infantile constipation is dietary change, specifically transitioning from breast milk to formula or the addition of solid foods. Of note, iron in formula as a cause of constipation has been disproved by multiple double-blind studies. Other dietary changes include transitioning from formula to cow's milk. Some normal breast-fed infants older than 6 weeks may have very infrequent soft stools (<1/week). This is not abnormal unless the child is uncomfortable or has abdominal distention.

Constipation in childhood is most often a functional issue, occurring during developmental transitions.

Specifically, these developmental transitions center on a loss of privacy, as commonly happens around the time of starting daycare, arrival of a new sibling, an all-day school, as well as toilet training. Childhood constipation can progress to encopresis and even enuresis, rendering the child ineligible for daycare, school, and other social functions.

Clinical presentation and differential diagnosis

In infants and children, constipation can present in a myriad of ways. Neonatal constipation, particularly if the neonate fails to pass stool in the first 24 h, is never normal. A thorough workup should be performed for Hirschprung's disease, cystic fibrosis, spinal cord abnormality, hypothyroidism, or congenital anorectal malformation. The differential diagnosis in infants is the same as in the neonate, with the added consideration of dietary changes. Childhood constipation usually presents with the signs and symptoms mentioned above; however, it can also present solely with poor appetite or weight loss, abdominal pain or vomiting, encopresis, or enuresis. The differential diagnosis still includes neonatal and infantile causes; however, the EP must keep in mind the more common psychosocial and dietary issues that often prevail in this age group.

Diagnosis

The workup of constipation in an infant requires information about birth, passage of meconium, and tolerance of early feeds. For children, a diet history is key, as are any transitions the child has been experiencing related to school, family life, and toilet training. It is important to note the characteristics of the stool and associated signs and symptoms, including anorexia, tenesmus, and/or abdominal pain. Family history should identify family members with thyroid disorders, metabolic disorders, or GI anomalies. Allergies to food and medication, as well as the medications currently being taken by the patient, should be noted. Physical examination should focus on the abdominal examination, including tenderness to palpation, distention, organomegaly, other masses, or palpable stool. A rectal examination is always necessary and should include noting a patent anus, checking the rectal tone and the rectal ampulla, and, lastly, looking for fissures and tears.

Most cases of constipation present to the ED as abdominal pain. The history, abdominal examination, and rectal examination

A Practical Guide to Pediatric Emergency Medicine: Caring for Children in the Emergency Department, ed. N. Ewen Amieva-Wang (associate eds. Jamie Shandro, Aparajita Sohoni, and Bernhard Fassl). Published by Cambridge University Press.

Table 62.1. Medications used for constipation.

Medication	Treatment side effects and comments
Lubricant	Risk of aspiration
Flax seed oil (PO): 1–3 ml/kg daily or divided BID	May chill or give with juice or yoghurt (mixes much better); do not recommend mineral oil as there is a risk of aspiration and pneumonitis
Glycerine suppository	Best for infants; avoid overly judicious use as it has been associated with mucosal breakdown
Biscodyl suppository	Prompt response for toddlers and older children
Fleets (pediatric for <2 years and adult for > 2 years) enema (PR)	Only given in ED
Osmotic laxative	Minimal side effects, can titrate at 3-day intervals for desired stool consistency
Milk of Magnesia (PO): 1–3 ml/kg daily	Minimal side effects
Polyethylene glycol powder (17 g/240 ml water or juice): 1 g/kg daily given in divided doses BID (15 ml/kg per day)	Can be easily titrated to effect; minimal side effects
Stimulants	Would not prescribe in an ED setting in general
Senna (PO)	
Enema (per rectum): pediatric phosphate for <2 years, adult phosphate >2 years	For children in acute discomfort

can be reassuring in cases of constipation. Although a flat plate, one-view, abdominal film is sensitive enough to confirm stool in the colon, it is not specific. Further imaging and laboratory testing should be directed by physical examination and history.

Management

In mild cases, treatment for constipation involves parental reassurance or dietary recommendations. In the infant, adding non-digestible sugar such as fructose, sorbitol, or lactulose that comes in fruit juice will serve well. Specifically, for infants, parents can add 1–2 teaspoons of karo syrup to each bottle. Parents can feed infants older than 3–4 months strained apricots, peaches, pears, and other fruits. For older children, recommendations should include increasing fruits and vegetables in the diet, and prune juice. Parents should be encouraged to keep a symptom diary for 5–7 days to follow up with the primary care clinician.

Pearls and pitfalls: constipation

Pearls

1. Constipation is the most common cause of abdominal pain in children.
2. Constipation can be a life-altering problem for children and their families.

Pitfalls

1. Failure to pass stool in the first 24 h of life is never normal.
2. Never send a child diagnosed with constipation home without a stool plan.

In moderate or long-standing constipation, medical treatment may be indicated. Treatment of constipation has different mechanisms:

- lubricant: lubrication of hard stool
- osmotic laxative: retains water in the stool, adding bulk and hydration to hard stool
- stimulant: increases effectiveness of colonic and rectal muscle contractions.

Table 62.1 lists the options for medications with these properties. Polyethylene glycol (Miralax), an osmotic laxative, is a pharmacologic intervention of choice that can safely be used in infants older than 6 months as well as children and can be titrated to effect. In the child or older infant presenting with constipation, it is important to determine if the stool pattern is abnormal and constipation is an isolated finding associated with other systemic signs and/or symptoms. Once the intervention is successful in the ED and the infant or child has stooled, the parents should be encouraged to keep a symptom diary for 5–7 days to follow up with the primary care clinician.

In mild cases, reassurance should first be given to the parents followed by instructions for home intervention. In more moderate or long-standing constipation, prescribing polyethylene glycol is recommended. In severe cases, a cleanout from below with a pediatric fleets enema is warranted in addition to medication initiation and dietary changes. Hospitalization is often warranted for GI and/or psychiatric intervention. Childhood constipation can often be a vicious cycle as secondary liquid stooling/soiling can develop from fecal impaction, worsening the retention as well as the constipation. Overly enthusiastic use of suppositories or enemas can also lead to constipation.

Gastroesophageal reflux

Non-obstructive, non-infectious vomiting in the neonate or infant is most often due to gastroesophageal reflux (GER). This is the passage of gastric contents into the esophagus or even the oropharynx owing to an incompetent lower esophageal sphincter. It is most commonly apparent around 4 months of age; however, it can start in the neonatal period and persist throughout the first year of life. Most cases of GER resolve by 1 year of age, if not sooner. The symptoms of GER exist along a continuum. Infants with GER are often described as "happy but spitty" babies, while gastroesophageal reflux disease (GERD) is GER that negatively affects the infant.

With GERD, it is believed that the neonate or infant may refuse feeds. This can subsequently cause disturbances in feeding, resulting in poor weight gain, weight loss, or otherwise poor health. Beyond infancy, GERD persists in 5–10% of affected children.

Clinical presentation

Gastroesophageal reflux may present as a chief complaint of vomiting, or frequent spitting up, that is often more concerning to the parent than to the infant. However, GERD presents with subtle signs and symptoms, including irritability, anorexia, anemia, weight loss, failure to thrive, painful or difficult swallowing, and, lastly, arching of the back and/or neck with feeds, the so-called Sandifer syndrome. Controversial associations include reactive airway disease, recurrent pneumonia, or stridor. Both GER and GERD can present solely as an episode of prolonged apnea (apparent life-threatening event) in an infant caused by the vasovagal response from reflux itself. Affected older children may complain of chest or epigastric pain, dysphagia, food impaction, or heartburn. As with infants, affected children may present with a respiratory illness characterized by persistent cough, reactive airway disease, or recurrent pneumonias.

Diagnosis

A thorough history and physical examination is required to diagnose GERD. Key questions in the history include the timing of the vomiting, association with meals, whether or not the infant is bothered by the vomiting, whether or not the infant arches their back or even refuses feeds, and if the infant is gaining weight: GERD is a diagnosis of exclusion. The vomitus must be non-bilious and non-bloody (suspect malrotation and GI bleed, respectively) and not projectile (pyloric stenosis). The infant should not have pain in between feeds, and the infant cannot be lethargic (intussusception, sepsis). Physical examination should rule out organomegaly, abdominal tenderness, a palpable olive, or signs of injury inconsistent with the presentation. Initial laboratory studies may include a CBC, basic metabolic panel, urinalysis and abdominal radiograph.

Pyloric stenosis, malrotation, volvulus and intussusception should always be considered in the differential diagnosis, as well as other non-GI conditions, including non-accidental trauma, intracranial processes, endocrine or metabolic conditions. If the differential diagnoses are seriously considered, further studies and imaging must be sought out.

Once the patient is admitted to the wards, workup will then include an upper GI radiographic series with swallow of dye to rule out anatomic abnormalities, including malrotation, tracheoesophageal fistula, or volvulus. A pH and/or impedence probe will further quantify the reflux. Endoscopy with biopsy will further qualify the reflux. Should pharmacotherapy not alleviate the reflux, a Nissen procedure would ultimately be considered.

Management

Management of GER/GERD is often initiated by the ED physician and followed by the primary care clinician. In the case of GER, parental reassurance is often the best medicine, with the primary care clinician follow-up as a close second. Reflux precautions, described below, may also be recommended.

Pharmacotherapy for GERD should be cautiously initiated in the ED. Initial pharmacotherapy involves acid suppression with histamine H_2 receptor antagonists. Antacids are also used as they neutralize the gastric acid that the stomach produces; however, they are not recommended for young infants because they can result in high levels of aluminum, which can be neurotoxic, and they may leave the infant at high risk for osteopenia. Ranitidine, in addition to the reflux precautions suggested above, is typically the pharmacotherapy of choice in the ED. Proton pump inhibitors are not recommended as initial therapy. Prokinetic agents are also sometimes used by gastroenterologists in the theory that they enhance esophageal peristalsis and accelerate gastric emptying. Should these interventions fail and the infant not thrive despite significant medical management, the physician may consider admission at this point for a hastened evaluation to determine if surgical intervention with G-tube and/or Nissen procedure is warranted. The provider should be aware that $<0.5\%$ of infants with GERD have symptoms warranting surgery.

Pearls and pitfalls: gastroesophageal reflux

Pearls

1. Gastroesophageal reflux is a self-limiting condition. Parental reassurance is often the best medicine.
2. Gastroesophageal reflux disease may warrant pharmacotherapy. In very rare instances, it even warrants surgical intervention.

Pitfalls

1. Subtle presentations of pyloric stenosis, malrotation, and volvulus have been mistaken for gastroesophageal reflux and should always remain in the differential, in addition to non-GI causes such as non-accidental trauma, intracranial processes, endocrine disorders, and metabolic disorders and metabolic disturbances.

Disposition

The majority of infants with GER do not need hospitalization and, after much parental reassurance and education, can safely be discharged home. Further recommendations upon discharge include positional techniques during and immediately following feeds, decreasing volume and increasing frequency of feeds, and burping more often. Positioning or "reflux precautions" includes holding the infant upright at a 30% angle during and after feeds. Bottle propping should always be discouraged. In the older child, discussing lifestyle changes with the parents including weight loss; dietary changes to eliminate chocolate, caffeine and spicy foods; as well as avoiding parental alcohol and cigarette smoking. Should these interventions not help, the ED physician may then start a trial of medical treatment. If the infant or child has already had a trial of appropriately maximized medical treatment, the ED physician may then consult a specialist to consider admission for pH/impedance probe study and possible endoscopy as a workup for possible surgical intervention with a G-tube and/or Nissen procedure.

Selected references

Abi-Hanna A. Constipation and encopresis in children. *Pediatr Rev* 1998;**19**:23.

Barganza S. Gastroesophageal reflux. *Pediatr Rev* 2005;**26**:304–305.

Barkin R, Rosen P. *Emergency Pediatrics: A Guide to Ambulatory Care.* St. Louis, MO: Mosby, 1999.

Reynolds AL. Diagnosing abdominal pain in a pediatric emergency department. *Pediatr Emerg Care* 1992;**8**:126–128.

Chapter 63

Gastrointestinal bleeding and inflammatory bowel disease

David H. Salzman and Michael A. Gisondi

Bleeding

Introduction

Gastrointestinal bleeding in a pediatric patient is an uncommon presentation with numerous potential etiologies. Just as with adults, childhood diseases associated with GI bleeding range from benign, self-limiting conditions to those that are life threatening. Priorities of care include resuscitation and a subsequent search for the source of bleeding. Classically, the source of bleeding in the GI tract has been divided into an upper GI bleed (UGIB) if located cephalad to the ligament of Treitz or a lower GI bleed (LGIB) if caudad. The incidence of GI bleeding in children has been reported as approximately 10% UGIB, 33% in the small intestine, and 50% in the colon or rectum. The diagnosis can often be further simplified by focusing on common etiologies of bleeding based on patient age and findings on physical examination such as organomegaly, purpura, telangiectasias, polyps, fissures, or skin discoloration (Table 63.1).

Management

Presumed GI bleeding should be confirmed and differentiated from food products or medications that can also cause red, maroon, or black stools (bismuth [Pepto-Bismol], iron containing compounds, or foods with red dye) with the use of bedside Hemoccult or Gastroccult testing. If confirmed, the patient's hemodynamic status should be urgently assessed and prompt fluid resuscitation begun. Intestinal transit in children is accelerated compared with that in adults; consequently a nasogastric lavage can be useful to help to localize the source of bleeding and determine if ongoing bleeding is occurring. In UGIB without active bleeding, the patient can be treated with proton pump inhibitors to decrease gastric acidity and should be admitted for monitoring and upper endoscopy. In a patient with ongoing bleeding, treatment includes a proton pump inhibitor, consideration of octreotide or vasopressin, and urgent consultation with a gastroenterologist for upper endoscopy. A stable patient with significant hematochezia and a negative gastric aspirate should be admitted for monitoring, serial CBCs, and evaluation by a gastroenterologist for a possible sigmoidoscopy or colonoscopy.

Specific causes of bleeding

Neonatal gastrointestinal bleed

Swallowed maternal blood

The neonate can ingest maternal blood either during birth or while nursing from an irritated, bleeding nipple. Newborns present with signs mimicking a true GI hemorrhage, with stool

Table 63.1. Differential diagnosis of gastrointestinal bleed in children based on age and location of bleeding

Type/age group	Causes
Upper gastrointestinal bleeding	
Neonate	Swallowed maternal blood, bleeding diathesis, hemorrhagic stress ulcer, gastritis, vascular malformation
Infant	Mallory–Weiss tear, gastritis or peptic ulcer disease, foreign body, esophagitis
Child/adolescent	Esophagitis, Mallory–Weiss tear, gastritis or peptic ulcer disease, foreign body, esophageal varices, nose bleed
Lower gastrointestinal bleeding	
Neonate	Necrotizing entercolitis, cow's milk allergy, malrotation with volvulus, swallowed maternal blood, anal fissure
Infant	Anal fissure, cow's milk allergy, infection, Meckel's diverticulum, intussusception
Child/adolescent	Infection, Meckel's diverticulum, Henoch–Schönlein purpura, polyp, inflammatory bowel disease, hemorrhoid, intussusception

A Practical Guide to Pediatric Emergency Medicine: Caring for Children in the Emergency Department, ed. N. Ewen Amieva-Wang (associate eds. Jamie Shandro, Aparajita Sohoni, and Bernhard Fassl). Published by Cambridge University Press.

that is often maroon or black. The Apt test historically has been recommended to differentiate maternal blood from fetal blood; however, it requires liquid blood samples, which are usually not available.

Bleeding diathesis

Once a common cause of neonatal morbidity and mortality, hemorrhagic disease of the newborn caused by vitamin K deficiency has all but disappeared since the introduction of routine vitamin K administration following birth. Vitamin K deficiency as a cause of hemorrhage is still observed with home births, in those who do not receive vitamin K, those with liver disease, and in infants who are primarily breast-fed. Hemorrhage is not isolated to the GI tract and is often associated with bleeding from lungs, skin (umbilicus), and genitourinary sources (circumcision). Newborns have vitamin K deficiency as there is a near complete placental barrier to transportation of this vitamin; this results in a depletion of vitamin K-dependent coagulation factors II, VII, IX, and X. Further aggravating this deficiency, the half-life of vitamin K is only 24 h and maternal breast milk is low in vitamin K.

Hemorrhagic disease of the newborn is described based on the time of presentation. Early bleeding is very rare and presents within the first 24 h of life in neonates born to mothers taking anticonvulsant and antituberculosis medications that interfere with vitamin K metabolism (phenytoin, barbiturates, carbamazepine, rifampin, isoniazid). This bleeding may be prevented by antenatal administration of vitamin K to the mother. Classically, bleeding occurs between 1 and 5 days of life, with a reported incidence of up to 1.5% in infants not receiving prophylactic vitamin K at birth. Late bleeding occurs with an incidence of approximately 4–10.5/100 000 in infants between 1 week and 6 months old who are exclusively breast-fed and did not receive prophylactic vitamin K. Diagnosis is made by evaluation of the coagulation profile with measurement of the PT.

Vitamin K treatment should be initiated in patients suspected of vitamin K deficiency and with persistent bleeding even before confirmatory tests.

Rapid institution of vitamin K treatment decreases the risk of intracranial hemorrhage. Transfusion with fresh frozen plasma or whole blood may be indicated for children with severe hemorrhage.

Mallory–Weiss syndrome

A Mallory–Weiss tear is a mucosal injury resulting in UGIB. The patient presents with hematemesis preceded by nausea and retching. The vomiting causes a linear tear in the esophageal mucosa near the gastroesophageal junction, which bleeds. Published studies have found the presence of a Mallory–Weiss tear in 13% of children presenting with UGIB. The same study found that unlike the disease in adults, which is often related to vomiting associated with inebriation, etiologic factors in children include gastritis, duodenitis, gastroesophageal reflux disease, asthma, and pregnancy.

Stress ulcers

The development of ulcers in children is predominantly secondary to stress associated with burns, trauma, surgery, elevated intracranial pressure, NSAID use, infection, multiorgan system dysfunction, or foreign bodies. The initial trauma resulting in mucosal injury is compounded by continued mucosal ischemia in the presence of an acidic environment that leads to further damage. Prophylaxis with acid-reducing medications should be instituted in children admitted to the ICU to minimize the risk of rapid development of hemorrhagic stress ulcers.

Necrotizing entercolitis

Necrotizing entercolitis is a disease that primarily affects newborns. Over 90% of affected infants are preterm, with increasing risk based on extent of prematurity and decreasing birth weight. While this is primarily a disease encountered in the special care nursery, infants born at term or neonates discharged from the hospital may still present with symptoms. Multiple factors appear to contribute to the pathophysiology, including intestinal prematurity, abnormal bacterial colonization, hypoxic–ischemic injury, and feeding. Neonates may present with feeding intolerance, abdominal distention, decreased gastric emptying, vomiting, bloody stools, or shock. The degree of bleeding can vary from occult blood to grossly positive stools or even hematemesis. Radiographic findings include dilated loops of bowel and, in more advanced stages, pneumatosis intestinalis or portal venous gas. Once there is concern for necrotizing entercolitis, standard laboratory tests should be obtained, including blood cultures. The patient is given nothing by mouth and is started on broad-spectrum antibiotics; gastric decompression is considered. All patients with necrotizing entercolitis should be admitted. Surgical consultation should be considered in most cases.

Malrotation with volvulus

Malrotation occurs in approximately 1 in 500 live births. During embryonic development, the duodenum and cecum fail to properly rotate and instead come to lie in close proximity without their usual attachments. This allows for twisting around their common vascular supply, the superior mesenteric artery, which creates both a distal duodenal obstruction as well as vascular compromise. An estimated 75% of cases present with volvulus in the first month of life. Clinically, infants present with sudden onset of bilious vomiting and abdominal distention. However depending on the proximity of the obstruction, physical examination findings may be completely normal early in the presentation; a high index of suspicion is required to correctly make the diagnosis. After 1–2 h of vascular compromise, the bowel begins to necrose. As ischemia worsens, perforation occurs leading to shock. Several diagnostic strategies can assist with diagnosis. Abdominal radiography may demonstrate non-specific findings including a paucity of distal gas, a double-bubble sign, or air–fluid levels suggesting obstruction. The diagnostic test of choice is the upper GI radiographic series, which demonstrates a corkscrew appearance of the duodenum as it lies in its abnormal position twisted around the superior mesenteric artery. Once the diagnosis of malrotation with volvulus is considered, supportive therapy with fluid resuscitation, broad-spectrum antibiotics, and gastric decompression is commenced. Most importantly, consultation with a pediatric surgeon should be obtained for definitive management and surgical reduction of the volvulus to prevent further bowel necrosis.

Henoch–Schönlein purpura

Henoch–Schönlein purpura (HSP; Ch. 85) is the most common vasculitis of childhood, with an estimated incidence of 10 cases per 100 000 children.

Henoch–Schönlein purpura may present with cutaneous purpura, arthritis, abdominal pain, GI bleeding, and nephritis.

The symptoms are manifested through a leukocytoclastic vasculitis caused by IgA deposition. The syndrome has a nearly equal distribution between boys and girls, with 90% of cases occurring in children 10 years or younger (average age of 6 years). Essential for the diagnosis is the presence of thrombocytopenic palpable purpura located predominantly in the buttocks and lower extremities (see Fig. 85.3, p. 381). Arthritis occurs in nearly 75% of patients; GI involvement occurs slightly less frequently, in only 50–75% of patients. Of these patients, abdominal pain is the most frequent complaint, with GI bleeding the next most common finding (in approximately one-third of patients). One in ten patients will have gross bleeding and one in four will have occult bleeding. The blood loss results from vasculitis and edema in the bowel wall. Nephritis occurs in approximately 40% of patients and should be evaluated with urinalysis, serial blood pressure measurements, and a serum creatinine. Children with HSP complicated by nephritis should be admitted for IV steroids and further monitoring. With normal renal function, the family can be discharged and instructed to have a repeat urinalysis every week while the disease is active. Associated arthritis and abdominal pain can be treated with corticosteroids; however, no randomized controlled trial supports their use in HSP; steroids do not change the rate of recurrence. Intussusception is not rare and imaging is indicated in patients with HSP and severe abdominal symptoms. Prognosis is dependent on the presence or absence of nephritis, with approximately 1% progressing to end-stage renal disease. Parents should also be aware that the disease may recur in one-third of patients.

Meckel's diverticulum

Meckel's diverticulum is a remnant of the omphalomesenteric duct that can present with GI bleeding. This has classically been described using the rule of 2's:

- found in 2% of the population
- only 2% of those affected will become symptomatic
- approximately 50% will present by age 2
- the diverticulum is often 2 cm long
- the diverticulum is often found within 2 feet of the ileocecal valve.

The diverticulum contains heterotopic tissue most commonly involving gastric mucosa. This heterotopic gastric mucosa creates an acidic environment, which leads to ulceration and bleeding. Clinically, the child will present with painless bleeding, which is tarry or red depending on the rapidity of the bleeding. The diagnosis is made by radionuclide scan (99m-technetium), which is 90% sensitive in patients with active bleeding. Treatment includes appropriate resuscitation with blood products for massive bleeding and surgical consultation for a positive radionuclide scan, peritoneal signs, or unstable vital signs.

Anal fissure

Anal fissures most often occur in children <1 year of age; they are reported as the most common source of LGIB in this population. Injury and bleeding occur following the passage of a large hard stool. After hard stool, infants may actively withhold stool to prevent another painful episode. Physical examination with gentle spreading of the buttocks demonstrates a tear, most often located in the posterior midline. Treatment includes stool softeners such as colace or mineral oil, perianal care, and application of ointments to prevent excoriation. Consistent treatment often results in painless bowel movements and healing of injury in 6–8 weeks. Patients with diarrhea can develop excoriation of the anal area, with some bleeding. These patients require careful cleaning and barrier ointments to protect excoriated skin.

Milk protein allergy

Milk protein allergies usually manifest by 3 months of age but can be delayed in infants not exposed to cow's milk early in life. Allergies can also appear in exclusively breast-fed infants with proteins passed through the mother's milk. The incidence has increased since the 1960s, with widespread availability and use of cow's milk formula, to range between 0.5% and 7.5% of infants. Mechanisms are poorly understood. Symptoms can manifest as diarrhea, vomiting, or weight loss. The diarrhea presents as colitis in an otherwise well-appearing infant, with loose stools, associated mucus, and streaks or specks of blood. The amount of blood can range from asymptomatic occult GI bleeding to rare profuse bloody diarrhea. Blood loss is generally minimal and anemia is rarely present. Diagnosis is based on a thorough history of newly introduced antigens. Further diagnosis can be accomplished through the use of specific allergy testing and endoscopy as needed. The goals of treatment involve avoidance of the allergen while maintaining adequate nutrition.

Intussusception

Intussusception is one of the most common causes of intestinal obstruction in children and can also present with GI bleeding. Symptoms arise as a proximal portion of bowel telescopes into the adjacent distal segment.

The classic triad of colicky abdominal pain, currant jelly stools, and vomiting is only present in 20–30% of patients.

Nearly 75% of patients will present with two of these complaints. Physical examination during a period of pain demonstrates an inconsolable infant with legs drawn up to the abdomen in considerable pain. A sausage-like mass might be palpated in the RUQ, representing the intussusception. A paucity of bowel contents in the RLQ is referred to as Dance's sign; although relatively pathognomonic for intussusception, it is uncommon. Diagnostic imaging begins with plain abdominal radiographs to screen for signs of obstruction, free air, or mass effect appearing as a target sign or meniscus sign. Definitive imaging with ultrasonography has a sensitivity of 98–100% and a specificity of 88%. The gold standard for diagnosis and treatment is the barium enema. Recent studies have demonstrated equal efficacy using air enema, with a decreased risk of complications should perforation occur. Prior to reduction, fluid resuscitation and analgesia are administered, and a surgical consultation made in preparation for potential perforation or failure of reduction. All children with a confirmed and reduced intussusception should be admitted for observation to monitor for recurrence, which can occur in 2–10% of cases depending on the method of reduction.

Polyps

Polyps are easily diagnosable lesions that present with painless rectal bleeding. Several variants exist, ranging from benign to preneoplastic conditions. For all polyposis syndromes, the patient should be referred to gastroenterology for endoscopy and tissue diagnosis.

Juvenile polyps. These are most common in the first decade of life, more common in boys, and are most often found in the rectosigmoid colon. The polyp is covered with normal colonic mucosa and is not thought to have neoplastic potential. Over two-thirds of patients will present with painless rectal bleeding but they can also demonstrate prolapse of the polyp through the anus.

Familial adenomatous polyposis. An autosomal dominant mutation of the gene *APC* (adenomatous polyposis coli) results in innumerable polyps in the large colon, which carries a virtually 100% lifetime risk of malignant degeneration. Symptoms can include rectal bleeding, abdominal pain, and mucus discharge from the rectum. Given the predisposition for colon cancer, treatment is total colectomy.

Peutz–Jeghers syndrome. This manifests as a combination of polyps and skin pigmentation. Numerous pedunculated hamartomatous polyps, primarily in the small bowel, generally cause symptoms early in adolescence. Patients often present with bleeding (20%) and abdominal pain, and can experience bowel obstruction from intussusception. Additionally, patients have characteristic mucocutaneous pigmentation, most commonly near the lips, which usually develops in infancy. Refer at-risk patients for urgent follow-up, as there is an approximately 50% risk of developing cancer in both the intestinal tract and other organ systems.

Hemangiomas and arteriovenous malformations

Abnormal vascular formations can be present throughout the GI tract but are usually located in the sigmoid colon and rectum. Associated cutaneous telangiectasias are associated with Osler–Rendu–Weber syndrome. Laboratory studies may demonstrate a thrombocytopenia caused by platelet trapping within the malformation.

Inflammatory bowel disease

Inflammatory bowel disease refers to the related clinical conditions of Crohn's disease and ulcerative colitis (Table 63.2). Patients often have crampy abdominal pain associated with loose, sometimes bloody, stools. Extraintestinal manifestations can include, but are not limited to, weight loss, delay in growth and puberty, perianal disease, stomatitis, mouth ulceration, pyoderma gangrenosum, erythema nodosum, and arthritis. Eye symptoms such as uveitis or episcleritis occur much less frequently in children than adults. The exact etiology is unknown but is thought to be a combination of environmental and genetic factors. The peak age of incidence for both forms of inflammatory bowel disease appears to be within the second to third decades of life. When observed in younger children, there is a slightly increased incidence of Crohn's disease in males; ulcerative colitis affects both males and females equally.

Table 63.2. Comparison of ulcerative colitis and Crohn's disease

Feature	Ulcerative colitis	Crohn's disease
Depth of involvment	Mucosal and submucosal	Transmural
Area affected	Isolated to the colon and rectum	Terminal ileum most commonly affected, but lesions can be anywhere in GI tract
Neoplastic risk	High	–
Lesion type	Loss of haustral markings ("lead-pipe" appearance)	Skip lesions, frequent fistulae

Ulcerative colitis

Unlike in adults, ulcerative colitis in children has a higher probability of pancolitis and proximal extension. Children commonly present with abdominal pain and diarrhea; however, other findings such as bloody stools, weight loss, anorexia, and growth delay may be present. Laboratory abnormalities include anemia, leukocytosis, electrolyte abnormalities, and hypoproteinemia. Abdominal radiographs may demonstrate perforation or toxic megacolon. Contrast enemas may reveal a loss of the haustral markings, resulting in the classic "lead-pipe" appearance. Diagnosis is confirmed with endoscopy and biopsy. Treatment with 5-aminosalycilic acid (5-ASA) reduces inflammation; steroids are often used concominantly, particularly during acute flares. Maintenance therapy in more severe cases includes an immunosuppressive agent such as 5-ASA or 6-mercaptopurine. If medical therapy fails, total proctocolectomy can be curative.

Crohn's disease

Crohn's disease differs from ulcerative colitis in that intestinal inflammation can occur at any point in the GI tract. The classic transmural lesions can lead to perforation, strictures, or fistulae. Diagnosis may be delayed in children because of variations in disease presentation; however, the majority of patients seek care for increasingly frequent diarrhea. Elevations in inflammatory markers such as CRP, ESR, white blood cell count (WBC), as well as abnormalities in platelet count and the presence of fecal leukocytes help support presumptive diagnosis. Crohn's disease is confirmed with endoscopy and biopsy. Immunosuppressive therapy is the mainstay of treatment, although children benefit from nutritional modifications and psychological support as well. Surgery does not have a primary role in the treatment of Crohn's disease but may be required for complications, including hemorrhage, strictures, intra-abdominal abscess, or perianal disease.

Celiac disease

Celiac disease is an immune-mediated enteropathy that presents in genetically susceptible individuals exposed to gluten proteins. The disease has a prevalence of around 1% with a peak incidence in early childhood.

Classically, children present after the introduction of gluten into the diet between 6 and 24 months of age. However, onset can be at any age. Impaired growth, diarrhea, abdominal distention, apathy, anorexia, muscle wasting and irritability are common features. Other findings may include dermatitis herpetiformis, iron-deficiency anemia, arthritis, aphthous stomatitis, short stature, vomiting, seizures, electrolyte abnormalities, osteopenia, and hepatitis. Serologic markers can aid in diagnosis; the standard test is the anti-endomysial IgA antibody, which approaches a specificity of 100%. Diagnostic criteria established by the European Society for Pediatric Gastroenterology state that the child must have characteristically abnormal intestinal mucosal biopsy in the presence of gluten and resolution of such findings upon complete elimination of gluten from diet. Duodenal biopsies confirm the diagnosis. The only accepted treatment for celiac disease is the life-long elimination of gluten-containing substances such as wheat, rye, and barley from the diet. Response is often rapid – symptom resolution can be seen in weeks to months, with histological improvement occurring several months later. Complications include an elevated risk of small bowel carcinoma. Children presenting with signs and symptoms concerning for advanced celiac disease marked by electrolyte abnormalities, failure to thrive, or dehydration should be admitted for stabilization and confirmatory diagnostic testing. Other well-appearing children can be referred to gastroenterology for outpatient evaluation.

Pearls and pitfalls

Pearls

1. Consider intussusception in any infant with altered mental status, abdominal pain, and Hemoccult-positive stools.
2. Meckel's diverticulum: remember the rule of 2's.
3. Evaluate renal function in patients with presumed Henoch–Schönlein purpura.
4. An acute onset of bilious emesis in the neonate suggests obstruction and volvulus. Maintain a high clinical suspicion for these entities, as necrosis of the bowel wall will ensue within 1–2 h.

Pitfalls

1. Failure to differentiate true GI bleeding from ingestion of other substances that can change the color of the stool.

Selected references

Cuffari C, Darbari A. Inflammatory bowel disease in the pediatric and adolescent patient. *Gastroenterol Clin North Am* 2002;**31**:275–291.

D'Agostino J. Common abdominal emergencies in children. *Emerg Med Clin North Am* 2002;**20**:139–153.

Fox VL. Gastrointestinal bleeding in infancy and childhood. *Gastroenterol Clin North Am* 2000; **29**:37–66.

Green PH, Cellier C. Celiac disease. *N Engl J Med* 2007;**357**:1731–1743.

McCollough M, Sharieff GQ. Abdominal pain in children. *Pediatr Clin North Am* 2006;**53**: 107–137.

Ponsky T, Hindle A, Sandler A. Inflammatory bowel disease in the pediatric patient. *Surg Clin North Am* 2007;**87**:643–658.

Squires Jr. RH. Approach to the child with upper or lower gastrointestinal bleeding. In Rudolph CD (ed.) *Rudolph's Pediatrics*. New York: McGraw-Hill, 2003, pp. 1371–1375.

Chapter 64

Hepatitis

Anita Kulkarni and Aparajita Sohoni

Introduction

Pediatric hepatitis, defined by inflammatory destruction of hepatocytes, is most commonly caused by a viral infection. Within the USA, hepatitis A, B, and C viruses (HAV, HBV, and HCV, respectively) are the most common identified causes of viral hepatitis. The epidemiology, route of transmission, incubation period, common presentation, and prognostic factors for these viruses are presented in Table 64.1. Of note, the incidence of HAV and HBV infections has significantly decreased with the implementation of nationwide vaccination programs. These viruses, along with hepatitis D virus (HDV) and hepatitis E virus (HEV), are known as hepatotropic viruses because of their preference for replication within hepatocytes. A number of other, non-hepatotropic, viruses are responsible for up to 10% of cases of viral hepatitis. Aside from viruses, other infectious agents such as bacteria or parasites, drugs, metabolic disorders, or autoimmune diseases can also result in hepatitis.

Clinical presentation

Patients with an acute viral hepatitis present similarly, regardless of etiology. Younger children, in general, present less severely than adolescents and adults. The most frequent symptoms include abdominal pain, nausea, vomiting, fever, and decreased appetite or anorexia.

Most young children infected with hepatitis A virus remain asymptomatic or have only mild fever, nausea, and abdominal pain.

However, approximately 40–70% of older children and adults will become jaundiced and have more severe symptoms. Infection with HDV and HEV is relatively rare amongst the general population and exceedingly rare in children. Chronic hepatitis is rare in the pediatric population. These patients with chronic hepatitis, normally caused by HBV or HCV, have a variety of presentations ranging from mild abdominal discomfort and nausea to fulminant hepatic failure, based on the level of viral replication ongoing.

Diagnostic studies

Laboratory studies will confirm the clinical diagnosis of hepatitis. Specifically, AST, alanine transaminase (ALT), alkaline phosphatase, and total bilirubin levels should be checked. A fractionated and unfractionated bilirubin level should also be obtained if the total bilirubin is elevated to help in differentiating an obstructive versus a hemolytic process. Coagulation studies (PT, PTT, and INR) and albumin levels should also be obtained to screen for overall hepatic function. A hepatitis panel should be checked, although the results of this are frequently delayed at most hospitals. Notably, the exact contents of a "hepatitis panel" are institution-specific and should be reviewed to include the assays most relevant to the particular patient. The appropriate viral and antibody levels to include in a complete hepatitis panel are presented in Table 64.2. Hepatitis D and E viruses are not normally included in routine testing for hepatitis.

If clinical suspicion for overall dehydration or other organ damage (such as renal dysfunction or pancreatitis) exists, serum electrolytes, creatinine, BUN, and lipase levels should be checked. The interpretation of laboratory studies in a patient with chronic hepatitis is more complex, as liver enzyme levels will vary with the amount of viral replication or may be persistently elevated. For patients with minimal viral replication, all laboratory results may be normal and they will generally be asymptomatic. In patients with persistent viral replication, serum ALT or AST levels may be elevated, as will levels of HBV DNA or HBeAg (HBV e antigen). These patients are at increased long-term (10–20 year) risk for developing cirrhosis or hepatocellular carcinoma and should be referred to a GI specialist for further evaluation, possible liver biopsy, and follow-up.

Management

The majority of patients who present with acute hepatitis will require supportive care with IV fluids, antiemetics, or

A Practical Guide to Pediatric Emergency Medicine: Caring for Children in the Emergency Department, ed. N. Ewen Amieva-Wang (associate eds. Jamie Shandro, Aparajita Sohoni, and Bernhard Fassl). Published by Cambridge University Press.

Table 64.1. Overview of hepatitis A/B/C viruses

	A	B	C
Epidemiology	0.7 cases per 100 000 population for children <5 years; 1.4 cases per 100 000 for ages 5–14 years	0.02 cases per 100 000 population in children <15 years	0.37 cases per 100 000 population aged 15–24 years; almost no cases reported in those <15 years
Route of transmission	Fecal–oral	Parenteral, sexual, vertical, horizontal	Parenteral, sexual, vertical, horizontal
Incubation	2–6 weeks	4–20 weeks	2–26 weeks
Clinical presentation	Fever, malaise, nausea, vomiting, anorexia, abdominal pain, jaundice		
Duration of symptoms	2 weeks to several months	2–3 months	
Treatment	Supportive care	Acute phase: supportive care Chronic phase: consult GI specialist	Acute phase: supportive care Chronic phase: consult GI specialist
Mortality prognosis in 2006 (all ages)	0.3%	0.8%	0.2%
Complications	Pancreatitis, renal failure, fulminant hepatitis, liver failure, death	Chronic hepatitis, cirrhosis, hepatocellular carcinoma	Chronic hepatitis, cirrhosis, hepatocellular carcinoma
Chronic state	None	Based on age at infection; 90% of neonates and 25–50% of adolescents will progress to chronic infections	60–80% of those infected will develop a chronic disease state
Vaccination	Whole-virus vaccine IM at 12 months and 18 months	Recombinant vaccine IM at birth, 1–2 months, and 6–12 months	None

Source: adapted from *Koslap-Petraco et al.*, 2008.

analgesics. Care should be taken to avoid prescribing medications metabolized by the liver, such as acetaminophen. Long-term therapies for treatment of chronic HBV or HCV, such as interferon-alpha, lamivudine, or ribavirin, should only be initiated by a pediatric gastroenterologist.

Disposition

Patients with mild symptoms who appear well clinically may be discharged with 24 h follow-up. Moderate or severe symptoms, specifically an inability to take oral intake, any change in mental status, or an INR of >1.5 warrant admission to the hospital for ongoing supportive care and observation for potential development of fulminant hepatitis or liver failure.

Table 64.2. Hepatitis panel results and interpretation for hepatitis A/B/C infections

Virus	Test
HAV	Immunoglobulin M (IgM) antibody to HAV (anti-HAV)
HBV	
Acute infection	IgM antibody to HBV core antigen (anti-HBc) or HBV surface antigen (HBsAg)
Chronic infection	Positive: HBsAg, anti-HBc IgG Negative: anti-HBs, IgM anti-HBc
Immunity	Anti-HBV surface antibody (HBsAb) positive
HCV	Serum ALT >7 upper level of normal plus anti-HCV antibody positive or positive HCV RNA nucleic acid testing

Source: adapted from Koslap-Petraco *et al.*, 2008.

Non-infectious causes of hepatitis

Total parenteral nutrition (TPN), along with drug and environmental hepatotoxins, are known to cause liver damage in the pediatric population. Prolonged use of TPN can lead to cirrhosis and liver failure. End-stage liver disease is the leading cause of death in TPN-dependent infants with short bowel syndrome. Preterm infants with immature bowel often require prolonged TPN feeds and are, therefore, most susceptible to developing cholestasis and associated liver disease. Although treatment options are not well defined, the use of medications to decrease cholestasis along with the introduction of enteric feeding have been shown to be beneficial. Patients with cystic fibrosis often experience cholestasis and have chronic low-grade hepatitis. Not uncommonly, this progresses to chronic liver damage and cirrhosis.

Drug-associated hepatotoxicity is relatively uncommon in the pediatric population. The most commonly implicated hepatotoxic drugs include acetaminophen, phenytoin, and several antibiotics. Acetaminophen toxicity is prominent and well described in the pediatric population. Phenytoin and sulfasalazine are also unpredictable hepatotoxins. Antibiotics such as erythromycin and trimethoprim–sulfamethoxazole can cause hepatic injury in the pediatric population. Minocycline, used in adolescents for treatment of acne, is associated with autoimmune hepatitis while oral contraceptives are associated with hepatic vein thrombosis and liver tumors.

In general, patients present with non-specific symptoms common to other liver diseases and may have a range of laboratory abnormalities, such as elevated liver enzymes or coagulopathy. Withdrawal of the offending agent is paramount, as the remainder of treatment is mainly supportive care. Few antidotes, other than *N*-acetylcysteine for acetaminophen toxicity, exist for hepatotoxic ingestions. Multiple factors, such as the specific nature of the drug, the dosage, the patient's age, gender, and genetic predisposition, determine the degree of liver injury and the likelihood of evolving into hepatic failure. If liver failure is suspected, transfer should be arranged to a liver-transplant center for further evaluation.

Pearls and pitfalls

Pearls

1. Vaccinations have dramatically reduced the incidence of viral hepatitis in the USA.
2. For patients with chronic hepatitis, referral to a pediatric gastroenterologist is key for coordination of long-term care.
3. Total parenteral nutrition, along with drug and environmental hepatotoxins, is known to cause liver damage in the pediatric population.
4. The single most important laboratory test in acute hepatitis is the international normalized ratio (INR).

Pitfalls

1. Failure to realize that a variety of medications, environmental exposures, or infectious etiologies can result in liver failure.

Selected references

Hsu EK, Murray KF. Hepatitis B and C in children. *Nat Clin Pract Gastroenterol Hepatol* 2008;**5**:311–320.

Koslap-Petraco MB, Shub M, Judelsohn R. Hepatitis A: disease burden and current childhood vaccination strategies in the United States. *J Pediatr Health Care* 2008;**22**:3–11.

Wasley A, Grytdal S, Gallagher K. Surveillance for acute viral hepatitis: United States, 2006. *MMWR Surveill Summ* 2008; **57**:1–24.

White FV, Dehner LP. Viral diseases of the liver in children: diagnostic and differential diagnostic considerations. *Pediatr Dev Pathol* 2004;7: 552–567.

Chapter 65

Organomegaly and abdominal masses

Marcela P. Mendenhall and N. Ewen Amieva-Wang

Introduction

In pediatrics, it is common to palpate a liver or a spleen in early infancy. As the child ages, hepato- and/or splenomegaly becomes less common. This chapter will first focus on the pathologic enlargement of the liver and the spleen before describing abdominal and pelvic masses.

Hepatomegaly

In infants and young children, it can be normal to palpate a liver edge beyond the costal margin.

A liver edge greater that 3 cm beyond the costal margin in infants and 2.5 cm in a child of 1–2 years is considered hepatomegaly.

By 10 years of age, the liver edge is usually tucked under the ribs and any extension beyond, is considered hepatomegaly. While palpating for a liver edge is easy to do, it is often not entirely accurate. To evaluate hepatomegaly effectively, the EP must rely on percussion of the liver to delineate the upper margin and ultimately define the liver span. A hepatic ultrasound would be indicated if liver span is difficult to determine. A normal liver span in an infant up to 2 months of age is 3.5–7.2 cm, and by 5 years of age, a range of 6.5–10 cm is considered normal.

Liver enlargement can occur secondary to inflammation, congestion and obstruction, storage disorders and infiltrative processes. In children, the most common cause by far is inflammation by Epstein–Barr virus or another similar mononucleosis-like illness such as CMV infection.

Diagnosis

It is as important to be as thorough as possible in obtaining a history as with the physical examination. Obtaining all information regard chronicity, associated symptoms, past medical history, birth history, family history and possible exposures, in addition to the overall clinical picture, will help to elucidate the etiology of the hepatomegaly. In general, children <2 years of age are more likely to have a congenital or metabolic problem than an older child or adolescent. Ultimately, the clinical picture of the child is going to guide the workup. The workup may range from obtaining CBC, LFTs, and monospot, to include electrolytes, glucose, ammonia, coagulation studies, inflammatory markers or viral studies. Ultrasound is usually the imaging modality of choice, unless recommended otherwise by subspecialty consultation.

Management

The differential is broad; therefore, management is based on clinical diagnosis and condition. Viral hepatitis has no specific therapy in an otherwise stable child. Patients with conjugated hyperbilirubinemia, dehydration secondary to vomiting, or severe liver dysfunction should be admitted for workup and management.

Splenomegaly

The spleen is normally felt in up to 30% of infants up to 1 year of age; however, this falls to less than 1% in adolescents. Specifically, the spleen can normally protrude 1 cm beyond the costal margin in infants. If it extends beyond 2 cm, then a diagnostic workup should be initiated. Splenomegaly is usually secondary to a systemic or liver process. Splenomegaly can be caused by the same pathologies that cause hepatomegaly: inflammation, infiltration, obstruction, and storage disease. It is also caused by autoimmune diseases, trauma, hemolysis, and extramedullary hematopoesis. Portal venous obstruction can cause relatively asymptomatic splenomegaly in childhood. Last, it is possible to confuse a spleen in a lower position (visceroptosis) with a truly enlarged spleen.

Diagnosis

As with hepatomegaly, the history, associated symptoms, and physical examination can guide workup. If the spleen extends farther than 2 cm below the costal margin, or is associated with other symptoms, then a diagnostic workup should be initiated.

A Practical Guide to Pediatric Emergency Medicine: Caring for Children in the Emergency Department, ed. N. Ewen Amieva-Wang (associate eds. Jamie Shandro, Aparajita Sohoni, and Bernhard Fassl). Published by Cambridge University Press.

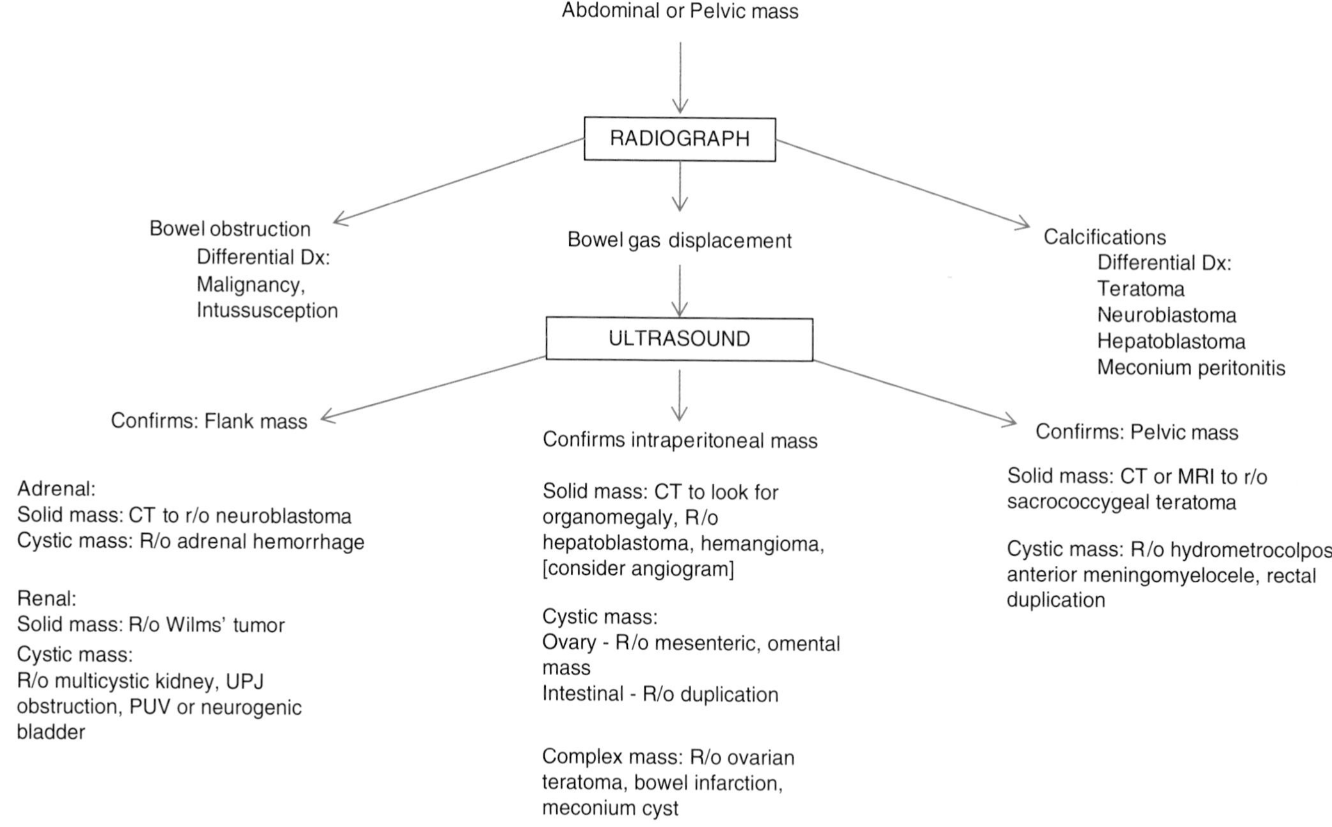

Figure 65.1 Algorithm to evaluate abdominal mass in a child. PUV posterior urethral valve; R/o rule out; Tx therapy; UPJ ureteropelvic junction.

Again, the most common etiology is inflammatory viral infection; however, an infiltrative process such as leukemia must also be considered. Basic workup should include a CBC with a differential, inflammatory markers, lactate dehydrogenase, uric acid and viral studies.

Management

A healthy child with a palpable spleen can be referred for outpatient follow-up. An unstable child, one with hemolytic anemia, or one with other associated symptoms, in addition to a palpable spleen, should be admitted for further workup.

Abdominal mass

Abdominal mass can be the presenting complaint to the ED. They are always concerning if not secondary to stool as abdominal masses are neoplastic until proven otherwise. In the neonatal period and early infancy, constipation, bladder distention, or organomegaly can be confused for an abdominal mass. However, if an abdominal mass is present and not clearly benign, imaging is warranted to rule out neoplasm. A review of neonatal abdominal masses shows varying frequency of occurrence by the organ or system of origin: 55% renal, 15% genital tract, 15% GI, 10% retroperitoneal, and 5% liver, biliary tract or spleen (Table 65.1).

In childhood, abdominal masses are more likely to be malignant.

Neuroblastoma and hepatoblastomas are more common in children younger than 2 years of age, whereas Wilms' tumor, hepatocellular carcinoma, rhabdomyosarcoma of the genitourinary tract, and ovarian germ cell tumors are more common in older children. Leukemia and lymphoma with lymph node as well as liver and spleen involvement occurs at an older age. Malignant diseases are slightly more common in boys than in girls.

Clinical presentation and diagnosis

Initial evaluation should be for pertinent symptoms (Fig. 65.1). Is the infant irritable or somnolent? Is there vomiting and is it bilious? Is the infant urinating? On physical examination, determining the exact location and characterization of the mass is always helpful. Is the mass solid or compressible? Is the mass fixated or mobile? Is the surface of the mass smooth

Table 65.1. Types of abdominal mass in children

Age group/type	Masses
Neonates	
Genitourinary	50% of masses
Renal	Hydronephrosis, multidysplastic kidney, mesoblastic nephroma (most common solid renal tumor in neonates), renal vein thrombosis, polycystic kidney disease, Wilms' tumor, rhabdoid tumor
Pelvic	Ovarian cyst, hydrocolpos, hydrometrocolpos, GI duplication
Children	
Retroperitoneal	Neuroblastoma, pheochromoblastoma, Wilms' tumor, lymphoma
Liver	Hepatoblastoma, hepatocellular carcinoma, embryonal sarcoma
Gastrointestinal	Duplication, Meckel's diverticulum, fecal mass
Pelvic	Ovarian mass (cyst or tumor)

or irregular? Is there tenderness with palpation? Are there peritoneal signs?

Initial laboratory evaluation from the ED should include CBC, inflammatory markers, comprehensive metabolic panel, urinalysis, human chorionic gonadotropin (beta-HCG), lactate dehydrogenase, uric acid and urinalysis. Further evaluation typically always involves an abdominal radiograph looking for bowel gas, air–fluid levels, organomegaly, free fluid or air, and calcifications, which can suggest neuroblastoma, hepatoblastoma, or meconium peritonitis. If no obvious source is discovered on radiograph, abdominal ultrasound is the next study of choice. Ultrasound, while a benign and inexpensive study, has the advantage of distinguishing solid from cystic masses, as well as further defining the organ of origin.

In the female pubescent population, one must never forget the pelvis. One of the most overlooked organs is the ovary. Ovarian masses are usually divided into two groups: functional cysts and tumors, including germ cell, epithelial and sex cord stromal tumors. Ovarian masses present at a median age of 9.9 years with abdominal pain in 73%, as well as increased abdominal girth, back pain, dysuria, and leg pain. Ovarian masses are less common than appendicitis; however, they are very often misdiagnosed as appendicitis.

Management and disposition

Specialty consult should be obtained for an abdominal mass newly diagnosed in the ED. Patients should be admitted for expedient definitive diagnosis and treatment.

Pearls and pitfalls

Pearls

1. Abdominal masses are neoplastic until proven otherwise.
2. The kidney accounts for more than 50% of neonatal abdominal masses.

Pitfalls

1. Failure to consider pelvic pathology in the female pubescent population.

Selected references

Brodeur A. Abdominal masses in children: neuroblastoma, Wilms' tumor and other considerations. *Pediatr Rev* 1991;**12**:196–206.

Louie J. Essential diagnosis of abdominal emergencies in the first year of life. *Emerg Med Clin North Am* 2007;**25**:1009–1040.

Pomeranz AJ, Sabnis S. Misdiagnoses of ovarian masses in children and adolescents. *Pediatr Emerg Care* 2004;**20**:172–174.

Schwartz M. Abdominal masses in the newborn. *Pediatr Rev* 1989;**11**:172–179.

Chapter 66

Intussusception

Aparajita Sohoni

Introduction

Intussusception, referring to the telescoping of one portion of the intestines (the intussusceptum) into an adjoining segment of intestine's lumen (the intussuscipiens), is the most common cause of the acute abdomen in infancy. Intussusceptions are classified by which segment of the bowel is affected, with the most common form being the ileocolic type (Fig. 66.1). Other types of intussusception include ileoileal, colocolic, or combinations such as ileoileocolic. The invagination of one portion of bowel into another compromises first the venous outflow, resulting in acute venous congestion and edema of the bowel wall, followed by decreased arterial supply to the affected bowel. The ischemic bowel is at risk for infarction and eventually perforation. In one study of deaths from intussusception, 61% were found to be avoidable; errors included delay in diagnosis, insufficient resuscitative care with fluids and antibiotics, or failure to detect a persistent intussusception after an attempt at reduction was made. Prompt identification and appropriate management of intussusception is critical, as failure to recognize this condition can result in significant morbidity and mortality.

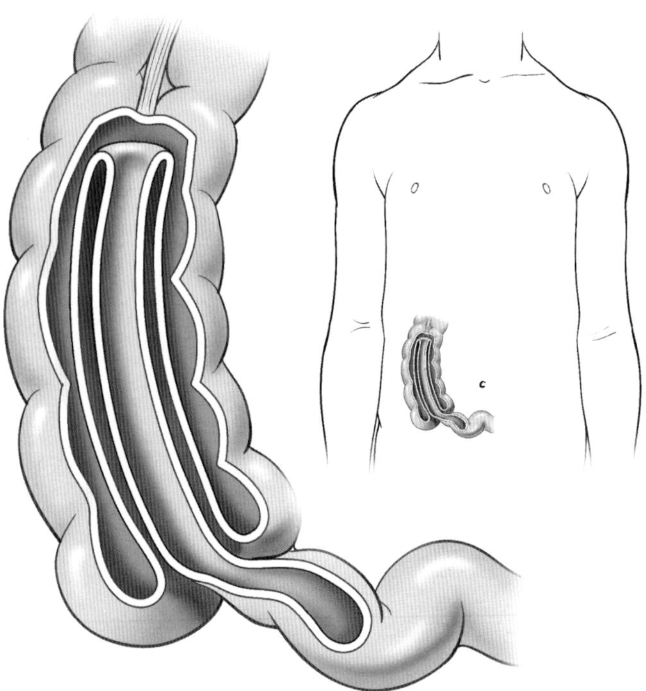

Figure 66.1 Ileocolic intussusception classically occurs in children (90%). (Copyright Chris Gralapp.)

Children <3 years of age are at highest risk of developing intussusception, with the peak incidence occurring between 5 and 10 months.

Intussusception is exceedingly rare in children <3 months old but 75% of cases occurs in children <2 years of age. Males are more frequently affected than females, with a ratio of 2–4:1. The global incidence of intussusception is approximately 0.3–4/1000 live births, with higher rates in developing countries.

The etiology of intussusception remains unknown in 90% of cases. Given the increased incidence of cases in the fall and spring seasons, a common hypothesis is that viral infections cause lymphoid hyperplasia, which subsequently serves as a lead point for intussusception. The remaining 5–10% of cases are commonly caused by Meckel's diverticulum, intestinal polyps, cysts within the intestinal mesentery, other intra-abdominal masses such as lymphoma, or hematomas associated with other conditions such as Henoch–Schönlein purpura.

Clinical presentation

The clinical presentation of intussusception varies. The classic triad of colicky abdominal pain, currant-jelly stools, and a palpable abdominal mass, while very specific, is a late sign, present in only 50% of patients. Currant-jelly stools are a late finding in intussusception, suggesting bowel ischemia has already occurred.

Patients may be relatively asymptomatic or present with generalized abdominal discomfort, pain, abdominal cramping, altered mental status, lethargy, dehydration, or severe shock.

A Practical Guide to Pediatric Emergency Medicine: Caring for Children in the Emergency Department, ed. N. Ewen Amieva-Wang (associate eds. Jamie Shandro, Aparajita Sohoni, and Bernhard Fassl). Published by Cambridge University Press.

Diagnosis

Diagnosing intussusception is challenging because of the range of clinical presentations, as well as the young age of the average patient with this condition. While the history and physical examination combined are always key in evaluating a pediatric patient, providers should keep in mind the range of complaints that may suggest intussusception, from transient abdominal pain to ALOC to bloody stools.

The choice of imaging modality for diagnosing intussusception should be determined by the stability of the patient. Patients who are clinically unstable with suspected intestinal perforation should be seen by pediatric surgery immediately. A screening plain film of the abdomen may be done to evaluate for an obvious intestinal obstruction and or perforation; however, the absence of free air on the radiograph does not preclude the existence of a small perforation.

Patients who are hemodynamically stable can be assessed with a combination of plain films and ultrasound. While historically these patients would have received diagnostic enemas, the advent of ultrasound has all but eliminated enemas as a diagnostic option. Any patient with evidence of peritonitis, shock, or intestinal perforation should not be given a diagnostic enema.

Plain films, taken in both supine and upright positions, may show a variety of signs that suggest intussusception (Fig. 66.2). The "target" and "meniscus" signs are considered most specific for intussusception but are also seen in other disease processes. The target sign refers to a rounded soft tissue mass with a central lucency that is created by the mesenteric fat within the intussusception. This sign has been seen in as many as 63% of those with intussusception, but it has also been found in other disease states. The meniscus sign is formed by gas within the apex of the intussusception forming a crescent and has been found in as many as 30% of those with intussusception. Non-specific signs that may suggest intussusception include evidence of small bowel obstruction, an absence of air in the RLQ, or a soft tissue mass in the RUQ. Overall, plain films "will be diagnostic in 50% of intussusceptions". None of these radiographic signs is sensitive or specific enough to rule out or make the diagnosis of intussusception. In patients for whom there is a high degree of suspicion for intussusception, normal plain films should not preclude further workup with abdominal ultrasound. Abdominal ultrasound is the most commonly used technique for diagnosing intussusception, with a negative predictive value of 100%.

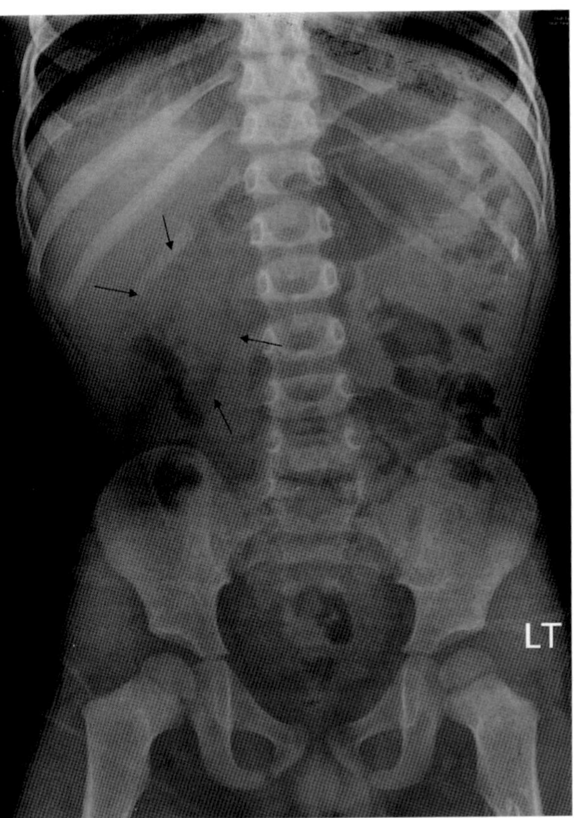

Figure 66.2 Radiograph with paucity of RUQ gas and soft tissue opacity (arrowed).

Management

The additional benefit of using ultrasound to diagnose intussusception is the immediate availability of ultrasound-guided pneumatic or hydrostatic reduction. The non-surgical reduction of intussusception has been in practice since the late 1800s and has evolved to include hydrostatic or pneumatic reduction under fluoroscopy, or ultrasound-guided administration of an air or saline-based enema. While ultrasound-guided and fluoroscopic-guided pneumatic reduction have similar success rates (70–95%), hydrostatic reduction under fluoroscopy has a wider range of success, from 55–90%. Which technique is employed will be determined by the comfort of the radiologist and the facilities available. In general, a maximum of three attempts are performed for reduction before the procedure is deemed unsuccessful. In general, patients with the following characteristics are less likely to have a successful non-surgical reduction, either with failure to reduce or with development of a perforation:

- age <3months or >5 years old
- symptom duration >48 h
- bloody stools
- dehydration
- small bowel obstruction.

The risk of perforation associated with non-surgical reduction is <1%. As always, a patient with peritonitis, perforation, or shock should not undergo non-surgical reduction.

Any patient who has failed non-surgical reduction, and any patient found to have perforated bowel, peritonitis, or shock, should be evaluated by a pediatric surgeon immediately. Surgical intervention for manual reduction of the intussusception, repair of a perforation, or management of an identified lead point (i.e., Meckel's diverticulum) is the next step. Patients suspected to have peritonitis, perforation, or shock should be given antibiotics to cover bowel flora. Metronidazole in combination with a cephalosporin is appropriate for mild–moderate disease, while piperacillin–tazobactam, or metronidazole in combination with gentamicin or clindamycin should be given to penicillin-allergic patients with severe illness. Supportive care with IV fluids and analgesics should also be administered.

Disposition

Patients who have had successful non-surgical reduction should be admitted and observed for any recurrence or other complication for a period of 24–48 h.

The recurrence rates range from 5.2 to 20% for the various non-surgical reduction techniques. Overall, approximately 10% of children who have had successful non-surgical reduction will have a recurrence. The majority of children will have only one recurrence in the immediate post-reduction time period. The decision of how best to manage an immediate recurrence of an intussusception is guided by the patient's clinical condition and should be made by the pediatric surgeon in conjunction with the radiologist.

Pearls and pitfalls

Pearls

1. Acute or chronic hepato- or splenomegaly is a contraindication to participate in sports (especially contact sports) and needs primary care or subspecialty physician clearance prior to participation.
2. Pulmonary hyperinflation can cause pseudohepatosplenomegaly.
3. Intussusception may present as an altered level of consciousness or non-specific abdominal pain.
4. Obtain a screening abdominal radiograph in any child with clinical suspicion of perforation.
5. Consult pediatric surgeons and radiology early to determine the best mode of diagnosis and treatment of intussusception.

Pitfalls

1. Relying on currant-jelly stools for a diagnosis of intussusception; this is a late finding and signifies severe bowel damage.

Selected references

Daneman A, Navarro O. Intussusception. Part 2: An update on the evolution of management. *Pediatr Radiol* 2004;**34**:97–108; quiz 87.

Ko HS, Schenk JP, Troger J, Rohrschneider WK. Current radiological management of intussusception in children. *Eur Radiol* 2007;**17**: 2411–221.

Sorantin E, Lindbichler F. Management of intussusception. *Eur Radiol* 2004;**14**(Suppl. 4):L146–L154.

Stringer MD, Pledger G, Drake DP. Childhood deaths from intussusception in England and Wales, 1984–9. *Br Med J* 1992;**304**:737–739.

Chapter 67

Jaundice

Aparajita Sohoni

Introduction

The term "jaundice" refers to a "yellowish or yellowish-greenish hue" present in the mucous membranes, skin, or sclera caused by the accumulation of serum bilirubin. This yellowing can usually be detected clinically when the serum bilirubin levels have exceeded 5 mg/dl (normal serum bilirubin is <1 mg/dl); however, in children, levels >2 mg/dl may produce clinical jaundice. In contrast with neonatal jaundice (see Ch. 154), jaundice in an older child or adolescent is never normal and always warrants a full workup.

Bile is composed of a variety of compounds, including water, bile salts, and bilirubin (bile pigment). The secretion of bile by the liver enables removal of toxins, management of cholesterol, and digestion and absorption of fats and fat-soluble vitamins within the intestinal tract.

Bilirubin is produced by the metabolism of heme. Within the reticuloendothelial system, heme is converted by heme oxygenase to biliverdin, and then by biliverdin reductase to bilirubin. Bilirubin travels from the reticuloendothelial system to the liver bound to albumin. The liver takes up bilirubin via an albumin receptor and transfers the bilirubin into the hepatocyte. Within the hepatocyte, bilirubin is conjugated into a water-soluble form. This conjugated (direct) bilirubin is excreted into the bile ducts, from where it travels to the intestine. Within the intestines, conjugated bilirubin is converted to urobilinogen and stercobilin by the gut flora. Total bilirubin includes both the conjugated (direct) and unconjugated (indirect) bilirubin levels.

Clinical presentation

A patient with jaundice may present with a range of symptoms, based on the type of hyperbilirubinemia and the etiology. For example, dark urine, pruritus, and pale stools usually suggests conjugated hyperbilirubinemia, while pallor may suggest a hemolytic (unconjugated) process. All patients with jaundice outside of the neonatal period should have a full laboratory evaluation carried out, as none of the physical examination findings reliably indicate either the level of hyperbilirubinemia or the etiology. A full history and review of systems, including medications and family history should be obtained, including all social habits, such as drug use, as viral hepatitis may present with jaundice. A thorough physical examination is carried out, starting with a neurological assessment to evaluate for any confusion or altered mental status that may suggest hepatic encephalopathy. The abdomen is examined for any evidence of hepatomegaly or abdominal pain.

Diagnosis

In a child with jaundice, the first diagnostic step should be to determine if the hyperbilirubinemia is conjugated or unconjugated. Once this is known, the differential diagnosis for each type can be considered:

- **unconjugated**
  - hemolytic anemia
  - Gilbert syndrome
- **conjugated**
  - viral infections (hepatitis A–E, Epstein–Barr, CMV, herpes simplex)
  - Metabolic liver disease (Wilson's disease, α_1-antitrypsin deficiency, cystic fibrosis)
  - biliary tract disorders (cholelithiasis/cholecystitis, choledochal cyst, sclerosing cholangitis)
  - autoimmune liver disease
  - hepatotoxins (acetaminophen, antibiotics, anticonvulsants, oral contraceptives, alcohol)
  - vascular disorders (veno-occlusive disease, Budd–Chiari syndrome).

In general, *conjugated hyperbilirubinemia* (conjugated bilirubin >2 mg/dl) indicates either an obstructive process blocking the usual drainage of bile or an inflammatory process within the hepatocyte causing intrahepatic cholestasis. *Unconjugated hyperbilirubinemia* is generally a hemolytic process, resulting in overproduction of bilirubin in its unconjugated form, or a

A Practical Guide to Pediatric Emergency Medicine: Caring for Children in the Emergency Department, ed. N. Ewen Amieva-Wang (associate eds. Jamie Shandro, Aparajita Sohoni, and Bernhard Fassl). Published by Cambridge University Press.

Box 67.1. Diagnostic workup for unconjugated and conjugated hyperbilirubinemia

Workup for unconjugated hyperbilirubinemia

1. CBC.
2. Reticulocyte count.
3. Peripheral blood smear.
4. Direct and indirect Coombs' test.
5. Serum haptoglobins.
6. Hemoglobin electrophoresis.

Workup for conjugated hyperbilirubinemia

1. Liver function tests
   - enzymes: AST, ALT, alkaline phosphatase, gamma-glutamyl transpeptidase
   - synthetic activity: PT, total protein, albumin, cholesterol, glucose, ammonia.
2. Viral tests
   - viral hepatitis panel
   - monospot and Epstein–Barr virus titers.
3. Abdominal ultrasound.
4. Autoimmune workup
   - serum IgG
   - autoantibodies: anti-nuclear antibody (ANA), anti-smooth muscle antibodies (ASMA), liver–kidney microsomal antibodies.
5. Alpha-1-antitrypsin level and phenotype.
6. Serum ceruloplasmin and 24 h urinary copper excretion.

deficiency within the hepatocyte of a normal mechanism for conjugating bilirubin. To further evaluate conjugated or unconjugated hyperbilirubinemia, laboratory tests should be sent (Box 67.1).

While a full review of each disease entity is beyond the scope of this chapter, we will provide an overview of several common conditions.

Unconjugated hyperbilirubinemia

Hemolytic anemias. These are most often the cause of unconjugated hyperbilirubinemia in an older child or adolescent. Hemolytic anemias can result from either an intrinsic red blood cell defect causing increased hemolysis (e.g., hereditary spherocytosis, glucose-6-phosphate dehydrogenase deficiency, or pyruvate kinase deficiency) or an inherited hemoglobinopathy (e.g., sickle cell anemia [Ch. 81] or thalassemia). Whichever the mechanism, the increased hemolysis leads to more heme being metabolized and circulated as bilirubin in unconjugated form.

Gilbert syndrome. An autosomal recessive disorder caused by a mutation in the gene *UGT1* results in an impaired UDP-glucoronyltransferase enzyme. This condition is present in 5% of the population. In these patients, fasting, physical stress, or other illness may cause a flare in their condition and produce jaundice. No other abnormalities should be seen on laboratory evaluation, and the patients should appear well overall.

Conjugated hyperbilirubinemia

Viral hepatitis. Any hepatotropic virus is capable of producing jaundice through intrahepatic cholestasis (see Ch. 64).

Inborn errors of metabolism. A variety of metabolic syndromes may present with jaundice in the older child or adolescent (e.g., defects in glucose and fatty acid metabolism and amino acid disorders).

Wilson's disease. An autosomal recessive disorder affecting the usual metabolism of copper. Excess copper can accumulate in the liver, cornea, brain, or other organs such as the heart. Within the liver, copper deposits may cause mild, chronic hepatitis or fulminant hepatic failure. Other classic signs of Wilson's disease, such as Kayser–Fleischer rings in the cornea, are usually present when neurologic or psychiatric symptoms develop. These symptoms may develop independently of liver symptoms, making it important to consider this diagnosis even in the absence of evidence of other organ involvement. A serum ceruloplasmin level and a 24-hour urinary copper collection are the diagnostic tests of choice. Obviously, these tests are difficult to arrange from the ED, and the primary care clinician or specialist should be consulted to determine the best way to arrange for these tests.

Alpha-1-antitrypsin deficiency. This is an autosomal codominantly inherited condition that may present with conjugated hyperbilirubinemia at any age.

Cystic fibrosis. Although this is a metabolic condition that can cause conjugated hyperbilirubinemia, it rarely presents as isolated cholestasis outside the neonatal period. As patients with cystic fibrosis are living longer, the prevalence of hepatic disease associated with the disorder, ranging from steatohepatitis to cholecystitis, is becoming better understood.

Biliary tract disorders. These can obstruct bile drainage and result in a conjugated hyperbilirubinemia. Abdominal ultrasound is useful for evaluating for gallstones or choledochal cysts. Cholangiography is useful for detecting the "beading and stenosis" pattern of the intrahepatic bile ducts that is classic for primary sclerosing cholangitis.

Hepatotoxins. There is a variety of drugs or other substances that can cause liver failure and resultant hyperbilirubinemia. Acetaminophen overdose is the leading cause of fulminant hepatic failure in older children and adolescents. The toxicity of acetaminophen results from glutathione depletion, thereby shunting metabolism of excess acetaminophen to the hepatic P450 system, which produces a hepatotoxic metabolite, *N*-acetyl-*p*-benzoquinoneimine (NAPQI). The patient will present with nausea and vomiting that then progresses to acute hepatic dysfunction, followed by failure. *N*-Acetylcysteine (NAC) is the antidote for acetaminophen ingestions.

Management/disposition

The management of a child with jaundice, and their ultimate disposition, depends entirely on their appearance, results of diagnostic tests, and reliability for follow-up. Most often, a child or adolescent who presents with first-time jaundice will be admitted. In particular, when the etiology of jaundice is unknown, inpatient observation while the workup is completed is prudent. At times, a liver biopsy may also be needed, which should be coordinated during the inpatient stay. Obviously, any child who is clinically unstable or ill-appearing should be transferred to a facility with pediatric specialists in both gastroenterology and liver transplant. Close contact with the primary care clinician, as well as with these consultants, should be initiated from the ED to determine a plan of care. Worrisome signs in a patient with jaundice include bilirubin levels >18 mg/dl, clinical suspicion for cerebral edema or hepatic encephalopathy, elevation of the PT, hypoglycemia, ascites, or an elevated creatinine suggesting multiorgan involvement or hepato-renal syndrome. Jaundice in a older child or adolescent may be the first sign of fulminant liver failure, and these patients should be assessed carefully.

Pearls and pitfalls

Pearls

1. Abdominal ultrasound is the test of choice for evaluating conjugated hyperbilirubinemia.
2. Infants <3 months of age with direct bilirubin >2 mg/dl, need urgent pediatric GI consultation.
3. In general, increased direct (conjugated) hyperbilirubinemia is indicative of obstructive process; increased indirect (unconjugated) hyperbilirubinemia is indicative of hemolysis.

Pitfalls

1. Failure to determine whether the hyperbilirubinemia is conjugated or unconjugated.
2. Failure to consult appropriate specialists regarding the management of these patients, or for close follow-up.

Selected references

Harb R, Thomas DW. Conjugated hyperbilirubinemia: screening and treatment in older infants and children. *Pediatr Rev* 2007;**28**:83–91.

Pashankar D, Schreiber RA. Jaundice in older children and adolescents. *Pediatr Rev* 2001;**22**:219–226.

Chapter

68 Fulminant hepatic failure

Bill Schroeder

Introduction

Acute liver failure (ALF) also known as fulminant hepatic failure is a rare but important cause of pediatric morbidity and mortality. It can be caused by different, relatively rare pathologies (Table 68.1), with variation with age. Overall, children with acute liver failure have a better spontaneous survival and better success rate after liver transplant than do adults.

Acute liver failure is defined as the onset of signs of hepatic failure (specifically clotting abnormalities, PT >15 s [INR ≥1.5], and any degree of mental alteration, referred to as encephalopathy) within 26 weeks of onset of an illness affecting the liver. The definition in children is more complicated given that many children, even with severe ALF that leads to death and/or liver transplant, never develop encephalopathy. In addition, it is very difficult to recognize encephalopathy in children, particularly infants (Table 68.2). Therefore, the Pediatric Acute Liver Failure Study Group defines acute liver failure as children with

- biochemical evidence of acute liver injury
- no known evidence of chronic liver disease, and
- a hepatic-based coagulopathy that does not correct with vitamin K.

It defines coagulopathy as

- a PT ≥15 s or INR ≥1.5 in the presence of encephalopathy, or
- a PT ≥20 s or INR ≥2.0 regardless of the presence or absence of clinical encephalopathy.

Clinical presentation

Acute liver failure can be a difficult diagnosis to make as it has many different etiologies. Although many children present with jaundice, the first symptoms are often vague and include a prodrome of malaise, nausea, vomiting, and poor appetite. Other symptoms include progressive jaundice, asterixis, tremors, poor sleep, fetor hepaticus, and encephalopathy. Fetor hepaticus is the breath odor produced as a result of the damaged liver's inability to metabolize and detoxify mercaptans produced by gut bacteria; it has been described as musty, fruity, or reminiscent of garlic. It is an inconsistent and late finding in ALF.

Pathophysiology and management

Children with ALF can present in shock from hypovolemia and hypotension secondary to a state of high cardiac output and vasodilatation similar to sepsis. Correction of this physiology may help to prevent the progression of multiorgan failure, particularly renal failure. Although children eventually need fluid restriction to help to prevent progression of cerebral edema, initially they are usually dehydrated and require careful rehydration. This is because most patients have had some degree of poor fluid intake, vomiting, and or diarrhea. Use of both crystalloid and colloid may be needed to restore the circulating volume. Because of the delicate fluid balance of these patients, early invasive monitoring is often required.

Coagulation defects are an important by-product of ALF. Reduced production of clotting factors and platelets, as well as increased consumption of both in disseminated intravascular coagulation, causes the coagulopathy. Unless the patient requires a life-saving invasive procedure or has a life-threatening hemorrhage (which is uncommon), the coagulopathy should not be corrected for two important reasons. First, the progression of the coagulopathy provides important prognostic information. Second, it could complicate listing the patient for a liver transplant. However, IV administration of vitamin K is always indicated as many patients are deficient as a result of cholestasis.

One of the most devastating complications of ALF is cerebral edema, which is found in up to 80% of the patients who die. The exact mechanism for cerebral edema is unknown.

A Practical Guide to Pediatric Emergency Medicine: Caring for Children in the Emergency Department, ed. N. Ewen Amieva-Wang (associate eds. Jamie Shandro, Aparajita Sohoni, and Bernhard Fassl). Published by Cambridge University Press.

Table 68.1. Age-based differential diagnosis for acute liver failure

	Infant	Child	Adolescent
Toxin/drug			
Most common	Acetaminophen (Tylenol) misadventure	Acetaminophen	Acetaminophen
Other		Valproic acid, isoniazid, halothane, phosphorus, acetylsalicylic acid, vitamin A toxicity	Mushrooms, monoamine oxidase inhibitor, *Bacillus cereus* toxin, tetracycline, Ecstasy
Infectious			
Most common	Herpes simplex, enterovirus	Epstein–Barr virus	Hepatitis A virus
Other	Echovirus, adenovirus, Epstein–Barr virus, hepatitis B virus, parvovirus, measles, human herpesvirus 6	Hepatitis A/B/C/D/E viruses, leptospirosis	Hepatitis B/C/D/E viruses, yellow fever, Dengue fever, Lassa fever
Immune/metabolic			
Most common	Fatty acid defects, mitochondrial defects, natural killer cell dysfunction	Autoimmune disease	Wilson's disease, autoimmune disease
Other	Galactosemia, tyrosinemia, neonatal hemachromatosis, fructose intolerance, hemophagocytic syndrome, Neimann–Pick type C	Fatty acid oxidation defects, leukemia, hemophagocytic syndrome, natural killer cell dysfunction, Wilson's disease, mitochondrial defect	Fatty liver of pregnancy, protoporphyria, fatty acid oxidation defects
Shock/ cardiovascular	Hypoplastic left heart, asphyxia, myocarditis	Heart surgery, cardiomyopathy, Budd–Chiari syndrome, myocarditis	

Table 68.2. Adjusted encephalopathy scale for children: birth to 3 years

Grade	Clinical	Reflexes/ neurologic
Early (I and II)	Confusion, inconsolable crying, sleep reversal, inattentiveness, mood changes	Possible asterixis, normal or hyperreflexia
Mid (III)	Somnolence and follows commands or stuporous but arousable, combative	Possible asterixis, hyperreflexia
Late (IVa and b)	IVa: comatose but arouses to pain IVb: comatose and not arousable	Absent reflexes/ asterixis, decorticate or decerebrate posturing

Children who develop grade III or IV encephalopathy usually require intubation (Table 68.2). Propofol is a good choice for sedation as ALF does not affect its pharmacokinetics and it is neuroprotective. Other strategies that have been suggested to help to manage increased intracranial pressure and severe encephalopathy include to raise the head of the bed to 30 degrees, to induce hypothermia (34–36°C) and hypernatremia (145–155 mEq/l), to give mannitol or hypertonic saline boluses, and to provide continous venovenous hemofiltration.

Refractory hypoglycemia may also occur because there are decreased gluconeogenesis and glycogen stores. Hypertonic glucose solutions via central line may be required because as much as 10 to 15 mg/kg per min of glucose may be needed to correct hypoglycemia. Other frequent electrolyte derangements are hypokalemia, hypophosphatemia, and acid–base disorders. These include respiratory alkalosis from hyperventilation, respiratory acidosis from respiratory failure, metabolic alkalosis from hypokalemia, and metabolic acidosis from shock or hepatic necrosis.

Superimposed sepsis is often present in hepatic decompensation. After obtaining appropriate cultures, broad-spectrum antibiotic administration should be considered.

For ALF secondary to acute acetaminophen hepatotoxicity, *N*-acetylcysteine (NAC) is both very successful and well known to both pediatricians and adult ER physicians. Caution must be used when giving IV NAC to young children, given the risk of iatragenic hyponatremia. There is even preliminary evidence that NAC may be helpful in non-acetaminophen-induced acute liver failure. Presumed benefits are increased hepatic oxygen delivery, consumption, and extraction, as well as improved coagulopathy and decreased progression of encephalopathy.

Pearls and pitfalls

Pearls

1. The definition and causes of acute liver failure in children differ from those in adults.
2. Severe coagulopathy is a more universal sign of acute liver failure in children then hepatic encephalopathy.
3. When using IV *N*-acetylcysteine (NAC), use a more concentrated NAC solution to prevent hyponatremia, particularly in children <20 kg.
4. A 1 liter 3% NAC solution can be made by adding 30 g NAC (150 ml of a 20% solution) to 850 ml D5W.

Pitfalls

1. Failure to realize that hepatic encephalopathy is not required for the diagnosis of acute liver failure in children.
2. Failure to realize that asterixis, tremors, and fetor hepaticus, which are common in adult liver failure, are often absent in children.
3. The only signs of hepatic encephalopathy may be irritability, poor feeding, vomiting, and changes in sleep (particularly reversal of day-night sleeping), particularly in the very young.

Selected references

Acute Liver Failure Study Group. http://acuteliverfailure.org/ (accessed 28 April 2010).

Bernal W, Auzinger G, Sizer E, Wendon J. Intensive care management of acute liver failure. *Semin Liver Dis* 2008;**2**:188–200.

Brush DE, Boyer EW. Intravenous *N*-acetylcysteine for children. *Pediatr Emerg Care* 2004;**20**:649–650.

Cochran JB, Losek JD. Acute liver failure in children. *Pediatr Emerg Care* 2007;**23**:129–135.

Squires Jr. RH, Shneider BL, Bucuvalas J, *et al.* Acute liver failure in children: the first 348 patients in the pediatric acute liver failure study group. *J Pediatr* 2006;**148**:652–658.

Chapter 69

Pancreatitis

Aparajita Sohoni

Introduction

Acute and chronic pancreatitis are rare in the pediatric population and chronic pancreatitis is even more rare than acute pancreatitis. There are "no reliable estimates" of the true prevalence of either condition. In adults, the two most common causes of acute pancreatitis are alcohol abuse and biliary disease such as gallstones. The causes of pancreatitis in pediatric patients are often more varied and complex: idiopathic (23%), trauma (22%), structural anomalies (15%), multisystem disease (14%), drugs and toxins (12%), viral infections (10%) and other congenital or metabolic conditions.

Pathophysiology

Acute pancreatitis is defined as abdominal pain of sudden onset in conjunction with an elevation in serum or urine pancreatic digestive enzymes, with or without corresponding radiographic changes. In acute pancreatitis, pancreatic inflammation is triggered by any of a range of mechanisms, including trauma to the pancreas, obstruction to pancreatic flow, toxin exposure, metabolic abnormalities, or increased permeability of the pancreatic duct. Traumatic events frequently involve handlebar-injuries, motor vehicle accidents, or child abuse. Several viruses, including mumps, hepatitis A, CMV, rubella, enterovirus, and coxsackievirus have been found to cause acute pancreatitis. Many medications, such as valproic acid, furosemide, thiazides, thiopurines (azathioprine and 6-mercaptopurine), and steroids, are also known to cause pancreatitis. Biliary tract obstruction by stones or sludge, choledochal or duodenal cysts, or other congenital conditions such as pancreas divisum or stenosis of the sphincter of Oddi can also give rise to pancreatitis. Generally, acute pancreatitis resolves without affecting function of the pancreas. In fulminant pancreatitis, the initial inflammatory cascade is begun within the pancreas; the acinar cells become damaged and can produce edema, necrosis, hemorrhage, or ischemia of the entire gland. These inflammatory changes can spread to involve the peritoneal space or cause multisystem organ failure.

Chronic pancreatitis results from persistent inflammation causing irreversible damage to the gland, evidenced by fibrosis, islet cell and acinar cell loss, and inflammatory cell infiltration. Currently, it is postulated that chronic pancreatitis evolves from repeated episodes of acute pancreatitis, leading to fibrosis and resultant malfunctioning of the gland. Cystic fibrosis is the most common genetic cause of chronic pancreatitis. Another genetic etiology of pancreatitis is hereditary pancreatitis, thought to result from mutations in the gene for trypsinogen. These patients generally present at around 10 years of age but can present as early as 1 year old. A family history of pancreatitis is classic. Genetic testing is available to confirm the diagnosis.

Clinical presentation

The majority of pediatric patients complain of abdominal pain, nausea, and decreased appetite during an episode of pancreatitis. The location of the pain need not be solely epigastric, and the duration and intensity of the pain may vary significantly. While adults more classically complain of epigastric pain radiating to the back, pediatric patients generally do not complain of radiation of pain. Less commonly observed signs of pancreatitis in pediatric patients include fever, hypotension, jaundice, tachycardia, guarding, or decreased bowel sounds. Cullen's sign and Grey Turner's sign, both manifestations of hemorrhagic pancreatitis, are rarely observed.

Diagnosis

Pancreatitis is diagnosed by a combination of history, physical examination, laboratory, and radiographic findings. Serum amylase, cleared by the kidneys, remains the mainstay of laboratory evaluation of pancreatitis. Amylase levels rise within 2–12 h after the inflammatory process has begun and remain elevated for as long as 5 days. The absolute value of the amylase does not correlate with severity of the pancreatitis, and a level greater than three times normal is thought to be significant for causing pancreatitis.

Amylase has a lower sensitivity in pediatric patients than in adults.

A Practical Guide to Pediatric Emergency Medicine: Caring for Children in the Emergency Department, ed. N. Ewen Amieva-Wang (associate eds. Jamie Shandro, Aparajita Sohoni, and Bernhard Fassl). Published by Cambridge University Press.

An incidence as high as 40% of cases of pancreatitis in pediatric patients with a normal amylase has been reported. Lipase levels are generally elevated for a longer period of time than amylase levels. Lipase, like amylase, is secreted from a variety of places in the body and can be falsely elevated. Combined elevations of amylase and lipase are thought to be a more sensitive/specific measurement than either alone; however, there is still considerable controversy surrounding this issue.

Additional laboratory testing that contributes to predicting the severity of pancreatitis includes serum glucose level, hypocalcemia, leukocytosis, elevated bilirubin, alkaline phosphatase, and gamma-glutamyl transpeptidase.

While imaging is not always required for pancreatitis, particularly in the ED, imaging studies for the diagnosis of pancreatitis include ultrasound, CT, MRI, magnetic resonance cholangiopancreatography, or endoscopic retrograde cholangiopancreatography. Findings on ultrasound include peripancreatic fluid collections and decreased echogenicity of the pancreas. Disadvantages of ultrasound include operator variability. The modality of choice for detecting acute pancreatitis is CT, particularly in traumatic cases where other intra-abdominal injuries can be identified. It has a sensitivity of 91% and specificity of 78% for pancreatitis. The major disadvantage is the radiation required.

Management

The mainstay of management for acute pancreatitis is supportive care while allowing the pancreas to "rest." Supportive care includes aggressive IV hydration, repletion of electrolytes, pain control, and enteric fasting. The major complications of pancreatitis include the development of pancreatic necrosis (usually seen within 2 weeks of the acute injury) or the formation of a pseudocyst (seen after 2 weeks). Necrotic pancreatitis is a rare but rapidly life-threatening condition, with a pediatric mortality rate of 15–50%. Early recognition is key as surgical intervention may be needed.

The most common complication of pancreatitis is formation of a pseudocyst. This complication is more frequently seen after trauma-induced pancreatitis. Options for management of a pseudocyst include observation for possible spontaneous resolution or resorption (successful in 30% of pseudocysts), drainage by interventional radiology, or surgical drainage. The management strategy should be determined in conjunction with a consulting surgeon. Less common complications include jejunal infarction, splenic vein thrombosis, pancreatic insufficiency, or diabetes mellitus. Offending medications should be discontinued and substituted after discussion with the prescribing physician. Chronic pancreatitis should be managed similarly, with the overall goal of elucidating the etiology and moving towards pancreatic enzyme supplementation as fibrosis of the pancreas progresses.

Disposition

Pediatric patients with acute pancreatitis should be admitted for workup, supportive care, and therapeutic intervention (if indicated). If the patient is stable and appears well and has chronic pancreatitis of known etiology, outpatient management is a viable option provided that close follow-up with a pediatrician can be arranged. Extensive return precautions should be provided to patients and their caregivers.

Pearls and pitfalls

Pearls

1. Acute pancreatitis in children is rare.
2. Causes of pancreatitis in pediatric patients are more varied than in adults and include trauma, structural anomalies, viral infections, drugs, and toxins.
3. Children with pancreatitis can present with non-specific abdominal pain; often they do not describe pain radiating to the back.

Pitfalls

1. Failure to include cystic fibrosis in the differential diagnosis of abdominal pain in a child with recurrent pancreatitis.
2. Failure to consider pancreatitis in children on medications known to cause pancreatitis.

Selected references

Benifla M, Weizman Z. Acute pancreatitis in childhood: analysis of literature data. *J Clin Gastroenterol* 2003;**37**:169–172.

Greenfeld JI, Harmon CM. Acute pancreatitis. *Curr Opin Pediatr* 1997;**9**:260–264.

Jackson WD. Pancreatitis: etiology, diagnosis, and management. *Curr Opin Pediatr* 2001;**13**:447–451.

Lerner A, Branski D, Lebenthal E. Pancreatic diseases in children. *Pediatr Clin North Am* 1996;**43**: 125–156.

Lowe ME. Pancreatitis in childhood. *Curr Gastroenterol Rep* 2004;**6**:240–246.

Chapter 70

Rectal complaints

N. Ewen Amieva-Wang and Aparajita Sohoni

Perianal itching

Perianal itching is not an uncommon complaint in children. Common causes include:

- fecal irritation: poor hygiene, diarrhea or poorly formed stools
- anorectal disease: fissures, hemorrhoids
- dermatologic pathology: contact dermatitis, atopic dermatitis
- infections: pinworm (*Enterobiasis*), scabies, candida, *Staphylococcal aureus*
- dietary irritants.

While anal itching can be caused by dermatologic or anorectal disease, in children it is usually caused by fecal irritation secondary either to diarrhea or, usually, poor hygiene. Chapter 26 discusses diaper dermatitis.

Pinworms

Pinworms are one of the most common parasitic infections in North America. Children commonly develop infection because of fecal oral contamination.

Children with pinworm infestation usually have pruritus at night, when the adult pinworms migrate to the anus to lay eggs.

History and examination can usually narrow the differential diagnosis. The "scotch tape test" is used to detect eggs (Box 70.1). Sometimes adult worms can be seen (approximately 1 cm in length) but visualization of worms is not necessary for diagnosis. Treatment is with either mebendazole (100 mg in one dose) or albendazole (100 mg dose if <2 years of age otherwise 400 mg). A second dose of either drug in 2 weeks prevents reinfection. Although treatment is highly effective, reinfection is not uncommon. The entire family should be treated and sheets and clothes washed to prevent reinfection. Because the eggs can accumulate under the fingernails and then be reinnoculated orally, fingernails should be clipped and handwashing encouraged.

Box 70.1. Scotch tape test

1. Apply scotch tape to anal area at night or first thing in the morning.
2. Microscopic examination will show bean-shaped eggs approximately 50 μm× 25 μm in size.
3. Three samples are diagnostic in 90% of cases.

Anal fissures

Anal fissures most often occur in children <1 year of age; they are reported as the most common source of lower GI bleeding in this population.

Injury and bleeding occur following the passage of a large hard stool. After a hard stool, infants may actively withhold stool to prevent another painful episode. Physical examination with gentle spreading of the buttocks demonstrates a tear, most often located in the posterior midline. Treatment includes stool softeners such as colace or mineral oil, perianal care, and application of ointments to prevent excoriation. Consistent treatment often results in painless bowel movements and healing of injury in 6–8 weeks. Patients with diarrhea can develop excoriation of the anal area with some bleeding. These patients require careful cleaning and barrier ointments to protect excoriated skin.

Rectal prolapse

Rectal prolapse is the protrusion of the rectal mucosa, a red mass, through the external anal sphincter (Fig. 70.1). It presents as a red mass protruding from the rectum during straining and can also reduce spontaneously. The description can be sufficient to make the diagnosis. Also examining the child while straining or squatting can reproduce the prolapse. Prolapse is usually painless or only mildly uncomfortable. Digital examination will demonstrate that the mucosa is continuous with the perianal skin. Anal tone can be decreased, which is usually temporary.

Rectal prolapse occurs in children usually under 4 years of age with underlying predisposition. Predisposing conditions include diarrheal disease, increased intra-abdominal pressure (constipation, chronic coughing), cystic fibrosis, decreased pelvic muscle tone as occurs in neurologic disorders, and

A Practical Guide to Pediatric Emergency Medicine: Caring for Children in the Emergency Department, ed. N. Ewen Amieva-Wang (associate eds. Jamie Shandro, Aparajita Sohoni, and Bernhard Fassl). Published by Cambridge University Press.

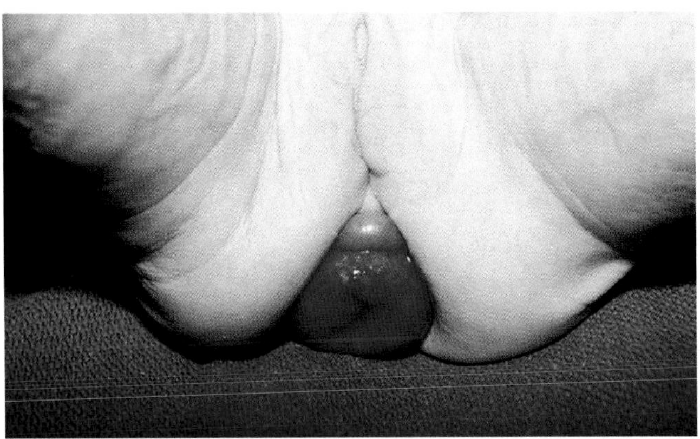

Figure 70.1. Rectal prolapse. Note the bright red tissue extruding from the anus. Causes include constipation, diarrhea, and cystic fibrosis. Rectal prolapse can be confused with intussusception. (Reproduced with permission from Zitelli BJ, Davis HW. *Atlas of Pediatric Physical Diagnosis* 5th edn. Philadelphia, PA: Mosby Elsevier, 2007. © 2007 Mosby Inc., an affiliate of Elsevier Inc.)

malnutrition. Rectal prolapse occurs in a quarter of children with cystic fibrosis and was a common presenting symptom prior to implementation of newborn screening.

All children who present with rectal prolapse without obvious predisposition should be screened for cystic fibrosis.

Intestinal parasites such as *Ascaris lumbercoides* and *Trichuris trichuria* (whip worm) are common cause of rectal prolapse in children in developing countries. Abuse must also be considered.

Other differential diagnoses include ileocecal intussusception, rectal hemorrhoids, and prolapsed rectal polyp. Children with intussusception are usually systemically ill with intermittent colicky pain. The intussusception is also separate from, instead of continuous with, the anal skin. Polyps and hemorrhoids can also be differentiated from rectal prolapse on physical examination. Children with trichuriasis will often have worms visible in the mucosa of the rectum. Definitive diagnosis can be made with stool examination for eggs.

Rectal prolapse can usually be manually reduced with firm even pressure to the prolapsed mucosa. Sometimes a finger in the rectum can guide the reduction. Rectal examination should be done afterwards to confirm reduction. Pressure dressing of lubricant and gauze should be applied. The underlying cause of the prolapse should be addressed. If manual reduction fails, surgical reduction should be performed promptly to avoid complications such as rectal ulcers. The majority of children will recover with conservative treatment. Treatment for trichuriasis is mebendazole 100 mg PO daily for 3 days or albendazole 400 mg for 3 days.

Selected references

American Academy of Pediatrics. Pinworm infection (*Enterobius vermicularis*). In Pickering LK (ed.) *Red Book: 2009 Report of the Committee on Infectious Diseases*, 28th edn. Elk Grove Village, IL: American Academy of Pediatrics, 2009. pp. 519–520.

American Academy of Pediatrics. Trichuriasis (whipworm infection). In Pickering LK (ed.) *Red Book: 2009 Report of the Committee on Infectious Diseases*, 28th edn. Elk Grove Village, IL: American Academy of Pediatrics, 2009. pp. 675–676.

Chapter 71

Umbilical lesions

Marcela P. Mendenhall and N. Ewen Amieva-Wang

Introduction

The most common umbilical lesions are secondary to trauma, infection, and congenital defects. Most patients with umblical lesions are neonates. The umbilical stump may be macerated or bleeding, with granulomatous tissue or a polyp. Omphalitis while rare, is a life-threatening infection. In older infants and children, except for umbilical hernia, umbilical masses are extremely rare.

Inflammatory lesions

Normal umbilical stump

The umbilical cord is clamped at birth and over the course of 7–14 days, it detaches. In developed countries, normal cord care consists of aseptic clamping and cutting the cord at birth and then gentle cleaning with water or alcohol at each diaper change. Topical antibiotics are not needed as a routine part of umbilical cord care to avoid infection.

It is not uncommon for parents to come to the ED because of concerns about the umbilical stump. Often the stump is macerated (by the diaper) with some bleeding; it can have some discharge and odor without signs of skin infection. Reassurance and demonstration of cleaning techniques as well as covering the cord stump with cotton gauze usually is sufficient care. Treatment with topical antibiotics is not known to affect outcome.

Umbilical granuloma

Umbilical granuloma is the most common cause of an umbilical mass. It develops in the first weeks of life after the cord has separated and is thought to be caused by inflammation of the cord. Umbilical granulomas are a friable, pink mass of granulation tissue up to a centimeter in size. Treatment is cautery with silver nitrate, and it usually requires multiple treatments, which can be done by the pediatrician. If the granuloma does not resolve after multiple treatments, the diagnosis should be reconsidered (umbilical polyp).

Umbilical polyp

Umbilical polyps are rare and result from vestiges of the omphalomesenteric or urachal ducts. These lesions are larger, firmer, and fleshier than umblical granulomas. They must be surgically removed. Pathology can differentiate a granuloma from a polyp if the diagnosis is in question.

Infection

Omphalitis

Omphalitis or infection of the umbilicus and the surrounding skin is rare in areas with aseptic umbilical care. It is a disease of the neonate. The umbilicus often has purulent discharge with a surrounding cellulitic-appearing area (red, indurated, and tender). Systemic signs such as fever, and lethargy indicate spread of infection. Diagnosis is clinical, although the purulent drainage should be cultured. Patients with omphalitis regardless of systemic signs must have a full workup to exclude sepsis. Treatment is with antistaphylococcal penicillin and aminoglycoside agents to cover Gram-positive and Gram-negative organisms. Additional anaerobic coverage is warranted in the sicker neonate with concern for necrotizing fasciitis. Neonatal necrotizing fasciitis and death are rare complications of omphalitis.

Congenital defects

Umbilical hernia

After birth, and the cutting of the umbilical cord, the umbilical ring in the infant's abdominal wall closes by the growth and joining of the rectus abdominus muscles. The peritoneal and fascial layers fuse at the umbilicus. Thus all infants have an umbilical hernia and most are resolved by 5 years of age. The majority of umbilical hernias are asymptomatic, very rarely become incarcerated or strangulated, and will spontaneously resolve. Unless the hernia is incarcerated, reassurance is the best management. Incarcerated umbilical hernias require prompt surgical repair to avoid strangulation.

A Practical Guide to Pediatric Emergency Medicine: Caring for Children in the Emergency Department, ed. N. Ewen Amieva-Wang (associate eds. Jamie Shandro, Aparajita Sohoni, and Bernhard Fassl). Published by Cambridge University Press.

Omphalomesenteric duct and urachal anomalies

Incomplete involution of the omphalomesenteric duct can cause a spectrum of symptoms, from an umbilical polyp to intestinal drainage from the umbilicus. Tissue can persist at the umbilicus with no intestinal connection (umbilical polyp); tissue can persist at the ileum with umbilical connection (Meckel's diverticulum is most common [Ch. 63]) or the duct can persist with no umbilical or ileal connection (omphalomesenteric duct cyst). Fibrous connections between the umbilicus and ileum can cause a small bowel obstruction. A complete connection leads to a persistent omphalomesenteric duct, with leakage of bowel contents from the umbilicus. Treatment is surgical excision.

Incomplete involution of the urachus between the umbilicus and the bladder leads to a similar spectrum of symptoms but is relatively rare. An umbilical polyp, bladder cyst, or urachal cyst can present as an abdominal mass, infection, or with draining of bladder contents via the umbilicus. Diagnosis is with renal ultrasound and treatment is surgical excision. The urologist or primary care physician should obtain renal ultrasound and voiding cystogram since urachal anomalies are associated with other genitourinary abnormalities.

Conclusions

Umbilical lesions can be inflammatory, infectious, or congenital. In the majority of cases they will be benign. Umbilical granulomas can be cauterized and umbilical hernias will usually resolve with time. The EP must consider omphalomesenteric duct and urachal anomalies, including umbilical polyps, in order to obtain the correct treatment for patients with these disorders.

Pearls and pitfalls

Pearls

1. The most common cause of an umbilical mass in the neonate is the umbilical granuloma.
2. Umbilical granulomas can be treated with silver nitrate. Umbilical polyps must be surgically excised.
3. All infants have an umbilical hernia, which is asymptomatic and which gradually closes by 5 years of age.
4. Failed involution of the omphalomesenteric and urachal ducts can cause a spectrum of rare umbilical disorders.

Pitfalls

1. Failure to recognize an incarcerated umbilical hernia.
2. Failure to recognize and aggressively treat omphalitis, a rare polymicrobial infection that starts in the umbilicus and can spread to the abdominal wall.

Selected reference

Pomeranz A. Anomalies, abnormalities, and care of the umbilicus. *Pediatr Clin North Am* 2004;**51**:819–827.

Chapter

72 Gastrointestinal foreign bodies

Aparajita Sohoni

Introduction

Foreign body ingestions in the pediatric patient differ from adult ingestions primarily in the type of object ingested and the motivation behind the ingestion (i.e., intentional versus accidental or recreational). Pediatric patients most frequently ingest coins, toys, needles or pins, batteries, and food-related items (e.g., chicken bones).

Approximately 80% of all foreign body ingestion cases occur in children <3 years of age.

Clinical presentation

The clinical signs and symptoms following foreign body ingestion vary with the type of object ingested, its location, size, and amount of time elapsed since ingestion. In pediatric patients, foreign bodies generally lodge at the upper esophageal sphincter or thoracic inlet (60–70%), just proximal to the lower esophageal sphincter (20%), or in the mid-esophagus (at the aortic notch) (Figure 72.1). Patients may complain of dysphagia, chest pain, odynophagia, or respiratory symptoms if there has been tracheal compression. On clinical examination, drooling or choking behavior may be seen, as well as posterior oropharyngeal erythema. The most severe complications of foreign body ingestion generally occur with longer and sharper objects or after ingestion of more than one magnet, and include GI perforation, fistula formation, or tracheal erosion. In these cases, severe abdominal pain, GI hemorrhage, or chest wall crepitus may be seen.

Diagnosis

The diagnosis of foreign body ingestion is generally made by history. The nature of the object, including size and composition (i.e., lead content) should be determined. Radiographs are helpful to visualize the current location of the foreign body and should be obtained if the object ingested is a coin or other radiopaque object.

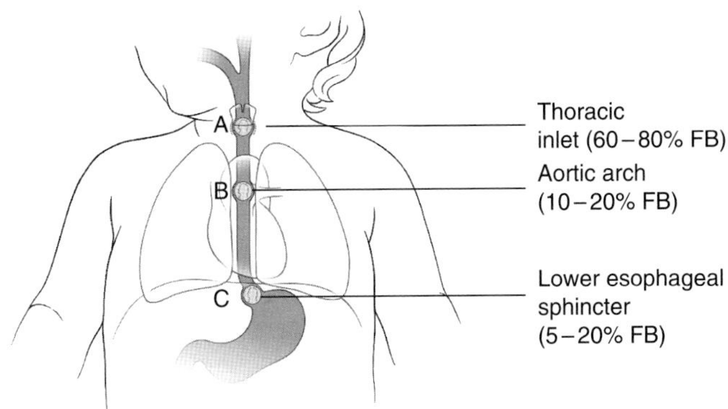

Figure 72.1 In pediatric patients, foreign bodies (FB) generally lodge at the thoracic inlet, upper esophageal sphincter (A), in the mid-esophagus (at the aortic arch, right main stem bronchus) (B), or just proximal to the lower esophageal sphincter (C). (Copyright Chris Gralapp.)

Coins in the esophagus appear "enface" on anterior–posterior chest radiographs, while the edge of the coin is seen on the lateral view.

Figure 72.2 shows a coin in the esophagus. In comparison, coins aspirated into the trachea appear "enface" on the lateral view and show the thin edge on the anterior–posterior radiograph. If there is any concern for lodging of a foreign body in the stomach or lower, abdominal series radiographs may be obtained.

Management

All esophageal foreign bodies warrant urgent removal. This is usually done by rigid or flexible endoscopy by either ENT or GI services (depending on hospital tradition). Objects that are not batteries, sharp, long, or magnetic can usually be managed with observation and radiographic follow-up. Those objects that have already passed beyond the proximal duodenum will usually pass without complications.

Coins

If a patient is severely symptomatic (i.e., unable to tolerate secretions or with severe respiratory distress) from an ingested

A Practical Guide to Pediatric Emergency Medicine: Caring for Children in the Emergency Department, ed. N. Ewen Amieva-Wang (associate eds. Jamie Shandro, Aparajita Sohoni, and Bernhard Fassl). Published by Cambridge University Press.

A

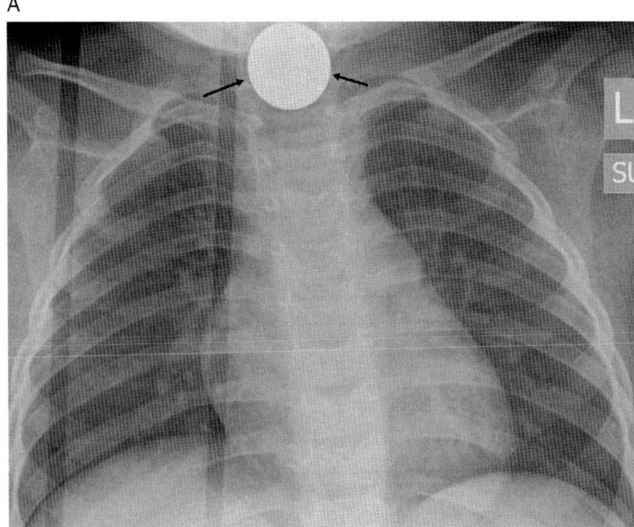

B

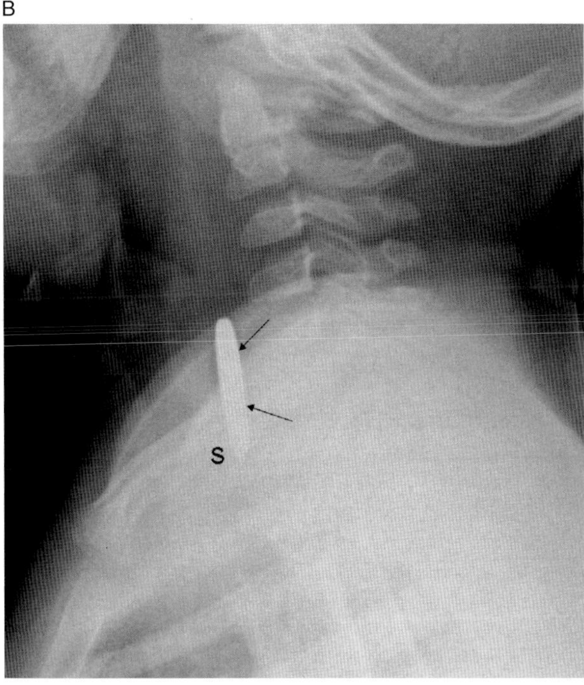

Figure 72.2 Coin in the esophagus in a 2-year-old boy. Chest radiographs with a coin lodged in the esophagus seen (A) flat on the frontal view (arrowed) and (B) on-edge on the lateral view (arrowed). Soft tissue thickening between the trachea and the esophagus on the lateral view suggests subacute or chronic inflammatory reaction (S). The tracheal air column is focally narrowed in this location.

esophageal coin, endoscopic removal should be arranged immediately. Asymptomatic patients should have the object removed within 12 to 24 h to allow for appropriate preoperative management. Glucagon has not been found to be effective for coin ingestion. Once a coin has passed into the stomach and past the pylorus, it will generally traverse the remainder of the GI tract without any adverse event. Coins being observed for passage can be followed with abdominal radiographs at 2–3 weeks and 4–6 weeks post-ingestion. The stool should be strained to ensure detection of the coin. If the coin does not spontaneously pass by 6 weeks, endoscopic removal should be arranged.

Batteries

Button batteries are the most common type of battery ingested by children. The danger of battery ingestions is from their content of concentrated alkali or sodium/potassium hydroxide. These alkali substances mimic a lye ingestion by causing liquefaction necrosis and can result in deep burns or perforation of the esophagus. If there is any history suggesting an ingested battery, radiographs must be taken to locate the battery.

Immediate endoscopic removal of a button battery is warranted.

Esophageal perforations can occur as early as 6 h following ingestion. Once passed into the stomach, batteries are generally able to pass through the remainder of the GI tract. Prolonged presence in the stomach can cause gastric ulceration. If a battery is in the stomach, serial radiographs should be done and close follow-up arranged with a gastroenterologist in case removal is needed.

Sharp or long objects

Pins or other sharp objects should be removed because of the risk of perforation or bleeding. Objects in the mouth should be removed with Magill's forceps. Sharp objects in the esophagus or stomach or those longer than 5 cm benefit from endoscopic retrieval in consultation with GI/ENT service.

Magnets

With the advent of magnetic toys, it has been found that ingestion of more than one high-power field magnet can lead to the formation of a fistula between the stomach and the intestines or between the intestines themselves. Magnets should be removed via endoscopy if they are within the stomach. If not, the stool should be monitored for passage, and serial abdominal radiographs taken to ensure that they have been removed safely.

Food bolus impaction

Esophageal food impaction is generally a consequence of underlying structural pathology of the esophagus, including narrowing of the esophagus from peptic ulcer disease, postoperative strictures, or eosinophilic esophagitis, an increasingly recognized condition. Any symptomatic patient (i.e., unable to tolerate their secretions) should have endoscopy carried out within 12 h. Asymptomatic patients can wait 12 h for endoscopy. The most common food associated with impaction is a meat bolus. Meat tenderizer should never be used as it can adversely affect the esophageal lining.

Disposition

Children who have ingested a foreign body may be sent home once the appropriate diagnostic workup and management is complete. Patients who have endoscopic removal of the object may be able to go home immediately. Patients who have ingested objects that warrant observation either before or after removal of the object should be admitted. Consultation with ENT/gastroenterologists will guide the disposition of these patients. Close follow-up for serial radiographs and return precautions should be explained to caregivers.

Pearls and pitfalls

Pearls

1. Urgent endoscopic removal of an ingested foreign body should be arranged for any symptomatic patient, or for a button battery that has not passed the pylorus.
2. Objects larger than 15 mm are unlikely to pass the pylorus and will need endoscopic removal.
3. In pediatric patients, foreign bodies generally lodge at either the upper esophageal sphincter (60–70%), just proximal to the lower esophageal sphincter (20%), or in the mid-esophagus (at the aortic notch).
4. Glucagon has not been shown to be helpful in esophageal foreign bodies in children.

Pitfalls

1. Administration of meat tenderizer for an impacted meat bolus.
2. Failure to consult GI early for possible caustic ingested foreign bodies.
3. Failure to realize that ingestion of two or more high-power field magnets can cause formation of a fistula between adjacent loops of bowel.

Selected references

Kay M, Wyllie R. Pediatric foreign bodies and their management. *Curr Gastroenterol Rep* 2005;7:212–218.

Litovitz TL, Klein-Schwartz W, White S, *et al.* 2000 Annual Report of the American Association of Poison Control Centers Toxic Exposure Surveillance System. *Am J Emerg Med* 2001;**19**:337–395.

Chapter

73 Tutorial: What imaging study should I get?

Teresa S. Wu

Diagnostic dilemmas in abdominal imaging

Of the numerous causes of acute abdominal pain in children, there are four that may present diagnostic dilemmas once the decision has been made to obtain an imaging study and these are discussed here. Modality selection will vary somewhat based on personal and institutional preferences, but it is important to be cognizant of the multiple options that currently exist.

Ultrasound provides a non-invasive means by which to quickly assess the pediatric abdomen in the absence of ionizing radiation. Correlation of the sonographic images with a complete history and physical examination allows for the safe and effective evaluation of common pediatric ailments (see Ch. 170).

Imaging options for appendicitis

A child presenting with appendicitis typically complains of periumbilical pain that migrates down into the RLQ as the inflammation progresses. Early distension of the appendiceal lumen causes visceral irritation and produces pain that is dull, aching, and poorly localized. With time, the inflamed appendix begins to stimulate the adjacent parietal peritoneum, and patients begin to notice localized intense RLQ pain. In patients who present with the classic features of anorexia, fever, and an elevated WBC, abdominal imaging is not required. Unfortunately, atypical presentations are common, and the push towards minimizing false-negative surgical rates has prompted many clinicians to rely more heavily upon diagnostic imaging.

For the evaluation of appendicitis, CT scans carry a reported sensitivity between 72 and 89% and a specificity approaching 100% (Table 73.1). In many institutions, CT scans are still used as the initial imaging modality of choice in the setting of an atypical clinical presentation.

Table 73.1. Computed tomography findings in the evaluation of appendicitis

Feature	Normal appendix	Appendicitis
Diameter (mm)	≤6	>6
Wall thickness (mm)	≤3	>3
Appendiceal lumen	Empty, containing gas or filled with oral contrast material	Appendicolith
Periappendiceal fat density	Normal	Increased secondary to edema
Periappendiceal appearance	Normal	Inflammation and fluid collections from abscess or phlegmon formation; air indicating perforation; thickened terminal ileum; peritoneal free fluid
Lymph nodes	Normal	Lymphadenopathy

The scanners vary in the technique utilized to obtain images (helical versus conventional), the thickness of the image slices (5 mm or thinner), and the form of contrast used to enhance the images (oral, IV, or rectal). When obtained in a timely manner, CT scans have been shown to be very useful not only in the diagnosis or exclusion of appendicitis but also in the evaluation of other sources of abdominal pathology that could be contributing to the patient's pain.

A Practical Guide to Pediatric Emergency Medicine: Caring for Children in the Emergency Department, ed. N. Ewen Amieva-Wang (associate eds. Jamie Shandro, Aparajita Sohoni, and Bernhard Fassl). Published by Cambridge University Press.

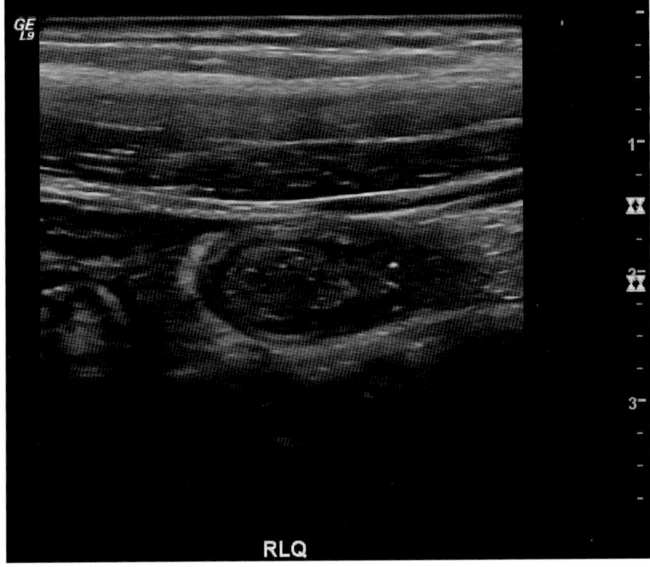

Figure 73.1 Ultrasound of appendicitis: a tubular non-compressible structure is seen.

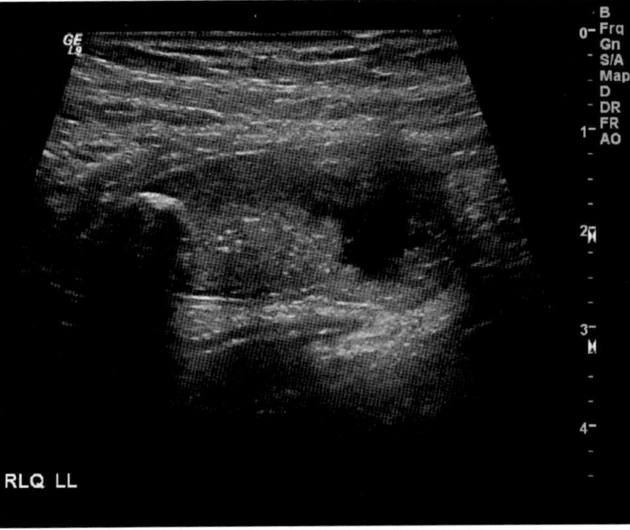

Figure 73.2 Ultrasound of an appendicolith: the hyperechoic appendicolith is seen casting a shadow farfield (posteriorly). The appendicolith is within the body of the appendix (hypoechoic longitudinal tubular structure).

Recent studies have begun supporting the use of ultrasound in the diagnosis of suspected appendicitis. With a reported sensitivity between 75 and 94% and specificity between 78 and 100%, ultrasound provides a quick, non-invasive evaluation of the appendix without exposing the child to ionizing radiation. Features of appendicitis are:

- non-compressible tubular structure lying under the point of maximal tenderness on examination
- appendiceal diameter >6 mm on cross-section
- periappendicial fluid or loculation
- presence of an appendicolith visible in the lumen of the appendix.

Furthermore, if the appendix appears normal on ultrasound, the scan can be expanded to examine the pelvic organs, renal system, and biliary tracts for another explanation for the pain.

On ultrasound, a normal appendix will appear as a small, compressible tubular structure lying within the RLQ. A normal sized appendix measures <6–9 mm in width at its greatest diameter. During the scan, the ultrasound probe is placed over the point of maximal tenderness on the patient's abdomen. A non-compressible tubular structure that measure >6 mm on ultrasound is highly suggestive of appendicitis (Fig. 73.1). Often times, an appendicolith will be visible within the lumen of the appendix. On ultrasound, an appendicolith appears as a bright white hyperechoic structure casting a dark acoustic shadow farfield from the lumen of the appendix (Fig. 73.2). Periappendiceal fluid is often visible on ultrasound and may represent inflammation or the early stages of abscess formation.

The sonographic evaluation for appendicitis is ideal in thin patients where subcutaneous fat is unlikely to interfere with sound wave transmission. In addition to body habitus, other limitations in the ultrasound evaluation of appendicitis include the sonographer's experience, patient discomfort during the graded compression of the RLQ, and the time required to adequately scan the abdominal contents. It is also important to note that a retrocecal appendix and an early, mildly inflamed non-perforated appendix are more difficult to evaluate via ultrasound. Despite these limitations, many centers have started incorporating ultrasonography into their imaging algorithm for suspected appendicitis. If an imaging study is recommended, patients receive an ultrasound first. Those with a positive sonogram proceed to surgery, and those with an equivocal scan and high index of suspicion undergo either a CT scan or an expedited surgical consult. This proposed algorithm not only saves many patients from radiation exposure during a CT scan but also shortens the time to radiographic confirmation and decreases the chance of perforation.

If the clinical suspicion for appendicitis is low, and a normal appendix is visualized on ultrasound or CT scan, the patient may be discharged home following a careful evaluation for other potentially catastrophic etiologies. All patients discharged from the ED with abdominal pain should receive detailed follow-up instructions and education about the signs, symptoms, and risk of developing appendicitis later. If the clinical suspicion for appendicitis is moderate to high, and the imaging obtained is equivocal, a surgical consult should be obtained with the option for admission and serial examinations.

Imaging options for intussusception

The diagnosis of intussusception should be considered in any child between 2 months and 36 months of age presenting with intermittent, colicky, abdominal pain. In intusssusception, the proximal bowel (the intussusceptum) telescopes into the distal bowel (the intussuscipiens). With each peristaltic wave, the intussusceptum tunnels deeper into the intussuscipiens, causing bowel wall stretching and crampy abdominal pain. Inflammation and edema of the bowel wall can lead to vascular compression, ischemia, and sepsis if the condition is not caught early enough. Although most childhood intussusceptions are idiopathic in nature, lead points from lymphoma, polyps, Meckel's diverticulum, and enlarged lymphoid tissue are not uncommon. Children presenting with suspicious symptoms in combination with a palpable abdominal mass or bloody stools should undergo a radiographic study to evaluate for intussusception. The presence of bloody stools is often a late finding and should prompt more aggressive and timely management.

Traditionally, diagnostic and therapeutic enemas are performed in cases where intussusception is suspected; such suspicious findings are:

- presence of an intraluminal mass highlighted by air, barium, or contrast
- reduction of the mass once air, barium, or contrast is injected
- barium highlighting the edematous mucosal folds of the intussusceptum in a "coiled ring" appearance
- rounded apex of the intussusceptum protruding into the column of contrast material ("the meniscus sign").

Enemas can be performed with air, a water-soluble contrast material, or with barium. The therapeutic efficacy of air or liquid contrast has been shown to be approximately 75–82%, with complication and perforation rates reported to be as low as 1% in most studies. Air or liquid contrast enemas have been shown to be safe in most patients in the absence of signs suggesting perforation or peritonitis (Table 73.2). Disadvantages to the use of an enema as the initial diagnostic modality include patient discomfort, the risk of perforation, and the resources and time required to perform the procedure. In many institutions, a nurse must accompany the patient during the enema in order to monitor for perforation, and a surgery consult must be obtained before the procedure is performed.

Ultrasound's ability to rapidly detect intussusception in a non-invasive manner has prompted many hospitals to replace enemas with ultrasound as the initial screening modality. Although the accuracy of ultrasound to detect intussusception is dependent upon the operator and sonographic equipment available, studies have shown a sensitivity of 95–100% and specificity of 88–100%. Findings on ultrasound suggestive of intussusception are:

Table 73.2. Non-surgical therapeutic options for intussusception reduction

	Success rate (%)	Risk for perforation (%)
Barium enema + fluoroscopy	55–95	0.39–0.7
Air enema + fluoroscopy	70–95.6	0.14–2.8
Water-soluble contrast enema + ultrasound	76–95.5	0.19–0.26

- a large mass with central echogenicity, surrounded by muscularis layers and edema ("loop-within-a-loop", "target sign," or "donut sign")
- the intussusceptum can be seen tunneling into the intussuscipiens on longitudinal imaging of the bowel
- decreased color Doppler in the walls of the entrapped intussusceptum.

The ability of ultrasound to simultaneously exclude other potential etiologies and to rapidly discover additional pathology has given it a favorable edge. Once the diagnosis of intussusception has been made via ultrasound, pneumatic or hydrostatic reduction can then be attempted under ultrasound guidance.

On ultrasound, intussusception appears as a large mass surrounded by a hypoechoic region of edema encompassed by a thick outer hyperechoic layer (Fig. 73.3). This characteristic "loop-within-a-loop" appearance has been termed the "target sign" or the "donut sign" on ultrasound. When the bowel is visualized in a longitudinal plane, the intussusceptum can often be seen extending directly into the intussuscipiens. Once an intussusception has been confirmed on ultrasound, color Doppler can be applied to assess for the degree of blood flow through the entrapped intussusceptum. Reduction via an enema or operative intervention can then be scheduled accordingly. In many institutions, patients who are risk for an intussusception are now initially screened with ultrasound, with the option of ultrasound-guided pneumatic or hydrostatic reduction readily available as the next therapeutic step. If the ultrasound findings are equivocal, and reduction attempts are not usually performed under ultrasound guidance, a traditional air, contrast, or barium enema should be obtained, along with an urgent pediatric surgery consultation.

Imaging options for hypertrophic pyloric stenosis

For every 1000 patients presenting with non-bilious vomiting before 1 year of age, two to three will have hypertrophic pyloric stenosis as the cause of their vomiting. The onset of vomiting may occur as early as the first week of life, but it may

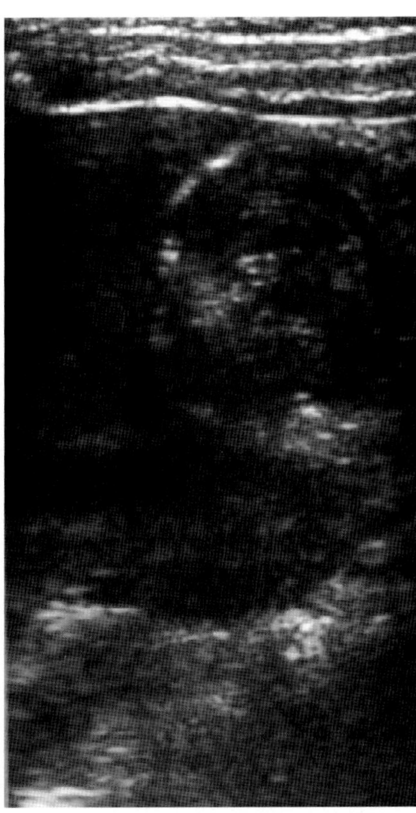

Figure 73.3 Ultrasound of intussusception.

be delayed to as late as 5 months of age. With protracted vomiting, these patients are at risk for profound electrolyte disturbances and metabolic alkalosis secondary to their fluid losses. It is essential that the diagnosis of pyloric stenosis be made early, so that endoscopic dilatation or surgical pyloromyotomy can be scheduled for definitive treatment.

In patients with pyloric stenosis, the pyloric channel narrows and elongates secondary to thickening of the circular muscle layers. As the muscle layers hypertrophy, obstruction occurs at the gastric outlet, causing distension and retrograde propulsion of stomach contents. Patients typically present with projectile, non-bilious vomiting because the gastric contents have not had a chance to mix with bile secreted distal to the gastric outlet obstruction.

Following a careful history and physical examination, the clinician must decide what type of imaging study should be obtained in patients at low to moderate risk. For many years, patients with a suspicious story and a peristaltic mass palpable in their epigastrium underwent a surgical pyloromyotomy based on clinical suspicion alone. The push for a lower incidence of false-negative laparotomies has prompted many centers to obtain a diagnostic imaging study first. Two options are available for diagnosing pyloric stenosis. Before the advent of ultrasound, an upper GI radiographic series with swallow of dye was considered the gold standard. It has a sensitivity of 89–92% and a specificity of 9%–100%. Findings are:

Table 73.3. Ultrasound findings in the evaluation of pyloric stenosis

Feature	Normal pylorus	Abnormal pylorus
Canal length (mm)	<15	≥15
Transverse pyloric diameter (mm)	<11	≥11
Muscle wall thickness (mm)	<2.5	≥2.5
Pylorus relaxation	Pylorus relaxes	Pyloric canal does not open
Gastric peristalsis	Normal, anterograde	Abnormal, retrograde

- delayed gastric emptying
- cephalic orientation of the pylorus
- filling defect at the antrum created by prolapse of the hypertrophic muscle, otherwise known as "shouldering"
- the "mushroom sign" or "umbrella sign": thickened muscle of the pyloric channel indenting the duodenal bulb
- the "double track sign": redundant mucosa in the narrowed pyloric lumen causes separation of the barium column into two channels
- the "string sign": barium passing through the narrowed pyloric channel causes a thin, markedly attenuated and elongated track
- pyloric tilt: muscle hypertrophy causing an outpouching and distortion of the lesser curve of the stomach
- retained gastric secretion and retrograde peristalsis, seen in the series.

In 1977, Teele and Smith introduced the concept of using ultrasound to diagnose pyloric stenosis. Since then various technical and technological improvements have been made, and subsequent studies have highlighted the advantages of obtaining a rapid ultrasound in the early evaluation of pyloric stenosis. Ultrasound is able to detect pyloric stenosis with a sensitivity of 89–97% and specificity of 72–99%. The ultrasound features distinguishing a normal pylorus from an abnormal one have been clearly described and validated by numerous studies (Table 73.3).

High-risk patients with a history and physical examination highly suspicious for pyloric stenosis should receive a surgical consult to determine if radiographic confirmation is deemed necessary. For patients who require radiographic confirmation, ultrasound is a rapid, non-invasive, and radiation-free option. Because the procedure is still highly operator dependent, it is important to bear in mind the limitations of this application. Patients who are considered moderate risk should undergo a careful scan by an experienced sonographer evaluating both the pyloric measurements and peristaltic behavior of the pylorus during the examination. If sonographic signs of an abnormal pylorus are not noted in a patient with moderate or high suspicion of pyloric stenosis, admission for IV fluids, serial examinations, and a repeat scan may be warranted.

Imaging options for intestinal malrotation and volvulus

Comprehension of the embryological development of the GI tract is important in the evaluation of children with suspected intestinal malrotation. The GI tract develops during the first 6–12 weeks of fetal life. Following the physiologic herniation of gut contents through the umbilicus at 6 weeks, the developing intestines rotate 180 degrees counter-clockwise around an axis surrounding the superior mesenteric artery (SMA). By the 10th to 12th week of fetal development, the intestines return into the abdominal cavity and complete the last portion of their full 270-degree counter-clockwise rotation. This last stage is accompanied by the attachment of the intestines to the posterior abdominal wall. The duodenal–jejunal loop becomes fixed just to the left of the aorta at the ligament of Treitz, and the cecum affixes to the right iliac fossa. Interruptions in development at any of these stages can alter the final anatomical placement of the abdominal organs, weaken or hinder physiological fixation, and leave the bowel at high risk for complete torsion or volvulus.

Most patients who suffer from intestinal malrotation will present within the first year of life, although some will not present with a concerning clinical picture until late childhood or adulthood. Because the venous and lymphatic systems operate under lower intravascular pressures, they are the systems affected first. When intestinal malrotation causes impedance of lymphatic drainage, chylous ascites may develop. Vascular congestion from venous insufficiency can lead to bowel edema, transluminal bleeding, and intestinal malabsorption. In severe cases of intestinal malrotation, a volvulus may develop. This form of complete obstruction occurs as the mesentery twists around the pedicle of the SMA. When rotation of the bowel creates high enough pressures to cause arterial compromise, ischemia, necrosis, perforation, and sepsis are imminent. Patients presenting with signs and symptoms suggestive of volvulus require aggressive resuscitation and emergency operative management.

The diagnosis of intestinal malrotation should be considered in any pediatric patient presenting with abdominal pain, distension, bilious vomiting, bloody stools, dehydration, or weight loss. Historical symptoms and physical signs will vary depending on the age of the patient, the degree of malrotation, and the amount of vascular or lymphatic insult that has occurred. In stable patients with findings suspicious for malrotation, plain film radiographs can be ordered as the initial screening modality. The radiographic interpretation is maximized by obtaining three views of the abdomen (supine, upright, and lateral decubitus).

With malrotation, a double bubble may be seen on plain radiograph. Obstruction at the level of the duodenum causes distension of the proximal gastric bubble and the prominent duodenal bulb. Note that the gastric bubble may not be evident in patients who have vomited recently.

The plain radiograph should also be evaluated for the presence of gas in the lower GI tract. With intestinal obstruction from malrotation, plain radiographs will show decompression of the distal bowel and a paucity of intra-abdominal gas. Dilated proximal bowel with numerous air–fluid levels is indicative of distal bowel obstruction. In patients where the clinical suspicion for malrotation is moderate or high, normal plain films should not be used to exclude the diagnosis. In this subset of patients, an upper GI radiographic series and surgical consult should be obtained as an emergency.

Patients receiving an upper GI radiography series will need to receive barium orally or through a nasogastric tube in order to evaluate for malrotation and potential volvulus. This technique has a sensitivity of 85–95% and specificity of 92–98%. The findings suggestive of intestinal malrotation are:

- abnormal displacement of the duodenal–jejunal junction towards the right of midline
- abnormal duodenal course noted on a lateral view
- abnormal positioning of the jejunum to the right side of the abdomen
- dilated fluid-filled duodenum
- proximal small bowel obstruction
- proximal jejunum spirals downward in the mid or right upper abdomen (corkscrew pattern, "apple peel sign," or "barber pole sign")
- abrupt termination of contrast noted
- a "beak" noted in the contrast column
- bowel wall edema and thickening.

Since the end of the 1990s, studies have suggested that ultrasound can be used to aid in the rapid diagnosis of malrotation by evaluating the relative positions of the SMA and superior mesenteric vein (SMV). This approach has a sensitivity of 85–92% and a specificity of 92–98%. The findings are:

- vertical or inverted SMA–SMV relationship; the SMV should lie to the right of the SMA on a normal longitudinal scan of the upper abdomen
- hyperdynamic or pulsating SMA
- distal SMV dilatation
- the "whirlpool sign," when the small bowel and mesenteric vessels are seen swirled around a central pedicle
- a truncated SMA ending abruptly next to an intestinal mass.

In 1992, Weinberger *et al.* published a paper describing how an SMV lying anterior or to the left of the SMA was highly suggestive of malrotation. Findings in 337 children were corroborated by results from upper GI series. Since then, several other authors have reported similar findings, although cases have been reported where reversal of the superior mesenteric vessels can be a normal variant. Just as an abnormal SMA–SMV relationship does not definitively indicate malrotation, a normal SMA–SMV relationship does not exclude malrotation. An upper GI radiographic series remains the imaging gold standard and should be obtained in cases where there is moderate to high suspicion for malrotation.

Conclusions

Hundreds of thousands of pediatric patients will present to an ED each year with complaints of non-traumatic abdominal pain. Recent technological advances and improving resource availability have expanded our imaging options, making the decision to obtain radiographic imaging one of the most challenging and evolving aspects of current emergency care. When attempting to differentiate between children in whom emergency radiographic imaging is warranted, it is important to recognize the various imaging modalities currently available and to acknowledge the limitations of each study. No one study can ever replace the value of a good, thorough history and physical examination, but when used appropriately in conjunction with a sound clinical assessment, imaging studies such as CT, upper GI radiographic series, and ultrasound can significantly augment clinical practice and improve patient care.

Selected references

Brennan GDG. Pediatric appendicitis: pathophysiology and appropriate use of diagnostic imaging. *CJEM* 2006; **8**:425–432.

Ko HS, Schenk JP, Troger J, *et al.* Current radiological management of intussusception in children. *Eur Radiol* 2007;**17**: 2411–2421.

Sabiha KP, Guelfguat JC, Leonidas JC, *et al.* Acute appendicitis in children: comparison of clinical diagnosis with ultrasound and CT imaging. *Ped Rad* 2004;**30**:94–98.

Swischuk LE. Emergency pediatric imaging: changes over the years. *Emerg Radiol* 2005;**11**:253–261.

Teele RL, Smith EH. Ultrasound in the diagnosis of idiopathic hypertrophic pyloric stenosis. *N Engl J Med* 1977;**296**: 1149–1150.

Vasavada P. Ultrasound evaluation of acute abdominal emergencies in infants and children. *Radiol Clin North Am* 2004;**42**:445–456.

Weinberger E, Winters WD, Liddell RM, Rosenbaum DM, Krauter D. Sonographic diagnosis of intestinal malrotation in infants: Importance of the relative positions of the superior mesenteric vein and artery. *AJR Am J Roentgenol* 1992; **159**:825–828.

Section

11

Gynecologic emergencies

Expert reviewer: Sophia Yen

Approach to the prepubertal genital examination

N. Ewen Amieva-Wang and Aparajita Sohoni

Introduction

An examination of the genitalia in children can be disconcerting for both the practitioner and the patient. In this chapter, we briefly discuss prepubertal anatomy and physiology as well as the appropriate approach to the pediatric genital examination in the ED.

Prepubertal and pubertal genital anatomy is distinct (Figure 74.1). In the prepubertal child, the labia majora are small and provide less protection to the underlying structures in the case of trauma and irritation. Lack of estrogen in the prepubertal vaginal tissues causes the tissue to be atrophic, thin, and friable. The prepubertal vaginal mucosa is also a

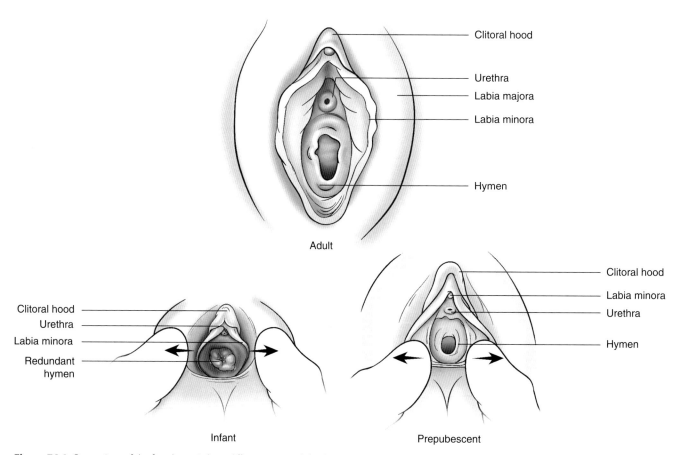

Figure 74.1 Comparison of the female genitalia at different stages of development. In the infant, the hymen is redundant and circumferential. In the prepubertal girl, there are no labia majora, scant labia minora, and a thin hymen. In the pubertal girl, the labia minora increased in size and the hymen is thickened. NB Drawings do not indicate relative sizes. (Copyright Chris Gralapp.)

A Practical Guide to Pediatric Emergency Medicine: Caring for Children in the Emergency Department, ed. N. Ewen Amieva-Wang (associate eds. Jamie Shandro, Aparajita Sohoni, and Bernhard Fassl). Published by Cambridge University Press.

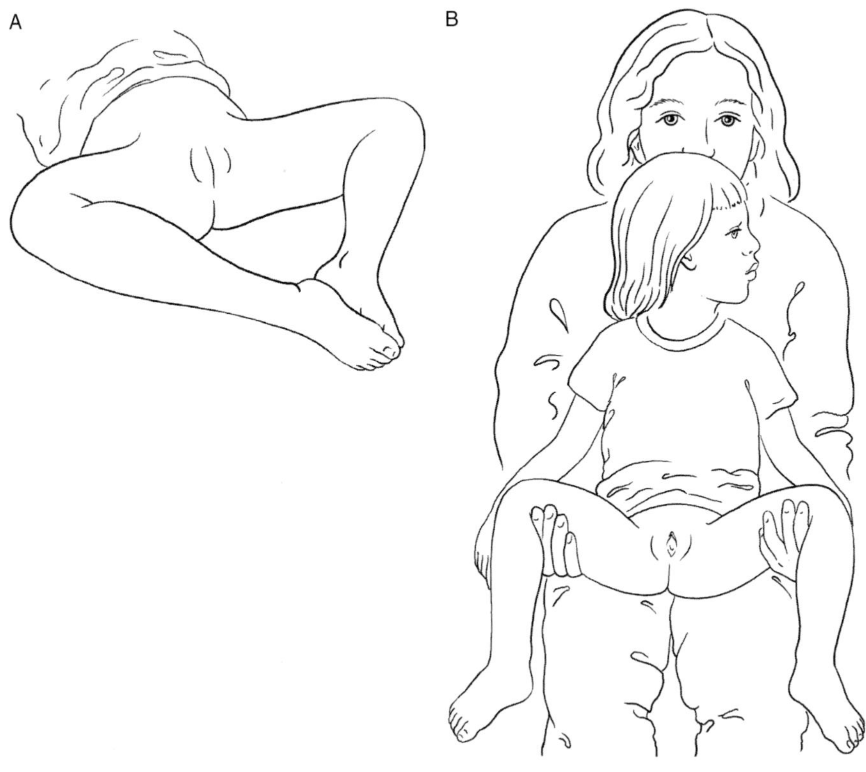

Figure 74.2 Supine frog leg position. (A) Standard frog leg position. (B) The examination can also be carried out on a caretaker's lap. (Copyright N. Ewen Wang.)

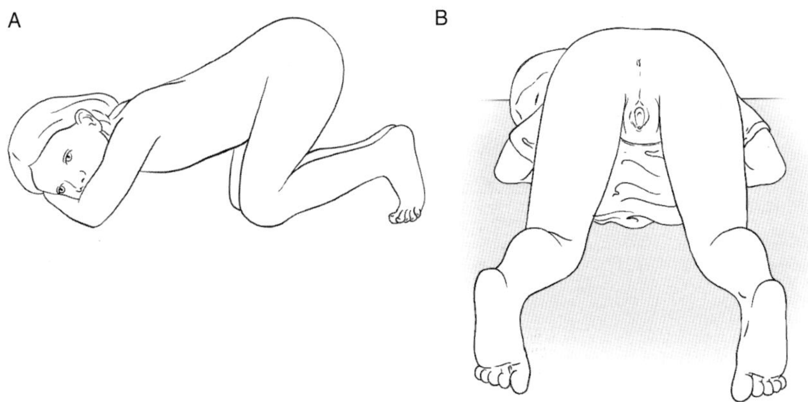

Figure 74.3 Knee chest position. (A) Lateral view. (B) Visualization of genitalia obtained by knee–chest position. (Copyright N. Ewen Wang.)

brighter red compared with the pale pink estrogenized vaginal mucosa. The prepubertal mucosa has a neutral pH of 6.5–7.5.

The prepubertal hymen can be redundant, making assessment difficult. It also has many documented shapes. This chapter is a guide for assessing normal prepubertal anatomy. Detailed assessment of anatomic findings in pediatric sexual abuse is beyond the scope of this book.

Approach to the genital examination

The genital examination should be done as part of a thorough physical examination. The child should be reassured that the examination is part of a thorough check to be sure she is healthy overall. It should be done after auscultation of heart sounds and lungs as the practitioner gains trust with the child. Examination of the genitalia should be done in the most non-threatening situation possible and usually will take less than a minute. For toddlers this may be done as "part of a diaper change." For older children, examination without completely removing the underwear by pulling the crotch to the side may be more acceptable. External examination in the prepubertal child is usually sufficient for ambulatory complaints. If an internal examination is judged necessary, it should be performed under anesthesia.

The best visualization is obtained in frog leg position or knee–chest position (Figures 74.2 and 74.3). A child can sit on the parent's lap in a frog leg position. Labial separation or

A

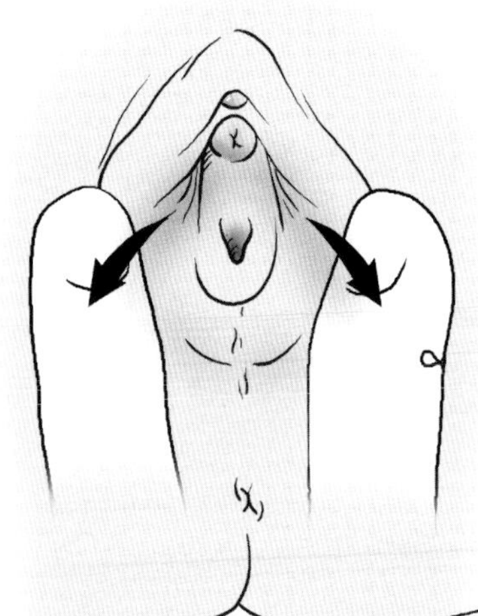

B

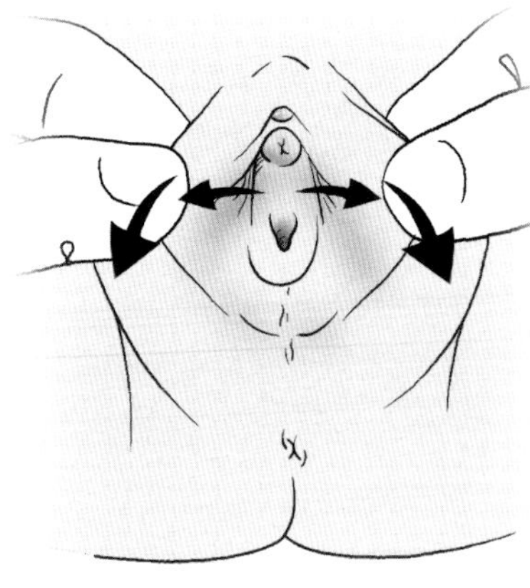

Figure 74.4 Vulvar inspection techniques. (A) Labial separation using gentle traction with the second and third digits. (B) Labial traction; the thumb and index fingers grasp the labia majora and pull laterally, downward, and outward. (Copyright Chris Gralappe.)

traction with the fingers on the labia majora is not painful and avoids the sensitive underlying tissues (Figures 74.4). The knee–chest position provides a vantage point for assessing the anus as well as for vaginal foreign bodies.

The provider should establish a rapport with the family and the patient to facilitate palpation (i.e., of a lump, a foreign body, or a laceration). Careful instructions should be given to the caregivers and the patient regarding what the provider is going to do, and all efforts should be taken to make the genital examination a calm and minimally stressful experience for all involved.

Once well positioned, the examination should proceed in a systematic fashion that includes assessment of the skin, the external genitalia, and the internal genitalia. With a prepubertal or pubertal child, the majority of the examination is dependent on appropriate visualization. The provider should keep in mind that the prepubertal genitalia are very sensitive and physical manipulation is often not necessary and should be minimized.

Of note, a common concern raised by caregivers and adolescent patients is that having a genital examination will "take away" the patient's virginity. Caregivers should be educated that virginity is generally defined as sexual abstinence and not as the presence or absence of an intact hymen and an "imperforate hymen" causes pathology. Usually the hymen is often torn as a result of normal physical activity by the time the first menstrual cycle is completed. Use of a small speculum causes very little trauma to the hymen. While a pelvic examination is definitely more uncomfortable for those who have never had sexual intercourse, being a virgin does not preclude having a pelvic examination. Internal examinations in prepubertal patients should be performed under general anesthesia or sedation.

The prepubertal genital examination can be difficult for practitioners because of lack of training as well as developmental differences between prepubertal and pubertal females. This chapter is meant to serve as an introduction for the basic prepubertal genital examination.

Pearls and pitfalls

Pearls

1. Prepubertal and pubertal genital anatomy and physiology are different.
2. Examination of the genitalia should be done as part of a complete physical examination.
3. Thorough examination of external genitalia can be accomplished in less than a few minutes.

Pitfalls

1. Failure to perform the prepubertal genital examination in a non-threatening manner.

Selected references

Christian CW, Decker JM. Prepubertal genital examination. In King C, Henretig FM (eds.) *Textbook of Pediatric Emergency Procedures*, 2nd edn. Philadelphia, PA: Lippincott Williams & Wilkins, 2008.

Kass-Wolf JH, Wilson EE. Pediatric gynecology: assessment strategies and common problems. *Semin Reprod Med* 2003; **21**:329–338.

Stukus KS, Zuckerbraun NS. Review of the prepubertal gynecologic examination: techniques and anatomic variation. *Clin Ped Emerg Med* 2009; **10**:3–9.

Sugar N, Graham EA. Common gynecologic problems in prepubertal girls. *Pediatr Rev* 2006; **27**:213–223.

Chapter 75

Breast disorders

Barbie J. Barrett

Introduction

The most common presentations to the ED for evaluation of pediatric breast disorders are pain, discharge, abnormal growth, and masses. Breast pain, as an isolated complaint, is a relatively unusual presentation in pediatric patients; it is more often one of a number of symptoms and, as such, must be addressed empathetically and promptly. Nipple discharge is either physiologic or pathologic; differentiation can be usually made by careful history and physical examination. Breast enlargement can be symmetric or asymmetric.

On evaluation, ask about breast trauma and family history of breast or ovarian malignancy. Examine the patient for developmental stage, breast masses, nipple discharge, signs of skin infection, and lymphadenopathy.

Breast disorders in prepubertal children

Physiologic hypertrophy of breast tissue in the male and female newborn is not uncommon and results from maternal estrogen stimulation. Females can more rarely develop galactorrhea (witch's milk), as well as clitoral hypertrophy and vaginal bloody discharge. Most symptoms will resolve within 4 weeks.

Neonatal mastitis may present as cellulitis or abscess. Mastitis neonatorum requires a septic workup and antibiotic coverage. Staphylococci are the most common causative agents. If an abscess needs drainage, it should be done by a surgeon, as breast bud damage and breast disfiguration can occur.

Older prepubertal females may also develop breast abscesses. Staphylococci are again the most common organisms, with an increasing prevalence of community-acquired methicillin-resistant *Staphylococcus aureus*. These abscesses may require drainage and antibiotic coverage.

Benign premature thelarche (breast development) can occur between 6 months and 9 years. Development is usually isolated to the breast. If breast development is associated with other signs of precocious puberty, the patient should have a prompt workup by her primary care clinician for CNS and ovarian disorders.

Breast disorders in adolescent girls

Breast pain can occur premenstrually, during exercise, and pregnancy. Careful history should be able to identify when the pain occurs. Developing girls may develop pain during exercise because of lack of appropriate support bras.

Juvenile breast hypertrophy may develop at thelarche. This is characterized by one breast developing before or more rapidly than the other. Breast asymmetry is more apparent as the adolescent is rapidly growing and developing. Usually the asymmetry resolves when development is complete. Once a mass is excluded, reassurance and follow-up with a pediatrician is appropriate. Anti-inflammatory drugs may alleviate symptoms.

Breast "masses" in girls are usually a direct function of thelarche. Fibroadenomas are the most common breast masses and are benign. These are smooth, mobile, and well circumscribed. Fibrocystic disease of the breast is both benign and common in adolescent females. It presents cyclically as painful masses or lumps in the breast. Nipple discharge may be present. Malignant breast masses are rare. Ultrasonography is the study of choice to evaluate a pediatric breast mass.

Breast abscesses are also seen in adolescent females. Lactating females are most vulnerable. Antibiotics, moist warm compresses, and ultrasound-guided drainage are therapeutic.

Benign breast disorders in males

Postpubertal gynecomastia is a benign condition occuring in 50 to 60% of boys during early adolescence. Other etiologies of

A Practical Guide to Pediatric Emergency Medicine: Caring for Children in the Emergency Department, ed. N. Ewen Amieva-Wang (associate eds. Jamie Shandro, Aparajita Sohoni, and Bernhard Fassl). Published by Cambridge University Press.

gynecomastia can include hypogonadism, pharmacologic agents (cimetidine, cannabis), lung and adrenogenital tumors, metastatic disease (liver, thyroid and renal), familial predisposition, and obesity. After these causes have been effectively ruled out, treatment consists of reassurance and/or referral back to their pediatrician.

Conclusions

The emergency provider must be able to distinguish emergency breast-related conditions (neonatal mastitis) from those requiring prompt primary care follow-up (thelarche, masses, gynecomastia, cysts).

Pearls and pitfalls

Pearls

1. The vast majority of breast masses in the pediatric population are benign.
2. Breast asymmetry is common during breast development.

Pitfalls

1. Failure to consider possible sexual abuse when evaluating breast complaints.
2. Failure to do a workup for sepsis in neonatal mastitis.
3. Failure to consider a hormone-secreting tumor as a possible cause of bilateral breast enlargement.

Selected references

Cady B, Steele Jr. GD, Morrow M, *et al.* Evaluation of common breast problems: guidance for primary care providers. *CA Cancer J Clin* 1998;**48**:49–63.

Simmons PS. Diagnostic considerations in breast disorders of children and adolescents. *Obstet Gynecol Clin North Am* 1992;**19**: 91–102.

Templeman C, Hertweck SP: Breast disorders in pediatric and adolescent patents. *Obstet Gynecol Clin North Am* 2000;**27**:19–34.

Chapter 76

Vaginal bleeding

Barbie J. Barrett, Jamie Shandro, and Sophia Yen

Introduction

Vaginal bleeding is a common presentation in the emergency setting. The EP must rapidly differentiate the stable from the unstable patient. The possibility of sexual abuse must be considered and documented in all patients presenting with vaginal bleeding. Vaginal bleeding is not as much dependent on age as it is on pubertal development. Causes are different for the premenarchal versus the postmenarchal population (Table 76.1).

History helps to guide the differential diagnosis of vaginal bleeding, including menstrual and sexual history, history of trauma or foreign body insertion, medication exposures, past episodes of unusual bleeding, and a careful review of systems (Table 76.2). (See Ch. 158 for how to take a careful history in an adolescent patient.) Approach the pediatric gynecologic examination with sensitivity, and carefully explain to both parents and patients all steps of the examination. Very young girls are most comfortable with a parent present during the examination, and it may help to have the parent hold the child. Speculum examinations are rarely indicated in the premenarchal female.

Table 76.1. Age-based causes of vaginal bleeding

Age	Causes
Premenarchal	Neonatal bleeding, precocious puberty, urethral prolapse
Postmenarchal	Anovulatory uterine bleeding, pregnancy-related (including ectopic, threatened abortion), menses
Age-independent	Foreign body, trauma, infections, dermatologic disorders, medications

Table 76.2. Most common causes of vaginal bleeding in the child

Type	Causes
Physiologic	Neonatal menarche, pregnancy related, ectopic pregnancy
Structural lesions	Urethral prolapse, condyloma accuminata, trauma, foreign body
Endocrine	Precocious puberty, primary pituitary disease, polycystic ovarian syndrome
Infections/ inflammation	Pelvic inflammatory disease, vaginitis/ cervicitis, sexually transmitted diseases, human papilloma virus
Hematologic	Von Willebrand disease, platelet abnormalities
Medications	Hormonal agents, oral contraceptive pills, intrauterine devices, NSAIDs

Premenarchal vaginal bleeding

Neonatal vaginal bleeding

Neonatal vaginal bleeding is caused by maternal hormone exposure during pregnancy. These maternal hormones are abruptly withdrawn at the time of birth. Neonatal vaginal bleeding can be a frightening experience for the parents. It is entirely normal and presents soon after birth as a "mini period" in females. It will resolve, usually lasting less than a day, and is painless. Parental reassurance and routine pediatric follow-up is all that is required.

Precocious puberty

Early puberty may be a variation of normal development, related to gonadal or adrenal disease, or caused by abnormal hormone exposure. True precocious puberty is mediated by pituitary gonadotropins. There will be a growth spurt, acne, advanced bone age, thelarche (breast development), and adrenarche (pubic hair growth) prior to vaginal bleeding. Specific CNS causes include pituitary tumors, trauma, irradiation, hydrocephalus, and phacomatosis. Primary hypothyroidism should also be in the differential for precocious puberty. Evaluation for precocious puberty includes a careful

A Practical Guide to Pediatric Emergency Medicine: Caring for Children in the Emergency Department, ed. N. Ewen Amieva-Wang (associate eds. Jamie Shandro, Aparajita Sohoni, and Bernhard Fassl). Published by Cambridge University Press.

examination (including Tanner staging) and management includes outpatient follow-up with the patient's pediatrician and possibly an endocrinologist.

Urethral prolapse

Although rare, urethral prolapse is an annular bright red protrusion of the distal urethra through the external meatus (Fig. 76.1). It is most common in Black prepubertal females. Most cases are asymptomatic and discovered incidentally. Parents will bring their daughters to the ED with worry of trauma and abuse as well as unexplained vaginal bleeding and/or dysuria. Hematuria is uncommon. Sitz baths are the treatment of choice for asymptomatic and mildly symptomatic patients. The patient should be referred promptly to a urologist for follow-up and further evaluation.

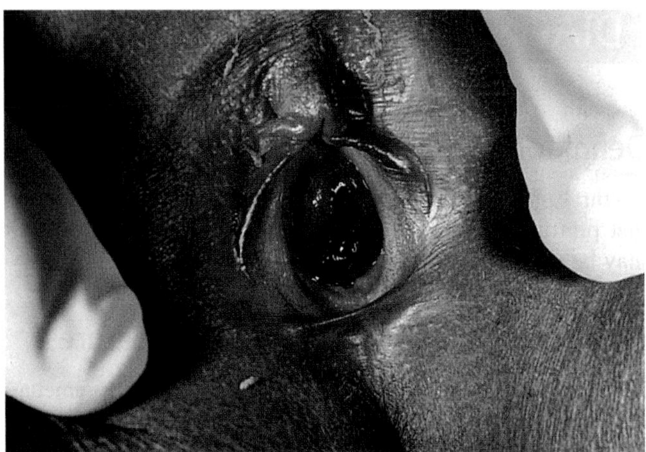

Figure 76.1 Urethral prolapse. This child was referred for evaluation for possible sexual abuse. Painless bleeding or spotting on the underwear is the most common symptom of urethral prolapse. A doughnut-shaped, edematous mass with hemorrhagic mucosa obscuring the vaginal introitus is seen in a 4-year-old African-American girl. (Reprinted with permission from Shah BR, Lucchesi M (eds). *Atlas of Pediatric Emergency Medicine*. New York: McGraw Hill, 2006.)

Postmenarchal vaginal bleeding

Anovulatory uterine bleeding

Several terms have been used to describe anovulatory bleeding, including dysfunctional uterine bleeding. Anovulatory uterine bleeding is caused by unopposed estrogen production and is defined as non-cyclic menstrual flow, which may range from scant to hemorrhagic. During the menstrual cycle, estrogen causes proliferation of the endometrial lining, while progesterone stabilizes it. In the adolescent, sporadic ovulation causes decreased progesterone levels and bleeding occurs. This occurs in the absence of pathology, medical illness, or structural abnormality. Multiple terms are used to characterize the variable bleeding patterns encountered in normal and anovulatory bleeding (Table 76.3).

The diagnosis of anovulatory bleeding is one of exclusion, although anovulatory cycles are normal/common during the first 2 years after menarche. Evaluation for a specific cause is mandatory (Table 76.2). History should include a family history of bleeding disorders and personal history of bleeding gums or easy bruising. Physical examination should include careful inspection for petechiae, purpura, ecchymosis, hirsutism, striae, obesity, thyroid masses, galactorrhea, pregnancy, and sexual abuse. Laboratory testing should include pregnancy testing, CBC, coagulation studies, thyroid-stimulating hormone (TSH), and von Willebrand panel. Referral to primary care clinician or gynecologist for further workup may be indicated.

Table 76.3. Definitions of postmenarche vaginal bleeding patterns

	Bleeding	Duration	Interval	Blood loss
Menstruation	Regular cyclic uterine flow, predictable	2–6 days	21–35 days	25–80 ml
Menorrhagia	Prolonged or excessive	7 days	21–35 days	>80 ml
Metrorrhagia	Irregular	Variable	Greater frequency than normal interval	
Menometrorrhagia	Prolonged or excessive, frequent	Irregular	Greater frequency than normal interval	>80 ml
Intermenstrual bleeding (spotting)	Variable amounts		Occurring between regular menses	
Polymenorrhea	Frequent		Every 21 days or less; regular	
Oligomenorrhea	Variable		35 days to 6 months	
Amenorrhea	No bleeding		Delay of menarch beyond age 16 (primary) or cessation of menstruation for ≥ 3 cycles or 3–6 months (secondary)	

Table 76.4. Gradation of vaginal bleed

Grades	Features	Treatment
Mild (Hb normal)	Longer period and shortened cycles for > 2 months	Referral to primary care clinician, keep menstrual calendar, iron supplements
Moderate (Hb 10–12 mg/dl)	Prolonged and frequent menses every 1–3 weeks with moderate to heavy bleeding	Referral to primary care clinician, keep menstrual calendar, iron supplements; progesterone therapy or combined hormonal contraceptives can be started to stabilize endometrium
Severe bleeding (Hb <10 mg/dl)	Asymptomatic but with irregular heavy bleeding	Volume resuscitation if symptomatic Give 30–35 μg ethinylestradiol + progesterone OCP QID If patient unwilling to take OCP, then start 10 mg medroxyprogesterone acetate PO for 10 days Also give iron supplementation and follow up with primary care clinician
	Low blood pressure, high heart rate, orthostatic, syncope; or actively bleeding with low Hb	Volume resuscitate; consider transfusion, admit to adolescent medicine ward/team Start Premarin (conjugated estrogens) 2.5–5 mg PO q. 4–6 h + medroxyprogesterone acetate PO 10 mg BID *or* IV estrogen 25 mg q. 4 h for two or three doses + medroxyprogesterone acetate PO 10 mg BID or Ethinylestradiol + norgestrel (Ovral) 50 μg PO q. 4 h until bleed stops Also give an antiemetic

Hb, haemoglobin; OCP, oral contraceptive pill.

The degree of dysfunctional bleeding can be categorized as mild, moderate, or severe. Most adolescents with anovulatory uterine bleeding will respond to medical management (Table 76.4). Once profuse hemorrhage and other emergency conditions have been ruled out, patients may be referred back to their pediatrician and/or adolescent medicine specialist/gynecologist for further evaluation and treatment, including consideration of hormonal contraceptive therapy to regulate the periods.

Dysmenorrhea

Dysmenorrhea is not uncommon in the adolescent patient. If the patient is stable with normal CBC and coagulation studies and a negative pregnancy test, treatment consists of NSAIDs (ibuprofen 800 mg PO three times a day [TID] with food, for a maximum of 5 days) and referral back to their pediatrician (for dysmenorrhea) and/or adolescent medicine specialist/gynecologist (endometriosis). Primary care providers may also provide oral contraceptives to control symptoms.

Pregnancy and complications

Any adolescent with vaginal bleeding must be considered pregnant, since the differential diagnosis and the treatment are utterly different for vaginal bleeding with pregnancy and without. Usually a urine pregnancy test is adequate to identify pregnancy from 1 day to 1 week after missed menses. If there is any suspicion for ectopic pregnancy despite a negative urine pregnancy, a serum human chorionic gonadotropin (HCG) level must be obtained. Although urine testing is now very sensitive, false-negative urine test may result if testing is done too soon after conception, urine specimen is dilute, or there is a low HCG owing to fetal demise or ectopic placement. Serum HCG levels correlate with size and age of a normal pregnancy. The quantitative level of HCG varies in ectopic pregnancy and low levels may occur.

If the patient is pregnant, the most important diagnosis to rule out is ectopic pregnancy: 60 to 80% of ectopic pregnancies present with vaginal bleeding. An ectopic pregnancy occurs when a fertilized ovum implants at a site other than the endometrial lining of the uterus. Females with a history of intrauterine devices, previous ectopic pregnancy, pelvic inflammatory disease or surgery, or anatomic abnormalities are at a high risk for ectopic pregnancy. Adolescents are at increased risk secondary to the high incidence of pelvic inflammatory disease. Ectopic pregnancies are the etiology for 10% of all maternal deaths.

Classically, ectopic pregnancy presents with a history of amenorrhea and either abdominal pain or vaginal bleeding, although it presents clinically in a wide variety of ways. History may include late or delayed menses, syncope, and shoulder, abdominal, and/or pelvic pain. Vaginal bleeding may be mild or absent. Physical examination is unreliable. Clinical shock may occur after rupture. Adnexal masses are rarely palpable. No constellation of physical findings may reliably exclude this diagnosis.

Ultrasound and serum HCG levels can be used to diagnose ectopic pregnancy. Serum HCG is usually detectable 8–9 days after ovulation. It doubles every 48 h with an intrauterine pregnancy and in only one-third of ectopic pregnancies. The rule of 10s is:

- HCG 100 IU/l at missed menses
- 100 000 IU/l at 10 weeks
- 10 000 IU/l at term

The elimination half-life of HCG is 1 day.

Use of ultrasound in conjunction with serum HCG levels can aid in diagnosis. Intrauterine pregnancy should be apparent by abdominal ultrasound if HCG is 5000–6000 IU/I and by vaginal ultrasound if HCG is 1500–2000 IU/I. If intrauterine pregnancy is not apparent, an ectopic pregnancy should be assumed until proven otherwise.

Early obstetrical consultation is necessary for all patients with ectopic pregnancy. Treatment may range from pharmacologic intervention to emergency laparoscopy/laparotomy.

Spontaneous, threatened, and incomplete abortion

Spontaneous abortion (miscarriage) is the spontaneous loss of a pregnancy before a viable gestational age. A threatened abortion is defined by bleeding with an early intrauterine pregnancy and a closed cervix. A threatened abortion may progress to a pregnancy with a viable outcome. Incomplete abortion, or inevitable abortion, is characterized by bleeding during early pregnancy with cervical dilatation, cramping, and passing of some but not all products of conception.

All of these conditions present with vaginal bleeding. Evaluation includes a pelvic examination to assess the cervix and look for evidence of passage of products of conception. Laboratory evaluation includes a quantitative beta-HCG, CBC, coagulation studies, Rhesus type to see if Rh_0(D) immunoglobulin (Rhogam) is indicated, and a von Willibrand panel. Unless complete products of conception are visualized, pelvic ultrasound is indicated to assess for intrauterine pregnancy, retained products of conception, or ectopic pregnancy. Obtain obstetrical consultation on all ectopic pregnancies and for those patients with ongoing bleeding with incomplete abortions.

Septic abortion

A septic abortion is an abortion that is complicated by infection. Infections involve the endometrium and retained products of conception and may progress to peritonitis and sepsis. Patients may present with fever, vaginal discharge, bleeding, abdominal pain and recent pregnancy. Laboratory evaluation should include CBC, HCG, electrolytes, coagulation studies, blood type and screen, blood culture and sensitivity, endocervical cultures for aerobes, anaerobes, *Neisseria gonorrhoeae*, *Chlamydia* sp., and Gram stain. Ultrasound of the abdomen to evaluate for retained products of conception and/or radiographs to identify free air are indicated.

Consult an obstetric/gynecology specialist on emergency basis and begin IV fluids, oxygen, Foley catheterization, and broad-spectrum antibiotics. Watch for signs of septic shock and disseminated intravascular coagulation.

Age-independent causes of vaginal bleeding

Foreign bodies and trauma

Vaginal foreign bodies and trauma are the most common causes of pediatric vaginal bleeding.

Perineal or rectal bleeding may present as vaginal bleeding. Anal fissures are often not recognized by the parent and blood may be present in the diaper.

Children may insert a foreign body into the vagina during normal exploration of the body. Often, they do not tell their parents and present to the ED with a vaginal bleed, discharge, or odor. A chronic foul-smelling vaginal discharge is the hallmark of a foreign body. The differential diagnosis of a vaginal foreign body should include sexual abuse and psychiatric disorders.

A trauma history may include straddle injuries, impalement, falls off bicycles, sexual assault, or sexual activity. If trauma is suspected, the severity of the injury may not be readily apparent. Narrow penetrating objects can damage abdominal viscera, bladder, or rectum. A patient with possible penetrating injury needs emergency, careful vaginal examination. This may require conscious sedation or general anesthesia.

Laboratory evaluation should include a CBC and urinalysis to screen for hematuria, which may indicate urethral or bladder injury or foreign body. Suspect a foreign body if there are white blood cells in the urine with a negative culture. Because the most common foreign bodies are toilet paper and condoms, radiographs are not helpful in diagnosis.

If a foreign body is discovered, treatment consists of removal, followed by a irrigation with dilute povidone-iodine (Betadine). Ring forceps may be helpful. If the young patient's vagina cannot be visualized when she is in the knee–chest position, gentle lavage may evacuate the foreign body. If this is unsuccessful, general anesthesia or procedural sedation may be indicated.

Infections and dermatologic vaginal bleeding

Bleeding and pruritus suggest chronic dermatitis, psoriasis, or seborrhea. Skin, once damaged by pruritus, leads to bleeding. Systemic diseases, such as varicella and measles, may present with bleeding. Pelvic inflammatory disease, genital warts, and pinworm may present with bleeding (see Chs. 77 and 96).

Coagulopathies

Over 10% of patients with menorrhagia have an inherited bleeding disorder. A history of increased bruising, epistaxis, prolonged bleeding, hematuria, or menorrhagia suggest dyscrasia. Physical examination includes special attention to skin, oropharynx, nasopharynx, liver, spleen, pelvis, and rectum. Suspected bleeding disorders should include determination of hemoglobin and hematocrit, a platelet count, and coagulation studies. Note that normal menstrual bleeding should not cause anemia.

Medications

Any pharmacologic agent that disrupts the hypothalamic pituitary ovarian axis may cause vaginal bleeding, particularly in the postmenarchal patient. Hormonal contraception, steroids, thyroid replacement, and anticoagulation drugs are potential causative factors. Question the preadolescent and adolescent patient privately as to the possible use of oral contraception or illegal drugs such as stimulants and presence of anorexia nervosa or bullemia, which may cause abnormalities in ovulation. Before discontinuing any prescription medication, consult with the prescribing physician.

Conclusions

Approach the pediatric patient with vaginal bleeding in a systematic fashion, considering the age and hormonal (premenarchal or postmenarchal) status of the patient when developing a differential diagnosis. Check a pregnancy test on all females of reproductive age with gynecologic complaints. Once profuse hemorrhage and other emergency conditions have been ruled out or treated, the majority of cases of vaginal bleeding can be referred for outpatient follow-up.

Pearls and pitfalls

Pearls

1. Causes of vaginal bleeding differ significantly between the premenarchal and postmenarchal population.
2. Always check a pregnancy test in reproductive aged females.
3. Once emergency conditions have been ruled out, the majority of cases of vaginal bleeding can be referred for outpatient follow-up.

Pitfalls

1. Failure to consider sexual abuse in the differential in all patients with vaginal or abdominal complaints.
2. Failure to realize that some patients will not be truthful about their sexual activity history.
3. Vaginal bleeding in every female of child-bearing age must be considered as ectopic pregnancy until ruled out.

Selected reference

Bravender T, Emans SJ. Menstrual disorders. Dysfunctional uterine bleeding. *Pediatr Clin North Am* 1999;**46**:545–553, viii.

Chapter 77

Common genitourinary complaints: vulvovaginitis, vaginal foreign bodies, and prolapsed urethra

Barbie J. Barrett and Aparajita Sohoni

Introduction

Vaginal complaints in the pediatric age group are diverse, ranging from vaginal foreign bodies to trauma to urethral prolapse to vulvovaginitis. This chapter will review some of the more common vaginal complaints in the pediatric age group (vulvovaginitis and vaginal foreign body), as well as urethral prolapse, which is an uncommon genitourinary complaint, but one that ED providers may need to identify and diagnose.

Vulvovaginitis

Vulvovaginitis is an inflammation of the vulva and vagina. In premenarchal girls, it is the most common gynecologic complaint. It may be a result of poor hygiene, irritation, foreign body, infection, or a change in vaginal pH. Common causes in postmenarche females are bacterial vaginosis, trichomoniasis, and candida infection (Table 77.1).

The prepubertal female is susceptible to vulvovaginitis because there is lower estrogen and vaginal secretions at this age and lack of genital hair conferring protection. Consequently, bowel flora may contaminate this area. Normal prepubertal flora includes *Escherichia coli*, diphtheroid, *Staphylococcus epidermis*, beta-hematolytic streptococci, and lactobacilli. Infectious etiologies include *Shigella* sp., group A streptococci, *Neisseria gonorrhoeae*, *Candida albicans*, and human papilloma virus.

History should be age directed to explore the suspected etiologies listed above. The patient should be asked about the use of soaps and bubble bath in the premenarche population, and about the use of tampons, vaginal hygiene products, and sexual activity in the adolescent population.

Physical examination of the genital area in the prepubertal girl may be all that is indicated. Parents should be at the bedside if appropriate. Young girls can best be examined in the knee–chest position while prone, with gentle external evaluation of the labia and vagina (see Fig. 74.3, p. 325).

Laboratory evaluation in the premenarchal female is not routinely necessary. Group A beta-hematolytic streptococci and urine cultures may be indicated. If abuse is suspected, follow local protocols for possible sexual assault evaluation. If pinworm is suspected, transparent tape may be applied to the perineum for microscopic evaluation the next morning.

In postmenarche females, a complete pelvic examination is indicated including wet mount and cervical cultures, as well as urinalysis. Yeast vaginitis without preceding antibiotic use should prompt investigation into diabetes mellitus.

Complications of vulvovaginitis may include labial adhesions and ascending infection (see pelvic inflammatory disease

Table 77.1. Causes of vulvovaginitis by age

	Premenarche	Postmenarche
Non-specific irritation, vaginitis	Bubble bath use, poor hygiene	Douche, spermicides, sexual activity
Medications	Antibiotics	Antibiotics, spermicides
Foreign body	Toilet paper	Tampons
Infection	Group A streptococci (after upper respiratory tract infection), enteric pathogens, pinworm	Gonorrhea, chlamydia, bacterial vaginosis, candidla, human papillomavirus, herpes, trichomoniasis
Dermatologic	Eczema, lichen sclerosis, Stevens–Johnson syndrome	Eczema, psoriasis, Stevens–Johnson syndrome
Endocrine	Thyroid, diabetes, lack of estrogen	Thyroid, diabetes

A Practical Guide to Pediatric Emergency Medicine: Caring for Children in the Emergency Department, ed. N. Ewen Amieva-Wang (associate eds. Jamie Shandro, Aparajita Sohoni, and Bernhard Fassl). Published by Cambridge University Press.

in Ch. 96). Labial adhesions may result from chronic irritation, and most will resolve with topical estrogen applications. The EP should not try to forcefully separate these adhesions as this may cause recurrence. These patients require outpatient follow-up.

Treatment of vulvovaginitis is based on the initial diagnostic impression and laboratory results. Irritants and medications that may be a cause of symptoms should be discontinued. For non-specific vaginitis, the patient should be encouraged to wear looser-fitting underwear and pajamas, and to take daily sitz baths (without soap). The patient should be instructed about the importance of front-to-back wiping after bowel movements. Any vaginal foreign bodies, if discovered, should be removed and any infections treated as indicated. Sexual abuse must be considered in any pediatric patient with a sexually transmitted infection or evidence of vaginal irritation. The vast majority of patients with vulvovaginitis may be treated as outpatients with primary care follow-up.

Vaginal foreign body

Vaginal foreign bodies are not infrequent in young girls. Patients usually present with vaginal discharge that has been present for days–weeks, foul-smelling odor in the genital area from secondary inflammation or infection of the vagina. They may also have vaginal spotting or bleeding that is intermittent or progressive in nature. Vaginal foreign bodies are often detected on inspection of the genitalia; if the object is easy to visualize, it should be removed using ring forceps or another appropriate tool. If a foreign body cannot be visualized but the suspicion exists, a vaginal ultrasound should be performed, and removal will likely need to occur under conscious or general sedation.

Following removal of the foreign body, antibiotics are not normally needed as the secondary infection usually resolves after the nidus has been removed. Close follow-up should be arranged, and if the secondary inflammation fails to resolve, antibiotics should be administered. The likelihood of a vaginal foreign body resulting in ascending infection of the genitourinary tract is rare – the majority of cases are in well-appearing patients and resolve with removal of the foreign body. Of course, in any ill-appearing patient, antibiotics should be given and the patient should be observed in the ED with a low threshold for admission.

Urethral prolapse

Urethral prolapse is an annular bright red protrusion of the distal urethra through the external meatus (Fig. 76.1, p. 330). It is most common in Black prepubertal females. Most cases are asymptomatic and discovered incidentally. Although rare, ED providers should be familiar with this entity, as parents will bring their daughters to the ED with worry of trauma and abuse as well as unexplained vaginal bleeding and/or dysuria. Hematuria is uncommon. Sitz baths are the treatment of choice for asymptomatic and mildly symptomatic patients. The patient should be referred promptly to a urologist for follow-up and further evaluation.

Pearls and pitfalls

Pearls

1. Causes of vulvovaginitis differ greatly between the premenarche and postmenarche population.
2. Non-specific irritant vulvovaginitis is the most common cause of vulvovaginitis in prepubertal girls.
3. A vaginal foreign body should be considered in a young girl with a vaginal complaint.

Pitfalls

1. Failure to consider that vaginal candidiasis may be a sign of undiagnosed diabetes.
2. Failure to consider sexual abuse when dealing with pediatric vaginal complaints.

Section

12

Hematology and oncology emergencies

Expert reviewers: Wendy B. Wong, Bertil Glader, and Gary V. Dahl

Chapter 78

Childhood anemia

Wendy B. Wong and Bertil Glader

Introduction

Medical providers in ED are likely to encounter anemia in their pediatric patients either as a chief complaint or as a finding noted upon evaluation of a sick child.

Normal hemoglobin levels vary with age during childhood.

The normal variation in hemoglobin must be kept in mind when determining whether a child is anemic (Table 78.1). While most childhood anemia detected in the ED can be managed as an outpatient, the EP must recognize anemia that needs urgent workup and treatment.

Clinical presentation

History

A detailed medical history and physical examination can guide the diagnostic workup and determine the urgency for completing the evaluation and treatment necessary in the ED. Many patients with complex medical histories have accompanying anemia. Inflammatory disorders can result in anemia of chronic disease. Medications and infections can cause bone marrow suppression or induce a hemolytic anemia. A bleeding history is important to rule out any obvious source of blood loss. In adolescent girls, it is important to elicit their menstrual history to evaluate for menorrhagia. Dietary history is helpful to assess for nutritional deficiencies. Nutritional problems are uncommon in healthy children except for iron deficiency, which is still prevalent in the toddler years. Nutritional deficiencies also need to be considered in medically complex patients who rely on alternative modes of nutrition (e.g., total parenteral nutrition) or have alterations in their GI tracts resulting in malabsorption. Environmental exposure to lead or other heavy metals should be questioned when obtaining the history. A family history of anemia, gallstones, or splenectomy at a young age may reveal the presence of a genetic red cell disorder causing hemolysis.

Table 78.1. Red blood cell hematologic characteristics in children

Age	Normal hemoglobin (g/dl)	Normal mean corpuscular volume (fl)
Birth	14–20	100–130
0.5–1 year	11–13	70–85
1–4 years	11–13	70–85
4 years to puberty	11–13	75–90
Pubertal female	12–16	80–100
Pubertal male	14–18	80–100

Signs and symptoms

Common symptoms of anemia in children are similar to adults, including pallor, decreased energy level, exercise intolerance, headache, and dizziness. Young children often cannot verbalize these complaints but may exhibit lassitude and poor feeding. Compared with adults, children tolerate a significant degree of anemia without the same degree of symptoms. For example, toddlers who develop severe iron-deficiency anemia over several months often appear well and have minimal hemodynamic changes. It is also important to ask about signs and symptoms of hemolysis. These include jaundice, sclera icterus, and dark (coca-cola) color urine.

The hemodynamic status of an anemic patient is the most important factor in determining how urgently a diagnosis needs to be sought and how urgently treatment is needed. In any patient complaining of dizziness, orthostatic vital signs should be performed. Physical examination should focus on looking for signs of other cytopenias and hemolysis. Are there petechiae or purpura to suggest thrombocytopenia? Is there organomegaly? Is there jaundice or scleral icterus?

Diagnostic studies

The initial approach to the diagnosis of anemia should assess whether there are other hematologic abnormalities in the CBC

A Practical Guide to Pediatric Emergency Medicine: Caring for Children in the Emergency Department, ed. N. Ewen Amieva-Wang (associate eds. Jamie Shandro, Aparajita Sohoni, and Bernhard Fassl). Published by Cambridge University Press.

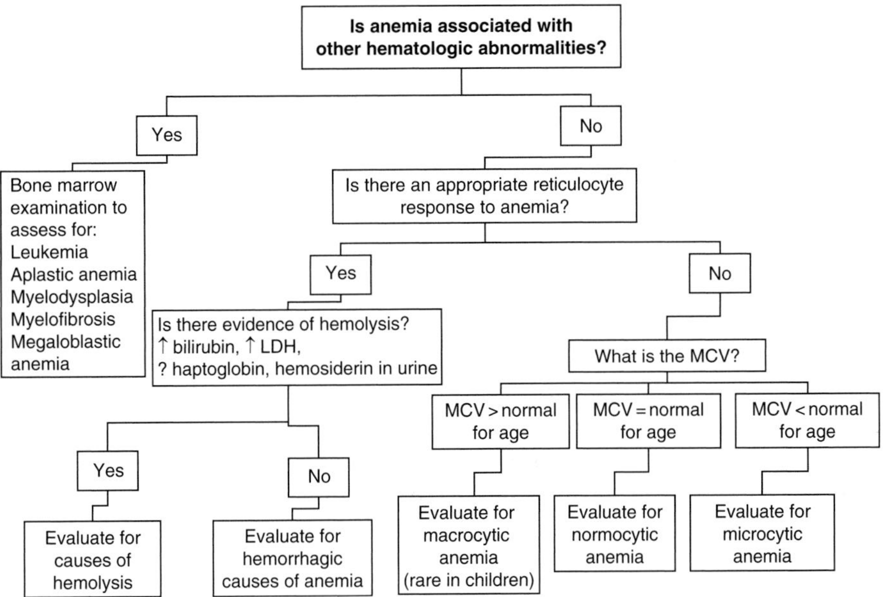

Figure 78.1 Initial approach to anemia. LDH, lactate dehydrogenase; MCV, mean cell volume.

(Figure 78.1). Pancytopenia suggests a primary bone marrow problem or an immunologic destructive process. The workup of these children should be done in consultation with a pediatric hematologist/oncologist.

The etiology of an isolated anemia in children is similar to adults. Anemia results from decreased red blood cell production, increased red blood cell destruction (hemolysis), or blood loss. Impaired production of red cells is characterized by a lower than expected reticulocyte response to the anemia. Laboratory studies suggesting hemolysis include unconjugated hyperbilirubinemia and elevated lactate dehydrogenase. Low serum haptoglobin and the presence of urinary hemosiderin also indicate hemolysis, but these tests are not readily available to help with diagnosis in the ED. In any anemic patient with jaundice or hemolytic markers, it is imperative to obtain a direct antiglobulin test, also known as the Coombs' test. Autoimmune hemolytic anemia is a true medical emergency and requires prompt diagnosis and treatment (see normocytic anemia, below). In the absence of hemolytic markers, a hemorrhagic cause for the anemia should be sought.

If there is no evidence of blood loss or hemolysis, further analysis of the red blood cell indices is useful. Mean corpuscular volume (MCV) measures the average red cell size and can be used to generate a differential diagnosis (Figure 78.1). Just like hemoglobin concentration, MCV also varies with age.

A simple rule of thumb, after 1 year of age, is that the lowest normal MCV is 70 + child's age in years.

Adolescent children have hemoglobin and MCV values similar to adults.

Types of anemia

Microcytic anemia

Microcytic anemia occurs with a deficit in the building blocks of the red blood cell, most commonly iron. The most common cause of microcytic anemia in children is iron deficiency, although the differential diagnosis for microcytic anemias includes thalassemia or thalassemia trait and anemia of chronic disease.

It is not uncommon that children with iron deficiency present with severe anemia (hemoglobin as low as 3 g/dl).

Nutritional anemia is typically seen in toddlers between the ages of 2 and 4 years whose diet consists almost exclusively of cow's milk.

Despite the magnitude of anemia, these children can be asymptomatic except for significant pallor. The diagnosis can be established with iron studies (low ferritin, low serum iron, high transferrin, and low transferrin saturation) but these studies are not always necessary in a child with a typical diet history and isolated microcytic anemia. Oral iron supplementation (ferrous sulfate 4–6 mg/kg daily of elemental iron) will generally correct the anemia within 1–2 months. Counseling the family about decreasing cow's milk intake and increasing iron-rich food is just as important as prescribing iron. It is particularly important to ensure that there is follow-up with the primary provider, to observe for improvement of anemia and compliance with oral iron regimen. In the ED, children with iron deficiency who have hemoglobin levels <5 g/dl and/or exhibit significant symptoms are candidates for slow transfusion of packed red blood cells (PRBC) and admission.

Anemia of chronic disease (ACD) occurs in children with chronic inflammatory disorders. This is usually a mild normocytic anemia but can be microcytic. The results of the iron studies in ACD are similar to iron deficiency except for elevated ferritin as an acute phase reactant and normal to low transferrin (ferritin is low and transferrin is elevated in iron deficiency anemia).

Thalassemia is an inherited condition resulting from decreased production of one of the normal globin chains. Significant thalassemia problems include hemoglobin H disease, homozygous β-thalassemia and hemoglobin E-β-thalassemia. Hepatosplenomegaly is a common finding on examination. These disorders result in a significant hemolytic anemia with increased reticulocytes and hemolytic markers. Nowadays, these thalassemic disorders are recognized early by newborn screening and are, therefore, unlikely to be a diagnostic problem for the emergency room. One exception is for children not born in the USA. Of note, α- or β-thalassemia minor/trait is associated with little to no anemia (hemoglobin 0–2 g/dl below normal). The newborn screen does not recognize α- or β-thalassemia minor/trait. If any thalassemia is suspected as the cause of the anemia, a hemoglobin electrophoresis should be obtained and the hematology service consulted for further specific studies.

Normocytic anemia

The reticulocyte count is used to aid the evaluation of normocytic anemia. The reticulocyte count reflects the body's ability to respond to decreased circulating red blood cells.

Normocytic anemia with reticulocytosis

A normocytic anemia with increased reticulocytes suggests a hemolytic or hemorrhagic cause for the anemia. History of jaundice and splenomegaly on examination and hemolytic markers on laboratory studies should direct the investigation towards hemolytic anemia. There are immune- and non-immune-related hemolytic anemias. Immune hemolytic anemias are characterized by positive direct antiglobulin test (DAT)/Coombs' test. The DAT test may be positive for IgG and/or C3.

Autoimmune hemolytic anemia can result in life-threatening anemia.

A child presenting with a first episode of DAT-positive hemolytic anemia requires hospitalization and hematologic consultation for further workup and treatment. Treatment generally includes IV steroids and PRBC transfusion. Because of the presence of antibody, cross-match of PRBC often is not possible. However, transfusion should not be withheld because of inability to find a cross-matched compatible PRBC unit. These patients should be given type-specific non-cross-matched PRBC with close monitoring for worsening hemolysis during transfusion. The management of these challenging transfusions often is facilitated by direct consultation with the transfusion medical director.

In hemolytic anemias that are not caused by antibody-mediated destruction (DAT negative), red cell destruction usually is secondary to a primary red blood cell problem such as hereditary spherocytosis, glucose-6-phosphate dehydrogenase deficiency, sickle cell anemia, or some other inherited red blood cell disorders. Children with a primary red blood cell defect usually have a chronic hemolytic anemia (anemia with reticulocytosis), except for children with glucose-6-phosphate dehydrogenase deficiency, who only experience intermittent hemolysis. Children with chronic hemolysis are at risk for aplastic or hemolytic crisis. Aplastic crises are caused by a temporary red cell aplasia, which develops in association with parvovirus B19 infection (see below). Hemolytic crises result from acceleration of red cell destruction from infections or drugs. Children who present with aplastic or hemolytic crisis often need PRBC transfusion when the anemia is severe or reticulocyte count is low.

Presence of microangiopathic changes on peripheral smear (schistocytes, burr cells, and helmet cells) are evidence of mechanical red cell damage. Microangiopathy is seen in disseminated intravascular coagulation), hemolytic uremic syndrome, and thrombotic thrombocytopenic purpura, as well as in toxin- or mechanically induced hemolytic anemias. Significant microangiopathic anemias almost always require hospitalization for treatment and consultation with hematology.

Hemorrhagic causes of anemia are often obvious on history and examination but one must also consider microscopic or intermittent blood loss, most commonly from the GI tract or during menses for adolescent girls.

Normocytic anemia with reticulocytopenia

A normocytic anemia without an appropriate increase in reticulocytes suggests decreased red cell production. This may reflect a primary bone marrow problem or may be secondary to renal, liver, or endocrine diseases. One of the most common presentations of anemia with reticulocytopenia in the ED is a hypoplastic crisis from parvovirus B19 infection in a child with previously diagnosed or undiagnosed chronic hemolytic anemia. This can be a life-threatening event and these patients invariably need PRBC transfusion in the ED and/or admission to hospital. These events are recognized by a decrease in hemoglobin concentration and reticulocyte count from previous measurements obtained when the child is well.

Primary bone marrow failures include pure red cell aplasia, aplastic anemia, and myelodysplastic syndrome. Infiltrative disorders such as leukemia, myelofibrosis, and metastatic solid tumors can also result in normocytic anemia and reticulocytopenia. Children with marrow failure and infiltration usually have abnormalities in their other blood cell lines and are found to have thrombocytopenia, neutropenia, and/or the presence of abnormal circulating white blood cells. The hematology/oncology service should be consulted for further workup and management of children with a decrease in more than one cell line.

Transient erythroblastopenia of childhood (TEC) is an acquired pure red cell aplasia occurring in children between 6 months and 3 years of age. This disorder is characterized by a normocytic anemia with a low reticulocyte count in an otherwise well child with normal physical examination, except for signs of anemia. This disorder often follows a viral illness and is caused by a transient immunologic suppression of erythropoiesis. It is not associated with parvovirus infection. The age of presentation and clinical picture often is similar to iron deficiency. The MCV is the most useful number to distinguish the two conditions; the MCV is normal in TEC but low in iron deficiency. There is no diagnostic test available for TEC. Affected children may have severe anemia and require PRBC transfusion. It is a self-limiting disorder and most children recover after one PRBC transfusion. Diamond Blackfan anemia, a congenital red cell aplasia, can present very similarly to TEC except that the anemia is usually macrocytic. Also, patients with Diamond Blackfan anemia usually present at an earlier age (birth to 1 year) and often have congenital anomalies (skeletal, cardiac, growth retardation).

The pediatric hematology/oncology service should be involved in the care of children who have significant anemia thought to be related to impaired red cell production.

Macrocytic anemia

Macrocytic anemia is rare in childhood and the least common type of anemia in children but will require thorough evaluation for etiology. False elevation of the MCV is seen with reticulocytosis because of the larger sizes of young red blood cells. Macrocytic anemias are categorized into megaloblastic anemias and non-megaloblastic macrocytic anemias. Non-megaloblastic macrocytic anemias are associated with liver disease and hypothyroidism. In addition, they also occur in bone marrow failure disorders, including Diamond Blackfan anemia and myelodysplasia.

Megaloblastic anemias result from alterations in DNA synthesis, which can affect all dividing cells. The peripheral blood smear reveals macroovalocytes and hypersegmented neutrophils (five or more lobes). The most common pediatric cause of megaloblastic anemia in the USA is vitamin B_{12} deficiency. Vitamin B_{12} deficiency can occur in infants born to vegan mothers. More commonly, this nutritional anemia is seen in children with a history of gastric surgery or bowel resection (removal of terminal ileum, such as in necrotizing enterocolitis). The gastric parietal cells produce intrinsic factor, which is a co-factor for B_{12} absorption, and the terminal ileum is the site for vitamin B_{12} absorption.

Macrocytosis is uncommon in childhood and, when it is real, it is often associated with other medical disorders. Any child with macrocytosis with or without anemia should be referred to hematology/oncology service for evaluation.

Management

Anemia. Anemias that might require emergency transfusion in ED include:

- anemia with reticulocytopenia from aplastic crisis in patients with chronic hemolytic anemia
- severe anemia (hemoglobin <6 g/dl) or symptomatic anemia from hemolytic crisis in patients with chronic hemolytic anemia
- severe anemia (hemoglobin <4.5 g/dl) or symptomatic anemia from iron deficiency
- symptomatic anemia from blood loss or if at risk for ongoing blood loss

Iron deficiency. Counseling is required regarding diet changes and patient discharge with iron supplementation.

Blood loss. This occurs from trauma and menorrhagia. Transfusions are given as necessary for hemodynamic stability. Later management includes obtaining a reticulocyte count. Transfusion should be considered if anemia is severe or moderate with inappropriately low reticulocyte count.

Autoimmune hemolytic anemia. If a DAT is positive, the patient should be admitted and consultation arranged with the hematology service for further management.

Non-immune hemolytic anemia. A blood sample for peripheral smear (red blood cell morphology), red blood enzyme measurement, or membrane testing is obtained prior to transfusion (one purple top will suffice).

Transfusion therapy

- In general, 10 ml/kg of PRBC transfusion will raise the hematocrit by 10% (hemoglobin by 3 g/dl)
- Transfusion of 10–15 ml/kg of PRBC over 4 h is generally safe. An exception is the case of a chronic, slowly developing severe anemia such as iron deficiency. In these situations, smaller amounts (e.g., 5 ml/kg) should be given over several 4 h sessions and the patient should be monitored for fluid overload.
- In any immunodeficient patient (infant <4 months, children on chronic steroid or other immunosuppressive medications, children on chemotherapy or after bone marrow transplant, children with primary immunodeficiency syndrome), all blood products should be irradiated prior to transfusion. They might also benefit from leukoreduced or CMV-negative products if they are available.

General indications for admission

- First episode of DAT-positive hemolytic anemia.
- Microangiopathic anemia.
- Anemia secondary to primary bone marrow problems or malignancy.
- Red blood cell aplasia in those with chronic hemolytic anemias.

Pearls and pitfalls

Pearls

1. For microcytic anemias, ask about iron intake and birthplace.
2. Use reticulocyte count to aid the evaluation of normocytic anemia.
3. Children can be asymptomatic from a severe anemia that develops gradually.
4. Most anemias can be worked up and treated as an outpatient with appropriate follow-up arranged.

Pitfalls

1. Failure to realize that normal hemoglobin level varies with age.
2. Failure to use symptoms as well as hemoglobin level to guide treatment of anemia.
3. Failure to identify hemolytic anemia.
4. Failure to carefully monitor blood transfusion in severe iron-deficiency anemia to avoid high-output cardiac failure.

Selected references

Glader BE. Hemolytic anemia in children. *Clin Lab Med* 1999;**19**:87–111, vi.

Hermiston ML, Mentzer WC. A practical approach to the evaluation of the anemic child. *Pediatr Clin North Am* 2002;**49**:877–891.

Means Jr. RT, Glader B. Anemia: general considerations. In Greer J, Foerster J, Rodgers GM, *et al.* (eds.) *Wintrobe's Clinical Hematology*, 12th edn, Vol. 1. Philadelphia, PA: Lippincott, Williams & Wilkins, 2009, pp. 779–809.

Richardson M. Microcytic anemia. *Pediatr Rev* 2007;**28**:5–14.

Chapter 79

Bleeding disorders in children

Ann Dahlberg and N. Ewen Amieva-Wang

Introduction

Bleeding disorders in children will usually present to the ED because of a history of prolonged bleeding (often mucocutaneous bleeding or menorrhagia), acute skin findings (petechiae), or in a child with a known bleeding disorder. Classification of these disorders by mechanism as well as by whether they are congenital or acquired can guide diagnosis, workup, and treatment.

Pathophysiology

Hemostasis involves three different systems: platelets, coagulation factors, and the vascular system (Table 79.1). Different disorders of hemostasis manifest differently (Table 79.2). Platelets create a plug at the site of vascular injury while coagulation factors are part of the glue that stabilizes the platelet plug with a more permanent fibrin clot. Von Willebrand factor (vWF) adheres platelets to each other as well as to the vascular subendothelium.

The coagulation cascade consists of the extrinsic and intrinsic pathways, which converge to a final common pathway (factors [F] II, V, VII, IX, X) that creates the cross-linked fibrin clot (Figure 79.1). In the extrinsic pathway, FVII is activated by vascular injury exposing subendothelial tissue factor. The intrinsic pathway (factors XII, XI, IX, VIII) amplifies this response. Von Willebrand factor is not only involved in platelet activation but also functions as a carrier protein for

Table 79.1. Causes of bleeding disorders in children

	Decreased production	Increased destruction	Poor function	Clinical manifestation	Helpful laboratory tests
Platelet disorders	Marrow failure (infection, aplasia, drug effect) Marrow infiltration (tumor, storage disorders)	Immune-mediated: idiopathic thrombocytopenic purpura Infection Consumptive (DIC) Microangiopathic processes (hemolytic uremic syndrome)	Drugs (acetylsalicylic acid) vWD	Mucocutaneous bleeding Petechiae Menorrhagia	Platelet count; bleeding time
Coagulation factors	Mutations in genes for factor production: hemophilia A (factor VIII), hemophilia B (factor IX) Liver disease (decreased synthesis of all factors except VIII)	vWD DIC	Vitamin K deficiency: hemorrhagic disease of newborn (neonate), malabsorption (cystic fibrosis), warfarin ingestion	Soft tissue bleeding Joint bleeding	Prothrombin time, partial thromboplastin time, international normalized ratio (INR)
Vascular problems		Vasculitis			

DIC, disseminated intravascular coagulation; vWD, von Willebrand disease.

Table 79.2. Clinical manifestations of disordered hemostasis[a]

Clinical characteristic	Bleeding disorder	
	Platelet defect	Clotting factor deficiency
Site of bleeding	Skin, mucous membranes (gingivae, nares, GI, genitourinary tracts)	Deeper soft tissues (joints, muscles)
Bleeding after minor cuts	Yes	Not usually
Petechiae	Present	Absent
Ecchymoses	Small, superficial	Large, palpable
Hemarthroses, muscle hematomas	Rare	Common
Bleeding after surgery	Immediate, mild	Delayed, severe

[a] These bleeding patterns are listed in their most general form, and may vary in individual patients.

FVIII, prolonging its half-life in the plasma. The final common pathway results in stabilization of the fibrin clot while endothelial repair occurs. Ultimately, the clot is then broken down by activated plasmin and associated enzymes.

All the coagulation factors except vWF are manufactured in the liver, and liver dysfunction will cause deficiencies in hemostasis.

Fat-soluble vitamin K activates clotting factors primarily in the extrinsic pathway (II, VII, IX, and X). Hemostatic disorders can result from decreased production, increased destruction, or poor quality platelets and/or coagulation factors.

Platelet disorders

Platelet disorders often manifest with mucocutaneous bleeding, such as epistaxis or bleeding of the gums, and petechiae.

Platelet disorders can be categorized as disorders of decreased quantity (decreased production or increased destruction) or decreased quality. Decreased platelet quantity can be either congenital and acquired. Congenital disorders with decreased platelets are rare and unlikely to present in the ED. Acquired disorders are more common. These disorders include immune-mediated idiopathic thrombocytopenia purpura (ITP), hemolytic uremic syndrome (HUS), marrow infiltration and failure, and consumptive processes such as disseminated

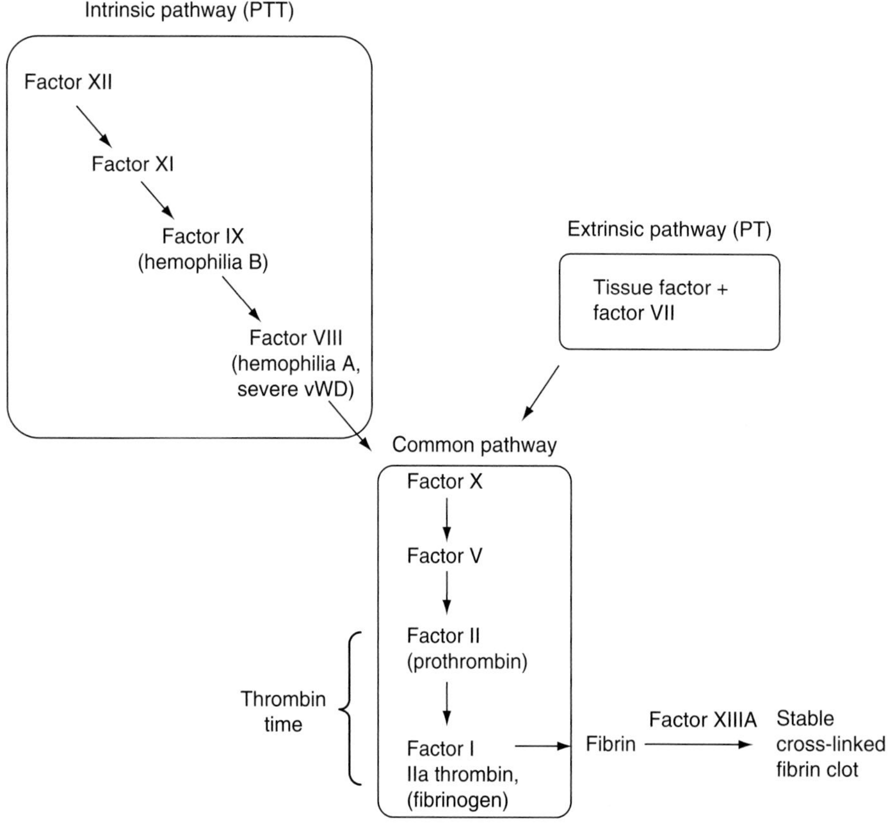

Figure 79.1 Coagulation cascade/secondary hemostasis. PT, prothrombin time; PTT, partial thromboplastin time; vWD, von Willebrand disease.

intravascular coagulation (consumptive coagulopathy). Marrow infiltration (most commonly by acute leukemia), will usually manifest with systemic symptoms and signs. Quantity of cells in all cell lines will be decreased; the smear should also reflect decreased production.

Immune idiopathic thrombocytopenic purpura

The most common cause of increased platelet destruction in previously healthy children is ITP. The annual incidence is estimated at 1/10 000, which is almost certainly an underestimation because of lack of diagnosis. Affected children are 2–10 years of age, with a peak incidence between 2–5 years. Often there is a history of a recent viral infection. Children usually are brought to medical attention because of bruising and petechiae and can be profoundly thrombocytopenic, although severe bleeding occurs in <1%. Diagnosis must confirm that the patient indeed has ITP and not oncologic disease.

Hemolytic uremic syndrome

Hemolytic uremic syndrome (Ch. 124) manifests with thrombocytopenia in addition to hemolytic anemia and renal failure.

Decreased platelet quality

Decreased quality of platelets can occur congenitally in von Willebrand's disease (vWD) or as an effect of drugs such as aspirin that inhibit platelet clumping. Von Willebrand protein plays a key role in platelet adhesion to damaged vessel walls. Patients with vWD will, therefore, have defective primary hemostasis.

Coagulation factor disorders

Von Willebrand's disease

Type 1 vWD is the most common inherited bleeding disorder. It is autosomal dominant disorder with a prevalence of in vitro identified disease of 1% in the USA, although clinically apparent disease occurs in 0.01% of the population. Since the majority of cases of vWD are mild, many patients may present without a previous diagnosis. Besides playing a role in platelet adhesion, vWF also stabilizes FVIII. Decreased level of vWF, therefore, can lead to low FVIII levels, resulting in prolongation of the PTT. However, some patients with low vWF will still have normal FVIII concentrations. Therefore, a normal PTT does not exclude vWD.

Hemophilia B

Hemophilia A and B are the most common inherited factor deficiencies (FVIII and FIX, respectively). They are X-linked disorders and affect approximately 1/5000 males. Historically this was a devastating disease; however, with the identification of the disease mechanism and the advent of recombinant factor replacement treatment, patients have decreased morbidity and mortality. Patients exposed to blood products and non-recombinant factor have an increased risk of infection with HIV and hepatitis C virus; some of these patients have developed factor inhibitors that can decrease the efficacy of transfused factor. Bleeding episodes are often treated at home; many hemophiliacs regularly use prophylactic factor and lead active lives. These patients may come to the ED when they have significant bleeding symptom or trauma and often they bring their factor with them.

Vitamin K deficiency

Vitamin K deficiency can be observed in newborns (decreased placental transfer, decreased initial level of clotting factors, and low levels of vitamin K in the breast milk) as well as in children with malabsorption syndromes (cystic fibrosis). Vitamin K inactivation by warfarin can cause hemorrhagic disease.

Liver dysfunction and other causes of bleeding diasthesis

Since all the coagulation factors except vWF are manufactured in the liver, liver dysfunction will cause deficiencies in hemostatic factors. A consumptive coagulopathy in children with widespread disease such as sepsis can develop with the uncontrolled formation and destruction of systemic clots; disseminated intravascular coagulation can result in both pathologic bleeding as well as clotting and infarction simultaneously.

Clinical presentation

History

A medical history detailing bleeding symptoms and family history is essential in determining the likelihood of an underlying bleeding disorder as well as focusing further workup. The age of the patient and past history of bleeding can initially guide the history and subsequent diagnosis. Patients presenting with new bleeding episodes should be questioned to determine the type of bleeding (i.e., mucocutaneous or deep tissue), duration, and amount (epistaxis greater than 15 min with adequate intervention and menses lasting greater than 7 days). If there is a known history of bleeding in the patient, then the nature of this disorder, specific medications, and past required interventions will guide current therapy. Many times these families actually have factor that should be administered promptly in conjunction with the family's expertise.

Physical examination

The physical examination is also important in the evaluation of a child with bleeding. For example, petechiae are almost pathognomonic for platelet-related bleeding whereas joint swelling or large intramuscular bleeds are more telling of coagulation disorder. Attention should be paid to the mucosal membranes in epistaxis, looking for signs of digital or other trauma.

If bruises are present, they should be examined for severity and location as the back and abdomen are unusual places for bruising in normal children. One must also pay close attention to the patterns of bruising as non-accidental trauma must also be considered on the differential. Finally, the overall health of the child must be considered, as children with underlying systemic disease should have other symptoms.

Diagnostic studies

The laboratory workup of a patient with unknown etiology of bleeding should be approached in a stepwise fashion focusing on the likely causes of bleeding given the history and physical examination. Obviously the acutely hemorrhaging child needs urgent laboratory analyses drawn and immediate intervention, but this is likely to be the exception rather than the rule in a child with an underlying bleeding disorder.

If a child arrives with stigmata of bleeding or prolonged bleeding and no prior diagnosis, an appropriate initial evaluation is a PT/INR, PTT, and CBC with smear. These three laboratory tests can be particularly helpful in narrowing the diagnostic possibilities and guiding further laboratory evaluation (Table 79.3).

The CBC in conjunction with a peripheral smear is useful to assess for thrombocytopenia as well as for abnormalities in other cell lines suggestive of marrow pathology, such as leukemia. Idiopathic thrombocytopenic purpura is a common cause of thrombocytopenia without other laboratory abnormalities. If the patient has isolated thrombocytopenia and the remainder of the CBC and smear are entirely normal, the patient can often be diagnosed with ITP without a bone marrow biopsy.

Function of the extrinsic pathway is measured by the PT or INR; the intrinsic pathway function is reflected by the PTT. An abnormal PT/INR or PTT will localize the bleeding problem to the extrinsic or intrinsic pathway. In general, a patient who is not systemically ill and who has an isolated prolongation of the PTT is likely to have an inherited bleeding disorder. Factor deficiencies can be further assessed with specific factor assays, with FVIII and FIX deficiencies being the most common. Pediatric hematology should be consulted in the workup of a child suspected of having hemophilia. If the child does not appear significantly ill and the bleeding is insignificant, it is important to remember that inhibitors (such as lupus anticoagulant) can cause clinically insignificant prolongation of the PTT or PT. Further studies can be done as an inpatient or outpatient.

The most common cause of bleeding in a patient with normal screening laboratory analyses is type 1 vWD (85% of all vWD).

Other bleeding disorders with normal screening laboratory analyses (FXIII deficiency, platelet dysfunction, and accelerated fibrinolysis) are much more rare but must also be considered in an urgent setting as they can cause more severe bleeding and require unique intervention. A useful additional screening test in patients with normal screening laboratory analyses and either borderline bleeding or severe mucocutaneous

Table 79.3. Screening for bleeding disorders

Test results	Differential diagnosis	Further testing
PT, PTT, platelet count normal	vWD, platelet function disorders, defect in fibrinolysis, factor XIII deficiency	Platelet function screen (PFA-100), vWD studies, specialized tests
PT, platelet count normal; PTT prolonged	PTT inhibitor, hemophilia A/B, heparin contamination, vWD type 2N/3, factor XI deficiency	PTT mixing study, factor assays, vWD studies, thrombin time
PTT, platelet count normal; PT prolonged	Early vitamin K deficiency, PT inhibitor, warfarin, factor VII deficiency	PT mixing study, factor assays
Platelet count normal; PT, PTT prolonged	Circulating inhibitor, liver disease, vitamin K deficiency, excess heparin, factor deficiency	PT/PTT mixing studies, thrombin/retiplase time, fibrinogen assay, factor assays
PT, PTT prolonged; platelet count low	DIC, liver disease	Thrombin time, fibrinogen/D-dimer, factor assays
PT, PTT normal; platelet count low	Acute or chronic ITP, spurious thrombocytopenia, collagen vascular disease, bone marrow failure, hemolytic uremic syndrome/thrombotic thrombocytopenic purpura	Blood smear, multiple tests for causes of chronic ITP, bone marrow aspirate if abnormal smear or chronic

DIC, disseminated intravascular coagulation; INR, international normalized ratio; ITP, idiopathic thrombocytopenic purpura; PT, prothrombin time; PTT, partial thromboplastin time; vWD, von Willebrand disease.

bleeding with no known personal or family history of a bleeding disorder is the platelet function screen (PFA-100). This is a rapid test that is available in most institutions and has replaced the bleeding time. It is a sensitive predictor of the most common platelet function disorders, which can be congenital or acquired (most commonly medication related). If a patient has borderline bleeding time and a normal PFA-100, a bleeding disorder is less likely whereas a severely abnormal test suggests vWD or other platelet function disorder. Further testing can usually be done with a subspecialist. In patients with a prolonged PT/PTT, drawing an extra blue top for further testing prior to giving fresh frozen plasma (FFP) or cryo infusion will facilitate workup.

Management

Most bleeding disorders have unique management strategies. Highlighted here are treatment plans for the most common inherited and acquired bleeding disorders (Table 79.4). It is important in treating any patient with a rare inherited disorder or an acquired disorder not due to an underlying systemic disease to consult with a hematologist as management strategies may differ at different institutions.

In emergency situations, blood products may be necessary as well as vitamin K administration if the bleeding is felt to be vitamin K dependent. The PT and PTT can be used to assess hemostasis during treatment.

Patients with pancytopenia from bone marrow failure or infiltration diseases can present with bleeding symptoms caused by thrombocytopenia. If a patient has pancytopenia, and leukemia is suspected, the EP should consult with a pediatric oncologist. A multitude of laboratory tests (CBC with differential, tumor lysis laboratory analyses, and viral titers), initiation of alkalinized fluids (center dependent), and possibly allopurinol may need to be commenced urgently in the ED. If the patient experiences significant symptoms from thrombocytopenia or anemia, packed red blood cells (PRBC) or platelet transfusion should be given for resuscitation. It is also important to remember that, if there is suspicion of a malignancy, steroids should not be given as this has the potential to cause a worse outcome in children with leukemia and other malignancies.

Idiopathic thrombocytopenic purpura

The treatment of ITP is controversial as there is no definitive evidence showing that medical therapy alters disease outcome. While ITP is generally a self-limited disease in most children resulting in only mild mucocutaneous bleeding, rare devastating cases of severe hemorrhage including intracranial hemorrhage can occur. This complication has led to the development of treatment guidelines for acutely increasing platelet counts to $> 20 \times 10^9$/l, a level felt to be protective against severe bleeding complications. Some centers may observe patients with mild bleeding symptoms regardless of platelet count, others may treat for a count $< 10 \times 10^9$/l or $< 20 \times 10^9$/l with bleeding. Treatment options include corticosteroids (different regimens range from a 21 day taper started at 2 mg/kg daily to a simple 3 day pulse of methylprednisolone [30 mg/kg daily]), Rh0 immunoglobulin (Rhogam; 50–75 μg/kg once). While IV immunoglobulin has been used to treat ITP, a hematologist should be consulted prior to use.

As ITP is very different in adults and children, it should be noted that teenagers may develop a more chronic form of ITP that requires ongoing follow-up by a hematologist and may be less responsive to therapy than their toddler counterparts. It is also very important not to start steroid therapy before discussion with a hematologist/oncologist as steroids can worsen outcomes in some malignancies (acute lymphoblastic leukemia in particular).

Von Willebrand's disease

The acute management of patients with vWD differs with the type of vWD and whether the disease has been previously diagnosed (Box 79.1). Desmopressin may be used in the patient with a known previous response who is not having a significant acute hemorrhage (it is commonly used in patients with type 1 vWD as

Table 79.4. Bleeding disorder and treatment

Bleeding disorder	Treatment	Emergency treatment
von Willebrand disease	Desmopressin	Platelets and factor VIII, FFP
Hemophilia A/B	Recombinant factor	FFP, blood
Idiopathic thrombocytopenic purpura	Steroids, immunoglobulin G	Platelets (supratherapeutic)
Unknown bleeding disorder/liver disease		Vitamin K, FFP, blood

FFP, fresh frozen plasma.

Box 79.1. Treatment for von Willebrand's disease

1. In the acute setting, desmopressin IV is the preferred choice.
2. The dose is 0.3 μg/kg to be given over 20–30 min.
3. An intranasal preparation (trade name Stimate) is also available. 150 μg (1 puff) should be given to patients < 50 kg and 300 μg (2 puffs) to those < 50 kg.
4. For more severe bleeds or von Willebrand's disease of unknown type, von Willebrand factor/factor VIII concentrate can be used: in general, 1 U/kg vWF will increase plasma concentration by 1.5 U/dl.

Stimate must not be confused with the desmopressin product that is used in patients with diabetes insipidus (DDAVP) and is a much lower concentration (DDAVP is 100 μg/ml; Stimate is 1500 μg/ml).

first-line therapy but may be not effective or even counterproductive in other types of vWD). Desmopressin can be given IV, IM, or intranasally. In the acute setting, IV is the preferred choice. Desmopressin rarely can cause tachyphylaxis, particularly in repeat administration within a short timeframe. Concentrates of vWF/FVIII are the other treatment option for patients with more severe bleeds or vWD of unknown type; vWF concentrate is a better treatment option in the acutely ill patient as all types of vWD should respond to this treatment modality. Some types of vWD may have associated thrombocytopenia and in the severe case need platelets as well. Platelet transfusion alone in these patients is insufficient.

Hemophilia

It is important first to clinically determine the severity of bleed. If the patient is the victim of a significant trauma and factor replacement is not immediately available, then packed RBCs and FFP may be necessary to acutely control bleeding. Use of FFP provides approximately 1 U of factor for 1 ml of product. The efficacy of this treatment can be monitored quickly by correction of the PTT, which normalizes when factor levels are approximately 30–40% of normal. The main problem in using FFP is volume overload, as 30–40 U/kg FFP will be needed to reach the level of 30–40% of normal. Therefore, treatment should be transitioned to factor concentrate or recombinant product as soon as possible.

Severe bleeding problems in hemophilia include retroperitoneal bleeding, muscle bleeds, and head injury. Retroperitoneal bleeds (spontaneous and traumatic) can result in a large volume of blood loss. Muscle bleeds can cause compartment syndrome. Ocular bleeding can occur after head trauma. If there is a suspicion of a severe bleed, treatment with factor prior to imaging is imperative. In the case of closed head injury, intracranial hemorrhage requires higher dose of factor infusion (50–75 U/kg of factor compared with 20–50 U/kg for hemarthrosis) and longer duration of treatment. Factor administration should always occur *first* followed by imaging. These patients may not demonstrate neurologic symptoms early in the course of a CNS bleed.

Concentrates of FVIII and FIX (from blood bank) or recombinant FVIII and FIX (from pharmacy) are readily available, and a patient with a bleeding history may have factor product at home and present to the ED for assistance in administration. A formula for determining the amount of FVIII necessary to achieve a desired level is:

$$\text{Dose (IU)} = \text{IU/dl (\%) desired rise in plasma FVIII} \times \text{body weight (kg)} \times 0.5$$

A similar formula is used for FIX except the 0.5 correction factor is excluded.

If the bleeding is not life threatening, it is important to determine what factor concentrate the patient has used in the past and if they have any known inhibitors. In a patient with significant inhibitors to FVIII or FIX, FFP will be ineffective. Patients may require a larger dose of factor concentrate or alternative therapy with agents such as FVIIa or prothrombin concentrates (PCC). Most patients, in concert with their hematologist, should be able to provide this information.

Disposition

There is no hard and fast rule on disposition of a patient with a bleeding disorder. Whether the patient's bleeding is adequately controlled and the likelihood of bleeding recurrence are essential questions in determining patient disposition. Patients with unstable vital signs or significant coagulopathy from underlying systemic disease obviously require admission for stabilization, administration of appropriate blood products, and management of their underlying disease. Patients with severe bleeding from factor deficiencies require admission to assist in continuous administration of factor replacement or for overnight observation. In the setting of concern for intra-abdominal or intracranial hemorrhage, the EP should have a much lower threshold to image and admit these patients than for a patient without a bleeding disorder. Factor should always be administered as quickly as possible and should never be delayed while waiting for imaging or other workup. Many families are able to administer factor at home; however, the patient may require supportive pain management with IV medications. Patients with newly diagnosed leukemia or marrow failure syndromes require admission after careful discussion of their workup and immediate care with the appropriate specialist.

Patients with ITP may require admission depending on their platelet count and clinical history. Patients with a platelet count $< 10 \times 10^9$/l require admission for observation and possible intervention. Patients with platelet counts 10×10^9/l to 20×10^9/l likely will be admitted for observation, with intervention varying depending on institution and history of bleed. Patients with platelet counts $> 20 \times 10^9$/l often will be observed as outpatients with clear instructions to avoid any physical activity or medications that increase bleeding risk. In addition, these patients should be advised to follow up with their primary care clinician the following day.

Patients with mild vWD likely can be discharged home if their bleeding is controlled, and they have not sustained clinically significant blood loss. Patients in whom there is concern for an underlying bleeding disorder but who do not meet admission criteria for persistent bleeding or hemodynamic instability should be referred to a pediatric hematologist–oncologist for further workup and management as an outpatient.

Thrombotic disorders

Thrombotic disorders are rare in children. When signs and symptoms suggest thromboembolic disease, the EP should consider disseminated infection (such as miliary tuberculosis) or immunologic disease (such as lupus). Workup and treatment should be carried out in conjunction with the pediatric subspecialist.

Pearls and pitfalls

Pearls

1. Platelet disorders typically manifest as mucocutaneous bleeding and petechiae.
2. Coagulation disorders typically manifest as soft tissue, joint, and intramuscular bleeds.
3. Vasculitis usually causes palpable purpura.
4. Idiopathic thrombocytopenic purpura in children presents very differently than in adults. It presents acutely and usually resolves spontaneously and fully.

Pitfalls

1. Failure to identify non-accidental trauma in patients with abnormal bruising or intracranial bleeds.
2. Confusing the desmopressin formulations used to treat von Willebrand's disease (Stimate) with DDAVP, which is used in patients with diabetes insipidus and is a much lower concentration (DDAVP is 100 μg/ml compared with Stimate, which is 1.5 mg/ml).
3. Failure to realize that while blood products are appropriate for acute patient stabilization, in most cases they will be insufficient to control bleeding from severe von Willebrand's disease and hemophilia, which will require specific factor administration.

Selected references

Allen GA, Glader B. Approach to the bleeding child. *Pediatr Clin North Am* 2002;**49**:1239–1256.

Berntorp E, Shapiro A, Astermark J, *et al.* Inhibitor treatment in haemophilias A and B: summary statement for the 2006 international consensus conference. *Haemophilia* 2006;**12**(Suppl. 6):1–7.

Blanchette V, Bolton-Maggs P. Childhood immune thrombocytopenic purpura: diagnosis and management. *Pediatr Clin North Am* 2008;**55**:393–420, xi.

Furie B, Limentani SA, Rosenfeld CG. A practical guide to the evaluation and treatment of hemophilia. *Blood* 1994;**84**:3–9.

Journeycake JM, Buchanan GR. Coagulation disorders. *Pediatr Rev* 2003;**24**:83–91.

Tarantino MD, Bolton-Maggs PH. Update on the management of immune thrombocytopenic purpura in children. *Curr Opin Hematol* 2007;**14**:526. [This article is an update to the article by George *et al.* in *Blood*, 1996.]

Witmer CM, Raffini LJ, Manno CS. Utility of computed tomography of the head following head trauma in boys with haemophilia. *Haemophilia* 2007;**13**: 560–566.

Chapter

80 Oncologic emergencies

Patrick M. Lank and Michael A. Gisondi

Introduction

Averaged across all pediatric age groups, cancer is cited as the second leading cause of death among American children. The most common cancers include leukemia, lymphoma, and intracranial tumors (Table 80.1). For a general appreciation of the incidence, unique characteristics, treatment, and prognosis of some of the more common childhood cancers, see Table 80.2 below. Two distinct populations of children with oncological problems will appear in the ED: children with an initial presentation suspicious for malignancy and children with a known diagnosis.

Clinical presentation and diagnosis

Many presenting symptoms of childhood cancer can mimic common conditions such as "viral syndrome" (e.g., fever, cough, vomiting, headache). At the time of diagnosis, the typical patient may have been seen by numerous physicians for vague complaints over a frustratingly long period of time. The EP may struggle with balancing anxious parents (sometimes with an unspoken agenda) with reasonable laboratory testing and radiographic imaging practices. Normal basic screening laboratory analyses and imaging, as discussed below, can be reassuring to parents who are primarily worried about cancer in their child. While approximately 8% of pediatric cancers are diagnosed in the ED, greater than 90% of pediatric cancer is diagnosed by a primary care physician. Close follow-up with a primary physician should be stressed if the initial ED workup is unremarkable.

In addition to chronic symptoms, constellations of specific symptoms should prompt evaluation for the most common pediatric cancers. Children with leukemia may present with low-grade fever, malaise, and/or lymphadenopathy; if the symptoms have been chronic and/or the child has additional symptoms and signs of bleeding/bruising, weight loss, bone pain, and hepatosplenomegaly, the EP should at least check a CBC with differential. Patients with lymphoma may present with similar symptoms. Painless lymphadenopathy (particularly prolonged or unresponsive to antibiotics) or persistent cough should precipitate investigation with CBC with differential and chest radiograph. Any palpable mass in the abdomen should prompt radiographic investigation (usually ultrasound) with surgical consultation. According to the Childhood Brain Tumor Consortium databank, 62% of children diagnosed with brain tumor experienced either chronic or frequent headaches. Worrisome symptoms associated with headache include pain associated with sleep, predominance of early morning headaches, absence of personal or family history of migraines, and a short duration of frequent headaches. These symptoms, as well as overt neurologic symptoms, should prompt evaluation with a head CT and close outpatient follow-up with further imaging if initial CT is negative.

The symptom complexes listed do not represent a comprehensive list, but should be used as a reminder to lower the threshold for testing in pediatric patients with confusing ED

Table 80.1. Most common pediatric cancer sites by age in the USA

<1 year	1–4 years	5–9 years	10–14 years	15–19 years
Neuroblastoma	Leukemia	Leukemia	CNS tumors	"Other" tumors[a]
Leukemia	CNS tumors	CNS tumors	Leukemia	Lymphoma
CNS tumors	Neuroblastoma	Lymphoma	Lymphoma	CNS tumors
Retinoblastoma	Renal tumors	Soft tissue tumors	Bone tumors	Leukemia
Germ cell tumors	Soft tissue tumors	Bone tumors	Soft tissue tumors	Germ cell/gonadal tumors

[a] Thyroid carcinoma, malignant melanoma, nasopharyngeal carcinoma, plus "unspecified" carcinomas.

A Practical Guide to Pediatric Emergency Medicine: Caring for Children in the Emergency Department, ed. N. Ewen Amieva-Wang (associate eds. Jamie Shandro, Aparajita Sohoni, and Bernhard Fassl). Published by Cambridge University Press.

Table 80.2. Description of most common pediatric cancers

Cancer	US incidence (per 1 000 000)	Description	Treatment	Prognostic information
Acute lymphocytic leukemia	33.4	*Symptoms*: fever, hepatosplenomegaly, lymphadenopathy, bleeding, anemia, increased WBC *Diagnosis*: bone marrow aspiration and biopsy	*Induction:* steroid with chemotherapy *Maintenance:* total ~2.5 years in girls, ~3 years in boys	Overall, ~80% 4-year EFS
Acute myeloid leukemia	8.2	Associated with ionizing radiation, chemical exposure (prenatal alcohol and tobacco), congenital conditions (e.g., Down syndrome, Fanconi anemia) *Symptoms*: fever, bleeding, increased WBC with functional neutropenia	*Induction*: often with cytarabine, 7+3 regimens (cytarabine + daunorubicin) *Consolidation/maintenance:* total ~6–12 months ± SCT	Overall, ~50% 4-year EFS
Chronic leukemias	1.6	Associated with Philadelphia chromosome (regional translocation t9;22) *Symptoms*: fever, splenomegaly, bone pain, or symptoms of hyperleukocytosis *Diagnosis*: median WBC 250 000/μl in children, thrombocytopenia	Combination chemotherapy with SCT, including hydroxyurea, busulfan: largely for symptomatic relief Imatinib, dasatinib SCT	Median survival 5–7 years; 80–85% 5-year EFS; 50% +10-year EFS
Hodgkin's lymphoma	11.3	*Symptoms*: commonly present with painless supraclavicular or cervical lymphadenopathy; two-thirds have mediastinal involvement; "B symptoms" include fever, weight loss, and drenching night sweats; unique symptoms are pruritus, alcohol-induced pain	Radiation; combination chemotherapy	Depends on stage at presentation, nodal bulk, and presence of "B symptoms" at presentation (worse prognosis)
Non-Hodgkin's lymphoma	8.4	Various types, including Burkitt's, diffuse large B cell, lymphoblastic lymphoma, and anaplastic large cell lymphoma *Presentation*: varies widely depending on type	Chemotherapy is the mainstay of treatment, with regimens completely dependent on type of lymphoma	Overall, ~80% cure rate
CNS tumors	37.2	Widely variable presentation and specific age distribution depending on tumor; generally peak in the first decade of life In childhood, greater incidence of posterior fossa tumors, so MRI is superior to CT for identification	Generally characterized by multidisciplinary approach including radiation, surgery (including shunting), chemotherapy	Prognostic indicators include age (worse if younger than 3 years), staging, resectability, biologic markers
Neuroblastoma	7.6	Most common solid tumor of childhood; found anywhere along the sympathetic chain; intra-abdominal most common (65%), also thoracic and cervical	Surgery: resection, aids in diagnosis and prognosis Radiation, chemotherapy	Prognostic indicators include age at diagnosis (better if < 1 year old), stage at presentation, and tissue pathology
Renal tumors	6.0	Wilms' tumor is the most common *Presentation*: abdominal mass, swelling, or pain; hematuria; fever; hypertension	Surgery: nephrectomy Radiation for greater stage tumors, chemotherapy	> 85% cure rate

Table 80.2. *(cont.)*

Cancer	US incidence (per 1 000 000)	Description	Treatment	Prognostic information
Osteosarcoma	5.2	Most common malignant bone tumor of childhood; found in metaphyses of most rapidly growing bones; early spread to lung and other skeletal structures	Surgery: local excision vs. amputation Chemotherapy - ± radiation	Prognosis depends on location; estimated > 50% cure rate with limb primaries without metastatic disease
Ewing sarcoma	2.6	Predilection to Caucasians; found in flat bones and diaphyses of long bones *Symptoms*: local pain that is less severe at night, fever, occasional palpable mass	Therapy depends on the tumor and its location; surgery, radiation, and chemotherapy can all be included in treatment protocols	In general, ~60% cure rate
Germ cell (gonadal)	11.8 (7.5)	Largely gonadal tumors, although extragonadal found along embryonal gonadal migration midline structures (sacrococcygeal most common) *Diagnosis*: serum markers and ultrasound are helpful in initial workup	Therapy usually includes combination platinum-containing chemotherapy and surgery (often after chemotherapy)	Prognosis is widely variable and depends on tumor pathology; ranges from 10–100% disease-free survival

EFS, event-free survival; SCT, stem cell transplant.

presentations. When cancer is suspected in the ED, parents will understandably have many questions about the treatment course and prognosis. It should be emphasized that these are widely variable and depend on studies (e.g., biopsy) that will not be performed in the ED. The child should be transferred to a center that specializes in the care of pediatric malignancies. The establishment of criteria for the formation of these centers, as well as the expert care provided at such regional institutions, has contributed to the increased survival of children with cancer.

Emergencies in children with cancer

Neutropenic fever

A child with a fever undergoing chemotherapy should be promptly assessed for neutropenia (low absolute neutrophil count [ANC]). Children who appear sick should have empirical antibiotics started while awaiting laboratory results. Others can await laboratory results with close observation prior to starting antibiotics unless the patient history or probability of neutropenia warrant empirical antibiotics.

Fever in the setting of neutropenia is usually defined as either a single temperature elevation ≥ 38.5°C (101.3°F) or an oral temperature of ≥ 38°C (100.4°F) for at least an hour, or two episodes over a 24-h period.

Clinically significant neutropenia is an absolute neutrophil count of < 500/μl (500 × 10^6 cells/l), or < 1000/μl if there is a anticipated fall to < 500/μl.

The ANC is calculated based on the WBC:

$$\text{WBC} \times [\text{segmented neutrophils } (\%) + \text{bands}(\%)]$$

For example, a WBC of 2.3 with Segs 48% and Bands 2% would be an ANC of 2300 × (0.48 + 0.02), which is 1150/μl. Of note, the risk of infection as well as the severity of infection increases as the neutrophil count falls below 1000 cells/μl (with highest risk of severe infection occurring at < 100/μl).

The timing of increased susceptibility to infection varies greatly depending both on the type of cancer and the phase of treatment. A majority of infections occur during maintenance and consolidation/intensification phases of chemotherapy for acute lymphocytic leukemia (ALL) and acute myeloid leukemia (AML). However, the most serious infections occur during the initial induction phases of therapy. Depending on the specific combination of chemotherapeutic agents used, the nadir of neutropenia typically is expected 7–10 days after myelotoxic drugs are given. Because of their therapy, most patients are immunosuppressed in addition to being neutropenic, when they present with fever.

It should be assumed that a child with fever and neutropenia has occult bacteremia. Evaluation for presumed bacteremia includes blood cultures from all indwelling catheter ports and a peripheral site, urinalysis (clean catch) with culture, and chest radiography. Empiric antibiotics and fluid resuscitation are required in parallel with diagnostic testing. As a rule, all patients with neutropenic fever should be admitted for IV antibiotics and close hemodynamic monitoring. Although decision rules exist that can identify "low-risk" pediatric neutropenic patients with fever, a patient should never be discharged home with only oral antibiotics unless this is specifically requested by the patient's oncologist.

While neutropenic fever is similarly treated in adults and children, there are a few characteristics unique to pediatric oncology. Although the ANC is, on average, lower in pediatric populations, children are less likely than adults to die from infection. Children are also less likely than adults to have an identified source of infection, and those recognized are more likely to be viral and from upper respiratory sources. Finally, although the incidence of isolated Gram-negative species is similar, children have more streptococcal bacteremia and less staphylococcal bacteremia than adults.

In pediatric oncology patients, bacteremia with Gram-positive organisms is, in general, more common than with Gram-negative species. The choice of empiric antibiotics, therefore, should reflect the preference of the patient's oncologist, hospital/community isolates, and drug resistance patterns. Most institutions use a parenteral third- or fourth-generation cephalosporin (e.g., cefipime) or a carbapenem (e.g., imipenem, meropenem) as monotherapy, unless there is an indication for IV antiviral or antifungal drugs.

Superior vena cava syndrome

Malignancies generally associated with superior vena cava syndrome (SVCS) in children include ALL and lymphoma, occurring in approximately 0.4% and 2%, respectively, at presentation. Mediastinal mass (with or without SVCS) is generally found at initial presentation. In children, SVCS usually presents as mild to moderate respiratory distress, which can progress rapidly. Because of the smaller size of the pediatric mediastinum and the higher compliance of the trachea and right mainstem bronchus, children presenting with SVCS typically have respiratory symptoms (e.g., dyspnea, cough, wheezing, orthopnea) more commonly than the plethoric and edematous face, jugular vein distension, and hoarse voice often associated with the syndrome in adults.

The management of respiratory distress in children with SVCS is challenging. Endotracheal intubation may be difficult or impractical to perform because of the extrinsic compression of a malignant mediastinal mass and should be avoided in almost all cases. Sedation must be avoided in SVCS patients, as either sedation or intubation could cause an irreversible compromise of the fragile airway. Pediatric oncologists should be consulted for all children with respiratory distress and a mediastinal mass identified on chest radiography. Regardless of previous cancer diagnosis, airway stabilization may be best acquired through emergency radiation and/or chemotherapy.

Acute tumor lysis syndrome

Acute tumor lysis syndrome is a constellation of metabolic derangements most commonly associated with chemotherapy-sensitive hematologic malignancies with an initial high WBC in ALL or AML, or a large tumor burden as seen in Burkitt's lymphoma.

Children with tumor lysis syndrome typically present within 1–5 days after the initiation of chemotherapy.

The metabolic abnormalities that occur are a direct result of the cellular destruction of large masses of cancerous cells. Hyperkalemia results from cell lysis, hyperuricemia from nucleic acid breakdown, and hyperphosphatemia from destruction of phosphate-rich lymphoblasts. Hyperphosphatemia will, in turn, promote hypocalcemia through the formation of calcium phosphate.

Symptoms of acute tumor lysis syndrome are related to the patient's metabolic abnormalities and concomitant renal failure. These may include fatigue, nausea, and vomiting – symptoms common in patients actively undergoing chemotherapy. Findings of hypocalcemia include cramping, carpopedal spasms, tetany, and seizures.

The progression of acute tumor lysis syndrome to acute renal failure drives many of the therapeutic modalities that should be initiated in the ED (if not already begun as preventive measures by the oncologist). The most important contributors to renal failure are the development of an obstructive nephropathy caused by uric acid crystallization in tubules, adenosine-mediated reduction in glomerular filtration, and hypovolemia. Therefore the mainstays of treatment include

- hydration
- urine alkalinization (to dissolve uric acid crystals)
- allopurinol (to reduce the formation of uric acid).

In children, fluid resuscitation and alkalinization is best accomplished with D5¼NS + 40 mEq/l of sodium bicarbonate (without potassium) at 2–4× maintenance, with a goal urine pH of 7–7.5. Patients with large leukemic cell burden with or without hyperuricemia may be treated with rasburicase if they have no history of severe allergy (e.g., bronchial asthma requiring bronchodilators, atopic eczema), glucose-6-phosphate dehydrogenase deficiency, or ongoing pregnancy. Rasburicase is given at a dose of 0.1–0.2 mg/kg daily and may be given twice for the first 2 days with repeated doses as necessary. For all other patients not at risk of hyperuricemia, hydration and judicious use of alkalinization (keeping the urine pH between 6.5 and 7.5) may be sufficient. Compared with allopurinol and IV sodium bicarbonate, rasburicase is costly and, therefore, judicious use of the medication is warranted.

Hyperkalemia is treated in the usual fashion with sodium polystyrene sulfonate (Kayexalate), insulin/glucose, and calcium gluconate as needed (see Ch. 55). Hyperphosphatemia can be treated with an oral phosphate binder, aluminum hydroxide 50 mg/kg PO. Finally, dialysis can be considered for any severe electrolyte abnormalities when conservative treatment is inadequate and there are signs of fluid overload (e.g., pleural or pericardial effusions), or in oliguria/anuria.

Hyperleukocytosis

Hyperleukocytosis is defined as a WBC >100 000/μl. Hyperleukocytosis can be seen in up to 20% of children with leukemia and is itself a poor prognostic indicator. Although most often seen at the time of initial diagnosis of leukemia, it can continue even after initiation of therapy. An oversimplification of the complex pathophysiology associated with hyperleukocytosis describes the process as "leukostasis," or a congestion of leukemic blasts in cerebral and pulmonary microcirculation, with associated increased blood viscosity particularly at those locations.

Although hyperleukocytosis is frequently asymptomatic, the clinical presentation in children can involve neurologic or respiratory symptoms as a result of its effect on cerebral and pulmonary microcirculation, or it can present as persistent bleeding because of the thrombocytopenia and coagulopathy associated with acute leukemia. Neurologic symptoms may range from headache and visual changes to mental status changes, seizure, or coma. Pulmonary leukostasis may present as hypoxemia, dyspnea, heart failure, or acute respiratory failure.

Management of hyperleukocytosis in the ED involves immediate stabilization with IV hydration and transfusions as needed. Similar to acute tumor lysis syndrome, hydration should be started with D5¼NS with sodium bicarbonate. Allopurinol or rasburicase may also be initiated in consultation with a pediatric oncologist. General recommendations also include transfusions for platelet counts $<20 \times 10^9$/l (to prevent cerebral hemorrhage), correction of coagulopathies with fresh frozen plasma and/or vitamin K, and avoidance of transfusion of packed red blood cells as this may increase blood viscosity. The use of exchange transfusion and leukophoresis are management strategies that may be considered by the pediatric oncologist after the above initial management steps are performed. All children with hyperleukocytosis will begin therapy appropriate for their specific type of leukemia as soon as clinically stable with good urine output.

Antibiotics should be considered in any child with hyperleukocytosis and fever, as they will have a "functional" neutropenia.

Malignant hypercalcemia

Malignant hypercalcemia is a rare complication in children, occurring with only approximately 0.4% of pediatric cancers (versus 20% of adult cancers). Hypercalcemia can complicate different pediatric malignancies, but it is most commonly associated with ALL. There are various physiologic etiologies for hypercalcemia, including an association with bony metastases (secondary to increased bone resorption) and direct release by the tumor.

Symptoms of hypercalcemia are popularly remembered by the phrase: "stones [nephrolithiasis], bones [pathologic fractures], groans [GI symptoms], and psychiatric overtones." In children with mild hypercalcemia (12–14 mg/dl), GI symptoms will predominate and may include polyuria and generalized weakness. Severe hypercalcemia (> 14 mg/dl) places patients at risk for bradyarrhythmias and ECG changes, including shortened QT intervals and prolonged PR intervals.

Hypercalcemia is treated in the ED with "forced diuresis": IV hydration for the profound dehydration and furosemide to promote the renal excretion of calcium.

Furosemide acts by blocking resorption of calcium at the loop of Henle. A recommended strategy for this "forced diuresis" includes giving normal saline at 2–3 times the maintenance, with furosemide 2–3 mg/kg every 2 h, with very close electrolyte monitoring. Other calcium-lowering strategies focus on decreased calcium release from bone using steroids, calcitonin, mithramycin, and bisphosphonates – all of which should be administered in consultation with a pediatric oncologist.

Cardiac tamponade

While malignant effusions are the most common cause of cardiac tamponade in adults with cancer, in children, pericardial effusions leading to tamponade are generally associated with infectious pericarditis in neutropenic patients and are very rarely the initial presentation of malignancy. Aside from this pathophysiologic difference, the clinical features, diagnosis, and management of children with tamponade are similar to those for adults with tamponade. Stabilization initially includes hydration and optimizing oxygenation. Children should then have percutaneous pericardial catheters placed with echocardiographic or fluoroscopic guidance by a pediatric surgeon. Placement of a percutaneous catheter, when compared with more invasive maneuvers such as pericardial windows and pericardiectomies, has been shown to be as effective and associated with minimal complications. Emergency bedside pericardiocentesis performed by the EP is reserved for children in extremis.

Neurologic emergencies

Common neurologic complaints of children with cancer – headache, mental status changes, and back pain – can be manifestations of chronic illness or can represent the first symptoms of a true oncologic emergency. Spinal cord compression, increased intracranial pressure, and herniation are the most worrisome neurologic complications in children with cancer.

In general, children with cancer who present with back or radicular pain should be assumed to have spinal cord compression until proven otherwise. The most common tumors causing cord compression are Ewing's sarcoma, neuroblastoma, and lymphoma.

Children with neurologic deficits should receive IV dexamethasone 1–2 mg/kg, followed by an emergency MRI to evaluate for a primary tumor or spinal metastases with cord compression.

Children without focal neurologic deficits but with new back pain should have a smaller dose of oral dexamethasone (e.g., 0.5 mg/kg), oral analgesics, and urgent MRI as an inpatient.

Further management of a child with diagnosed metastasis and/or cord compression should be arranged in consultation with a pediatric oncologist and neurosurgeon.

The clinical findings of increased intracranial pressure associated with childhood malignancies vary with the degree of accumulated pressure, location of the tumor, and age of the patient. Especially in older children, the most recognized symptom of increased intracranial pressure is headache. Other symptoms, including lethargy, vomiting, neurologic deficits, and seizures, should alert the EP to the possibility of increased intracranial pressure in children with brain tumors. A CT scan of the brain is the initial imaging modality of choice for children stable for the scanner. The use of IV fluids should be limited and dexamethasone given (0.5–1 mg/kg IV). The child should be closely monitored in the ED. Other treatment modalities including mannitol, acetazolamide, and antiepileptics should be given in consultation with a pediatric oncologist and/or pediatric neurosurgeon.

Disposition

The treatment of children with cancer is multidisciplinary and constantly evolving. The management of these children is out of the expected scope of training of the general EP. The care of these children should be coordinated in a pediatric cancer center. Any child diagnosed with cancer or with an emergency complication of cancer should be transferred to one of these centers as soon as possible after stabilization. The pediatric EP at a tertiary care center may be expected to have more advanced knowledge about specific cancers, their treatment, and the complications of their treatment, although a majority of treatment interventions will take place under the guidance of a pediatric oncologist.

Special population: bone marrow transplant

Patients who have undergone bone marrow transplantion as a treatment for malignancy are at special risk for infections as well as for graft versus host disease. Infections can be characterized as:

- pre-engraftment: 0–3 weeks
- immediate post-engraftment: 3 weeks to 3 months
- late after engraftment.

Patients suspected of infection within the first 3 months of a bone marrow transplant should be treated with broad-spectrum antibiotics, although during the post-engraftment period, reactivation of viruses including Epstein–Barr virus, CMV, and varicella are increasingly frequent. Patients with allogeneic (not autologous) transplants are at risk for late post-engraftment disease usually secondary to ongoing immunosuppressive treatment for graft versus host disease.

Patients with allogeneic transplants are at risk for graft versus host disease. This can manifest with various skin lesions, GI problems such as abdominal pain and diarrhea, and liver abnormalities with increased jaundice and LFT abnormalities. Additionally, pulmonary complaints are not uncommon. The patients' oncologist should always be consulted regarding diagnostic tests, treatment and disposition.

Pearls and pitfalls

Pearls

1. Patients and parents usually know their disease. Whenever possible, follow their wishes relating to treatment practices (e.g., anesthetics at port site prior to accessing).
2. Promptly assess the child with possible fever and neutropenia.

Pitfalls

1. Failure in administration of appropriate IV fluids: metabolic derangements associated with pediatric cancer will always benefit from monitored IV fluid.
2. Be cautious of the airway in children with suspected superior vena cava syndrome – avoid sedation and have a high threshold for intubation, as the intubation may cause hemodynamic instability or simply be impossible.

Selected references

Heron M. *National Vital Statistics Reports*, Vol. 20: Deaths: Leading Causes for 2004. Atlanta, GA: National Center for Health Statistics, 2007.

Hughes WT, Armstrong D, Bodey GP, *et al.* Guidelines for the use of antimicrobial agents in neutropenic patients with cancer. *Clin Infect Dis* 2002;**34**:730–751.

Kelly K, Lange B. Oncologic emergencies. *Pediatr Clin North Am* 1997;**44**:809–830.

Pizzo PA, Poplack DG (eds.). *Principles and Practice of Pediatric Oncology*, 5th edn. Philadelphia, PA: Lippincott Williams & Wilkins, 2006.

Young D, Toretsky JA, Eskenazi AE. Recognition of common childhood malignancies. *Am Fam Physician* 2000;**61**: 2144–2154.

Chapter

81 Sickle cell emergencies

Claudia R. Morris

Introduction

Sickle cell disease (SCD) is an inherited hemolytic anemia that affects approximately 100 000 individuals in the USA, primarily African-Americans, and millions more worldwide, while 8% of African-Americans carry the sickle cell gene (giving rise to hemoglobin HbS). Sickling conditions are also common in individuals from Mediterranean countries, Turkey, the Arabian Peninsula and India and are rapidly increasing among those of Hispanic ethnicity. This disease represents a group of genetic disorders in which there is a mutation resulting in an amino acid substitution of valine for glutamic acid in the sixth position of the beta subunits of hemoglobin. Sickle cell anemia is homozygous HbSS. Other milder variants of SCD exist, including HbSC and S-β-thalassemia, where the gene for HbS and that for β-thalassemia is carried, one HbS chain (HbSC). In S-β-thalassemia, the gene for HbS and that for β-thalassemia are carried. Sickle cell disease is variably characterized by anemia, severe pain, and potentially life-threatening complications such as bacterial sepsis, splenic sequestration, acute chest syndrome (ACS), stroke, and chronic organ damage.

The clinical features of the disease result from intracellular polymerization of hemoglobin under conditions of hypoxia and dehydration. Sickled red blood cells are less deformable than normal cells and fragment in the circulation, resulting in shortened red blood cell (RBC) survival of only 10–12 days compared with 120 days for normal erythrocytes. Oxidative stress, chronic endothelial damage, and hemolysis initiate a cascade of events that results in episodic vaso-occlusion and subsequent ischemia–reperfusion injury.

All children with SCD should be considered immunocompromised as a result of developing abnormal splenic function.

With age, progressive renal, pulmonary, liver, neurological, and cardiac damage occurs. Acute occlusion of larger vessels results in sudden vaso-occlusive symptoms such as pain, stroke, acute splenic sequestration crisis, and pulmonary infarction, while occlusion of capillaries and small vessels results in chronic and often asymptomatic organ damage.

Patients with SCD have a shortened life expectancy, and death in infancy and childhood is still a significant risk, with approximately 15% mortality in US patients with homozygous HbS prior to 20 years of age, peaking between 1 and 3 years of age. Sepsis is the primary cause of death, most commonly associated with streptococcal pneumonia. Acute anemic complications, ACS, and stroke are also significant causes of mortality and morbidity in children. After age 10, cerebrovascular accidents and traumatic events surpass sepsis as the major causes of death. Early recognition of complications and aggressive treatment initiated in the ED can dramatically improve patient survival. Rehydration, oxygen, antibiotics, and attention to respiratory status, and urgent packed red blood cell (PRBC) transfusion for those with precipitous drops in hemoglobin can be critical life-saving interventions. This chapter summarizes emergency management approaches to common complications encountered in children with this debilitating condition.

Sickle cell trait

Sickle cell disease is an autosomal recessive condition. Sickle cell trait (Hb-AS) is not regarded as a disease state. Complications occurring in HbAS are uncommon, but certain conditions such as high altitude or vigorous exercise, which cause hypoxia, acidosis, dehydration, hyperosmolality, hypothermia, or elevated erythrocyte 2,3-diphosphoglutarate can transform silent sickle cell trait into a syndrome resembling SCD.

Emergency complications

Symptoms of SCD can start to show at as early as 4 to 6 months of age, but more typically manifest between the ages of 1 and 2 years.

The etiology, clinical presentation, differential diagnosis, evaluation, and management of common complications of SCD are summarized below. Obtaining vital signs, and a thorough history and physical examination are a crucial part of the evaluation regardless of the presenting complaint. Early consultation

A Practical Guide to Pediatric Emergency Medicine: Caring for Children in the Emergency Department, ed. N. Ewen Amieva-Wang (associate eds. Jamie Shandro, Aparajita Sohoni, and Bernhard Fassl). Published by Cambridge University Press.

with a pediatric hematology specialist should always be considered when evaluating a child with SCD in the ED.

Fever/infections

Patients with SCD, particularly infants and young children, are at high risk for serious bacterial infection. These patients are immunocompromised. Most have absent splenic function, defects in alternate complement pathways, and low nitric oxide bioavailability. *Streptococcus pneumoniae, Haemophilus influenzae, Escherichia coli, Salmonella* spp, and Mycoplasma are common culprits. Vaccination for *H. influenzae* type b (Hib) and *S. pneumoniae* has significantly reduced the incidence of sepsis, as has the institution of prophylactic penicillin. Often penicillin prophylaxis is discontinued after 5 years of age because of a lack of evidence demonstrating continued benefit past this age.

Fever (>38.0°C) is often the only sign of serious infection. Sepsis is the leading cause of death in young children with SCD.

Among febrile children with SCD, 2–6% will have bacteremia. Other symptoms of concern include unusual sleepiness, irritability, rapid breathing, pale color, vomiting, and diarrhea. The occurrence of ACS is discussed under pulmonary complications. Patients with SCD are at increased risk of osteomyelitis, and *Salmonella* sp. and *Staphylococcus aureus* are common pathogens. Osteomyelitis causes fever, pain, and swelling over a bone; this may appear similar to a pain episode, but the child usually is sicker than expected.

Diagnostic studies

The following studies are required:

- CBC with differential, and reticulocyte count
- blood culture
- chest radiography (antero–posterior and lateral)
- urinalysis, urine culture
- stool culture (if diarrhea is present)
- lumbar puncture in any patient with symptoms of meningitis (strongly consider in <1 year with slightest indication)
- evaluation for osteomyelitis: if high fever and localized bone pain, consider bone scan, skeletal films, early orthopedic consultation
- type and hold/cross-match blood if there is extreme pallor, respiratory or neurological symptoms, or acute splenic enlargement.

Management

Box 81.1 gives the management of fever.

Box 81.1. Management of fever/presumptive infection

1. Immediate dose of ceftriaxone IV/IM (50 mg/kg), while awaiting laboratory results.
2. Cefuroxime (50 mg/kg IV dose q. 8 h) + oral erythromycin or azitromycin for acute chest syndrome/pneumonia
3. Admission for acute chest syndrome (see Disposition/indications for admission criteria).

Acute anemic complications

Steady-state hemoglobin in SCD typically ranges between 6 and 9 g/dl. Hemoglobin can fall acutely or chronically. Acute anemia resulting from a sudden drop in hemoglobin can result from splenic sequestration of RBCs, a transient aplastic crisis, a hyperhemolytic crisis, or ACS. It is, therefore, important to determine an individual patient's steady-state hemoglobin during an ED visit.

Acute splenic sequestration crisis

It is very important to assess splenic size in young children.

Splenic sequestration is the second most common cause of death in children over 5 years of age with SCD.

Viral infections often precede the episode. Peak incidence is between 1 and 2 years, with a 30% probability of having an event by age 5, prior to complete splenic autoinfarction. There is up to a 50% recurrence rate within 2 years. An acute sequestration crisis develops rapidly, with sudden engorgement of the child's spleen (i.e., new splenomegaly more than 2 cm from baseline). This develops as the spleen suddenly traps a large number of RBCs, with pooling of peripheral blood. Severe anemia can result, as hemoglobin falls by 20% or more. Mild thrombocytopenia may also occur. Hypovolemic shock may follow, and a high mortality rate is associated with severe sequestration crisis (15% per event). Clinical findings are sudden weakness, pallor, increased respiratory rate, abdominal engorgement, and splenomegaly. A major crisis is life threatening, and hemoglobin can precipitously fall to <2 g/dl, resulting in rapid death.

Aplastic crisis

Impaired RBC production in the bone marrow can result in a rapid reduction in hemoglobin and profound anemia. Increased fatigue and shortness of breath are common clinical signs. The hallmark of an aplastic crisis is a low hemoglobin, and absent reticulocytes (<2%). Aplastic crisis is more common in children than adults and is often associated with viral triggers, particularly parvovirus B19 (80%). Typically, it will spontaneously resolve in 1–2 weeks, and treatment is symptomatic; transfusion of PRBCs is used for low hemoglobin (<5 g/dl) or cardiopulmonary compromise.

Hyperhemolytic crisis

Acceleration of an already rapid rate of RBC destruction can compound underlying anemia. Hemolysis-associated complications result from erythrocyte release of free hemoglobin during RBC rupturing, which consumes nitric oxide (potent vasodilator), and simultaneous RBC release of the arginine-consuming enzyme arginase, which rapidly consumes the substrate for nitric oxide production, contributing to vasoconstriction and SCD complications. Recent studies suggest that a hyperhemolytic subphenotype exists in SCD that is associated with pulmonary hypertension, stroke, leg ulcers, and priapism. Acute hyperhemolytic crises often occur during a vaso-occlusive episode or ACS event. They can also be triggered by infection or co-existence of glucose-6-phosphate dehydrogenase deficiency after taking certain medications (sulfa drugs, nitrofurantoin). Clinical manifestations include fatigue, pain, increased scleral icterus, and jaundice.

Diagnostic studies

Diagnostic studies include CBC with differential and reticulocyte count. Blood should be typed and held/screened for possible PRBC transfusion.

Management

Management varies depending on the type of crisis (Box 81.2).

Box 81.2. Management of splenic sequestration crisis

Acute splenic sequestration crisis

1. Transfuse to hemoglobin of 9–10 g/dl:
   - with no signs of cardiopulmonary distress, give two separate transfusions using furosemide in-between to prevent fluid overload.
2. Exchange transfusion (in pediatric ICU) with signs of cardiopulmonary distress (hypoxemia, respiratory distress, clinical evidence of shock):
   - remove 75% blood volume and replace with packed RBC/normal saline (50/50)
   - regular transfusion while preparing for exchange transfusion if there is going to be a significant delay as this is a life-threatening complication
3. Splenectomy if patient age >2 years or patient age <2 years with no evidence of splenic function.
4. A pitted RBC count (pit count) is a non-invasive measure of splenic function; while the gold standard analysis is a technetium scan of the spleen, this is not typically determined in an ED setting.
5. Chronic transfusion program until age 2 years; maintain HbS <30% if patient is <2 years and splenic function is intact.

Aplastic crisis

1. Treatment is symptomatic; typically resolves in 1–2 weeks.
2. Close follow-up in asymptomatic patient.
3. Transfuse with packed RBCs for severe anemia (hemoglobin <5 g/dl) or for associated cardiopulmonary compromise.

Hyperhemolytic crisis

1. Evaluate for and treat underlying cause or trigger (including infection, vaso-occlusive event, acute chest syndrome).
2. Transfusion packed RBCs for severe anemia (10 ml/kg over 3–4 h).
3. Reduction of HbS to <30% of total circulating RBCs will effectively prevent further sickling; exchange transfusion may be needed based on severity of crisis.

Pulmonary complications

Acute pulmonary disease is estimated to be hundreds of times more frequent for those with SCD than for the general population (overall incidence 10.5/100 patient-years). Abnormal pulmonary function has been identified in >80% of adults and children with SCD. Pulmonary symptoms in the ED carry a fairly large differential diagnosis. Overview and management of the most common pulmonary complications are summarized below.

Acute chest syndrome

Acute chest syndrome is the second most common complication of SCD, one of the most frequent conditions at time of death, and carries a 3% mortality rate.

Acute chest syndrome is defined as a new infiltrate on chest radiography (lobar consolidation, excluding atelectasis) in a patient with SCD, and at least one of the following: fever, cough, sputum production, tachypnea, dyspnea, or new hypoxia.

The pneumonia can be occult, so clinical suspicion should be high. Progression to hypoxia, decreasing hemoglobin, and multilobar pneumonia is a common scenario for ACS.

Children tend to present with fever and cough, and often a normal lung examination, while adults tend to present with chest or extremity pain.

An acute worsening of obstructive disease and an "asthma-like" syndrome develops in many children with ACS and responds to bronchodilators. The condition may also manifest as abdominal pain. Duration of illness can be prolonged, often 10 to 12 days, and mechanical ventilation is required in 13% of patients. The etiology of ACS is varied; infection is a more common trigger in children, while pain and pulmonary fat emboli are more common in adults. Acute chest syndrome is often accompanied by a falling hemoglobin level and a significant increase in the WBC. Complications are common and include respiratory failure, neurologic events (11% of hospitalizations), altered mental status, seizures, and death.

Asthma

Asthma is a common co-morbidity in SCD, identified in 30–70% of children. It is notoriously underdiagnosed and undertreated in patients with SCD. It may be associated with pulmonary hypertension in children. Symptoms and triggers are typical for asthma in children generally. Asthma is associated with other complications of SCD and should be aggressively managed based on US National Institutes of Health guidelines. It is very difficult to clinically differentiate an asthma exacerbation from ACS in children. Therefore, treatment should be for both.

Pulmonary hypertension

Pulmonary hypertension is an increasingly recognized complication of chronic hemolytic anemias including SCD. Approximately a third of adults with SCD have an abnormally elevated tricuspid regurgitant jet velocity (>2.5 mg/s) measured by Doppler echocardiography at steady state, suggestive of pulmonary hypertension. This is associated with a 10-fold risk of early mortality. Advancing age is a clinical risk factor for pulmonary hypertension; however, it also develops in approximately 20% of children, even those as young as 3 years of age, and is associated with decrease exercise tolerance and low oxygen saturation. Since pulmonary artery pressure rises acutely during vaso-occlusive pain episodes, and even more so during acute chest syndrome, it is an important complication to consider in a patient with SCD and respiratory distress.

Diagnostic studies

The following studies are required:

- chest radiography (antero-posterior and lateral)
- CBC with differential, and reticulocyte count
- blood culture if fever is present or suspect ACS
- type blood and hold in patients with moderate/severe respiratory distress, if ACS is suspected or if a pneumonia is identified on chest radiography, even without respiratory symptoms, as hemoglobin can fall unexpectedly during ACS
- for ACS, consider: acute and convalescent serology, studies for *Mycoplasma pneumoniae*, *Chlamydia pneumoniae*, *Legionella pneumophila*, parvovirus B19, Epstein–Barr virus (optional)
- arterial blood gas on room air if hypoxic with respiratory distress (venous blood gas is not sufficient)
- ventilation–perfusion ($\dot{V}/\dot{Q}$) scan when significant chest symptoms exist with normal chest radiography
- ECG (prolonged QTc has been reported in children and adults with SCD)
- Doppler echocardiography to screen for pulmonary hypertension for unexplained hypoxemia or respiratory distress.

Management

For any pulmonary manifestation, oxygen should be used for respiratory distress or hypoxemia (oxygen saturations <92%). The routine use of oxygen is not indicated without signs of hypoxia or respiratory distress. Early consultation with pulmonary and hematology specialists is important given the mortality associated with pulmonary complications. Box 81.3 gives the management protocol

Box 81.3. Management of pulmonary complications

Acute chest syndrome

1. *Respiratory*. Supplemental oxygen as clinically indicated, bronchodilators, incentive spirometry every 2 h for patients with chest pain (reduces progression of pulmonary infiltrates and reduces atelectasis).
2. *Antibiotics*. Use local bacterial patterns and culture results to guide therapy. Empiric recommendation: second- or third-generation cephalosporin (immediate IV cefuroxime 100–150 mg/kg daily ideal) and an oral macrolide.
3. *Fluids*. Rehydrate as appropriate for clinical state. Maintain hydration (IV + PO) at 1.5× maintenance rate; avoid overhydration, which can contribute to pulmonary edema.
4. *Transfusion*. Simple transfusion for moderate or severe anemia, tachycardia, fatigue; exchange transfusion for evolving impending respiratory, neurological findings, tachycardia/hypotension, falling hemoglobin, or evidence of multiorgan involvement.
5. *Pain control*. It is important to attain adequate pain relief to allow deep breaths but to avoid over-narcotized hypoventilation; see pain management for vaso-occlusive episodes.

Asthma exacerbation

1. Treat asthma based on NIH *Asthma Guideline 75*.
2. Liberal use of inhaled steroids for persistent asthma symptoms, and consider other controller medications such as leukotriene inhibitors (montelukast).
3. Admit and consult pulmonary or hematology specialist if placing the patient on corticosteroids.
4. Close monitoring and follow-up is essential.

Pulmonary hypertension

1. Supplemental oxygen.
2. Consult a cardiopulmonary expert who has experience of SCD and pulmonary hypertension
3. Acute benefit from L-arginine hydrochoride (0.1 g/kg IV) and inhaled nitric oxide have been reported and are under investigation. Use of sildenafil in SCD has been associated with increased pain episodes, and it should be used only in consultation with hematology and cardiolopulmonary specialists.

Vaso-occlusive episodes

Pain is the most frequent reason patients with SCD seek care in an ED, and it is the most common cause of hospitalization. The pain is often excruciating and debilitating and is a true medical emergency. Pain is often managed at home using acetaminophen with codeine, fluids, rest, and hot packs; the ED visit is often the final resort after conservative outpatient measures have failed. Pain can occur in children as young as 6 months but typically manifests after 1 year of age (before which fetal hemoglobin is protective). The frequency of vaso-occlusive episodes is extremely varied. Only a subset of patients with SCD are the most frequent utilizers of the ED. Studies support the contention that those who are high utilizers of the ED tend to have more severe disease, including lower hemoglobins, lower quality of life, more pain episodes, and more transfusions than those without frequent ED visits. When controlling for the severity of their disease, high utilizers did not use more opioids than those with fewer ED visits. Prompt and adequate pain management in the ED will decrease need for hospitalization.

Table 81.1. Differential diagnosis by location of pain masquerading as vaso-occlusive episodes

Location	Differential diagnosis
Bones, joints, extremities	Osteomyelitis, septic arthritis, dactylitis, osteonecrosis/avascular necrosis of joint (mainly hip or shoulder)
Head/skull	Stroke, meningitis
Ribs/chest	Acute chest syndrome/pneumonia, asthma, pulmonary embolism, fat embolus, costochondritis, gastroesophageal reflux
Abdomen	Acute chest syndrome/pneumonia, gallstones/cholecystitis, appendicitis, ovarian torsion, pregnancy, pelvic inflammatory disease, renal colic/calculi, urinary tract infection, acute splenic sequestration

The differential diagnosis associated with vaso-occlusive episodes is extensive and varies depending on the location of pain (Table 81.1). Severe pain is often the harbinger of life-threatening conditions. The challenge for the EP is deciphering uncomplicated sickle cell pain from more serious complications. Initial assessment should include the duration of the pain episode and current treatment regimen: time, type, and dose of last pain medication. A description of the pain episode should be elicited including usual sickle cell pain, unusual location or intensity or unusual presentation for the current vaso-occlusive episode. The child's description of the pain should be obtained. Etiology for conditions other than vaso-occlusion should be sought through a thorough review of systems, and physical examination to rule out a medical emergency or other etiology.

Dactylitis (hand-foot syndrome)

Dactylitis may be the earliest manifestation of SCD, and prior to newborn screening was often the event that led to a diagnosis. This vaso-occlusive episode typically occurs in infants <6 months old but can occur up to age 4 years. It involves painful swelling of the infant's hands and feet, fever, and an elevated WBC and ESR; it is associated with increased disease severity. Initial radiographs are normal but may reveal periosteal elevation several days after the onset of symptoms. Care for dactylitis is supportive, and symptoms are usually self-limited. Management includes analgesia similar to the approach for other forms of vaso-occlusive episode, hydration, and warm compresses. Antibiotics should be given empirically to any infant or child with a vaso-occlusive episode associated with fever.

Diagnostic studies

The following studies are required:

- CBC with differential, and reticulocyte count
- urinalysis, urine culture
- chest radiography, when clinically indicated (fever, chest pain, abdominal pain).

Normally a child's hemoglobin should be unchanged during a vaso-occlusive episode, therefore a fall in hemoglobin below baseline should alert the evaluating physician to a possible acute anemic complication. Any additional diagnostic workup is dictated by individual symptoms and specific areas of pain.

Symptoms of dehydration: serum electrolytes.

Fever: diagnostic studies for fever. Aggressively evaluate for infection.

Chest pain: evaluate for ACS and asthma.

Bone pain: consider osteomyelitis if clinically indicated.

Abdominal pain: most with abdominal pain require no diagnostic imaging. However, localized tenderness or peritoneal signs (particularly with fever) warrant surgical consultation and/or diagnostic imaging (abdominal CT).

Caution is warranted when obtaining a CT with contrast, as the contrast material can trigger acute sickling and hemolysis. Contrast studies should be obtained in consultation with a pediatric hematologist, as transfusion may be needed prior to administration of contrast.

Additional studies for abdominal pain may include a urinalysis and culture, urine pregnancy test evaluation for possible pelvic inflammatory disease in fertile females (urine screen for gonorrhea/chlamydia PCR), abdominal films, LFTs (for RUQ pain), ultrasound to evaluate for appendicitis (or ovarian torsion in females) or gallstones/gallbladder disease.

Severe headache: consider evaluation for stroke if not improving. Headache can be the only clinical manifestation of a stroke early on in SCD.

Management

Adequate and timely treatment of pain is essential. Analgesic therapy should be titrated to provide prompt relief. Therapy choice is based on pain severity. Opioids are the drug of choice for pain management in the ED (Box 81.4). Avoid the pain pendulum by giving opioids at fixed intervals rather than waiting for pain to recur after relief.

Central nervous system complications

Stroke, seizure, and meningitis are common in SCD, with a prevalence of 15%. Of these, stroke remains one of the most devastating complications of SCD and will be the focus of this section.

Stroke

Stroke is a leading cause of death in both adults and children, affecting 6–8% of patients with SCD. Children between 2 and

Box 81.4. Pain management in the emergency department

1. Morphine (0.1–0.15 mg/kg IV dose every 1–3 h; max. 10 mg/dose) or hydromorphone (0.01 to 0.015 mg/kg IV dose) as initial therapy is the best choice for parenteral narcotics.
2. Ketoralac (0.5 mg/kg IV to max. 30 mg); this is a synergistic adjunct with narcotic-sparing effects.
3. NSAIDs in patients with normal renal function or acetaminophen are suggested for the use of mild-to-moderate pain and outpatient management (acetaminophen/codeine or acetaminophen/hydrocodone (Vicodin) as discharge medicine for vaso-occlusive episode).
4. Hydration IV (1–1.5 time maintenance rate, D5 ½) should be administered to treat dehydration, which promotes sickling; however, oral hydration is preferred if tolerated. It is important to balance fluids and avoid fluid overload, which can lead to pulmonary edema and acute chest syndrome. Routine use of IV fluids during vaso-occlusive episode is not indicated without signs of dehydration.
5. Diphenhydramine (1–2 mg/kg q. 4 h) is usually needed as an antihistamine if morphine is used. Some patients experience significant urticaria from morphine-induced histamine release, which is partially alleviated by antihistamines.
6. A histamine H_2 blocker such as ranitidine (1 mg/kg IV single dose) is given if more than one dose of ketorolac is given as there is GI irritation associated with ketorolac.
7. Consider an antiemetic, ondansetron (0.15 mg/kg IV single dose), for nausea or vomiting.
8. Use warm packs on sites of pain.
9. Inhaled nitric oxide.

Avoid

1. Meperidine (1–1.5 mg/kg dose q. 3 h; max. 100 mg/dose). As there is an increased incidence of seizures, this should not be used in patients with renal or neurological disease, and is not an ideal choice for pain management.
2. Fentanyl has a short duration of action limit, which limits its utility in SCD.
3. Oral pain medication in ED is less effective than IV.

Modified with permission from *Best Practices Clinical Guidelines*, created by the Department of Hematology, Children's Hospital and Research Center, Oakland, USA.

10 years of age are at highest risk. Younger children are at risk for infarction, while the incidence of hemorrhagic stroke increases with age. The majority of stroke in children results from occlusion of the large cerebral arteries. Rapid identification and treatment of stroke is necessary.

Diagnostic studies

Emergency head CT (without contrast) and head MRI if available. A lumbar puncture can be performed if meningitis is suspected.

Management

Box 81.5 outlines the management of CNS complications

Box 81.5. Management of central nervous system complications: stroke

1. Parenteral hydration is started immediately.
2. Emergency exchange transfusion is commenced, with the goal of lowering HbS to 30%.
3. Simple transfusion is not recommended because of issues of hyperviscosity.
4. Neurosurgical and neurological consultation should occur early.
5. Long-term chronic transfusion is necessary.
6. Thromboembolic agents for ischemic stroke have not been studied in SCD: they are controversial in SCD and not currently recommended.

Ocular emergencies

Ophthalmologic complications including proliferative and non-proliferative retinopathy are common in SCD but are not typically a pediatric problem. The most important ocular emergency is a hyphema, or blood in the anterior chamber of the eye, which is usually the result of trauma or surgery. In fact a sickledex preparation to rule out sickle cell trait should be ordered on every hyphema, regardless of ethnic background. This is a known complication in sickle cell trait as well as SCD. Low Po_2 and low pH in the aqueous humor triggers sickling of RBCs containing HbS and is a potential complication in patients with trait as well as SCD itself. The sickled cells block the flow of aqueous humor, and this may lead to sharp increases in intraocular pressure and acute glaucoma. The eye should be tested for visual acuity and to determine intraocular pressure. Box 81.6 gives the management of ocular emergencies.

Priapism

The diagnosis of priapism is usually self-evident. A history of over 4 to 6 h of priapism is a poor prognostic indicator. Patients should be hydrated, treated for pain, and admitted to hospital; consult hematology and urology specialists for treatment recommendations.

Special situation: transfusion therapy

Transfusion is one of the most common treatments for SCD complications. The two primary goals of transfusion are to correct the low oxygen-carrying capacity caused by severe anemia and to improve microvascular perfusion by decreasing the proportion of sickle red cells in the circulation, which will improve blood flow. Routine transfusion in SCD is not indicated outside of specific circumstances, which include the following: respiratory, cardiac or CNS dysfunction associated with hemoglobin <5 g/dl, stroke, acute splenic sequestration,

Box 81.6. **Management of ocular emergencies**

1. Place the patient in a supine position with the head elevated 30–45 degrees and an eye shield in place to prevent further trauma.
2. Treat for acute angle closure glaucoma if intraocular pressure is ≥24 mmHg with timolol 0.5% ophthalmic BID. Pilocarpine 2% one drop every 15 min should also be used.
3. The patient should be admitted to hospital and an emergency ophthalmologic consultation arranged.
4. Management for persistent elevation of intraocular pressure should be determined in consultation with the ophthalmologist.

Box 81.7. **Admission and discharge criteria for patients with sickle cell anemia and fever or vaso-occlusive episode**

Fever

Admission criteria

- Clinical signs or suspicion of serious bacterial infection or systemic toxicity.
- All children with temperature >40°C (104°F).
- WBC >30 000 or <5000/μl.
- Evidence of additional acute complication.
- Evidence of dehydration.
- Concerns about compliance.
- All infants <6 months.
- Strongly recommended in young children <5 years with temperature >38.3°C (101°F).

Outpatient management has been expanded for older children with fever who appear well; however, this decision should be made in consultation with a hematologist

Discharge criteria

- Healthy appearing non-toxic older child or adult.
- Normal vital signs.
- Reliable family and available for 24 h follow-up by phone or in ED/clinic.

Vaso-occlusive episode

Admission criteria

- Abnormal vital signs including fever >38.3°C (101°F).
- Pain not controlled in the ED.
- Abnormalities on physical examination including sign of significant infection, acute abdomen, or new CNS finding.
- Laboratory or radiograph abnormalities, including abnormal chest radiograph, acute fall in hemoglobin >1 g/dl and acidosis.
- Pregnancy.

Discharge criteria

- Pain is under control.
- No evidence of significant concomitant disease.
- Follow-up with primary care physician or hematologist within 1–2 days.
- Adequate oral analgesia as outpatient prescription.

Box 81.8. **Specific blood-ordering requirements for transfusion in sickle cell disease**

1. Before transfusion, a history of transfusion reactions and alloantibodies should be sought.
2. Phenotypic matching (for antigens E, C and Kell at minimum).
3. Test for HbS: Sickledex (a 5-min test for HbS) negative.
4. Washed cells eliminate febrile reactions in patients receiving recurrent transfusions.
5. Transfuse 10 ml/kg packed RBCs for acute anemia; repeat CBC, consult hematology, consider furosemide if a second transfusion is indicated.
6. A post-transfusion hemoglobin goal is between 9 and 10 mg/dl since a higher values theoretically causes hyperviscosity, which is dangerous to sickle cell patients.

Pearls and pitfalls

Pearls

1. Fever is a more common presentation of acute chest syndrome in children with sickle cell disease (SCD), while pain is more common in adults.
2. Splenic sequestration is a life-threatening cause of acute anemia in young children with hemoglobin SS prior to spleen autoinfarction.
3. Young infants and children ≤5 years old are at high risk for sepsis, pneumonia, meningitis, and osteomyelitis because of functional asplenia.
4. Any patient with sickle cell disease presenting with headaches and neurological symptoms should trigger a careful evaluation for stroke.
5. Dactylitis is one of the earliest manifestations of SCD; it is typically seen in infants <6 months but can occur up to age 4.

Pitfalls

1. Failure to use caution when considering the use of radiographic contrast media given the common occurrence of renal dysfunction in this population.
2. Failure to realize that asthma is very common in children with SCD; loss of reversibility and restrictive lung disease develops in adulthood.
3. Failure to realize that fever may be the only symptom of serious bacterial infection or pneumonia in children with SCD.
4. Patients with SCD are not "sicklers." This term is offensive and should be avoided.

and aplastic crisis. Transfusion may be indicated for diagnostic procedures requiring contrast, and preoperatively for surgery. Exchange transfusions should be performed in an ICU setting with close monitoring. It is not generally an ED intervention. Exchange transfusion requires central venous access and avoids potential problems with increased blood viscosity that can occur with simple transfusion. A special type of blood is needed when transfusing a patient with SCD in order to decrease febrile transfusion reactions, allo-immunization to the human leukocyte antigen, and CMV transmission (Box 81.8).

Disposition in sickle cell disease

Disposition from the ED depends on severity of illness. The child's social situation is also a consideration, in particular the ability to return to hospital and access to a phone or car. Indications for admission and discharge for fever and vaso-occlusive episode are summarized in Box 81.7.

Selected references

Freeman L. Sickle cell disease and other hemoglobinopathies: approaches to emergency diagnosis and treatment. *Emerg Med Pract* 2001;**3**:1–24.

Gladwin MT, Vichinsky E. Pulmonary complications of sickle cell disease. *N Engl J Med* 2008;**359**:2254–2265.

Miller ST, Sleeper LA, Pegelow CH, *et al.* Prediction of adverse outcomes in children with sickle cell disease. *N Engl J Med* 2000;**342**:83–89.

Steinberg MH. Management of sickle cell disease. *N Engl J Med* 1999;**340**:1021–1030.

Stuart MJ, Nagel RL. Sickle-cell disease. *Lancet* 2004;**364**:1343–1360.

Section 13

Immunologic emergencies: vasculitis and rheumatology

Expert reviewer: Hayley A. Gans

Chapter 82

Approach to emergency department diagnosis of pediatric rheumatologic disease

Andrew S. Zeft

Introduction

Systemic rheumatologic conditions are disorders of an overactive immune system. Patients present in various clinical states of systemic inflammation (Table 82.1). Rheumatologic diseases have a multifactorial etiology. Risk is associated with the subject's genetic susceptibility as well as their previous exposure to environmental risk factors. Family history of rheumatic disorders and identification of recent environmental triggers is important when assessing children with a suspected rheumatic disease. A number of rheumatic conditions present solely in the pediatric age group, while others are primarily adult disorders.

Patients with rheumatologic disease can present with fever and dermatologic and/or musculoskeletal symptoms. Rheumatologic disease often becomes a part of the differential diagnosis when a patient presents with a combination of these symptoms. This chapter provides a rubric for the EP to formulate a differential diagnosis and workup for children presenting with arthralgia or arthritis, prolonged fever, possible vasculitides, and chronic musculoskeletal pain. The following chapter highlights the emergency conditions associated with specific rheumatologic diagnoses as well as complications associated with treatment.

Arthralgia and arthritis

Arthralgia or joint pain is not an unusual complaint in children. While arthralgias can be a precursor of arthritis, often they resolve. Arthritis is characterized by one or more inflamed joints with swelling or joint effusion, pain on range of motion, and/or tenderness. Typically arthritis is characterized by morning stiffness. While radiography or joint ultrasound may aid in the detection of a joint effusion, gadolinium-enhanced MRI detects synovial proliferation, the hallmark of arthritis. In the end, however, arthritis is a clinical diagnosis.

Arthritis should be distinguished from enthesitis and apophysitis.

Both enthesitis and apophysitis typically have signs of tender points on palpation

Table 82.1. Typical age of presentation of childhood rheumatologic disorders, listed in order of frequency of occurrence

Disease	Symptoms	Age
Juvenile arthritis	Arthritis, fever and rash Different forms have different prognosis	<16 years of age
Systemic lupus erythematosus	Rash, constitutional symptoms, multisystem disease Similar to adults, may be more severe	Typically teenager, but peak onset is in those aged 20–30 years; rare in those <5 years of age
Juvenile dermatomyositis	Inflammation of muscles, skin, and GI	Variable, mean 8 years
Scleroderma	Localized, affects focal areas of skin and subcutaneous tissue Systemic disease with diffuse sclerosis	School age
Raynaud phenomenon	Fingers and toes turn white/blue/purple after exposure to cold	

A Practical Guide to Pediatric Emergency Medicine: Caring for Children in the Emergency Department, ed. N. Ewen Amieva-Wang (associate eds. Jamie Shandro, Aparajita Sohoni, and Bernhard Fassl). Published by Cambridge University Press.

Table 82.2. Bacterial septic arthritis

	Features
History	Recent antibiotic use (possible resistant organism), recent trauma (possible nidus for infection), sexually active (disseminated gonococcal infection)
Examination	90% of infected joints in children involve knees, hips, ankles, elbows Often painful, erythematous, febrile
Diagnosis:	Joint aspiration and culture to direct therapy Typical synovial fluid WBC >100 000/µl (50 000–300 000) with >75% polymorphonuclear leukocytes
Management	After joint fluid and blood culture sent, start IV antibiotics tailored to Gram stain, culture results, and patient age and history
Disposition	Admit for IV antibiotics

Table 82.3. Neoplastic process

	Features
History	Weight loss, painful joint, awaking at night
Examination	Focal pain, non-specific findings of organomegaly and lymphadenopathy?
Diagnosis	If suspected order laboratory tests: CBC (for cytopenia), lactate dehydrogenase, or uric acid (elevated representing high cell turnover) After plain films consider bone scan or MRI to further differentiate; osteosarcoma has characteristic appearance on plain film

- **enthesitis** describes an inflammatory focus of pain at the enthesis or sites of tendon, ligament, fascia, or capsule insertion to bone; it is characteristic of the juvenile idiopathic arthritis (JIA) subtype enthesitis-related arthritis
  - often presents at *multiple* sites
  - often has morning stiffness similar to arthritis
  - may occur in children with acute reactive arthritis or during a flare of psoriatic arthritis or inflammatory bowel disease
- **apophysitis** describes local irritation at sites of tendon insertion on growth cartilage from stress-related injury (Ch. 106)
  - Osgood–Schlatter disease
  - Sever disease.

Before a rheumatologic etiology is entertained, it is important to first determine if the child has septic arthritis (Table 82.2) or neoplasm (Table 82.3).

Arthritis can be reactive and associated with other infections such as parvovirus B19, *Mycobacterium pneumoniae, Chlamydia trachomatis.*

Recurrent or chronic large joint arthritis should initiate a consideration for Lyme disease.

Gastrointestinal infection by *Salmonella, Shigella, Campylobacter,* or *Yersinia* spp. with or without a recent diarrhea history is associated with reactive arthritis. The underlying infection should be appropriately treated. The pain of the arthritis can be treated with NSAID therapy.

With arthritis, other diagoses to consider include acute rheumatic fever (p. 368), and juvenile idiopathic arthritis.

Juvenile idiopathic arthritis is the new classification nomenclature for juvenile rheumatoid arthritis. It is a chronic and idiopathic arthritis. If JIA is suspected, the patient should be referred to pediatric rheumatology, as well as to ophthalmology for slit lamp examination as soon as possible regardless of ocular symptoms.

Patients with juvenile idiopathic arthritis can develop a vision-threatening yet relatively asymptomatic uveitis.

Patients can be started on long-acting NSAIDs during workup since it takes 3 weeks to achieve optimal efficacy. In possible JIA, it is reasonable to order CBC with differential, comprehensive metabolic panel, ESR, CRP, and antinuclear antibody (ANA).

Of note, systemic-onset JIA may present without arthritis; fever and rash are characteristic:

- initially, fever should be present for >2 weeks, and commonly ocurs in the evening or early morning
- patients may have lymphadenopathy, hepatosplenomegaly, serositis including pericarditis, leukocytosis, anemia, and thrombocytosis
- patients can spiral into a septic-like state of consumptive coagulopathy called macrophage activation syndrome; despite pronounced systemic inflammation, the disseminated intravascular coagulation-like pathophysiology of macrophage activation syndrome may normalize the ESR and platelet count.

Indications for admission

The following would be reasons to admit a patient presenting to ED:

- needing IV antibiotics for suspected septic arthritis
- acute rheumatic fever with carditis
- fever of unknown origin
- possible systemic JIA, to exclude possible infectious and oncologic etiologies
- non-ambulatory
- systemic JIA with macrophage activation syndrome.

Fever

Patients with rheumatic conditions may present with fever, but should have other signs or symptoms to direct further diagnostic workup. Fever of unknown origin (FUO; Ch. 87) is a chronic fever where, as the name implies, no other signs or symptoms are present to suggest a diagnosis. The initial evaluation in any patient with prolonged fever should include a thorough examination for possible infectious or oncologic etiologies. Acute rheumatic fever and vasculitis syndromes of childhood should be in the differential diagnosis (Ch. 85).

Whenever vasculitis is suspected, indicators of systemic inflammation should be examined: CBC, ESR, LFTs, urinalysis, CRP.

Periodic fever syndromes characteristically have recurrent, periodic episodes of fever. These may be hereditary or idiopathic as in periodic fever, apthous stomatitis, adenitis, and pharyngitis (PFAPA) syndrome. When suspecting a periodic fever syndrome:

- all possible infectious etiologies should be ruled out
- a careful family history should be obtained and families instructed to record a fever and symptom diary to aid their pediatrician at future outpatient visits
- screen for neutropenia may be needed
- follow up typically with rheumatology and infectious disease departments.

Acute rheumatic fever

Acute rheumatic fever is a complication of streptococcal pharyngitis. It is an acute self-limited inflammatory condition:

- patients are typically >6 years of age
- it is more common in patients with certain ethnic backgrounds such as Polynesian or Indian
- USA incidence is 0.5–3.0/100 000 children.

The diagnosis is made by application of the Jones criteria (Box 82.1) when considering this diagnosis. The diagnosis requires:

- culture documentation of recent group A streptococcal pharyngitis (typically 2–3 weeks) *or*
- high anti-streptolysin O (ASO) and/or anti-DNase B (DNase B) titers.

The specificity of ASO or DNase B is 80% or if ordered together 90% in identifiying an ARF streptococci-related immune process. These antibodies peak 6 weeks after an acute infection and often remain elevated for around 2 months. The signs of ARF typically occur after signs of streptococcal pharyngitis have resolved, so a throat culture is not necessary when considering ARF, potentially giving false-positive information if the child is a chronic carrier of streptococci. Arthritis is the most common but least specific manifestation of ARF, making screening for streptococci-associated antibody titers inappropriate in every child presenting with arthritis.

Fever is characteristic of ARF, and one of the minor Jones Criteria for diagnosis (Box 82.1).

Box 82.1. Jones criteria for acute rheumatic fever

Major criteria

- Polyarthritis during acute episode: painful, migrates <24 h, large joints.
- Carditis during acute episode: mitral > aorta.
- Erythema marginatum: intermittent pink rings on the trunk and inner surfaces of the limbs.
- Sydenham's chorea: later finding (>3 weeks, more at 8–14 weeks).
- Subcutaneous nodules on joint extensor surfaces.

Minor (less-specific) criteria

- Fever.
- Arthralgia.
- ESR, CRP raised.
- Prolonged PR interval.

Box 82.2. Management of acute rheumatic fever

1. Primary: penicillin V 250 mg TID for 10 days; erythromycin 20–40 mg/kg daily, divided BID or QID, for 10 days; benzathine penicillin G as a single dose of 1×10^5 to 1.2×10^6 U IM.
2. Secondary: penicillin V 250 mg BID, erythromycin 250 mg BID, benzathine penicillin G as a single dose of 1×10^5 to 1.2×10^6 U IM IM q. 4 weeks.
3. Arthritis pain commonly responds to a NSAID. Aspirin is the traditional, classic treatment for arthritis in acute rheumatic fever.
4. Corticosteroids for significant cardiac involvement.
5. Admit for carditis or concern with chorea.
6. Close follow-up is mandatory.

Treatment

Box 82.2 gives the treatment protocol for ARF.

Musculoskeletal pain

Patients with rheumatic disorders may present with pain, but more specific signs and symptoms should be present to direct further workup. A chief complaint of musculoskeletal pain should carry a broad differential diagnosis.

Focal pain not palliated by NSAID therapy is concerning for an infectious or oncologic etiology. A nuclear medicine bone scan may be necessary to screen for focal areas of infectious osteomyelitis, osseous tumor, or metastases.

Children with amplified pain syndromes often complain of diffuse musculoskeletal pain: pain around the periscapular region or other musculoskeletal trigger points is characteristic. Amplified pain syndromes are best treated with graduated physical therapy programs utilizing desensitization techniques, reassurance, and psychological counseling when appropriate.

Regional neurovascular dystrophy can present as a painful, swollen, cyanotic-appearing distal extremity and has characteristic bone scan findings. It often improves with directed physical therapy and reassurance.

Active hypermobile children often complain of arthralgias and can be clinically screened for genetic syndromes of hypermobility such as Ehler–Danlos syndrome.

Mechanical musculoskeletal etiologies of arthralgia are common and include misalignment secondary to pes planus.

Patellofemoral pain is common in teenage females and is best treated with physical therapy to improve flexibility and medial quadriceps strength.

Apophysitis describes areas of local injury at the site of tendon insertion on immature non-ossified bone.

Low-back pain in young children (see also Ch. 107) requires a careful evaluation for focal disorders such as diskitis or an infiltrating mass such as a teratoma. Bone scan imaging is often necessary to evaluate for these conditions.

Pearls and pitfalls

Pearls

1. Arthritis should be differentiated from enthesitis and apophysitis.
2. The differential diagnoses in pediatric joint pain and/or swelling includes septic arthritis, reactive arthritis, and rheumatologic disorders.

Pitfalls

1. Failure to rule out septic arthritis before considering a rheumatologic cause of arthritis.

Chapter 83

Emergency presentations in patients with underlying rheumatic disease

Andrew S. Zeft

Introduction

Pediatric rheumatologic disease can present as an emergency in a patient with a known diagnosis or as the initial presentation. This chapter describes the rheumatologic diseases that are most common in the pediatric population and discusses their emergency presentations and treatment: juvenile arthritis, systemic lupus erythematosus (SLE), juvenile dermatomyositis and scleroderma. The vasculitides Henoch–Schönlein purpura and Kawasaki disease will be discussed in Ch. 85.

Juvenile arthritis

Juvenile arthritis is the most common pediatric rheumatologic disease, with a prevalence of approximately 150/100 000 in the USA. Juvenile rheumatoid arthritis has been reclassified as the juvenile idiopathic arthritides (JIA). Subtypes have different clinical manifestations and complications (Table 83.1)

Macrophage activation syndrome

Macrophage activation syndrome (MAS) is a relatively rare but potentially fatal complication of children with systemic-onset JIA. It is a state of cytokine storm.

The trigger can be a viral illness (Epstein–Barr virus), by medications (Sulfa), or it can be idiopathic. Signs and symptoms include fever; hepatosplenomegaly; lymphadenopathy; emesis and rash; encephalopathy, which may progress to seizures and coma; and possible myocarditis or pericarditis. Patients are in a disseminated intravascular coagulation-like state with diffuse microthrombosis, hemophagocytosis (cytopenias), hepatitis, and possible hemorrhage.

Diagnostic studies

Laboratory evaluation of MAS includes the features of disseminated intravascular coagulation: anemia, thrombocytopenia, increased D-dimer, WBC low, ESR normal or low, CRP elevated. Diagnosis is clinical but can be confirmed by bone marrow biopsy.

Management

Treatment of MAS involves supportive care of the disseminated intravascular coagulation, empiric coverage with antibiotics, and consultation with rheumatologic subspecialists to give pulse steroids and cyclosporine.

Cervical spine involvement

A patient with JIA and atlantoaxial subluxation or cervical stenosis from chronic cervical spine arthritis has an increased risk of cervical spinal cord injury.

Atlantoaxial subluxation (Ch. 144) should be suspected in a patient with JIA who has distal upper extremity paresthesia and weakness. Patients should have lateral neck flexion/extension radiographs to initially evaluate their disease. In patients needing intubation, cervical spine immobilization and in-line stabilization must be maintained. Intubation with flexible larynoscopy should be considered.

Iritis/uveitis

Patients with oligoarticular or polyarticular JIA can have chronic uveitis, which may cause irreversible visual damage; these patients can have an improved prognosis with early regular ophthalomology screening for uveitis. While uveitis can present typically with photophobia, conjunctival erythema, and decreased visual acuity, in these patients it often is asymptomatic and can present in advanced stages with posterior synechia, band keratopathy, cataracts, or fixed pupil.

Arthritis

First-line treatment of pain from arthritis is NSAIDs. Methotrexate, corticosteroids, and other therapies should be initiated by the pediatric rheumatologist.

Acute systemic lupus erythematosus

Systemic lupus erythematosus is the second most common pediatric rheumatologic disease in the USA. It is a chronic systemic inflammatory disease that presents with diverse

A Practical Guide to Pediatric Emergency Medicine: Caring for Children in the Emergency Department, ed. N. Ewen Amieva-Wang (associate eds. Jamie Shandro, Aparajita Sohoni, and Bernhard Fassl). Published by Cambridge University Press.

Table 83.1. Classification of juvenile idiopathic arthritides

Subtype	Percentage of patients	Peak age (years)	Female: male ratio	Diagnostic clues	Prognosis	Complications/ emergencies
Systemic onset	10–15	Variable; 1–5	1:1	Fever, rash, arthritis, pericarditis Increased WBC (15 000–30 000 cells/μl)	Untreated active disease may be disabling and inhibit growth	Macrophage activation syndrome
Polyarticular	30–35	Variable; 2–4, 6–12	3:1	>5 inflamed joints	Untreated arthritis may be disabling and affect growth	Subacute uveitis in up to 10%, which can progress to blindness if left untreated
Oligoarticular	40–50	2–4	4–5:1	<5 symmetric small joints	Minority of patients progress to destructive arthritis If uveitis is left untreated, vision loss occurs	Subacute uveitis in 10–20%, which can progress to blindness if left untreated
Enthisitis-related arthritis	10–15	7–16		Large joints, frequently enthesitis Associated with inflammatory bowel disease	Variable, can develop into classic ankylosing spondylitis	Acute symptomatic anterior uveitis

symptoms in children as in adults. There are 5/10 000 children in the USA affected, with a greater incidence in Asians, Blacks, and Hispanics than in Whites. Onset is usually after 5 years of age. Female to male ratio is 4:1 before puberty and 8:1 after puberty. Incidence peaks at 20–30 years of age.

Skin, musculoskeletal, and renal systems are the most common organ systems involved. Most patients with lupus nephritis also have constitutional symptoms, including malaise and anorexia. The classic malar rash is absent over two-thirds of the time and renal disease and small-joint arthritis may go undiagnosed. Initial manifestations can require emergency treatment as it can affect all organ symptoms (Table 83.2). The differential diagnosis for SLE includes systemic infection such as infectious mononucleosis and streptococcal infections, lymphoid neoplasm, and other rheumatologic disorders. Drugs can induce lupus (minocycline among others).

Patients with SLE have many autoantibodies. Anti-double-stranded DNA and anti-Smith antibodies are highly specific for the disease and 98% of those with SLE have antinuclear antibody (ANA). Many of the manifestations of SLE result from deposition of immune complexes. Without appropriate treatment, approximately 30% of children with SLE progress to end-stage renal disease. However, with current treatment, there is a 90% survival rate after 15 years.

In general, patients with SLE are acutely managed with corticosteroids. Cyclophosphamide and mycophenelate mofetil has been used with success to treat severe lupus and lupus nephritis. The EP must be aware of the side effects and complications these medications can cause (Ch. 84).

Sepsis

Patients with SLE and other rheumatic disease who are treated with steroids and immunosuppressive medications are at risk for infectious disease, which can rapidly spread systemically. These patients are immunosuppressed and should be treated as such with broad-spectrum antibiotics and careful observation.

Antiphospholipid syndrome

Antiphospholipid syndrome is an acquired hypercoagulation state in children; SLE is the most common autoimmune disease associated with it. Many common childhood bacterial and viral infections can increase antiphospholipid syndrome transiently with no clinical manifestations. These cases have been most commonly associated with parvovirus B19, CMV, HIV, varicella zoster and mycoplasma pneumonia. Children with antiphospholipid syndrome can present with thrombotic symptoms such as deep vein thrombosis, pulmonary embolism, and stroke.

Patients with antiphospholipid syndrome who have had evidence of a clot are treated initially as other patients with thrombotic syndromes, with heparin followed by warfarin or SC heparin. Pulse solumedrol and plasma exchange should be initiated in conjunction with rheumatology.

Table 83.2. Signs and symptoms of systemic lupus erythematosus (SLE), in frequency of occurrence

	Signs and symptoms	Comments
Rash	Malar, purpuric, vasculitic, alopecia; oral and nasal ulcers	
Constitutional	Fever, weight loss, fatigue	
Cardiac	Pericarditis, myocarditis; myocardial infarction from thrombosis	
Pulmonary	Pneumonitis ± pleural effusion	Pneumonitis: chest radiograph shows diffuse alveolar infiltrate (unilateral or bilateral) Pleural effusion: consider infection, tap fluid and consider bronchoalveolar lavage or biopsy
	Acute alveolar hemorrhage ± hemoptysis (secondary to underlying vasculitis and possible concomitant infection)	
	Pulmonary hypertension	Secondary vasculitis or thrombosis of pulmonary vasculature
	Pulmonary embolus	
Renal	Glomerulonephritis, nephrosis, hyptertension, renal insufficiency	
Hematologic	Anemia ± autoimmune bleeding (positive Coombs' test), hypercoagulability; macrophage activation syndrome (rare in SLE)	If acute fall in hemoglobin consider internal hemorrhage; hemolytic anemia is treated with steroids
Raynaud phenomenon	Vasospasm of distal digits when cold	
CNS	Cerebritis, seizures, cerebrovascular accident, peripheral neuropathy, movement disorders	Consider infection, evaluate with imaging and lumbar puncture
Gastrointestinal	Pancreatitis, mesenteric vasculitis, microperforation, exudative ascites	

Acute catastrophic antiphospholipid syndrome

Acute catastrophic antiphospholipid syndrome, while rare, describes progressive multiple clot formation and often involves the CNS vasculature; systemic involvement can lead to multiorgan failure. Patients can present with venous and/or arterial thrombotic events. Involvement of the CNS (stroke, seizure, transverse myelitis, mononeuritis), renal (renal vein thrombosis [acute flank pain]), cardiac (valvular heart lesions), pulmonary (pulmonary hyptertension), and vascular (digital ischemia) systems can occur.

Thrombotic thrombocytopenia purpura (TTP)

Thrombotic thrombocytopenia purpura has a high mortality in SLE. It is microangiopathic hemolytic anemia with thrombocytopenia and renal and CNS abnormalities. Patients present with hemolytic anemia, mental status changes, coma, fever, gross hematuria, and rash. Evaluation demonstrates shistocytes and nucleated red blood cells, hemolytic anemia, and raised lactate dehydrogenase. Treatment is supportive plus plasma exchange and steroids in conjunction with rheumatology or hematology consult.

Juvenile dermatomyositis

Juvenile dermatomyositis is a vasculitis which manifests as skin and muscle inflammation. It is slightly more common in girls than boys and can manifest at any time during childhood. The pediatric disease has features of a vasculitis with small-vessel and capillary involvement. If the disease is well managed, permanent remission often occurs after approximately 5 years.

Onset can be insidious over years or acute over weeks. Constitutional symptoms such as fever, weight loss, or anorexia may occur. Muscle pain is usually mild to moderate. Important differential diagnosis includes muscular dystrophy and neurologic disease. Abnormal muscle enzymes are present in the majority of patients although the diagnosis may be difficult because of the subtle dermatologic signs. Scleroderma and SLE also have elements of inflammatory myopathy.

Complications can occur as a result of disease progression as well as secondary to treatment. Patients are susceptible to aspiration and atelectasis and subsequent pneumonia. Patients rarely develop pneumothorax, with advanced interstitial lung disease and pulmonary hypertension. Nasal or esophageal regurgitation with recurrent aspiration and secondary venopalatine weakness can occur. Vasculitis can cause GI bleed and perforation. Cardiac involvement is rare. Patients also have poor wound healing, secondary vasculitis, and poor circulation. Corticosteroid treatment increases susceptibility to infection.

Scleroderma

Children can have localized scleroderma, limited to focal areas of the skin and subcutaneous tissues (the more common form), and diffuse scleroderma, similar to the adult disease. While juvenile-onset systemic scleroderma is rare, the children affected have high morbidity. The disorder is characterized by a symmetrical fibrosis of the skin with concomitant fibrosis of the internal organs caused by autoimmune stimulation of fibroblasts.

Systemic scleroderma has an insidious and slow onset in childhood and may not be diagnosed initially. Raynaud syndrome is one of the earliest symptoms of systemic scleroderma, although it can also occur in otherwise healthy individuals. Patients develop pulmonary hypertension, and pneumothorax secondary to interstitial fibrotic lung disease. The GI complications include acute abdomen secondary to viscus perforation, severe malabsorption and reflux and aspiration secondary to distal esophageal dysmotility. Patients can develop congestive heart failure with restrictive cardiomyopathy (dyspnea, orthopnea, fatigue). Hypertension or renal crisis can occur with sudden blood pressure elevation up to 150–200 mgHg diastolic, with headache as the only symptom. Possible triggers include vasospasm (emotional stress, cold exposure), physical trauma, steroids, nicotine, and hypovolemia.

Treatment is initially with an ACE inhibitor. Steroids may worsen symptoms.

Pearls and pitfalls

Pearls

1. Macrophage activation syndrome is a state of cytokine storm that can occur and progress rapidly in children with a diagnosis of systemic-onset juvenile idiopathic arthritis (JIA).
2. Treat febrile patients with systemic lupus erythematosus where a bacterial source is suspected (particularly if the absolute neutrophil count is $<1000/\mu l$) with broad-spectrum antibiotics.
3. In patients with systemic scleroderma, lower blood pressure judiciously to preserve renal perfusion and prevent further crisis.

Pitfalls

1. Failure to consider cervical spine disease in patients with JIA with upper extremity muscle weakness and sensory symptoms.
2. Failure to arrange for prompt ophthalmologic consult in patients with JIA.
3. Failure to diagnose and empirically treat broadly for infection in an immunosuppressed patient with systemic lupus erythematosus and a possible infection.

Chapter 84

Tutorial: Pharmacy of rheumatology

Andrew S. Zeft

Medication-related complications

The lists below indicate the main complications with the therapeutic options used in treating rheumatic disorders.

Non-steroidal anti-inflammatory drugs

- Reye syndrome with exposure to varicella or influenza: emesis and altered mental status.
- Gastrointestinal hemorrhage (significant NSAID gastropathy rare in children).
- Hepatotoxicity, nephrotoxicity (proteinuria and renal papillary necrosis).
- Anaphylaxis.

Disease-modifying agents

- Sulfasalazine hypersensitivity reaction (Stevens–Johnson syndrome).
- Methotrexate: low doses for rheumatologic disease so toxicity profile low:
  - hepatic fibrosis
  - lymphopenia or pancytopenia, secondary bone marrow suppression
  - pulmonary hypersensitivity (first 6–12 months, rare in children)
  - dyspnea, cough, fever, fluffy infiltrates on chest radiograph; discontinue methotrexate and start corticosteroids if side effects have been distinguished from infectious pneumonitis.

Corticosteroids

- Pituitary–adrenal axis hypofunction with chronic use in previous year:
  - "stress coverage" required during acute infection, trauma, surgery: can use hydrocortisone 1 mg/kg daily in four or six divided doses (adult dose 100 mg IV q. 8 h).
- Side effects secondary to chronic use include:
  - avascular necrosis: painful, femoral head and vertebrae are common sites
  - osteopenia: increased fracture risk
  - pseudotumor cerebri: headache, check lumbar pressure for opening pressure; treatment is gradual periodic removal of CSF to lower pressure, and taper steroids
  - GI hemorrhage.

In a child taking glucocorticoids:

- fever may be absent during infective illness; therefore, judicious use of antibiotics will be needed
- susceptibility to herpes viruses (disseminated varicella) and intracellular pathogens (mycobacteria, listeria) will increase.

Intravenous immunoglobulin

- Acute hypersensitivity reaction, anaphylactoid or anaphylaxis during infusion.
- Signs and symptoms of hypersensitivity reaction: fever, rash, nausea, hypotension, shortness of breath, hoarseness, cough, bronchospasm, arrhythmia, sense of impending doom.
- Treatment:
  - premedicate with diphenhydramine PO (1.25 mg/kg, max. 50 mg) and acetaminophen (10 mg/kg IM)
  - anaphylaxis protocol: ABCs, epinephrine (0.01 mg/kg, 0.3 mg max.), diphenhydramine, ceterizine/histamine H_1 blocker 0.25 mg/kg to 10 mg, ranitidine/histamine H_2 blocker 1 mg/kg to 50 mg IV, solumedrol (1–2 mg/kg to 12.5 mg IV) or prednisone PO (1 mg/kg to 75 mg).

Immune-suppressant medications

- Azathioprine, mycophenolate mofetil, cyclophosphamide, cyclosporine (aplastic anemia): increase infection risk, including *Pneumcystis jirovecii* infection (was *P. carinii*).

Biologic agents

- Avoid live vaccines (MMR, varicella).
- Generally withhold during febrile illness.

A Practical Guide to Pediatric Emergency Medicine: Caring for Children in the Emergency Department, ed. N. Ewen Amieva-Wang (associate eds. Jamie Shandro, Aparajita Sohoni, and Bernhard Fassl). Published by Cambridge University Press.

- Tumor necrosis factor inhibitors (etanercept, infliximab, adalimumab) make the patient more more susceptible to infections from:
  - mycobacteria (tuberculosis)
  - bacteria (sepsis, cellulitis, pneumonia)
  - herpes
  - histoplasmosis.
- Manifestations of latent infections include secondary development of:
  - systemic lupus erythematosus-like syndrome with positive serologies (antinuclear antibody, anti-double-stranded DNA antibody)
  - rare CNS disorders (multiple sclerosis, optic neuritis)
  - acute serum sickness.
- Anti-CD20 monoclonal antibody (rituximab) can cause:
  - susceptibility to bacterial infections
  - cases reported of visceral varicella zoster, parvovirus B19 with pure red cell aplasia, enterovial meningitis, CMV.

Plasmapheresis

Plasmapheresis may be indicated when an acute critical disease process is driven by pathologic autoantibodies such as in thrombotic thrombocytopenia purpura, systemic lupus erythematosus, Wegener's granulomatosis, microscopic polyangiitis, and acute antiphospholipid syndrome.

Pearls and pitfalls

Pearls

1. Corticosteroids can decrease the adrenal stress response.

Pitfalls

1. Failure to realize that medications used in rheumatologic disease modulate the immune response and so patients are at risk for sepsis.

Chapter 85

Vasculitis syndromes

Theresa M. van der Vlugt, Andrew S. Zeft, and Cynthia J. Wong

Vasculitis syndromes often present with fever and rash in addition to other multisystemic symptoms, which are dependent on the size of the involved blood vessels.

The major childhood vasculitides presented in this section are Kawasaki disease (KD), Henoch–Schönlein purpura (HSP), and serum sickness (a subset of hypersensitivity vasculitis). An overview of the more common childhood vasculitis syndromes is presented in Table 85.1.

Ischemic complications from small or medium vessel vasculitis are an emergency issue if there is imminent risk of damage to vital organ systems. Whenever the EP suspects

Table 85.1. Differential diagnosis of childhood vasculitis

	Vessels affected	Incidence	Age/sex ratio	Typical presentation	Complications
Henoch–Schönlein purpura	Small vessel	10–22 in 100 000	Peak ages 2–6 years; M>F	Palpable purpura on dependent areas, abdominal pain, arthritis	GI bleeding, intussusception, nephrotic or nephritic syndrome; overall often mild/benign course
Kawasaki disease	Medium vessel	17–18 in 100 000 in USA (greater in Asia)	1–2 years; 90% in those <5 years; M>F	Fever ≥5 days, diffuse rash, non-purulent conjunctivitis, mucous membrane changes, unilateral cervical lymph node swelling	Coronary artery aneurysm with thrombosis or rupture, myocardial infarction, myocarditis/pancarditis, atrioventricular block
Takayasu arteritis	Large vessel	1–3 per 1 000 000 in the USA; greater in Asia/Africa	10–40 years; 80–90% F	Early: fatigue, fever, weight loss, lower leg rash Late: claudication, decreased pulses, syncope, chest pain, hemoptysis, dyspnea	Myocardial and mesenteric ischemia, cardiac valvular insufficiency, vertigo, seizure, dementia
Wegner's granulamatosis	Small vessel	1–2 in 1 000 000 children	15% <19 years	Nasal/oral ulcers, bloody/purulent nasal discharge, cough, hemoptysis, dyspnea; also rash	Glomerulonephritis, renal insufficiency, arthritis, pulmonary nodules (occasionally cavitary) and infiltrates, ocular complaints
Polyarteritis nodosa (PAN)	Small/medium vessel	Infantile (IPAN): rare, Typical (TPAN): 2–33 in 1 000 000 Benign cutaneous (BCPAN): most common form in children	IPAN: <2 years TPAN: usually late middle age, occasionally seen in adolescence. BCPAN: case reports ages 2 to adult	IPAN: congestive heart failure, severe systemic illness TPAN: subcutaneous nodules, muscle pain, weight loss, hypertension, neuropathy, testicle pain BCPAN: red tender nodules on lower extremities, ulcers, urticaria, livedo	IPAN: often diagnosed by autopsy TPAN: renal insufficiency/infarct, mesenteric ischemia, myocarditis, skin necrosis or gangrene BCPAN: peripheral gangrene

A Practical Guide to Pediatric Emergency Medicine: Caring for Children in the Emergency Department, ed. N. Ewen Amieva-Wang (associate eds. Jamie Shandro, Aparajita Sohoni, and Bernhard Fassl). Published by Cambridge University Press.

vasculitis, indicators of involvement and systemic inflammation should be sent: CBC, ESR, LFTs, urinalysis, CRP.

A Kawasaki disease

Theresa M. van der Vlugt and Andrew S. Zeft

Introduction

Kawasaki disease, also called mucocutaneous lymph node syndrome, is a systemic vasculitis of children. Peak incidence of cases is between 1 and 2 years of age and 90% of cases occur in children under 5 years of age. Incidence in the USA is estimated at 18/100 000 children <5 years old. Pacific Islanders, Asians, African-Americans, and Hispanics have a higher incidence than Caucasian children, and boys have 50% higher incidence than girls.

Coronary artery aneurysm is the significant complication of KD and can occur in up to 25% of untreated patients.

With treatment, the occurrence of coronary artery aneurysm falls to 4–6%.

The etiology KD is unknown, but is possibly infectious.

Disease course

Kawasaki disease is usually a self-limiting illness that resolves locally after approximately 10–14 days if untreated. Morbidity and mortality is caused by coronary artery aneurysms, carditis, and their sequellae, such as myocardial infarction and congestive heart failure. During the first 10 days after the onset of fever, generalized microvasculitis occurs throughout the body, with a predilection for the coronary arteries. Coronary artery aneurysms develop in 15–20% during the acute phase. The aneurysms tend to develop most frequently in the proximal segment of the major coronary arteries and may assume fusiform, saccular, cylindrical, or a beads-on-a-string appearance. The elevated platelet count seen in this condition contributes to a hypercoagulable state, which contributes to coronary artery thrombosis and subsequent myocardial infarction. During the acute phase, there is a pancarditis. Inflammation of the atrioventricular conduction system, myocardium, pericardium, and endocardium can produce atrioventricular block, myocardial dysfunction and congestive heart failure, pericardial effusion, and aortic and mitral valve dysfunction, respectively. Late changes consist of healing and fibrosis in the coronary arteries, with thrombus formation and stenosis in the post-aneurysmal segment as well as myocardial fibrosis after myocardial infarction.

Clinical presentation

The clinical presentation of KD starts with several days of high fever unresponsive to antipyretics or antibiotics, along with other signs of systemic vasculitic inflammation: bilateral non-purulent conjunctivitis, erythema of lips and oral mucosa, rash, extremity changes, and lymphadenopathy that is not diffuse, usually characterized by a unilateral large cervical node (Table 85.2). Fever is the most common symptom, lymphadenopathy the least common. Oral mucous membrane changes include red, fissured, or crusted lips and strawberry tongue. The conjunctivitis often includes limbal sparing, with a white/uninvolved ring around the outer border of the iris. Extremity changes include hand and foot erythema and edema, with fusiform swelling of the digits and late desquamation starting around the nail beds (Figure 85.1). The rash of KD occurs in 90% of children with typical disease and is usually a polymorphous diffuse erythematous macular and papular eruption, worse in the groin or other skin fold areas (Figure 85.2).

Table 85.2. Diagnosis of Kawasaki disease

Criteria	Frequency (%)	Comments
Absolute criteria		
Fever >38.3°C (101°F) for 5 days plus four of the five clinical criteria below		Patients with fever of at least 5 days but <4 clinical criteria can be diagnosed with Kawasaki disease when coronary artery abnormalities are detected on 2D echocardiography or angiography
Clinical criteria		
Polymorphous erythematous diffuse exanthema	>90	Rash is not vesicular
Bilateral non-purulent bulbar conjunctivitis	80–90	Conjunctivitis often has limbic sparing; not purulent
Orophayngeal mucous membrane changes including erythema, cracked lips, strawberry tongue	80–90	Oral mucosa changes are not vesicular or bullous, discrete ulcers not present; pharyngitis is not exudative
Changes in extremities: erythematous; edematous hands and feet, with subacute periungual peeling of fingers and toes, then palm and sole desquamation	80	Desquamation occurs late in disease
Cervical lymphadenopathy ≥1.5 cm in diameter, usually unilateral	50	Not suppurative or diffuse

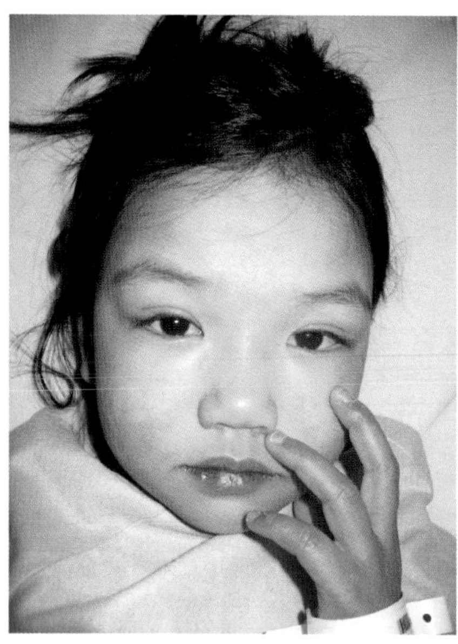

Figure 85.1 Kawasaki disease. Conjunctival changes with limbic sparing, mucosal changes of the lips, and extremity erythema and swelling are noted. (Courtesy of T. M. van der Vlugt).

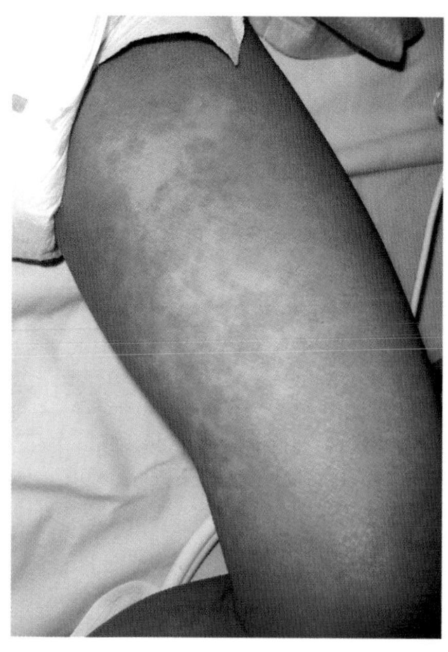

Figure 85.2 Kawasaki disease. Rash is polymorphous, diffuse, erythematous macular papular eruption worse in the groin or other skin fold areas. (Courtesy of T. M. van der Vlugt).

Table 85.3. Differential diagnosis of Kawasaki disease (KD)

Disease	Similarity to KD	Difference from KD
Stevens–Johnson syndrome (SJS)	Mucosal involvement	Frank blistering/ulceration of mucosa in SJS; only erythema and cracking in KD; KD has strawberry tongue
Rocky Mountain spotted fever (RMSF)	Fever; extremity changes of non-blanching rash that spreads centrally during acute disease	Extremity with erythema and edema; desquamation on palms and soles 2 weeks into the disease; prominent headache with RMSF but not KD
Systemic group A streptococcal infections and staphylococcal toxic shock syndrome (TSS)	Fever and rash	Lack of ocular involvement; hypotension and multisystem organ involvement in TSS
Enteroviral exanthem (particularly caused by adenovirus), Epstein–Barr virus, rubeola	Fever, rash, elevated inflammatory markers	Often lack extremity findings; diffuse lymphadenopathy (not in KD), adenoviral conjunctivitis is purulent, KD is not
Systemic-onset juvenile idiopathic arthritis (soJIA) and Reiter syndrome	Conjunctivitis, rash	Acute, painful conjunctivitis, with or without episodes of reactive arthritis and/or urethritis; lack oral findings of KD; Diffuse adenopathy with soJIA; patients may be older (Reiter), often do not meet KD diagnostic criteria
Mercury toxicity (acrodynia)	Fever, rash, swelling and desquamation of hands and feet	Rare in the developed world; requires convincing history of mercury exposure
Mycoplasma pneumonia	Fever, rash, mucosal changes	Pneumonia/bronchitis, ulcerative stomatitis (ulcers not seen in KD)
Morbilliform drug eruption/allergy	Diffuse rash, palm and sole involvement, malaise, fever, arthralgia, late superficial desquamation	Mucous membrane involvement rare, diffuse adenopathy (not in KD), necessary drug ingestion (antibiotic, antifungal, anticonvulsant, NSAID) in prior 7–14 days

NSAID, non-steroidal anti-inflammatory drug.

Myocarditis develops in 50% of patients within the first 2 weeks of disease. Patients with giant coronary aneurysms (>8 mm) have the highest risk of coronary stenosis, thrombosis, or aneurysm rupture, which usually occurs during the convalescent state. Common peripheral aneurysm sites include subclavian, brachial, axillary, iliac, and femoral arteries.

While the differential diagnosis of KD includes many diseases presenting with fever and rash (Table 85.3), probably the most difficult differentiation is with a viral syndrome such as that seen with adenovirus.

However the specific signs of KD should not mimic common viral and bacterial syndromes, as does systemic-onset juvenile idiopathic arthritis.

In the influenza season, care must be taken to rule out influenza prior to aspirin administration for presumed KD, because of aspirin's association with Reye syndrome in this setting. The following features should lead a clinician to suspect a diagnosis *other* than Kawasaki disease:

- exudative conjunctivitis
- exudative pharyngitis
- discrete intraoral lesions
- bullous or vesicular rash
- generalized lymphadenopathy.

Incomplete KD is defined as fever >5 days with less than four of the five diagnostic criteria. Incomplete KD has the same risk for cardiac and coronary abnormalities but a worse prognosis owing to delayed diagnosis. Infants, particularly those under 6 months, have an increased incidence of incomplete KD, possibly because of the circulating maternal antibodies. Laboratory tests are suggested when incomplete KD is suspected, as is early echocardiography. Presence of two-dimensional echo-proven coronary artery aneurysm in the setting of prolonged fever with two or three diagnostic criteria is sufficient to institute treatment, as is prolonged fever, plus two or three diagnostic criteria and with three or more laboratory abnormalities.

Diagnostic studies

The American Heart Association (AHA)/AAP recommended laboratory studies to evaluate for KD are CBC, CRP, ESR, ALT, serum albumin, and urinalysis. Clean catch or bag urinalysis is preferred to catheter specimen because the sterile pyuria associated with KD is urethral in origin and will be missed on catheter specimen or suprapubic tap. Laboratory abnormalities suggestive of Kawasaki disease include

- elevated CRP ≥3.0 mg/dl or ESR ≥40 mm/h
- WBC ≥15 000/μl
- normocytic normochromic anemia for age
- pyuria: WBC ≥10/high-power field
- serum ALT ≥50 U/l
- serum albumin ≤3.0 g/dl
- platelets ≥ 450 000/μl.

The presence or extent of cardiac involvement can be further assessed with ECG and echocardiography.

Management

Treatment for KD requires admission for IV immunoglobulin (IVIG) and aspirin and expedient echocardiography. If the diagnosis of KD is probable, IVIG and aspirin can be administered without echocardiography results. The IVIG should be administered in consultation with a specialist in an effort to prevent coronary artery aneurysms. Use of IVIG will also normalize serum lipoprotein abnormalities that might otherwise persist for years, as well as potentially reverse depressed myocardial contractility. Note that IVIG is most efficacious in preventing coronary artery aneurysms if given in the first 10 days, and if possible in the first 7 days. Children diagnosed after day 10 but with persistent fever or elevated inflammatory markers are also candidates for IVIG. The AHA/AAP guidelines recommend high-dose aspirin at 80–100 mg/kg daily in the acute phase of illness divided QID. When fever has been absent for 48 h, patients are switched to low-dose aspirin (3–5 mg/kg daily).

Pearls and pitfalls: Kawasaki disease

Pearls

1. Kawasaki disease is the most common cause of acquired heart disease in children.
2. It is unlikely in the presence of exudative conjunctivitis, exudative pharyngitis, discrete intraoral lesions, bullous or vesicular rash, or generalized lymphadenopathy.
3. Prompt treatment with IV immunoglobulin and aspirin within 7–10 days of the disease onset can decrease morbidity greatly.
4. Patients at highest risk for aneurysm development are male, <1 year of age, with prolonged fever, raised CRP, raised band count, decreased albumin.
5. If poor response to two doses of IV immunoglobulin, an infectious etiology or another auto-inflammatory disease (systemic-onset juvenile idiopathic arthritis, Reiter syndrome) should be considered.

Pitfalls

1. Failure to realize that incomplete presentations of Kawasaki disease can occur at age extremes, resulting in delayed diagnosis and worse outcomes.
2. Myocarditis may be present early in the disease's acute phase; but coronary artery abnormalities may not be noted until the second or third week of illness.

B Henoch–Schönlein purpura

Theresa M. van der Vlugt and Cynthia J. Wong

Introduction

Henoch-Schönlein purpura, also called anaphylactoid purpura or cutaneous necrotizing venulitis, is the most common systemic vasculitis of children, with a peak in children 2–6 years of age. It is more common in boys than girls and is a self-limited condition with few sequellae in the majority of cases.

Henoch-Schönlein purpura is a small-vessel vasculitis that primarily involves four systems: skin, joints, kidneys, and GI tract.

The cause is not known, but vessel damage is immune-mediated and involves deposition of IgA immune complexes in affected organs. Onset of HSP often follows an upper respiratory infection or viral acute gastroenteritis. Although HSP will usually resolve over 2–6 weeks, 30–40% of children will have at least one recurrence, usually within the first several months.

Almost all long-term morbidity or mortality is attributable to renal disease.

Clinical presentation

Symptoms of HSP are given in Table 85.4. Skin involvement is present in 100%, but it is the presenting feature in only half to three-quarters of cases. The rash is classically palpable purpura with normal platelet counts and normal PT/PTT. The rash can begin as an urticarial eruption that progresses to erythematous macules and papules and then purpura. Purpura occur classically on the legs and buttocks (and scrotum in boys) but can occur anywhere, particularly in dependent areas and pressure points. Younger children can develop marked edema of hands, feet, face, or scalp. Non-deforming arthritis or arthralgia is present in about 80% of US cases but is the presenting complaint in only 15%; it commonly involves knees and ankles, less commonly elbows and wrists.

Table 85.4. Symptoms of Henoch–Schönlein purpura

Symptom	Characteristics	Frequency (% affected)
Rash	Palpable purpura on areas of pressure, classically buttocks	100%; presenting symptom in 50–75%
Arthritis		80%; presenting symptom in 15%
Gastrointestinal disturbance	Colicky abdominal pain with nausea and vomiting	40–75%; can precede rash
Renal	Nephrotic or nephritic syndrome	One-third develop nephrotic or nephritic syndrome

Gastrointestinal symptoms occur in 38–75% of children with HSP and usually consist of colicky abdominal pain, worse with eating, and nausea/vomiting. Complications of GI involvement in HSP include ileo-ileal intussusception (2% of those with GI involvement), GI bleeding (hematochezia or hematemesis), and, more rarely, bowel perforation, visceral infarction, pancreatitis, or cholecystitis. The GI symptoms can precede the rash in 15–35% of cases, making diagnosis difficult.

Most children have mild renal disease. Renal involvement develops in about one-third, and in two-thirds of these patients is limited to hematuria or proteinuria on the urinalysis; the remaining patients develop nephrotic syndrome. Children with normal urinalysis and creatinine at 6 months appear to have essentially no risk of long-term renal sequellae or renal failure.

Diagnosis

Diagnosis is clinical. The classic presentation would be a young child with non-thrombocytopenic palpable purpura on the back of the legs and buttocks in addition to joint and or abdominal pain (Figure 85.3). Laboratory tests should include platelet count and clotting factors (should be normal for HSP), serum creatinine, and urinalysis. Complement levels and antinuclear antibody (ANA) may be checked to rule out other immune-mediated causes including lupus. Children with significant abdominal pain should be evaluated with ultrasound for intussusception, as ileo-ileal intussusception will not be revealed on barium enema. Stool occult blood testing should be performed.

Differential diagnosis in the advent of low platelets and abnormal coagulation profile includes sepsis, hemolytic uremic syndrome, neoplasm, and vasculitides (systemic lupus erythematosus, Wegner's granulomatosis, hypersensitivity vasculitis, septic vasculitis), which may have purpura but will have different laboratory and associated clinical findings. The rash on the buttocks and legs can raise the suspicion of child abuse in those without a classic history and examination. Severe abdominal pain occurring prior to other symptoms can mimic appendicitis.

Management

Treatment for mild cases (common in younger children) includes NSAIDs for joint pain, leg elevation, and maintaining hydration status in the setting of GI symptoms. There is no evidence that NSAIDs worsen GI symptoms or GI bleeding in HSP.

While steroids are often advocated for relief of severe abdominal pain, no controlled clinical trials have been done demonstrating benefit. Doses used are 1–4 mg/kg daily of oral glucocorticosteroids (in divided doses) or equivalent methylprednisolone IV. Care should be taken to taper slowly (around 4 weeks) so as not to precipitate a disease flare. Targeted therapy for GI complications includes management of intussuception as

A

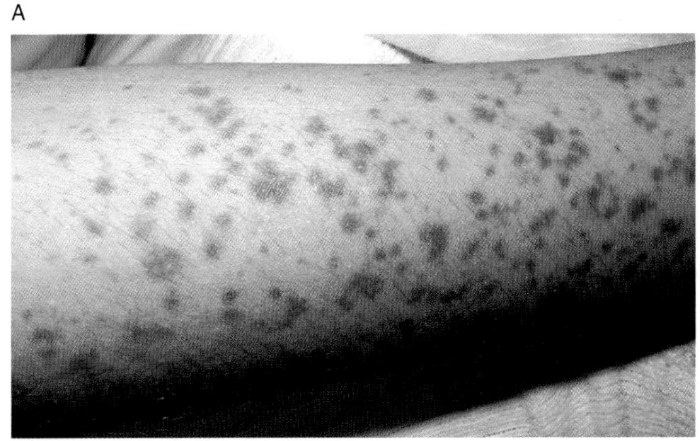

B

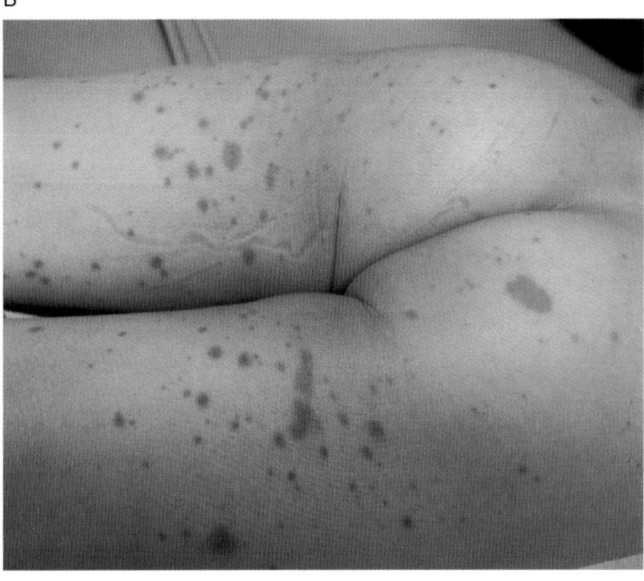

Figure 85.3 Henoch–Schönlein purpura: Urticarial, purpuric papules and plaques classically on the extremities (A) and buttocks (B). (A, courtesy Dr. Mehran Mosely; B, courtesy Dr. Paul Matz.)

well as surgery as necessary for bowel obstruction, perforation, or infarction. Often non-obstructive intussusception with no evidence of ischemia or infarction is managed non-operatively.

Nephrotic syndrome is treated with various immunosuppressive drugs, plasmapheresis, antiplatelet agents, and anticoagulants, with no therapy showing significant efficacy in controlled trials.

Pearls and pitfalls: Henoch–Schönlein purpura

Pearls

1. Henoch–Schönlein purpura is more common in children than adults.
2. It is a small-vessel vasculitis that primarily involves four systems: skin, joints, kidneys, and intestines.
3. Renal and GI diseases are less common in children <2 years of age, but edema is more common in this age group.
4. More severe renal and extrarenal involvement may occur in adults and adolescents than in young children.

Pitfalls

1. Children may develop rash first then renal involvement; therefore, urine must be monitored for development of hematuria and proteinuria.
2. Failure to realize that in children GI symptoms (nausea/vomiting/abdominal pain) can precede rash in 15–35% of cases, and arthritis precedes rash in 15%, thus delaying diagnosis.

Disposition

Patient with classic mild symptoms can be discharged with close follow-up. Those with severe abdominal pain warrant admission for observation, further testing, and pain control. Children with hypertension, proteinuria, or elevated creatinine warrant referral for nephrology consultation.

Given that HSP symptoms can last up to 2 weeks and often recur, and that children are at risk for renal disease for up to a year after presentation, patients should have close follow-up. Patients should specifically receive repeated blood pressure and urine analysis checks (biweekly for 1 week, weekly for 2 weeks, alternating weeks for 4 weeks, monthly for 2 months, *then* alternating months for 4 months).

C Hypersensitivity vasculitis/ serum sickness

Theresa M. van der Vlugt

Introduction

Hypersensitivity vasculitis of which serum sickness is a subset, classically presents as variably purpuric rash, fever, and polyarthritis 1–2 weeks after first exposure to the causative agent. Patients can be acutely ill and uncomfortable during the acute febrile stage, although the prognosis is excellent once the responsible drug is stopped. Drugs are the cause of approximately 10% of childhood cutaneous vasculitis. Serum sickness-like drug reaction (SSLDR, see Ch. 24), which is *not* a vasculitis, can mimic true serum sickness.

Hypersensitivity vasculitis is characterized by immune-mediated inflammation and necrosis of small blood vessels. It presents with typical cutaneous findings but in serum sickness also with fever, arthralgia, lymphadenopathy, splenomegaly, hypocomplementemia, proteinuria, renal dysfunction, and GI symptoms.

True serum sickness, mediated by immune-complex deposition, occurs only with vaccines or serum preparations. Drug-induced vasculitis occurs with many drugs, most commonly antibiotics such as penicillins and sulfa-drugs.

Clinical presentation

Hypersensitivity vasculitis begins 7–21 days after ingestion/absorbtion of the inciting agent with an erythematous, blanching eruption of macules and papules, centered on the legs or dependent areas, evolving to palpable purpura. Urticaria can co-occur, as can blistering of purpura. The small-vessel damage can be limited to skin or can affect kidney, liver, GI tract, or the CNS.

Management

The inciting agent should be stopped. In patients with mild symptoms, antihistamines and NSAIDs may be sufficient to treat pruritis, fever, and rash. Patients with severe symptoms can be treated with steroids.

Pearls and pitfalls: hypersensitivity vasculitis and serum sickness

Pearls

1. True serum sickness is rare nowadays.
2. Medications are the cause of 10% of childhood cutaneous vasculitis.

Pitfalls

1. Failure to search for and stop an inciting medication.

Selected references

Narchi H. Risk of long term renal impairment and duration of follow-up recommended for Henoch–Schönlein purpura with normal or minimal urinary findings: a systematic review. *Arch Dis Child* 2005;**90**:916–920.

Newburger JW, Takahashi M. Gerber MA, *et al.* Diagnosis, treatment, and long-term management of Kawasaki disease: a statement for health professionals from the Committee on Rheumatic Fever, Endocarditis, and Kawasaki disease, Council on Cardiovascular Disease in the Young, American Heart Association. *Circulation* 2004;**110**:2747–2771.

Ting TV, Hashkes PJ. Update on childhood vasculitides. *Curr Opin Rheumatol* 2004;**16**:560–565.

Primary immunodeficiency disease in the emergency department

Naresh Ramarajan and N. Ewen Amieva-Wang

Introduction

There are more than 500 000 children living with a primary immunodeficiency (PI) in the USA today.

In children, primary immunodeficiencies are more common than leukemia and lymphoma combined.

Children with PI differ from those with secondary immunodeficiencies (malignancy, HIV, etc.) as PI is genetically based and often undiagnosed until the first or second major illness. Children with PIs can also present to the ED with mild symptoms of common diseases yet have severe, complicated courses with fatal outcomes. Despite the diverse pathophysiologic basis of the many PI syndromes, the ED approach to these patients is fairly uniform. Emergency physicians must have a basic familiarity with warning signs of PI in children and treatment strategies for these patients. Such an approach has the potential to improve outcomes and quality of life. In addition, detection of PI makes family genetic counseling and prenatal counseling possible through the primary care clinician. This chapter will focus on when to suspect a PI, common and lethal presentations of children with PI, and an early treatment algorithm for patients with known PI.

Pathophysiology

An intact immune system is composed of the innate immune system and the adaptive immune system.

The innate immune system consists mainly of phagocytes (neutrophils, monocytes and macrophages) and complement, circulating proteins synthesized by the liver that are activated to attack bacteria. The innate immune system is the first line of defense against pathogens, poised to attack common bacterial epitopes such as lipopolysaccharide (endotoxin) and other microbial components. Phagocytes, particularly, patrol the skin, gut, soft tissues, and reticuloendothelial system (lymph nodes, spleen, liver) and hence defects in phagocyte number or function predispose children to bacterial and fungal infections and abscesses in these areas. The complement system is particularly active against encapsulated pathogens such as *Streptococcus pneumoniae*, *Haemophilus influenzae* type b, and *Neisseria meningitidis*. Children with complement deficiencies can present with bacteremia and meningitis as well as recurrent sinopulmonary infections.

The adaptive immune system comprises T and B cells, which are activated by exposure to specific antigens and mount a tailored response to individual microorganisms. T cell populations include cytotoxic (or CD8) T cells, which are essential in recognizing and killing intracellular viral infections as well as in maintaining surveillance against common opportunistic fungi (*Candida* spp., *Pneumocystis jirovecii* [was *P. carinii*]) and tumor cells in the body. Helper (or CD4) T cells, are responsible for providing cell-mediated immune responses, supporting memory responses as well as stimulating T cell-dependent B cell responses. Isolated primary T cell deficiencies (though rare) present with severe, protracted viral infections, chronic diarrhea, and failure to thrive. These must be considered in any children with a clinical presentation consistent with AIDS but HIV negative.

B cells, with the stimulation of helper T cells, mature into plasma cells in the lymph nodes over a period of 3–7 days and produce antibodies specific to various microorganisms. Antibodies are particularly important in the opsonization, phagocytosis, and killing of encapsulated organisms such as *Streptococcus pneumoniae*, *H. influenzae* type b, and *N. meningitidis*. In addition, children with B cell disorders tend to present with recurrent sino-pulmonary infections as *S. pneumoniae* and *H. influenzae* colonize the sinuses. B cell disorders also often have associated autoimmune manifestations such as autoimmune hemolytic anemia, thrombocytopenia, and thyroiditis as there is dysregulation of antibody production resulting in autoantibody formation. The clustering of recurrent sinopulmonary infections in a child and/or autoimmune manifestations may be the EP's first sign to screen for such deficiencies to prevent devastating attacks of meningitis in the future. Meningitis from any of the encapsulated organisms or enterovirus is a serious concern in children with B cell deficiencies.

A Practical Guide to Pediatric Emergency Medicine: Caring for Children in the Emergency Department, ed. N. Ewen Amieva-Wang (associate eds. Jamie Shandro, Aparajita Sohoni, and Bernhard Fassl). Published by Cambridge University Press.

In summary, the type of pathogen and the location of the infection may give valuable insight into the nature of the immunologic defect:

- neutrophil defects: bacterial infections of the skin and gut
- complement deficiencies: bacteremia and meningitis, specifically *Neisseria* spp.
- T cell defects: viral and fungal infections
- B cell defects: encapsulated bacteria and enterovirus infections.

Differential diagnoses

An approach to the patient in the ED in whom a PI is suspected, is based on the presentation and age of the child (Table 86.1).

Children who present with life-threatening infections in the first few months of life often have combined T and B cell disorders.

The combined T and B cell disorders include severe combined immunodeficiency (SCID) and other genetic syndromes (e.g. Wiskott–Aldrich, DiGeorge syndrome, ataxia–telangiectasia). In addition, disorders of the innate immune system (typically neutrophils and complement) tend to present in young infancy with bacterial infections, which can be severe.

In contrast, children who present with infections after 5 to 7 months of life often have primary B cell deficiencies and become symptomatic as they lose protective maternal antibody. Some PIs present later in childhood or early adulthood, such as common variable immunodeficiency (CVID) (Table 86.1).

While the differential diagnosis for presentations of PI is extensive, in the vast majority of cases, the symptoms of PI can be narrowed to specific parts of the immune system, which helps to guide treatment strategies.

Clinical presentation

For patients with known PI presenting to the ED with a new complaint, a focused history of their disorder, prior infections, current exposures (particularly by patients or family members to live vaccines), therapies used including dates of last IVIG infusion, and contact information for their immunologist and pediatrician are vital. In all other patients, the diagnosis of PI should be considered if any of the the warning signs are present:

- eight or more new infections within 12 months
- two or more serious sinus infections or pneumonias within 1 year
- two or more episodes of sepsis or meningitis
- 2 or more months of antibiotics with little effect
- need for IV antibiotics and/or hospitalization to clear infections
- failure to gain weight or grow normally
- resistant superficial or oral candidiasis, after 1 year of age
- recurrent soft tissue or organ abscesses
- infection with an opportunistic organism
- complications from a live vaccine
- family history of immunodeficiency or unexplained early death
- unexplained autoimmunity
- lymphopenia in an infant.

In addition to suspecting PI, physicians must attempt to rule out other causes of recurrent infections on history and examination, particularly localizing to the same anatomic region. Common "mimickers" of PI include hidden foreign bodies, inadequately treated resistant organisms, continuous reinfection (travel, endemic source or contaminated water/food supply), anatomic defect (congenital bronchial abnormality, vesicoureteral reflux, etc.), allergic triad (eczema, rhinitis, and asthma) as well as rare causes of chronic infections such as fistulae.

Diagnostic studies

The following tests may be ordered in the ED.

Complete blood count

CBC with a manual differential is particularly useful as it evaluates quantitative levels of different cell lines affected by PI.

Lymphopenia is often seen in SCID, primary T cell immunodeficiencies and HIV, and it should never be ignored even if the total WBC is normal.

However, normal levels of the main components of the CBC do not preclude deficiencies in cellular subsets, such as low CD4 cell counts in HIV with high CD8 cells. Picking up a diagnosis of SCID in an infant based on lymphopenia in the CBC may prevent life-threatening infections. Thrombocytopenia with small platelets is a pathognomonic feature of Wiskott–Aldrich syndrome, and autoimmune thrombocytopenia and hemolytic anemia are common features of CVID disorders. Neutropenia is associated with hyper-IgM syndrome while leukocytosis is often baseline in disorders of neutrophil function such as chronic granulomatous disease and leukocyte adhesion deficiency.

The smear may reveal evidence of hyposplenism (Howell-Jolly bodies) contributing to PI, such as congenital asplenism, asplenia secondary to hemoglobin disorders, after splenectomy.

Quantitative immunoglobulins

Quantitative immunoglobulins (QIg) and complement levels are send-out tests and results will not be available to ED physicians. However, it is useful to know how these tests are used. Quantitative immunoglobulins are useful if there is suspicion of a B cell disorder such as CVID or X-linked agammaglobulinemia. The test is a measurement of total IgG, IgM,

Table 86.1. Aged-based differential diagnosis for primary immunodeficiency (PI)[a]

Characteristic features	Antibody disorders (B cell)	Combined disorders (B and T cell)	Innate immune system disorders (complement, phagocytes)
Age	Usually 5–7 months; CVID usually presents in second to third decade of life	Early infancy	Can appear from infancy to early childhood
Common diagnoses	XLA, CVID, IgA deficiency	SCID, WAS, AT	CGD, complement deficiency
Inheritance/ family history	XLA affects boys in the family; selective IgA deficiency and CVID are typically sporadic but family history can reveal autoimmune diseases	Usually autosomal recessive so may skip generations; consanguinity may be important	CGD and properdin deficiencies are X-linked; complement defects tend to have autosomal dominant family histories
Site of infections	Sinopulmonary infections (chronic or recurrent), enteroviral meningitis, unexplained bronchiectasis, recurrent gastroenteritis, failure to thrive	Severe protracted bacterial or viral infections along with opportunistic infections; failure to thrive	*Neutrophil defects*: deep abscesses of skin, lung, gut; periodontitis; poor wound healing *Complement defects*: meningitis, sepsis
Associated symptoms	Idiopathic thrombocytopenic purpura, autoimmune hemolytic anemia, autoimmune hepatitis	Thrombocytopenia with small platelets (WAS); failure to thrive and delayed developmental milestones	Delayed separation of umbilical cord (lymphocyte adherence deficiency); angioedema, autoimmunity (complement)
Common pathogens	Encapsulated bacteria (*Streptococcus pneumoniae, Haemophilus influenzae* B, *N. meningitidis*), enterovirus, *Giardia* spp.	In addition to *S. pneumoniae* and *H. influenzae* type b, viral (CMV, varicella zoster virus, herpes simplex virus) and opportunistic pathogens (CMV, *Candida*, PCP)	*Neutrophil defects*: *Staphylococcus aureus, Aspergillus, Candida* spp., Gram-negative rods, mycobacterium *Complement defects: N. meningitidis, S. pneumoniae*
Screening laboratory tests	CBC with differential, quantitiative immunoglobulins, LFTs (total gammaglobulin)	CBC with differential, quantitative immunoglobulins, HIV	ANC, CH50, AP50
Incidence within PI	Most common	Common	Rare

ANC, absolute neutrophil count; AP50, alternative pathway hemolytic complement activity; AT, ataxia–telangiectasia; CGD, chronic granulomatous disease; CH50, total classical pathway hemolytic complement activity; CMV, cytomegalovirus; CVID, common variable immunodeficiency; PCP, *Pneumocystis jiroveci* (was *carinii*) pneumonia; SCID, severe combined immunodeficiency; WAS, Wiskott–Aldrich syndrome; XLA, X-linked agammaglobulinemia.
[a] Isolated T cell disorders are very rare, even within PI and have not been presented in the above table. Many of them are severe, and present in early infancy (e.g., DiGeorge syndrome) as B cells are also functionally incapable as they lack T cell help. These children also tend to have other congenital defects and immunodeficiency. Similarly, cytokine deficiencies (interleukins 2 and 7) have not been discussed as they are extremely rare. However, the warning signs of PI and general approach in this chapter are relevant for all PI that will be encountered in the ED setting.

and IgA levels and looks at total immunoglobulin levels but not the ability to make specific antibodies.

The total hemolytic complement (CH50) is the screen of choice if the history and physical examination points to a complement deficiency, particularly in the case of a severe first presentation or recurrent presentation of meningococcemia in a child.

Specialized immunologic and gene testing

Specialized immunologic testing, including flow cytometry for specific T and B cell markers (e.g., CD40 ligand expression in activated T cells), and specific gene testing is usually undertaken in the context of the pediatrician and the immunologist involved in the child's care and is not in the scope of tests performed in the ED.

Inflammatory markers

Tests should be carried out for markers of inflammation (ESR, CRP), leukocytosis/leukopenia, or abnormal antibody levels based on the illness and presentation of the child.

Microbial studies

Microbial studies may be warranted based on the illness and presentation of the child. Sick children with known history or suspicion for PI should have samples taken for for bacterial, viral, and fungal cultures, with special consideration paid to identifying opportunistic pathogens. This should be done even in the absence of inflammatory markers as these markers may be unreliable in children with PI. For details on how to send specific cultures and sources, see Ch. 104.

Imaging

Imaging studies are particularly important in children with PI presenting with abdominal pain. Many PIs have been associated with Crohn's and ulcerative colitis, granuloma formation, and intra-abdominal abscess formation (CVID, chronic granulomatous disease, and other neutrophil defects). In addition, imaging may be used to assess for non-abdominal chronic or "cold" abscesses, which may need IV antibiotics or admission for surgical debridement. Chest radiography may also be useful for evaluation of the thymus size in an infant with a presentation suspicious for SCID. It is also very important for any child with known or suspected PI and no source for fever.

Management

The key to managing these patients is the recognition that an individual may have a PI since there is a high possibility of rapidly evolving sepsis even in routine sick visits/complaints. For children with known PI, triage to an isolation room with rapid assessment and contact with a primary immunologist is warranted. For children with suspected PI on the basis of history and physical examination features, an aggressive approach with rapid isolation, screening diagnostics, and immunology consult is needed. Early antimicrobial therapy or surgical debridement is the mainstay of therapy in these children.

The primary goals of treatment in the ED setting are isolation, physiologic stabilization, early administration of antibiotics, symptom relief, and, in some cases, prompt referral and preparation for surgical debridement.

Antimicrobial therapy

Antimicrobial therapy should be administered early with broad-spectrum antibiotics in children with known PI in consultation with immunologists or infectious disease specialists to include appropriate antibacterial, antiviral, and antifungal coverage. This aggressive approach is needed to have an impact on survival for children with PI, as they present with life-threatening illness that evolves very quickly with rare pathogens. In the ED, given the likely pathogens for the immune defect, as broad a coverage as possible should be started, which can later be narrowed to specific sensitivities on culture results.

Blood products

Blood products must be leukocyte depleted, irradiated, and CMV negative before transfusion to children with PI. Clinicians must be alert to the fact that blood products (including IVIG) may cause an anaphylactic reaction in children with IgA deficiency.

Urgent intravenous immunoglobulins

Urgent IVIG therapy should be considered for any sick child with PI on maintenance, long-term IVIG therapy, if possible in consultation with the child's immunologist. Baseline IgG levels should be obtained before giving additional therapy.

Disposition

Sick children with known PI require immediate evaluation by an appropriate specialist (e.g., pediatric intensivist, immunologist, infectious disease specialist or surgeon) in the ED. Known or suspected PI and severe illness requiring admission always require specialty consultation in the ED. However, other cases of suspected PI may be suitable outpatient management with telephone consultation and close immunology follow-up.

Pearls and pitfalls

Pearls

1. Be sensitive to red flags for primary immunodeficiency (PI) when evaluating a child with autoimmune conditions, family history of unexplained deaths or autoimmune diseases, thrombocytopenia, lymphopenia and recurrent sepsis, and infections with unusual pathogens.
2. Diseases that tend to be subacute in adults with immunodeficiencies, such as *Pneumocystis jirovecii* pneumonia (PCP), tend to present as an emergency in children with PI.
3. Children with PI have distinct susceptibilities and clinical presentations depending on the immune system component that is compromised (see text).
4. There is the potential for high morbidity and mortality, so early empiric broad-spectrum antimicrobial therapy, early and aggressive surgical debridement of abscesses, inpatient admission, and management and close immunologic follow-up are particularly important.

Pitfalls

1. Giving blood products to a child with PI without ensuring that they do not have a T or B cell dysfunction, and that the blood is CMV negative, irradiated, and leukocyte reduced.
2. Failure to realize that the vast majority of recurrent infections in the same location are a result of anatomic abnormalities rather than immunodeficiencies.
3. Ignoring lymphopenia in an infant.
4. Failure to realize that infections in children with PI still need to be treated aggressively even if the infection is not unusual in pathogen or severity.

Admission is also considered for children with known PI if they need parenteral antibiotics, IVIG treatment, and further workup and stabilization of their condition. In addition, patients with unclear diagnoses, chronic infections, unreliable follow-up, or an unstable social situation may require inpatient management by an appropriate specialist or a primary care provider.

Selected references

Blaese, RM, Winkelstein, JA. *Patient and Family Handbook for Primary Immunodeficiency Diseases.* Towson, MD: Immune Deficiency Foundation, 2007, www.primaryimmune.org (accessed 28 April 2010).

Braskett M, Roberts RL. Evaluation and treatment of children with primary immune deficiency in the emergency department. *Clin Pediatr Emerg Med* 2007;**8**:96–103.

Buckley RH. *Diagnostic and Clinical Care Guidelines for Primary Immunodeficiency Diseases.* Towson, MD: Immune Deficiency Foundation, 2007, www.primaryimmune.org (accessed 28 April 2010).

Jeffrey Model Foundation. *National Primary Immune Deficiency Resource Center* www.Info4pi.org (accessed 28 April 2010).

Section

14

Infectious disease emergencies

Expert reviewers: Manuel Amieva and Kathleen M. Gutierrez

Chapter

87 Approach to child fever

Irma T. Ugalde and Aparajita Sohoni

A Fever without a source

Irma T. Ugalde and Aparajita Sohoni

Introduction

Fever is a common cause of pediatric visits to EDs. Fever is usually caused by a clinically obvious bacterial infection or a on physical examination self-limited viral infection. A small but significant subset of children with fever without an obvious source on physical examination have a serious bacterial infection. Children <3 years of age are more susceptible to serious bacterial illness because of an immature immune system. Neonates and infants 1–3 months of age are at increased risk of serious bacterial illness from perinatally acquired and late-onset perinatal infection, respectively. Also, the younger the child, the more difficult it is to rule out a serious bacterial infection on physical examination alone. Different organisms cause infection and disease at different ages (Tables 87.1 and 87.2). This chapter addresses the management of a non-toxic-appearing child 0–36 months of age with a fever without an obvious source. The management of fever of unknown origin (FUO), a distinct entity defined as more than 8 days of fever without an identified source is discussed separately later in the chapter.

Table 87.1. Infectious sources for bacteremia and bacterial meningitis by age

0–3 months	3 months to 5 years	>5 years
Group B streptococci, *Escherichia coli*, *Enterococcus* spp., *Listeria monocytogenes*	*Streptococcus pneumoniae*, *Neisseria meningitidis*, *Haemophilus influenzae*	*S. pneumoniae*, *N. meningitidis*

Epidemiology

Prior to the availability of *Haemophilus influenzae* type b conjugate (Hib) vaccine in 1991 and the heptavalent pneumococcal conjugate vaccine (Prevnar) in 2000, the rate of occult bacteremia was 5% in well-appearing children with fever in the USA. *Streptococcus pneumoniae* and *H. influenzae* type b bacteremia made up 80% and 20% of these cases, respectively. The Hib vaccine has virtually eradicated bacteremia from *H. influenzae* type b in the USA. Similarly, the incidence of pneumococcal bacteremia has declined to <1% in well-appearing children with fever. In 2003, it was estimated that nearly 30 000 cases of invasive pneumococcal disease caused by vaccine serotypes were prevented through routine immunization. However, while the rates of invasive pneumococcal disease have decreased overall, the incidence remains greater among certain high-risk populations including HIV-positive children; those with anatomic or functional asplenia; cochlear implant recipients; children with immunodeficiency; and African-Americans, Native Americans, and Alaskan Natives. There has also been a

Table 87.2. Infectious sources for pneumonia (bacterial) by age

Birth to 1 month	1–3 months[a]	3 months to 5 years[a]	>5 years[a]
Group B streptococci, Gram-negative enteric bacteria, *Staphylococcus aureus*, *Listeria monocytogenes*	Group B streptococci, *Enterococcus* spp., *Staphylococcus aureus*, *Streptococcus pneumoniae*, *Chlamydia trachomatis*	*S. pneumoniae*, *S. aureus*, *Mycoplasma pneumoniae**	*M. pneumoniae*, *Chlamydia pneumoniae*

[a]Viral infections causing pneumonia are most commonly respiratory syncytial virus, influenza virus, adenovirus, parainfluenza virus.

A Practical Guide to Pediatric Emergency Medicine: Caring for Children in the Emergency Department, ed. N. Ewen Amieva-Wang (associate eds. Jamie Shandro, Aparajita Sohoni, and Bernhard Fassl). Published by Cambridge University Press.

concurrent rise in invasive disease caused by non-vaccine strains, particularly serotypes 19A, 15, and 33, although the significance of this remains to be seen.

In this setting, *Escherichia coli*, *Staphylococcus aureus*, *Salmonella spp*, *Neisseria meningitidis*, and *Streptococcus pyogenes* are increasingly identified as causes of bacteremia. Furthermore, the concurrent false-positive blood culture rate is more than double the rate of true bacteremia (<1%).

In the case of fever and recognizable viral illness, such as hand, foot, and mouth disease or herpes stomatitis, the incidence of serious bacterial illness is considerably less than in children with fever without a source. Studies have been conducted to find out the association of specific viral illness, such as bronchiolitis and influenza, with concomitant serious bacterial infection, and the impact of rapid viral testing on the management of children with febrile illness. It has been shown that hospitalized children with bronchiolitis still have a significant incidence of urinary tract infection. The results of these studies are not sufficient to change management of very young febrile infants at this time.

Definition of fever and when to initiate a workup

Fever is defined as a rectal temperature of at least 38.0°C (100.4°F). Rectal temperatures in infants, and oral temperatures in older children, are recommended as the sensitivity of tympanic and axillary temperatures is poor. When an elevated temperature is thought to be caused by bundling, the child may be unbundled and the temperature rechecked in 15–30 min. However, a temperature greater than 38.5°C should never be attributed to bundling, teething, or vaccinations. Tactile or subjective fever has been shown to be a sensitive measure of fever. Severity of infection is not reflected by height of fever or response to antipyretics.

In infants from birth to 3 months of age, a laboratory workup is indicated for a fever >38.0°C (100.4°F.) In those aged 3–36 months of age, a workup should be considered for a fever greater than 39.0°C (102.2°F).

History

Present illness and symptoms

The history should include the sequence of development of symptoms, and elicit the parents' major concerns. A child's oral intake and urine output are important to assess for hydration status. Specific questioning about the timing and dosing of antipyretic drugs can identify under- and overdosing of these medications.

Past medical and social history

Birth and prenatal history, prior hospitalizations, previous and recent febrile illnesses, and antibiotic use are important. For young children, family history of significant infections may help to detect familial immunodeficiency syndromes as well as exposure risks. Immunization status, sick contacts, daycare, and travel history are also helpful. Children with underlying chronic disease such as sickle cell disease or malignancy fall outside the routine guidelines and require special attention.

Physical examination

A complete examination will involve a review of vital signs and identification of any subtle indications of focal infection.

Children who are alert, smiling, and interactive rarely are septic.

Management guidelines

Current guidelines for management of fever without a source in young children have evolved from initial guidelines published in the early 1990s. These guidelines take into account the widespread introduction of the Hib and pneumococcal conjugate vaccines into the childhood vaccination series. The approach to children with fever without a source is typically categorized by patient age. These guidelines address the non-toxic child with a fever without a source. The approach is divided by the child's age: 0–28 days, 29–90 days, and 3 months to 3 years of age (Figs. 87.1 and 87.2). While management of fever without a source in the age categories of 0–28 days and 3–36 months are fairly standard, the recommended management of children 28–90 days of age is controversial; these children are essentially unvaccinated and have variable levels of social development.

In a toxic child of any age, a bacterial illness should be suspected and a complete workup with resuscitation and antibiotic treatment should be immediately begun in the ED.

In a toxic neonate, neonatal herpes infection should also be considered and acyclovir given concurrently with antibiotics.

While neonatal herpes infection usually presents during the first 4 weeks of life, it can occur much later after birth.

Infants less than 28 days old

In neonates with a fever, a complete workup should be obtained even if a recognized viral illness or focal bacterial infection is present (see also Ch. 157). This complete workup includes:

- CBC, blood culture
- urinalysis and urine culture (catheterized)
- CSF studies including cell count, glucose, protein, Gram stain and culture
- chest radiograph if respiratory symptoms
- stool culture and abdominal radiography if abdominal symptoms
- CRP is often obtained to follow response to inpatient treatment in infants 0–60 days of age.

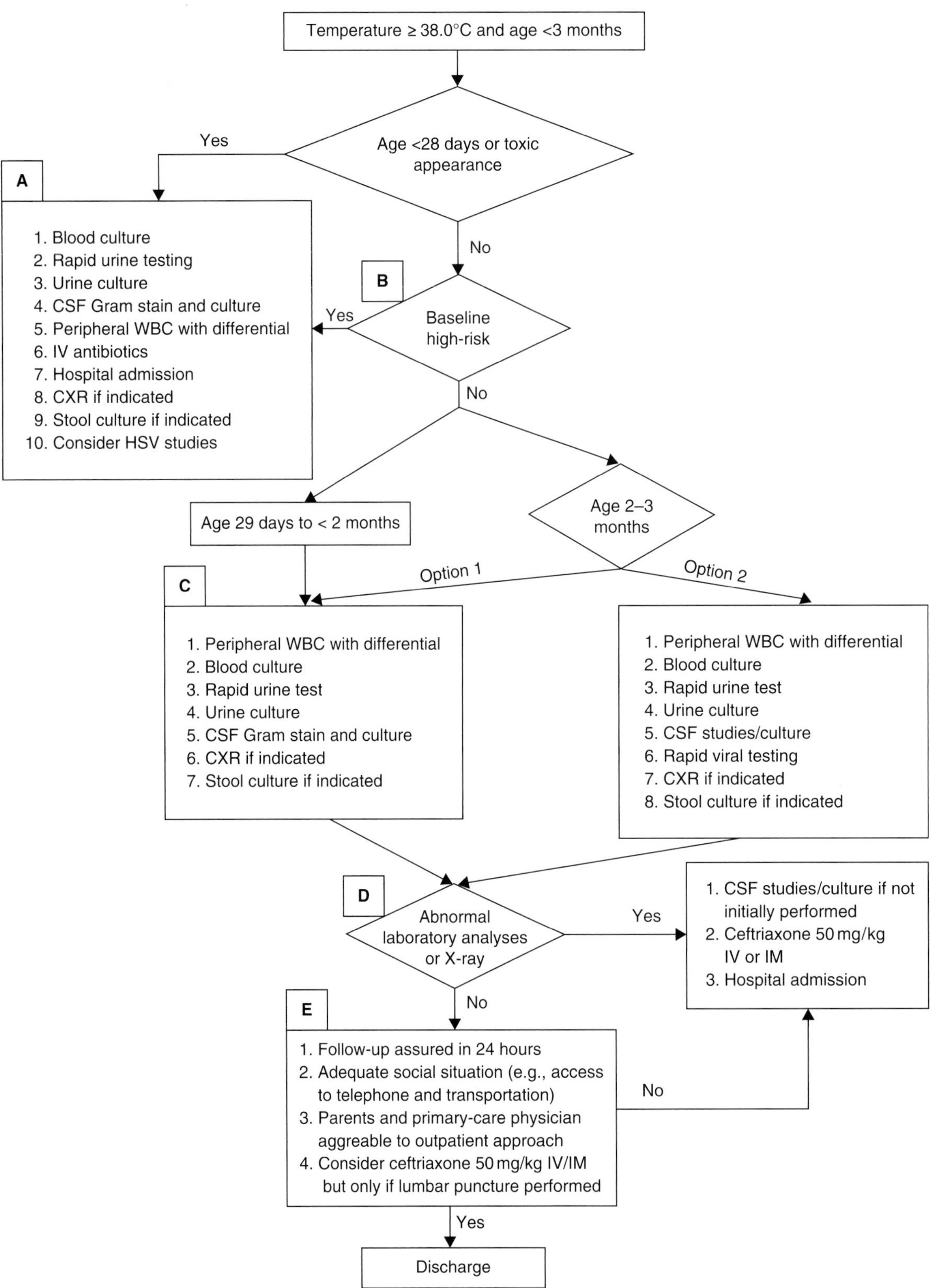

Figure 87.1 Approach to fever without a source for children <3 months of age. CSF, cerebrospinal fluid; CXR, chest radiography; HSV, herpes simplex virus. (Adapted with permission from Ishimine P. Fever without source in children 0–36 months of age. *Pediatr Clin North Am* 2006;53:167–194.)

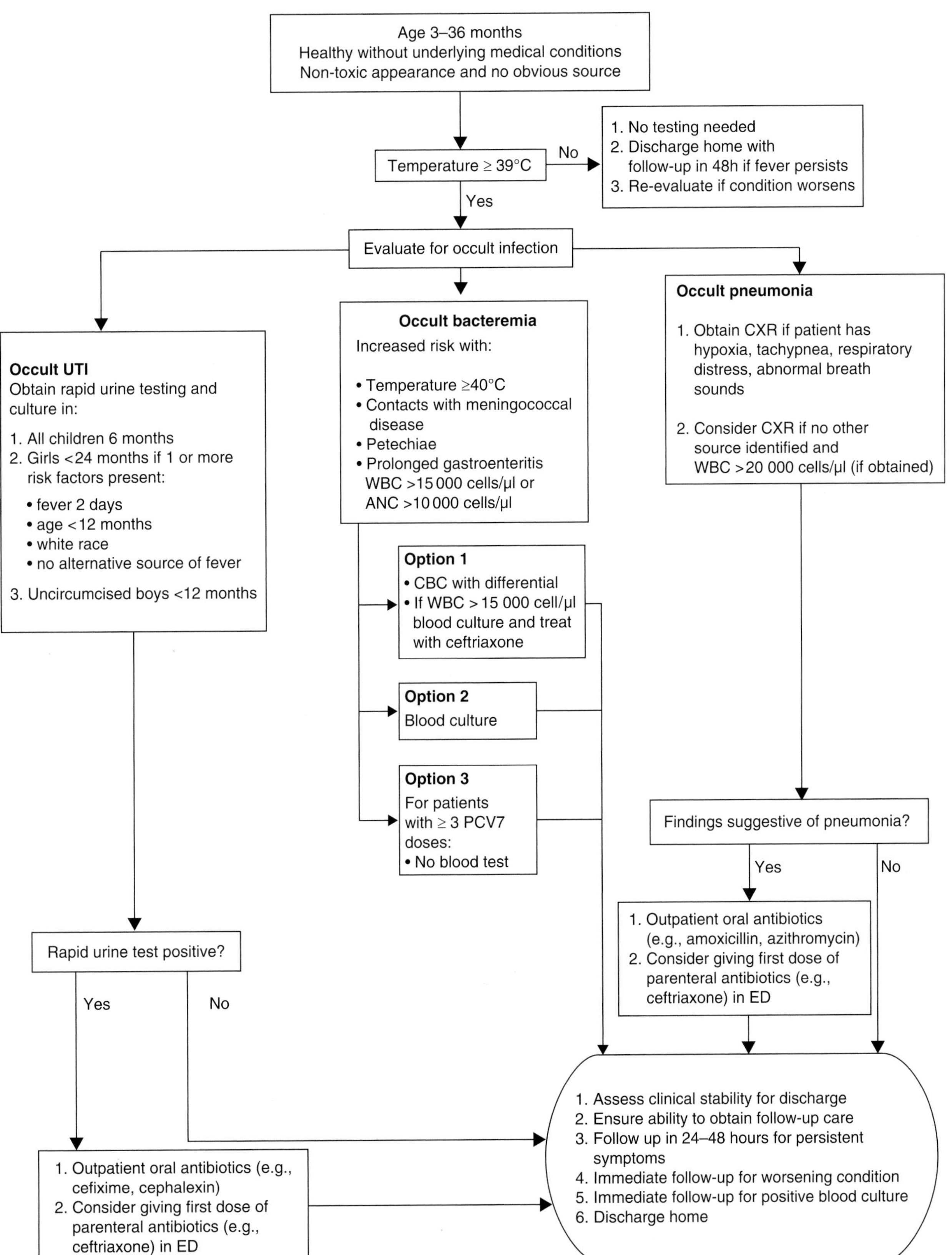

Figure 87.2 Approach to fever without a source for children 3 months to 3 years of age. ANC, absolute neutrophil counts CXR, chest radiography; PCV7, pneumococcal conjugate vaccine; UTI, urinary tract infection. (Adapted with permission from Ishimine P. Fever without source in children 0–36 months of age. *Pediatr Clin North Am* 2006;53:167–194.)

All neonates should be hospitalized and given empiric antibiotic treatment pending culture results. Treatment is with ampicillin (50 mg/kg IV) plus cefotaxime (50 mg/kg IV) *or* gentamicin (2.5 mg/kg IV). Note that ceftriaxone is not recommended for neonates. If meningitis is suspected, meningitic doses of antibiotics should be given.

Infants 1 to 3 months of age

In febrile well-appearing infants 1–3 months of age (Fig. 87.1), workup includes:

- blood culture
- CBC
- catheterized urine analysis and culture
- CSF studies.

If the clinician finds the clinical examination reassuring for the child not having meningitis (i.e., the child is well appearing), the clinician may defer the lumbar puncture. However, if empiric antibiotics are going to be given, a lumbar puncture should be performed to avoid the risk of partially treating a meningitis.

Patients with a WBC >15 000/μl or <5000/μl, urinalysis suggesting a urinary tract infection (positive nitrites or leukocyte esterase or WBC >5/high-power field), pneumonia, CSF pleocytosis, or laboratory values consistent with serious bacterial illness should be admitted and treated with antibiotics until culture results are available. Children with a suspected infection should be treated with ceftriaxone 50 mg/kg IV. Children <2 months old should be admitted to the hospital. Children 2–3 month of age may be discharged home with reliable parents and 12–24 h follow-up of clinical status and blood cultures.

Children 29 days to 3 months of age with negative workup, appearing well, feeding and voiding normally, and who have reliable caretakers, can be discharged without antibiotics and followed within 12–24 h.

Age 3 to 36 months

In well-appearing fully-vaccinated children aged 3–36 months with fever >39°C, blood studies are not usually necessary (Fig. 87.2). However the risk of urinary tract infection as the source of fever is high in girls <24 months of age, uncircumcised boys <12 months of age, and circumcised boys <6 months of age, as well as in children with a prior history of urinary tract infection. In these groups, a catheterized or clean catch (if toilet trained) urinalysis and urine culture should be obtained (see also Ch. 100). If a urinalysis shows evidence of probable infection, and a presumptive diagnosis of urinary tract infection is made, antibiotic treatment can be initiated on an outpatient basis unless the child is not tolerating oral medications or fluids. Because of growing antibiotic resistance, empiric antibiotic therapy should be tailored to local bacterial epidemiology. Cultures must be followed and antibiotics changed as needed. The duration of therapy should be from 7 to 14 days.

If the urinalysis is normal, and the CBC shows a WBC >20 000/μl, further evaluation for an occult pneumonia may be warranted. Children with a CBC with a WBC >20 000/μl or absolute neutrophil count >10 000/μl, blood culture pending, and reliable social situation may be treated with a dose of IM ceftriaxone and next day follow-up.

Conclusions

The approach to fever is one that will continue to evolve. While guidelines in the treatment of fever without obvious source have been created to guide the ED approach, each case is unique. The neonate with fever should have a full workup and admission to the hospital. The older, immunized child may not warrant any laboratory studies but will usually warrant close follow-up and extensive return precautions.

B Fever of unknown origin

Irma T. Ugalde

Introduction

The length of time for FUO is generally defined as 8 consecutive days of fevers without an etiology. Fever may also show periodicity, occurring at regular intervals (Table 87.3). Typically, parents of these patients may come to the ED in frustration after a negative workup by the primary care physician. While most cases can be worked up as an outpatient, the ED physician must determine which patients require inpatient workup.

An extensive history can guide differential diagnosis and workup: travel history and exposure to insects, pets, or sick contacts can help in making a diagnosis. Recurrent fever associated with a combination of rash, arthralgia, or arthritis suggests rheumatologic disease. A history of a periodic fever, one occurring at regular time intervals, should suggest a periodic fever syndrome (Table 87.3). Fever associated with weight loss, malaise, and lymphadenopathy should be worked up to exclude malignancy.

Initial screening laboratory analyses include a CBC with peripheral smear, urinalysis/urine culture, comprehensive metabolic panel (chemistry 23), ESR, CRP, blood culture, chest radiograph, and tuberculin skin test, with additional tests driven by examination, history, and age of patient. These initial laboratory analyses reflect the common etiologies of FUO, which are, in order of frequency, infection, connective tissue disease, and malignancy. Typhoid fever and malaria should be high on the differential in children with recent travel to locations with endemic disease (Ch. 98).

Further laboratory analyses and imaging should be led by the prominent constellation of symptoms and usually do not

Table 87.3. Familial periodic fever syndromes: autoinflammatory diseases

Disease	Age of onset (years)	Inheritance	Ethnicity	Length of fever (days)	Symptoms	Treatment
Familial Mediterranean fever	<20	AR	Sephardic and Ashkenazi Jews, Armenians, Turks, Arabs	1–3	Abdominal pain, pleurisy, arthralgia, arthritis, scrotal swelling, erysipeloid rash	Cochicine
Tumor necrosis factor alpha receptor 1 associated syndrome	<20	AD	Irish, Scottish, other	>5	Conjunctivitis, abdominal pain, regional myalgia, arthralgia, arthritis, rash	Glucocorticoids
Hyperimmunoglobulin D syndrome	<1	AR	Dutch, French, other		Cervical LAN, abdominal pain, arthralgia/arthritis, rash, splenomegaly	NSAIDs, glucocorticoids
PFAPA	<5	Unknown	Unknown		Cervical LAN, aphthous stomatitis	Glucocorticoids, cimetidine, tonsillectomy
Cyclic neutropenia	Child/adult (child more common; wide spectrum of disease)	Appears familial	Unknown	On average severe neutropenia of 1 week duration every 21 days; prone to fever at this time	Neutropenia 3–5 days out of several consecutive cycles; when febrile with neutropenia can develop severe infection	Mostly supportive: antibiotics during febrile, neutropenic episodes; consider G-CSF in children with recurrent severe infections; regular dental care

AD, autosomal dominant; AR, autosomal recessive; G-CSF, granulocyte colony-stimulating factor; LAN, lymphadenopathy; NSAID, non-steroidal anti-inflammatory drug; PFAPA, periodic fever with aphthous stomatitis, pharyngitis, and cervical adenitis.

need to be completed in the ED unless the clinical situation warrants. For example, stool cultures or examination for ova and parasites should be considered in those with loose stools or recent travel. Disposition should be based on the severity of disease, social situation, and assurance of appropriate follow-up. Children younger than 1 year of age, with increased length of FUO should strongly be considered for admission. Children who are ill appearing or have failure to thrive should also be admitted.

Pearls and pitfalls

Pearls

1. Febrile children 0–3 months of age are at increased risk for serious bacterial illness.
2. Neonates with fever >38.0°C should have blood, urine, and CSF testing and be admitted for IV antibiotics pending culture results.
3. In children who are completely immunized with pneumococcal conjugate and *Haemophilus influenzae* type b vaccines, the risk of a false-positive blood culture is greater than a true positive.

Pitfalls

1. Attributing a temperature >38.5°C to environmental causes such as bundling, teething, and vaccinations.
2. Failure to realize that young children may have a urinary tract infection despite a negative urinalysis.
3. Failure to have a low threshold for fever workup, antibiotics, and admission in children with underlying chronic illness or immunosuppression.

Selected references

Bachur RG, Harper MB. Predictive model for serious bacterial infections among infants younger than 3 months of age. *Pediatrics* 2001;**108**:311–316.

Baker MD, Bell LM, Avner JR. Outpatient management without antibiotics of fever in selected infants. *N. Engl JMed* 1993;**329**:1437–1441.

Givens T. Fevers caused by occult infections in the 3–36 month old child. *Pediatr Emerg Med Pract* 2007;**4**:1–24.

Ishimine P. Fever without source in children 0–36 months of age. *Pediatr Clin North Am* 2006;**53**:167–194.

Infectious disease associated with systemic exanthems and enanthems

Theresa M. van der Vlugt and Aparajita Sohoni

Introduction

The term exanthem is derived from the Greek *exanthema* meaning "a breaking out," which itself is from the Greek *anthos* meaning flower, comparing these syndromes to plants bursting into flower in the spring. An enanthem is a syndrome with mucosal lesions. Many of the classic viral exanthems such as rubeola (measles) and rubella are now rare or non-endemic in the USA, or becoming more rare with vaccination, such as primary varicella.

While infections with cutaneous manifestations are caused by bacteria, viruses, fungi, and protozoa, it is not so important to make a definitive diagnosis as to identify those rashes that represent potentially fatal disease (Rocky Mountain spotted fever, meningococcemia), and those that have a potential to cause significant disease in a subset of the population (congenital rubella infection, neonatal HSV infection). Recognition of the classical exanthems associated with particular virus or bacteria can alleviate worry, avoid inappropriate antibiotic treatment of a viral syndrome, promote appropriate screening for contacts at risk, and lead to appropriate antibiotic treatment.

While the next sections have an artificial separation of viral, bacterial, and tick-borne infectious diseases, it is intended as a means to compare and contrast these syndromes in order to diagnose and appropriately treat these patients.

Viral exanthems can be polymorphous and are often never definitively diagnosed. Enteroviral and adenoviral exanthems account for the majority of viral exanthems frequently encountered in the USA. Enteroviral infections with coxsackievirus and echovirus strains have been known to cause the classic hand-foot-mouth disease, with painful vesicular lesions on the palms, soles, and/or mucous membranes plus herpangina (vesicular lesions on the posterior pharynx). It is difficult to distinguish between viral exanthems and a drug-induced eruption from antibiotics.

Table 88.1 compares the classic viral infections with rash, which mostly warrant supportive treatment; Figures 88.1 to 88.6 illustrate these rashes. Table 88.2 discusses rashes that cause vesicular disease (Figs. 88.7–88.9) and Table 88.3 discusses rashes thought to be viral in origin (Figs. 88.10–88.12). While these rashes are less common than the others discussed, they are distinct enough that visual diagnosis can alleviate worry and lead to appropriate follow-up and management.

A Practical Guide to Pediatric Emergency Medicine: Caring for Children in the Emergency Department, ed. N. Ewen Amieva-Wang (associate eds. Jamie Shandro, Aparajita Sohoni, and Bernhard Fassl). Published by Cambridge University Press.

Table 88.1. Classic viral infections with rash

Disease	Measles	Rubella	Erythema infectiosum	Roseola
Illustration	Figures 88.1, 88.2	Figure 88.3	Figures 88.4, 88.5	Figure 88.6
Synonyms	First disease, rubeola, red measles	Third disease, German measles, 3-day measles	Slapped cheek disease, fifth disease	Exanthem subitum, sixth disease
Etiologic agent	Measles virus	Rubella virus	Parvovirus B19	Human herpes virus type 6 or 7
Epidemiology	Affects unvaccinated, highly contagious, spread by respiratory droplet	Affects unvaccinated, endemic and congenital disease eliminated in USA, spread by respiratory droplet	School-age children, infection more common in winter and spring, by spread respiratory droplet	Children 6–24 months
Incubation period	1–2 weeks	2–3 weeks	3–5 days	2–5 days
Clinical syndrome	Fever, characterized by "3 Cs": cough, coryza, conjunctivitis; cervical LAN; child appears ill	Low-grade fever, malaise, lymphadenopathy; pharyngitis in adolescents; generally appear well, 50% asymptomatic	Usually afebrile or low-grade fever, first sign of illness is rash	Possibly 50% of infections are asymptomatic; 3–5 days of high fever in generally well-appearing children
Rash	Begins after 2–4 days of fever Maculopapular confluent rash, starts at face and spreads to feet; fades in 5–10 days in order of appearance; enanthem occurs 1–2 days before exanthem; pathognomonic Koplik spots are 1-mm white spots "grains of sand" on intensely erythematous buccal mucosa	Rash 7–10 days after infection (may be absent in up to 40% of cases) Faint "rose-pink" macules, starts on the face and spreads to the trunk and proximal extremities; fades in 2–3 days in order of appearance; enanthem of erythematous papules on soft palate can occur	Rash has three stages: (1) starts with fiery-red facial erythema sparing the nasal bridge and perioral area, resembling "slapped cheeks" for 1–4 days; (2) symmetric, lacy, reticulate erythema mostly on the extremities (1–3 weeks), can involve palms and soles and can be pruritic; (3) exanthem fades over 2–3 weeks but often reoccurs or is exacerbated with exercise, sunlight, or warmth	Rash occurs within 12–24 h of defervescence. Discrete pink macules and papules that blanch with pressure; start on trunk and spread to extremities, face and neck; fades in 1–3 days, sometimes within hours
Diagnosis	Clinical diagnosis Virus isolation and serologic testing should be sent in suspected cases Reportable disease	Difficult to diagnose clinically; IgM diagnostic Reportable disease	Clinical diagnosis Polymerase chain reaction and serologies available if necessary	Clinical diagnosis Usually retrospective after the rash has occurred
Management	Supportive; age-dependent vitamin A doses for all confirmed cases	Supportive	Supportive	Supportive
Complications	Pneumonia, otitis media, acute gastroenteritis, myocarditis, encephalitis, subacute sclerosing panencephalitis Morbidity is increased for children <5 years and immunosuppressed[a]	Congenital rubella infection is most devastating complication[a]	Can precipitate transient aplastic crisis in sickle cell disease, and other hemolytic anemias Risk of hydrops in fetuses of newly infected pregnant women	Accounts for approximately one-third of febrile seizures in children under 2 years old

[a] Virus-specific immunoglobulin is available for post-exposure prophylaxis in susceptible contacts.

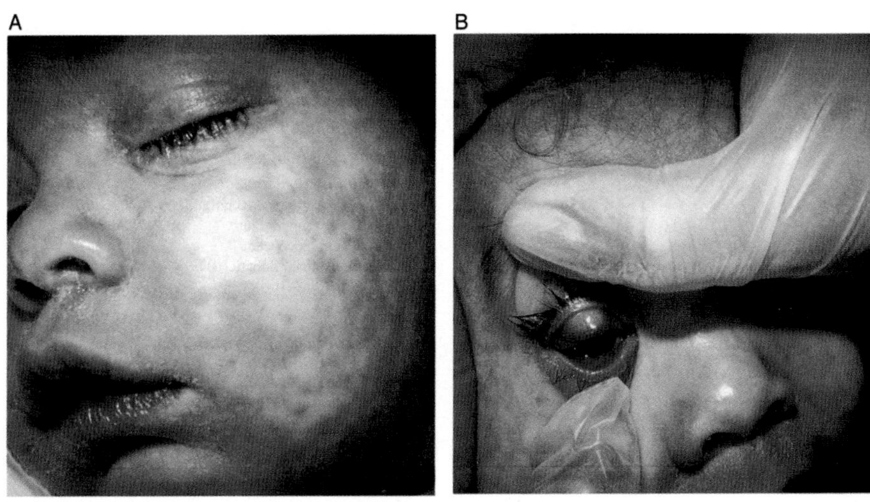

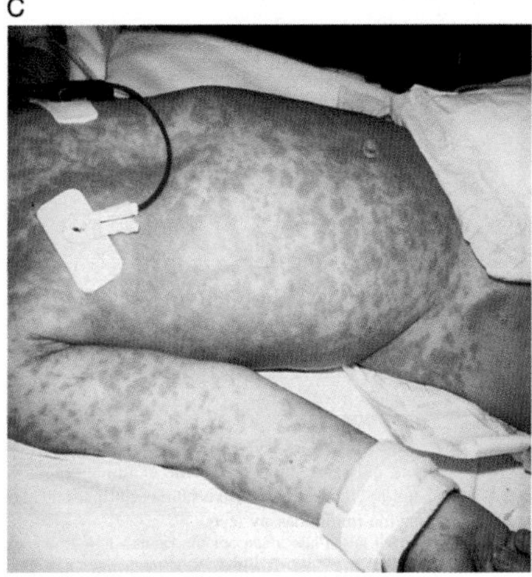

Figure 88.1 Rubeola/measles in an 8-month-old child with fever, coryza, and marked conjunctivitis associated with intense photophobia. Confluent, erythematous maculopapular rash on the face developed on the 5th day of fever. The rash spreads cephalocaudally. (Reprinted with permission from Shah BR, Lucchesi M (eds). *Atlas of Pediatric Emergency Medicine*. New York: McGraw Hill, 2006.)

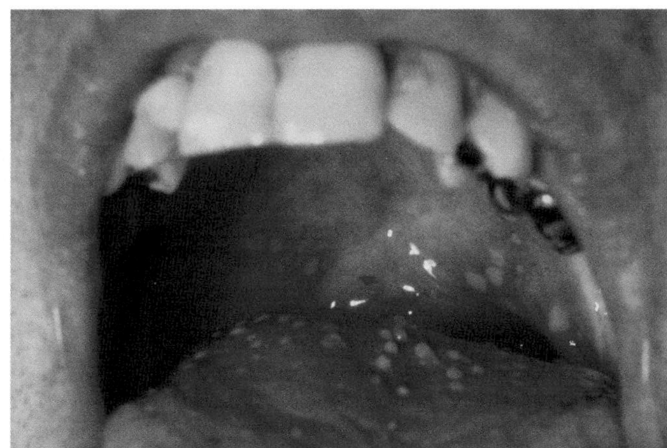

Figure 88.2 White (Koplik's) spots on the hard palate of a person with measles. (Reproduced with permission from Kane KS, Lio PA, Stratigos AJ, Johnson RA (eds). *Color Atlas and Synopsis of Pediatric Dermatology*, 2nd edn. New York: McGraw Hill Medical 2009.)

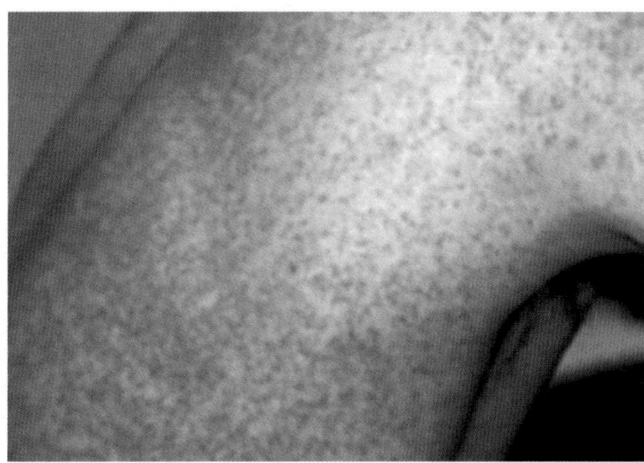

Figure 88.3 Rubella. Non-specific "rose-pink" macules and papules on the trunk of an adolescent male with German measles. (Reprinted with permission from Paller, AS, Manicini AJ (eds.) *Hurwitz Clinical Pediatric Dermatology: A Textbook of Skin Disorders of Childhood and Adolescence*, 3rd edn. Philadelphia, PA: Elsevier Saunders, 2006. © 2006 Saunders Inc., an affiliate of Elsevier Inc.)

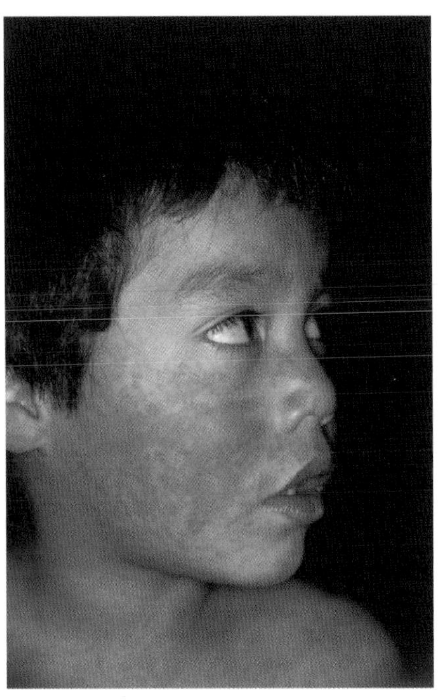

Figure 88.4 Slapped-cheek appearance of a child with parvovirus B19 infection (erythema infectiosum). (Reproduced with permission from Weston WL, Lane AT, Morelli JG. *Color Textbook of Pediatric Dermatology*, 4th edn. Philadelphia, PA: Mosby Elsevier, 2007. © 2007 Elsevier Inc.)

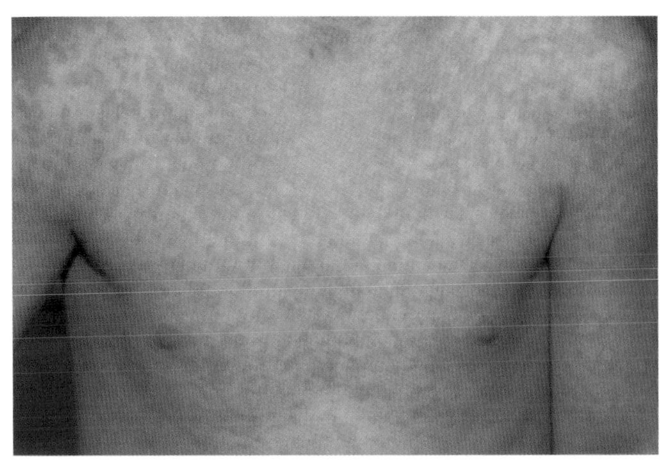

Figure 88.5 Erythema infectiosum: lacy pink eruption on chest and upper abdomen. (Reproduced with permission from Weston WL, Lane AT, Morelli JG. *Color Textbook of Pediatric Dermatology*, 4th edn. Philadelphia, PA: Mosby Elsevier, 2007. © 2007 Elsevier Inc.)

A

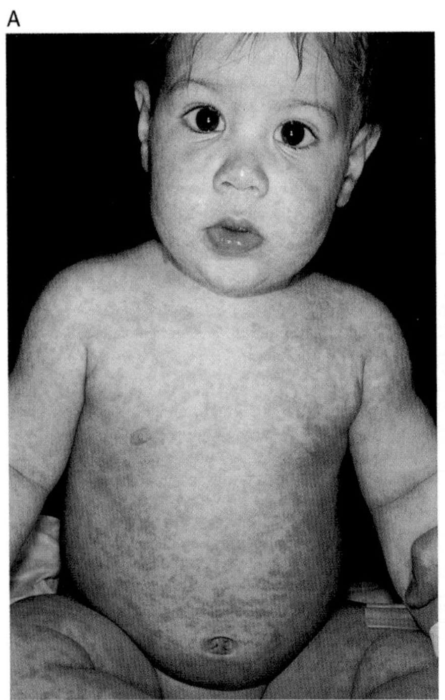

B

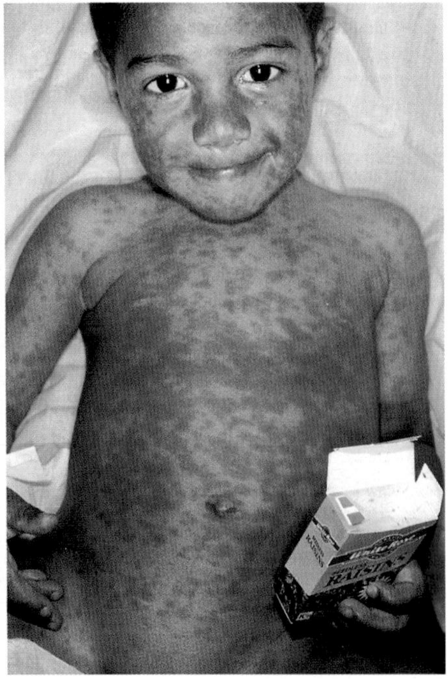

Figure 88.6 Erythematous maculopapular eruptions (presumed to be roseola). (A) Diffuse erythematous maculopapular eruptions developed after 3 days of intermittently high fever in this well-appearing 8-month-old child. (B) Diffuse erythematous maculopapular eruption that developed after 4 days in this happy 18-month-old toddler. The rash appeared when he was afebrile. (Reprinted with permission from Shah BR, Lucchesi M (eds). *Atlas of Pediatric Emergency Medicine*. New York: McGraw Hill, 2006.)

Table 88.2. Other viral infections with vesicular rash

Disease	Hand-foot-mouth disease	Herpangina	Herpes simplex	Varicella (chickenpox) and herpes zoster (shingles)	Small pox
Illustration	Figure 88.7			Figures 88.8, 88.9	
Etiologic agent	Multiple: coxsackievirus A, echovirus	Multiple: coxsackievirus A, echovirus	Herpes simplex virus types 1 and 2	VZV	Variola virus
Epidemiology	Common in ages 3–10 years; epidemics in summer or early fall	Young children	Young children and young adults	School-age children; decreased incidence secondary to vaccine; herpes zoster rare in immunocompetent children	Eradicated; patients infectious only after rash has started; very contagious
Clinical syndrome	Low-grade fever, anorexia, malaise, abdominal pain, diarrhea	High fever with primary infection	High fever with primary infection; foul breath with primary herpetic gingivostomatitis; tender cervical or groin adenopathy	*Varicella*: 1–2 days of fever, anorexia, malaise, sore throat, headache; commonly no prodrome in children; *Herpes zoster*: a prodrome of burning shooting, or stabbing pain or itching in the affected dermatome precedes skin lesions for 2–3 days (up to a week)	Severe prodrome including high fever, headache, backache, abdominal pain, and malaise
Rash	*Enanthem*: red macules on buccal mucosa, palate, tongue, and tonsillar pillars, progress to fragile vesicles that rupture to form shallow ulcers on an erythematous base; painful *Exanthem*: erythematous papules on palms, fingertips, interdigital webs, soles of feet, buttocks/genital area; knee and elbow lesions are common	*Enanthem*: multiple grey–white vesicles and shallow erythematous erosions on posterior pharynx, palate, uvula, and tonsillar pillars; no labial involvement *Exanthem*: none	*Enanthem*: grouped vesicles on erythematous base *Exanthem*: cheeks, lips, mouth, fingers, genitals; involvement of mucous membranes	Different stages of rash present at same time; may involve mucous membranes *Varicella*: maculopapular eruption evolves into vesicles, "dewdrop on a rose petal"; starts on face, scalp, and upper trunk and spreads to the extremities; vesicles dry and shed, leaving a shallow ulcer *Herpes zoster*: lesions occur unilaterally in 1–2 sensory dermatomes and do not cross the midline; usually persist 7–10 days	*Exanthem*: erythematous macules that progress to papules, vesicles, then pustules over 4–7 days; starts on face and extremities and spreads inward to trunk; all lesions in the same stage of development; palm and sole lesions are common; lesions crust and scar after 10 days

Table 88.2. *(cont.)*

Disease	Hand-foot-mouth disease	Herpangina	Herpes simplex	Varicella (chickenpox) and herpes zoster (shingles)	Small pox
Diagnosis	Clinical	Clinical Serology or PCR available if necessary	Clinical PCR, DFA, culture of unroofed vesicle available if necessary	Clinical DFA, PCR or culture of unroofed vesicle; Tzank non-specific for VZV/HSV	PCR of vesicular fluid; notifiable for suspected cases (CDC in USA)
Management	Supportive care	Supportive care; "magic mouthwash" can be helpful	Supportive care; early acyclovir can decrease severity	Supportive care; acyclovir can decrease severity if started <24 h after rash; VariZIG for post-exposure in non-immune subjects at high risk for complications (see below)	Supportive care
Complications	Rare	Dehydration; other complications rare	Eczema herpeticum or neonatal herpes; CNS complications	Pneumonitis, CNS, group A beta-hemolytic streptococci superinfection; immunocompromised, neonates and pregnant women can get severe disease	Bacterial superinfection

CDC, US Centers for Disease Control and Prevention; DFA, direct fluorescent antibody; PCR, polymerase chain reaction; VZV, varicella zoster virus.

A

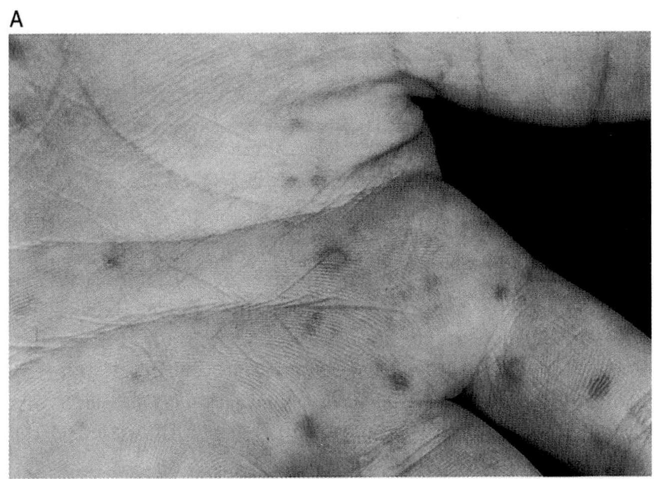

B

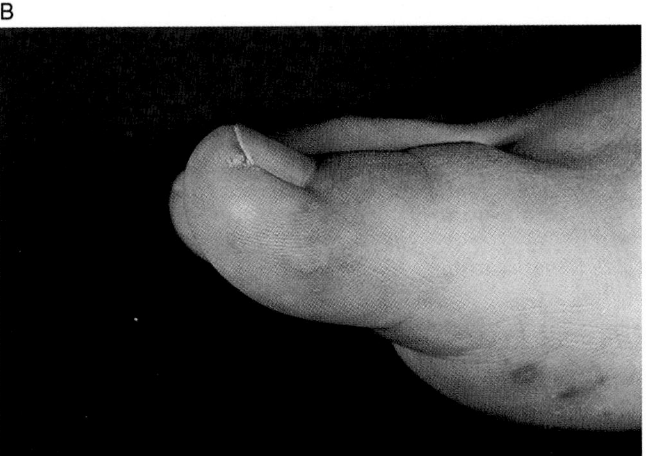

C

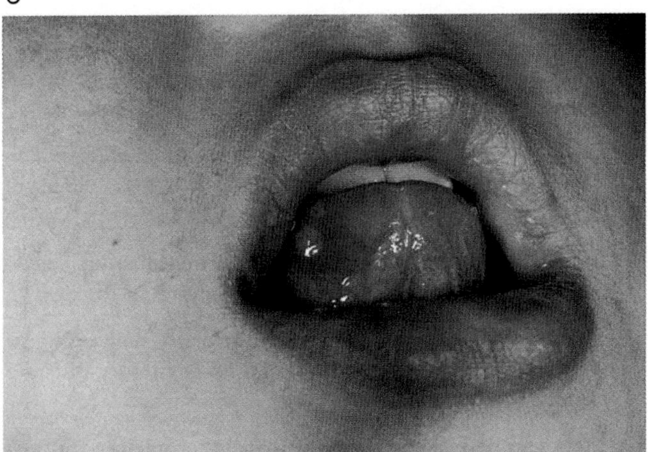

Figure 88.7 Hand-foot-mouth disease. (A,B) Typical elliptical or oval-shaped papulovesicular lesions with erythematous rims are seen on the hand and foot. (C) Ulcers surrounded by a rim of erythema are seen in the mouth. (Reprinted with permission from Shah BR, Lucchesi M (eds). *Atlas of Pediatric Emergency Medicine*. New York: McGraw Hill, 2006.)

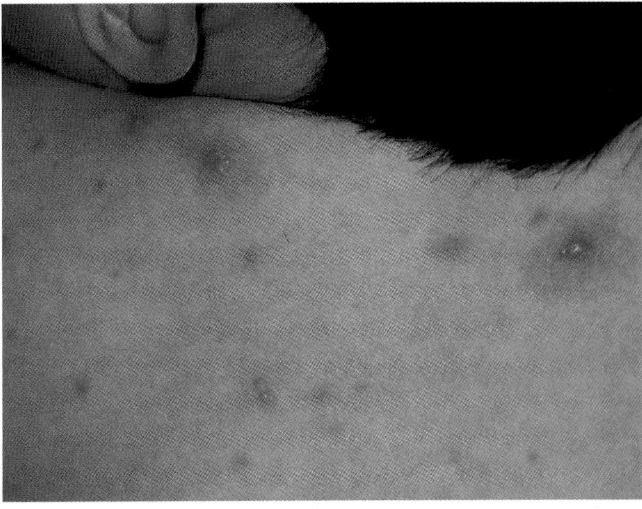

Figure 88.8 Lesions in primary varicella/chickenpox. Note the clear vesicles on an erythematous base. The lesions start centrally and are in different stages of development. (Courtesy of T. M. van der Vlugt.)

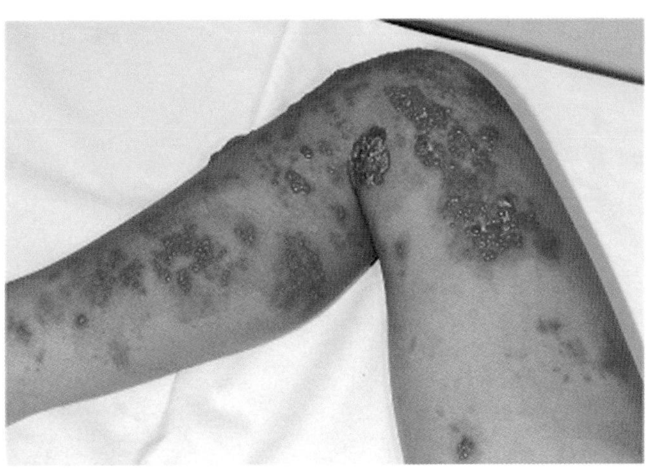

Figure 88.9 Herpes zoster. Confluent vesicles and bullae with erythema in a dermatomal distribution. (Reprinted with permission from Paller, AS, Manicini AJ (eds.) *Hurwitz Clinical Pediatric Dermatology: A Textbook of Skin Disorders of Childhood and Adolescence*, 3rd edn. Philadelphia, PA: Elsevier Saunders, 2006. © 2006 Saunders Inc., an affiliate of Elsevier Inc.)

Table 88.3. Unique exanthems thought to be viral, or with varying viral causes

Disease	Papular purpuric gloves and socks syndrome (PPGSS)	Eruptive pseudoangiomatosis	Unilateral laterothoracic exanthem	Papular acrodermatitis of childhood (PAC), Gianotti–Crosti syndrome
Illustration	Figure 88.10		Figure 88.11	Figure 88.12
Agent	Parvovirus, coxsackievirus, human herpes virus 6, Epstein–Barr virus	Suspected viral; reported following flea/mosquito bites	Suspected viral	Multiple viruses, including Epstein–Barr virus; also occurs following vaccines
Epidemiology	Young adults (no children), spring and summer; infectious when rash appears	Young children	6 months to 10 years, Caucasian, spring, not apparently contagious	1–6 years of age
Clinical syndrome	Mild prodrome of fever and arthralgia	Fever, malaise, headache, GI or respiratory complaints; can be asymptomatic	Low-grade fever, diarrhea, or rhinitis; localized lymphadenopathy is often present in the originally affected axilla or groin	Upper respiratory tract infection prodrome, cough and fever; occasionally lymphadenopathy, hepatomegaly, splenomegaly
Rash	*Enanthem*: oral erosions, vesicles, swollen lips and petechiae of hard palate, pharynx and tongue *Exanthem*: edema and erythema of hands and feet with associated purpura and petechiae; sharply marginated at wrists and ankles but may extend to dorsal surfaces; burning and pruritis	Widespread bright red pinpoint papules similar to hemangiomas often with a surrounding rim of pallor	Erythematous, polymorphous eruption of papules and macules; lesions often spread to become bilateral, but retain a predominance on the original side	Occurs the week after the viral prodrome. Symmetric, homogenous papules distributed on cheeks, extensor extremities and buttocks
Diagnosis	Clinical	Difficult to diagnose clinically	Clinical	Clinical
Management	Supportive; resolves over 1–2 weeks	Supportive; resolves in 2–6 days	Supportive; resolves in 3–6 weeks	Supportive; resolves in 2–8 weeks

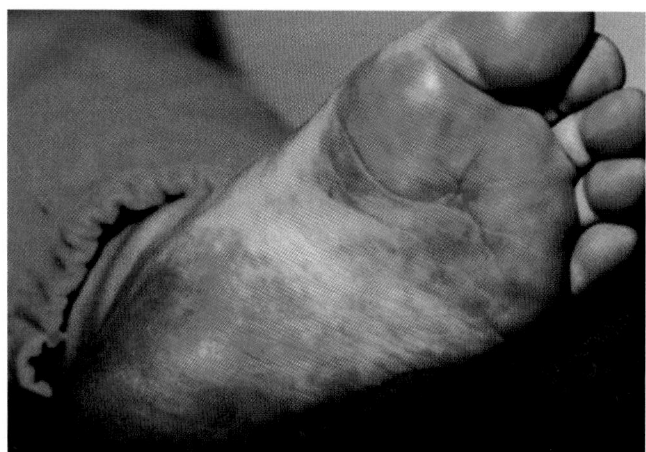

Figure 88.10 Purpuric glove and stocking syndrome. Erythema and petechiae of the plantar feet were accompanied by pruritus and sore throat in this young girl with parvovirus B19 infection. (Reprinted with permission from Paller, AS, Manicini AJ (eds.) *Hurwitz Clinical Pediatric Dermatology: A Textbook of Skin Disorders of Childhood and Adolescence*, 3rd edn. Philadelphia, PA: Elsevier Saunders, 2006. © 2006 Saunders Inc., an affiliate of Elsevier Inc.)

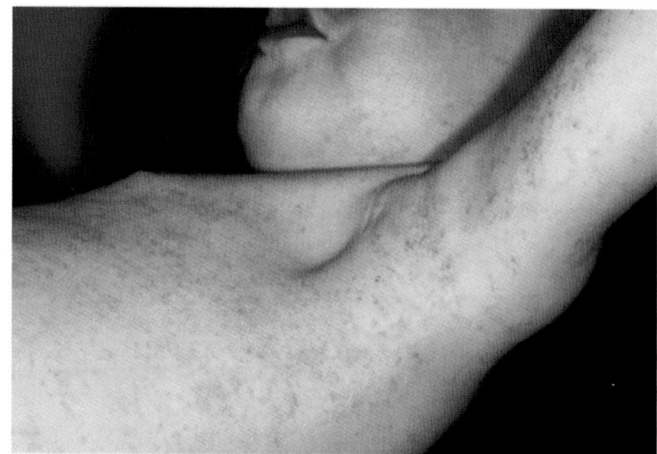

Figure 88.11 Unilateral thoracic exanthem. Early involvement shows erythematous macules and papules localized to the lateral trunk, axilla, and proximal inner arm in this patient. (Reprinted with permission from Paller, AS, Manicini AJ (eds.) *Hurwitz Clinical Pediatric Dermatology: A Textbook of Skin Disorders of Childhood and Adolescence*, 3rd edn. Philadelphia, PA: Elsevier Saunders, 2006. © 2006 Saunders Inc., an affiliate of Elsevier Inc.)

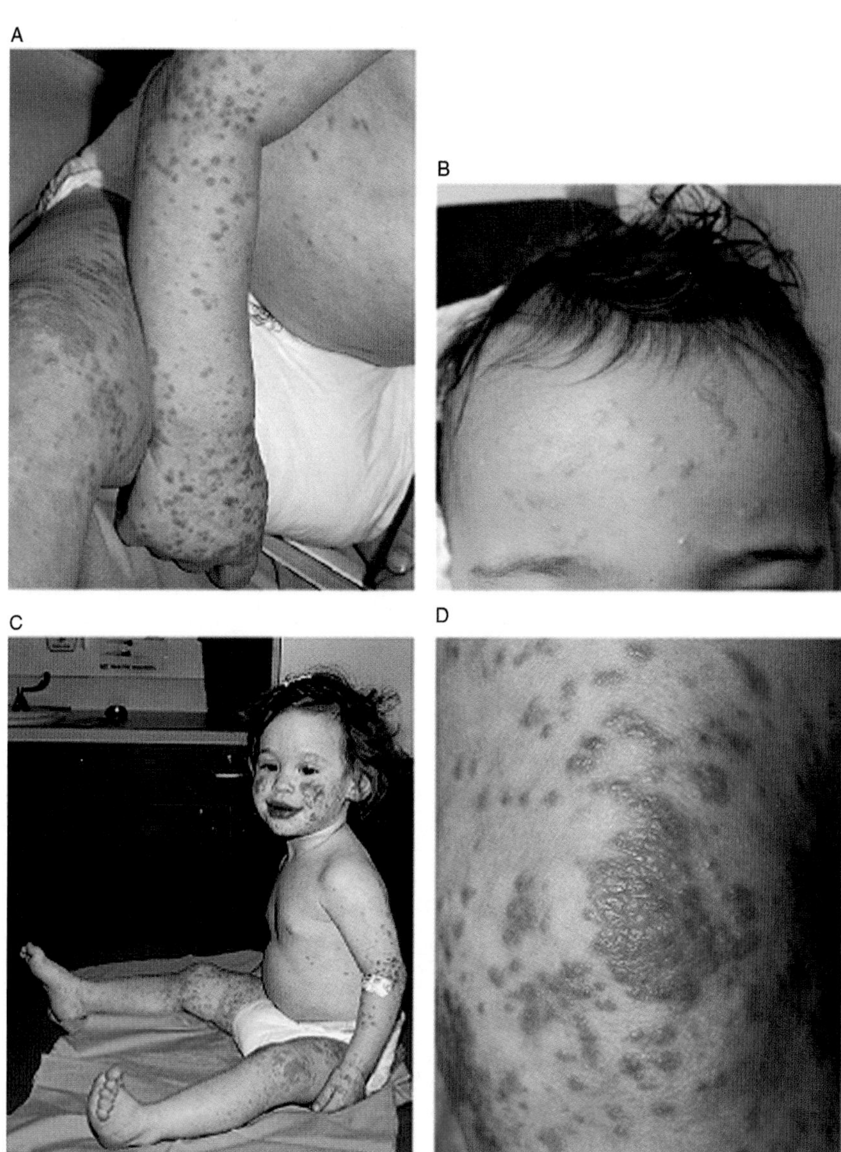

Figure 88.12 Papular acrodermatis of childhood/ Gianotti–Crosti syndrome. (A,B) Lesions consist of raised lichenoid papules with flat tops that appear in crops and tend to remain discrete. (C) This child shows the characteristic acral distribution, with lesions involving the extremities and face but with relative sparing of the trunk. (D) Lesions can become confluent over pressure points such as the knee. (Reproduced with permission from Zitelli BJ, Davis HW *Atlas of Pediatric Physical Diagnosis*, 5th edn. Philadelphia, PA: Mosby Elsevier, 2007. © 2007 Mosby Inc., an affiliate of Elsevier Inc.)

Pearls and pitfalls

Pearls

1. Viral and bacterial exanthems can appear similar; the history, physical examination and overall appearance of the child will largely guide management.
2. Rashes that the provider is unable to identify warrant closer follow-up and strict return precautions.
3. The majority of viral exanthems are treated with supportive care.

Pitfalls

1. Failure to identify a life-threatening rash, a highly contagious rash such as measles, or a potentially teratogenic infectious disease with a pathognomonic rash.
2. Failure to warn of possible complications of parvovirus, measles or varicella zoster virus infection in immunocompromised or pregnant family members of children with possible infection.

Selected references

Dayan G, Redd S, LeBaron C. Measles: United States, 2004. *MMWR Morb Mort Wkly Rep* 2005;**54**:1229–1231.

Dyer JA. Childhood viral exanthems. *Pediatr Ann* 2007;**36**:21–29.

Hambleton S. Chickenpox. *Curr Opin Infect Dis* 2005;**18**:235–240.

Kimberlin DW. Herpes simplex virus infections in neonates and early childhood. *Pediatr Infect Dis* 2005;**16**:271–281.

Powell KR. *Challenging Cases in Pediatric Infectious Disease*, Vol. 1. Elk Grove Village, IL: American Academy of Pediatrics, 2007.

Vaquez M. Varicella infections and varicella vaccine in the 21st century. *Pediatr Infect Dis J* 2004;**23**:871–872.

Young NS, Brown KE. Parvovirus B-19. *N Eng J Med* 2004;**350**;586–597.

Chapter 89

Bacterial infections with rashes

N. Ewen Amieva-Wang, Theresa M. van der Vlugt, Aparajita Sohoni, and Jennifer R. Reid

Introduction

Some bacterial organisms cause systemic disease with a systemic rash. The division between viral and bacterial disease is not particularly helpful when a clinician is evaluating a rash de novo; however, three bacterial infections are described here that cause recognizable syndromes. This chapter will review toxic shock syndrome (TSS), meningococcemia, and streptococcal scarlet fever (Table 89.1). Tick-borne diseases are discussed in Ch. 90.

Scarlet fever

Scarlet fever is a relatively benign childhood exanthem, although historically virulent epidemics have occurred and outbreaks of toxic cases may still occur. Scarlet fever occurs most commonly in children aged 2–10 years and is caused primarily by strains of group A beta-hemolytic streptococci (*Streptococcus pyogenes*; often referred to as group A streptococci or GABHS) producing a pyrogenic exotoxin.

Table 89.1. Comparison of three bacterial rashes

Disease	Toxic shock syndrome	Meningococcus	Scarlet fever
Etiologic agent	*Staphylococcus aureus*; group A beta-hemolytic streptococci	*Neisseria meningitidis*	Group A beta-hemolytic streptococci
Incubation	2 days	<24 h	3–8 days
Prodrome	Fever, chills, abdominal pain, hypotension, myalgias, erythroderma	Fever, rash, neck stiffness, altered mental status, severe myalgias	Fever
Lesions	Diffuse, red, macular rash (erythroderma), resembles a sunburn; strawberry tongue; desquamation of palms/soles 1–3 weeks later	Angular petechial lesions which start on the extremities; rash evolves with hemorrhagic bullae formation and purpura fulminans, with mucous membrane involvement	Erythematous macules and papules, feels like sandpaper; petechial palatal rash; white strawberry tongue that denudes to red strawberry tongue; peripheral desquamation from days 5 to 7
Distribution	Diffuse, involves palms, soles, mucous membranes	Starts on trunk and lower extremities; spreads diffusely	Neck, upper chest; spreads to trunk and limbs. Spares palms, soles, and perioral areas.
Diagnosis	Clinical CDC definition: fever, hypotension, erythroderma, desquamation, three organ systems involved	Clinical Blood cultures, CSF cultures, or skin biopsy	Clinical Pharyngeal swab or culture for streptococci
Treatment	Supportive care; antibiotics (clindamycin and vancomycin or linezolid); remove foreign bodies	Supportive care; antibiotics	Penicillin G IM single dose or 10-day course of penicillin V

A Practical Guide to Pediatric Emergency Medicine: Caring for Children in the Emergency Department, ed. N. Ewen Amieva-Wang (associate eds. Jamie Shandro, Aparajita Sohoni, and Bernhard Fassl). Published by Cambridge University Press.

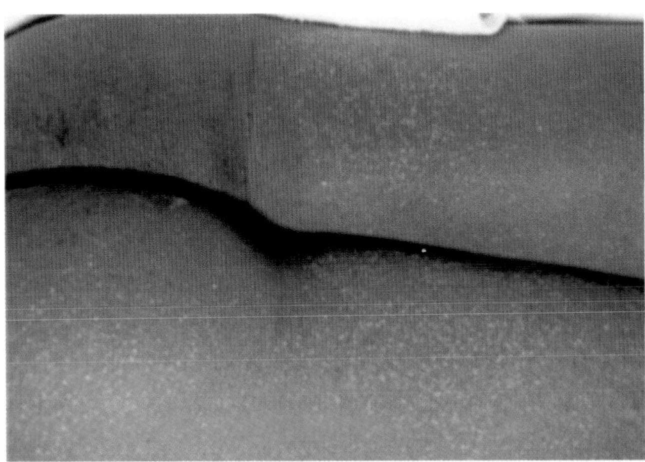

Figure 89.1 Scarlet fever. Diffuse erythema with small, punctuate papules. This eruption has a sandpapery texture to palpation. (Reprinted with permission from Paller, AS, Manicini AJ (eds.) *Hurwitz Clinical Pediatric Dermatology: A Textbook of Skin Disorders of Childhood and Adolescence,* 3rd edn. Philadelphia, PA: Elsevier Saunders, 2006. © 2006 Saunders Inc., an affiliate of Elsevier Inc.)

Clinical course

The exanthem of scarlet fever starts 24–48 h after the onset of fever and begins on the neck and upper chest as tiny discrete erythematous macules and papules; these spread down the trunk and limbs and have a "sandpapery" feel. Palms and soles are typically spared. In dark-skinned individuals, the erythroderma may be difficult to appreciate and the exanthem may resemble non-transient "goose pimples" (Fig. 89.1). Perioral sparing creates circumoral pallor, and petechiae can appear in flexural lines in the axilla, antecubial fossa, and groin (Pastia's lines). The rash becomes a brownish skin discoloration in 3–5 days and a fine desquamation follows on days 5–7, centered on hands, feet, and knees. Occasionally there is early desquamation in the perineal area at the time of acute infection.

The enanthem of scarlet fever consists of petechial macules of the palate and a white-coated tongue with red papillae protruding through the coating ("white strawberry tongue"). The coating peels off in 4–5 days to reveal a glistening "red strawberry tongue" with prominent red papillae (Fig. 89.2).

Children commonly complain of throat pain, headache, and chills, and children with a pharyngeal source will have a classic "strep throat" with tonsillar and posterior pharyngeal edema, erythema, and exudates, often with tender anterior cervical adenopathy.

Diagnosis

Differential diagnosis includes viral exanthems (Ch. 88), drug eruptions, early Kawasaki disease or TSS, staphylococcal scalded skin syndrome, rubella or rubeola. Pharyngeal rapid strep swab or throat culture (or wound culture from a skin source) can be diagnostic for streptococcal scarlet fever. Sparing of palms and soles, lack of oral involvement or erosions other than the specific enanthem of strawberry tongue, petechiae, posterior pharyngitis/tonsillitis, and general non-toxic appearance should point to scarlet fever.

Management

Treatment of choice is 10 days of penicillin V or a single dose IM of penicillin G. Macrolides (erythromycin, clarithromycin, azithromycin) are recommended in penicillin-allergic patients. Amoxicillin is often prescribed, but it has no microbiological advantage over penicillin.

Complications

Scarlet fever will improve without antibiotics, but antibiotics prevent the complication of acute rheumatic fever. It is recommended that antibiotics be started within 9 days of onset of GABHS pharyngitis to prevent acute rheumatic fever. The risk of post-streptococcal glomerulonephritis, a rare complication of the GABHS infection, is not reduced by antibiotics.

Toxic shock syndrome

Toxic shock syndrome is characterized by abrupt onset of fever, rash, hypotension, and multiorgan dysfunction in an otherwise healthy individual. It was first described in children in the late 1970s but received increased attention in 1980 with a large number of cases related to super-absorbent tampons. Menstrual TSS has declined sharply and now menstrual and non-menstrual cases are reported approximately equally. Between 1979 and 1996, 50 cases of TSS were reported, with more than half being in children 2 years old or younger.

Toxic shock syndrome is usually caused by *Staphylococcus aureus* expressing a superantigen toxin, although it can be caused by invasive GABHS; it is then termed streptococcal TSS. Non-menstrual TSS is associated with skin wounds and foreign bodies such as nasal packing.

Diagnosis

Toxic shock syndrome is a clinical diagnosis. The formal case definition from the CDC is shown in Table 89.2. A *probable case* is a case meeting the laboratory criteria and in which four of the five clinical findings are present. A *confirmed case* is a case meeting the laboratory criteria and all five of the clinical finding categories. Clinically, TSS begins after a 24–48 h prodrome of fever, chills, and malaise, followed by myalgias, vomiting, diarrhea, muscle tenderness, and mental status changes. Initial physical examination may reveal fever, tachycardia, tachypnea, low blood pressure, diffuse erythroderma, conjunctival hyperemia, and beefy red mucous membranes. Muscle tenderness often occurs in conjunction with edema and peripheral cyanosis.

The rash of TSS begins after 24–48 h as a diffuse macular erythroderma that is sometimes accentuated in the skin fold of the neck, axillae, and groin. The erythroderma tends to be most intense around the site of infection. In menstrual causes, this includes the inner thighs and perineum. In non-menstrual causes, this includes the area surrounding the site of infection.

A

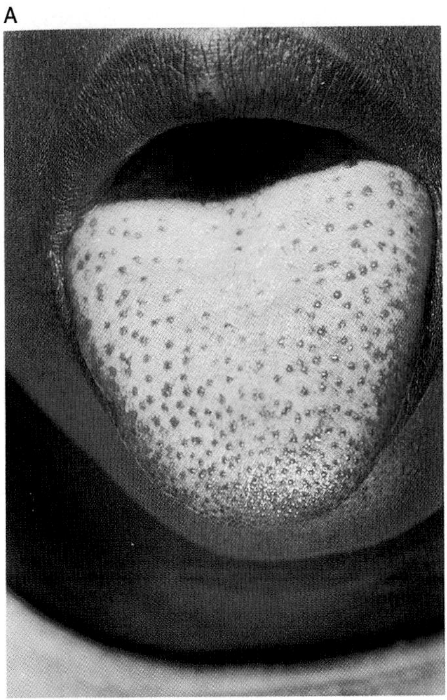

B

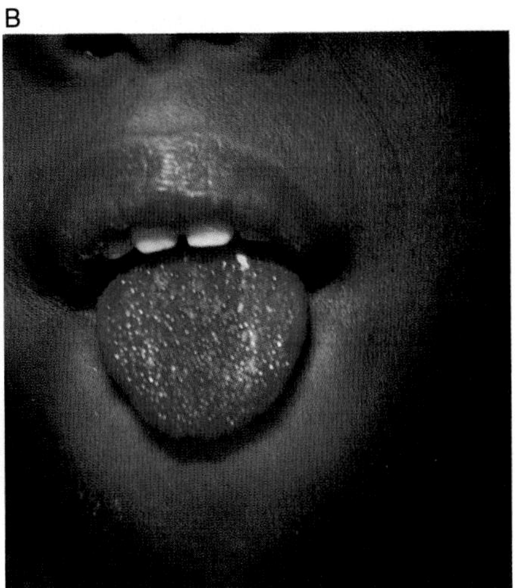

Figure 89.2 Strawberry tongue. This finding is found in scarlet fever, toxic shock syndrome, and some other syndromes. (A) White strawberry tongue (edematous red papillae projecting through white-coated tongue; seen on the 2nd day of illness in a child with scarlet fever. (B) Red strawberry tongue (as white coating disappears, the red tongue studded with prominent papillae appears; seen on the 3rd day of illness in a child with scarlet fever.) (Reprinted with permission from Shah BR, Lucchesi M (eds). *Atlas of Pediatric Emergency Medicine.* New York: McGraw Hill, 2006.)

The erythdroderma also involves the palms and soles. Strawberry tongue (Fig. 89.2), mucous membrane hyperemia, palatal petechiae, and conjunctival infection are usually present, and swelling of hands, feet, and face may occur. Desquamation follows in 1–2 weeks and is most prominent in the palms and soles; patients can shed their hair and fingernails weeks later.

Differential diagnosis includes scarlet fever, Kawasaki disease, staphylococcal scaled skin syndrome, drug reaction, atypical measles, or other viral exanthematous illnesses.

Hypotension is unusual with these differential diagnoses and should always lead the physician to suspect toxic shock syndrome.

Blood cultures are positive for *S. aureus* only 5% of the time, although *S. aureus* is often recovered from suspected sources of infection in patients with TSS. In streptococcal TSS, up to 50% of blood cultures will be positive for GABHS. Laboratory studies for both forms of TSS will reflect multiorgan system dysfunction and disseminated intravascular coagulation.

Management

Treatment is initially supportive with attention to correcting hypotension, as the rate of organ dysfunction is related to hypoperfusion (Box 89.1). Ongoing crystalloid boluses to correct hypotension are the mainstay of therapy, as are IV vasopressors to maintain end-organ perfusion. Ventilator support requirements are common, and ICU admission is the rule.

Tampons or foreign bodies must be removed, abcesses drained, and any necrotic wound or tissue debrided aggressively and immediately.

Empiric parenteral antibiotic treatment should be started immediately to cover both methicillin-resistant *S. aureus* and GABHS. Clindamycin should never be used alone empirically as some GABHS is resistant.

Meningococcal infection

Meningococcal disease is caused by the Gram-negative bacteria *Neisseria meningitidis*. With the advent of the vaccines for *Haemophilus influenzae* type b and the pneumococcus (*Streptococcus pneumoniae*) in the USA, meningococcal disease has become one of the leading causes of meningitis in the USA. There has been little change in disease mortality since the 1950s. In the USA, there are 2500–3500 cases annually, with a case fatality of 6–12%. Predominant serogroups causing infection in the USA are B, C, and Y. In Africa and Asia the predominant serotypes are mostly A and also C.

N. meningitidis can live as a commensal bacteria in humans. Nasopharyngeal carriage rates increase with overcrowded

Table 89.2. Diagnosis of toxic shock syndrome

Feature	Characteristics
Fever	Temperature ≥38.9°C
Rash	Diffuse macular erythroderma
Desquamation	1–2 weeks after onset of illness, particularly on palms/soles
Hypotension	Systolic blood pressure <90 mmHg for adults, or <5th percentile by age for children <16 years; orthostatic syncope, dizziness, or change in diastolic blood pressure ≥15 mmHg from lying to sitting
Multisystem involvement	Three of more of the following: GI: vomiting or diarrhea Muscular: myalgias or elevated creatine phosphokinase (>2× ULN) Mucous membranes: vaginal, oropharyngeal, or conjunctival hyperemia Renal: BUN or creatinine at least 2× ULN, or urinary sediment with pyuria (>5 leukocytes per high-power field) in the absence of urinary tract infection Hepatic: total bilirubin, ALT, or AST at least twice the ULN Hematologic: platelets <100 000/µl CNS: disorientation or altered level of consciousness without focal neurologic signs when fever and hypotension are absent
Laboratory criteria (if obtained)	Negative blood/throat/CSF cultures (blood can be positive for *S. aureus*); rise in titer to Rocky Mountain spotted fever, leptospirosis, or measles

Source: Centers for Disease Control and Prevention (CDC) http://www.cdc.gov/ncphi/disss/nndss/casedef/toxicsscurrent.htm (accessed 14 August 2009).

Box 89.1. Key points for treatment of toxic shock syndrome

1. Drain the source of toxin production and irrigate.
2. Conduct sensitivity testing of the organism: culture and check sensitivities from source sample.
3. Administer antimicrobial therapy for *S. aureus*: empiric treatment is with vancomycin and clindamycin.
4. Consider antitoxin in severe cases, consulting with an infectious diseases specialist.
5. Treat the systemic effects of the toxins with fluid resuscitation and vasopressors; consider IV immunoglobulins and steroids.

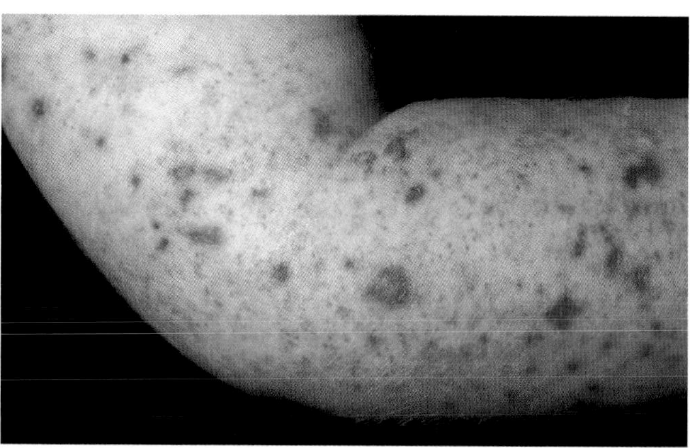

Figure 89.3 Meningococcemia. Erythematous and angular petechiae and purpura with central skin necrosis. (Courtesy of Logical Images, Inc.)

conditions as well as with increasing age: 2% in children <2 years; 5% in children <17 years; 20–40% in young adults. Meningococcal disease commonly affects children <5 years of age and adolescents living in institutional settings. The disease rate is 10 times higher in children <2 years old than in the overall population.

Individuals with inherited or acquired terminal complement deficiencies are at increased risk of meningococcal infection.

Meningococcal disease is a spectrum from transient bacteremia, meningococcemia with or without meningitis, and meningoencephalitis alone. The mortality rate of meningococcemia without meningitis is 20–30%; with meningitis alone, it is 2–10%. Severe disease can result in purpura fulminans, including fulminant sepsis and death within hours.

Clinical presentation

Meningococcal disease often follows a upper respiratory infection. Patients can have non-specific signs, such as headache, nausea, vomiting, myalgias, and arthralgias, that are difficult to distinguish from a viral syndrome. Not all patients appear toxic.

Skin lesions occur in 70%. A petechial rash is the most common sign (Fig. 89.3), with the majority of lesions appearing on the extremities (as opposed to benign petechiae, which occur above the nipple with a history of increased intrathoracic pressure). The lesions are angular (Fig. 89.3). They can develop a necrotic center and become gangrenous.

Patients can rapidly go into septic shock with mental status changes, disseminated intravascular coagulation, and multi-organ failure. Poor prognostic factors include hypotension, hypothermia, leukopenia, thrombocytopenia, absence of meningitis, purpura fulminans, and petechiae <12 h prior to presentation.

Differential diagnosis

Differential includes TSS and Rocky Mountain spotted fever (Ch. 90), which are other causes of classic hypotension, rash, and fever. Other diseases on the differential include bacterial sepsis, endocarditis, viral illness, and leptospirosis.

Management

The key to reduced morbidity and mortality is prompt recognition, stabilization and immediate broad-spectrum antibiotics such as: cefotaxime (200 mg/kg daily) or ceftriaxone (100 mg/kg daily). Treatment should be started without waiting for the results of diagnostic testing if meningococcemia is strongly suspected. Management of ABCs is imperative.

Prophylaxis

Risk of disease in close contacts is 300–400 times that of the general population.

Close contacts should receive prophylaxis within 24 h of diagnosis. Close contact is defined as household contacts, child care, or nursery school exposure or someone who has frequently eaten or slept with the patient. Healthcare workers generally are not considered close contacts unless they came into contact with the patient's respiratory secretions.

Prophylactic regimens include rifampin 600 mg every 12 h for 2 days (adults) or 10 mg/kg every 12 h for 2 days (children); a single dose of ceftriaxone 125 mg in those <12 years and 250 mg in those >12 years; ciprofloxacin 500 mg single dose in contacts >18 years of age.

Pearls and pitfalls

Pearls

1. Early diagnosis and prompt treatment of streptococcal syndromes has led to a marked decrease in the incidence of acute rheumatic fever.
2. Scarlet fever historically has been virulent; however presently in the USA, it causes limited disease.
3. Meningococcemia is one of the three hallmark diseases that cause rash, fever and hypotension.
4. Acute meningococcemia can mimic a virus-like illness, initially presenting with fever, myalgias, headache, weakness, and pharyngitis.
5. Transient non-pruritic maculopapular rash mimicking a wide variety of viral exanthems may be a presenting sign of meningococcemia.
6. Toxic shock syndrome occurs in children and even neonates.

Pitfalls

1. Failure to take into account family history of death from overwhelming infection in suspected meningococcal infection.
2. Failure to provide prophylaxis to close household contacts in cases of meningococcal infection.
3. Failure to search for and remove foreign bodies or debride wounds in toxic shock syndrome.

Selected references

Aber C, Connelly EA, Schachner LA. Fever and rash in a child: when to worry? *Pediatr Ann* 2007;**36**:30–38.

Chuang Y-Y, Huang Y-C, Lin T-Y. Toxic shock syndrome in children, epidemiology, pathenogenesis, and management. *Pediatr Drugs* 2005:7:11–25.

Hajjeh RA, Reingold A, Weil A, *et al.* Toxic shock syndrome in the United States: surveillance update, 1979–1996. *Emerg Infect Dis* 1999; 5;807–810.

Pickering LK, Baker CJ, Kimberlin DW, Long SS (eds.). *The Red Book: 2006 Report of the Committee on Infectious Diseases*, 27th edn. Elk Grove Village, IL: American Academy of Pediatrics; 2006.

Chapter 90 Tick-borne disease

Theresa M. van der Vlugt

Introduction

This chapter addresses a variety of tick-borne diseases including Rocky Mountain spotted fever (RMSF), Lyme disease, typhus, and ehrlichiosis (Table 90.1). These diseases are common within the USA and are frequently difficult to diagnose in pediatric patients who are unable to provide a full history. Even in adults, a history of a tick bite is frequently difficult to elicit. Still, these diseases may have complicated long-term sequelae if not detected and treated appropriately.

Rocky Mountain spotted fever

Introduction and epidemiology

Rocky Mountain spotted fever classically presents with rash, fever, and headache, and is caused by *Rickettsia ricketsii*, an intracellular parasite transmitted by the bite of an infected tick, although history of tick bite is only elicited in 50–60% of cases. The organism replicates in endothelial cells and causes widespread vasculitis. Important vectors are American dog ticks (*Dermacentor variabilis*), and wood ticks (*Dermacentor andersoni*). Two thirds of cases occur in children under the age of 15, and 15% of deaths are in children under the age of 10; 90% of reported cases of RMSF occur between April and September. Cases have been reported in all 48 contiguous states, but five states (North Carolina, South Carolina, Tennessee, Oklahoma, and Arkansas) account for more than 50% of cases. Rocky Mountain spotted fever is also endemic in countries in Central and South America.

Clinical presentation

Rocky Mountain spotted fever commonly presents with symptoms 2–14 days after tick exposure, mimicking a non-specific viral illness: fever, headache, nausea or vomiting, generalized malaise, and anorexia. The rash begins on days 2–5 and the classical petechial rash develops on days 5 or 6 (Fig. 90.1).

The rash starts as small non-specific erythematous blanching macules around feet, ankles, wrists, and hands (including palms and soles); it rapidly progresses to the trunk and head.

Clinical presentation initially is similar to rubeola or disseminated meningococcal disease. Children at this time are systemically ill and often have mental status changes. Differential diagnosis at this time includes meningococcemia, viral syndrome with rash, erythema multiforme, drug reaction, and secondary syphilis.

As many as 15% of children never develop a rash.

Diagnostic studies

There is no widely available laboratory study to confirm early RMSF. Laboratory studies can show hyponatremia and thrombocytopenia, as well as elevated AST and ALT. The CSF can be normal or show a mononuclear pleocytosis or mild hyperproteinemia.

Even in areas where awareness of RMSF is high, 60–75% of patients receive an alternative diagnosis on their first visit for medical care. Acute titers of serum IgG and IgM are usually not detectable until day 7 of the illness. Direct immunofluorescence assay of tissue samples (including biopsy of skin rash) can be useful in the first week.

Management

Treatment of choice for children of all ages is doxycycline 2–4 mg/kg divided BID, PO or IV, up to 100 mg BID. Treatment is continued for 3 days after defervescence or clinical improvement. Fluoroquinolones or chloramphenicol are alternative therapies, but chloramphenicol does not cover ehrlichosis and is not available in oral form in the USA. Poor outcomes are associated with delayed administration of appropriate antibiotics, and the risk of death triples if antibiotics are not started by days 5 or 6. Patients with glucose-6-phosphate dehydrogenase deficiency are also at high risk for fulminant

A Practical Guide to Pediatric Emergency Medicine: Caring for Children in the Emergency Department, ed. N. Ewen Amieva-Wang (associate eds. Jamie Shandro, Aparajita Sohoni, and Bernhard Fassl). Published by Cambridge University Press.

Table 90.1. Tick-borne diseases

Disease	Rocky Mountain spotted fever	Lyme disease	Endemic typhus	Human monocytic ehrlichiosis
Tick vector/host	*Dermacentor variabilis* (American dog tick), *Dermacentor andersoni* (Rocky Mountain wood tick)	*Ixodes scapularis* (blacklegged tick), *Ixodes pacificus* (Western blacklegged tick)	*Xenopsylla cheopsis* (rat flea), *Ctenocephalides felis* (cat flea)	*Amblyomma americanum* (Lone Star tick)
Infectious agent	*Rickettsia ricketsii*	*Borrelia burgdorferi*	*Rickettsia typhii*	*Ehrlichia chaffeensis*
Geographic location	All 48 contiguous US states, with increased prevalence in southeastern and south central states	Majority of cases in northeast and mid-western states (*I. scapularis*); fewer cases in western states (*I. pacificus*)	Texas, California, Hawaii	Southeast, southcentral, mid-Atlantic states
Incubation	2–14 days	7–14 days	6–14 days	7–14 days
Prodrome	Fever, headache, malaise, nausea, anorexia	Fatigue, anorexia, headache, neck pain, myalgias, arthralgias, lymphadenopathy, fever	Fever, fatigue, myalgias, headache	Fever, fatigue, myalgais, headache
Disease	Fever, rash, abdominal pain; can progress to seizures, confusion, mental status changes, bleeding, or gangrene of extremities	*Focal disease*: rash, fever, myalgia, arthralgia, headache *Early or late disseminated disease*: meningitis, cranial nerve palsies, radiculopathy, neuropathy, heart block, carditis, conjunctivitis, persistent arthritis	Rash, viral syndrome; rarely may progress to pulmonary, hepatic, cardiac, or renal involvement	Fever, viral syndrome, rash; rarely may progress to seizures, coma, heart failure, respiratory failure
Lesions	Erythematous blanching macules until day 5, then evolves into diffuse petechial rash	Erythema migrans (erythematous ring with central clearing and necrotic center), may be uniformly erythematous	Erythematous, macular, diffuse May be petechial or maculopapular	Macular, maculopapular, or petechial lesions
Distribution	Initially feet, ankles, wrists, hands, palms and soles; spreads to face and trunk	Axilla, inguinal region, belt-line, popliteal fossa; may enlarge over weeks	Trunk; spreads peripherally, sparing palms and soles; significant variability in presence and distribution of rash	Diffuse
Diagnosis	Clinical IgG and IgM titers; skin biopsy in first 7 days	Clinical Serologic testing unreliable early, with false positives secondary to cross reaction; recommend testing with consultation with a infectious disease specialist	Clinical Serologic testing for antibody titers during acute and convalescent phase	Clinical Peripheral blood smear; serologic testing for antibody titers during acute and convalescent phase
Treatment	Doxycycline, broad-spectrum antibiotics	Doxycycline for children >7 years; amoxicillin or cefuroxime for all ages; IV ceftriaxone or penicillin for CNS or cardiac symptoms, or severe arthritis; supportive care	Doxycycline, supportive care	Doxycycline, supportive care

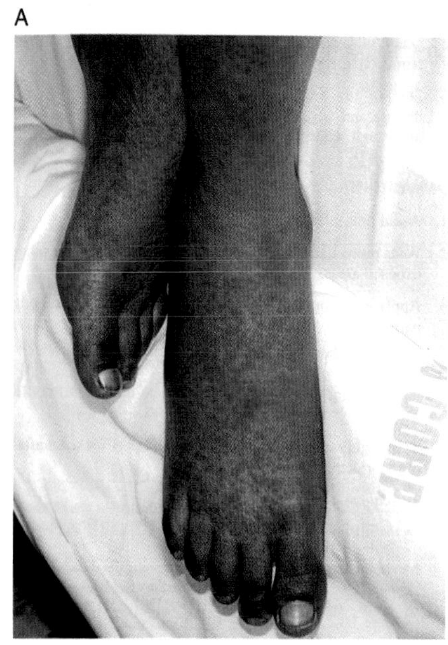

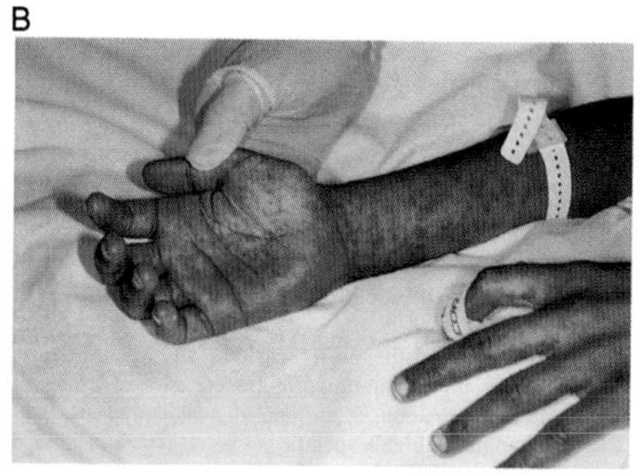

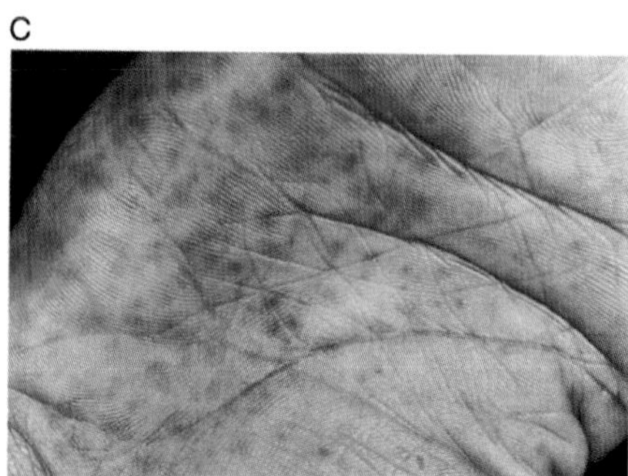

Figure 90.1 Rocky Mountain spotted fever. This erythematous maculopapular eruption started on the distal extremity and subsequently became petechial in a 12-year-old boy. He also had fever, severe headache, and myalgia. He gave a history of camping outdoors during his summer vacation in North Carolina 12 days prior to onset of this rash. These photographs were taken on the 5th day of his illness. As seen here, the palms and soles are nearly always affected. He also had edema of both hands and feet. (Reprinted with permission from Shah BR, Lucchesi M (eds). *Atlas of Pediatric Emergency Medicine*. New York: McGraw Hill, 2006.)

course of disease in RMSF. Treatment with sulfa drugs appears to worsen outcomes from RMSF.

Antibiotics to cover menigococcal infection should usually be started concomitant with doxycycline for suspected RMSF because the illnesses can be indistinguishable in the early stages.

Conversely, consider adding doxycycline to broad-spectrum antibiotics given for febrile rash with suspected sepsis, because RMSF is insensitive to most broad-spectrum antibiotics.

Lyme disease

Introduction and epidemiology

Lyme disease is the leading tick-borne illness in North America and Europe. The disease is endemic in three USA regions: the northeast (most commonly in coastal areas from Maryland to northern Massachusetts), the upper mid-west (Wisconsin and Minnesota), and the far west (California and Oregon). The disease has been reported from every part of the world, including most of the USA. It is caused by the spirochete *Borrelia burgdorferi*, carried by hard-bodied ticks (e.g., *Ixodes dammini*).

Clinical presentation

The spirochete initially produces a characteristic skin lesion (erythema chronicum migrans) (Fig. 30.2, p. 161) and then spreads through the lymphatics and bloodstream and disseminates to other organs, including the heart, the CNS, and the peripheral nervous system. Cardiac manifestations occur in approximately 10% of patients with confirmed Lyme disease. They generally appear 4 to 8 weeks after the initial illness, but appearance can vary from 4 days to 7 months. The most common cardiac manifestation is varying degrees of atrioventricular block, occurring in up to 87% of cases. Over 95% of these patients show first-degree atrioventricular block at some time in their course. Up to 50% develop complete heart block, and some of them develop permanent heart block. First-degree atrioventricular block can rapidly progress to complete heart block.

Diagnostic studies

Testing in early disease is controversial, as antibodies to *B. burgdorferi* are not detected in most individuals in the first few weeks. Because of testing controversies and risk of false positives and negatives, testing should be done by an infectious disease specialist, not from the ED.

Management

Doxycycline 100 mg BID for 14–21 days is the drug of choice for children 8 years and older with early localized disease. Amoxicillin 50 mg/kg daily divided TID (max. 1.5 g daily) or cefuroxime 100 mg/kg daily divided BID for 14–21 days can also be used in all age groups as first-line treatment. The same agents are used for a 21–28 day course for early disseminated disease. Carditis, meningitis, encephalitis, and persistent or recurrent arthritis are treated with IV penicillin or IV/IM ceftriaxone for 14–28 days. Close follow-up should be arranged with the pediatrician to monitor for long-term complications of Lyme disease.

The AAP does not recommend routine prophylaxis of tick bites, even confirmed deer ticks in endemic Lyme areas.

Risk of transmission from non-engorged ticks is very low but increases in engorged ticks, particularly if attached >72 h.

Testing of removed ticks has poor predictive value and is not recommended. In hyperendemic areas, with discovery of engorged ticks with prolonged attachment, a single dose of doxycyline 200 mg or 4.4 mg/kg for weight under 45 kg has been shown to be useful in prevention but has not been studied in children under 12 years.

Human monocytic ehrlichiosis

Introduction and epidemiology

Human monocytic ehrlichiosis is a tick-borne illness (*Ehrlichi chaffeensis*) with the same geographic concentration, seasonal timing, and clinical presentation as RMSF. It is more common in adults than children, but more children are likely to have rash with HME (66%).

Clinical presentation

Children with HME have fever, headache, myalgia, and nausea, with a rash primarily on the trunk and extremities that may be macular, maculopapular, or petechial. Leukopenia, anemia, and hepatitis are more common with HME than with RMSF. Vasculitic damage is less prominent, and the overall clinical course less severe in HME.

Diagnostic studies

Diagnosis is made by peripheral blood smear showing intracytoplasmic morulae along with a single immunofluorescence assay result $\geq$64, or by acute and convalescent serum immunofluorescent antibody titers. As with RMSF, antibodies are usually not detectable at first presentation. Subclinical disease is also probably more prevalent than has been diagnosed, with 12.5% of children testing seropositive for previous infection in a study of endemic areas.

Management

Treatment is the same as for RMSF, with doxycycline 4 mg/kg daily divided BID, up to 100 mg BID, for 10 days.

Endemic (murine) typhus

Introduction and epidemiology

Murine typhus is caused by *Rickettsia typhii*, transmitted to humans from rats, house mice, opossums, skunks, and cats by the bite of a rat flea (*Xenopsylla cheopsis*) or a cat flea (*Ctenocephalides felis*). It is prevalent worldwide and previously endemic in the southeastern and Gulf states. It is now primarily reported in south Texas and southern California, with a recent increase in Hawaii.

Clinical presentation

The incubation period is 6–14 days, after which all affected children develop fever (39°C or lower): 66–80% of children have rash, and 50% have the classic triad of fever, headache, and rash. The rash appears on day 4 or later of illness and is generally erythematous, macular, and diffuse, but it can be maculopapular or occasionally petechial. In younger children, the disease can be quite mild and is probably underdiagnosed.

Diagnostic studies

Diagnosis can be made by testing antibody titers to *R. typhii* in acute and convalescent serum with direct immunofluorescence assay, enzyme immunoassay, complement fixation or latex agglutination. The CDC can perform molecular diagnostic assays on whole blood or tissue samples.

Management

Fever usually resolves 1–3 days after the child receives an appropriate antibiotic (doxycycline 2.2 mg/kg every 12 h, maximium 300 mg daily, continued for 3 days after fever abates, usually 5–10 days). However, fever will resolve spontaneously in 2–3 weeks in children who are not treated. Disease in children usually has no complications, and deaths are quite rare.

Pearls and pitfalls

Pearls

1. Lyme disease is the leading tick-borne disease in North America and Europe.
2. Doxycycline is appropriate for use in children of all ages with highly suspected or documented Rocky Mountain spotted fever (RMSF).
3. Doxycycline provides coverage for all common tick-borne or flea-borne rickettsial diseases causing fever (RMSF, human monocytic ehrlichiosis, murine typhus, human granulocytic anaplasmosis, and *Ehrlichia ewingii* infection.)
4. The majority of tick-borne diseases should be diagnosed clinically, as laboratory testing is delayed and frequently unreliable.
5. Lyme disease is a difficult diagnosis to make serologically. Testing should be done by a pediatric infectious disease specialist using a reliable laboratory.
6. Prophylaxis for Lyme disease is not routinely recommended after a tick bite.

Pitfalls

1. Failure to consider tick-borne disease when there is lack of insect bite history in a child with exposure, non-specific symptoms, and a rash.
2. Failure to initiate appropriate therapy for RMSF while awaiting serologic testing.
3. Failure to consider source control, where appropriate, such as animal decontamination.

Selected references

Centers for Disease Control and Prevention. Diagnosis and management of tickborne rickettsial diseases: Rocky Mountain spotted fever, ehrlichioses, and anaplasmosis – United States. *MMWR Morb Mort Wkly Rep* 2006;**55**: 1–27.

Dumler JS, Walker DH. Rocky Mountain spotted fever: changing ecology and persisting virulence. *N Engl J Med* 2005;**353**:551–553.

Feigin RD, Cherry JD, Demmler GJ *et al. Textbook of Pediatric Infectious Diseases*, 5th edn. Philadelphia, PA: Saunders, 2004.

Fergie JE, Purcell K, Wanat D. Murine typhus in South Texas children. *Pediatr Infect Dis J* 2000;**19**:535–538.

Pickering LK, Baker CJ, Kimberlin DW, Long SS (eds.). *The Red Book: 2006 Report of the Committee on Infectious Diseases*, 27th edn. Elk Grove Village, IL: American Academy of Pediatrics, 2006 (also Red Book Online, last updated 5 January 2009).

Chapter 91 Botulism

Laura W. Kates

Introduction

Botulism is a rare but devastating disease that affects cholinergic synapses to cause bulbar paralysis and ultimately respiratory failure. Initially recognized in the eighteenth century in Europe, the clinical syndrome was thought to be associated with sausage ingestion and the word "botulinum" is derived from the German word for sausage. There are four forms of clinically significant botulism in humans: food-borne, adult intestinal colonization, wound, and infant. The focus of this chapter is on infant botulism.

Infant botulism typically affects infants between the ages of 2 months and 1 year. Classically, it is thought to be secondary to ingestion of spores from foods such as honey.

The majority of cases of infant bolulism are now thought to be secondary to inhalation of spores from dust.

First described in 1976, infant botulism makes up the majority (60%) of clinical botulism cases (approximately 75 cases per year) in the USA. In 2004, 87 cases of infant botulism were reported in patients aged 6 days to 61 weeks old. Of these, 57% were concentrated in the western USA, with California seeing most cases.

Pathophysiology

Clostridium botulinum is a Gram-positive anaerobic spore-forming bacillus. The bacteria is heat resistant and is found ubiquitously in soil, improperly canned foods, corn syrup, and (as noted prominently in medical school texts) honey. *C. botulinum* produces the most potent neurotoxin known and is, therefore, of great interest both as an infectious pathogen and as a potential bioterrorism agent. Merely 0.3 ng of *C. botulinum* spores can cause clinically significant disease.

Incubation periods vary for the different forms of botulism (Table 91.1). Food-borne transmission has the shortest time to symptoms as the toxin is preformed and directly ingested. Although older children and adults likely ingest clostridial spores without adverse effects, infants younger than 12 months of age are prone to in vivo toxin formation due to a lack of GI motility and competitive bacterial flora.

The clinical range of botulism is wide, from mild hypotonia, which may manifest as a weak suck, to complete paralysis, loss of cranial nerve function, and respiratory failure. As such, the differential diagnosis is wide and is varied depending on the age of the patient.

Clinical presentation

Botulism is a rare disease and potentially missed unless healthcare providers keep it in their differential of ill-appearing infant patients.

Infants with botulism predominantly present with fatigue, malaise, poor energy, poor feeding, weak cry, and constipation.

As the disease progresses, caregivers and clinicians may note the infant is hypotonic, has lost facial expressions, and eventually develops descending weakness and respiratory distress. A source of exposure is rarely known and is unlikely to change clinical management.

Physical examination of infants presenting with symptoms of botulism should remain focused on rapid assessment of airway and ventilatory status and intervention as necessary. The child should be carefully examined for physical signs of sepsis, as meningitis is a much more likely cause of the patient's complaints than botulism. Typically, a child with botulism is afebrile and has normal skin. Particular attention should be directed towards a careful neurologic evaluation. Reflexes (including the suck reflex), quality of the infant's cry, quality of facial expression, and overall muscular tone

Table 91.1. Incubation period of different forms of botulism

Form of botulism	Incubation period
Food-borne	12–48 h
Wound	4–14 days
Infant	3–30 days

A Practical Guide to Pediatric Emergency Medicine: Caring for Children in the Emergency Department, ed. N. Ewen Amieva-Wang (associate eds. Jamie Shandro, Aparajita Sohoni, and Bernhard Fassl). Published by Cambridge University Press.

should raise clinical suspicion for botulism. More advanced cases may present with loss of the gag reflex, loss of extraocular movements, respiratory distress, and apnea.

Diagnosis

Definitive diagnosis of botulism is not possible in the ED yet early suspicion of botulism is critical to timely acquisition of antitoxin.

Ultimately, a child with botulism will have had an extensive workup to exclude other more common diseases in the differential. Usually patients with botulism will have normal laboratory electrolyte panel, LFTs, and hematology panel, a normal urinalysis, and normal ECG. Often these patients have had a lumbar puncture as part of their evaluation. The CSF will most likely be normal or show slightly elevated protein levels, in contrast to normal levels seen in patients with Guillain–Barré syndrome.

Confirmatory stool testing for the *C. botulinum* toxin is available but takes several days to result. A minimum of 25 ml is required for testing, which is often difficult to obtain given the clinical constipation that accompanies botulism. Serum and urine assays are also available and the CDC and local health departments can help to coordinate sample testing.

Management

Care in the ED should be supportive, with particular focus on airway and respiratory management. Once botulism emerges as the primary diagnosis, clinicians caring for the child should acquire and administer the antitoxin.

In 2003, a human-derived immune globulin was approved by the FDA specifically for the treatment of infant botulism. The "BabyBIG" antitoxin is available through the California Department of Health Services (24 h service). The cost is high ($45 000 per dose in 2004 dollars) and because it is derived from humans it carries a risk of allergic reaction, although has been proved to be highly effective at treating infant botulism. Patients with food-borne or wound botulism should receive equine-derived antitoxin available through state health departments or the CDC. The equine-derived antitoxin should not be given to infants, even if the Baby BIG is not easily available, because of the high rates of hypersensitivity reactions.

Antimicrobial therapy should be limited as there is a risk of increasing toxin release and worsening the patient's condition. However, during the ED phase of treatment patients will often receive empiric doses of antibiotics. This is appropriate care for the undifferentiated toxic-appearing infant but should be stopped once meningitis and encephalitis are excluded and botulism diagnosed.

Healthcare providers are legally required to report all suspected and confirmed cases of botulism to their local public health department or directly to the CDC. Most state health departments and the CDC have a 24-h phone line available for reporting and these agencies will undoubtedly serve as an invaluable resource in coordinating the care of patients with botulism. As there is an environmental component to botulism, once a case is diagnosed in a geographic area the ED staff should remain alert for other potential cases. Early recognition, support, and treatment with antitoxin are key to improving clinical outcomes.

Disposition

Botulism can advance quickly and unpredictably and, given the delay in definitive diagnosis, *all* patients with suspected botulism should be admitted to an intensive care setting for close monitoring and ventilatory support. The average duration of required ventilatory assistance for patients with infant botulism is 2–8 weeks. Patients should be transferred using critical care transport to a center that can provide this care in the form of a pediatric ICU. Serious consideration should be given to securing the patient's airway prior to transport.

Pearls and pitfalls

Pearls

1. Consider infantile botulism when evaluating hypotonia in constipated infants.

Pitfalls

1. Failure to consider requesting antitoxin from the state health department/CDC.
2. Underestimating the potential for rapid progression of disease.

Selected references

Arnon SS, Schecter R, Maslanka SE, Jewell NP, Hatheway CL. Human botulism immune globulin for the treatment of infant botulism. *N Eng J Med* 2006;**354**:462–4671.

California Department of Public Health, Division of Communicable Disease Control. *Infant Botulism Treatment and Prevention Program.* www.infantbotulism.org (accessed 27 April 2010).

Centers for Disease Control and Prevention, Division of Bacterial and Mycotic Diseases. *Botulism in the United States, 1899–1996: Handbook for Epidemiologists, Clinicians, and Laboratory Workers.* Atlanta, GA: Centers for Disease Control and Prevention, 1998.

Fox CK, Keet CA, Strober JB. Recent advances in infant botulism. *Pediatr Neurol* 2005;**32**:149–154.

Long SS. Clostridium botulinum (botulism). In Long SS (ed.)

Principles and Practice of Pediatric Infectious Diseases, 2nd edn, Ch. 204. 2003: Philadelphia, PA: Churchill Livingstone.

Pickering LK, Baker CJ, Kimberlin DW, Long SS (eds.). Botulism and infant botulism (*Clostridium botulinum*). In *The Red Book: 2006 Report of the Committee on Infectious Diseases*, 27th edn. Elk Grove Village, IL: American Academy of Pediatrics, 2006, pp. 257–260 (also Red Book Online, last updated 5 January 2009).

Thilo EH, Townsend SF, Deacon J. Infant botulism at 1 week of age: Report of 2 cases. *Pediatrics* 1993;**92**:151–153.

Thompson JA, Filloux FM, van Orman CB, *et al.* Infant botulism in the age of botulism immune globulin. *Neurology* 2005;**64**: 2029–2032.

Torrens JK. *Clostridium botulinum* was named because of association with "sausage" poisoning. *Br Med J* 1998;**316**:151.

US Department of Health and Human Services, Public Health Services, Centers for Disease Control and Prevention. 2005 *Annual Summary of Notifiable Diseases*. Atlanta, GA: Centers for Disease Control and Prevention, 2005, www.cdc.gov/ncphi/disss/nndss/annsum/2005/05graphs.htm (accessed 28 April 2010).

Chapter 92

Central nervous system infection

Kathleen Ann Jobe

Introduction

Meningitis refers to inflammation of the meninges surrounding the brain as well as inflammation of the subarachnoid space. Meningitis is usually caused by hematogenous spread of organisms from the upper respiratory tract as well as other sites of infection. Inflammation and neurologic sequelae are the result of the host's inflammatory response. Pathogens in the CNS replicate quickly and release cell wall or membrane-associated compounds. This bacterial lysis causes the release of cytokines and other inflammatory mediators, which increase the permeability of the blood–brain barrier and result in injury to the vascular epithelium. The inflammatory process leads to cerebral edema, increasing intracranial pressure (ICP), as well as alteration of brain metabolism and of cerebrovascular autoregulation.

Aseptic meningitis refers to a non-pyogenic cellular response, with no specific cause of meningitis identified after initial evaluation. Often these cases are reclassified as viral meningitis when additional results become available.

Encephalitis represents infection and inflammation of the brain parenchyma. Viral agents are usually responsible and spread may be hematogenous or through neuronal routes. The most common cause is HSV-1 in the USA. In neonates, either HSV-1 or HSV-2 can be implicated. Hematogenous spread, direct extension through the cribiform plate, or spread through neuronal pathways have all been postulated as mechanisms of spread causing encephalitis.

Epidemiology

In the USA, bacterial meningitis affects approximately 3/100 000 people per year, and viral meningitis affects approximately 10/100 000 people per year. Worldwide, the incidence and etiology varies by age, immunologic status, and vaccination status (Table 92.1).

Bacterial meningitis has a significant mortality and morbidity. Neonates have the highest mortality, up to 30%, and 15–20% of children have long-term neurologic sequelae including seizures, developmental delay, and sensironeural hearing loss.

Bacterial meningitis is most likely to occur in the first month of life.

The major causes of bacterial meningitis in healthy children are the pneumococcus (*Streptococcus pneumoniae*) and the meningococcus (*Neisseria meningitidis*). Since the widespread use of *Haemophilus influenzae* type b vaccine, the pneumococcus is now the most common cause of invasive bacterial infection in children in the USA and other developed nations. Children <24 months old are now routinely vaccinated, decreasing the incidence of invasive pneumococcal disease, including meningitis, by 90%. In comparison, unvaccinated children <2 years have the highest rate of pneumococcal meninigitis (approximately 20/10 000). Of note, patients with cochlear implants have a 30-fold increase in the risk of pneumococcal infection if unvaccinated.

Annually 1400–3000 cases of invasive meningococcal disease occur in the USA. Death occurs in 10–14% of these, and significant sequelae in 11–19%. The incidence of invasive meningococcal disease peaks among infants younger than 1 year and adolescents 15–18 years of age. While the incidence of disease is highest in infants, the case fatality rate in adolescents is increased, at approximately 20%, compared with 5–11% in infants. The AAP now recommends vaccination for children aged 11–12 years, students entering high school or age 15 years and above, and college freshman living in dormitories.

H. influenzae type b infection is a disease of infancy. Babies in the first year of life have the highest rate, most occurring in children 3 months to 3 years of age.

H. influenzae infection is unusual in the first 3 months of life because the baby carries maternal antibodies. In areas where vaccination is common, diseases related to *H. influenzae* have been virtually eliminated in the pediatric population but occur sporadically in older unvaccinated individuals.

Viral meningitis is diagnosed when there is evidence of meningitis without bacterial pathogens in the CSF. In general,

A Practical Guide to Pediatric Emergency Medicine: Caring for Children in the Emergency Department, ed. N. Ewen Amieva-Wang (associate eds. Jamie Shandro, Aparajita Sohoni, and Bernhard Fassl). Published by Cambridge University Press.

Table 92.1. Epidemiologic, clinical, and pathogenic data for common viruses causing meningitis

Virus	Transmission	Age	Associated syndromes	Frequency	Pathway to CNS
Piconavirus–enterovirus, coxsackievirus, echovirus	Person to person: oral–fecal, inhalation	All ages; more common in children	Encephalitis, myocarditis, neonatal sepsis, poliomyelitis	Common	Blood
Arboviruses	Direct inoculation by vectors: mosquitoes, ticks	All ages	Encephalitis	Common	Blood
Rabies	Direct innoculation by bite of a rabid animal, transplant or inhalation	All ages	Encephalitis	Rare	Neuronal
Influenza	Person to person: inhalation	All ages	Encephalitis	Infrequent	Unknown
Herpes viridae	Person to person				
Herpes simplex	Vertical or horizontal	More common in neonates	Meningoencephalitis	Common	Blood, neuronal
Varicella zoster	Respiratory	Any age following primary infection	Cerebellitis, encephalitis, myelitis	Infrequent	

prognosis is good. Viral meningitis accounts for 26 000–42 000 hospitalizations in the USA each year. It affects predominantly infants <1 year and children 5–10 years of age and is caused by enteroviruses in 85–95%. In temperate climates, infection occurs during the warmest months of the year. In the tropics the incidence is without seasonal variability.

Clinical manifestations

Clinical manifestations of meningitis depend on age. The classic manifestations present in older children and adults are rarely seen in infants. Generally, the younger the child, the more subtle and atypical the presentation. A full fontanelle and normal neck flexion are the rule for infants presenting with meningitis. Symptoms are often subtle in infants; the most common clinical signs are temperature instability, irritability, poor feeding, and vomiting. While meningitis classically presents with fever, chills, photophobia, headache, and vomiting, signs in infants include fever, apnea, seizures, bulging fontanelle and rash. Seizures are the presenting complaint in one-third of cases of bacterial meningitis in children. Delirium and coma may develop with disease progression. With increasing inflammatory response in the CSF, nuchal rigidity develops and is the most consistent finding in older children and adults. Petechial and purpuric rash usually indicates meningiococcemia but can be present with any bacterial meninigitis.

Diagnosis

Treatment of the patient with suspected bacterial meningitis requires early recognition, rapid diagnosis, early aggressive antimicrobial therapy, and adjunctive therapy. Empiric antibiotics should be administered prior to definitive diagnosis for patients strongly suspected of having meningitis.

Delayed administration of antibiotics is associated with higher morbidity and mortality.

Consider starting antiviral therapy pending CSF results (Table 92.2).

Recommended laboratory studies include two blood samples for aerobic culture, CBC with differential and platelets, chemistry, and creatinine. If purpura is present, coagulation studies should be ordered. Antibiotic therapy should be initiated and adjunctive measures begun prior to lumbar puncture if the patient is unstable or there will be any significant delay in obtaining CSF, such as obtaining a CT scan. Blood cultures should be obtained prior to antibiotic therapy. There may be decreased sensitivity of CSF Gram stain and culture after antibiotics are given, but CSF findings of elevated WBC, decreased glucose, and increased protein will be unaffected. If the patient has been taking oral antibiotics previous to presentation, the sensitivity of the Gram stain and culture is decreased from 50–90% to 7–41%. The glucose will be elevated and the protein decreased compared with untreated patients. The Bacterial Meningitis Score cannot be applied to patients who have been taking antibiotics previously. Cytochemical studies are not affected.

A CT scan should be obtained prior to lumbar puncture in any patient with suspected increased ICP based on focal neurologic findings, papilledema, hemodynamic instability, history of CNS disease, immunocompromise, ALOC or sustained new-onset seizure activity.

Table 92.2. Cerebrospinal fluid findings in meningitis

Agent	Opening pressure (mmHg)	WBC (per μl)	Glucose (mg/dl)	Protein (mg/dl)	Microbiology
Bacterial meningitis	200–300	100–5000; >80% polymorphonuclear leukocytes	<40	>100	Specific pathogen demonstrated in 60% of Gram stains and 80% of cultures
Viral meningitis	90–200	10–300; lymphocytes	Normal; reduced in lymphocytic choriomeningitis and mumps	Normal but may be slightly elevated	Viral isolation, PCR assays
Tuberculous meningitis	180–300	100–500; lymphocytes	Reduced, <40	Elevated, >100	Acid-fast bacillus stain, large volume culture, PCR
Cryptococcal meningitis	180–300	10–200; lymphocytes	Normal, reduced in some	50–200	Cryptococcal antigen, culture
Aseptic meningitis	90–200	10–300; lymphocytes	Normal	Normal but may be slightly elevated	Negative findings on workup
Normal values	80–200	0–5; lymphocytes	50–75	15–40	Negative findings on workup

Ultimately, any patient with suspected CNS infection requires a spinal tap. Definitive diagnosis depends on Gram stain and culture of the CSF. The CSF analysis should also include WBC, glucose, and protein concentrations. While acid-fast and fungal stains are often not helpful, they may be useful in the immunocompromised host or in patients with basilar meningitis (suggestive of tuberculosis or fungal CNS infection). For patients with suspected HSV or enterovirus, PCR is most useful. Specific CSF analyses should be sent as indicated by patient's presentation, exposure history, and underlying medical condition. Additional CSF tubes may be held in the laboratory for further testing if initial evaluation does not lead to definitive diagnosis. Opening pressure in conjunction with WBC and differential can be helpful in discriminating between bacterial and viral or aseptic meningitis.

Current guidelines do not support the routine use of additional diagnostic testing such as latex agglutination, PCR, CSF procalcitonin, and CSF lactate concentration in bacterial meningitis. Normal CRP has a high negative predictive value for bacterial meningitis in patients with negative Gram stains in whom the physician is considering withholding antibiotics. In patients with suspected enteroviral meningitis, reverse transcription PCR has been shown to be more sensitive than CSF culture in detecting enterovirus. A rapid (<3 h) PCR for enteroviral RNA has been approved by the FDA. It has a sensitivity of 97% with 100% specificity and may be useful to ED decision making. Other viral PCR studies (e.g., West Nile virus) are not rapid and should be ordered on the basis of the patient's specific risks and local public health recommendations. A CSF sample for HSV PCR should be sent if encephalitis is suspected based on the presence of altered mental status or a focal neurologic examination.

Encephalitis in a neonate should be treated with acyclovir until proven not to be secondary to herpes.

Results of CSF studies can be difficult to interpret, as they vary depending on whether the child is evaluated early or late in the disease. In the neonate, a CSF WBC of >30/μL, CSF protein >100 mg/dl, and CSF glucose <30 mg/dl are consistent with bacterial meningitis.

The Bacterial Meningitis Score is a prediction tool for children with CSF pleocytosis. Children are considered to have a very low likelihood of bacterial meningitis if they *lack* all of the following:

- positive CSF Gram stain
- CSF neutrophil count <1000/dl
- CSF protein >80 mg/dl
- serum absolute neutrophil count of ≥10 000/dl
- history of seizure.

Aseptic meningitis

There is overlap of clinical and laboratory findings of bacterial meningitis with meningitis from other causes such as viruses, mycobacteria, fungi, or protozoa. If the CSF and blood cultures are negative for bacteria, aseptic meningitis should be considered with the aim of identifying treatable

Table 92.3. Age-based treatment based on organism

Age	Organisms	Treatment
<1 month	Group B streptococci, Gram-negative enteric bacteria, *Escherichia coli, Listeria monocytogenes* (zoonotic outbreaks), *Klebsiella, Enterobacter, Salmonella* spp.	Ampicillin plus cefotaxime or aminoglycoside
1–23 months	*Streptococcus pneumoniae, Neisseria meningitidis, Streptococcus agalactiae, Haemophilus influenzae* type b (unvaccinated)	Vancomycin plus a third-generation cephalosporin
>2 years	*S. pneumoniae, N. meningitidis*	Vancomycin plus a third-generation cephalosporin
Immunocompromised	Staphylococci, Gram-negative enteric bacteria, *Pseudomonas aeruginosa*	Cefotaxime or ceftriaxone plus vancomycin plus aminoglycoside if Gram-negative infection is suspected
Post-neurosurgery	*P. aeruginosa, Staphylococcus aureus, Staphylococcus epidermidis*	Vancomycin plus cefepime; vancomycin plus ceftazidime; vancomycin plus meropenum
CSF shunt	Coagulase-negative staphylococci, *S. aureus, P. aeruginosa*	Vancomycin plus cefepime; vancomycin plus ceftazidime; vancomycin plus meropenum
Basilar skull fracture	*S. pneumoniae, H. influenzae,* group A beta-hemolytic streptococci	Vancomycin plus ampicillin plus a third-generation cephalosporin
Penetrating trauma	*S. aureus*, coagulase-negative staphylococci, *P. aeruginosa*	Vancomycin plus cefepime; vancomycin plus ceftazidime; vancomycin plus meropenum

pathogens. These would include viruses such as HSV, which can cause meningoencephalitis, CMV, enterovirus, rubella, lymphocytic choriomeningitis virus, and varicella zoster virus. If the initial diagnosis of bacterial meningitis is in question, the patient should be treated with IV acyclovir until CSF results are complete. Parasitic infections such as toxoplasmosis or Chagas' disease can be considered if the patient has had appropriate exposure. Fungal infections should be considered in the immunocompromised patient. Spirochete infections such as Lyme disease (*Borrelia burgorferi*) or syphilis would also be in the differential if the child had risk factors.

Management

Use of dexamethasone in children with bacterial meningitis has caused controversy for many years. A recently published retrospective cohort study of 2780 children with bacterial meningitis showed no benefit in mortality or time to discharge in patients treated with corticosteroids.

The choice of initial antibiotic therapy should be guided by the patient's age and any premorbid conditions, such as immunocompromise or neurological procedure (Table 92.3). Patients with CSF shunt infections may require direct infusion of the antibiotic into the shunt reservoir or external ventriculostomy. Neurosurgical consultation is appropriate. Acyclovir should be used in addition to antibiotics pending the initial results of the lumbar puncture if there is concern for encephalitis. Altered mental status and focal neurologic findings are key features of encephalitis. Treatment can be further refined once these and other results are available.

Supportive treatment

Additional therapy should be directed at maintaining adequate oxygenation, preventing hypoglycemia, controlling seizure activity, decreasing intracranial pressure and preventing fluctuation of cerebral blood flow. Controlling fever, maintaining normal systemic blood pressure, raising the head of the bed 30°, correcting hyponatremia and SIADH should be standard therapy for patients with evidence of increased ICP or cerebral edema on CT. Use of mannitol and high-dose barbituate therapy may be considered. Hyperventilation to PCO_2 of 25–30 mmHg is no longer recommended because of the risk of lowering ICP at the expense of reducing cerebral blood flow.

Disposition

Pediatric patients with suspected bacterial meningitis should be admitted to hospital for IV therapy and monitoring. Patients with hemodynamic instability, ALOC, prolonged seizure activity, coma, or significant co-morbidities should be admitted to the pediatric ICU. Patients with aseptic meningitis may be discharged if they are stable and there is reliable follow-up. There remains variation in the management of patients with CSF that reveals mildly elevated WBC but other findings

Pearls and pitfalls

Pearls

1. The younger the child the less likely that classic symptoms of meningitis will be present.
2. Bacterial meningitis is most likely to occur in the first month of life.
3. Obtain a CT scan on any patient suspected to have a mass lesion or increased intracranial pressure; CNS disease; prolonged seizure activity; or with papilledema or focal neurologic findings.
4. Encephalitis in a neonate should be treated with acyclovir until proven not to be secondary to herpes.
5. The CSF of children with early bacterial meningitis can be equivocal; these children should be observed and/or treated until the diagnosis is definitive.
6. Children with viral meningitis may require supportive hydration and pain management.

Pitfalls

1. Failure to initiate antibiotic treatment in the very ill child awaiting CT or lumbar puncture. Delay in initiation of therapy is associated with increased morbidity and mortality.
2. If dexamethasone is used it must be given prior to or in conjunction with antibiotics.

consistent with viral meningitis. The patient may be admitted with ongoing antibiotics pending culture results, or discharged home with an empiric dose of an antibiotic with a long half-life (e.g., ceftriaxone), with close follow-up and strict return precautions. The family's reliability and social supports should be considered in the disposition plan.

Selected references

Fitch MT, Abrahamian FM, Moran GJ, Talan DA. Emergency department management of meningitis and encephalitis. *Infect Dis Clin North Am* 2008;**22**:33–52.

Mongelluzzo J, Mohamad Z, Ten Have TR, Shah SS. Corticosteroids and mortality in children with bacterial meningitis. *JAMA* 2008;**299**:2048–2055.

Nigrovic LE, Malley R, Masias CG, *et al.* Effect of antibiotic pretreatment on cerebrospinal fluid profiles of children with bacterial meningitis. *Pediatrics* 2008;**122**:726–730.

Tunkel AR. Practice guidelines for the management of bacterial meningitis. *Clin Infect Dis* 2004;**39**:1267–1284.

van de Beek D, de Gans J, McIntyre P, Prasad K. Corticosteroids for acute bacterial meningitis. *Cochrane Database Syst Rev* 2007;(1):CD004405.

Chapter 93

Gastroenteritis and diarrheal disease

Kimberly Schertzer

Introduction

Worldwide, there are an estimated 3–5 billion cases of acute gastroenteritis yearly, which contribute to the deaths of approximately 2 million children <5 years of age. Current reports suggest that 1 out of every 26 children in the USA will be hospitalized for diarrheal illness prior to age 5 years.

Mortality with gastroenteritis is typically related to dehydration rather than disease progression.

Gastroenteritis is a general term that involves irritation or infection of the GI tract and is typically characterized by nausea, vomiting, and diarrhea. There are several factors that make the treatment of pediatric diarrhea unique:

- it is more likely to be infectious in etiology
- children are more likely to become significantly dehydrated
- specific treatments that are employed for adults are not applicable to children with diarrheal illness.

Pathophysiology

Most pediatric diarrhea is caused by viruses, specifically rotavirus or norovirus strains, and bacteria make up a minority of cases (Table 93.1). Spread is usually fecal–oral and most often affects children 6 months to 2 years of age. Because of their close association with other diaper-wearing children, those who attend daycare are at increased risk for diarrheal illness and may be affected by local outbreaks. Immunocompromised children are at special risk for opportunistic infections.

In general, diarrhea can be categorized as osmotic, mechanical, secretory, or inflammatory:

- osmotic diarrhea is the result of poorly absorbed molecules shifting water into the intestinal lumen
- mechanical diarrhea is caused by increased bowel motility, often seen postoperatively or in disorders such as irritable bowel disease
- secretory diarrhea occurs when increased amounts of fluid are secreted into the bowel lumen
- inflammatory diarrhea is the result of decreased fluid resorption because of bowel wall inflammation.

Most pathogens cause a secretory or inflammatory diarrhea through direct action on the bowel itself. Pathogens that produce diarrhea through toxin production follow a relatively predictable time course, often causing diarrhea within 6–12 h. Bloody diarrhea tends to be the result of invasive organisms (Table 93.2).

Non-infectious causes of acute pediatric diarrhea include dietary disturbances (e.g., food allergies, lactose intolerance, vitamin or mineral deficiency), antibiotic use, intussusception, hemolytic uremic syndrome, inflammatory or irritable bowel disease and malabsorption.

The usual presentation of gastroenteritis is nausea and vomiting, followed by diarrhea. Isolated vomiting can be caused by multiple etiologies and while it can be an "early gastro," without a diarrheal component, the diagnosis of gastroenteritis should be made with caution. The major complication from gastroenteritis is dehydration. Most cases of acute gastroenteritis are mild and self-limited. However, several invasive pathogens, such as *Escherichia coli* O157:H7, can be deadly, and providers should carefully assess for a toxic-appearing child.

Table 93.1. Aged-based differential diagnoses of common infectious causes of pediatric diarrheal illness in North America

Infant/ toddler	Child (5–12 years)	Adolescent
Rotavirus	Norwalk virus	Norwalk virus
Adenovirus	*Giardia* sp.	*Campylobacter* sp.
Salmonella sp.		Enterotoxigenic *Escherichia coli* (ETEC)
Campylobacter sp.		Enterohemorrhagic *E. coli* (EHEC)
Yersinia sp.		*Salmonella* sp.
Giardia sp.		*Shigella* sp.

A Practical Guide to Pediatric Emergency Medicine: Caring for Children in the Emergency Department, ed. N. Ewen Amieva-Wang (associate eds. Jamie Shandro, Aparajita Sohoni, and Bernhard Fassl). Published by Cambridge University Press.

Table 93.2. Typical diarrheal pathogens and disease

Infectious agent	Incubation period	Main symptoms	Exposure	Diagnosis	Treatment
Non-invasive (toxin mediated)					
Staphylococcus aureus	1–6 h	Nausea, vomiting, loss of appetite, abdominal cramps; symptoms may appear more intense than with other pathogens	"Creamy foods" such as mayonnaise, cream puffs, potato salad; food that has been improperly stored	Clinical	Supportive; generally subsides after 1–2 days
Bacillus cereus (preformed toxin)	2–14 h	Vomiting early on; diarrhea and abdominal cramps may occur	Fried rice, vegetables, meats, gravies	Clinical	Supportive; usually resolves in <24 h
Invasive					
Entertoxigenic *Escherichia coli*	24–72 h	Abdominal cramps, low-grade fever, non-bloody diarrhea that may be prolonged (2–3 weeks)	Fecal–oral, contaminated surfaces, unsanitary water	Clinical	Supportive
E. coli O157:H7	3–8 days	Severe abdominal pain and tenderness, bloody diarrhea, often afebrile	Spinach, ground beef, processed food contaminated with livestock feces	Special stool culture (usually assessed at central/county level, although screening may be done at institution first); CBC for hemolysis or thrombocytopenia; renal function checked with BUN/creatinine	Supportive; avoid antibiotics as they predispose to thrombotic thrombocytopenic purpura/hemolytic-uremic syndrome
Campylobacter jejuni	2–5 days	Watery or hemorrhagic diarrhea	Contaminated food, undercooked poultry, wilderness water, birds	Stool culture	Supportive; usually resolves 5 days
Clostridium difficile	5–14 days	Fever, foul-smelling watery diarrhea (up to 10 times per day), abdominal cramps	Antibiotic-associated colitis in hospitalized children; may be spread easily.	*C. difficile* toxin is identified in the stool	Highly contagious; initial treatment in mild cases is to stop offending antibiotics; in more severe cases (e.g., when febrile), treatment is with antibiotics Infants <1 year usually colonized with *C. difficile*, do not get colitis
Giardia intestinalis	1–3 weeks	Watery diarrhea, steatorrhea, flatulence	Rural areas with poor sanitation and inadequate drinking water treatment, swallowed recreational water, daycare centers	Stool ova and parasite testing or stool antigen or antibody testing	Metronidazole

Table 93.2. *(cont.)*

Infectious agent	Incubation period	Main symptoms	Exposure	Diagnosis	Treatment
Rotavirus	24–72 h	Watery diarrhea, nausea/vomiting; may be febrile early in disease course	Seen particularly in winter months in children 6–24 months; spread is fecal–oral, common at daycare centers	Clinical, although special tests exist	Supportive; dehydration may occur quickly
Norovirus	24–72 h	Nausea, vomiting, abdominal cramps; may have associated headache and fever/chills	Seen in adults and older children, fecal–oral spread person to person; aerosolized emesis, "ready to eat" cold foods (salads, sandwiches), hotels, cruise ships, camps	Clinical	Supportive
Shigella spp.	24–48 h	Bloody, painful diarrhea, high fever; malaise and anorexia common	Person–person spread, poor hygiene, water-borne		Initially supportive; if prolonged, may consider antibiotics after excluding *E. coli* O157:H7 by testing first
Salmonella spp. (see Ch. 98 *S typhi* and typhoid fever)	8–24 h	Less vomiting seen than with other pathogens; may have mild fever, fatigue, myalgia; may cause a bloody diarrhea	Grade A eggs, poultry, unpasteurized milk, domestic pets	Generally clinical, although may test for stool culture on special agar Check blood cultures in infants as there is increased risk for bacteremia with salmonella-associated gastroenteritis	Supportive; antibiotics in high-risk patients including children <1 year
Yersinia enterocolitica	12–48 h	Diffuse, vague abdominal discomfort common; arthritis may occur	Contaminated food, water, milk, person–person spread,	Yersinia-selective agar	Supportive

Source: adapted from Bitterman, 2002; Centers for Disease and Prevention, 2008.

Clinical presentation

A detailed history of the duration of diarrheal illness, number and character of stools per day, ability to tolerate PO intake, and presence of vomiting is important. Breast-feeding status, recent travel, ill contacts, and attendance at daycare centers are also relevant historical items. Immunization status is important, as some children may have received immunization against a common pathogen, rotavirus.

The physical examination of a child with diarrheal illness should focus on the child's general appearance and estimated degree of dehydration.

Diagnostic studies

In general, no routine laboratory testing is indicated for children with diarrheal illness. Exceptions to this include severe dehydration, in which case electrolytes are useful. Stool cultures are of little benefit unless the stool is bloody or the diarrhea is prolonged, there has been recent foreign travel, or there is suspicion for a community outbreak. Stool cultures should be sent for immunocompromised children, who are also at special risk for *Entamoeba histolytica, Cyclospora* and *Cryptosporidium* spp. infections. These three pathogens are not identified by culture. Testing for ova and parasites is necessary to identify *E. histolytica*; special stains are needed to identify *Cryptosporidium* and *Cyclospora* spp. Pathogen-specific testing is indicated in cases of suspected *C. difficile* or giardia-associated diarrhea. Although a clinical diagnosis of rotavirus infection is usually sufficient, it may be helpful to definitively identify rotavirus as the responsible pathogen in children for whom it may change management.

Bloody diarrhea should be evaluated for the presence of *E. coli* O157:H7, which can cause hemolytic uremic syndrome. Screening is performed using stool cultures on a special MacConkey–sorbitol agar. Suspicious samples are then sent on to county or other agencies for further typing. Bloody diarrhea should also be cultured for *C. difficile*, as an associated pseudomembranous colitis may be seen in children who received prior antibiotic therapy. There is a higher likelihood of these illnesses in afebrile children, although children with significant *C. difficile* colitis will be febrile and appear ill. Febrile children with bloody diarrhea should have routine stool cultures sent for *C. difficile*, *E. coli* O157:H7, and *Shigella*, *Salmonella*, and *Campylobacter* spp. They should have samples drawn for CBC and BUN/creatinine drawn to screen for hemolytic uremic syndrome/thrombotic thrombocytopenic purpura and blood cultures to screen for bacteremia. They also warrant a referral to the outpatient pediatrician, as these symptoms may represent a first presentation of inflammatory bowel disorder.

Management

Regardless of etiology, the mainstay of treatment for children with diarrheal illness is the prevention and treatment of dehydration. Rehydration can occur orally, via nasogastric tube, or IV.

Oral rehydration therapy

Oral rehydration therapy (ORT) is the preferred method of rehydration for children who are mildly to moderately dehydrated. Commercial solutions are the preferred method. Other beverages are not recommended for use as rehydration solutions because they do not contain adequate ratios of electrolytes and their high osmolality may exacerbate diarrhea. Oral rehydration therapy is composed of two distinct stages. The first is rehydration, with a goal of rapidly replacing lost fluids and electrolytes over 3–4 h. This is accomplished by providing 50–100 ml/kg oral rehydration solution over 3–4 h. The second stage is maintenance fluids.

Intravenous rehydration therapy

Severely dehydrated children may benefit from IV fluid therapy. For otherwise healthy children, guidelines recommend an initial bolus of either normal saline or lactate Ringer's solution at a rate of 20 ml/kg. Multiple boluses may be required and following the results of an electrolyte panel may be of use. One exception to this principle is that frail or malnourished infants require a smaller starting bolus (10 ml/kg) because of their limited ability to increase their cardiac output. After an initial bolus of lactated Ringer's solution or normal saline, solutions containing dextrose are recommended, theoretically, to stop the catabolic cycle.

Medications

Antiemetic therapy

Historically, antiemetic use has been controversial because the side effects of older medications confounded the clinical examination. Newer serotonin antagonists (such as ondansetron) have been used successfully to augment ORT in pediatric populations without the sedative and extrapyramidal effects of older medications. The dose of oral ondansetron for pediatric gastroenteritis is 1.6 mg at ages 6 months to 1 year, 3.2 mg at 1–3 years, and 4 mg at 4–12 years. Approximating these doses may require splitting the orally dissolving tablet. Dose frequency is every 8 h regardless of age, and ORT may begin as soon as 15 min after administration. Other agents, such as dexamethasone, have not been shown to be effective. Despite the potential for decreasing hospitalizations, the CDC does not recommend routine use of antiemetics because of a fear of shifting focus away from rehydration and nutritional therapy. Nevertheless, a discharge prescription for oral ondansetron may enable parents to more effectively accomplish rehydration at home and should be strongly considered for all children >6 months of age with gastroenteritis-related vomiting.

Antidiarrheal agents

Antidiarrheal agents are contraindicated for all children because of the potential for significant morbidity and death.

Antidiarrheal agents should be reserved only for adults without fever or mucoid/bloody diarrhea and should not be prescribed for children.

Antibiotics

Antibiotics generally have a minimal role in pediatric diarrheal illness. First, most cases are viral in etiology. In addition, antibiotics cause complications in some kinds of diarrheal illness.

There is concern that the risk of development of hemolytic uremic syndrome may be increased in children with *E. coli* O157:H7 infection who are treated with antibiotics.

Providers should generally avoid prescribing antibiotics for diarrheal disease. Exceptions to this include children with presumptive traveler's diarrhea, children with significant co-morbidities, suspicion for sepsis, or high likelihood of giardiasis, shigella, or cryptosporidium infection. Children who receive antibiotics should have stool cultures performed as well as close follow-up arranged.

Dietary therapy

Dietary therapy plays a large role in discharge planning once dehydration is corrected. While many practitioners recommend a BRAT diet (bananas, rice, applesauce, toast) it may unnecessarily restrict nutrient intake. Instead, children are encouraged to return to their standard diets as soon as possible. Infants who are breast-fed should continue to nurse, those who are formula-fed should continue to receive their regular (non-diluted) formula, and those receiving solid foods should be encouraged to resume a relatively unrestricted diet. Foods containing high levels of simple sugars (sodas, juices, candy) may exacerbate diarrhea because of their high osmotic load and should be limited initially. For acute diarrheal illness, there is no indication for lactose restriction, although it may be considered for patients with diarrheal illness lasting several weeks.

Disposition

In most cases, diarrheal illness may be successfully treated at home once any initial dehydration has been corrected. Prior to discharge, parents should be educated about signs of dehydration, how to properly continue ORT at home and about using good hand hygiene to limit the spread of disease and reinfection. Further ED observation is useful in children with moderate dehydration to ensure fluid intake is tolerated and to monitor parental techniques for ORT.

Inpatient admission is warranted in severe dehydration, failure of ORT (including inadequate intake of oral rehydration solution or continued vomiting), if dehydration persists despite oral rehydration therapy, in the presence of another complicating illness, or when parents or caregivers are unable to provide adequate home care. Social concerns may also play a role in hospital admission.

Referral to a patient's pediatrician for further testing is indicated for children with diarrhea lasting more than 14 days or for those with a history of travel or freshwater stream exposure. These children should have stool sent for culture and ova and parasite analysis; while stool studies may be sent from the ED, results may take several days before they are available. Diarrhea lasting more than 14 days in immunocompetent children is less likely to be infectious and primary care evaluation is warranted to explore functional causes of frequent, loose stools.

Pearls and pitfalls

Pearls

1. Differing from adults, there is no role for antimotility therapy in pediatric diarrhea.
2. Most acute diarrheal illness in children is viral.
3. As a general rule, there is no role for antibiotic therapy.
4. Bloody diarrhea requires workup for *Escherichia coli* 0157:H7 testing and stool cultures.
5. Antiemetic therapy with serotonin antagonists may increase the success of oral rehydration therapy and decrease rates of hospitalizations.
6. Routine laboratory studies are seldom indicated in healthy children without signs of clinical dehydration.
7. Including glucose in rehydration fluids may stop the cycle of catabolism.

Pitfalls

1. There is no specific dietary recommendation for children with diarrhea. The commonly used BRAT diet has not been shown to impact the course of disease.
2. Failure to realize that children <1 year of age are regularly colonized with *Clostridium difficile* and in general do not develop *C. difficile* colitis.

Selected references

Bitterman RA. Gastrointestinal system: acute gastroenteritides. In Marx JA, Hockberger R, Walls R (eds.) *Rosen's Emergency Medicine: Concepts and Clinical Practice*, 5th edn, Vol. 2. Philadelphia, PA: Mosby. 2002.

Centers for Disease Control and Prevention. Managing acute gastroenteritis among children: oral rehydration, maintenance, and nutritional therapy. *MMWR Morb Mort Wkly Rep* 2003;**52**:1–16.

Centers for Disease Control and Prevention. Prevention of specific infectious diseases. *Yellow Book: Health Information for International Travel*, Ch. 4. Atlanta, GA: Centers for Disease Control and Prevention, 2008 http://wwwn.cdc.gov/travel/ybToc.aspx (accessed 1 June 2010).

Elliot EJ. Acute Gastroenteritis in Children. *Br Med J* 2007;**334**:35–40.

Ramaswamay K, Jacobson K. Infectious diarrhea in children. *Gastroenterol Clin North Am* 2001;**30**:611–624.

Ramsook C, Sahagun-Carreon I, Kozinetz CA, Moro-Sutherland D. A randomized clinical trial comparing oral ondansetron with placebo in children with vomiting from acute gastroenteritis. *Ann Emerg Med* 2002;**39**:397–403.

Chapter 94

Human immunodeficiency virus

Renee Y. Hsia, Joan Hwang Dunlop, and Benjamin R. Cohen

Introduction

In contrast to the devastation caused by HIV among children in the developing world, HIV now affects relatively few children in the USA as a result of increased screening of pregnant mothers and the introduction of prophylactic regimens of highly active antiretroviral therapy (HAART). The number of newly infected infants per year decreased to fewer than 100 in 2003. As of 2005, the CDC reported 6726 children under the age of 13 infected with HIV (only includes individuals living in the the 33 states and dependent areas with confidential name-based HIV/AIDS infection reporting). The rate of HIV among adolescents, however, continues to increase, and approximately 50% of new HIV infections in the USA occur among people between 13 and 24 years of age.

Infection may be transmitted by sexual contact, by percutaneous exposure, or by mother-to-child transmission perinatally and postnatally through breast-feeding. Mother-to-child transmission of HIV now accounts for almost all new infections in preadolescent children. The median age of onset of symptoms for untreated perinatally infected infants in the USA is approximately 12 to 18 months. However, some children may remain asymptomatic for 5 years and a rare few may delay symptoms until adolescence. Without therapy, two patterns of symptomatic infection in untreated children have been recognized. Rapid progressors are those 15–20% of children who manifest symptoms early on and die before 4 years of age. Most other untreated children have delayed onset of symptoms and survive beyond 5 years of age.

The diagnosis and management of HIV/AIDS in pediatric patients is complicated by four factors: (1) the difficulties confirming the diagnosis of HIV in early infancy; (2) the rapid disease progression in infants with vertically acquired infection; (3) the immature and naive immune system of pediatric patients, which influences disease expression differently in children compared with adults; and (4) the adverse effects of HIV on the developing nervous system and normal linear growth and weight gain. Before the introduction of HAART, median survival of children infected with HIV was 9 years. Now, studies show greater than 95% survival to 16 years of age.

This chapter addresses two aspects of the pediatric patient in respect to HIV as it relates to EPs in the diagnosis and management: (1) when to suspect HIV in a pediatric patient, and (2) how the diagnosis of HIV affects evaluation of common pediatric complaints.

New diagnosis

Manifestations of pediatric HIV infection are often non-specific. The diagnosis of HIV should be considered in a pediatric patient in certain cases including:

- history/physical consistent with opportunistic infection
- candidal thrush at >1 year of age; recurrent fungal and yeast infections
- maternal risk factors
- adolescent risk factors
- failure to thrive
- unexplained lymphadenopathy
- acute retroviral syndrome (a flu-like illness in the first 2 weeks of infection): may occur in adolescents but is rare in perinatally acquired HIV.

These primary manifestations of HIV and the development of opportunistic infections are now rare with the introduction of early testing and HAART, and most diagnoses will not be made in the ED. However, the EP should consider HIV testing in patients with one or more of the above symptoms and risk factors. It is important to note that the diagnosis of HIV infection in infants is complicated and strict guidelines for diagnosis exist and a pediatric virologist should dictate the workup. Perinatal transmission of the virus in pregnant women with HIV infection can be greatly decreased by initiating and adhering to perinatal treatment guidelines.

Known HIV infection

Prior to the widespread availability of HAART, the most common opportunistic infections among HIV-positive

A Practical Guide to Pediatric Emergency Medicine: Caring for Children in the Emergency Department, ed. N. Ewen Amieva-Wang (associate eds. Jamie Shandro, Aparajita Sohoni, and Bernhard Fassl). Published by Cambridge University Press.

children in the USA were serious bacterial infections (most commonly pneumonia and bacteremia), herpes zoster, disseminated *Mycobacterium avium* complex (MAC), *Pneumocystis jirovecii* pneumonia (PCP), and candidiasis (esophageal and tracheobronchial disease). Less commonly observed opportunistic infections included CMV disease, cryptosporidiosis, tuberculosis (TB), systemic fungal infections, and toxoplasmosis.

While there are limited data on infection rates in the post-HAART era, the EP should possess an expanded differential for common complaints of HIV-infected children (Box 94.1). In summary, children with HIV who are taking HAART are still likely to have an element of immunodeficiency despite normal CD4 cell counts. Immunologic monitoring of HIV-infected children differs from that in adults and depends on age-based criteria. Response to childhood vaccinations may be inadequate and HIV-infected children may still be susceptible to vaccine-preventable diseases. Also, remember that, like adults, teenagers can be non-compliant with medications and that children who rely on their parents to give them their medications may also be at risk for non-compliance.

Box 94.1. Expanded differential for common complaints in children with HIV

Chief complaint: cough

Differential for non-HIV-infected children still applies but also consider:

1. Slightly different predominance of bacterial pneumonia, e.g. the most common cause of bacterial pneumonia aged 3 weeks to 4 months is *Chlamydia trachomatis* (treated by macrolides), but HIV-positive counterparts have *Streptococcus pneumoniae* as the most common etiology (and should thus be empirically treated with a second- or third-generation cephalosporin).
2. *Pseudomonas* pneumonia, which is almost always nosocomial in the pediatric population, can be community-acquired in children with HIV
3. Tuberculosis is more likely to present as overwhelming, systemic-type infections.
4. *Pneumocystis jirovecii* (previously *P. carinii*) pneumonia (PCP) (this infection peaks at age 4 months and CD4 cell counts cannot be relied upon to determine a child's susceptibility to this infection; *every child* with suspected HIV infection should at least have a pulse oximetry documented at triage, even if their chief complaint is not respiratory in nature).
5. Histoplasmosis.
6. Coccidiomycosis (in endemic areas, such as the southwestern USA).

Follow-up

- Obtain TB exposure history.
- Check oxygen saturation for increased risk of *Pneumocystis jirovecii* pneumonia.
- Check radiograph.

Box 94.1. *(cont.)*

Chief complaint: fever

Differential for non-HIV-infected children still applies.

1. Children with HIV have a higher incidence of serious bacterial infection.
2. In neonates <1 month, hold particular suspicion for HSV (HSV) infection, as HIV-infected mothers with HSV have a higher rate of vertical transmission of the virus and may also be asymptomatic.

Considerations in workup and disposition

If performing lumbar puncture on a neonate, obtain PCR for HSV and give acyclovir IV.

HIV-positive children with normal CD4 cell count and fever who are clinically well-appearing can be discharged home with observation *if* they are followed closely by their physician; this practice will differ according to their infectious disease physician; others may prefer to take laboratory findings and if these are normal and the child is still well-appearing, then discharge home with close follow-up

Chief complaint: altered mental status

Differential for non-HIV-infected children still applies.

Consider:

- bacterial meningitis
- cryptococcal meningitis/meningoencephalitis (more commonly adolescents rather than infants)
- toxoplasmosis (usually congenitally acquired in infants; rarely acquired in young adults)
- tuberculosis
- HIV encephalopathy.

Considerations in workup and disposition

- Lower threshold for lumbar puncture.
- Consider studies for cryptococci in adolescent with altered mental status.

Chief complaint: diarrhea

Differential for non-HIV-infected children still applies but also consider:

- protozoal etiologies (particularly cryptosporidium and microsporidium)
- viral causes (such as CMV)
- medication side effects.

Considerations in workup and disposition

Send stool for ova and parasite screen, cryptosporidium, and viral studies

Chief complaint: rash

Differential for non-HIV-infected children still applies but also be aware of possibility of Stevens–Johnson syndrome, as trimethoprim–sulfamethexazole use becomes more common for PCP prophylaxis.

Considerations in workup and disposition

Examine mucous membrane involvement.

Special situation: co-infection with tuberculosis

While it is beyond the scope of this chapter to discuss the laboratory diagnoses of each HIV-associated disease listed in Box 94.1, several important points will be made here regarding TB in HIV-infected children:

- Because of the inability of most children to produce adequate sputum specimens, diagnosis is usually made by linking the child to an adult with proven TB infection, or by skin test. If the child is young, has evidence of pulmonary disease on chest radiography, and cannot produce sputum, three early morning gastric aspirate samples can be obtained to isolate the organism from culture. Unfortunately, 10% of children will have negative skin tests secondary to the short duration between exposure and active infection in HIV-positive children. Therefore, with a high index of suspicion based on history and physical examination, HIV-positive children should be presumed to have TB until proven otherwise, despite a negative acid-fast sputum stain.
- Younger children are more likely to present with disseminated disease rather than isolated cough, and TB must remain on the differential diagnosis for younger children presenting with fever, even if cough is not a prominent component.
- Importantly, TB is found in children with HIV infection without regard to degree of immunologic suppression. This may be because HIV-infected children usually reside with HIV-infected adults, who have a higher rate of TB and have a higher degree of infectivity.

Age-based management

This section discusses the treatment and management of children with suspected or confirmed HIV infection.

HIV-exposed infants

Only approximately 30% of HIV-positive infants will have a positive HIV PCR test at 48 h of age; 93% have a positive test by 2 weeks of age, and almost all HIV-infected infants have a positive PCR result by 1 month of age. Because HIV infection cannot be properly excluded until 1 month of age, an infant born to an HIV-positive mother (even if she has been taking antiretroviral drugs) should be considered HIV positive (even if the test at birth is negative) until the 1-month HIV PCR testing comes back.

Consequently, any HIV-exposed infant younger than 6 weeks presenting with fever, tachycardia, cough, or any other symptoms should be evaluated with a heightened level of suspicion for serious disease, with a low threshold to check blood, urine, CSF, and chest radiography for possible sources of infection. Because a small number of infants with perinatal exposure to HIV under zidovudine prophylaxis may become significantly anemic, a CBC can also screen for anemia.

Antimicrobial therapy should include coverage for bacterial infection, and an IV antiviral drug (e.g, acyclovir) should be strongly considered after CSF has been obtained for bacterial culture and HSV PCR.

Table 94.1. Degree of immunosuppression based on CD4 cell count by age

Immunosuppression	CD4 cell count (cells/μl)		
	<12 months	1–5 years	6–12 years
No evidence	>1500	>1000	>500
Moderate	750–1499	500–999	200–499
Severe	<750	<500	<200

Source: modified from Centers for Disease Control and Prevention 1994.

Pearls and pitfalls

Pearls

1. Children with HIV have a higher rate of serious bacterial infection than those without HIV, particularly in children <2 years of age.
2. The EP should have a low threshold for considering tuberculosis in any HIV-positive infant with risk factors and supporting clinical history, despite CD4 cell count.
3. Any HIV-exposed infant <4 weeks should be assumed HIV positive (and, in the ED setting, treated with heightened suspicion for more severe illness) until proven otherwise by PCR.
4. Consult pediatric ID for any child with HIV (known or highly suspected) if in doubt of workup and disposition.
5. Immune reconstitution syndrome with initiation of antiretroviral therapy does happen in children and has the potential to be more severe than that of adults, as they have an earlier and more significant increase in naive T cell subsets compared with adults.

Pitfalls

1. Using CD4 cell counts exclusively in HIV-positive children to stratify risk for complaints; these are not as reliable and are highly age dependent.
2. Opportunistic infection in children tends to reflect primary infection, rather than reactivation of latent disease. Therefore, diseases such as tuberculosis are more likely to present as extrapulmonary or disseminated disease rather than isolated cough.

Infants in whom HIV infection has been reasonably excluded

Infants older than 4 months who have received regular pediatric care, whose physicians have discontinued zidovudine and trimethoprim–sulfamethoxazole prophylaxis, can be treated as normal infants.

HIV-infected children and adolescents

The CD4 cell count should be obtained, ideally on the day of presentation, but more likely from recent records. Patients should be classified according to the degree of immunosuppression (Table 94.1). Patients with no evidence of immunosuppression should be treated as ordinary patients; however, TB, serious bacterial infections, and herpes zoster have been found across the spectrum of immune status, so they must be considered even if a patient has no other evidence of immunocompromise.

Disposition

Pediatric patients who would require hospitalization (e.g., fever in a neonate <1 month, hypoxemic patients) regardless of an HIV diagnosis should be admitted. Other criteria to consider for a child with HIV, however, include:

- severely immunologic suppression and fever, or suggestion of opportunistic infection
- hypoxemia
- inability to comply with or tolerate PO medications.

Selected references

American Academy of Pediatrics and Canadian Paediatric Society. Evaluation and treatment of human immunodeficiency virus-1-exposed infant. *Pediatrics* 2004;**114**:497–505.

Centers for Disease Control and Prevention. Guidelines for the use of antiretroviral agents in pediatric HIV infection. *MMWR Morb Mort Wkly Rep* 1998;**47**(RR-4):1–51.

Centers for Disease Control and Prevention. 1994 Revised classification system for HIV infection in children <13 years of age. *MMWR Morb Mort Wkly Rep* 1994;**43**(RR-12):1–10.

Centers for Disease Control and Prevention. *HIV/AIDS Surveillance Report, 2003.* Atlanta, GA: Centers for Disease Control and Prevention, 2004, pp. 1–46.

Pickering LK, Baker CJ, Kimberlin DW, Long SS (eds.). Human immunodeficiency virus. In *The Red Book: 2006 Report of the Committee on Infectious Diseases*, 27th edn. Elk Grove Village, IL: American Academy of Pediatrics, 2006 (also Red Book Online, last updated 5 January 2009).

Pickering LK, Baker CJ, Kimberlin DW, Long SS (eds.). Infection. In *The Red Book: 2006 Report of the Committee on Infectious Diseases.* 26th edn. Elk Grove Village, IL: American Academy of Pediatrics, 2006, pp. 378–401 (also Red Book Online, last updated 5 January 2009).

University of California at San Francisco. www.Hivinsite.com (accessed 28 April 2010).

US Department of Human Services. www.Aidsinfo.nih.gov (accessed 28 April 2010).

Working Group on Antiretroviral Therapy and Medical Management of HIV Infected Children. *Guidelines for the Use of Antiretroviral Agents in HIV-infected Adults and Adolescents.* Rockville, MD: National Pediatric and Family HIV Resource Center of the Health Resources and Services Administration, 2000.

Chapter 95

Musculoskeletal infections

Patrick Coleman and Michael A. Gisondi

Introduction

Pediatric musculoskeletal infections are a source of great morbidity if not promptly recognized and treated. The differential for a child presenting with joint or extremity pain is extensive (see also Ch. 106). The clinical challenge is to identify those patients who have osteomyelitis or septic arthritis. This chapter will focus on the diagnosis and management of the child who presents to the ED with fever and either joint or extremity pain, with emphasis on these two high-risk entities.

Clinical presentation

History

Pediatric osteomyelitis and septic arthritis most often arise from an underlying bacteremia. Patients may initially exhibit only constitutional signs and symptoms, such as fever, lethargy, malaise, decreased appetite, and irritability. Osteomyelitis, in particular, may present with systemic symptoms days before the joint or extremity pain begins. Septic arthritis typically progresses faster than osteomyelitis, classically with a recent onset of fever and a painful, swollen joint.

It is critical to inquire about all elements of a child's pain: location, duration, chronology, severity, and quality. If the patient is non-verbal, it is important to ask the family member why they believe their child is in pain. Common associated complaints may include limping, refusal to move an extremity, or refusal to bear weight. Children and parents should be asked about any antecedent trauma, which can often predispose children to musculoskeletal infections.

Given the vague symptoms associated with pediatric musculoskeletal infections, one must consider various other diagnoses (Table 95.1). For patients with joint pain, determine the number of joints involved.

The likelihood of septic arthritis decreases with the number of affected joints.

Polyarticular involvement is more commonly the result of an inflammatory etiology, such as juvenile rheumatoid arthritis (JRA) or acute rheumatic fever. Preceding enteritis or urethritis in the setting of joint pain suggests possible reactive arthritis. A history of tick exposure could hint at Lyme arthritis as a cause of joint pain.

Table 95.1. Causes of pediatric musculoskeletal pain

	Causes
Infectious	Septic arthritis, osteomyelitis, pyomyositis, Lyme disease, cellulitis, septic bursitis
Traumatic	Fractures, dislocations, traumatic synovitis
Neoplastic	Bone tumors, leukemia, metastases
Inflammatory	Juvenile idiopathic arthritis, acute rheumatic fever, reactive arthritis, transient synovitis
Hematologic	Sickle cell disease, hemophilia (hemarthrosis)
Other	Legg–Calvé–Perthes disease, slipped capital femoral epiphysis

Physical examination

The general appearance of a child with a musculoskeletal infection may range from well to systemically toxic. Fever may or may not be noted at the time of ED presentation. The affected limb or joint should be evaluated for localized tenderness, edema, erythema, or decreased range of motion. Physical signs are more focal and easily identified in older children. While the patient may complain of a specific pain, a thorough head to toe examination is particularly valuable in younger patients to assess for other sources of infection.

In the patient with a septic arthritis, ranging the affected joint or applying an axial force may elicit significant pain. The joint should be palpated to assess for the presence of an effusion. Observe if the patient limps secondary to pain.

In neonates, clinical signs are decreased extremity movement, edema, and erythema; ranging the affected limb may elicit more pain than in older children, reflecting the propensity of acute hematogenous osteomyelitis to cause a concurrent septic arthritis in this population.

A Practical Guide to Pediatric Emergency Medicine: Caring for Children in the Emergency Department, ed. N. Ewen Amieva-Wang (associate eds. Jamie Shandro, Aparajita Sohoni, and Bernhard Fassl). Published by Cambridge University Press.

Osteomyelitis

Osteomyelitis refers to progressive bone inflammation and destruction by a pyogenic organism. Non-specific symptoms and diagnostic tests result in delays in diagnosis and treatment of this clinical entity, which can ultimately produce substantial morbidity. Less common in children than adults, osteomyelitis accounts for roughly 1% of pediatric hospitalizations. Osteomyelitis has typically been characterized as:

- acute <2 weeks
- subacute 2–6 weeks
- chronic >6 weeks.

Pathogenesis

The pathogenesis may be through:

- hematogenous seeding of the bone
- direct inoculation
- spread from a contiguous infection.

Acute hematogenous osteomyelitis affects children, with the highest incidence among patients 3 months to 16 years of age. Boys are affected twice as often as girls. The infection follows an episode of bacteremia, during which the bone is inoculated. Long-bone metaphyses are most often the sites of infection, with the tibia and femur being the two most common locations of seeding. Infections of the spine or other axial skeleton are less common.

The inciting organism induces a suppurative process within the bony trabeculae and subcortical bone, which subsequently spreads laterally to the cortex through the Haversian systems and Volkmann canals. As purulence expands through vascular channels, resultant edema and infectious mediators raise intraosseous pressure and occlude local blood flow, ultimately leading to ischemia and necrosis. As bone cortex is more loosely attached in children, peripheral spread of disease can lift the cortex to form a subperiosteal abscess. Involvement of the periosteum stimulates vigorous compensatory growth of new periosteum, termed involucrum. As the infection propagates within the bone, pain becomes more localized to the affected area.

The unique blood supply of newborns accounts for different features of disease in this population. In these patients, nutrient arterial vessels from the metaphysis perforate the epiphyseal growth plate. This vasculature can facilitate the spread of infection to the adjacent joint space, resulting in a concomitant septic arthritis. Around the first year of life, these metaphyseal capillaries atrophy, in effect sealing off the joint space from contiguous spread of osteomyelitis. As the skeleton further matures, the bony cortex and periosteum become thicker and denser. As a result, the infection is more contained and less likely to rupture through the periosteum to the surrounding soft tissues.

Uncommon pathogenic mechanisms of osteomyelitis in children include direct inoculation through trauma and the spread of infection from a contiguous structure. Infection from a contiguous structure is more common in the adult population, occurring within the context of such predisposing states as diabetes and peripheral vascular disease. Infection spreads inward towards the bone marrow, as opposed to the outward propagation of acute hematogenous osteomyelitis.

Table 95.2. Common causes of musculoskeletal infections by age

	Osteomyelitis	Septic arthritis
Neonates	*Staphylococcus aureus*, group B streptococci, enteric Gram-negative rods	*S. aureus*, group B streptococci, enteric Gram-negative rods
Children[a]	*S. aureus*, *Kingella kingae*, *Streptococcus pyogenes*	*S. aureus*, *K. kingae*, *S. pyogenes*, *Streptococcus pneumoniae*
Adolescents	*S. aureus*, *S. pyogenes*	*S. aureus*, *S. pyogenes*, *N. gonorrhoeae*

[a] *H. influenzae* type b or *S. pneumoniae* may cause osteomyelitis and septic arthritis in unimmunized or incompletely immunized children.

The principle offending organism in pediatric acute hematogenous osteomyelitis is *Staphylococcus aureus*, which is responsible for 40–80% of infections. Common precipitants of neonatal sepsis such as group B streptococci and *Escherichia coli* are more likely to cause osteomyelitis in neonates (Table 95.2). The fastidious Gram-negative organism *Kingella kingae* is increasingly identified as a cause of osteomyelitis in children under 5 years of age. *Haemophilus influenzae* type b is no longer a common cause of osteomyelitis since the development of the highly effective Hib vaccine. More recently, community-associated methicillin-resistant *S. aureus* (CA-MRSA) has emerged as a prime inciting agent in certain areas. The prevalence of CA-MRSA within specific communities now virtually dictates the choice of empiric therapy for any skin or soft tissue infection.

Other specific patient populations are at risk for bone infections from specific pathogens. Osteomyelitis caused by puncture wounds to the feet is most often caused by *Pseudomonas aeruginosa* and *S. aureus*. Teenagers who are intravenous drug users are also at risk for *Pseudomonas* bone infections. The presence of orthopedic hardware may serve as a nidus for infection by *S. aureus*, *Staphylococcus epidermidis*, or *P. aeruginosa*. Children with sickle cell disease are predisposed to osteomyelitis from *Salmonella* spp., which accounts for up to 60–80% of cases in this particular population. Animal bites, particularly those from cats and dogs, can potentially lead to osteomyelitis from *Pasteurella multocida*.

Diagnostic studies

Laboratory tests for suspected osteomyelitis should include a white blood count, ESR, CRP, and blood cultures. Leukocyte count may be normal or elevated. Both ESR and CRP are sensitive markers frequently elevated in bone infections, but each lacks specificity. Blood cultures are positive in roughly 50% of cases.

Imaging tests are the primary means of diagnosing osteomyelitis. The initial study should include plain radiographs of the affected area. Radiographic changes consistent with osteomyelitis can take up to 1 to 2 weeks to manifest. Characteristic findings on plain radiographs include osteolysis, periosteal hypertrophy and elevation, and sequestra.

A CT scan can better define the anatomic area of involvement. Unfortunately, it suffers from the same lag time as plain radiographs. For early detection, MRI and radionuclide skeletal scintigraphy (bone scanning) are more sensitive imaging modalities; MRI is emerging as the test of choice, as it achieves the highest resolution of all available tests, clearly defining the affected anatomic structures. Bone scans are quite sensitive for osteomyelitis and can detect bone infection after 2–3 days; these are particularly useful for patients without localizing findings. However, false-positive scans can result from soft tissue infection, trauma, or tumors.

After admission, direct tissue diagnosis through percutaneous needle aspiration or bone biopsy can help to guide specific antibiotic therapy. Real-time PCR is also emerging as a potential means of identifying the inciting pathogen.

Management

Initial empiric parenteral broad-spectrum antibiotic therapy is given in all cases of presumptive osteomyelitis. Antibiotic regimens should treat likely etiologic agents given the patient's epidemiologic factors. If possible, blood cultures should be obtained prior to antibiotic therapy for use in guiding later treatment. Most antibiotic regimens are 4 to 6 weeks in length.

For neonates and infants, empiric therapy should consist of an antistaphylococcal agent (e.g., nafcillin or vancomycin) and a third-generation cephalosporin (e.g., cefotaxime). Depending on the local prevalence of CA-MRSA, older infants and children may be treated with nafcillin, clindamycin, or vancomycin. A third-generation cephalosporin should be added to the treatment regimen for patients who have not received Hib immunization. Patients with sickle cell disease should also receive a third-generation cephalosporin to cover *Salmonella* sp. Osteomyelitis resulting from puncture wounds through a shoe should include coverage for *Pseudomonas* with either a quinolone in teenagers (e.g., ciprofloxacin) or a third- or fourth-generation cephalosporin (e.g., ceftazidime or cefipime).

Surgical debridement is often necessary for patients who fail antimicrobial therapy or for chronic osteomyelitis.

Septic arthritis

Septic arthritis refers to pyogenic invasion and subsequent destruction of the joint space. Early diagnosis and prompt treatment are vital to avoid osteonecrosis, abnormal bone growth, and impaired joint mobility. Most cases of pediatric septic arthritis occur in children under age 5 years. The cumulative incidence for septic arthritis and osteomyelitis in children under age 12 years is approximately 1/10 000 per year.

Pathogenesis

Septic arthritis in children occurs most often as a result of hematogenous deposition of bacteria into the vascular synovial membrane. However, like osteomyelitis, it may also result from direct inoculation from penetrating trauma. In children, it is most often a monoarticular process.

Septic arthritis may occur in concert with osteomyelitis, as an infection of either the bone or the adjacent joint may spread to the other structure. This phenomenon is particularly prevalent in newborns because of the existence of the metaphyseal arteries, which perforate the epiphysis and facilitate the spread of infection from bone to joint. The knee and the hip are most commonly affected in children. Predisposing conditions include joint trauma, hemoglobinopathies, host phagocytic defects (chronic granulomatous disease), and intravenous drug use and/or sexual activity in the teenage population.

The vascular synovial tissue lacks a limiting basement membrane, thereby allowing blood-borne bacteria to seed the synovial space. Once gaining access to the joint space, the bacteria proliferate and trigger an acute inflammatory response. If the infection is not quickly cleared, the immune response can result in joint destruction. The accumulation of fluid within the joint may also result in pressure necrosis.

The most prevalent etiologic agent in pediatric septic arthritis is *S. aureus*. As with osteomyelitis, septic arthritis from CA-MRSA is increasing in prevalence. Neonates are susceptible to infections from group B streptococci and Gram-negative enteric bacilli. In children younger than 2 years, group A streptococci and *K. kingae* are also fairly common pathogens. *S. aureus* and group A streptococci continue to predominate in older children (Table 95.2). Older children are also prone to septic arthritis from *Neisseria gonorrhoeae* as they become sexually active. *H influenzae* type b, once a common cause of infectious arthritis, has declined in prevalence since the advent of the Hib vaccine.

Diagnostic studies

Joint fluid analysis is the cornerstone of the diagnosis of septic arthritis. Blood tests are inconsistent. Routine tests in suspected cases should include a WBC, ESR, CRP, and blood cultures. Both ESR and CRP are fairly sensitive and may be used to monitor treatment response.

As the majority of cases of pediatric septic arthritis result from hematogenous seeding during an episode of bacteremia, the EP must investigate for causes of the initial infection. This search may mandate culturing other body fluids, obtaining urine, throat, sputum, cervical, or urethral cultures as necessary. Blood cultures are positive in 50% of cases. Synovial tissue biopsy during subsequent arthroscopy may have a greater yield than synovial fluid culture, for example in gonococcal disease.

Patients with suspected septic arthritis should undergo arthrocentesis as soon as possible both in an effort to isolate the causative organism and to potentially remove the purulent material. Joint fluid should be analyzed for culture and Gram stain, leukocyte count, glucose, protein, and lactate. Culture sensitivity ranges from 30 to 90%. Septic arthritis has classically been associated with a joint WBC >50 000/μl with a predominance of polymorphonuclear leukocytes; however, this cutoff value lacks the sensitivity to adequately exclude septic arthritis. Synovial fluid may have a low glucose and an elevated protein and lactate.

In the child with a limp and hip pain, it is crucial to distinguish potential septic arthritis from the more common and more benign transient synovitis of the hip. A recent prospective study comparing these two diseases found a fever >38.5°C to be the best predictor of septic arthritis, followed in order by an elevated CRP, an elevated ESR, refusal to bear weight, and an elevated serum WBC. Patients with all five predictive factors had a 98% chance of having septic arthritis; those with four had a 93% chance, and those with three had an 83% chance.

Plain radiographs are mostly useful to exclude other causes of joint pain (e.g., fractures) but may identify soft tissue swelling or joint space widening resulting from joint effusion. Ultrasound can be used both diagnostically to confirm the presence of joint fluid and therapeutically as a guide during arthrocentesis. Use of MRI readily establishes all surrounding anatomy and is quite sensitive for the early detection of joint fluid.

Management

A strong suspicion of septic arthritis mandates prompt initiation of appropriate IV antibiotic therapy. In neonatal septic arthritis, empiric therapy must include coverage for *S. aureus*, group B streptococci, and Gram-negative enteric bacilli. A good initial regimen consists of a beta-lactamase-resistant antistaphylococcal penicillin, such as nafcillin, combined with an aminoglycoside or third-generation cephalosporin, such as cefotaxime.

Outside of the neonatal age group, empiric antibiotic therapy may include a third-generation cephalosporin and nafcillin, vancomycin or clindamycin, depending on the local prevalence of MRSA. Antibiotic choices can later be adjusted based on culture susceptibilities. Uncomplicated septic arthritis is treated for 3 to 4 weeks.

Early orthopedic consultation is always advisable to determine whether the infection necessitates open surgical drainage and irrigation. Some experts advocate surgical drainage for all infants and children with septic arthritis. Others espouse a more conservative approach, saving operative management for hip or shoulder disease, lack of clinical improvement, large amounts of purulence, or concomitant osteomyelitis.

Disposition

Any patient with a musculoskeletal infection should be admitted for IV antibiotics. Orthopedics should be promptly consulted to assist in management and to decide whether the particular patient would benefit from operative intervention.

Patients with a clinical appearance suggestive of septic arthritis but equivocal findings on arthrocentesis should be admitted for observation and antibiotics. Patients with vague symptoms and joint fluid findings not consistent with septic arthritis may be discharged with follow-up. Children with inconsistent examination findings and low inflammatory markers can also be discharged. The guardians of any discharged patient should be advised to return to the ED or contact their primary physician for progressive or worsening symptoms, or recurrent fevers.

Pearls and pitfalls

Pearls

1. Musculoskeletal infections in pediatric age groups most often arise from hematogenous seeding; consider why this patient has bacteremia in the first place.
2. Polyarticular involvement is more suggestive of an inflammatory etiology, such as juvenile rheumatoid arthritis or acute rheumatic fever, rather than an infectious source.
3. In newborns, the metaphyseal blood vessels cross the epiphyseal growth plate, allowing for concurrent osteomyelitis and septic arthritis.
4. Osteomyelitis is primarily diagnosed radiographically. Septic arthritis is primarily diagnosed through synovial fluid analysis.

Pitfalls

1. Failure to realize that plain films, blood tests, and physical examination findings all lack specificity in the diagnosis of musculoskeletal infections.
2. Failure to maintain a high index of suspicion for musculoskeletal infections in neonates; signs are often not well localized.
3. Failure to realize that a synovial fluid WBC <50 000/μl is not sensitive enough to exclude septic arthritis. Many cases will be missed with strict reliance on this cutoff value.

Selected references

Caird MS, Flynn JM, Leung YL, *et al.* Factors distinguishing septic arthritis from transient synovitis of the hip in children. *J Bone Joint Surg Am* 2006;**88**:1251–1257.

Chometon S, Benito Y, Chaker M, *et al.* Specific real-time polymerase chain reaction places *Kingella kingae* as the most common cause of osteoarticular infections in young children. *Pediatr Infect Dis J* 2007;**26**:377–381.

Lew DP, Waldvogel FA. Osteomyelitis. *N Engl J Med* 1997;**336**:999–1007.

Li SF, Cassidy C, Chang C, *et al.* Diagnostic utility of laboratory tests in septic arthritis. *Emerg Med J* 2007;**24**:75–77.

Chapter 96

Sexually transmitted diseases

Stephanie Cooper

Introduction

Adolescents are the population most at risk for acquiring sexually transmitted diseases (STDs) relative to all other age groups. Sexual activity and experimentation often begin during the teenage years; approximately 50% of high school students report having engaged in intercourse. In fact, almost half of the annually reported 19 million STD infections are acquired among those aged 15 to 24 years. This chapter will focus on risk factors, symptoms, and the EP's role in treating gonorrhea, chlamydia, syphilis, and human papillomavirus (HPV) within adolescent populations.

Adolescent risk

Teenagers may be particularly vulnerable to contracting STDs for a variety of reasons. They may not understand which behaviors transmit STDs, and they may experience obstacles to gaining further knowledge. In addition, young adults may encounter barriers to accessing healthcare, such as lack of transportation and lack of insurance/ability to pay. Concerns about confidentiality may discourage adolescents from seeking treatment. When young adults do encounter health practitioners, they may lack the language to report their symptoms or may not understand what their symptoms signify.

Teenagers may be more likely to engage in sex without barrier contraception, and to have sexual encounters with multiple partners. In addition, physiologic susceptibility to infection – such as increased ectopy of the teenage cervix – may lead to increased incidence of STDs among young people. For these reasons and others, the incidence of many STDs is highest among adolescents.

If an STD is discovered in a non-sexually active child, it should prompt concern for sexual abuse, and child protective services should be immediately involved. Gonorrhea, chlamydia, and syphilis acquired after the neonatal period are almost always indicative of sexual contact.

Chlamydial infection

Chlamydia trachomatis is the most common STD among adolescents, and a significant cause of infertility.

The incubation period for genital tract chlamydia is 1 to 3 weeks after exposure. *C. trachomatis* is transmitted through sexual activity but can also be spread vertically from mother to newborn.

Incidence

The rates of both chlamydia and gonorrhea are highest among adolescents aged 15 to 19 years. One in five sexually active females are carriers of chlamydia. Rates are higher among minorities and socioeconomically disadvantaged young adults. Compared with all other age cohorts in the US population, chlamydia is most prevalent in those aged 15–24 years.

Risk factors

Risk factors predictive of chlamydial infection include unprotected sex, history of STD, multiple sex partners, age 15 to 24 years, low socioeconomic class, and exchange of drugs for sex or money.

Chlamydia in newborns

The transmission rate from infected mothers to neonates is approximately 50–66%. Chlamydia in newborns can present as chlamydial pneumonia, or as chlamydial conjunctivitis. The incubation period of the neonatal chlamydial infection can take weeks to months (Ch. 155).

Complications/morbidity

Chlamydia can lead to pelvic inflammatory disease (PID), which may cause scarring of fallopian tubes and consequent ectopic pregnancy. As such, chlamydia is a major cause of infertility. The infection may progress to salpingitis, tubo-ovarian abscess, and possible abscess rupture, leading to peritonitis and even sepsis.

A Practical Guide to Pediatric Emergency Medicine: Caring for Children in the Emergency Department, ed. N. Ewen Amieva-Wang (associate eds. Jamie Shandro, Aparajita Sohoni, and Bernhard Fassl). Published by Cambridge University Press.

Clinical presentation

Most carriers of chlamydia are asymptomatic. However, females infected with chlamydia may present with cystitis, urethritis, cervicitis, dyspareunia, and increased or malodorous vaginal discharge. The infection may ascend to the upper genital tract, causing abdominal pain. Males may present with dysuria, urethral discharge, abdominal pain, proctitis, epididymitis, orchitis, and rectal discharge.

Diagnostic studies

Practitioners should obtain urethral cultures in males and cervical cultures in females. When available, urine DNA probes can be utilized. Urine should be obtained in both sexes, and a pregnancy test is mandatory for females. The presence of white blood cells in the urine of asymptomatic males should direct further diagnostic testing for STDs. Asymptomatic partners of culture-proven patients can be presumptively treated. Because of the silence of its symptoms, the severity of potential sequelae, and the incidence of chlamydia in young people, the CDC recommends screening all sexually active women <26 years.

Management

The drug of choice for isolated lower genital tract chlamydial infection is azithromycin 1 g PO once (for patients >45 kg). This one-time treatment is advantageous as it avoids the potential for medication non-compliance. Doxycycline 100 mg BID for a week is a reasonable second option. Fluoroquinolones should be avoided because of increasing resistance. Patients should also be treated for gonorrhea, given the 20–40% incidence of co-infection. Sexual partners should also be treated to prevent repeat infection.

Gonorrhea

Neisseria gonorrhoeae (gonococcus) is an intracellular Gram-negative diplococcus spread by sexual contact. Gonorrhea is second to chlamydia as the most commonly reported STD, and frequently infects sexually active adolescents. The incubation period is usually 2 to 7 days after exposure. Gonorrhea can also be acquired neonatally, in vertical transmission during childbirth.

Incidence

The incidence of gonorrhea is higher in women 15–19 years of age than in all other female age cohorts. Within the teenage cohort, rates are higher in African-Americans than in other racial and ethnic groups. An estimated 1–5% of sexually active females are asymptomatic carriers of gonorrhea.

Risk factors

Risk factors for gonorrhea include multiple sex partners, lack of barrier contraception, history of STDs, low socioeconomic status, early age of sexual activity, and substance use.

Complications/morbidity

Infertility in both males and females is the most feared consequence of gonorrheal infection. In females, gonorrhea can progress to PID, causing salpingitis, tubo-ovarian abscess, tubal scarring, and ectopic pregnancy. Not surprisingly, the likelihood of infertility correlates with repeated infection. In males, infertility can result from long-term epididymitis and orchitis. In both sexes, gonorrhea can lead to disseminated gonococcal infection, with signs including fever, rash, arthralgias, polyarthritis, septic arthritis, and meningitis. Gonococcal conjunctivitis can rapidly progress to blindness.

Clinical presentation

Adult symptoms of gonorrheal infection are similar to chlamydial infections. Males may present with dysuria, penile discharge, urethritis, or epididymitis. Females may present with vaginal discharge, dysuria, cystitis, dyspareunia, and abdominal pain. Both sexes may present with sore throat and joint pain.

Management

Based on the growing incidence of resistance (6.7% of all cases), 2007 CDC guidelines no longer recommend fluoroquinolones. Instead, cephalosporins are the drug of choice.

Pelvic inflammatory disease

Both the gonococcus and *C. trachomatis* are leading causes of PID, an ascending infection of the female reproductive tract that occurs when bacteria spread from the vagina to the uterus, fallopian tubes, and ovaries. An estimated 10–20% of untreated gonorrhea and chlamydial cervicitis may progress to PID. Less frequently, PID may develop from bacteria introduced to the vagina and/or cervix during IUD placement and other gynecological procedures. Pelvic inflammatory disease is common and serious and may evolve into salpingitis, tubo-ovarian abscess, and peritonitis.

Risk factors

Risk factors associated with PID include sexually active woman under 25 years, multiple sex partners, history of STDs, lack of barrier protection, and frequent vaginal douching (which alters the normal vaginal flora). Treatment of sexual partners is crucial to avoid reinfection.

Clinical presentation

Signs and symptoms of PID are widely variable but include pelvic pain, malodorous vaginal discharge, vaginal bleeding, chills, fever, nausea, dyspareunia, low back pain, and dysuria. Lower abdominal pain is the most common presenting complaint. However, PID may present asymptomatically.

Diagnosis

Pelvic inflammatory disease may be elusive to diagnose because of its varied presentation (Box 96.1). Minimal criteria include uterine or adnexal tenderness (often bilateral) and

Box 96.1. Criteria for clinical diagnosis of pelvic inflammatory disease

Minimum criteria

Empiric treatment of pelvic inflammatory disease (PID) should be initiated in sexually active young women and others at risk of sexually transmitted infections if the following **minimum criteria** are present and no other cause(s) for the illness can be identifed:

- uterine or adnexal tenderness
- cervical motion tenderness.

Additional criteria

More elaborate diagnostic evaluation often is needed because incorrect diagnosis and management might cause unnecessary morbidity. These additional criteria may be used to enhance the specificity of the minimum criteria above. Additional criteria that support a diagnosis of PID include the following:

- oral temperature greater than 38.3°C (101°F)
- mucopurulent cervical or vaginal discharge
- presence of white blood cells on saline microscopy of vaginal secretions
- increased ESR
- increased CRP
- laboratory documentation of cervical infection with *Neisseria gonorrhoeae* or *Chlamydia trachomatis.*

Most women with PID have mucopurulent cervical discharge *or* evidence of white blood cells on a microscopic evaluation of a saline preparation of vaginal fluid. If the cervical discharge appears normal *and* no white blood cells are found on the wet preparation, the diagnosis of PID is unlikely, and alternative causes of pain should be sought.

Most specifc criteria

The most specific criteria for diagnosing PID include:

- endometrial biopsy with histopathologic evidence of endometritis
- transvaginal ultrasonography or MRI showing thickened, fluid-filled tubes with or without free pelvic fluid or tubo-ovarian complex
- laparoscopic abnormalities consistent with PID.

A diagnostic evaluation that includes some of these more extensive studies may be warranted in selected patients.

Source: adapted from Pickering *et al.*, 2006; Centers for Disease Control and Prevention, 2006. The CDC website (http://www.cdc.gov/std/treatment) contains the latest recommendations.

cervical motion tenderness. Additional criteria which support the diagnosis are listed in the box. The diagnosis of PID may be confirmed via laparoscopy and transvaginal ultrasound, revealing tubo-ovarian abscess or thickened, fluid-filled fallopian tubes.

Management

The majority of patients with PID can safely be treated as outpatients. Recommended oral antibiotic regimens are listed in Table 96.1.

Treating STDs early in their course can prevent PID. Treatment of partners is essential to avoid repeat infection. Partners should be treated empirically for gonorrhea and chlamydia if they have had sex with the patient within 2 months of onset of PID symptoms. Sex should be avoided until all partners fully complete the recommended antibiotic regimen. Additionally, patients should be cautioned to seek testing for other STDs, including HIV, and should be educated about barrier protection and other methods to reduce risk of STD transmission and reinfection.

Complications

Because of the potential for tubal infection and scarring, PID is a significant cause of infertility, ectopic pregnancy, and chronic pelvic pain. Incidence of infertility increases with prior PID infections; an estimated 1 in 10 women with PID become infertile. Other complications include tubo-ovarian abscess formation, Fitz-Hugh–Curtis syndrome (perihepatitis) and complications to the fetus, including growth retardation and septic abortion.

Disposition

Hospitalization is indicated for PID in certain circumstances:

- toxic appearance (high fever, ongoing nausea and vomiting)
- tubo-ovarian abscess
- no response to, or unable to take, oral medications
- inability to rule out another surgical condition (e.g., appendicitis)
- pregnancy
- immunocompromise
- concerns about loss of follow-up and inability to complete the treatment regimen.

Human immunodeficiency virus

In 2004, the CDC reported 4883 people aged 13 to 24 diagnosed with HIV/AIDS, accounting for 13% of total diagnoses. The prime spread of HIV is through sexual contact (70%) and by intravenous drug use. Of consequence to the adolescent population, inflammatory STDs such as gonorrhea and chlamydia facilitate transmission of HIV. Screening and/or referral for HIV screening should be considered with all adolescent patients, particularly those with other STDs.

Syphilis

Syphilis is a genital ulcerative disease. Primary syphilis appears as a painless chancre. Secondary syphilis can present in many forms, including a mucocutaneous rash and generalized lymphadenopathy. Tertiary syphilis, occurring years to decades after acquisition of the disease, can lead to devastating cardiovascular and neurological sequelae.

Table 96.1. Recommended treatment of pelvic inflammatory disease[a]

Regimen type	Contents	Comments
Parenteral regimens	Parenteral therapy may be discontinued 24 h after a patient improves clinically; continuing oral therapy should consist of doxycycline (100 mg PO, BID) or clindamycin (450 mg PO QID) to complete a total of 14 days of therapy	Hospitalization is recommended for severe illness, pregnancy, or inability to tolerate or follow ambulatory regimens
Regimen A	Cefotetan 2 g IV q. 12 h or cefoxitin 2 g IV q. 6 h; plus doxycycline 100 mg PO or IV q. 2 h to complete 14 days	Standard
Regimen B	Clindamycin 600–900 mg IV q. 8 h plus gentamicin loading dose IV or IM (2 mg/kg), followed by maintenance gentamicin 1.5 mg/kg q. 8 h; single daily dosing may be substituted	Alternative parenteral regimens include ampicillin–sulbactam plus doxycycline
Ambulatory regimen	Ceftriaxone 250 mg IM once or cefoxitin 2 g IM and probenecid 1 g PO in a single dose concurrently once, or other parenteral third-generation cephalosporin (e.g., ceftizoxime or cefotaxime); plus doxycycline 100 mg PO BID for 14 days ± metronidazole 500 mg PO BID for 14 days	Patients with inadequate response to outpatient therapy after 72 h should be re-evaluated for possible misdiagnosis and should receive parenteral therapy; because of widespread fluoroquinolone-resistant GC; fluoroquinolones are not recommended for PID in the USA
Alternative ambulatory regimens	If parenteral cephalosporin therapy is not feasible, use of fluoroquinolones may be considered if community prevalence and individual risk of gonorrhea is low (www.cdc.gov/std/treatment)	Tests for GC must be performed before instituting therapy GC nucleic acid amplification test positive, parenteral cephalosporin recommended GC culture positive, treatment based on susceptibility results GC isolate quinolone resistant or susceptibility cannot be assessed, parenteral cephalosporin recommended

[a]For further alternative treatment regimens, see Centers for Disease Control and Prevention, 2006 (www.cdc.gov/std/treatment has updated treatment regimens). Data to indicate whether expanded-spectrum cephalosporins (ceftizoxime, cefotaxime, ceftriaxone) can replace cefoxitin or cefotetan are limited. Many authorities believe they also are effective therapy for PID, but they are less active against anaerobes.
GC, gonococci; PID, pelvic inflammatory disease.
Source: adapted from Pickering *et al.*, 2006.

Incidence

Syphilis rates in adolescents have been rising in recent years. In 2006, there were 2.3/100 000 adolescents aged 5–19 years. Highest incidence was in the south of the USA, in urban areas, and among men who have sex with men. Rates of congenitally acquired syphilis in 2005 were 8.0/100 000 live births.

Management

Syphilis is treated with 2.4×10^6 U (2.4 million) IM benzathine penicillin. Doxycycline is an alternative in the non-pregnant, penicillin-allergic patient.

Human papilloma virus

Human papilloma viruses cause epithelial tumors of the skin and mucous membranes. Types 16 and 18 are linked to cervical and anogenital cancers and are considered "high-risk" subtypes. Types 6 and 11 cause genital warts and have low oncogenic potential. The virus is transmitted via sexual contact.

Since sexual experience often begins in adolescence, teenagers are at high risk for acquiring HPV. In those aged 14–19 years, prevalence of HPV types 16 and 18 is 35% higher than all other age cohorts. Infection with HPV correlates with early age of first intercourse and increased number of sexual partners.

Vaccine

In June 2006, a vaccine targeting HPV types 6, 11, 16, and 18 was licensed for use in the USA. The vaccine is administered in a three dose intramuscular series. Recommended age for vaccination is 11–12 years, and "catch up" vaccination is recommended for females 13 to 26 years who have not been previously vaccinated.

Special adolescent populations

Men who have sex with men

In recent years, rates of syphilis, gonorrhea, chlamydia, and hepatitis B have increased among men who have sex with men. Clinicians should inquire about the sex of the partner and specific sexual activities so they can better assess risk characteristics and thereby provide appropriate testing and treatment. Practitioners should ask about symptoms such as urethral discharge, anal and genital ulcers, dysuria, inguinal lymphadenopathy, skin rash, and anorectal pain. Among men who have sex with men, the CDC recommends annual testing for HIV, gonorrhea, chlamydia, and syphilis.

Juvenile justice inmates

Both male and female adolescents entering juvenile justice facilities have high rates of gonorrhea and chlamydia. Among those aged 12–18 years entering juvenile correction facilities, the overall chlamydial positivity for males was 6.4%, and for females 14.3%. In this cohort of adolescents, gonorrhea positivity was 1.3% for men and 5.2% for women. These high rates of STD infection among juvenile justice inmates should prompt clinicians to inquire about pertinent symptoms. Additionally, clinicians should consider PID as a possible diagnosis for abdominal pain in this high-risk population.

Legal issues

In all 50 US states, adolescents can consent to STD diagnosis and treatment without parental consent or awareness. In most states, adolescents can consent to HIV testing. Some states, however, require parental consent for vaccination services. Healthcare providers should be aware of their state laws in order to provide STD treatment with utmost confidentiality (see Ch. 159).

The role of the emergency department

Screening

Since the ED may be an adolescent's portal into the healthcare system, there may be a role for ED screening of STDs in young adults. Several studies investigating the utility of ED screening for gonorrhea and chlamydia found that between 10 and 15% of young adults who accepted free screening tested positive.

The clinician

Emergency medicine clinicians should incorporate awareness of the frequency of adolescent STDs into their encounters with teenage patients. Since adolescents may seek emergency services for exactly these reasons, healthcare providers should be comfortable in discussing about sexual behavior.

Past STD diagnosis has been associated with increased risk of current STDs. In fact, a significant percentage of women diagnosed and treated for STDs are reinfected within 6 months. Consequently, the practitioner should not assume that because the person was treated in the recent past that they are disease free in the present. Practitioners should recognize their role as educators, provide counseling about risky behaviors, and encourage preventative behavioral change.

Pearls and pitfalls

Pearls

1. Adolescents are at greatest risk for acquiring sexually transmitted diseases (STDs) compared with all other age groups. Pelvic inflammatory disease should be considered as a cause of abdominal pain in adolescent women.
2. In all 50 US states, teenagers may seek treatment for STDs without parental consent.
3. Since 2006, a human papillomavirus (HPV) vaccine has been available for adolescent females.

Pitfalls

1. Failure to ask teenage patients about their sexual practices, sexual orientation, and possible STD symptoms.
2. Failure to treat sexual partners of teenagers being treated for STDs.
3. Failure to understand state-specific laws regarding parental consent for HPV vaccination and teenage HIV testing.

Selected references

Centers for Disease Control and Prevention. *HIVAIDS.* Atlanta GA: Centers for Disease Control and Prevention.

Centers for Disease Control and Prevention. *Special Populations: STD Treatment Guidelines* 2006. Atlanta GA: Centers for Disease Control and Prevention, 2006 http://www.cdc.gov/STD/treatment/2006/specialpops.htm (accessed 27 April 2010).

Centers for Disease Control and Prevention. *Updated Recommended Treatment Regimens for Gonococcal Infections and Associated Conditions: United States, April 2007.* Atlanta GA: Centers for Disease Control and Prevention, 2007 http://www.cdc.gov/std/Treatment/2006/updated-regimens.htm (accessed 27 April 2010).

Centers for Disease Control and Prevention. *Sexual Risk Behaviors.* Atlanta GA: Centers for Disease Control and Prevention, 2008. http://www.cdc.gov/HealthyYouth/sexualbehaviors/ (accessed 27 April 2010).

Centers for Disease Control and Prevention. *Special Focus Profiles:Adolescents and Young Adults.* Atlanta GA: Centers for Disease Control and Prevention, 2008.

Centers for Disease Control and Prevention. *CDC Fact Sheet: Sexually Transmitted Diseases, Pelvic Inflammatory Disease* Atlanta GA: Centers for Disease Control and Prevention, Centers for Disease Control and Prevention, 2008. http://www.cdc.gov/std/PID/STDFact-PID.htm (accessed 27 April 2010).

Dicelemente RJ, Wingood GM, Sionean C, *et al.* Association

of adolescents' history of sexually transmitted disease (STD) and their current high risk behavior and STD status: a case for intensifying clinic-based prevention efforts. *Sex Transm Dis* 2002;**29**:503–509.

Fiscus LC, Ford CA, Miller WC. Infrequency of sexually transmitted disease screening among sexually experienced US female adolescents. *Perspect Sex Reprod Health* 2004;**36**:233–238.

Markowitz L, Dunne E, Saraiya M, *et al.* Quadrivalent human papillomavirus vaccine. Recommendations of the Advisory Committee on Immunization Practices (ACIP). *MMWR Recomm Rep* 2007; **56** (RR-02):1–24.

Mehta SD, Hall J, Lyss SB, *et al.* Adult and pediatric emergency department sexually transmitted disease and HIV screening: programmatic overview and outcomes. *Acad Emerg Med* 2007;**14**:250–258.

Peterman TA, Tian LH, Metcalf CA, *et al.* High incidence of new sexually transmitted infections in the year following a sexually transmitted infection: a case for rescreening. *Ann Intern Med* 2006;**145**:564–572.

Pickering LK, Baker CJ, Kimberlin DW, Long SS (eds.). *The Red Book: 2006 Report of the Committee on Infectious Diseases*, 27th edn. Elk Grove Village, IL: American Academy of Pediatrics, 2006 (also Red Book Online, last updated 5 January 2009).

Chapter 97

Skin and soft tissue infections

Eva Delgado

Introduction

Skin and soft tissue infections are a common presenting complaint to EDs. This chapter will cover superficial skin infections, such as impetigo, ecthyma, and cellulitis (Fig. 97.1), as well as covering the appropriate management of a skin abscess. It will also briefly review methicillin-resistant *Staphylococcus aureus* (MRSA).

Impetigo and ecthyma

These skin infections are commonly caused by *Staphylococcus aureus* or group A beta-hemolytic streptococci (GABHS).

Impetigo involves invasion of the superficial dermis. Impetigo is the most common skin infection in children between the ages of 2 and 5 years. Impetigo is common on the face (nares and perioral), hands, forearms and neck. Impetigo has a high attack rate and spreads rapidly through contact inoculation and fomites in preschools or crowded environments. Bullous impetigo is more common in infants and neonates; it is usually seen on the trunk, thighs, and diaper area and is almost always caused by a type of *S. aureus* elaborating exfoliative exotoxins (as in staphylococcal scalded skin syndrome).

Ecthyma is a skin infection, also usually from GABHS, that extends through the mid-dermis.

Erysipelas is a less common skin infection caused by inoculation with GABHS; it occurs within the dermis above the subcutaneous space, with progression to the superficial lymphatics.

Clinical presentation

Impetigo usually does not cause systemic symptoms. Lesions of impetigo begin as erythematous papules, which become thin-walled vesicles that rupture easily to become shallow erosions; the resultant serum dries to form the classic "honey crusts" (Fig. 97.2). Lesions are quickly spread locally through autoinoculation, and sometimes central clearing will cause gyrate or annular lesions. Satellite lesions are common. Bullous impetigo has flaccid, translucent bullae that quickly unroof to tender shallow erosions with an outer rim of desquamated skin (residual blister roof.) Often only the erosions are seen (see Fig. 97.3).

Ecthyma presents as a well-circumscribed, firm, dark, dry crust with a raised, red, tender margin (Fig. 97.4). Purulent material can sometimes be expressed from underneath the crust. When removed, a punched-out or saucer-shaped ulcer remains. Ecthyma may have associated fever and systemic illness.

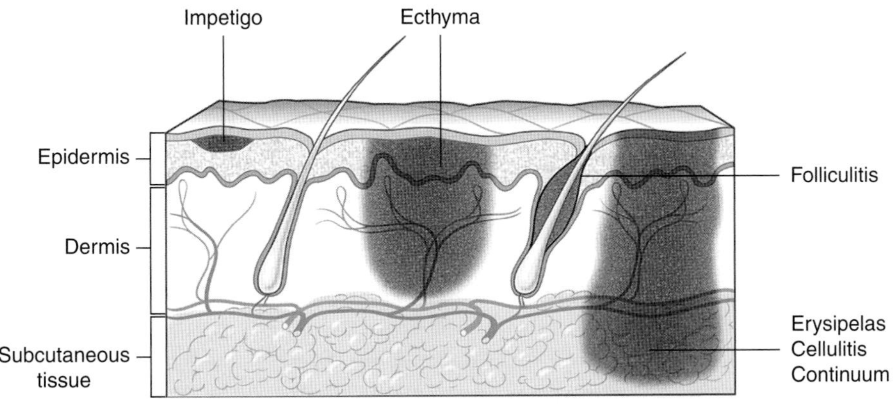

Figure 97.1 Schematic of different skin and soft tissue infections. (Copyright Chris Gralapp.)

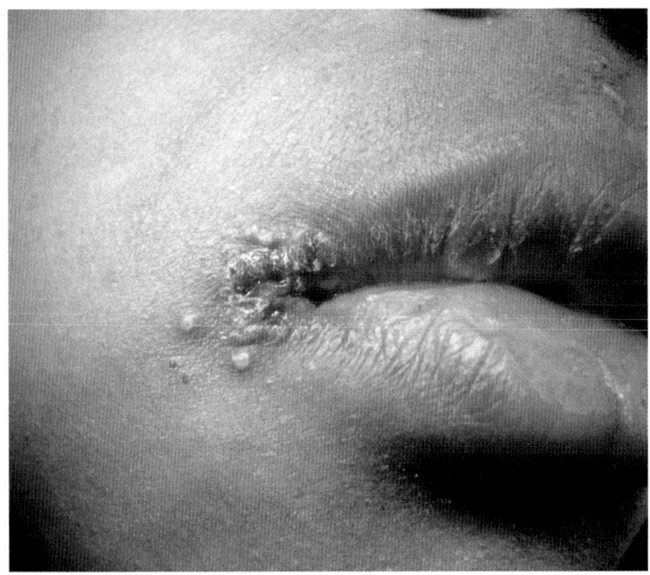

Figure 97.2 Impetigo. Honey-crusted lesions often starting out as small vesicles in exposed areas of face and extremities in young children. (Courtesy Dr. Hans Kersten.)

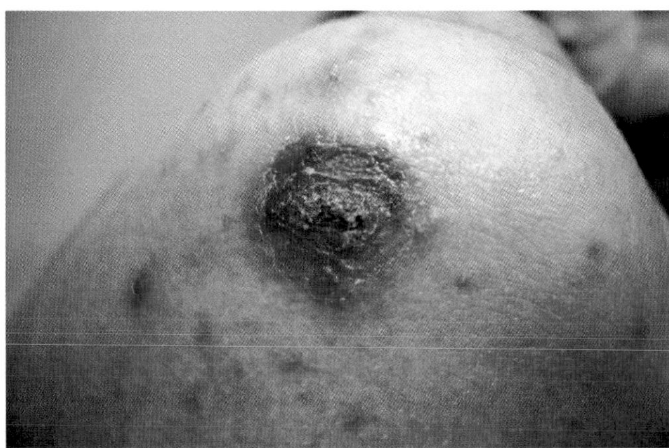

Figure 97.3 Bullous impetigo. Blisters on an erythematous base which often rupture and develop into erosions with crusting. (Courtesy Dr. Hans Kersten.)

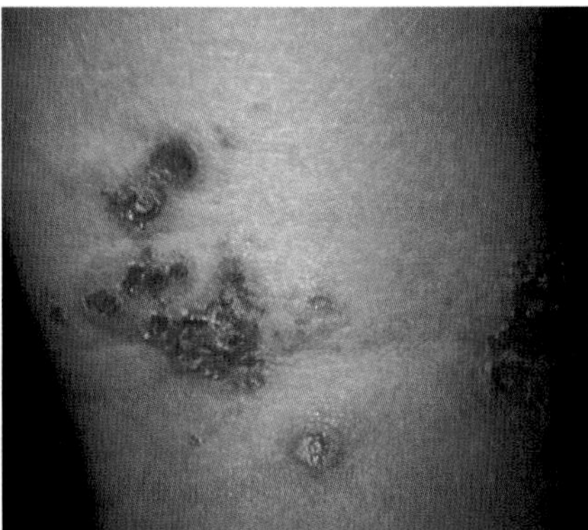

Figure 97.4 Ecthyma. Discrete, round lesions with a dark crust in the center often surrounded by a rim of shallow ulcerations. (Courtesy of Logical Images, Inc.)

Erysipelas, presents with a warm, tender, edematous, bright red or pink plaque usually with a well-demarcated or raised border. Skin edema in erysipelas can cause a shiny or "peau d'orange" appearance. The face ("butterfly" distribution, unilateral or bilateral), neck, hands, or lower legs are common sites of involvement. If systemic symptoms precede the development of a circumscribed area of erythematous plaque with a raised border and marked tenderness, it may be reasonable to obtain a throat culture for GABHS, the causative agent of erysipelas.

Diagnosis

The differential diagnosis for impetigo includes herpetic lesions, such as primary herpes or herpes zoster, Stevens–Johnson syndrome/toxic epidermal necrolysis, and dermatitis; clinical examination and biopsy can differentiate.

Management

Therapy for impetigo, bullous impetigo, ecthyma, and erysipelas has grown more complex as local antibiotic resistance patterns cause general recommendations to be potentially inaccurate.

Methicillin-resistant *S. aureus* now accounts for 70–80% of isolates from childhood impetigo in some areas of North America.

For localized, limited infections of impetigo, a 1–2 week course of topical mupirocin or fusidic acid (not available in the USA) two or three times daily can be used. Retapamulin ointment (twice daily for 5 days) has been recently approved in the USA for use in primary impetigo in children <9 months of age. Topical agents should never be used in widespread disease, in disease secondary to superinfection of atopic dermatitis or other chronic underlying skin conditions, or for diseases known or suspected to be from GABHS (ecthyma, erysipelas). Duration of topical therapy should also be limited. Topical agents other than mupirocin and fusidic acid are not recommended as they can prolong infection through achieving only a partial response and this encourages a carrier state. Mupirocin resistance has been reported in some communities; again, checking local isolate sensitivities is of paramount importance in deciding any oral or topical treatment.

Primary impetigo, erysipelas, and ecthyma can be treated with a 10 day course of oral penicillinase-resistant penicillins (cloxacillin, dicloxacillin, amoxicillin/clavulanate), 10 days of a first- or second-generation cephalosporin, or a newer macrolide (azithromycin or clarithromycin). Communities with high rates of MRSA should begin with trimethoprim–sulfamethoxazole or clindamycin for impetigo; quinolones can be considered for adolescents if local resistance patterns allow. Trimethoprim–sulfamethoxazole should never be used alone for erysipelas or ecthyma in children, as it does not clinically cover GABHS infections despite activity in vitro; it should be paired with a cephalosporin or other GABHS treatment. Additionally, more and more GABHS are resistant to macrolides, and local sensitivities should always guide in consideration of macrolide use. Warm compresses aid in loosening crusts of ecthyma or severely crusted impetigo. The skin should *not* be scrubbed, as this has *not* been shown to help.) Non-clearance or rapid recurrence of impetigo after treatment should prompt culture of any open or purulent areas. Acute rheumatic fever is not known to occur after skin infection with GABHS; however antibiotic treatment does not prevent post-streptococcal glomerulonephritis.

Disposition

Patients with primary impetigo, ecthyma, and erysipelas can usually be managed on an outpient basis. As always, any ill-appearing, immunocompromised, or otherwise concerning child should be admitted for management. Close follow-up with the primary doctor for assessing improvement of the rash is key, particularly given the risk of antibiotic-resistance. Thorough return precautions should be provided to caregivers.

Cellulitis

Cellulitis is defined as subcutaneous infection and inflammation, often sparing the epidermis. Typically, there is a break in the skin from a prior trauma that allows entry of infectious organisms; alternatively, an underlying lesion may provoke the inflammation. Children are particularly at risk given their propensity for cuts, scrapes, and insect bites. Even more at risk are those with eczema, lymphatic stasis, or immunocompromise. Most cellulitis is attributed to GABHS or *S. aureus,* but *Haemophilus influenzae* type b is possible in the incompletely immunized and the immunocompromised (particularly those with sickle cell disease). *S. aureus* and GABHS infections are sometimes distinguishable based on appearance alone, with GABHS capable of rapid progression along the lymphatics as is seen in erysipelas. *S. aureus* causes a more localized area of inflammation with a greater likelihood of suppuration, a characteristic that can complicate the differentiation of cellulitis from abscess formation. Cellulitis that erupts following a human or animal bite may be caused by oral anaerobes or *Pasteurella* sp., respectively. *S. aureus,* GABHS, oral anaerobes, *H. influenzae,* and *Streptococcus pneumoniae* are all possible causative agents of preseptal and orbital cellulitis (see Ch. 119).

Clinical presentations

Examination findings necessary for diagnosis with cellulitis include erythema, warmth, and edema, with pain and tenderness at a site marked by indistinct lateral margins. Fever and fatigue may also be present, but such systemic symptoms do not indicate bacteremia in an otherwise healthy and immunized child. The entire affected extremity or body part should be carefully examined for any erythematous streaking marks, consistent with lymphangitic streaking. This erythema, along with enlarged draining lymph nodes, indicates spread of the infection and should lead to aggressive treatment with antibiotics. Necrotizing fasciitis, a potentially fatal skin and soft tissue infection, starts similarly to cellulitis with swelling and erythema, usually of an extremity. Clinical clues to suggest necrotizing soft tissue infection include exquisite tenderness to palpation/intense pain, rapid progression, bullae or necrosis, possible crepitus, lack of prompt response to antibiotics, and toxic appearance.

Diagnostic studies

Studies have shown that routine blood cultures for routine cellulitis are not indicated as they will rarely yield an organism or change treatment. However, in an immunocompromised or toxic-appearing child, or in one with possible joint or orbital involvement, cultures should be sent to guide further treatment. In neonates, the diagnosis of cellulitis or erysipelas should prompt consideration of further laboratory studies to evaluate for sepsis.

Management

Treatment for cellulitis should target both *S. aureus* and GABHS, with attention to local antibiotic resistance patterns. In children with no personal or family history of MRSA, a first-generation cephalosporin is appropriate. If the cellulitis is related to a bite or if it occurs on the face, augmentin is a better first-line agent to target anaerobes. If there is concern for MRSA, clindamycin may be a good choice depending on the local sensitivity profile. Trimethoprim–sulfamethoxazole provides good *S. aureus* coverage, even in populations with resistance, but may be better paired with a cephalosporin since this alone will not treat GABHS. Any cellulitis that threatens a joint or the orbit warrants admission for IV antibiotic therapy, as does a cellulitis with rapid progression or failure to improve within 24–48 h of oral outpatient therapy. Therefore, close follow-up after initial diagnosis is imperative.

Folliculitis

Folliculitis is superficial infection of a hair follicle caused by occlusion of the follicle, poor hygiene, or exposure to bacterial pathogens in a hot tub.

Clinical presentation

The infected follicles usually develop into small, dome-shaped pustules, most commonly on the scalp, buttocks, or extremities. In hot-tub folliculitis, the lesions predominate in areas covered by a bathing suit, and they typically erupt within 8–48 h of hot tub use. Diagnosis is made primarily by appearance on examination.

Diagnostic studies

Examination of the fluid drained from the lesions often identifies the causative organism as the pustules contain a high yield of infectious bacteria.

Management

S. aureus is the most likely pathogen responsible for folliculitis but this varies depending on the origin of the infection and the patient's past medical history. If there are no systemic symptoms and *S. aureus* is expected, a chlorhexidine wash may be sufficient treatment. A first-generation cephalosporin such as cephalexin is another option. Adolescents with acne and a history of systemic antibiotic use are at risk for Gram-negative bacteria such as *Escherichia coli*, or *Pseudomonas, Klebsiella,* and *Enterobacter* spp., so close attention to wound culture results is required to determine optimal treatment. Hot-tub folliculitis, often caused by *Pseudomonas* sp. will resolve within a few weeks. Treatment with ciprofloxacin is an option for uncomfortable adolescents but is not routinely recommended in younger children.

Abscesses, furuncles, and carbuncles

Furuncles and carbuncles are larger, suppurative progressions of an underlying folliculitis or perifollicular nodule. Carbuncles that coalesce into fluctuant areas can become abscesses. An abscess is an infection in the dermis or subcutaneous space that promotes necrosis within an area of induration and tenderness. Provoked by regional trauma or bacterial colonization, an abscess is also identified by inflammation, erythema, and progression to fluctuance. As an abscess is evolving, the distinction between abscess and cellulitis may require further evaluation. Eventually, suppuration promotes rupture of these lesions with expulsion of the inner, necrotic debris. Children at risk include those with eczema, frequent insect bites, obese body habitus, and history of prior *S. aureus* skin infection, particularly MRSA, as it is the most common causative agent of any abscess.

Management

Incision and drainage is necessary for both diagnosis and treatment of an abscess. Several studies of both adult and pediatric populations have determined that incision with adequate drainage provides sufficient treatment in an otherwise healthy patient, as subjects given inappropriate therapy for the sensitivity profile of their infecting organism still improved following incision and drainage. This may be the only therapy necessary in an abscess <5 cm in diameter in an immunocompetent child with minimal systemic symptoms. Larger abscesses warrant antibiotic therapy in addition to incision and drainage, and in some cases, admission for IV antibiotics. Abscess location is another point to consider, as an abscess over a joint or near the orbit might be more likely to require IV antibiotics for full penetration.

The pathogen usually responsible for abscesses is *S. aureus*. Treatment choice should be based on local sensitivities, and the understanding that MRSA is the leading cause of penetrating skin and soft tissue infections that present to the ED. The age of the child, history of prior skin infections, body habitus, ethnicity, demographic information, and exposures are important to consider when assessing for the possibility of MRSA infection. Even in a child with no perceived risk factors, empiric treatment for MRSA with trimethoprim–sulfamethoxazole or clindamycin is best (doxycycline is an option in children >8 years) while waiting for identification of the bacterium from culture. If the organism is MSSA, it is appropriate and recommended to transition to a first-generation cephalosporin. If the organism is MRSA, careful attention to the sensitivity profile is important, as is close follow-up.

Methicillin-resistant *Staphyloccus aureus*

Methicillin-resistant *S. aureus* is resistant to beta-lactam antibiotics, including methicillin, oxacillin, nafcillin, and cephalosporins. First detected in the 1960s, MRSA was primarily known as a hospital-associated (nosocomial) infection. In the mid-1990s, MRSA was found responsible for the deaths of a handful of children not previously exposed to a hospital environment. This community-associated form has even more virulence factors than the hospital-related MRSA form, which makes it increasingly evasive to treatment. Infants, children, and adolescents harbor the majority of community-acquired MRSA (CA-MRSA) infections, and 80% of these are localized to the skin. Overall, ED visits for skin and soft tissue infections have tripled since the identification of CA-MRSA, and its prevalence continues to increase.

Children under 2 years are at increased risk for MRSA (and all *S. aureus* infections).

This increased risk may occur from the increased potential for breaks in the skin, allowing infection in MRSA-endemic environments or from difficulty maintaining careful hygiene.

Of MRSA infections, 15% will recur in the same host, and parents will often describe these children as prone to recurrent "spider bites."

The lesions often start with a central pustule, which resembles a puncture wound or spider bite.

There also seems to be a predilection for MRSA infection among Pacific Islanders. Geographic isolation in the past may have conferred genetic traits that increase susceptibility to these organisms. At the same time, Pacific Islanders in the USA also tend to have several characteristics outside of ethnicity that pose independent risk factors for MRSA: large family size with possible overcrowding, poverty, decreased access to care, obesity, and more diabetes, with related immunocompromise.

Since most abscesses grow CA-MRSA when cultured, treatment of any suppurative lesion, from bug bite to carbuncle, should target CA-MRSA to prevent progression to more invasive infection. As noted above, following incision and drainage, empiric treatment with trimethoprim–sulfamethoxazole or clindamycin is best, depending on local sensitivity data. Most laboratories now perform the D-test, which detects inducible resistance to clindamycin following exposure of an in vitro isolate to erythromycin. If resistance is inducible, the area of clearing surrounding clindamycin resembles the letter "D." When parenteral therapy is necessary because of the severity or location of the infection, vancomycin is usually the antibiotic of choice, but resistance is emerging to this potent antibiotic as well. With susceptibility constantly changing, it is very important to obtain a wound culture and guaranteeing follow-up.

Pearls and pitfalls

Pearls

1. Topical and oral antibiotics for impetigo or ecthyma should cover methicillin-resistant *Staphylococcus aureus* (MRSA).
2. Incision and drainage of a suppurative infection is the key to proper treatment; send a swab for Gram stain and culture; ensure follow-up.
3. Know where to find the local *S. aureus* and group A beta-hemolytic streptococci sensitivity profile.
4. Children <2 years have an increased risk for *S. aureus* infection in general, as well as MRSA, compared with others.

Pitfalls

1. Failure to recognize impetigo or ecthyma as bacterial in etiology.
2. A well-appearing child may still warrant admission based on size of abscess (>5 cm diameter) or location of skin infection (proximity to joint or face).
3. Failure to recognize that trimethoprim–sulfamethoxazole, a first-line antibiotic choice for skin infections in adults, will not treat group A beta-hemolytic streptococci, which are a common co-contaminant in pediatric skin infections.

Selected references

Centers for Disease Control and Prevention. Community-associated methicillin-resistant *Staphylococcus aureus* infections in Pacific Islanders, Hawaii 2001–2003. *MMWR Morb Mort Wkly Rep* 2004; **53**:767–770.

Gorwitz RJ. Community-associated methicillin-reistant *Staphylococcus aureus*: epidemiology and update. *Pediatr Infect Dis J* 2008;**27**: 925–926.

Hasty MB, Klasner A, Kness S, *et al.* Cutaneous community-associated methicillin-resistant *Staphylococcus aureus* among all skin and soft-tissue infections in two geographically distant pediatric emergency departments. *Academy Emerg Med* 2007;**14:** 35–40.

Konig S, van der Wouden JC. Treatment for impetigo. *Br Med J* 2004;**329**: 695–696.

Lee MC, Rios AM, Aten MF, *et al.* Management and outcome of children with skin and soft tissue abscesses caused by community-acquired methicillin-resistant *Staphylococcus aureus. Pediatr Infect Dis J* 2004;**23**:123–127.

Moran GJ, Krishnadasan A, Gorwitz RJ, *et al.* Methicillin-resistant *S. aureus* infections among patients in the emergency department. *N Engl J Med* 2006;**355**:666–674.

Chapter 98

Travel and tropical disease management in the emergency department

Kathleen Ann Jobe

Introduction

Travel to exotic and underdeveloped areas presents specific problems to the pediatric patient. More than 50 million people visit the developing world each year. Of these only 4% are children, but 25% of travel-related hospitalizations occur in the pediatric population. Children are more susceptible to the effects of dehydration from diarrheal illnesses and less likely to have received appropriate travel-specific vaccinations. The antibiotics commonly prescribed for traveler's diarrhea are not appropriate for children and children of certain ages cannot receive some recommended travel vaccinations for increased risk of complications (e.g., yellow fever). This chapter will discuss diarrhea, fever, and skin conditions in returning pediatric travelers.

In evaluating illness in the returning traveler attention should be paid to the following:

- specific information obtained regarding travel including countries and regions, duration of travel and activities while traveling, time of return
- pretravel and routine vaccination history
- malaria prophylaxis and compliance
- use of prophylactic and therapeutic medications
- timing of symptom onset
- specific exposures (freshwater, animals, mosquitos and other insects, large gatherings).

Diarrheal illness

Traveler's diarrhea is the leading cause of morbidity in travelers. There are few published data regarding the disease in children, but existing data suggest that the etiology of pediatric traveler's diarrhea is predominantly bacterial, which is consistent with patterns seen in adult travelers. The limited data that exist regarding traveler's diarrhea in infants and children suggest that children <3 years are at high risk for acquiring it and generally have a more severe course than do adults. This is likely because of the child's active 'oral' exploration, lack of previous immunity, and the higher innoculum per body weight in young children.

Etiology

Causes of traveler's diarrhea in children are similar to those in adults. *Campylobacter jejuni*, enteropathogenic *Escherichia coli*, *Clostridium difficile*, and *Shigella*, *Salmonella*, *Vibrio*, *Aeromonas*, and *Plesiomonas* spp. are the most commonly identified causes of acute traveler's diarrhea (50–75%). The common organisms vary based on the travel destination:

- bacteria
  - enterotoxigenic *E. coli*
  - Other *E. coli* types (e.g., enteroaggregative *E. coli*)
  - *C. jejuni*
  - *Salmonella* (non-typhoid)
  - *Shigella dysenteriae*, *S. flexneri*, *S. sonnei*
  - *Aeromonas* spp.
  - *Vibrio* (non-cholera)
- parasites
  - *Giardia intestinalis*
  - *Entamoeba histolytica*
  - *Cyclospora cayetanensis*
  - *Cryptosporidium parvum*
- viruses
  - rotavirus
  - noroviruses.

Organisms in each category are listed by the most common causes; however, the prevalence of specific pathogens may vary significantly based on travel destination. Only 1–5% of cases are related to parasitic infection.

Clinical presentation

Invasive enteropathy should be considered in patients with bloody diarrhea, those with both diarrhea and fever, and patients with white blood cells in the stool.

The average onset of diarrhea in travelers occurs at 8 days; the median duration is 3–11.5 days in children and adolescents and 18–30 days in children under 3 years.

A Practical Guide to Pediatric Emergency Medicine: Caring for Children in the Emergency Department, ed. N. Ewen Amieva-Wang (associate eds. Jamie Shandro, Aparajita Sohoni, and Bernhard Fassl). Published by Cambridge University Press.

In children, the morbidity from traveler's diarrhea is caused by dehydration (for management see Ch. 53). Dysentery (fever and bloody diarrhea) predisposes children to bowel perforation and sepsis.

Management

The prevention and treatment of dehydration should begin immediately with the onset of traveler's diarrhea. Oral rehydration solution (ORS) is preferred for initial rehydration.

While empiric antibiotics have no role in the developed world in treating a child with diarrhea, they are reasonable in a child with a recent history of travel who presents with diarrhea and either fever or blood in the stool, or both.

There is clear evidence that use of antibiotics decreases the duration and severity of traveler's diarrhea in adults. Children tend to experience long and severe episodes and antibiotic use should decrease the severity and duration of illness.

Treatment with bismuth subsalicylate has been shown to be safe and effective in children with traveler's diarrhea and can be used as an adjunct to ORT. A dose of 20 mg/kg every 4 h has been shown to decrease the frequency and duration of diarrhea and reduce the amount of rehydration solution required. Pepto-Bismol liquid contains 262 mg of bismuth subsalicylate/15 ml. Avoid use of bismuth subsalicylate in patients with a history of aspirin or NSAID allergy, bloody stool, bleeding abnormalities, or recent viral upper respiratory tract infection symptoms. Loperamide has been associated with adverse affects such as paralytic ileus, vomiting, and drowsiness. The AAP does not recommend the use of antimotility agents in the treatment of acute diarrhea.

Currently recommended antibiotics for traveler's diarrhea in children include ciprofloxacin and azithromycin. Ciprofloxacin is felt to be safe in the pediatric population. Although it is not approved for pediatric use in the USA because of concerns regarding cartilaginous growth plate development, some travel medicine specialists recommend it as the drug of choice in the treatment of traveler's diarrhea in infants and children. Azithromycin is particularly effective against *Shigella* and *Campylobacter* spp., including campylobacter resistant to fluoroquinolones. Although ideal dosing has not been established, it has been shown to be effective as a single oral dose. Rifixamin is a poorly absorbed rifamycin drug that has been shown to be effective in treatment of traveler's diarrhea caused by non-invasive *E. coli*. It has been shown to have efficacy equal to ciprofloxacin.

Giardiasis is caused by the protozoan *Giarida intestinalis*. It is a common infectious agent in the developing world, with a prevalence of 15–20% in children <10 years. It is associated with person-to-person transmission and water-borne transmission. It is not associated with deaths except in infants with extreme dehydration. Symptoms generally manifest 2–3 weeks after infection. A minority of those infected experience explosive watery diarrhea, cramping and flatus, which lasts 3–4 days before resolving to a subacute syndrome. Most patients experience an insidious onset of watery diarrhea, and stools may become fatty and very malodorous. Some patients experience constipation with nausea, bloating, and abdominal cramping. Diagnosis is made on the basis of detection of *Giardia* antigen in the stool. These tests have a sensitivity of 85–98% and specificity of 90–100%. Stool examination may also result in the diagnosis of giardiasis. At least three stools taken at 2 day intervals should be examined for the presence of cysts or trophozoites. Fecal leukocytes will not be seen and stool cultures are not useful. Treatment consists of metronidazole 5 mg/kg TID for 5–7 days.

Amoebiasis is an unusual cause of diarrhea in children, even in less-developed countries. Treatment of amoebiasis should be reserved for those cases in which trophozoites are detectable in the stool.

Febrile illness without diarrhea

Onset of fever more than 3 weeks after return from travel largely eliminates dengue fever, yellow fever, and rickettsial disease as etiologies.

Malaria

Malaria is the most important cause of fever in the returning pediatric traveler. The *Anopheles* mosquito transmits the parasite. There are several species of *Plasmodium*, with a varied geographic distribution: 90% of patients with *P. falciparum* acquire it in sub-Saharan Africa and 90% become symptomatic within one month of return; 70% of *P. vivax* is acquired in either Asia or Latin America. *P. falciparum* infection can rapidly be fatal and must be ruled out in children returning from areas of possible exposure.

Clinical presentation

Clinical presentation includes recurring high fever, sweats, rigors, chills, headache, and GI symptoms. Physical examination may reveal splenomegaly. Thrombocytopenia may be seen, however leukocytosis is rare.

Diagnostic studies

Blood samples should be obtained for thick and thin films and, if negative, they should be repeated at 12–24 h.

Management

Antimalarial medication should be given parenterally if there is evidence of renal failure, seizure, ALOC, severe anemia, or if the *P. falciparum* load is greater than 4% of erythrocytes. Detailed recommendations for treatment of malaria in the pediatric patient are available from the CDC Malaria Hotline (770) 488–7788 (M-F 8a-4:30 p, EST), or (707) 488–7100 (after hours).

Disposition

All pediatric patients with presumptive *P. falciparum* infection should be admitted to hospital.

Dengue fever

Dengue is a common cause of fever in travelers to tropical and subtropical regions. The mosquito host *Aedes aegypti*, which lives in stagnant water in urban areas, transmits the virus.

Clinical presentation

Dengue (break bone fever) is characterized by fever, headache, and severe myalgias: 50% of patients will develop lymphadenopathy, diffuse erythema, or a non-specific maculopapular rash. Dengue shock syndrome and dengue hemorrhagic fever-are generally seen only in patients with a prior history of dengue infection.

Diagnostic studies

In Dengue fever, leukopenia, thrombocytopenia, and an elevated AST are common; CBC with platelets and LFTs should be tested.

Dengue is generally a clinical diagnosis. Acute and convalescent titers of IgM should be obtained to confirm the diagnosis. Hemagglutination inhibition testing is the gold standard for virus-specific antibodies. Dengue-specific enzyme-linked immunosorbent assay (ELISA) and a monoclonal-antibody ELISA (MAC-ELISA) are available but have poor sensitivity.

Management

Treatment is supportive. Vaccines for all four serotypes of dengue are currently in varying stages of development, with one vaccine in phase III trials (late 2010).

Rickettsial infections

Rickettsial diseases are transmitted by arthopods. Painless eschar is usually present in the case of African tick typhus (*R. africae*), Mediterranean tick typhus (*R. conorii*) and scrub typhus (*O. tsutsugamushi*).

Clinical presentation

Rickettsial diseases are characterized by headache, fever, and myalgias. Regional lymphadenopathy, rash, leukopenia, and thrombocytopenia may be seen.

Diagnosis

Diagnosis is clinical and treatment should be started while awaiting the results of serological studies.

Management

Doxycycline is the drug of choice for ricksettsial disease in the pediatric population. The duration of therapy is 7–14 days. There is little risk of tooth staining in children under 8 when doxycycline therapy is for 14 days or less.

Typhoid (enteric) fever

Salmonella typhi is a Gram-negative bacillus that is transmitted via human feces. Patients contract the infection via exposure to contaminated water in less-developed countries. (This is important to differentiate from other *Salmonella* spp., which are transmitted from animal feces and cause gastroenteritis.). Vaccines for typhoid are only partially protective.

Clinical presentation

Patients with typhoid fever have fever and headache of insidious onset without diagnostic features on physical examination, although lymphadenopathy may be present. Many patients complain of abdominal pain and constipation. Diarrhea is rare. Some may report dry cough.

Diagnostic studies

Laboratory testing should include cultures and sensitivities and may reveal leukopenia, thrombocytopenia and elevated LFTs. The diagnosis is confirmed by isolating *S. typhi* and non-typhi *Salmonella* serotypes from the blood. Serologic testing is unreliable.

Management

While treatment is effective, it has become complicated because of rapid spread of drug resistance. Individuals can also be cured and become carriers. Therefore, consultation with infectious disease unit is recommended. The initial drug of choice for management of typhoid fever in children is ceftriaxone 100 mg/kg IV for 7–14 days.

Young children with any *Salmonella* infection should be presumed to be septic and be admitted for full workup and IV antibiotics.

Supportive care includes hydration and, in severe cases, transfusion. There is a risk of bowel perforation requiring surgical intervention.

Helminthic infection

The presence of fever and eosinophilia in a returning traveler suggests helminthic infection. Patients with fever after travel should have a CBC with a differential ordered. Acute hookworm, *Ascaris*, or *Strongyloides* infection should be considered. Also in the differential diagnosis is acute schistosomiasis, visceral larva migrans, lymphatic filiarisis, and trichonosis.

Initial evaluation should include ova and parasite examination of the stool, examination of the peripheral smear for microfilariae and serologic testing for strongyloides, schistosomiasis, and other helminths.

Test results should guide treatment.

Skin disorders

There are a number of common skin complaints in returning travelers. Common causes are scabies and fungal infections such as *Tinea capitis*. Examination of KOH-treated skin samples is easy and helpful in diagnosing both these conditions. In addition, travelers are at risk for dermal myiasis and other larval infestations.

Travelers to the equatorial regions are at risk of dermal myiasis. Dermal myiasis is common in Central and South America caused by *Dermatobia hominis*; furuncular myiasis in Africa is caused by *Cordylobia anthropophaga*. The Latin American botfly attaches its eggs to a mosquito, which then feeds on a mammalian host and the fly larva is deposited in the dermis of the host. The larva breathes through a hole in the skin, which can be seen on close inspection. If not removed, the larva will emerge in roughly 30 days. The African tumbu fly lays eggs on laundry and the larva penetrate the mammalian host via the skin. Larvae emerge in 6 to 7 days. Patients generally present to the ED with botfly infestation when they feel movement under the skin. Botfly myiasis may be treated by asphyxiation of the larvae with petrolatum, raw bacon, or an occlusive dressing. The deceased larvae can then be removed with forceps.

Cutaneous larva migrans results from penetration of the epidermis by dog and cat hookworm. *Ancylostoma braziliense* is the most common cause, but many hookworms, roundworms, and *Strongyloides* spp. may cause the lesions. Children in tropical areas are at particular risk if they walk barefoot. The larvae cause pruritic, serpinginous lesions. Larvae will die if untreated in 2–8 weeks. Larval migration occurs at 2–20 mm per day. The diagnosis is made clinically based on exposure (usually walking barefoot in sand or gardens) and by the characteristic appearance of the lesion. Cutaneous larva migrans may be treated with ivermectin as a single dose administered PO:

- <15 kg: 3 mg
- 16–30 kg: 6 mg
- 31–45 kg: 9 mg.

Alternatively albendazole may be given, 10–15 mg/kg daily for 3–5 days.

Pearls and pitfalls

Pearls

1. Traveler's diarrhea should be treated promptly with antibiotics, which differs from diarrhea contracted in developed countries.
2. Malaria and typhoid should be top of the differential for a returning febrile child.
3. Consult the CDC website to assess pathogens of concern based on patient travel locations.

Pitfalls

1. Failure to elicit a detailed history of travel sites with explicit detail of regions, exposures, and activities.
2. Failure to consider non-travel-related causes of infectious symptoms.

Selected references

Centers for Disease Control and Prevention. http://www.cdc.gov/travel/regionList.aspx and http://www.cdc.gov/travel/contentDiseases.aspx (useful resource sites).

Christenson JC. Preparing children for travel to tropical and developing regions. *Pediatr Ann* 2004;**33**:676–684.

Halstead SB. Dengue. *Lancet* 2007;**370**:1644.

Mackell SM. Traveler's diarrhea in the pediatric population: Etiology and impact. *Clin Infect Dis* 2005;**41**:S547–S552.

Ryan E. Illness after international travel. *N Engl J Med* 2002;**347**:505–516.

Staat M. Traveler's diarrhea. *Pediatr Infect Dis J* 1999;**18**:373–374.

Stauffer WM. Illness after international travel. *N Engl J Med* 2002;**347**: 505–516.

Chapter 99

Tuberculosis

Aparajita Sohoni

Introduction

A confirmed case of pediatric tuberculosis (TB) is important from many standpoints. First, each case of pediatric TB serves as a "sentinel case," indicating recent transmission of TB from an actively infectious contact. Second, children infected with TB more commonly develop severe extrapulmonary forms of the disease, such as miliary disease or meningitis. Third, pediatric patients are capable of spreading TB within the home and in settings such as schools and daycare centers – although adults and adolescents are more likely to transmit disease than younger children. Finally, children with TB represent future "reservoirs of disease," making the detection and treatment of this condition a public health imperative. This chapter will briefly review the global and US burden of pediatric TB, the pathophysiology of infection, common presentations, system-based differentials and diagnostic approaches, treatment and management regimens for this important disease.

Epidemiology

An accurate assessment of the global incidence and prevalence of pediatric TB is complex. While current case detection and registry methods involve documenting each case of sputum smear-positive TB, almost 95% of pediatric TB is negative on this criterion. In 2000, there were approximately 8.3 million new cases of TB globally, of which 884 019 (10.7%) occurred in children. In general, countries with increased levels of poverty, population density, and malnutrition demonstrate a higher incidence of pediatric TB, with rates ranging from 2.7% to 25.3%. An increased prevalence of HIV infection is also correlated with higher incidences of pediatric TB. Within the USA, the incidence of pediatric TB is on the decline.

Pathophysiology

In humans, the majority of cases of TB are caused by *Mycobacterium tuberculosis*. This aerobic bacillus has a relatively long generation time of 15 to 20 h. The lack of a true outer membrane distinguishes the *Mycobacterium* genus from other Gram-negative bacteria. Mycolic acids comprising the cell envelope define this genus and are thought to enable the bacteria to resist lysis by lysozymes or oxygen radicals. Humans are the only natural reservoir for infection with *M. tuberculosis*.

Transmission of TB is determined by the nature of the bacillus, the environment, and the host. The mycobacterium is spread between humans via air-borne droplets. These tubercle-containing particles are capable of remaining air borne for minutes to hours; they are 1–5 μm in size and can penetrate to the pulmonary alveoli. Crowded environments with poor ventilation, such as homeless shelters, correctional facilities, schools, and airplanes, are areas of higher risk for transmission of TB. Prolonged exposure to the bacillus also increases rates of infection. Especially in cases of pediatric TB, household contacts are most often the source of infection. Children <5 years old and immunocompromised children are at highest risk of becoming infected with TB.

As children rarely cough with enough force to aerosolize tubercle bacilli, they rarely are the source of transmission to others.

Once in the alveolus, the bacillus replicates and spreads via lymphatics and the bloodstream. The cellular immune response causes granulomas, which contain the bacilli, to form. The initial granuloma formation, termed the Ghon complex, occurs at the site of the primary pulmonary infection, its draining lymphatics, and surrounding lymph nodes. The bacilli that are not killed within the granuloma enter into a state of latency. Approximately 95% of people who are infected primarily with *M. tuberculosis* contain the bacteria in granulomas and enter into a latent phase of infection. In this stage, granulomas hold the bacilli in an inactive form, incapable of reproducing, spreading, or causing further disease. Once in this latent stage, there is an approximately 10% lifetime risk of reactivation of the disease, at which point lymphohematogenous spread or pulmonary disease may develop. Factors increasing the likelihood of reactivation disease include chronic diseases such as

A Practical Guide to Pediatric Emergency Medicine: Caring for Children in the Emergency Department, ed. N. Ewen Amieva-Wang (associate eds. Jamie Shandro, Aparajita Sohoni, and Bernhard Fassl). Published by Cambridge University Press.

diabetes mellitus, chronic renal failure, or other immunosuppressive conditions such as malignancies, organ transplantation, or HIV infection. Age at time of infection also influences the risk of reactivation, with children infected at <5 years of age being at greater risk for developing reactivation disease.

Of the 5% of patients with a primary infection who are unable to sequester the bacillus into granulomas, primary progressive disease can develop. Children <5 years old have higher rates of developing more severe primary progressive manifestations of TB infection, including pulmonary, meningeal, or miliary disease. Children between 5 and 10 years of age have much lower rates of progression to active TB infection, and when they do progress, tend to develop less severe forms of disease (i.e., lymphatic involvement versus miliary and meningeal disease).

Clinical presentation

Pulmonary disease

The lungs are the most common site of infection in pediatric cases of both primary and reactivation TB. Children with pulmonary TB may be asymptomatic or symptomatic. Those who are asymptomatic are usually detected with a positive tuberculin skin test and then undergo a screening chest radiograph.

Children aged <5 years or >10 years are more likely to manifest symptoms of pulmonary TB. These symptoms are often indistinguishable from other forms of pneumonia and include fevers and cough in 80% of children. The classic signs of night sweats, weight loss, and hemoptysis are present in <50% of children. Systemic symptoms in children are difficult to assess but can include fever, cough, fatigue, anorexia, weight loss, or failure to thrive.

Chest radiographs in symptomatic patients demonstrate a wide range of findings, from lobar consolidation to multiple infiltrates and lymphadenopathy. Cavitary disease is most commonly seen in children older than 10 years of age.

The presence of cavitary disease connotes a high degree of infectivity.

Lymphatic disease

In children, lymphatic disease is the most common form of extrapulmonary TB.

The peak incidence of lymphatic TB occurs in children aged 1 to 6 years. The lymph nodes most frequently infected are the superficial nodes of the head and neck region, accounting for 90% of cases. Bilateral involvement is common. Infected lymph nodes enlarge slowly, generally over 2–3 weeks, and are non-erythematous, mobile, and non-tender. Associated symptoms of weight loss, fever, fatigue, or anorexia are found in <20% of children with lymphatic TB and concomitant pulmonary TB in 50–80%. If untreated, the lymph node develops a caseous center and an erythematous and fluctuant appearance; it finally ruptures, producing a draining sinus tract known as scrofula.

Central nervous system disease

Invasion of the CNS with TB generally results in either TB meningitis (which untreated is uniformly fatal) or the development of parenchymal lesions called tuberculomas. Tuberculous meningitis accounts for 9–16% of cases of extrapulmonary TB in children. The meningitis progresses through three clinical stages. In stage 1, symptoms include fever, headache, vomiting, irritability, drowsiness, or loss of developmental milestones in younger children. In stage 2, children become increasingly drowsy, disoriented, and stuporous; on examination, they may demonstrate signs of meningeal irritation, such as seizures, or manifest other neurologic deficits such as hemiparesis. In stage 3, children show signs of severely elevated intracranial pressure, such as decerebrate or decorticate posturing, and are generally comatose with hemi- or quadriplegia. Concomitant chest radiograph abnormalities are found in only 40–80% of children with TB meningitis.

Tuberculomas are isolated parenchymal lesions that can present with headache, seizures, ALOC, or new neurological deficit. Tuberculomas may temporarily increase in size following the initiation of anti-TB treatment. This enlargement is purportedly a result of an immune reaction to the bacterial antigens released during treatment. Steroids are effective in the treatment of tuberculomas.

Bone/joint disease

Bone and joint involvement is found in 5–6% of those with pediatric extrapulmonary TB. Symptoms generally present 1–3 years after infection. Tuberculous dactylitis, more common in young infants, can present within the first month following infection. More than 50% of cases involve the vertebral bodies, termed TB spondylitis, TB osteomyelitis, or Pott's disease. Usually, multiple vertebral bodies are affected, and lesions may not be in contiguous vertebrae. Given that the seeding of the vertebral bodies occurs via the bloodstream, the anterior portions of the vertebral bodies are more commonly affected than the posterior structures. If untreated, disease may progress to involve the disc. The surrounding soft tissues also frequently become infected. More than 90% of children with TB spondylitis have co-existing retropharyngeal or psoas abscesses, or epidural masses. Other highly vascular sites commonly infected with TB include the knee, hip, elbow, or ankle. In pediatric patients, infection and destruction of the epiphyseal growth plates frequently occurs. In TB osteomyelitis, concomitant pulmonary infection is generally absent.

Miliary disease and immunosuppressed patients

Miliary TB is generally found in younger infants or immunosuppressed children. Immunosuppression may be secondary to

Table 99.1. Recommended dosages and adverse effects of first-line anti-tuberculosis drugs in pediatric patients

Drug	Method of administration	Common dosages	Daily dose (mg/kg)	Twice a week (mg/kg)	Maximum in one dose	Adverse effects
Isoniazid	PO/IM/IV	100 or 300 mg	10–15	20–30	300 mg for daily; 900 mg for twice weekly	Hepatitis, peripheral neuritis, rash
Rifampin	PO/IV	150 or 300 mg capsules, syrup	10–20	10–20	600 mg	Orange discoloration of secretions, contact lenses, urine; rash; thrombocytopenia; drug interactions
Pyrazinamide	PO	500 mg tablets	20–40	50	2 g for daily; 4 g for twice weekly	GI upset, hepatitis, hyperuricemia, arthralgia
Ethambutol	PO	100 or 400 mg tablets	15–25	50	2.5 g	Optic neuritis, GI upset, decreased red–green color discrimination

malnutrition; concomitant infection such as HIV; prior exposure to measles, pertussis, or varicella; or from the use of chronic immunosuppressive therapies, such as corticosteroids in transplant recipients. The median age of children with miliary TB ranges from 11 months to 4 years, with rapid onset of disease, frequently within 6 months of the primary infection. Congenital infection with TB (acquired from a mother with miliary TB or contact with an infectious source in the perinatal period) is exceedingly rare, but may occur, and presents as failure to thrive, pneumonia, organomegaly, or feeding intolerance.

Common presenting signs include fever, cough, weight loss, decreased appetite, and fatigue. On examination, generalized lymphadenopathy and hepato- or splenomegaly is frequently seen. Chest radiographs show the classic millet seed pattern of diffuse pulmonary infiltrates characteristic of miliary TB. Significant respiratory distress may be present. Meningeal TB has been found in as many as 19–30% of patients at the time of presentation. Even with treatment, mortality rates range from 9 to 14%.

Diagnosis

In the ED, diagnosis will be presumptive. The country of birth, socioeconomic status, and exposure to known sources of TB should raise suspicion for the patient having TB. Also, ingestion of unpasteurized milk or cheese products should raise concern for *Mycobacterium bovis*. Although beyond the scope of this chapter, *M. bovis* infection usually results in abdominal or GI symptoms. The treatment for *M. bovis* is rifampin and isoniazid for 6 months.

Children with pulmonary TB who are asymptomatic are usually detected with a positive tuberculin skin test and then undergo a screening chest radiograph.

The chest radiograph in asymptomatic patients usually shows patchy peripheral infiltrates and hilar lymphadenopathy. In symptomatic patients, chest radiographs demonstrate a wide range of findings, from lobar consolidation to multiple infiltrates and lymphadenopathy. In miliary TB, the radiographs show the classic millet seed pattern of diffuse pulmonary infiltrates.

Management

Patients with suspected active disease should be placed in appropriate isolation and hospitalized for definitive workup and therapy in conjunction with pediatric infectious disease specialists. Unless an emergency, therapy can usually be started on an inpatient basis. Patients who present to the ED with possible TB recurrence should be questioned as to the length of previous treatment, and the number of drugs used.

Specific drug treatment

While EPs should probably not initiate treatment with antituberculous medication, it is important to understand the usual drug regimens used as well as their side effects (Table 99.1). The physician can determine generally if treatment has been with an appropriate number of drugs for the appropriate time period.

Latent infection

Latent TB should be treated with 9 months of daily isoniazid therapy. Transaminitis or symptomatic hepatitis is rare in pediatric patients. Concomitant pyridoxine administration (25 to 50 mg daily) is only recommended in children who are breast-feeding, have diets low in milk or meat, are malnourished, or have symptomatic HIV infection. In patients who do not tolerate isoniazid, daily rifampin therapy should be instituted for 6 months.

Active infection

The treatment of active TB is divided into an initiation phase, consisting of four drugs for 2 months, and a continuation phase, lasting 4 to 7 months, at which point antibiotics should be tailored based on culture sensitivities and disease response. Tuberculous meningitis should be treated for 9–12 months. For miliary TB, a total of 9 months of therapy should be instituted. In patients with HIV, therapy is complex and should be initiated in conjunction with a specialist. Steroids are indicated only for meningitis, pericarditis, and endobronchial disease and must be used only in concert with appropriate TB therapy. Prednisone daily doses of 1–2 mg/kg are sufficient. Cultures and sensitivities, or failure to respond with standard treatment, will suggest the presence of multidrug-resistant TB, at which point the medication regimen must be tailored appropriately.

Directly observed therapy (DOT) is recommended for all pediatric patients to ensure compliance. Regular follow-up with a primary medical doctor is paramount to ensure monitoring of therapy as well as screening for possible adverse drug effects.

Disposition

In general, the following guidelines apply in determining admission and follow-up for patients with suspected TB:

- any patient with concern for active pulmonary or extrapulmonary disease should be admitted
- household contacts should be referred for screening as well
- children with normal chest radiographs are considered not to be contagious
- patients with positive sputum smears are considered not to be contagious after completing 2 weeks of therapy
- the younger the patient is, the less likely it is that they are coughing with enough force to aerosolize infectious particles.

Pearls and pitfalls

Pearls

1. Suspect tuberculosis (TB) in children with suspected or known contacts, systemic illness, or non-specific systemic symptoms.
2. Referring suspected contacts for screening is key. If any contact is found to have TB, and is the likely source case, their cultures and sensitivities can guide treatment of the pediatric patient, for whom sputum cultures and sensitivities are more difficult to obtain.
3. Within the USA, suspect TB particularly in immigrant, Hispanic and non-Hispanic Black children, as they account for almost 75% of new cases annually.

Pitfalls

1. Failure to realize that children, particularly younger infants, are less able to report, or have undergone, "classic" signs and symptoms of TB.
2. Pediatric patients are less able to generate a forceful cough, making suspicion and diagnosis of pulmonary TB more difficult.
3. Failure to maintain a high index of suspicion for pulmonary and extrapulmonary TB in pediatric patients, as the majority of patients will be asymptomatic.

Selected references

American Thoracic Society (ATS) and Centers for Disease Control and Prevention. Treatment of tuberculosis. *MMRW Morb Mort Wkly Rep* 2003;**52**: 1–77 http://www.cdc.gov/mmwr/preview/mmwrhtml/rr5211a1.htm (accessed 1 June 2010).

Nelson LJ, Wells CD. Global epidemiology of childhood tuberculosis. *Int J Tuberc Lung Dis* 2004;**8**:636–647.

Nelson LJ, Schneider E, Wells CD, Moore M. Epidemiology of childhood tuberculosis in the United States, 1993–2001: the need for continued vigilance. *Pediatrics* 2004;**114**: 333–341.

Powell DA, Hunt WG. Tuberculosis in children: an update. *Adv Pediatr* 2006;**53**: 279–322.

Sharma SK, Mohan A, Sharma A, Mitra DK. Miliary tuberculosis: new insights into an old disease. *Lancet Infect Dis* 2005;**5**:415–430.

World Health Organization. *Global TB information, statistics, patient information handouts and treatment strategies*. Geneva: World Health Organization http://www.who.int/topics/tuberculosis/en/ (accessed 1 June 2010).

Chapter 100

Urinary tract infections

Joel T. Levis

Introduction

Urinary tract infections (UTI) are common throughout infancy, childhood, and adolescence, occurring in 3–5% of girls and 1% of boys. Infection can occur at any level of the urinary tract, including the bladder (cystitis), renal pelvis (pyelitis), or renal parenchyma (pyelonephritis). During the first year of life, the male:female ratio is 2.8–5.4:1. After 1–2 years, there is a female preponderance, with a male:female ratio of 1:10. In girls, the first UTI usually occurs by the age of 5 years, with peaks during infancy and toilet training. After the first UTI, 60–80% of these girls will develop a second UTI within 18 months. In boys, most UTIs occur during the first year of life. During this time, lack of circumcision increases the likelihood of development of a UTI in boys.

Enterobacteriaceae are the most common isolates from uncomplicated UTI, with *Escherichia coli* accounting for 70–90% of infections. Other Gram-negative organisms associated with UTI are *Klebsiella, Enterobacter, Proteus,* and *Pseudomonas* spp. The Gram-positive organisms occasionally encountered are *Enterococcus,* and group B streptococci in the neonatal period, and *Staphylococcus saprophyticus* in sexually active adolescents. Viral infections, particularly adenovirus, may also occur, particularly as a cause of cystitis.

Pathophysiology

In neonates, infection of the urinary tract is assumed to be from hematogenous spread rather than ascending infection.

After the neonatal period, the bladder is the initial primary locus of infection from perineal contaminants such as *E. coli*, with ascending disease of the upper tract (kidneys) and bacteremia as potential sequelae. Bacterial invasion of the bladder with overt UTI is more likely to occur if urinary stasis or low flow exists. Some causes of these conditions are infrequent or incomplete voiding, reflux, or other urinary tract abnormalities. The ascending route of infection helps to explain the gender difference because the shorter female urethra increases the frequency of UTI in girls.

Clinical presentation

School-age children with UTI may present with symptoms similar to those seen in adults (i.e., dysuria, frequency, urgency, hesitancy, small-volume voids, incontinence, fever, and suprapubic, lower abdominal, or flank pain). Infants more commonly present with non-specific symptoms such as fever, irritability, jaundice, vomiting, or failure to thrive. Fever is the most common presentation in young children. Unusual odor of the urine is not helpful in predicting UTI. Symptoms and signs found to be most predictive of UTI in infants with a fever include history of a previous UTI, temperature >40°C, and suprapubic tenderness. Among male infants, lack of circumcision increases the likelihood of a UTI.

Children with suspected UTI should be examined thoroughly to determine whether a source can be found to explain the fever. The external genitalia should be carefully examined to rule out any gross anatomic abnormalities, skin lesions, frank discharge, or foreign body. Suprapubic tenderness (suggestive of cystitis) and costovertebral angle tenderness (suggestive of pyelonephritis) should be assessed. Other conditions may mimic UTI symptoms. Acute urethritis or vulvovaginitis may be caused by various types of irritant, including chemical (e.g., bubble baths, soaps), physical (e.g., self-exploration), and biologic (e.g., pinworms). As sexually transmitted infections (STDs) are among the most common infectious diagnoses in adolescents, these infections should be considered in adolescent patients presenting with acute urethritis or vulvovaginitis (see Ch. 96).

Diagnostic studies

Guidelines for urine testing

The AAP recommends that a UTI should be ruled out in any child 2 months to 2 years of age with unexplained fever. Although no sign or symptom by itself is diagnostic of UTI in children, the presence of a temperature >40°C, history of a previous UTI, lack of circumcision, abdominal pain, back pain, dysuria, frequency, new-onset incontinence, and suprapubic tenderness increase the baseline likelihood of UTI two- to six-fold.

A Practical Guide to Pediatric Emergency Medicine: Caring for Children in the Emergency Department, ed. N. Ewen Amieva-Wang (associate eds. Jamie Shandro, Aparajita Sohoni, and Bernhard Fassl). Published by Cambridge University Press.

Improper collection of specimens leads to misdiagnosis and overtreatment. Bag specimen collection is not appropriate for diagnosis of UTI at any age because of the substantial rate of contamination. Spontaneously voided, clean-catch mid-stream urine may be used to evaluate older infants and children with suspected UTI, if the specimen is not contaminated. Suprapubic aspiration is considered the gold standard for UTI diagnosis, although is used uncommonly. Use of a urethral catheter also provides a reliable specimen for culture, is less invasive than suprapubic aspiration, and can be readily carried out by trained nursing staff. All urine specimens should be processed as expeditiously as possible.

Laboratory tests

Because urine culture typically requires at least 24 h of incubation, urinalysis and urine microscopy are the initial tests used to establish the presumptive diagnosis of UTI and to guide the initiation of empiric treatment. Leukocyte esterase testing detects enzymes generated by inflammatory cells; however, this test is neither more sensitive nor more specific than the detection of the cells themselves. Nitrite detection in urine is based on the observation that many urine pathogens convert nitrate to nitrite in the bladder. When the nitrite reaction is performed with a freshly voided specimen, a positive result is highly predictive of UTI.

Microscopy of a urine sample will enable the detection of white blood cells and bacteria. Pyuria is usually defined as the presence of a WBC >5–8/μl in uncentrifuged urine, representing more than 1/high-power field. The occurrence of more than 20 cells/high-power field usually correlates with significant bacteriuria of 100 000 colony-forming units (cfu) per milliliter of a clean-catch sample. While most patients with symptomatic UTIs will have pyuria, the presence of pyuria alone does not necessarily indicate the presence of a UTI. False-positive results may be caused by vaginal washout, chemical irritation, fever, viral infection, immunization, or glomerulonephritis. Finally, a Gram stain of uncentrifuged urine is a useful test for the presumptive diagnosis of UTI. Any of the following are suggestive of UTI

- positive results of a leukocyte esterase test
- positive results of a nitrite test
- WBC >5/high-power field of a properly spun specimen
- bacteria present on an unspun Gram-stained specimen.

Therefore, the combination of a negative leukocyte esterase, nitrite, and urine microscopy can rule out UTI in children beyond the neonatal period, while positive results can be used to guide empiric treatment while awaiting culture results. Because newborns and infants do not concentrate urine as their kidneys are immature, urinalysis alone may inaccurately reflect the absence of infection, thus necessitating urine culture testing in these patients.

A positive culture in properly collected urine specimens establishes the diagnosis of UTI and provides an isolate for susceptibility testing. The presence of organisms in any number is considered significant when obtained by suprapubic aspiration. When urine is collected by catheterization, a colony count greater than 1000 cfu/ml urine can be considered diagnostic. However, for infants, counts of 10 000 cfu/ml or greater have been obtained from catheterized specimens in the absence of other findings of UTI and may indicate the presence of asymptomatic bacteruria. For urine obtained by catheter, infections should be defined by a colony count >50 000 cfu/ml and pyuria with leukocytes of at least 10/μl. If the quantitative culture from a mid-stream sample reveals ≥100 000 cfu/ml urine, it also indicates the presence of significant bacteriuria.

Management

Multiple antibiotic options are available to the practitioner to treat uncomplicated lower UTIs (e.g., cystitis). Common choices, as a course over 7–10 days, include:

- trimethoprim–sulfamethoxazole (8 mg/kg daily divided q. 12 h)
- nitrofurantoin (5–7 mg/kg daily divided q. 6 h)
- cephalosporins, including cefixime (8 mg/kg daily divided q. 12–24 h)
- cephalexin (25–50 mg/kg daily divided q. 6–8 h)
- ampicillin (50–100 mg/kg daily divided q. 6 h)
- amoxicillin and amoxicillin/clavulinic acid (each 20–40 mg/kg q. 12 h).

Common uropathogens are increasingly resistant to trimethoprim–sulfamethoxazole and ampicillin. *E. coli* resistance has been noted to be as high as 32% in the western USA, while uropathogen resistance to ampicillin has ranged from 25% to 45% in recent years. Predictors of situations in which uropathogens will be more likely to be resistant to commonly used agents are diabetes, recent hospitalization, recent use of antibiotics (particularly trimethoprim–sulfamethoxazole), presence of urinary malformations, urethral catheters, and antimicrobial prophylaxis.

In general for pyelitis or pyelonephritis, the combination of ampicillin (50–100 mg/kg daily divided q. 6 h) or a cephalosporin (e.g., cefazolin [25–50 mg/kg daily q. 6–8 h] for infants >1 month) plus an aminoglycoside (e.g., gentamicin [7.5 mg/kg daily q. 8 h] for newborns >1 week) is adequate coverage for most uropathogens. Because of changing resistance patterns of uropathogens and a concern for nephrotoxicity, a single third-generation cephalosporin (e.g., ceftriaxone [50–75 mg/kg daily divided q. 12–24 h] or ceftazidime [90–150 mg/kg daily q. 4–6 h]) is increasingly being used as an alternative initial regimen. Several studies have demonstrated the efficacy of fourth-generation cephalosporins (e.g., cefepime [50 mg/kg q. 8–12 h]) in the parenteral treatment of pediatric UTI.

Disposition

A healthy young child with a presumed uncomplicated UTI who is non-toxic, is taking in fluids, has reliable caretakers, and is able to be followed up on a daily basis may be managed as an outpatient with oral antibiotics. It is recommended that a single dose of a parenteral or oral antibiotic be given in the ED or clinic before discharge to ensure adequate blood levels of an antibiotic to which more than 95% of common uropathogens are susceptible. Fever from UTI should resolve by 48–72 h with adequate therapy.

An acutely ill child, immunocompromised patient, or infant younger than 2 months of age with a UTI is assumed to have acute pyelonephritis or a complicated UTI. These patients should be managed with hospital admission, rehydration, and parenteral broad-spectrum antimicrobial therapy immediately after urine culture is obtained. Any patient with questionable compliance or difficulty with follow-up should be considered for inpatient management.

Imaging studies

The occurrence of a UTI in young children may indicate the presence of an anatomic abnormality. Vesicoureteral reflux (VUR) is believed to be present in $\leq$1% of normal children, although the incidence is likely to vary depending on the age of screening because VUR often resolves over time. Most VUR is diagnosed after occurrence of a UTI. In children with UTIs, the reported frequency of VUR varies from 20 to 40%. Boys and girls are equally likely to have VUR after a UTI, but boys are more likely to have higher-grade VUR. Girls are more commonly diagnosed with VUR because they are more likely to have a UTI.

Imaging of the urinary tract is recommended in every febrile infant or young child 2 months to 2 years of age with a first UTI to identify those with abnormalities that predispose to renal damage. The AAP guidelines state that infants and young children 2 months to 2 years of age with UTIs who do not demonstrate the expected clinical response within 2 days of antimicrobial therapy should undergo ultrasonography promptly, and either voiding cystourethrogram or radionuclide cystography should be performed at the earliest convenient time. Young children 2 months to 2 years of age with UTIs who have the expected response to antimicrobial drugs should have a sonogram and either voiding cystourethrogram or radionuclide cystography performed at the earliest convenient time. This imaging can be done as an outpatient with a primary care provider.

Conclusions

Urinary tract infections are one of the most common bacterial infections in children. Older children with UTI may present with symptoms similar to adults, while infants more commonly present with non-specific symptoms. While empiric treatment can be started based on urinalysis, a urine culture is necessary in the very young for confirmation of the infection and to guide antibiotic treatment. All young children with UTI require follow-up and imaging to rule out structural disease.

Pearls and pitfalls

Pearls

1. Fever is the most common presentation in young children with urinary tract infections (UTI).
2. A urine culture should be obtained in all infants and young children with a suspected UTI to confirm infection and guide antibiotic treatment.
3. During the first year of life, lack of circumcision increases the likelihood of developing a UTI in boys.
4. In neonates, UTI is assumed to result from hematogenous spread rather than ascending infection.

Pitfalls

1. Bag urine specimen collection is not appropriate for diagnosis of UTI at any age secondary to the substantial rate of contamination.
2. Failure to consider UTI in infants with non-specific symptoms such as fever, irritability, jaundice, vomiting, or failure to thrive.
3. Failure to assume that acutely ill children, immunocompromised patients, or infants <2 months have acute pyelonephritis or a complicated UTI and require hospital admission with parenteral antibiotics.

Selected references

Arrieta AC, Bradley JS. Empiric use of cefepime in the treatment of serious urinary tract infections in children. *Pediatr Infect Dis J* 2001;**20**:350–355.

Bergman DA, Baltz RD, Cooley JR, *et al.* American Academy of Pediatrics Committee on Quality Improvement. Practice parameter: the diagnosis, treatment, and evaluation of the initial urinary tract infection in febrile infants and young children. *Pediatrics* 1999;**103**:843–852.

Elder JS. Urinary tract infections. In Behrman RE, Kliegman RM, Jenson HB (eds.) *Nelson's Textbook of Pediatrics*, 17th edn. St. Louis, MO: Elsevier, 2004, pp.1785–1790.

Malhotra SM, Kennedy WA. Urinary tract infections in children: Treatment. *Urol Clin North Am* 2004;**31**:527–534.

Patel HP. The abnormal urinalysis. *Pediatr Clin North Am* 2006;**53**:325–337.

Shaikh N, Morone NE, Lopez J, *et al.* Does this child have a urinary tract infection? *JAMA* 2007;**298**:2895–2904.

Shortliffe LM. Urinary tract infections in infants and children. In Walsh P, Retik AB, Vaughn ED, *et al.* (eds.) *Campbell's Urology*, 8th edn. Philadelphia, PA: Saunders, 2002, pp. 1846–1884.

Chapter 101

Pediatric upper respiratory tract infections and influenza

Aparajita Sohoni

Introduction

The majority of pediatric upper respiratory tract infections (URIs) are self-limited, although the symptoms are frequently concerning enough to bring families to the ED. This chapter will cover the presentation and management of URIs and then specifically focus on the diagnosis and management of the influenza virus in the pediatric patient.

The common cold

The common cold in children usually manifests with fever, upper respiratory congestion, pharyngitis, and cough. "Colds" develop more frequently and last twice as long in children than in adults (six to eight episodes/year versus two to four episodes/year, and 14 days versus 7 days, respectively). While the vast majority of URIs are caused by rhinoviruses, there are many other etiologies, some of which cause specific and identifiable syndromes (Table 101.1). Transmission most often occurs when infected nasopharyngeal secretions are transferred to hands and inoculated into the nose, eyes, or mouth. Coughing and sneezing can also generate infectious droplets that can land on surfaces such as toys or directly on other's mucous membranes. While in adults, congestion is the main symptom and fever is absent, children often develop fever and systemic symptoms in addition to nasal congestion.

Children can develop complications from the common cold. In infants 0–3 months of age, fever with or without URI symptoms may warrant a "rule out sepsis" workup (see Ch. 157).

Since young infants are obligate nasal breathers, nasal congestion can, albeit rarely, cause significant respiratory distress.

Approximately a quarter of children with URI develop otitis media through eustachian tube dysfunction. Approximately 50% of acute asthma exacerbations are associated with viral URI. Secondary infections such as sinusitis and pneumonia are less common complications of URI in children.

While the treatment of a viral URI consists of symptomatic relief and support, there is an increasing interest in rapid testing for specific viruses. This testing can be required for admitted patients to avoid viral transmission. Viral test results in febrile children with possible URI can contribute to the overall workup and disposition of infants and children, or to the management of a child with serious co-morbidities Another useful role of viral testing is epidemiologic surveillance to define infectious seasons in a particular community.

Table 101.1. Syndromes for viral infections

Virus	Syndrome
Respiratory syncytial virus	Bronchiolitis <2 years
Parainfluenza virus	Croup
Coxsackieviruses	Herpangina, hand-foot-mouth disease
Adenoviruses	Pharyngoconjunctival fever

Management

There is no role for antibiotics in the treatment of a viral URI. Specific viral syndromes are covered in other chapters (croup, Ch. 134; bronchiolitis, Ch. 131; influenza is discussed below).

There is no role for the use of decongestants, antitussives, or expectorants in small children with UTIs.

In spite of this, approximately 39% of US households purchased such medications for use in pediatric patients in 2004–2007. Unfortunately, the use of such medications in pediatric patients is not evidence based. There are no well-designed randomized trials that have shown a difference in placebo versus active drug therapy in children younger than 12 years of age. This absence of efficacy, combined with the fact that dosages of these medications are frequently extrapolated from adult-based pharmacokinetics, makes the administration of these medications to pediatric patients particularly dangerous. The Poison Control Center logged 750 000 calls in 7 years related to the use of these medications in pediatric patients, and approximately 123 pediatric deaths have been attributed to

A Practical Guide to Pediatric Emergency Medicine: Caring for Children in the Emergency Department, ed. N. Ewen Amieva-Wang (associate eds. Jamie Shandro, Aparajita Sohoni, and Bernhard Fassl). Published by Cambridge University Press.

complications arising from the dose or administration of these medications. While the FDA has issued a black box warning regarding the use of these medications in children younger than 2 years old, it is important for medical providers to be aware that no data show that these medications are safe in children aged 2–11 years either.

Safer symptomatic therapy includes antipyretics, nasal irrigation, and the use of a humidifier. Beta-agonists often relieve cough, even in children without a "diagnosis" of asthma. First-generation antihistamines (diphenhydramine) may help in drying up secretions secondary to their anticholinergic effects. Vitamins and minerals such as vitamin C or zinc and other food supplements have not been proven helpful in adults or children. It is important to realize that young infants may require observation and hospitalization secondary to respiratory distress (particularly with bronchiolitis), and decreased ability to stay hydrated.

Influenza

Influenza virus is classified as type A, B, or C based on differences in the nucleocapsid protein. Type A is associated with more severe disease, causing epidemics or pandemics, and is capable of infecting animals and humans. Influenza A virus is subdivided into groups based on the surface neuraminidase (NA) and hemagglutinin (HA) proteins. The continuous mutation, or antigenic drift, of these proteins necessitates annual vaccine development, as the host's antibodies will only be effective against a particular strain of the virus. Type B strains do not infect most animals and cause less severe infection in humans. Type C strains will not be further mentioned here as they cause mild disease only.

Epidemiology

The epidemiology of influenza virus attacks is seasonal, with "influenza-season" referring to November to March annually. Aside from URIs, influenza is associated with acute otitis media and increased susceptibility for developing more severe bacterial pneumonias with either *Streptococcus pneumoniae* or *Staphylococcus aureus*. Influenza virus causes higher rates of infection, complications, and hospitalizations or death in children <5 years of age, in those >65 years of age, and in those who have pre-existing medical conditions. Children without high-risk co-morbidities are hospitalized at a rate of 100/100 000. The overall mortality rate for pediatric patients with influenza is approximately 3.8/100 000 population.

Transmission

Influenza virus is transmitted via respiratory secretions that become air borne (i.e., via coughing, sneezing, or talking) or by direct contact with secretions that are contaminated. The incubation period is 18–72 h. Hosts are infectious for approximately 24 h before symptoms begin and for as long as 5 days into the illness.

Table 101.2. Influenza versus common cold symptoms

Signs/symptoms	Influenza	Cold
Onset	Sudden	Gradual
Fever	High, lasting >3 days	Rare
Upper respiratory tract infection symptoms (congestion, sore throat)	Occasionally	Common
Cough	May become severe	Less common
Systemic signs (headache, myalgias, fatigue)	Prominent and prolonged	Mild

Clinical presentation

A child with influenza will typically present with an abrupt onset of fever, followed by myalgias, headache, malaise, rhinitis, sore throat, and a non-productive cough. These symptoms may evolve into pneumonia, either viral or from bacterial superinfection, or may result in concomitant sinusitis or otitis media. Influenza may also cause croup or bronchiolitis, exacerbations of underlying asthma, renal failure, myocarditis, or pericarditis. As mentioned above, children with other medical problems, such as asthma, or who are immunocompromised have higher rates of developing clinically severe infections or co-infections.

Clinically, distinguishing influenza from other causes of URIs can be challenging. Table 101.2 presents criteria that suggest influenza infection rather than other causes of the common cold.

Diagnosis

The diagnosis of influenza is based on clinical suspicion, as well as on detection of viral protein or viral RNA in respiratory secretions/washings of throat/nares specimens. The rapid viral diagnostic tests for detection of viral RNA protein have sensitivities ranging from 45 to 96% and specificities ranging from 52 to 100%. Viral culture and viral serologies both during the infection and 14 days post-infection can also be obtained to confirm the diagnosis.

Management

Currently, there are four antiviral drugs for the treatment of influenza infections. Amantadine, rimantadine, and oseltamivir are approved for use in pediatric patients (Table 101.3). These medications should be offered to any child >1 year of age who is experiencing either a severe influenza infection (i.e., influenza pneumonia), or who is at risk of serious complications from influenza. If initiated within 48 h of the onset of symptoms, these medications can shorten the duration of disease by approximately 1 day. Amantadine and rimantadine are effective against influenza A, while oseltamivir can reduce the duration of uncomplicated influenza A and B infections.

Table 101.3. Pediatric agents/dosages for treatment and prophylaxis of influenza

Drug	FDA-approved indication by age	Treatment dosage	Prophylaxis dosage
Amantadine	>*1 year*: treatment or prophylaxis of influenza A	<*10 years* or < 40 kg: 5 mg/kg daily in 1–2 doses (max. 150 mg) for 3–5 days, or for 24–48 h after asymptomatic >*10 years*: 100 mg BID for 3–5 days or for 24–48 h after asymptomatic	Same doses as for treatment but for at least 10 days or up to 6 weeks
Rimantadine	>*13 years*: treatment of influenza A >*1 year*: prophylaxis of influenza A	100 mg BID for 5–7 days	<*10 years*: 5 mg/kg daily (max. 150 mg) for 10 days or up to 8 weeks >*10 years*: 100 mg BID for at least 10 days or up to 8 weeks
Oseltamivir	>*1 year*: treatment of influenza A and B >*13 years*: prophylaxis of influenza A and B	*1–12 years* <*15 kg*: 2 mg/kg dose (max. 30 mg) BID for 5 days *15–23 kg*: 45 mg BID for 5 days *23–40 kg*: 60 mg BID for 5 days >12 years or >*40 kg*: 75 mg BID for 5 days	75 mg daily for at least 7 days or up to 6 weeks
Zanamivir	>*7 years*: treatment of influenza A and B	10 mg BID for 5 days	

Source: Pickering *et al.*, 2006.

Zanamivir (the other neuraminidase inhibitor) is approved for prophylaxis of influenza in children >5 years of age and for treatment in children >7 years of age. Guidelines for these medications vary with the influenza strain (see the CDC website for current guidelines).

The major side effects of amantadine and rimantadine consist of behavioral changes, delirium, agitation, or seizures. These effects are seen principally in people with underlying renal insufficiency, resulting in increased plasma levels of the drug, or in people with seizure or psychiatric disorders. Amantadine also has anticholinergic effects and, therefore, should not be used in patients with untreated acute angle closure glaucoma as it can cause mydriasis. Oseltamivir can cause nausea and vomiting, or occasionally transient neuropsychiatric events such as delirium. Zanamivir can also cause nausea and vomiting but may also cause diarrhea, sinusitis, cough, bronchitis, headache, or dizziness. These complications were reported in <5% of people, making zanamivir generally very well tolerated.

Immunization guidelines

Immunization is paramount in the protection from infection with influenza virus. Current guidelines for immunization are shown in Box 101.1. Between the ages of 6 months and 9 years, children who are vaccinated for the first time should receive two doses before the influenza season begins. The two forms of the influenza vaccine are the trivalent inactivated influenza vaccines (TIV) and the live attenuated influenza vaccine (LAIV). The two doses should be administered at least 4 weeks apart. Following vaccination with LAIV, viral shedding may occur for approximately 10 days; however, this viral shedding does not generally result in transmission of the virus, as the virus that is shed is the same attenuated version as that included in the vaccine. After receipt of either vaccine, pain at the site of injection, myalgias, fever, or malaise may occur. These vaccines should not be administered to anyone with an egg allergy, as both vaccines are grown in embryonic hen eggs.

Box 101.1. Vaccine recommendations for influenza 2009–2010

- All children healthy or otherwise age 6 months to 18 years.
- Adults ≥50 years.
- Children and adults with medical conditions at risk for complications including:
  - pulmonary disease (cystic fibrosis, asthma, emphysema)
  - cardiovascular disease
  - metabolic disease (diabetes)
  - renal dysfunction
  - hemoglobinopathies
  - immunosuppression.
- Household members and health providers of:
  - high-risk patients
  - healthy children <5 years of age.
- Pregnant women.
- Healthcare providers.

Note: These recommendations can change year to year; confirm on the CDC website http://www.cdc.gov/flu/about/season/index.htm.

Special situations: influenza H1N1

In 2009, a novel H1NI strain of influenza resulted in a pandemic, with the majority of cases reported from the USA,

Mexico, and Canada. As of June 2009, approximately 27 000 probable or confirmed cases were reported within the USA, with approximately 120 deaths. Initially termed "swine flu," the H1N1 virus resulted from a combination of pig, bird, and human flu viruses. The clinical presentation mimicked that of other influenza viruses, with fever, cough, runny nose, myalgias, headache, and fatigue being the predominant symptoms. Populations considered at increased risk from complications relating to infection with H1N1 are children <5 years of age, particularly those under 2 years; adults >65 years of age; immunosuppressed individuals; those with chronic pulmonary, cardiovascular, renal, hematological, hepatic, neurologic, or metabolic (including diabetes mellitus) disorders; pregnant women; and residents of nursing homes. The H1N1 strain of influenza was found to be sensitive to zanamivir and oseltamivir, but resistant to amantadine and rimantadine. Although the CDC recommendations regarding treatment for H1N1 evolve over the course of an outbreak, treatment is recommended for any high-risk patient (as defined above), and for all hospitalized patients with suspected or confirmed H1N1. Although oseltamivir has not been officially recommended for use in children <1 year old, given the higher morbidity and mortality of influenza infections in this age group, the CDC has recommended treating infants with confirmed or highly probably H1N1 with oseltamivir. Children <3 months should receive 12 mg twice daily; those aged 3–5 months should receive 20 mg twice daily, and those aged 6–11 months should receive 25 mg twice daily.

The indications for prophylaxis are unclear. In general, a high-risk patient who has been in contact with a confirmed case should receive oseltamivir prophylaxis. This information is from the CDC website (http://www.cdc.gov/h1n1flu) and is updated frequently. The CDC website should be checked for any further updates.

Pearls and pitfalls

Pearls

1. Children develop upper respiratory tract infections more frequently and with greater severity than adults.
2. Over-the-counter cough suppressants/antitussives/decongestants should never be prescribed for a child <2 years of age.
3. All children >6 months should receive vaccination against influenza, provided they do not have allergies to eggs.

Pitfalls

1. Failure to warn parents about the potentially dangerous side effects associated with over-the-counter cough and cold medicines.
2. Failure to recognize an immunosuppressed or otherwise high-risk child who may develop serious sequelae from influenza infection.
3. Failure to screen household members of pediatric patients diagnosed with influenza to determine need for prophylaxis or treatment.

Selected references

Committee on Infectious Disease. Policy statement recommendations for the prevention and treatment of influenza in children 2009–2010. *Pediatrics* 2009;**124**:1216–1226.

Meissner HC. Influenza vaccines: a pediatric perspective. *Curr Opin Pediatr* 2007;**19**:58–63.

Meissner HC. Reducing the impact of viral respiratory infections in children. *Pediatr Clin North Am* 2005;**52**:695–710.

Pickering LK, Baker CJ, Kimberlin DW, Long SS. (eds.) *The Red Book: 2006 Report of the Committee on Infectious Diseases*, 27th edn. Elk Grove Village, IL: American Academy of Pediatrics, 2006 (also Red Book Online, last updated 5 January 2009).

Sharfstein JM, North M, Serwint JR. Over the counter but no longer under the radar: pediatric cough and cold medications. *N Engl J Med* 2007;**357**:2321–2324.

Townsend KA, Eiland LS. Combating influenza with antiviral therapy in the pediatric population. *Pharmacotherapy* 2006;**26**:95–103.

Chapter 102

Tutorial: Ultrasound-guided lumbar puncture

Teresa S. Wu

Introduction

Lumbar punctures can usually be successfully completed using anatomic landmarks for guidance. Bedside ultrasound can be used to help to direct the lumbar puncture in patients where landmarks may be difficult to appreciate (e.g., patients who are obese, have scoliosis, or those who are unable to create a kyphotic lumbar curve for the procedure).

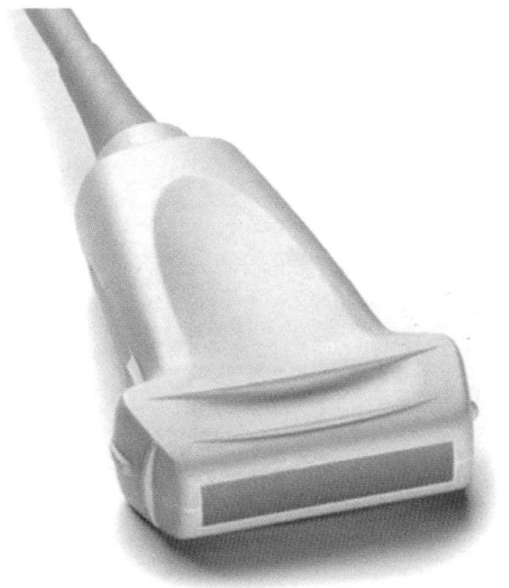

Figure 102.1 Linear array transducer. (Image courtesy of SonoSite, Inc.)

Method

1. Position the patient in a lateral decubitus fetal position or sit them upright with an exaggerated kypohotic lumbar curve.
2. Use the longest 5 MHz or 7.5 MHz linear probe available (Fig. 102.1).
3. Start by placing the transducer in a transverse plane over the midline of the patient's back at the level of the iliac crests (Fig. 102.2).
4. With the probe positioned perpendicular to the patient's spine, scan from the patient's left to right until a spinous process is found. In this view, the spinous processes will appear as a hyperechoic object casting a dark shadow farfield across the screen (Fig. 102.3).
5. Move the probe from the patient's left to right until the dark shadow is centered in the middle of the screen. When the spinous process shadow is visualized in the middle of the screen, it is centered directly under the middle of the probe.
6. Use a marker to identify this point as midline on the patient's back.
7. Scan and identify two more adjacent spinous processes. Extend a short line from cephalad to caudad connecting the adjacent spinous processes in order to clearly distinguish the midline.
8. Once the midline has been demarcated, rotate the transducer 90 degrees so that it lies parallel to the spine (Fig. 102.4). Scan along the line that was drawn to delineate midline along the patient's back.

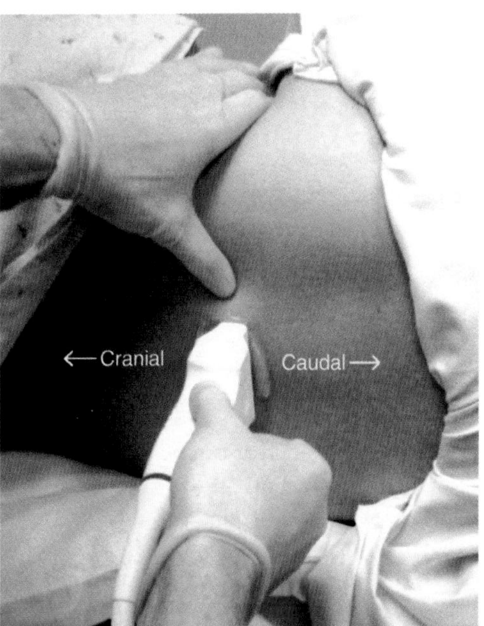

Figure 102.2 Transducer position to delineate midline. Place the transducer in a transverse fashion perpendicular to the patient's spine.

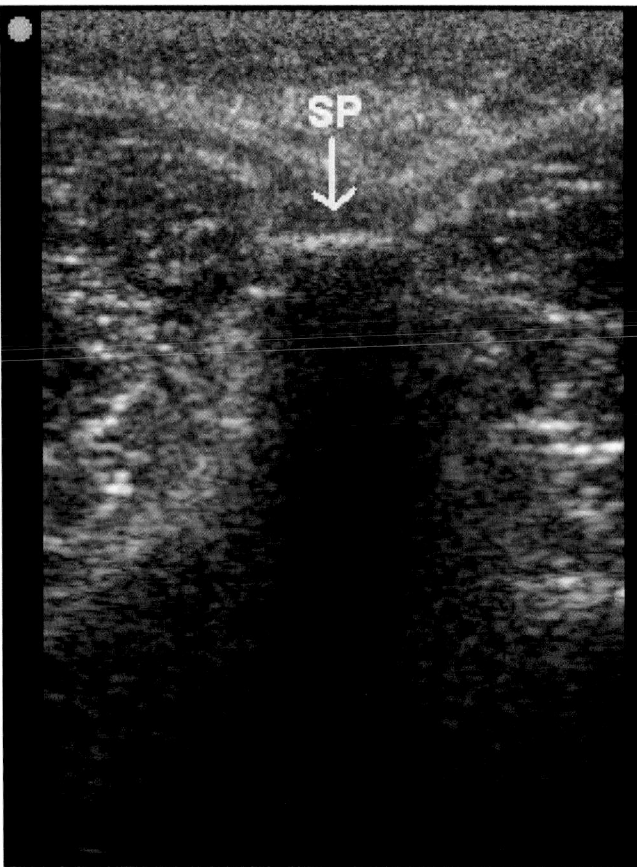

Figure 102.3 Sagittal (transverse) view of a spinous process (SP). Note the dark acoustic shadow farfield (posterior) to the spinous process.

9. The spinous processes in this view will appear as hyperechoic curves casting dark shadows farfield to the transducer (Fig. 102.5).
10. Center the transducer over the spinous processes and try to capture two spinous processes simultaneously. Scan from cephalad to caudad along the midline until the hypoechoic interspinous space is in the middle of the screen. The interspinous space is lying directly under the middle of the transducer.
11. Identify this spot with a marker or use a needle cap to gently indent the skin at this point. Direct the spinal needle towards the interspinous space identified.

An ultrasound-guided lumbar puncture can be performed in a static or dynamic manner, depending on the number of personnel available to help with the procedure. If the procedure is performed in a dynamic manner, remember to use sterile ultrasound gel and prep the ultrasound probe in a sterile fashion.

Ultrasound can be used to localize the interspinous space for lumbar punctures performed through the traditional interspinous space, or via the paraspinous approach.

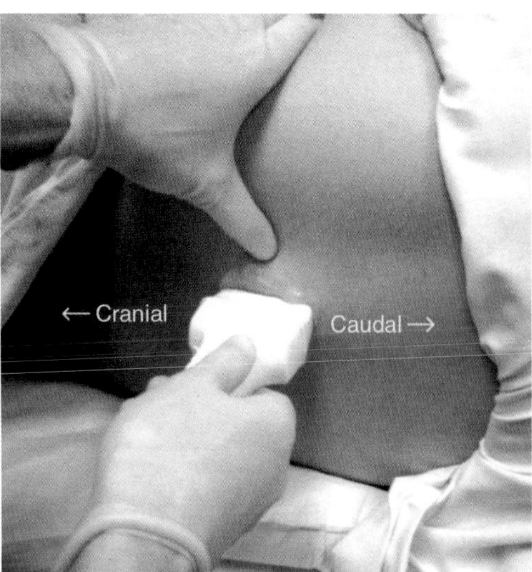

Figure 102.4 Transducer position to delineate the interspinous space. Place the transducer in a longitudinal fashion along the patient's spinous processes.

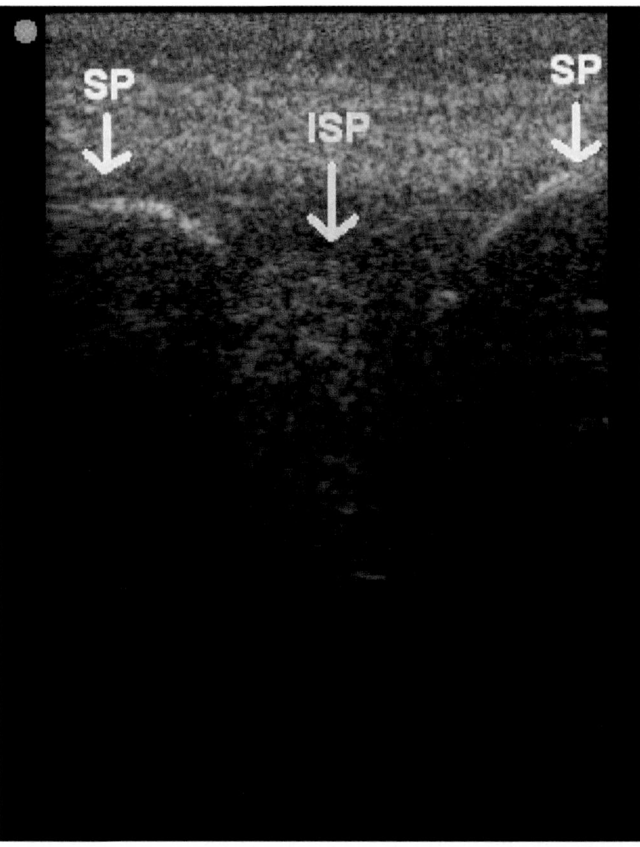

Figure 102.5 Axial (longitudinal) view of two spinous processes (SP) and the interspinous space (ISP).

Chapter

103 Tutorial: Laboratory tests for pediatric infectious disease

Zita Konik

Introduction

Laboratory tests for infectious diseases can aid with diagnosis, treatment, disposition, and public reporting in the ED. Whether to order a particular test in the ED, however, does not just depend on the clinical scenario but also on the impact the result will have on patient management: turnaround time, sensitivity, and specificity. This chapter will review the principles of basic laboratory infectious disease tests that can be ordered in the setting of clinical suspicion of pediatric infectious disease.

Most laboratory tests for infectious disease employ one of two approaches: bacteriologic, where the organism itself is identified using stains or cultures, or immunologic (serologic), where a patient's sample is tested for antibodies against the organism. While identification of the organism is usually the gold standard, and cultures should be obtained for confirmation of a suspected organism, the time interval required to obtain the result does not usually aid in ED management.

Serologic (antibody-based) tests

Antibodies are proteins produced by the immune system in reaction to a specific antigen that stimulated their production. Reactions between antibodies and antigens are highly specific and, consequently, are widely used to confirm suspicion of a specific infection. This type of testing is used to detect infectious disease and immunologic disease, as well as in blood typing.

There are five classes of immunoglobulin antibody: IgA, IgM, IgG, IgE, and IgD. In terms of testing for infection, IgM, IgG, and IgE are the most medically relevant.

IgE. This mediates anaphylactic reactions as well as acts as the main host defense against helminthic infection.

IgM. The main immunoglobin produced in the first exposure to an antigen is IgM; it is the first circulating antibody to appear after exposure. It can take the body 7–10 days to develop IgM antibodies after the primary exposure. IgM can stay positive anywhere from weeks to a year depending on the infectious cause.

IgG. The predominant antibody in the secondary response is IgG, which is important for the body's defense against bacteria and viruses. When the body is re-exposed to that antigen, antibody formation, in the form of IgG, occurs more rapidly through the action of memory B cells formed during the primary exposure. Presence of IgG does not necessarily signify current infection; rather it may signal previous infection.

Detection methods for antigen or antibody

In the case of infectious diseases, testing of a patient's serum for the presence of an antibody is carried out where the organism cannot be cultured (e.g., hepatitis B), when the organism takes too long to grow (e.g., *Mycoplasma*), or when a culture media does not exist (e.g., HIV). The titer, which is often reported, is the highest dilution of the specimen that gives a positive reaction.

Seroconversion, or the presence of antibodies toward an infection that was not previously present, does not necessarily indicate current infection. A rise in the titer of antibody to a virus or microbe, however, can indicate current infection. A serum sample is usually obtained during the suspected acute phase of infection, and a repeat sample is taken at 10–14 days. If the repeat titer is four-fold higher, the patient is considered to be infected.

In certain viral illness, however, the type of antibody present can give an indication of the current infection. For example, IgM to the core antigen of hepatitis B indicates current infection with hepatitis B. In certain infectious diseases, an arbitrary IgG antibody titer of sufficient magnitude is used to make a diagnosis (Box 103.1).

Nucleic acid-based methods

Polymerase chain reaction is a method of amplifying low levels of specific DNA sequences in a sample to reach the threshold of detection. In this method, two pieces of "primer" DNA specific for the pathogenic DNA are added to the sample and will attach to the ends of the pathogenic DNA, flanking each

A Practical Guide to Pediatric Emergency Medicine: Caring for Children in the Emergency Department, ed. N. Ewen Amieva-Wang (associate eds. Jamie Shandro, Aparajita Sohoni, and Bernhard Fassl). Published by Cambridge University Press.

Box 103.1. Antibody methods for diagnosis

Use of an immunoglobulin G titer

Infections typically identified/confirmed

Streptococcus spp., hepatitis A/B/C, measles, rubella, West Nile virus, Epstein–Barr virus, HIV.

Time to result

Two to three days.

Clinical indications

Serologic tests are useful in the ED in the diagnosis of illnesses with a prolonged incubation period, during which time the body has been able to develop antibodies, or when an antibody (IgM) is present at the same time as the symptoms.

Advantages

This approach can identify infectious agents that cannot be identified directly through culture and may be able to determine previous infection.

Disadvantages

Results are not back quickly and may be falsely negative early in disease.

Rapid tests

There are several rapid tests available for various infections; these can aid in diagnosis in the ED and may dictate further treatment in the patient, depending on the clinical scenario.

Infections typically identified

Influenza and respiratory syncytial virus (RSV). The rapid RSV and rapid influenza A/B tests are immunochromographic tests that can detect viral antigen in respiratory secretions. Anti-RSV or anti-influenza A/B antibody is attached to a color particle and impregnated in a line on a membrane paper. The patient's respiratory secretion sample is deposited at the base of the membrane paper. If antigen is present in the sample it will bind to the color-coded antibody and appear as a colored line on the paper.

Streptococcal pharyngitis. The rapid strep test is also an immunochromographic test that detects the presence of a carbohydrate specific for group A streptococci. The swab obtained from the patient is placed in an extraction material that removes the carbohydrate antigen specific to group A streptococci. The solution containing the antigen is then mixed with streptococcal antibodies that have been labeled with color particles. When the antigen and antibody complex forms, the color is activated and a blue line will appear.

HIV. Rapid HIV tests may be available in certain EDs. The FDA has approved four rapid HIV antibody tests, one of which uses a saliva sample. Two of the tests are available as point of care testing. All of the tests are interpreted visually. All positive rapid tests must be followed with confirmatory testing by Western blot.

Epstein–Barr virus or CMV. The Monospot test is used to diagnose mononucleosis, which can be caused by either the Epstein–Barr virus or CMV. This test is a latex agglutination test using horse red blood cells as the substrate. A patient's blood sample is mixed with the substrate and if the heterophile antibodies are present in the blood sample, the mixture will react to give a positive result. Because this test depends on the presence of antibody, it may be falsely negative early in the infection.

Time to result

Results available at the bedside or within minutes to hours from the laboratory

Clinical indications

Rapid tests are helpful in the ED as they allow rapid confirmation of a suspected disease-causing organism and may help in deciding which treatment is most appropriate.

Advantages

Results available rapidly, reduces cost by decreasing or preventing unnecessary treatments or further testing.

Disadvantages

The tests are not always available and sensitivity or specificity varies among tests.

Direct fluorescent antigen (DFA) test

The DFA test is used for detection of antigens using fluorescently labeled antigen-specific antibody. Fluorescent dyes, such as fluorescein, are attached to a specific antibody molecule and become visible when complexed with an antigen and placed under ultraviolet light. In the DFA test, the antibody–fluorescent dye complex interacts directly with the antigen in a patient's serum.

Infections typically identified/confirmed

Influenza, RSV, HSV, adenovirus, parainfluenza, *Bordatella pertussis*, varicella zoster virus.

Time to result

Results are available within hours or days depending on the test.

Clinical indications

Rapid tests allow rapid confirmation of a suspected disease-causing organism and may help in deciding which treatment is most appropriate.

Advantages

Tests are readily available in most EDs and results are rapid.

Disadvantages

Samples must be prepared and read by trained laboratory personnel

Enzyme-linked immunosorbent assay (ELISA)

The ELISA is a laboratory method that can be used to detect either antibody or antigen in a patient's sample using an enzyme linked to a known antigen or antibody. The patient's sample is then mixed with the enzyme–antibody (or antigen) complex. The corresponding antigen (or antibody) in the patient's sample then binds to the complex. The enzyme-specific substrate is then added to the mixture and the resultant reaction (specific to that enzyme) is looked for (i.e., color change).

Infections typically identified

HIV, *Clostridium dificile* toxin, *Escherichia coli* O157:H7, *Giardia* sp., rotavirus.

Time to result

One to three days.

Box 103.1. *(cont.)*

Clinical indications

The ELISA is not as useful in determining treatment or disposition for the patient in the ED as the results will not return rapidly, but it will help to determine future management.

Disadvantages

Samples must be prepared and read by trained laboratory personnel

Western blot

The Western blot is used to confirm a positive result on a screening immunologic test, usually done to confirm HIV or Lyme disease found on ELISA screening. In this method, the viral proteins are separated by electrophoresis in a gel. This gel is then blotted onto filter paper and the patient's serum is added to the paper. If antibodies are present in the serum, they will bind to the viral proteins. An antibody that binds to human IgG labeled radioactively or with an enzyme is added and can then be detected if specific viral proteins are present.

Infections typically identified

Confirmation for HIV or Lyme disease.

Time to result

One to three days.

Clinical indications

The Western blot is not as useful in determining treatment or disposition for the patient in the ED as the results will not return rapidly, but it will help to determine future management.

Advantages

Used in confirmation of disease found on screening test because of its high sensitivity.

Disadvantages

The test is time intensive to perform and the results are not rapidly available.

Box 103.2. Nucleic acid detection for diagnosis

Infections typically identified/confirmed

Hepatitis C, HSV, enterovirus, *B. pertussis, N. gonorrhoeae, Chlamydia* sp.

Time to results

One to three days.

Clinical indications

PCR is not as useful in determining treatment or disposition for the patient in the ED as the results will not return rapidly, but it does help to determine future management.

Advantages

PCR is highly sensitive, detecting small amounts of DNA or RNA that would not be identified by other methods.

Disadvantages

Time intensive.

end. Repeated cycles are done to make copies of this piece of DNA, with each cycle doubling the amount of DNA in the sample. A radioactively labeled segment of DNA that is complementary to the pathogenic DNA is then added to the sample and will pair to the pathogenic DNA. Electrophoresis is then performed to look for the radioactively tagged pathogenic DNA (Box 103.2). Viruses that use RNA as their genetic material are detected using reverse transcriptase PCR (RT-PCR), where the reverse transcriptase first converts the RNA to DNA.

Bacteriologic culture methods

Growing an offending organism on blood agar (blood culture) is considered the gold standard in diagnosing a disease-causing pathogen. Once identified, antibiotic testing is done to determine sensitivity, which aids further specific treatment. Most common bacteria will grow on blood agar; however, some atypical infections require specialized "selective/differential" material in order to grow (atypical cultures). Although there are immunologic methods of detection of viral infection, viral cultures are also available. These methods are outlined in Box 103.3

Box 103.3. Culture methods for diagnosis

Blood culture

The sensitivity of a blood culture is dependent on the amount of blood that is drawn. Sensitivity in detecting an organism increases from 60% for 2 ml of blood to >99% with 40 ml. In children, the optimal amount of blood needed to detect pathogens is 4% of the total blood volume. If <5 ml of blood is obtained, only one aerobic bottle should be used. If more is obtained, the blood should be divided between an aerobic and an anaerobic bottle (Routine blood culture bottle accepts 10 ml).

Infections typically identified

Bacterial infections such as streptococci, staphylococci. For less typical bacteria, specific agars need to be chosen (see below).

Time to results

One to three days.

Clinical indications

This is the gold standard for confirmation/identification of disease-causing bacteria. Although blood culture will not dictate acute management in the ED, it should be drawn and sent in the ED *prior* to initiating antibiotic therapy.

Advantages

Once an organism(s) is identified, sensitivity testing of various antibiotics can be performed to select the most effective antibiotic for the identified organism, which is relatively cost-effective.

Disadvantages

It may take days to a week to obtain results.

Box 103.3. *(cont.)*

Atypical culture

If the clinical suspicion exists for an atypical bacterial infection, isolator cultures can be made. This method uses media containing materials that selectively allow one organism to grow while also allowing for the differentiation of that organism based on specific reactions. When ordering cultures for atypical infections, the laboratory should be contacted with exactly which type of organism is suspected. When in doubt, the infectious disease service should be contacted for specific requirements to grow atypical organisms.

Infections typically identified

Brucella, *Bartonella*, or *Mycobacteria* spp.

Time to results

May take days to a week to obtain results.

Clinical indications

Same as for blood culture.

Advantages

Same as for blood culture.

Disadvantages

Must inform the laboratory of suspected organism to ensure plating on specific agar.

Viral culture

The growth of viruses requires cell cultures, as viruses grow and live inside living cells. Growth of the virus causes a cytopathic effect on the host cells. This change in appearance of the host cells is characteristic by virus and can help to give a presumptive diagnosis. If the virus does not cause a cytopathic effect, other methods of detection are employed such as ELISA and DFA (see Box 103.1).

Infections typically identified/confirmed

Herpes simplex virus.

Time to results

Time varies, from 2 to 14 days.

Clinical indications

May be used as confirmation of other tests such as PCR.

Selected references

Greenwald JL, Burstein GR, Pincus J, Branson B. A rapid review of rapid HIV antibody tests. *Curr Infect Dis Rep* 2006;**8**: 125–131.

Levinson W. *Review of Medical Microbiology and Immunology*, 10th edn, Ch. 64. New York: McGraw-Hill, 2006.

Nairn R. Immunology. In Brooks GF, Carroll KC, Butel JS, *et al.* (eds.) *Jawetz, Melnick & Adelberg's Medical Microbiology*, 23th edn, Ch. 8. New York: McGraw-Hill, 2004.

Chapter 104

Tutorial: Microbiology laboratory cheat sheet

Naresh Ramarajan and Zita Konik

Table 104.1 provides a quick guide to microbial testing.

Table 104.1. Microbiology laboratory cheat sheet

Site of infection	Suspected pathogen	Media of collection	Test	Time to result	Comments
Blood	Atypical bacteria or fungi (*Malassazia furfur, Brucella, Bartonella* spp., mycobacteria)	Blood culture bottle	Isolator cultures	2–4 weeks	Call laboratory to inform of organism suspected, ID consult may be necessary
	Hepatitis panel (screen)	Blood sample	Hepatitis A Ab IgM, HBsAg, HBcAb-IgM, hepatitis C Ab	2–4 days	
	Hepatitis A	Blood sample	Hepatitis A Ab IgM	2–4 days	
	Hepatitis B	Blood sample	HbsAg, HbeAg, HbcAb (IgM and IgG), HbsAb, HbeAb	2–4 days	
	Hepatitis C	Blood sample	Hepatitis C Ab, PCR (RNA)	7 days	
	HIV	Blood sample	ELISA HIV1/HIV2 Ab; if positive send Western blot for confirmation	Rapid 5–40 min; ELISA 1 day; Western blot 1–4 days	Rapid: sensitivity >99%, specificity 98–100% If positive on rapid, confirm with both ELISA and Western blot
	Measles, mumps and/or rubella	Blood sample	IgG and IgM	2–7 days	
	Mononucleosis (Epstein–Barr virus)	Blood sample	*<4 years*: IgM to antiviral capsid antigen (VCA) *>4 years*: Monospot	1 h (Monospot), 1 day (IgM)	Sensitivity 85%, specificity 100% Monospot not sensitive for <24 months and only 75% at 24–28 months
	Routine bacteria	Blood culture bottle	Gram stain and culture	Most pathogens positive by 8 h; STAT Gram stains within 1 h if positive; identity/sensitivity results, 2–4 days	Increased sensitivity with higher sample volume, ideally 4% of total body volume Weight <9 kg, 2 ml blood Weight 20–40 kg, 20–30 ml blood

A Practical Guide to Pediatric Emergency Medicine: Caring for Children in the Emergency Department, ed. N. Ewen Amieva-Wang (associate eds. Jamie Shandro, Aparajita Sohoni, and Bernhard Fassl). Published by Cambridge University Press.

Table 104.1. *(cont.)*

Site of infection	Suspected pathogen	Media of collection	Test	Time to result	Comments
CNS	*Cryptococcus*	Blood sample; CSF tube	*Cryptococcus* Ag; order both CSF and serum (CRAg)	Same day	
	Enterovirus	CSF tube, 1 ml	Enterovirus PCR	1–3 days	
	HSV-1 or HSV-2	CSF tube	PCR	1–3 days	
	Mycobacterium tuberculosis	CSF tube	Direct acid-fast bacilli and culture	Same day (direct); 2–4 weeks (culture)	
	Routine bacteria	CSF tube	Gram stain and culture	Same day (stain) Cultures usually positive in 2 days; identity/ sensitivity results 2–4 days; negative by 4 days	
	Fungi	CSF tube	Fungal stain and culture	2–4 weeks	
	West Nile virus (WNV), arbovirus	CSF tube, blood sample	Serum and CSF WNV IgM at presentation and IgG at end of first week of symptoms	2 days (serum), 3–5 days (CSF)	
Eye	HSV, adenovirus	Swab of eye in viral transport media	DFA	1 day	
	Routine bacteria	Swab of eye	Gram stain and culture	2 days	
Oropharynx	*Neisseria gonorrhoeae*	Throat swab	Gram stain and culture	2–3 days	
	Streptococcus spp.	Throat swab	Rapid streptococci and culture	<30 min (rapid), 2–3 days (culture)	Sensitivity 65–90%, specificity >95%; always send culture
	Streptococcus spp.	Blood sample	If suspicious for post-streptococcal glomerulonephritis or Henoch–Schönlein purpura order anti-streptolysin (ASO) Ab titer	Same day (ASO titer), 4–5 days (anti- DNase Ab)	
Respiratory	Adenovirus, parainfluenza	Nasopharyngeal swab, nasal washing	DFA panel	1 day	Sensitivity 60–95%
	Bordatella pertussis	NP swab	DFA, PCR; if positive, send serology (acute and convalescent)	1 day (DFA), 3–5 days (PCR), 1–3 weeks (serology)	Sensitivity <30% (DFA); sensitivity 61–95%, specificity 88% (PCR)
	Influenza A and B	Nasal swab	Rapid Flu A/B, DFA	1–2 h (rapid), I day (DFA)	Sensitivity 45–96%, specificity 52–100% (rapid)
	Respiratory syncytial virus	Nasal swab	Rapid Ag, DFA	Same day (rapid), 1 day (DFA)	Sensitivity and specificity >90% (rapid Ag)
Skin/ mucous membranes/ wound	Deep aspirate	Swab of aspirate or sample of fluid	Aspirate Gram stain and culture	Same day (stain); cultures usually positive in 2 days; identity/ sensitivity results 2–4 days; negative by 4 days	

Table 104.1. *(cont.)*

Site of infection	Suspected pathogen	Media of collection	Test	Time to result	Comments
	HSV-1, HSV-2, varicella zoster virus	Swab of unroofed lesion	Skin lesion: DFA and viral culture Mucous membrane lesion: viral culture or PCR	1 day (skin), 2–4 days (mucous membrane)	
	Routine bacterial or fungal	Swab of wound	Wound Gram stain and culture	Same day (Gram stain), 2–3 days (culture), 2–3 weeks (fungal culture)	
Stool	*Clostridium difficile*	Stool sample	ELISA toxin	Usually same day	Sensitivity 60–95%, specificity 99%; may need to send three consecutive samples to increase diagnostic yield
	Escherichia coli O157:H7	Stool sample	ELISA for Shiga-like toxin A&B, Culture	Varies (ELISA), 5–7 days (culture)	
	Giardia sp.	Stool sample	ELISA for Ag	2–3 days	Sensitivity 90–100%, specificity 95–100%
	Helicobacter pylori	Blood sample	Ag	2–3 days	
	Parasites	Stool sample	Stool ova and parasites	1–2 days	
	Rotavirus	Stool sample	PCR, ELISA	Usually 1–2 days (PCR), 1 day (ELISA)	Sensitivity 99%, specificity 98% (PCR) Rotazyme is commercial name of the ELISA tests
	Salmonella, Shigella, Campylobacter spp.	Stool sample	Culture	2–3 days	
Urogenital	*N. gonorrhoeae/ Chlamydia* spp.	Urine (first void) or urethral swab	Gonococcal chlamydial PCR; culture	2–3 days (PCR), 2–4 days (culture)	Sensitivity 56%, specificity 99% (PCR); specificity 100% (culture); PCR is more expensive than culture
	Bacteria and fungi	Urine	Urine analysis culture	1–3 days	

Ab, antibody; Ag, antigen; DFA, direct fluorescent antigen test; ELISA, enzyme-linked immunosorbent assay; GN, glomerulonephritis; HSV, herpes simplex virus; ID, infectious diseases; PCR, polymerase chain reaction.

Acknowledgements

The following laboratory personnel were extremely helpful in determining turnaround times for the various microbiology, virology, and special chemistry tests: Shao-Ching Tracy Chang, Shannon Sackett (Stanford University Medical Center Laboratory, CA), Vasundara Ramarajan, LaWanda Young (Kaiser Permanente Medical Group Laboratory, San Francisco, CA), and Thara Rangamannar (Merrimac Valley Hospital Laboratory, NH).

Selected references

Chernesky M, Castriciano S, Mahony J, DeLong D. Examination of the rotazyme II enzyme immunoassay for the diagnosis of rotavirus gastroenteritis *J Clin Microbiol* 1985;**22**: 462–464.

Pickering LK, Baker CJ, Kimberlin DW, Long SS (eds.). Respiratory syncytial virus. *The Red Book: 2006 Report of the Committee on Infectious Diseases*, 27th edn. Elk Grove Village, IL: American Academy of Pediatrics, 2006, p. 561 (also Red Book Online, last updated 5 January 2009).

Section

15

Musculoskeletal system

Expert reviewer: Andrew Man-Lap Ho

Chapter 105

Approaches to the musculoskeletal examination

Clinton J. Coil

Introduction

The musculoskeletal examination is usually performed to evaluate a specific injury or because of a complaint of pain or weakness. Pain and weakness are very different symptoms, and it is challenging for the medical provider and the patient to distinguish between the two (see Ch. 117). This chapter will discuss a general approach to the musculoskeletal examination, and a head to toe examination for a general musculoskeletal examination in an infant or young child brought to the ED with apparent new deformity, pain, or other musculoskeletal complaint.

The musculoskeletal examination in children presents two unique challenges for the EP. First, the musculoskeletal system changes dramatically during the course of development. Second, many of the findings depend on cooperation from the patient, which can be difficult if an injured child simply will not move or screams when examined.

There can be several strategies to overcome these challenges. Many important findings can be uncovered by observing the child from a distance. Providing toys or games and watching how the child interacts with siblings can increase or decrease suspicion of an injury depending on how the child moves and plays. The same strategy can be used close up, by having a child walk toward you to retrieve a toy, or grab a sticker (which is just out of reach) while the child's other hand is occupied. Childhood games like "Simon Says", holding a "jumping contest," or giving a "high five" are other ways to trigger specific movements.

For the anxious patient, allowing breaks during the examination can give them a greater sense of control. Avoid separation from parents or caregivers, who can be a source of comfort, because triggering separation anxiety can compound the problem. Touching the head and face can be particularly uncomfortable for the anxious child. Consider standing far from the child first, then moving nearer and speaking softly without making contact. Initiate touching with the patient's hands and feet first and slowly move more proximally as the child relaxes. Tickling can be intended as playful but can be uncomfortable and anxiety provoking so should be avoided.

If a child is afraid of instruments like a stethoscope or tongue depressor, ask the child to reach and grab the object first so that he/she can explore it on their own and become comfortable with it. Distracting the patient with other familiar people and objects can also be helpful. Demonstrating the proposed examination on a parent or older sibling can also help the child to form expectations that relieve anxiety. Reducing unknown elements and surprises as well as giving the child a degree of control over what happens is important (e.g., "which ear do you want to show me first?")

While the examiner is often more comfortable placing patients on an examination table, bed, or crib, the opposite may be true for the patient. Having the child rest in a caregiver's arms or lap may help to calm the patient, facilitating your examination. Avoid touching an obviously injured body part first. Start with apparently normal areas.

Musculoskeletal examination of the infant

History

Birth history can give important clues and focus attention as the child is examined. Birth trauma can cause injuries such as a clavicle fracture. Ask about any complications during the pregnancy or childbirth. Nerve damage or fractures that can occur from birth trauma can lead to persistent deformities. Reports that it is difficult to place diapers on the patient can be a clue to developmental hip dysplasia or other hip problems. Be alert to the history that does not match any injuries that are discovered. Treat all injuries as potential signs of child maltreatment.

General tone

General tone in a neonate is more flexed because of the constraints of the fetal position. As the child develops, more extensor tone will be expected. In contrast, premature infants can initially have more predominant extensor tone. Carefully lift the infant into a sitting position. Head control is expected by 3–4 months of age. Full control of the trunk in order to maintain a seated position is expected by 6–8 months of age.

A Practical Guide to Pediatric Emergency Medicine: Caring for Children in the Emergency Department, ed. N. Ewen Amieva-Wang (associate eds. Jamie Shandro, Aparajita Sohoni, and Bernhard Fassl). Published by Cambridge University Press.

Generalized hypotonia can signal a serious neuromuscular process, such as botulism.

Head and neck

Torticollis ("wry neck") in the infant can have any one of up to 80 causes, which can generally be categorized as congenital or acquired. Congenital torticollis can be the first manifestation of spinal malformation. There are varying opinions as to whether some cases of congenital torticollis are caused by birth trauma, resulting in scarring of one of the sternocleidomastoid muscles, or if trauma in utero is the primary event and contributes to a difficult delivery.

Acquired torticollis can sometimes be from benign causes of muscle strain and can follow an upper respiratory infection as a result of coughing. Other causes can be serious spinal abnormalities, such as subluxation or fracture. Sometimes the infant can present with torticollis from a spinal injury that occurred months earlier. Other causes of torticollis include infection or inflammation of nearby structures (i.e., mastoiditis, tonsillitis, or adenitis), or a dystonic reaction to medications.

Key examination elements include evaluation of the spine as well as the sternocleidomastoid muscles on both sides. A lump in the muscle may be palpable on the side opposite to the direction the head is turned and is more associated with congenital torticollis, also called pseudotumor of infancy. It is important to differentiate torticollis from nuchal rigidity. A complete neurological examination should be performed to identify any focal defects from spinal or brachial plexus injury.

Radiographic study of the cervical spine is indicated in all first time presentations of torticollis that is not paroxysmal in nature in order to exclude fracture, subluxation, or malformation.

Upper extremities

Inspect and palpate each upper extremity. Compare the length of the arms. Count the fingers and look for fingers that are joined together (syndactyly). Abnormalities of the digits may be a clue to other developmental disorders. A palpable mass over a neonate's clavicle is likely a callus from a healing clavicle fracture from birth trauma.

Spine

Obvious scoliosis may not be apparent in the spine of a young infant. A tuft of hair, discoloration, or mass over the lumbar spine can indicate occult spina bifida, meningocele, myelomeningocele, or tethered cord syndrome.

Lower extremities

Inspect and palpate the lower extremities. Examine active and passive range of motion. Compare the length of the leg and

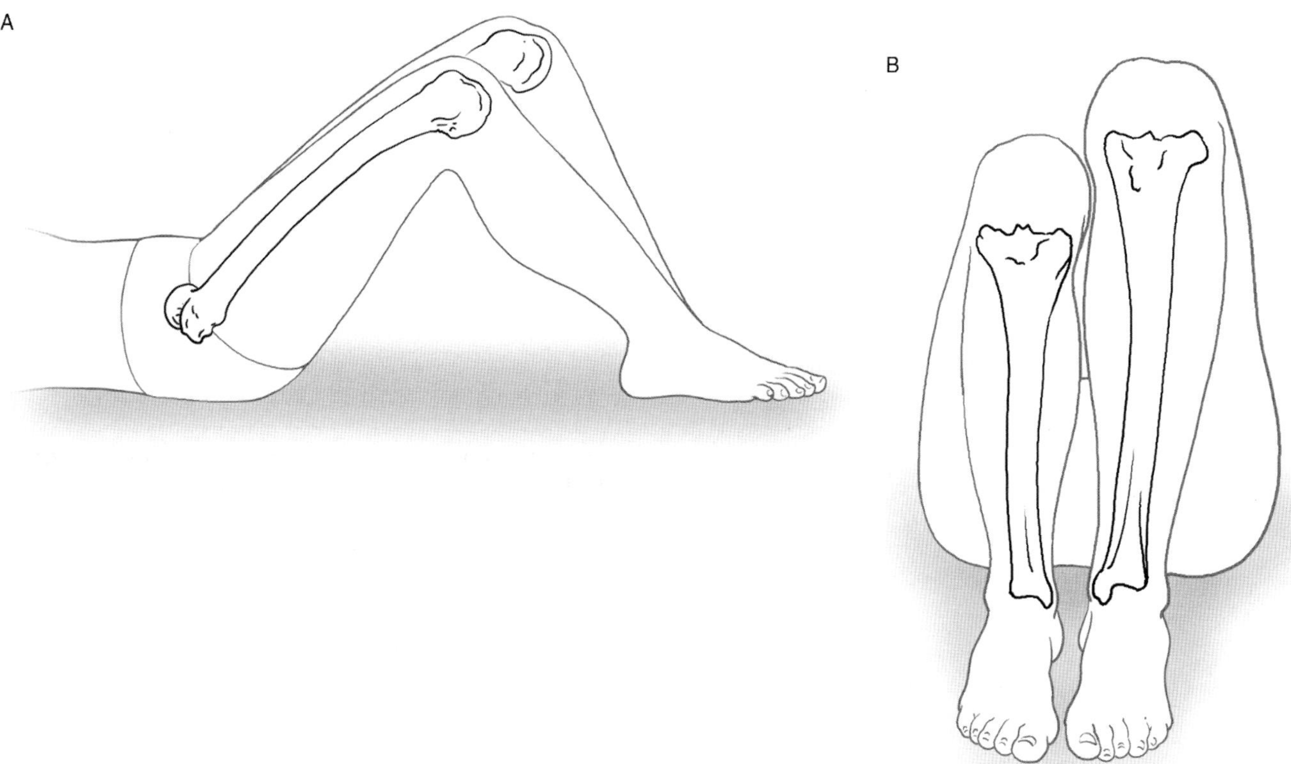

Figure 105.1 Examination techniques to demonstrate asymmetry of tibial and femoral length. (A) Femoral length discrepancy assessment (Galleazzi sign). (B) Tibial length discrepancy assessment (Ellis test). (Copyright N. Ewen Wang.)

count the number of toes. Check for short limbs, which may be a clue to an occult fracture, dislocation, or developmental dysplasia of the hip. The best way to measure the length of the femurs is to lie the patient on his/her back and hold the legs in adduction with the hips and knees both flexed to 90 degrees. In this position, the knees should be in the same location (a negative Galleazzi's sign) (Fig. 105.1A). In this same position, evaluate the length of the tibia by holding the knees medial malleoli together and checking the position of the knees (the Ellis test) (Fig. 105.1B). If limb lengths are abnormal, consider whether it is the longer or shorter limb that is pathological. An infant with a septic hip joint will classically hold the joint in flexion, abduction, and external rotation.

Look at the shape and angles of the joints. In the neonate and young infant, some degree of deformity can persist from the patient's compact position inside the uterus, and this usually resolves during the first year. Torsion of the ankle in the tibial direction and/or adduction of the forefoot is normal and usually resolves after several months of weight bearing. Flat footedness, in which the normal anterior–posterior and transverse arches are absent, is normal in infants and usually resolves once the child begins to walk. Many apparent abnormalities need only to be followed by a pediatrician and do not require any intervention. See below in the section on toddlers and school-aged children for more details on examination of joint positions and angles.

The hips should be assessed for stability using the Ortolani and Barlow tests (Fig 105.2). In the Barlow test, the examiner holds each femur in adduction and provides posterior pressure to observe a click as the hip is easily dislocated. This is followed by the Ortolani test in which the femurs are held in abduction

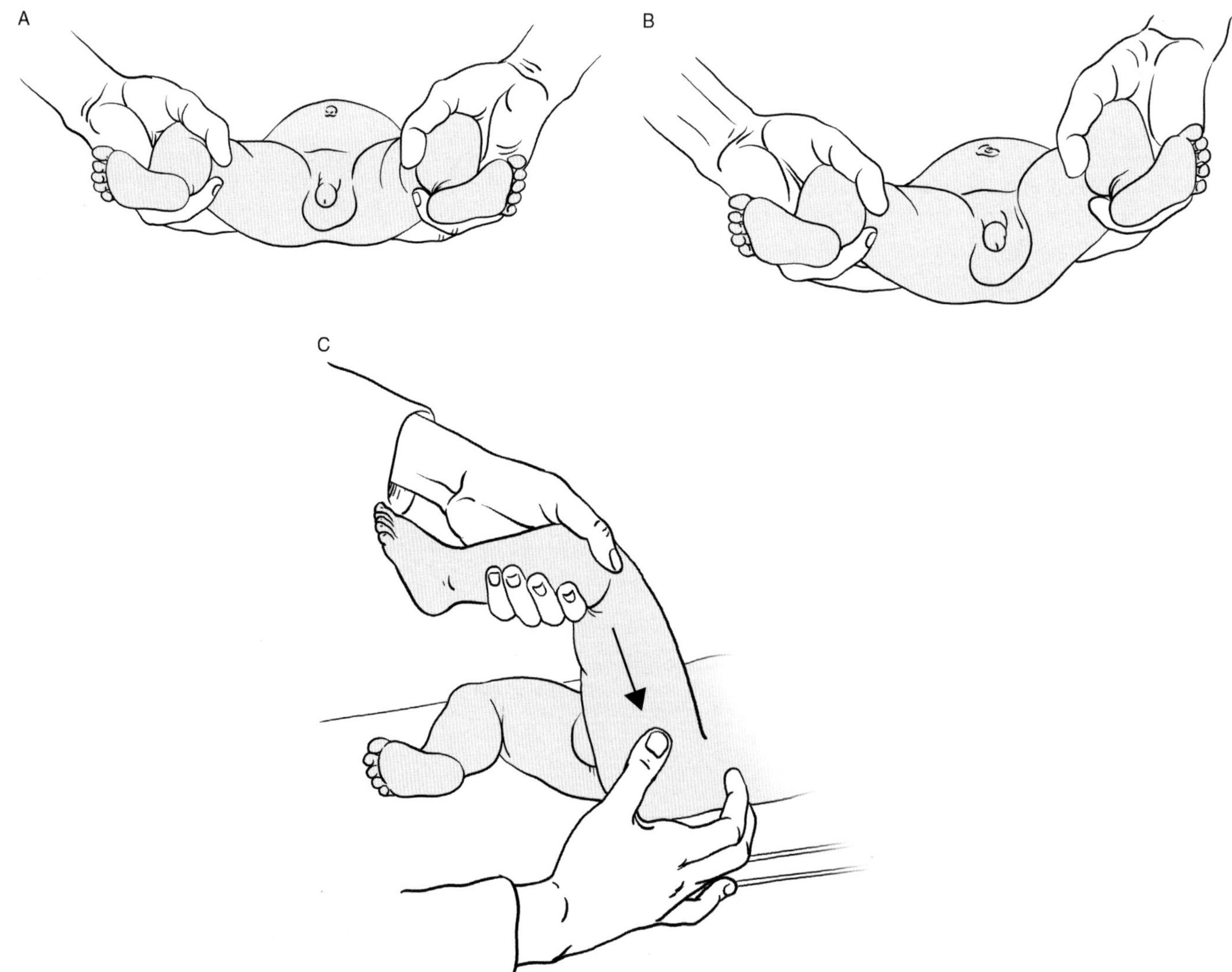

Figure 105.2 Tests for congenital hip dislocation in the newborn. (A) Typically, both hips can be equally flexed, abducted, and externally rotated (Ortolani test). (B) The involved hip is not able to be abducted as far as the opposite one and there is a "click" as the hip reduces. (C) The Barlow test: pushing the femur in the positive direction will result in a "clunk" as the hip dislocates. (Copyright N. Ewen Wang.)

and driven into the hip joint to observe a palpable click as a dislocated hip is reduced.

Because of adipose tissue, it may be difficult to assess the exact locations of the bones and joints. Skin folds however, should usually be symmetric bilaterally, including gluteal, inguinal, and popliteal creases. A lack of symmetry may indicate a congenital deformity or a dislocated joint and should prompt further investigation. However, lack of symmetric creases is non-specific and can be found in up to 30% of normal infants. Allis sign, which occurs when an examiner can easily push the tip of the finger into loose soft tissue between the trochanter and illiac crest, indicates a likely femoral neck fracture with soft tissue laxity owing to shortening of the thigh. This finding should prompt radiographic studies as there may not be any history of injury, in the case of a congenital deformity, mild occult trauma, or inflicted injury.

Examination of the toddler and school-aged child

History

The history related to the musculoskeletal system for the toddler and school-aged child should focus on any changes in the patient's usual activities, or failure to progress in development (Table 105.1). Participation in organized sports can be an important historical feature that can provide possible mechanisms for acute or chronic injury (see Ch. 111).

General tone

Tone can be assessed by passively ranging the elbow joint bilaterally to assess for development of spacticity or hypotonia.

Strength

Strength of each joint can be assessed directly using a five point scale. If the patient is having difficulty cooperating with a direct strength examination, sometimes observing more natural motions can give a good estimate of whether strength is normal or abnormal. For example, strength in the lower extremities can be assessed by having the child walk on his/her toes and heels, and stand up from a crouched position. For the upper extremities, reaching for objects can detect major strength defects but is not as precise as the lower extremity maneuvers described above.

Gower sign, when a child uses his/her upper body to stand up, can be a sign of generalized or lower extremity weakness.

Gait

Assessment of gait should be done as inconspicuously as possible. If the child refuses to walk, or it is possible that they are exaggerating a limp, try placing the child away from the parent and have the child walk toward the parent to retrieve a toy. Covert observation while the child is playing can also give valuable clues.

The normal gait consists of a stance phase, which begins when the heel strikes the floor and ends when the toes push off (Fig. 105.3). The swing phase begins with swinging of the hip forward and flexion of the knee and ends with dorsiflexion of the foot just before heel strike (Fig. 105.4).

Main types of gait disorders, including antalgic gait, Trendelenburg gait, and drop-foot (Figs. 105.5 to 105.7, respectively) gait are described in Table 105.2.

Examination of the child's footwear is a key part of investigating a limp or other gait disturbance. Look for wear patterns that are different on each side, or pronounced wearing of one part of the shoe and compare that with observation of the gait for abnormal touchdown at the end of the swing phase. Look for penetrating foreign bodies in the soles.

Upper extremities

Observe active and passive range of motion and then palpate the entire upper extremity. Be sure not to overlook the clavicle

Table 105.1 Some common historical features and their differential diagnoses

History:	Possible diagnoses
Lump over upper chest	Callus from healed clavicle fracture
Lateral epicondyle pain	Tennis elbow
Wrist pain	Overuse syndromes, sports related
Arm held in flexion and pronation, possibly without complaint of pain unless arm is supinated	Nursemaid's elbow
Hip pain	Septic joint, transient synovitis, sacroiliitis
Knee pain	Patellofemoral syndrome, growing pains, slipped capital femoral epiphysis
Shin pain	Osgood–Schlatter disease (proximal tibia), shin splints (tibialis anterior muscle)
Foot/ankle pain	Plantar fasciitis, Achilles tendinitis, Sever's disease

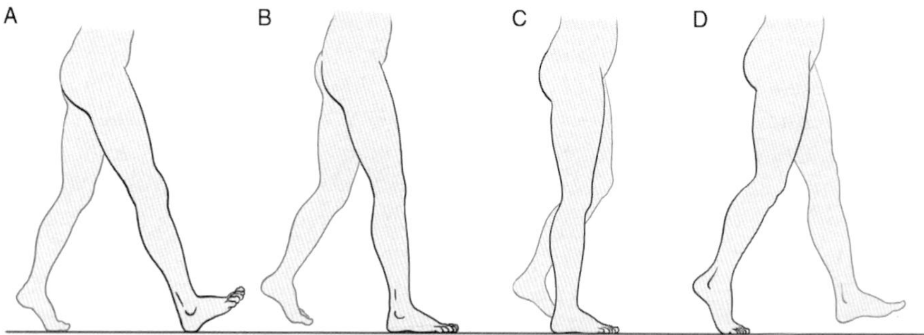

Figure 105.3 The different phases of the gait in stance phase: (A) heel strike; (B) foot flat; (C) mid-stance; (D) push-off. (Copyright N. Ewen Wang.)

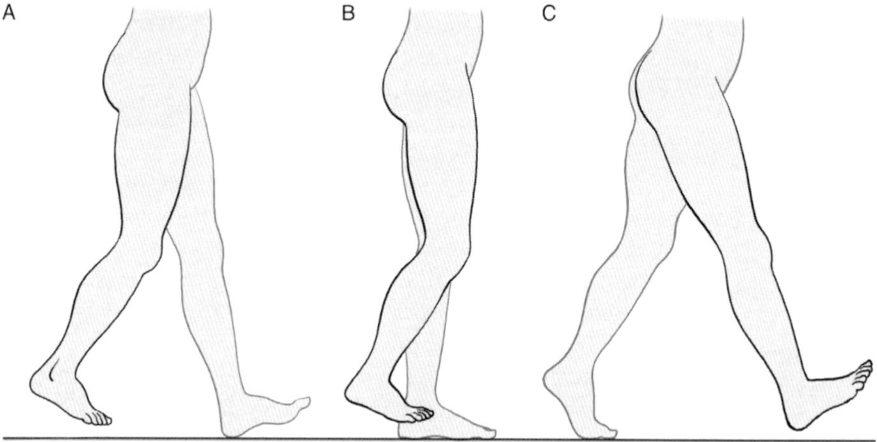

Figure 105.4 The phases of gait in swing phase: (A) acceleration; (B) mid-swing; (C) deceleration. (Copyright N. Ewen Wang.)

during the upper extremity examination – it is the most commonly fractured bone in the human body. Certain conditions, such as nursemaid's elbow, will only be elicited during pronation and supination of the forearm. Try to observe if the child is favoring one arm or the other during play, if necessary.

Spine

Undiagnosed scoliosis or kyphosis may be the underlying cause in new presentations of back, neck, hip, or leg pain, or gait disturbances. When standing erect, there should be 20–50 degrees of thoracic kyphosis and 30–60 degrees of lumbar lordosis. The apices of these curvatures should occur around T6–T7 and L3–L4. There should be no kyphosis or lordosis at the thoracolumbar junction. The appropriate curvature of the spine is best assessed by having the patient stand facing away from the examiner. First the spine and scapulae should be carefully observed for symmetry in the upright position, followed by asking the child to bend forward to touch the toes. Unequal height of the scapulae and/or deviation of the spine to one side is usually easy to discern as long as the patient is appropriately disrobed and undergoes the above maneuver. Having the child against a firm backrest and observing if the child must hold the hips unevenly to sit up straight can also be helpful. Observed scoliosis may be structural or functional. Structural scoliosis is of an unclear etiology and progresses during adolescence. Functional scoliosis may occur as a compensatory maneuver for unequal leg length, pain, or other deformities.

Lower extremities

Observe active and passive range of motion, and then palpate the entire extremity. A tender nodule at the insertion of the patellar tendon on the anterior surface of the tibia is suggestive of Osgood–Schlatter disease. Be aware that the location of the presenting complaint may not be the actual site of injury. For example, hip problems such as slipped capital femoral epiphysis can sometimes present as knee pain (Ch. 106). Occasionally problems can present as pain on the opposite side, as the affected leg is favored during walking. Palpate the posterior fossa of the knee to identify a Baker's cyst.

Check for undiagnosed deformities of the lower extremities as a cause of indolent or subacute pain that is worsening. Intoeing is also a common complaint that can be very concerning for caregivers, yet usually is benign and resolves without intervention. Differentiating between serious and minor cases of intoeing requires careful examination for specific rotational deformities. Pathological causes of intoeing include metatarsus adductus, internal tibial torsion, excessive femoral

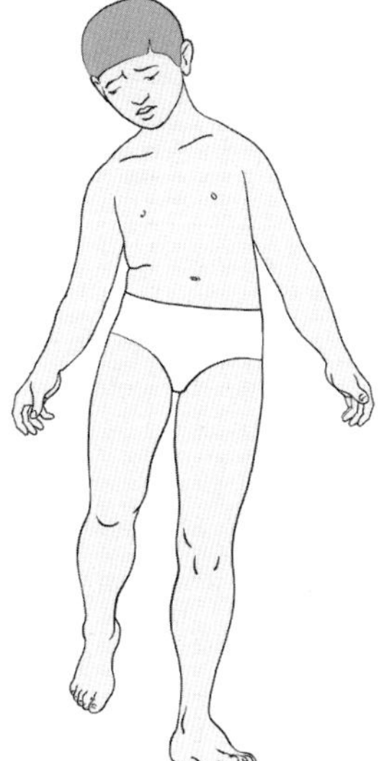

Figure 105.5 Antalgic gait results when the patient attempts to avoid the painful part of the gait. (Copyright N. Ewen Wang.)

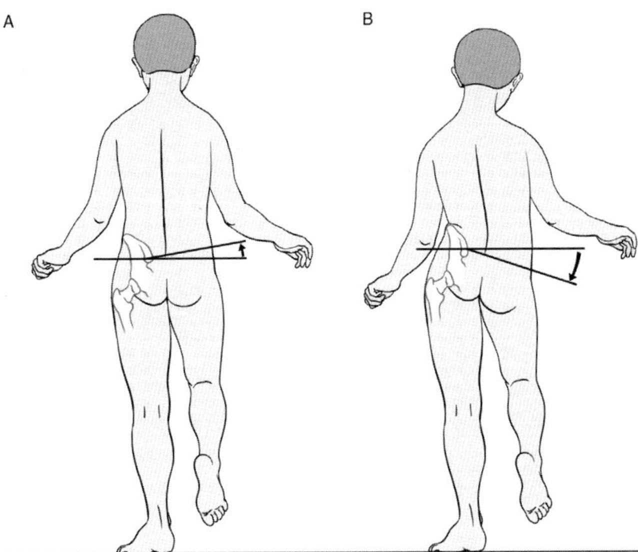

Figure 105.6 The Trendelenburg test assesses for strength of gluteus medius. Normally the superior iliac spines are level. (A) Normal. (B) Abnormal: pelvis descends. (Copyright N. Ewen Wang.)

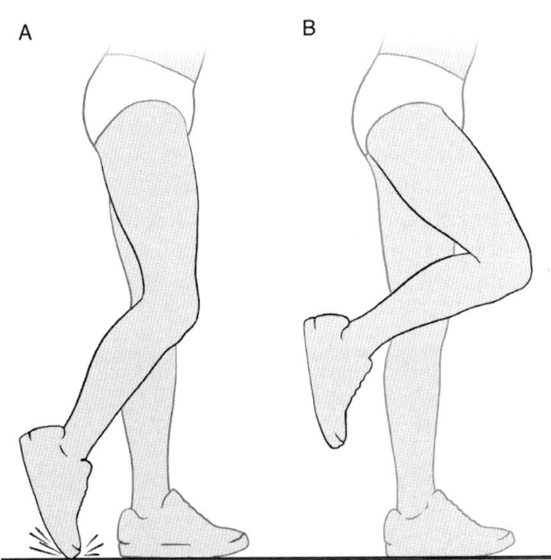

Figure 105.7 Ankle dorsiflexors. (A) When the ankle dorsiflexors are not working, the patient will be unable to elevate the toe and will scrape it on the floor. (B) The "steppage gait" occurs when the patient compensates by lifting the knee higher than normal so the foot will clear the floor. (Copyright N. Ewen Wang.)

anteversion, cerebral palsy, developmental dysplasia of the hip, rickets, and spina bifida.

To examine the child with intoeing, first look at the sole of the foot. The lateral border of the foot should be straight. A C-shaped curve is associated with metatarsus adductus. The severity of the disorder is then graded by holding the heel fixed and abducting the forefoot. A flexible deformity is less serious than one which is rigid or fixed. On a normal foot, the midline bisects the heel in a line extending to between the second and third toes. The further this line is displaced toward the fifth toe, the more severe the deformity.

Next, assess the degree of tibial torsion. The degree of external tibial torsion normally increases from 5 degrees at birth to 15–20 degrees at maturity. Tibial torsion can be measured by having the child sit with the knee bent to 90 degrees and the tibial tubercle pointing forward. The examiner places his/her hands on the medial and lateral malleoli and assesses the angle between the hands. Expected external torsion is 2–4 degrees in newborns, 9 degrees by age 5, and 15–20 degrees at maturation. Lesser degrees of external torsion make the diagnosis of internal tibial torsion. The thigh–foot angle can be assessed by having the child stand on one foot facing away and holding one knee in 90 degrees of flexion. The thigh–foot angle is the angle between the axis of the foot and the thigh. An external rotation is expected. The diagnosis can also be made more simply by carefully observing the positions of the feet and patellae during walking. In internal tibial torsion, the patellae will face forward while the toes point inward. Outlining the patellae in ink can make this examination easier.

Finally, assess the degree of femoral anteversion. Have the child lie prone with the knees flexed to 90 degrees. Observe the positions of the legs with internal and external rotation of the hips. With excessive femoral anteversion, internal rotation will be much more prominent than external rotation, ranging from 70 to 90 degrees. It may also be possible to see that both the patellae and toes are turned inward during ambulation.

Table 105.2 Gait disturbance features and differential diagnosis

Gait disturbance	Features	Possible diagnoses
Antalgic gait (Fig. 105.5)	Shortens stance phase on affected side and swing phase on unaffected side to miminize pain caused by bearing weight	Fracture, dislocation, septic joint, slipped capital femoral epiphysis, Legg–Calvé–Perthes disease, Osgood–Schlatter disease
Trendelenburg gait (Fig. 105.6)	Inability to maintain pelvis level because of unilateral weakness of trunk muscles	Developmental dysplasia of the hip
Shuffling gait	Small shallow steps; can be associated with peritoneal signs.	Acute appendicitis, pelvic inflammatory disease
Waddling gait	Can indicate bilateral pathology	Bilateral developmental dysplasia of the hip
Drop-foot (Fig. 105.7)	Pronounced lifting of the knee (steppage gait) to compensate for inadequate foot dorsiflexion at end of swing phase	Spinal nerve compression, peripheral nerve injury, central muscular palsy

Look for bowing of the knees, either valgus (inward) or varus (outward). It is normal for newborns to have 15 to 20 degrees of varus deformity at birth. This gradually develops into 10 degrees of valgus deformity by about age 3 and settles at a normal adult structure with around 5 degrees of valgus alignment by age 7. Because of these normal changes, most caregiver complaints of bowleggedness or knock-knees require only reassurance and will resolve during development. Varus and valgus deformities that do not conform to this expected progression may need further investigation.

One serious cause of varus deformity is Blount's disease, which has infantile and adolescent varieties. This disorder is caused by problems with endochondral ossification of the medial proximal tibial physis, causing varus deformity and internal tibial torsion. An abnormal "beaking" of the proximal tibial metaphysis may be palpable. In the infantile form, varus deformity is usually accompanied by medial tibial torsion, a limp or waddling gait, and posteromedial subluxation of the knee when held in partial flexion (Siffert–Katz sign). In the adolescent form, leg shortening is common, there is <20 degrees of varus deformity, and there may be mild laxity of the medial collateral ligament with lateral knee thrust during an antalgic gait. The derotation test can differentiate normal from pathologic varus deformity in the patient with suspected Blount's disease. With the patient sitting with the knee held in 90 degrees of flexion, the examiner steadys the femur with one hand and externally rotates the knee with the other hand. In a normal patient, any varus deformity will disappear with this maneuver. The intercondylar distance should also be measured by having the patient stand with medial malleoli touching. A distance between the femoral condyles of greater than 6 cm is abnormal.

Growing pains become a common concern as older children move into adolescence. Various aches and pains may come and go related to rapid, sometimes unbalanced, growth of bones, muscles, ligaments, and joints. These pains often manifest between the ages of 6 and 8 years. They can occur at night and wake the child from sleep. They can change positions over time. The patellofemoral joint is a particularly common location for aches and pains that may become worse with exertion, particularly with involvement in sports. It is important to make this diagnosis of exclusion only after more serious conditions have been considered. There is a patellofemoral pain syndrome that can be caused by foot deformities (such as flat footedness or high arches), weakness of the quadriceps muscles, or overuse. For this reason the entire extremity should be carefully examined, in addition to a focused knee examination.

Examine the foot for tenderness or morphologic abnormalities. Tenderness along the plantar aspect of the foot could be associated with plantar fasciitis. Tenderness at the base of the heel could be from inflammation of the achilles tendon, or from Sever's disease, an apophysitis of the calcaneus. Flat feet can be detected by having the child stand on his/her toes and observing for lack of curvature of the plantar surface.

Pearls and pitfalls

Pearls

1. The joints and bones above and below the area of injury should always be examined.
2. In order to facilitate a child's cooperation with the musculoskeletal examination, extra time should be spent establishing a rapport with the child, or turning the examination into a game or play.
3. Radiographic imaging of the cervical spine is indicated in all first presentations of torticollis that are not intermittent in nature.

Pitfalls

1. Failure to consider infection as a cause of acquired torticollis.
2. Failure to consider hip pathology (slipped capital femoral epiphysis, or Legg–Calvé–Perthes disease) in a patient with knee pain.
3. Failure to assess the gait in a child complaining of back or lower extremity pain.

Selected references

Seidel HM, Ball JW, Dains JE, Benedict GW (eds.). The musculoskeletal system. *Mosby's Guide to Physical Examination,* 4th edn, Ch. 19. St. Louis, MO: Mosby,1999, pp. 689–754.

McWuillen KK, Paul RI. Nontraumatic orthopedic emergencies. In Advanced Pediatric Life Support Steering Committee (ed.) *The Pediatric Emergency Medicine Resource,* 4th edn. Sudbury, MA: Jones & Bartlett for the American Academy of Pediatrics and the American College of Emergency Physicians, 2006, pp. 410–445.

Staheli LT. *Practice of Pediatric Orthopedics.* Philadelphia, PA: Lippincott, Williams, & Wilkins.

Zitelli BJ, Davis HW. *Atlas of Pediatric Physical Diagnosis.* New York: Gower Medical.

Chapter 106

Limp/hip pain

Steven H. Mitchell and Noel C. Hastings

Introduction

Limp is defined as an uneven, jerky, or laborious gait, usually caused by pain, weakness or deformity. The most common causes of limp in children are secondary to trauma or conditions that resolve spontaneously without long-term consequences, such as transient synovitis. The clinician, however, must pay careful consideration to less common conditions that may rapidly become life or limb threatening, such as neoplasm and septic arthritis. When evaluating the child with a limp, the EP must remember that patients with hip pathology may present without hip pain or may complain of pain elsewhere such as the mid thigh or knee. Distinguishing true emergencies requiring urgent evaluation and treatment from conditions that are safe for outpatient management is the primary task of the EP in the acute care setting (Table 106.1).

Table 106.1. Aged-based differential of limping child

Age	Causes
All ages	Septic arthritis, osteomyelitis, cellulitis, stress fracture, neoplasm (leukemia), neuromuscular, child abuse, soft tissue injury
1–3 years	Septic arthritis (hip >knee), developmental dysplasia of hip, osteomyelitis (<5 years), toddler's fracture, foot fracture
3–10 years	Legg–Calvé–Perthes disease, transient synovitis, juvenile rheumatoid arthritis/rheumatic disease

Traumatic and mechanical causes of limp

Most children with traumatic etiologies have a history of trauma that corresponds to their complaints. The history guides the evaluation and workup, looking for fractures and for ligamentous and soft tissue origins of the child's pain. Although children are often the victims of accidental traumatic injuries, maintaining a high level of suspicion for suspected cases of abuse is crucial.

Toddler's and CAST fractures

Toddler's fractures are an example of a subtle presentation of limp in a child, usually from an accidental trauma.

The trivial nature of the antecedent trauma and age of the child, often between 2 and 6 years, sometimes limits the useful history. Toddler's fractures are believed to be a subset of childhood accidental spiral tibial (CAST) fractures involving the distal half of the tibia. Toddler's and CAST fractures are most often the result of a low mechanism event resulting in the twisting of the ankle or tibia relative to the foot. On examination, the child will likely have pain with torsion applied to the lower tibia or dorsiflexion of the ankle and point tenderness along the distal half of the tibia. Radiological findings are often subtle and may not always be evident in a recent injury. Possible findings include a faint lucency that obliquely crosses the distal tibia and terminates medially. In children with evidence of a fracture on radiograph, casting of the affected limb is performed to include the ankle. Without obvious radiological fracture, observation is usually the best course of action. If the child continues to refuse to bear weight the radiograph and examination should be repeated.

Foot fracture

Foot fractures are another cause of limp with subtle examination findings in a child too young to effectively communicate the events that led to the injury. Parents often describe a child who preferentially crawls to avoid weight bearing on the foot. Radiographs are often negative and this may necessitate a bone scan if suspicion is high. Careful examination of the foot is essential. Stress fractures are caused by repetitive loading and overuse injuries and occur most commonly in the adolescent (11–16 years). Radiographs may be negative. Use of MRI or bone scan may be required to detect the fracture.

A Practical Guide to Pediatric Emergency Medicine: Caring for Children in the Emergency Department, ed. N. Ewen Amieva-Wang (associate eds. Jamie Shandro, Aparajita Sohoni, and Bernhard Fassl). Published by Cambridge University Press.

A

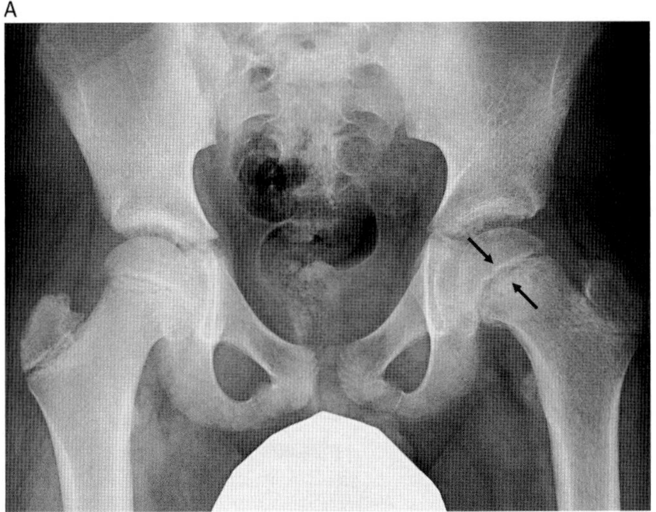

B

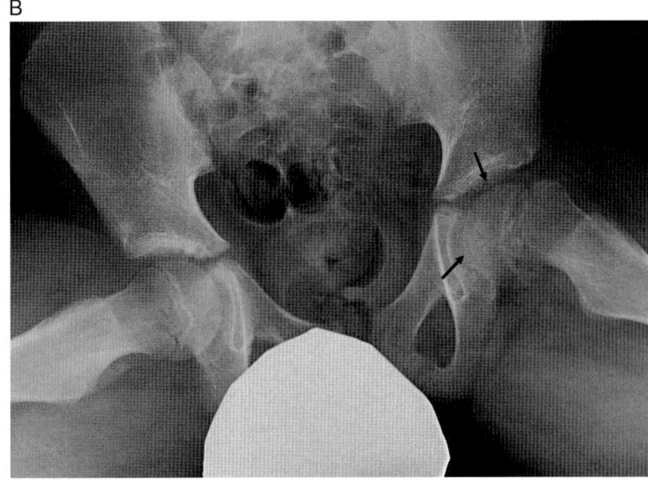

Figure 106.1 Slipped capital femoral epiphysis in a 12-year-old boy presenting with hip pain. (A) On the frontal view, there is subtle widening of the left femoral physis (arrows). (B) Frog lateral view demonstrates posteromedial slippage of the left femoral epiphysis (arrows).

Slipped capital femoral epiphysis

Slipped capital femoral epiphysis (SCFE) is a disorder where the femoral neck slips off the proximal femoral epiphysis. It is believed to be a mechanical condition because of its prevalence in obesity. Other risk factors include hypothyroidism, growth hormone deficiency, renal disease, and previous chemotherapy/radiation.

Slipped capital femoral epiphysis is most often seen in older children and adolescents who are obese.

The highest incidence occurs in boys ages 10 to 16. It is found bilaterally in 20–25% of patients and often presents as referred pain to the knee that occurs after activity. Pain may radiate to the groin or thigh and be insidious over several weeks. This often leads to a delay in diagnosis and increased risk of arthritis and osteonecrosis as the degree of epiphyseal slippage increases and the SCFE becomes unstable. On examination, the child may have localized hip tenderness, a shortened leg, decreased internal rotation, and a need to outwardly rotate the hip with flexion. All patients with a concern for SCFE merit radiographic evaluation. Initial views should include anteroposterior, lateral, and frog leg lateral projections (Fig. 106.1). The lateral view is the most sensitive for early slips but findings may be subtle and may require comparative views. Confirmation may be obtained by CT or MRI. Patients should be placed on crutches and instructed to avoid weight bearing pending urgent orthopedic follow-up. Management is concerned with avoiding further slippage by surgical stabilization.

Inflammatory and infectious causes of limp

Infectious causes of limp in a child are not dissimilar to those in an adult. Infectious etiologies include, in order of prevalence, septic arthritis, osteomyelitis, myositis, abscess, and discitis.

Septic arthritis

Of the infectious etiologies of limp, septic arthritis is the most commo. Long-term joint destruction can result without prompt diagnosis. The hip and knee are two of the most common sites of septic arthritis. The reduced rate of blood flow within vessels at the metaphysis makes this region more susceptible to hematogenous seeding of infection. Before the appearance of secondary ossification centers, the cartilaginous epiphyses receive their blood supply directly from metaphyseal blood vessels. The neonate is particularly susceptible to the development of infection in joints such as the hip, in which the metaphysis is intracapsular.

Children with septic arthritis typically appear toxic, refuse to bear weight, resist movement of the joint, and have a concurrent or recent history of fever. Risk factors most commonly identified are a history of fever >37.5°C, refusal to bear weight, an elevated WBC (11 000–12 000/μl), elevated ESR, elevated CRP, increased joint space on radiographs, and prior healthcare visits. Generally, greater than two risk factors increases the likelihood of septic arthritis and obviates the need for further investigation. The gold standard for diagnosis remains joint aspiration with evidence of bacteria on Gram stain and a WBC of >50 000/μl, although the WBC can vary greatly, even within the same sample.

Osteomyelitis

Osteomyelitis refers to infection of bone and/or bone marrow. In children of all ages, acute osteomyelitis has a gradual onset over several days to 1 week. Symptoms are often those of bacteremia, such as malaise and low-grade fever. As a result, the child may not present for medical care until symptoms referable to bone develop. Retrospective studies have identified fever, localized pain, and decreased mobility as the most likely clinical symptoms in osteomyelitis. There may also be a history of antecedent trauma, erythema, swelling, or frank cellulitis overlying the infected bone.

Laboratory findings in osteomyelitis are non-specific but may aid diagnosis. The ESR has been shown to be elevated in 92% of cases and CRP elevated in 98% of cases. The sensitivity of the WBC is much lower, being elevated in just 35–46% of cases.

A plain radiograph is performed initially in all patients with suspected osteomyelitis. A plain film may identify findings such as lytic sclerosis or periosteal reaction compatible with the clinical findings. Additional radiographic evaluations that aid diagnosis include MRI, scintigraphy, and CT.

Transient synovitis

Transient synovitis is a benign, often self-limited condition that can easily be confused with the infectious causes of limp. It usually presents between 3 and 8 years of age, with an average annual incidence of 0.2% and a lifetime risk of up to 3%. Most children have less than a week of symptoms and most present without fever. Transient synovitis affects males more often (2:1). The most common presentation is a child with pain and decreased range of motion in the affected hip. It has been proposed that this may represent a post-infectious immune response. Any child with risk factors of osteomyelitis and septic arthritis should have these entities ruled out. Transient synovitis generally has an excellent prognosis when treated conservatively with NSAIDs and rest.

Legg–Calvé–Perthes disease

Legg–Calvé–Perthes disease is a disease of idiopathic avascular necrosis of the proximal femoral epiphysis that occurs in children aged 4–12 years of age. It occurs most often in boys, with a prevalence of 4:1. Children with Legg–Calvé–Perthes disease may present with a painless limp or relate an insidious onset of pain and worsened limp. Increasing symptoms are attributed to worsening collapse of the femoral head. The pain is often referred to the knee or medial thigh. On examination, the child may have pain with internal rotation and abduction of the affected hip. Radiographic evaluation with antero-posterior, lateral, and frog leg plain views are indicated with clinical suspicion. The earliest radiographic signs are asymmetry in size of the femoral epiphysis, which may also show increased density on the involved side (Fig. 106.2). Therapy is based on age and is focused on containment of the femoral head within the acetabulum. Children should be made non-weight bearing until specialty consultation is obtained.

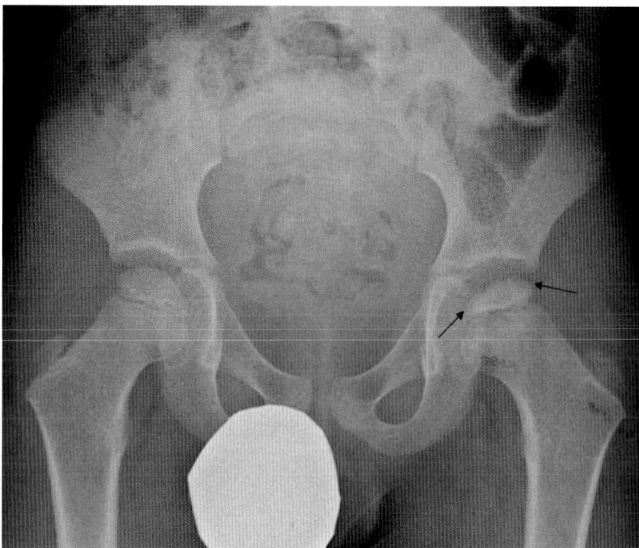

Figure 106.2 Legg–Calvé–Perthes disease. Frontal radiograph shows widening of the left hip joint space and a sclerotic flattened irregular left femoral head (arrows).

Developmental dysplasia of the hip

Developmental dysplasia of the hip consists of a group of disorders that are characterized by anatomic abnormalities in the relationship of the femoral head with the acetabulum. It is clinically diagnosed using the Ortolani or Barlow test (Fig. 105.2, p. 478), usually by primary care physicians in infancy and resolves spontaneously. When unrecognized however, it is a significant cause of childhood disability. While most children have no identifiable risk factors, risk factors include family history, female gender, large birth weight, and breech delivery. Diagnosis is made based on clinical examination which varies by age. When developmental dysplasia of the hip is unilateral, the limp will present as a wobbling gait noticed when walking begins. This is referred to as the Trendelenburg gait, where the child limps because of shortening of the limb, telescoping of femoral head on the pelvis, and a contralateral tilt of pelvis as a result of abductor muscle weakness. Ultrasound is the preferred modality for diagnostic confirmation, with plain radiography playing a limited role until bone maturation occurs in the child. Expert referral is indicated. Treatment goals vary depending upon age, stability, and severity of the condition but range from splinting to surgical repair.

Neoplastic causes of limp

Benign tumors

Fibrous dysplasia, osteoid osteomas, and various bone cysts are all non-malignant neoplastic causes of limp. Osteoid osteomas are one of the most common and present primarily in the teenage years. Osteomas occur primarily in the femur and are twice as common in boys. The history usually includes a description of night aches that respond well to the use of NSAIDs. Treatment is surgical and outcomes excellent.

On plain films or CT, these bone cysts appear as a visible lucency with a dense central core. The key to differentiating these slow-growing benign tumors from malignant tumors is close attention to the margins of the lesion. Slow-growing tumors demonstrate clear margins, whereas malignant, fast-growing tumors often display rough margins and "onion skinning" from repetitive periosteal reactions.

Malignant tumors

Malignant tumors that can cause bone pain and possibly a limp in children are rare compared with other more common causes of limp. Ewing's sarcoma, osteosarcoma, and leukemias are some of the most feared malignancies. Most malignancies usually begin with vague symptoms. Limp may be a late finding. Radiographs are a way to discriminate between malignant and benign tumor. Even with normal plain films, a child presenting with aching bone pain, particularly at night or if accompanied by bleeding abnormalities or adenopathy, is concerning for malignancy. A CBC with smear may reveal an anemia and/or thrombocytopenia, which are present in most leukemias. Concern for malignancy mandates expert referral for a complete workup.

Conclusions

Limp has a characteristic age-based differential diagnosis. All children must be taken seriously and examined systematically for infectious and mechanical causes of this common symptom.

Pearls and pitfalls

Pearls

1. Knee pain equals hip pain until proven otherwise in children.
2. A toddler with pain over the tibia and no identifiable fracture on radiograph should be splinted and scheduled for a repeat examination and radiograph if symptoms persist.
3. Consider septic arthritis in any ill-appearing child with a fever, irritability, and joint pain.

Pitfalls

1. Failure to consider non-accidental trauma in a child with a limp.
2. Failure to recognize rest or night pain as a worrisome symptom of neoplasm in a child with skeletal pain of uncertain etiology.
3. Hip pathology not correctly diagnosed may result in chronic conditions such as arthritis, limp, or change in gait, or require hip athroplasty if left untreated.

Selected references

Arnold SR, Elias D, Buckingham SC, *et al.* Changing patterns of acute hematogenous osteomyelitis and septic arthritis: emergence of community-associated methicillin-resistant *Staphylococcus aureus. J Pediatr Orthop* 2006;**26**:703–708.

Bache CE, Clegg J, Herron H. Risk factors for developmental dysplasia of the hip in the neonatal period. *J Pediatr Orthop B* 2002;**11**:212–221.

Chung SM. Identifying the cause of acute limp in childhood. Some informal comments and observations. *Clin Pediatr* 1974;**13**:769–772.

Clark M. Overview of the causes of limp in children. *UpToDate*, 2008 http://www.uptodate.com/patients/content/topic.do?topicKey=~ETlb3xPIrm_px9&selectedTitle=47~150&source= search_result (accessed 27 April 2010).

Coffey C, Haley K, Hayes J, Groner JI. The risk of child abuse in infants and toddlers with lower extremity injuries. *J Pediatr Surg* 2005;**40**:120–123.

Del Beccaro MA, Champoux AN, Bockers T, Mendelman PM. Septic arthritis versus transient synovitis of the hip: the value of screening laboratory tests. *Ann Emerg Med* 1992;**21**:1418–1422.

Do TT. Transient synovitis as a cause of painful limps in children. *Curr Opin Pediatr* 2000;**12**:48–51.

Frick, S. Evaluation of the child who has hip pain. *Orthoped Clin North Am*, 2006;**37**:133–140.

Gafur OA, Copley LA, Hollmig ST, *et al.* The impact of the current epidemiology of pediatric musculoskeletal infection on evaluation and treatment guidelines. *J Pediatr Orthop* 2008;**28**:777–785.

Goergens ED, McEvoy A, Watson M, Barrett IR. Acute osteomyelitis and septic arthritis in children., *J Paediatr Child Health* 2005;**41**:59–62.

Halsey MF, Finzel KC, Carrion WV, et al. Toddler's fracture: presumptive diagnosis and treatment. *J Pediatr Orthoped* 2001;**21**:152–156.

Haueisen DC, Weiner DS, Weiner SD. The characterization of "transient synovitis of the hip" in children. *J Pediatr Orthoped* 1986;**6**:11–17.

Jung S, Rowe S, Moon E, *et al.* Significance of laboratory and radiologic findings for differentiating between septic arthritis and transient synovitis of the hip. *J Pediatr Orthop* 2003;**23**:368–372.

Kocher M, Zurakowski D, Kasser J. Differentiating between septic arthritis and transient synovitis of the hip in children. An evidence-based clinical prediction algorithm. *J Bone Joint Surg Am* 1999;**81**:1662–1670.

Kocher M, Mandiga R, Zurakowski D, *et al.* Validation of a clinical prediction rule for differentiation between septic arthritis and transient synovitis of the hip in children. *J Bone Joint Surg Am* 2004;**86**:1629–1635.

Krogstad, P. Clinical features of hematogenous osteomyelitis in children. *UpToDate* May 2008. http://www.utdol.com/patients/content/topic.do?topicKey=~Q0V2MsZrZsI5 (accessed 27 April 2010).

Landin LA, Danielsson LG, Wattsgard C. Transient synovitis of the hip. Its incidence, epidemiology and relation to Perthes' disease. *J Bone Joint Surg* 1987;**69**:238–242.

Marx J, Hockberger R, Walls R. (eds.) *Rosen's Emergency Medicine: Concepts and Clinical Practice,* 6th edn. St. Louis, MO: Mosby Elsevier, 2006.

Mellick LB, Milker L, Egsieker E. Childhood accidental

spiral tibial (CAST) fractures. *Pediatr Emerg Care* 1999; **15**:307–309.

Offiah AC. Acute osteomyelitis, septic arthritis and discitis: differences between neonates and older children. *Eur J Radiol* 2006;**60**: 221–232.

Patel H. for the Canadian Task Force on Preventive Health Care. Preventive health care, 2001 update: screening and management of developmental dysplasia of the hip in newborns. *CMAJ* 2001;**164**:1669–1677.

Perron AD, Miller MD, Brady WJ. Orthopedic Pitfalls in the emergency department: slipped capital femoral epiphysis. *Am J Emerg Med* 2002;**20**:484–487.

Swan A, Amer H, Dieppe P. The value of synovial fluid assays in the diagnosis of joint disease: a literature survey. *Ann Rheum Dis*. 2002;**61:** 493–498.

Wheeless III CR (ed.). Physical exam of DDH. *The Wheeless' Textbook of Orthopaedics*. http://www.wheelessonline.com/ortho/physical_exam_of_ddh (accessed 27 April 2010).

Chapter 107

Back pain

Aparajita Sohoni

Introduction

Pediatric back pain is an increasingly recognized phenomenon for primary care and ED practitioners. While historic teaching was that back pain in every child was a "red flag" and should be evaluated thoroughly to uncover any organic cause (i.e., neoplasm, discitis, spondylolysis, or spondylolisthesis), more recent US-based studies have shown benign causes of back pain in as many as 78% of cases. This increase has been linked to a variety of lifestyle factors, from types of activity performed by children to the increased prevalence of childhood obesity. The EP should still approach the pediatric patient with back pain cautiously and rule out all serious pathologies before assigning the diagnosis of benign, or musculoligamentous, back pain. It is still generally felt that back pain in younger children may signify serious pathology.

Clinical presentation

History

History of pediatric patients with back pain should include general characteristics of the pain, such as time of onset, intensity, location, frequency, and duration. Ask about worsening of pain at night, or with specific movements; as well as modification of daily activities; history of trauma; associated symptoms such as fever, weight loss, limps, numbness or tingling; and any bowel or bladder changes. Review any medications used and relief associated with those medications. Elicit past medical history including history of similar pain, treatments tried. Table 107.1 shows the differential diagnosis of back pain by patient presentation. Table 107.2 presents a full differential diagnosis of back pain by system

Physical examination

The physical examination is commenced with the patient undressing and putting on a gown. Socks should be removed in order to fully assess gait and foot positioning. The spine is examined starting with overall posture, alignment, trunk balance, and skin changes. Hemangiomas or cysts may indicate underlying neurologic malformations. The EP should then have the patient bend forward to evaluate the spine in both forward flexion and recovery. Pain that worsens with hyperextension is likely spondylolysis or spondylolisthesis. During gait assessment, balance and coordination should be evaluated, followed by reflex testing and overall motor and sensory function. Asymmetric reflexes may indicate a spinal cord tumor or syringomyelia. Straight leg raise tests should also be done to evaluate for radiculopathy.

Diagnosis

The diagnostic evaluation of pediatric back pain is controversial with a variety of algorithms and advantages and disadvantages reported for plain films, CT, MRI, and bone scans. The overall diagnostic approach will be guided by the patient's appearance, examination, the history, and the provider's differential diagnosis. It is recommended that any patient with "red flags" on history (i.e., nighttime pain, radiculopathy, fevers), young age, or an abnormal neurological examination should receive laboratory studies and plain films of their spine. Radiology and laboratory test results coupled with the differential diagnosis should guide further workup.

Management

For adolescent patients with no red flags on history or physical examination, conservative therapy with pain medication and stretching coupled with close follow-up is recommended. The management of some of the most common causes of pediatric back pain is discussed below.

Spondylolysis and spondylolisthesis

Spondylolysis and spondylolisthesis are distinct traumatic disorders of the lower lumbar spine that commonly occur in children. In spondylolysis, a fracture of the pars interarticularis occurs, while in spondylolisthesis the instability caused by

A Practical Guide to Pediatric Emergency Medicine: Caring for Children in the Emergency Department, ed. N. Ewen Amieva-Wang (associate eds. Jamie Shandro, Aparajita Sohoni, and Bernhard Fassl). Published by Cambridge University Press.

Table 107.1. Differential diagnosis of pediatric back pain by presentation

Primary symptom	Associated symptoms	Diagnoses
Acute pain	Radicular pain, positive SLR	Herniated disk, slipped apophysis, spondylolysis
	Other injuries, neurologic loss	Vertebral fracture
	Muscle tenderness without radiation	Muscle strain
Pain with forward flexion	Radicular pain, positive SLR	Herniated disk
Pain with extension	Hamstring tightness	Spondylolysis, spondylolisthesis, posterior arch (pedicle or lamina) injury
Pain worse at night	Fever, weight loss, malaise	Tumor, infection
Pain with fever or generalized symptoms	Nighttime pain	Tumor, infection
Chronic pain	Rigid kyphosis	Scheuermann's kyphosis
	Morning stiffness, sacroiliac joint tenderness	Inflammatory spondyloarthropathy
Pain with new-onset scoliosis	Fever, malaise, weight loss, positive SLR	Tumor, infection, syrinx, herniated disk
	Patient >15 years of age	Idiopathic scoliosis
Other	Abnormal urinalysis, history of sickle cell disease, other bone pain	Pyelonephritis, sickle cell disease

SLR, straight leg raise.
Source: adapted from Bernstein and Cozen, 2007.

Table 107.2. Differential diagnosis of back pain by system

Type	Causes
Traumatic	Spondylolysis, spondylolisthesis, musculoligamentous strain, herniated nucleus pulposus
Neoplastic	Bony (osteoid osteoma, osteoblastoma, osteosarcoma), leukemia, lymphoma, eosinophilic granuloma, Ewing's sarcoma, neurogenic (glioma, neuroblastoma)
Inflammatory	Ankylosing spondylitis, enteropathic arthritis
Infectious	Discitis, sacroiliac joint infection, tuberculosis
Congenital	Tethered cord
Developmental	Scheuermann disease, iliac apophysitis
Extraspinal	Abdominal, renal, vascular
Psychogenic	

Source: With permission from Sponseller 1996.

the fracture leads the vertebra to slip (see Fig. 107.1). While the overall neurological examination in a child with spondylolysis is normal, usually hyperextension reproduces the pain. On examination, tight hamstrings are usually noted. Initial treatment is rest, pain control, and hamstring stretches. Back strengthening exercises should be started after the pain has resolved. A back brace may be needed only if symptoms are not controlled with analgesics or back-strengthening exercises. Children, particularly girls, and those in a "growth spurt" should be followed yearly to monitor for spondylolysthesis, which occurs in up to 3% of people with spondylolysis. Surgical fusion may be required if the slip is greater than 50% or if the back pain is severe despite supportive care.

Scheuermann disease

Scheuermann disease, thought to be caused by excessive heavy lifting or flexion of the spine, is a common cause of upper back or thoracolumbar pain. This diagnosis is made by plain films of the spine demonstrating growth disturbance, wedging, or irregularity on three successive vertebrae with narrowing of the intervertebral disc spaces. On physical examination, kyphosis is noted that worsens with forward bending. Tight hamstrings may also be seen. Kyphosis of greater than 60 degrees usually results in moderate symptoms (up to 45 degrees of kyphosis is normal in the thoracic spine). Mild cases are treated with back-strengthening exercises, specifically the thoracic extensor muscles, and hamstring stretching. Bracing can be used if the patient's posture is altered or if there is severe kyphosis.

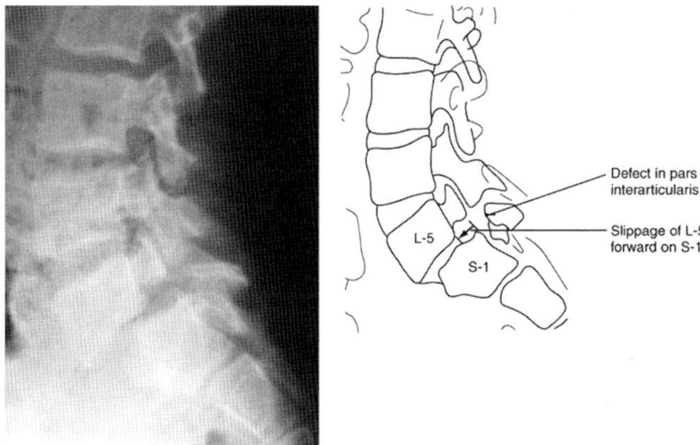

Figure 107.1 Spondylolisthesis. Radiograph of moderate isthmic spondylolisthesis in a 14-year-old boy and an illustration of the defect. The forward slippage of L5 on the sacrum was the result of a fatigue fracture of the pars interarticularis. (Reproduced with permission from Zitelli BJ, Davis HW. *Atlas of Pediatric Physical Diagnosis,* 5th edn. Philadelphia , PA: Mosby Elsevier, 2007. © 2007 Mosby Inc., an affiliate of Elsevier Inc.)

Discitis

Discitis is one of the most common infectious etiologies of back pain in a pediatric patient. Classically, children with discitis are 4–7 years of age. On examination, they will have a stiff back, resist flexion of the back, and have concomitant signs of illness, such as a fever or irritability. Patients may also present with hip pain or refusal to walk. Laboratory tests usually reveal an elevated ESR and leukocytosis. While plain films of the spine are usually normal at the time of diagnosis, MRI is the diagnostic test of choice. Appropriate treatment for a patient with discitis includes antibiotics to cover *Staphylococcus aureus*, rest, and use of a brace if the child has extreme pain. Intravenous antibiotics should be administered until the child is afebrile, well appearing, and any culture and sensitivity reports are obtained. Patients with discitis usually do well, and have a minimally increased risk of back pain in adulthood.

Epidural abscesses

Epidural abscesses in pediatric patients are rare but they have a great potential for morbidity and mortality. Medical literature regarding pediatric epidural abscesses is limited to case reports, with few comprehensive reviews. The average age of children with epidural abscesses is 9 years. Only approximately one-third of pediatric patients with epidural abscesses have associated medical conditions, such as leukemia or sickle cell disease, that predispose them to developing this disease, in contrast to adults who are more likely to have a predisposing condition such as intravenous drug abuse. Pediatric patients are more predisposed to developing epidural abscesses because their epidural spaces contain more fat and are more vascular than adult spines. *Staphylococcus aureus*, both methicillin resistant and sensitive, plays a significant role in epidural abscesses, even in the pediatric patient.

Children with back pain and fever have an imaging study even if neurologic findings are normal.

Sensitivity of CT to detect an epidural abscess is limited and MRI remains the diagnostic test of choice. The recommended therapy is a combined approach of surgical drainage and parenteral antibiotics. Patients who have developed classic backpain, fever, and paresis do poorly. However, appropriately managed, pediatric patients with epidural abscesses recover well and with appropriate treatment have minimal residual morbidity.

Tumors of the spine

Tumors of the spine may be benign or malignant. Tumors usually present with back pain that is worse at night, back stiffness, and mild scoliosis. Osteoid osteomas are small tumors that usually spontaneously resolve over years and do not require surgical removal unless the pain becomes too severe. Osteoblastomas are larger versions of osteoid osteomas. Malignant tumors of the spine include leukemias, Ewing's sarcoma, osteosarcoma, and neuroblastoma. The diagnostic test of choice for tumors is MRI, given that they are rarely seen on plain films.

Ankylosing spondylitis

Ankylosing spondylitis, a rheumatologic disorder, frequently presents with back pain. Generally, older children present with chronic back pain and have concomitant diseases such as psoriasis or inflammatory bowel disease, which also suggest a rheumatologic etiology. Patients will complain of chronic back stiffness. Radiographs may show narrowing of the sacroiliac joints, difficulty with forward flexion, and limitation of chest expansion. Rheumatology follow-up should be arranged to complete a full autoimmune workup and for long-term follow-up.

Disposition

The etiology of the patient's back pain will determine their disposition. For patients who are deemed to have non-specific back pain, follow-up with the pediatrician is recommended while starting a trial of pain medications and back-strengthening/stretching exercises. Return precautions should be provided to the patient and the caregiver.

Pearls and pitfalls

Pearls

1. The approach to the pediatric patient with back pain should be systematic to avoid missing a serious diagnosis.
2. Close follow-up with the pediatrician and good return precautions are key.

Pitfalls

1. Failure to treat back pain in a child seriously.
2. Failure to perform a thorough neurological examination, including reflexes and gait.
3. Failure to consider other infections (i.e., urinary tract infections) in a child with back pain.

Selected references

Afshani E, Kuhn JP. Common causes of low back pain in children. *Radiographics* 1991;**11**:269–291.

Auerbach JD, Ahn J, Zgonis MH, *et al.* Streamlining the evaluation of low back pain in children. *Clin Orthop Relat Res* 2008;**466**:1971–1977.

Auletta JJ, John CC. Spinal epidural abscesses in children: a 15-year experience and review of the literature. *Clin Infect Dis* 2001;**32**:9–16.

Bernstein RM, Cozen H. Evaluation of back pain in children and adolescents. *Am Fam Physician* 2007;**76**:1669–1676.

Bhatia NN, Chow G, Timon SJ, Watts HG. Diagnostic modalities for the evaluation of pediatric back pain: a prospective study. *J Pediatr Orthop* 2008;**28**:230–233.

Feldman DS, Straight JJ, Badra MI, Mohaideen A, Madan SS. Evaluation of an algorithmic approach to pediatric back pain. *J Pediatr Orthop* 2006;**26**:353–357.

King HA. Back pain in children. *Orthop Clin North Am* 1999;**30**:467–474, ix.

Sponseller PD. Evaluating the child with back pain. *Am Fam Physician* 1996;**54**:1933–1941.

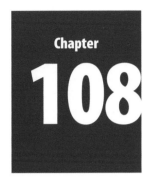

Chapter 108 Hand injury

Amritha Raghunathan

Introduction

Pediatricians and urgent care physicians will often see hand injuries as part of their practice. Crush injuries are common in infants and toddlers, and adolescents frequently sustain sports injuries. It is imperative to have a full understanding of when a referral to a hand surgeon is necessary to ensure optimal outcomes. Particularly in the pediatric population, it is crucial to properly diagnose and treat such injuries to avoid a lifetime of issues.

Basic anatomy

Hand injuries involve bones as well as tendons and ligaments (Figs. 108.1 and 108.2). Finger flexion is achieved mainly by two tendons, the flexor digitorum superficialis that flexes the proximal interphalangeal (PIP) joint and the flexor digitorum profundus that flexes the distal interphalangeal (DIP) joint. The intrinsic muscles assist in metacarpophalangeal (MCP) joint flexion. Finger extension is achieved by the dorsal extensor tendon (this tendon has two parts, the central slip that extends the PIP and the lateral bands that insert as the terminal tendon on the distal phalanx to extend the DIP). Finally, the volar plate, collateral ligaments, and the joint capsule stabilize the joints.

Fractures involving non-ossified epiphyses are radiographically invisible until healing begins. There is variable onset of ossification of the bones of the hand, but physeal closure usually occurs between 14 and 21 years of age.

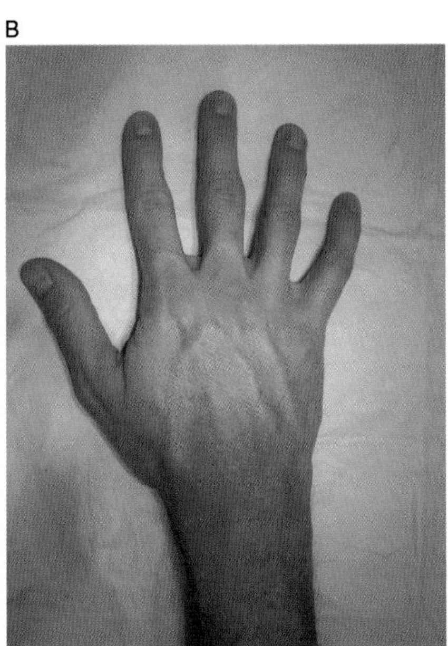

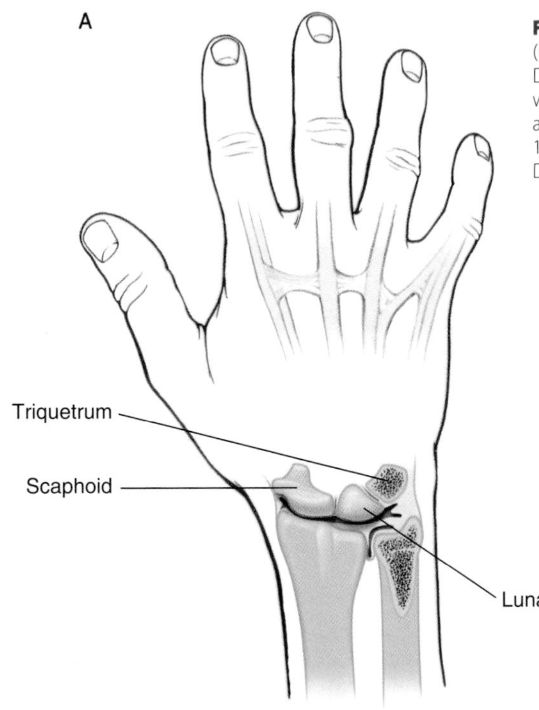

Figure 108.1 The wrist: (A) wrist anatomys; (B) surface structures. (Originally published in Daniels II JM, Zook EG, Lynch JM. Hand and wrist injuries: Part 1. Nonemergency evaluation. *Am Fam Physician* 2004; l69:1941–1948; A, copyright N. Scott Bodell; B, courtesy Dr. J. Daniels.)

A Practical Guide to Pediatric Emergency Medicine: Caring for Children in the Emergency Department, ed. N. Ewen Amieva-Wang (associate eds. Jamie Shandro, Aparajita Sohoni, and Bernhard Fassl). Published by Cambridge University Press.

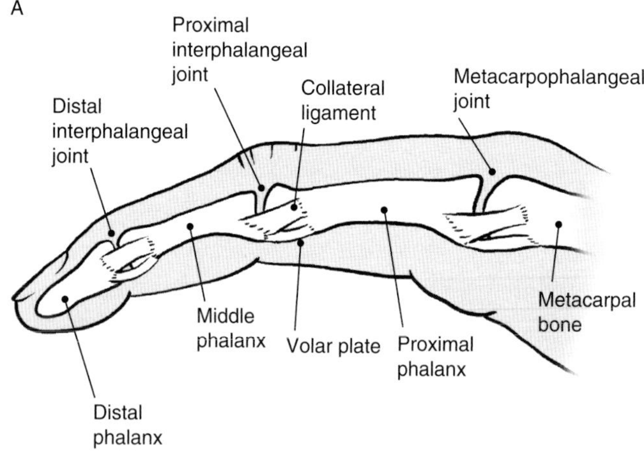

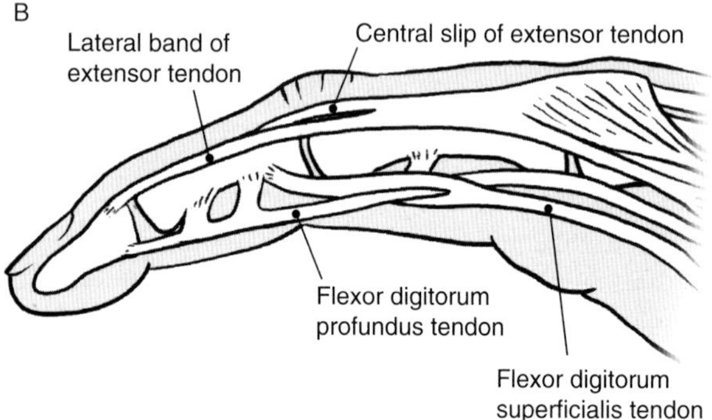

Figure 108.2 Anatomy of the finger tendons (A) and ligaments (B). (Copyright N. Ewen Wang.)

Anesthesia

In the infant or young child, it may be necessary to do procedural sedation in order to repair lacerations or reduce fractures (Ch. 152). Have a low threshold to consult the hand or plastic surgeon to perform the definitive repair.

Injuries

Table 108.1 summarizes the examination and treatment for hand injuries. The discussion below is grouped by whether bone, ligments, or tendons are affected.

Finger lacerations and amputations

Finger lacerations and amputations are the second most common hand injuries seen in children. As with adults, a thorough examination must be performed to check all tendons, digital artery, digital nerve, and to rule out fractures. Simple lacerations can be irrigated and repaired in the ED. Even with extensive soft tissue loss, irrigation and gauze covering with referral to hand surgery within the next 24 h is adequate. If injury to the tendons, artery, or nerves are present or suspected, however, a hand surgeon should be consulted as an examination under anesthesia and/or a skin graft/flap may be necessary.

In young children, simple skin lacerations can be closed with absorbable sutures such as chromic or plain gut in order to avoid the trauma of suture removal. Dermabond can be used for small lacerations or for increased strength over suture closure. Nailbed injury, subungual hematoma and fight bites are covered in Ch. 151 on wound care.

Paronychia

Paronychia is a soft tissue infection around a fingernail (Fig. 108.3). It is the most common hand infection. The major inciting risk factor is prolonged contact with water or skin irritants. A common cause in the pediatric population is finger sucking.

Acute paronychia is most common although chronic infection can also exist. Those with acute paronychia often have a history of trauma to the fingertip or nail. *Staphylococcus aureus* is the most common causative pathogen. Chronic paronychia is diagnosed when the patient has had 6 weeks or more of symptoms. The majority of cases of chronic paronychia are caused by *Candida albicans* with a bacterial superinfection.

Clinical presentation and diagnosis

Erythema and soft tissue swelling occur on the dorsal finger around the nail. Pus may also be present. A felon (a closed space infection of the fingertip pulp) can develop if a paronychia is left untreated.

Unlike most other hand injuries, radiologic studies have no role to play in the diagnosis of acute paronychia but may be useful in assessing the presence of underlying osteomyelitis in chronic or persistent cases.

Management

Early acute paronychia can be treated conservatively, with warm water soaks three to four times a day, and oral antibiotics. If purulence or a deep abscess is present, incision and drainage is required. Although this can be performed in the clinic setting, debridement in the operating room can allow a more thorough exploration under a controlled setting and should be considered with extensive infection. The patient should be counseled to avoid any manipulation of the nail (including finger sucking; parents may have to resort to mittens for infants and toddlers to protect them) until the infection is completely healed.

Chronic paronychia treatment consists of avoidance of the inciting factors, warm soaks, and topical or oral antifungal agents. Recalcitrant cases may require a surgical debridement with possible nail plate removal and marsupialization of the eponychium.

Table 108.1. Hand injuries, examination and treatment

Injury	Mechanism	Examination	Treatment	Notes
Paronychia: soft tissue infection around fingernail	Trauma, including finger sucking and nail biting	Erythema, soft tissue swelling, purulent drainage	*Acute*: warm soaks, oral antibiotics, I&D if abscess present *Chronic*: warm soaks, antifungals, I&D with nail plate removal and marsupialization	Emergency hand consultation for advanced infections
Scapholunate dissociation: injury to the scapholunate ligament	Repetitive motion in adolescents, trauma	Watson scaphoid test (see text); 3 mm space on radiograph between scaphoid and lunate	Orthopedic consultation; if well aligned then immobilization with long-arm cast for 6 weeks	No athletic activity for at least 3 months
Perilunate and lunate dislocation	Hyperextension injury to the wrist	Minimal tenderness to extreme swelling; radiograph shows "spilled teacup sign"	Emergency orthopedic referral for open reduction and internal fixation	Diagnosis requires a high index of suspicion
Scaphoid fracture	Fall on to an outstretched hand	Pain at the snuffbox or volar scaphoid tuberosity	Short-arm thumb spica casting	Diagnosis requires a high index of suspicion
Collateral ligament injury	Forced ulnar or radial deviation at DIP/PIP joint	Pain, swelling at the affected ligament	Buddy tape finger; orthopedic referral for young children	
Ulnar collateral ligament injury to first MCP joint (gamekeeper's or skier's thumb)	Valgus force on the thumb MCP joint; most common in skiers football, rugby players	Stress testing for joint instability	Thumb spica cast for 6 weeks if non-displaced or partial tear	If complete tear or displaced fracture of the ulnar collateral ligament, displaced fracture then orthopedic consultation
Trigger finger: stenosing tenosynovitis of flexor tendon sheath	Repetitive finger use; increased incidence in gymnasts, musicians	Pain with movement, snapping sensation during extension and flexion	Finger splinting, analgesics, steroid injection, surgery	
Mallet finger: injury to extensor tendon at DIP join	Forced flexion of the DIP joint with active extension; ball hitting an outstretched finger	Pain at dorsal DIP joint; unable to actively extend the joint; intact passive joint extension	Splinting for 8–10 weeks; avulsion fracture involving >25% of joint surface requires orthopedic referral	Crucial to *never* flex the joint during immobilization
Central slip rupture/extensor tendon injury	PIP joint is forcibly flexed during active extension, volar dislocation of the PIP joint; basketball players at risk	Tenderness over the dorsal middle phalanx; unable to actively extend the joint	Splinting for 8–10 weeks; avulsion fracture involving one-third of the joint requires orthopedic referral	Crucial to *never* flex the joint!
Distal phalangeal injury	Crush injury; basketball, volleyball players at risk	Tenderness, swelling in the distal phalanx	Splinting for 4–6 weeks; if nail bed laceration, fix with 6-0 abs suture; cephalosporin antibiotic 7–10 days	
Middle and proximal phalanx fracture	Crush injury	Swelling, tenderness; check for rotational deformity	Splint for 6 weeks	If rotational deformity, requires orthopedic referral within a week
Boxer finger: 5th metacarpal bone fracture	Boxing/punching	Deformity, loss of contour of 5th MCP joint	Reduction then ulnar gutter splint	

DIP, distal interphalangeal; I&D, incise and drain; MCP, metacarpophalangeal; PIP, proximal interphalangeal.

Ligamentous injuries

Scapholunate dissociation

Serious ligamentous injury that causes joint instability is rare in young children. Most cases of scapholunate dissociation occur secondary to trauma; however, scapholunate dissociation can occur secondary to repetitive motion (such as pitching a baseball) or trauma in adolescents.

Clinical presentation and diagnosis

The patient has pain during the Watson scaphoid test. The examiner's thumb is placed on the scaphoid tubercle when it is in the ulnar deviated position. When the patient's hand is then deviated radially and flexed, there is pain from subluxation of the scaphoid over the dorsal rim of the radial scaphoid facet. Release of thumb pressure sometimes produces a clunk as the subluxated scaphoid is reduced.

Radiographs show a scapholunate interval of >3 mm or a cortical ring sign as a result of the end-on projection of the rotated scaphoid and a dorsiflexed lunate.

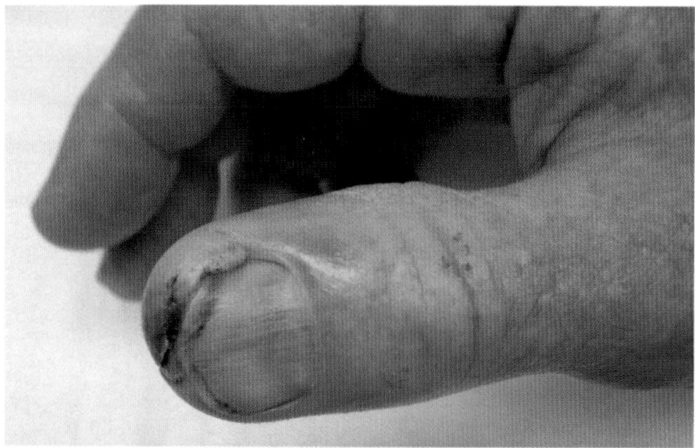

Figure 108.3 Paronychia. (Courtesy of Dr. Andrew Man-Lap Ho.)

Management

Consult a hand surgeon. Immobilization with a long-arm thumb spica cast for 6 weeks can be attempted. If symptoms persist or intercarpal instability occurs, then surgical management will be necessary. No athletic activity is recommended for at least 3 months after surgical repair.

Perilunate and lunate dislocation

Perilunate and lunate dislocations are among the most serious of wrist injuries. They are caused by a hyperextension injury to the wrist. High-energy trauma such as a fall from considerable height or a motor vehicle crash with the wrist struck against the dashboard cause this. Another primary cause is a fall on an outstretched hand (FOOSH), which can occur in sports injuries. Hyperextension causes the scaphoid to strike the dorsal lip of the radius, rupturing the radioscaphoid, scapholunate, and radiocarpal ligaments, and causing the lunate to be volarly displaced while the distal carpal row is dorsally displaced (Fig. 108.4).

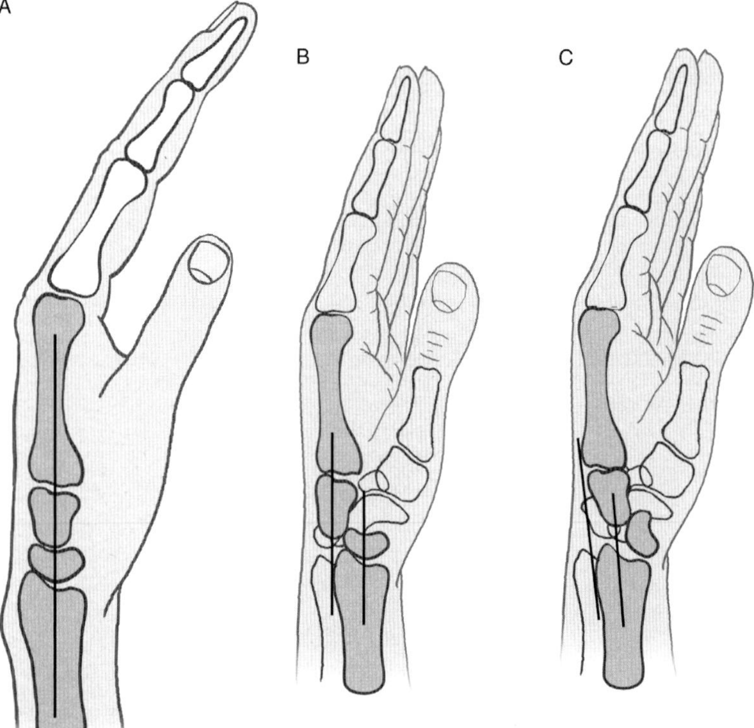

Figure 108.4 Alignment of the radius, capitate, and lunate. (A) With normal alignment, a line drawn through the mid-point of the radius and the capitate on the lateral view of the wrist traverses the mid-point of the lunate. The line will miss or only traverse a fragment of the bone if the lunate is displaced. (B) Lunate dislocation (volar). (C) Perilunate dislocation (dorsal). (Copyright N. Ewen Wang.)

Clinical presentation and diagnosis

There is great variability in clinical presentation, from extreme swelling and tenderness over the carpal bones to minimal tenderness with movement. The EP should have a high degree of suspicion for this injury as it is often missed, leading to chronic morbidity. During the examination, it is also important to test the median nerve as it is frequently injured or compressed due to this injury as well.

Radiographs show the dislocated lunate with the typical "spilled teacup sign."

Management

Closed reduction in the ED should be attempted if operative reduction is delayed. However, repeated attempts at closed reduction in the ED should be avoided as perilunate dislocations are often difficult to reduce, and excessive manipulation risks further trauma to the median nerve. Orthopoedic surgery (open reduction and internal fixation) is often required in order to stabilize the wrist.

Collateral ligament injury

Collateral ligament injury occurs with forced ulnar or radial deviation at the DIP or PIP joint. The PIP joint is most commonly involved.

Clinical presentation and diagnosis

Pain and swelling at the affected ligament is the most common symptom. Examine the joint by flexing the MCP joint at 90 degrees, holding the affected joint at 0 and 30 degrees flexion and then applying a varus or valgus force.

Radiography should be done to rule out a concomitant avulsion fracture.

Management

The finger should be "buddy taped" (wrapped snugly to the neighboring finger) to prevent movement and bending of the joints. While in adults, buddy taping the finger is enough and these injuries will heal without intervention, in children the growth plate is often involved so referral to an orthopedic surgeon is recommended. Patients can continue athletic activities as long as the finger is protected by the splint. Ligament repair or reconstruction may be needed for chronic injuries with persistent symptoms or instability.

Gamekeeper's or skier's thumb

In gamekeeper's or skier's thumb, there is chronic or acute injury to the ulnar collateral ligament of the thumb MCP joint. This injury occurs after a valgus force is directed on the joint. While any fall on an abducted thumb can cause it, this commonly occurs during skiing, when the skier lands on the ground with his thumb braced on a ski pole. It also occurs during football, rugby, or any game with the possibility of direct ball to thumb impact like volleyball or basketball.

Clinical presentation and diagnosis

The patient will have swelling and pain at the ulnar side of the MCP joint. A mass might be present, indicating the retracted portion of the ulnar collateral ligament. Before performing a full physical examination including stress testing for joint instability, it is important to rule out a displaced avulsion fracture (called a gamekeeper's fracture) by radiographs. A non-displaced avulsion fracture, however, is not a contraindication to stress testing. Test for instability with the thumb MCP joint at 0 and 30 degrees, while applying a valgus force. Opening of more than 30 degrees or 15 degrees more than the uninjured side suggests rupture of the ulnar collateral ligament.

Radiographs are crucial as in the pediatric population, there is often a fracture of the proximal phalanx of the thumb (Salter–Harris type III).

Management

For partial tears of the ulnar collateral ligament (no joint instability present), conservative or non-surgical treatment is recommended. This can be done with fractures when the proximal phalanx fracture is displaced by <2 mm as well. The thumb should be immobilized in a thumb-spica cast for 6 weeks. In 90% of cases, this results in complete recovery. The drug of choice for pain and inflammation is a NSAID.

For complete tears of the ulnar collateral ligament or where there is a displaced fracture segment or an interposed adductor pollicis aponeurosis (Stenner lesion), open reduction and fixation is recommended, necessitating a hand specialist. The patient should see a hand surgeon within a week.

A missed injury or improper treatment can result in chronic pain and chronic instability, leading to a weak pincer grasp or significant arthritis.

Tendon injuries

Trigger finger

Congenital trigger thumb is more common in children than classic trigger finger; however, congenital trigger thumb is not an acute emergency and will not be discussed here. Stenosing tenosynovitis of the flexor tendon sheath causes pain and difficulty with extension and flexion. The inflamed tendon nodule catches at the A1 pulley at the volar MCP joint. The finger usually "catches and locks" and is held in the flexed position in severe cases, leading to the name trigger finger. Repetitive finger use may be the cause for this syndrome but its etiology is unclear. It is common in gymnasts or musicians.

Clinical presentation and diagnosis

The primary complaint is pain with movement and a "snapping" sensation during both extension and flexion. A palpable nodule may be felt at the volar aspect of the MCP joint. In the classic case, there is a locking of the finger in flexion as the patient attempts to extend the fingers from the fisted position. This is a clinical diagnosis and radiographs are not necessary.

Management

Finger splinting and analgesics should be tried as first-line agents. There are many splints available for trigger finger, but any splint that limits flexion of the MCP and PIP joints will suffice. This splint can be worn either all the time or at nighttime only depending on how symptomatic the patient is. If there is continued pain and difficulty with movement after 6 weeks of conservative therapy, steroid injection into the tendon sheath can be attempted. Surgery with A1 pulley release may also be necessary in cases that do not respond to therapy.

Rugby or jersey finger

Rugby or jersey finger is injury to the flexor digitorum profundus tendon caused by forced extension of the DIP joint during active flexion. Often during athletics (classically while playing rugby), this occurs when a player's finger is caught on another's jersey (hence the name). In 75%, the ring finger is affected.

Clinical presentation and diagnosis

Pain at the volar portion of the DIP joint along with inability to flex the DIP joint is classic. With tendon retraction, a tender swelling may be felt at any level of the finger, or even at the palm depending on the level of retraction. Radiographs may demonstrate an associated avulsion fracture.

Management

Early diagnosis is key as delayed treatment worsens outcomes. Splint the joint in extension. *All* these injuries require urgent hand surgery consultation as early surgical repair is necessary. Patients should see a hand surgeon within 3 days.

Mallet finger

Mallet finger is injury to the extensor tendon at the DIP joint. It is the most common closed tendon injury in the fingers. It occurs with forced flexion of the DIP joint with active extension. Commonly, this happens when a ball has hit an outstretched finger.

Clinical presentation and diagnosis

The patient will have pain at the dorsal DIP joint. The DIP joint will be held in a flexed position, with an inability to actively extend the joint (Fig. 108.5). Passive joint extension should be intact. If not, there might well be bony or soft tissue entrapment necessitating operative repair. It is important to keep in mind that one-third of patients have bony avulsion fractures. The DIP joint has to be isolated (by holding the MCP and PIP joints of the same finger) to properly evaluate the extensor tendon. Radiography should be done to rule out an associated fracture or avulsion.

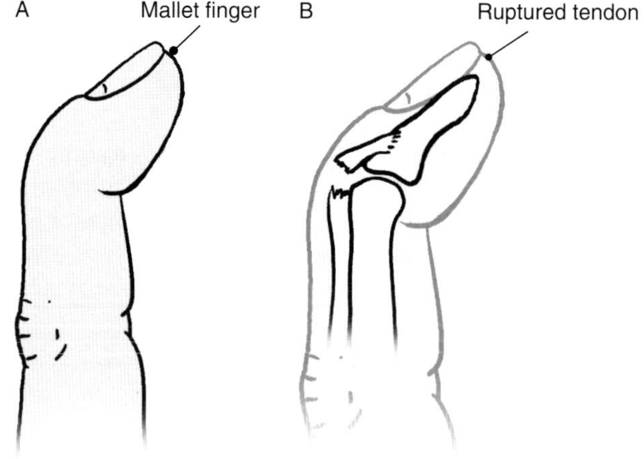

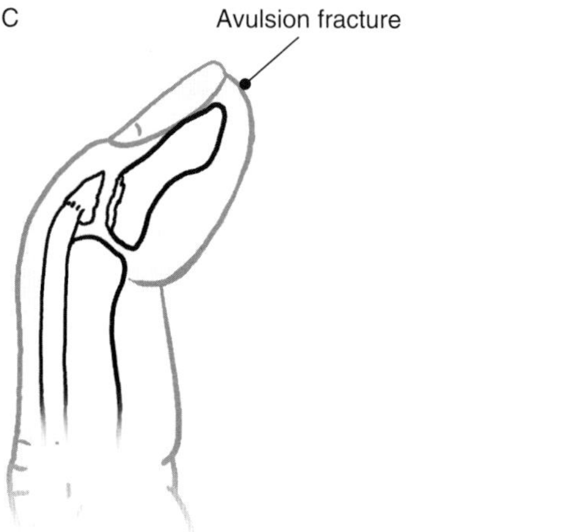

Figure 108.5 Injury to the joint extensor tendon at the distal interphalangeal joint (mallet finger). (A) The patient is unable to straighten the distal phalanx. (B) The tendon can be disrupted. (C) An avulsion fracture can result in mallet finger. (Copyright N. Ewen Wang.)

Management

Soft tissue and bony mallet injury involving <25% of the articular surface require finger splinting in neutral-to-mild hyperextension position for 8–10 weeks. Ensure that all other joints including the PIP joint are free. It is crucial that the patient *never* flexes the joint – if that occurs at any time during treatment, 6 more weeks of splinting is required. For an unreliable patient or one that cannot avoid flexing the joint, casting is recommended.

Bony avulsions involving <25% of the joint space or an incongruent DIP joint require a hand referral after splinting is initiated. Inability to achieve full passive extension (as mentioned above, this suggests bony or soft tissue entrapment) also necessitates referral for definitive treatment. They should see a hand surgeon within a week.

Central slip rupture extensor tendon injury

A central slip rupture extensor tendon injury is commonly seen in basketball players. Two different mechanisms cause a central slip extensor tendon injury: (1) when the PIP joint is forcibly flexed during active extension, and (2) with volar dislocation of the PIP joint.

Clinical presentation and diagnosis

Tenderness over the dorsal middle phalanx will be present. The patient will hold the joint in 15–30 degrees of flexion and should be unable to actively extend the joint. Passive extension should be intact. As with the other tendon injuries, radiography is recommended to evaluate for an associated avulsion fracture.

Management

Immediate splinting is necessary to prevent deformity, specifically called a boutonnière deformity. This is caused by volar migration of the lateral bands of the dorsal extensor tendon (Fig. 108.6). This deformity is usually progressive over time. Splinting is necessary for 6 weeks with the finger in full extension. No flexion is allowed. If flexion occurs, 6 more weeks of splinting is necessary (as in the mallet finger).

Refer to hand surgery for avulsion fractures involving one-third or more of the joint. Patients should see a hand surgeon within a week.

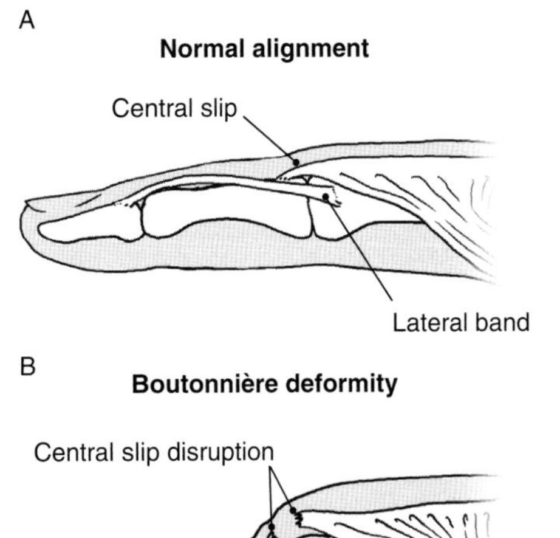

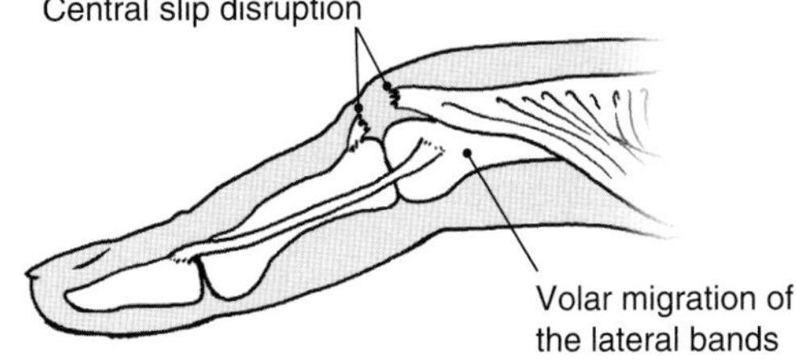

Figure 108.6 Central slip with (A) normal alignment and with (B) disruption (boutonnière deformity). (Copyright N. Ewen Wang.)

Fractures

Scaphoid fracture

Less than <0.5% of pediatric fractures are in the carpal bones. The scaphoid bone is the most commonly fractured carpal bone. These fractures occur almost exclusively in the adolescent population as a result of trauma.

Clinical presentation and diagnosis

Pain in the snuffbox or at the volar scaphoid tuberosity is suggestive of injury. Decreased range of motion of the wrist is also frequently seen. Radiographs may not demonstrate an acute fracture so a high index of suspicion should exist for a scaphoid fracture in anyone with typical symptoms. When in doubt, treat any suspected scaphoid fracture with cast immobilization and perform repeat clinical and radiographic follow-up.

Management

Immobilization with a short-arm thumb spica cast for 8 weeks is indicated for most non-displaced scaphoid fractures. Where no fracture is demonstrated in initial radiographs, presumptive treatment is with cast immobilization and repeat radiographs should be conducted in 2 weeks to re-evaluate. Non-displaced distal pole and tubercle fractures require 8 weeks of immobilization, and fractures through the proximal pole require a long-arm thumb spica cast for 4 weeks and then a short-arm thumb spica cast until bony union is demonstrated. Consult orthopedic surgery for all displaced fractures and chronic non-unions.

Distal phalangeal injury

Distal phalangeal injuries are common in children. In young children, a crush injury (frequently by a car door or window) causes this. In adolescents, this often is seen during sports such as basketball or volleyball and is caused by a direct blow onto the distal phalanx.

Clinical presentation and diagnosis

Tenderness and swelling over the distal phalanx is present. Subungual hematomas may also be present, indicating a nail bed laceration. Radiography should be done to evaluate for fracture.

Management

Pediatric distal phalanx soft tissue injuries heal very well. In the absence of significant soft tissue trauma or loss, a digital block, cleansing of the wound, and a finger extension splint for protection is all that is necessary for crush injuries. Oral antibiotics with a tetanus booster are indicated for open injuries. If a subungual hematoma is present involving >50% of the nail, hematoma evacuation with nail plate removal and nail bed repair may be required; if the nail bed is intact, trephination only may be appropriate. The patient should have wound checks every week or so to assess for infection. For complex wounds with significant soft tissue loss, local or regional flaps may be required for soft tissue coverage.

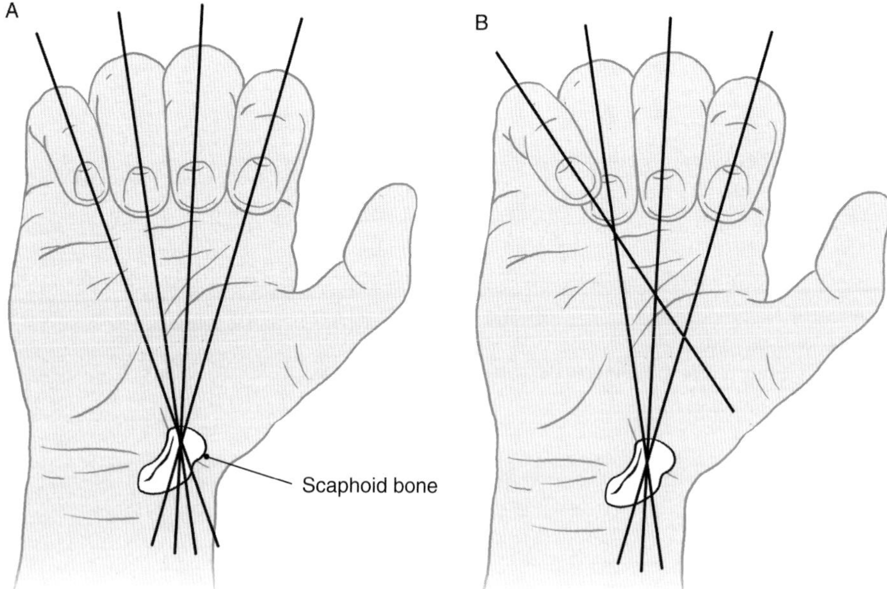

Figure 108.7 Middle phalanx fractures. (A) If no rotation is present, all fingertips will be on the same plane and pointing toward the scaphoid bone. (B) If rotation occurs, the affected finger will misalign. (Copyright N. Ewen Wang.)

For distal phalanx fractures, splinting and immobilization for 4–6 weeks is necessary for healing. Elevation and pain medication are also recommended. The patients should be counseled that tenderness may be present in a comminuted fracture for up to 2–3 months. When there is a nail bed laceration, this is considered an open fracture and a cephalosporin should be prescribed for 7 to 10 days. After thorough cleaning, the nail bed should be irrigated and sutured using a 6-0 absorbable suture material. Historically, the recommendation was to remove the nail in all such cases, but this recommendation is changing. Currently, as long as the remaining nail is intact and the nail fold is not involved, the nail need not be removed.

Middle and proximal phalanx fractures

Middle and proximal phalanx fractures are caused by a large number of mechanisms, including severe crush injuries. In the pediatric population, this often occurs when the child's finger is caught in a door or window.

Clinical presentation and diagnosis

Physical examination will show soft tissue swelling and tenderness at the site. Examination can also detect rotation. Evaluate the hand in the fist position. In the normal hand, all fingernails should be in the same plane, pointing towards the scaphoid bone with no scissoring of the digit rays (Fig. 108.7). Radiography should also be done to evaluate for displacement or rotation.

Management

Fractures with displacement but no rotation can be treated by the EP. It is important to achieve proper alignment through reduction. Once good alignment is achieved, splint with the MCP joint in flexion and the IP joints in extension ("position of safety") for 6 weeks, then re-evaluate. If a volar lip fracture is present (caused by an avulsion of the volar capsule plate), a hand surgeon should manage this potentially disabling fracture. The affected joint must be examined fluoroscopically through its full range of motion to assess for any joint subluxation or instability. The joint will then be immobilized in an extension block splint to prevent it from extending beyond the range of stability. The joint is reassessed weekly with advancement of extension block gradually in the next 6 weeks. Failure to maintain reduction in the splint will necessitate operative fixation.

If malrotation is present, the patient should be referred to an orthopedic surgeon for reduction and surgical fixation. Patients should see an orthopedic surgeon within a week.

Boxer's fracture

Boxer's fracture is a fracture at the neck of the fifth metacarpal bone and is the most common metacarpal bone fracture. The name stems from the fact that this is often caused by a missed punch. It is typically seen in the adolescent or young adult populations.

Clinical presentation and diagnosis

There is usually a significant deformity seen, with "loss" of the fifth knuckle (MCP joint) through volar displacement of the distal fracture fragment (Fig. 108.8). Malrotation is generally more common in metacarpal than phalangeal fractures and it is important to assess for rotation.

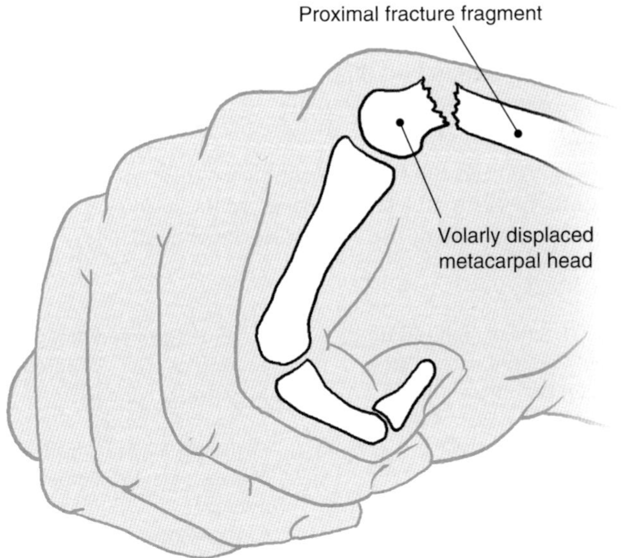

Figure 108.8 Boxer's fracture with volarly displaced metacarpal head. (Copyright N. Ewen Wang.)

Management

In Boxer's fractures with acceptable alignment and no malrotation, overall outcomes have been shown to be equally good for patients who received reduction and those who did not. Therefore, physicians can be reassured that the fracture will heal with no significant clinical deficits unless angulated at more than 50 degrees or malrotated. This being said, an attempt at reduction is recommended. A digital or hematoma block can help with pain control during reduction. Reduction is done by holding the hand with the MCP joint flexed to 90 degrees. Pressure should then be directed dorsally to the metacarpal head and volarly to the proximal fracture segment. The proximal phalanx or PIP joint can also be used to move the metacarpal head into position. The finger should placed in an ulnar gutter splint in 70–90 degrees of MCP flexion and interphalangeal extension for 6 weeks.

Radiography every 2 weeks should be carried out to check alignment and maintenance of reduction. Physiotherapy is very important and should be started after the 6-week splinting period.

Potential complications include post-traumatic arthritis, a stiff MCP joint, and chronic deformity.

Lunatomalacia: avascular necrosis of the lunate

Also known as Kienbock's disease, lunatomalacia is a rare condition in adults but is seen primarily in children. In children <10 years of age, this condition occurs spontaneously. However, in adolescents, it is seen with chronic overexertion. It is very common in gymnasts, for example, and other athletes.

Clinical presentation and diagnosis

Patients will have wrist pain, and a radiograph is often unrevealing. An MRI scan shows distinct edema of the lunate bone and often definite necrosis with collapsing of the bone structures.

Management

Athletic activities should be stopped immediately. Ibuprofen can be used for pain and the wrist should be immobilized. This measure should improve the pain within a matter of months. Referral to a hand surgeon should be done for longitudinal care and follow-up, and for consideration for surgical intervention such as revascularization with bone grafting or joint-leveling procedures.

Other serious pediatric hand injuries

There are a number of serious injuries of the hand and wrist that are, in general, managed similarly in children and adults. While they are uncommon, each hand injury should be carefully evaluated to rule out these potentially limb-threatening diagnoses.

Compartment syndrome

A high index of suspicion should occur for compartment syndrome. While rare, the consequences can be devastating

Pearls and pitfalls

Pearls

1. When examining the hand, always start with the uninjured extremity to see what the range of motion and tone are at baseline.
2. Elicit help from the parents to perform different hand maneuvers, or use an initial play period with age-appropriate toys to facilitate the physical examination.
3. Immobilize patients with possible scaphoid fracture in a thumb spica, even if no radiographic changes initially.

Pitfalls

1. Failure to correlate a child's developmental age with their functional abilities. For example, children under the age of 9 months have not yet developed the pincer grasp so a lack of coordinated thumb opposition is normal.
2. Failure to recognize that any amount of rotational malalignment in metacarpal or phalanx fractures can cause permanent disability.
3. Failure to recognize fractures involving the physis and non-ossified epiphyses as they are radiographically invisible until healing begins.

in the pediatric population. Check compartment pressures when necessary. This is a surgical emergency so have a low threshold for consulting hand surgery to further evaluate.

Flexor tenosynovitis

Flexor tenosynovitis is also a surgical emergency. Have a high index of suspicion and remember Kanavel's four cardinal signs:

- intense pain along tendon with extension
- pain with range of motion
- uniform (fusiform) swelling of entire finger
- tenderness to percussion along course of flexor tendon sheath.

An infection of the flexor sheath can rapidly spread to the palm and forearm if left untreated, so treat this as a true emergency and consult the hand surgeon immediately.

Selected references

Anderson BC. *Office Orthopedics for Primary Care: Diagnosis and Treatment*, 2nd edn. Philadelphia, PA: Saunders, 1999.

Cornwall R. The painful wrist in the pediatric athlete. *J Pediatr Orthoped* 2010; **30**:S13–S16.

Daniels II JM, Zook EG, Lynch JM. Hand and wrist injuries: Part I. Nonemergency evaluation. *Am Fam Physician* 2004;**69**: 1941–1948.

Leggit JC, Meko CJ. Acute finger injuries: part I. tendons and ligaments. *Am Family Physician* 2006; **73**:810–816.

Leggit JC, Meko, CJ. Acute finger injuries: part II. fractures, dislocations and thumb injuries. 2006;**73**:827–834.

Ong YS, Levin LS. Hand infections. *Plast Reconstr Surg* 2009;**124**:225e–233e.

Rettig AC. Athletic injuries of the wrist and hand. Part I: traumatic injuries of the wrist. *Am J Sports Med* 2003;**31**:1038–1048.

Rigopoulos D, Larios G, Gregoriou S, Alevizos A. Acute and chronic paronychia. *Am Fam Physician* 2008;**77**:339–346.

Staheli, LT. *Pediatric Orthopaedic Secrets.* Philadelphia, PA: Hanley & Belfus, 1998.

Waters, PM. The upper limb. In Morrissy, RT, Weinstein, SL (eds.) *Lovell and Winter's Pediatric Orthopaedics*, 6th edn. Philadelphia, PA: Lippincott Williams & Wilkins, 2006, p. 942–977.

Weiner DS, Jones K. *Pediatric Orthopedics for Primary Care Physicians*, 6th edn. Cambridge, UK: Cambridge University Press, 2006.

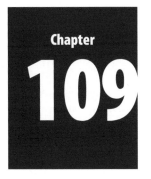

Chapter 109 Musculoskeletal trauma: fractures

Ram S. Duriseti

Introduction

Fractures seen in children differ from those in adults, in part because of anatomic differences between children and adults. This chapter will first discuss the description of pediatric fractures. It will then address the special types of fracture children experience, in particular Salter–Harris fractures of the growth plate. Lastly, it will cover specific pediatric fractures. This is not an all-inclusive account but rather will cover common pediatric fractures or fractures where the management may differ from adults. It is presumed all children will get adequate pain management. Fracture reduction will not be discussed here.

Pediatric bone

Because it is growing, pediatric bone is distinct from adult bone (Fig. 109.1). Bone components include:

- physis: growth plate
- epiphysis: secondary ossification site located at the ends of long bones
- apophysis: secondary ossification site at tendon insertions
- diaphysis: shaft of long bones
- metaphysis: bone adjacent to the physis.

Fracture description

Fracture description is similar to that of adults, with the exception that the child has an active growth plate or physis (Box 109.1, Figs. 109.1–109.3).

Children have strong, compliant ligaments and a thicker periosteum than adults. Also since children's bones have a growth plate, their bones are potentially weaker at the points of growth (active growth plate or physis). These qualities characterize the types of injury seen in children. Children tend not to dislocate or sprain a bone or joint. Rather, fractures are seen since the growth plate, as opposed to the ligament, is the weakest component of a musculotendenous/ligamentous unit. When bones do break, the tough periosteum can make fractures difficult to reduce. Pediatric bones remodel well and often tolerate more post-reduction deformity with good outcome

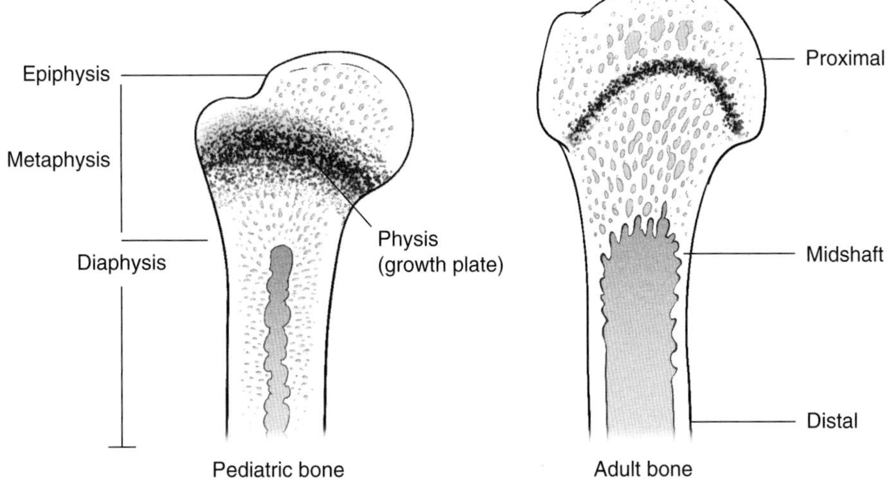

Figure 109.1 Anatomy of pediatric bone. Note the width of the physis: the cartilaginous growth plate. (Copyright Chris Gralapp.)

Box 109.1. The three main descriptive parameters for a fracture

Every fracture should be described using at least one element from each of the three features: type, displacement, and location.

Location (Fig. 109.1)

The position along the bone (Fig. 109.1):

- distal
- midshaft
- proximal.

Fracture type

Children's bones break in a distinctive way that reflects the fact that they are still growing (Fig. 109.2):

- oblique
- spiral
- comminuted
- open/compound
- greenstick
- transverse
- simple.

Fracture displacement

Displacement is described by three facets:

- *translation*: "sideways" motion of the fracture usually, described as a percentage of the diameter of the bone
- *angulation*: described by degrees relative to the apex position (Fig. 109.3)
- *shortening*: described in centimeters, includes description of "bayonet" apposition.

Example description

An open fracture of the distal tibia with 45 degree angulation of the distal relative to the proximal fragment and 5 cm of shortening.

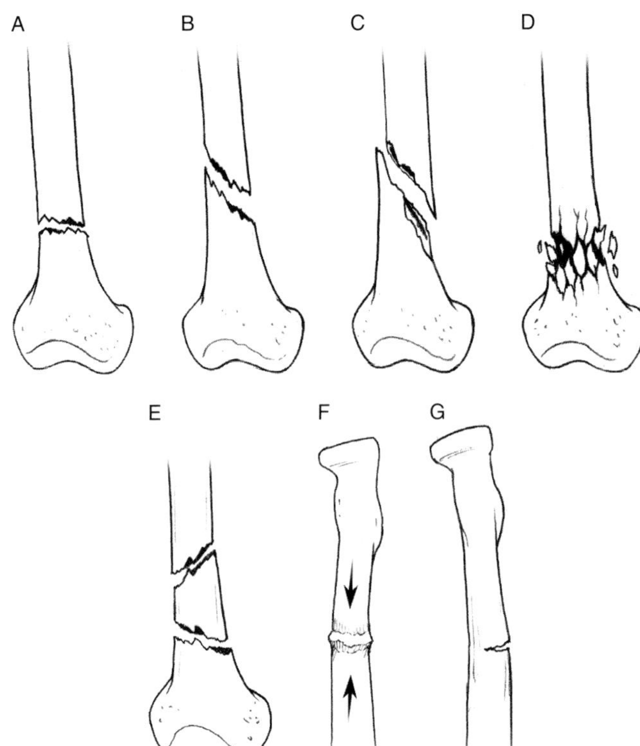

Figure 109.2 Types of pediatric fractures: (A) transverse, (B) oblique, (C) spiral, (D) comminuted, (E) segmental, (F) torus, (G) greenstick. (Copyright Chris Gralapp; reproduced with permission from Mahadevan SV, Garmel GM. *An Introduction to Clinical Emergency Medicine.* Cambridge, UK: Cambridge University Press, 2005.)

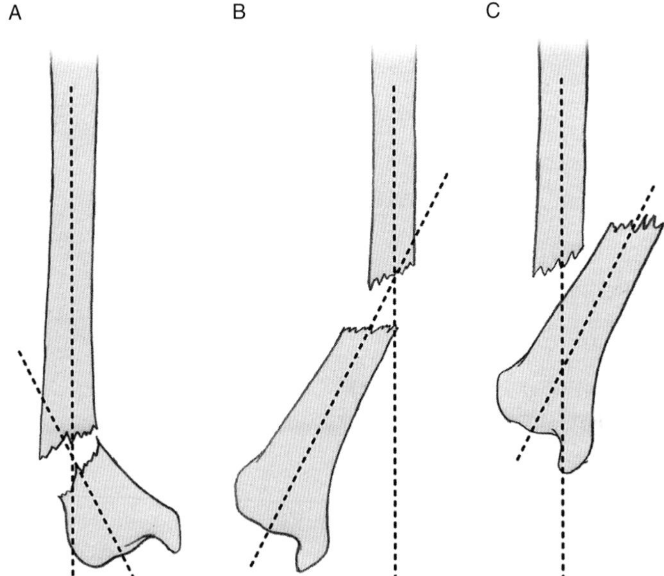

Figure 109.3 Angulation and displacement. (A) fracture with 30 degrees of lateral angulation. (B) Fracture with 30 degrees of medial angulation. (C) Fracture with 30 degrees of medial angulation, 100% displacement, and shortening of undetermined length. (Copyright Chris Gralapp; reproduced with permission from Mahadevan SV, Garmel GM. *An Introduction to Clinical Emergency Medicine.* Cambridge, UK: Cambridge University Press, 2005.)

than adults. Common fractures in children are outlined in Table 109.1. Figure 109.4 illustrates torus/buckling.

For the pediatric EP, it is important to always consider a growth plate injury when examining a child with an orthopedic injury. Pediatric physis injuries or fractures may present without a sprain of the adjacent joint because of a child's strong and compliant ligaments, and growth plate fractures are particularly worrisome because they can cause premature closure of the growth plate and focal bone growth arrest if unnoticed.

Salter–Harris classification

The Salter–Harris classification of growth plate periarticular pediatric fractures in the setting of an immature physis is the standard commonly used by practitioners (Fig. 109.5). In the Salter–Harris schema, the relative positions of *above* and *below* are referenced relative to the physis, with the joint aligned in the field of view such that the diaphysis is above the epiphysis. The treatment and outcome of Salter–Harris fractures are seen in Table 109.2.

Type I fractures involve the physis alone and can be displaced (diaphysis displaced relative to the metaphysis) or non-displaced. Type II fractures involve the area above the growth plate. Type III fractures involve only the metaphysis while type IV fractures involve the metaphyseal and diaphyseal bones.

As a general rule, the risk of epiphyhseal damage increases with the Salter–Harris type, and, therefore, increases the risk for growth disruption.

It is important to remember that a Salter–Harris I fracture can be displaced or non-displaced.

The most commonly involved bones in pediatric fractures are the clavicle, humerus (including the supracondylar region), the distal tibia/fibula, and the radius/ulna. Common pediatric

Table 109.1. Fractures commonly seen in children

Fracture type	Location, description
Torus/buckling (Fig. 109.4)	Distal radius fracture caused by compression of one side of the cortex
Greenstick	Through periosteum; one side of the bone breaks while the other side bends but stays intact
Bending/plastic/ bowing	Bone bends but remains intact
Growth plate	Through growth plate; categorized by Salter–Harris classification

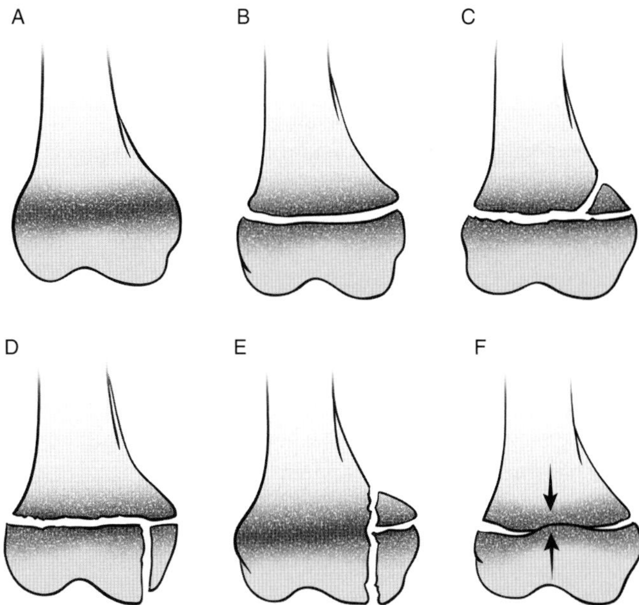

Figure 109.5 Salter–Harris classification. (A) normal. (B) Type I, the fracture is through the physis or epiphyseal plate. (C) Type II, fracture of the metaphysis and through the physis. (D) Type III, fracture of the physis extends to the epiphysis. (E) Type IV, the fracture is through the metaphysis, physis, and epiphysis. (F) Type V, fracture has crushed the physis. A mnemonic to remember the Salter–Harris classification is to describe the fracture in relation to the epiphyseal plate **SALTR**. Type I, **s**ame level; type II, **a**bove; type III, **l**ower; type IV, **t**hrough; type V, c**r**ush. (Copyright Chris Gralapp.)

A

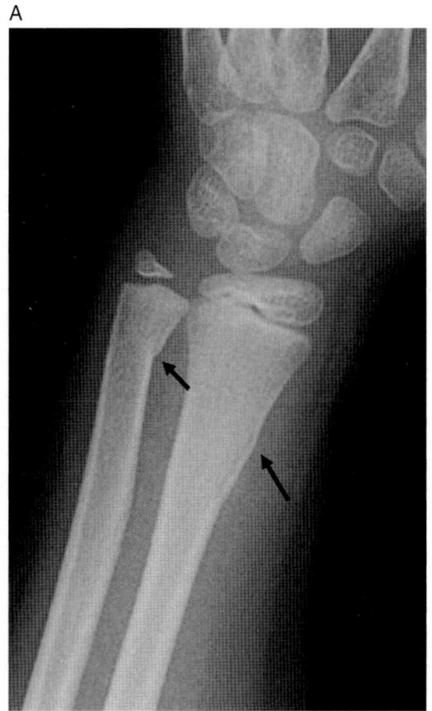

B

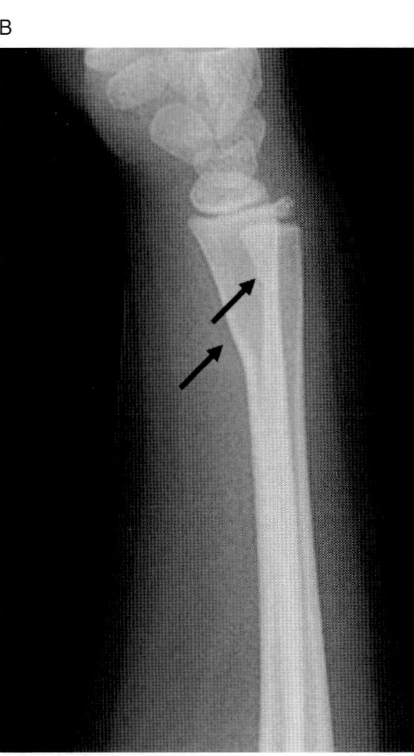

Figure 109.4 Radiographic representation of greenstick and buckle fracture (arrowed): (A) A-P view; (B) lateral view.

fractures of the upper and lower extremity are discussed focusing on fracture patterns that differ from adults as well as when management might differ.

In general, a splint is recommended for children with normal radiographs and injury because of the high frequency of clinically significant fracture upgrades that occur with more advanced imaging.

Clavicle fractures

The clavicle is one of the most frequently fractured bones in pediatric patients. In newborns, clavicle fractures usually occur by compression of the clavicle during birth. These fractures are usually greenstick fractures and can go unnoticed until a large callus has formed. In older children and adolescents, the usual mechanism of a clavicle fracture is from falling onto an outstretched hand, or from a direct blow to the clavicle.

Table 109.2. Treatment and outcome by Salter–Harris class

Type	Treatment	Prognosis
I	Splint immobilization; icing and elevation	Good
II	Splint immobilization if no angulation or displacement of fracture fragment	Good
III	Consult orthopedics; requires alignment of fracture	Generally good, depending on displacement of fracture fragment and impact on blood supply
IV	Consult orthopedics; requires alignment of fracture	Risk of growth disturbance depending on impact on blood supply
V	Consult orthopedics	Great risk of growth disturbance

Clinical presentation

These mechanisms usually result in pain, swelling, tenderness along the clavicle, and lowering of the affected shoulder. It is important to palpate the clavicle in every injured child since sometimes they cannot give a history of trauma.

Management

Clavicle fractures have a good prognosis. Newborns with clavicle fractures are treated supportively with handling precautions given to the parents. Infants with pain may have their arm splinted for 1–2 weeks. Children and adolescents with clavicle fractures are usually treated with a sling for 1–4 weeks. Surgical repair of pediatric clavicle fractures is exceedingly rare and only performed if the overlying skin is significantly deformed (tented or pierced), or if a concomitant posterior clavicle dislocation has occurred with mediastinal injury.

Elbow dislocation: radial head subluxation

Radial head subluxation, also known as nursemaid's elbow, is the most common pediatric dislocation. It is thought that the radial head becomes trapped distal to the annular ligament secondary to a traction force along the axis of the radius. This can occur via active traction or via the classic history of the child falling to the ground while a caregiver is holding the hand. The child usually presents with decreased motion of the affected arm and no apparent pain. No deformity is present on examination.

Clinical presentation

No radiographic investigation is necessary if the mechanism of injury is consistent with the injury. Atypical history, swelling, pain without manipulation, failed reduction, or ongoing immobility should trigger radiographs to assess for radial head or supracondylar fracture.

Management

There are two main reduction techniques: supination/flexion (classic) and hyperpronation (Fig. 109.6). Supination of the

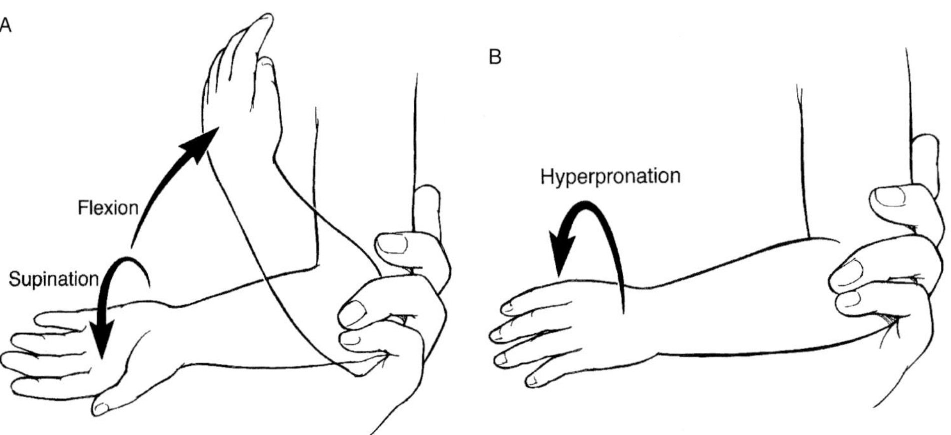

Figure 109.6 Reduction of radial head subluxation. (A) Supination and flexion approach. (B) Hyperpronation technique. (Reproduced with permission from Macias CG, Bothner J, Wiebe R. A comparison of supination/flexion to hyperpronation in the reduction of radial head subluxations. *Pediatrics* 1998;102:e10. © American Academy of Pediatrics.)

hand with flexion at the elbow has a reported 80–92% success rate. Hyperpronation has recently been shown to be superior. In both techniques, one hand is placed at the radial head, providing slight direct pressure. The EP's dominant hand holds firm traction on the forearm and performs the reduction maneuver. Often, but not always the EP and patient will feel the radial head reduce. Classically, it takes young children approximately 20 min to forget about the injury. The practitioner does well to leave the room and return to have the child use the affected arm to give a high five or reach for a popsicle. In 25% of patients with a history of radial head subluxation, there is a recurrence. Children with a first episode prior to 24 months of age are at higher risk for recurrence.

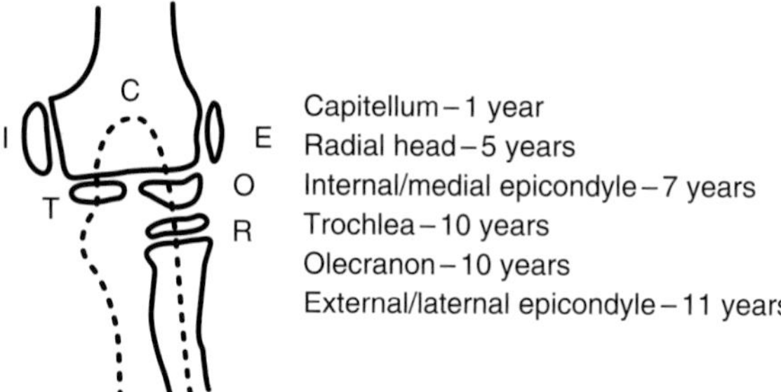

Figure 109.7 The six growth plates of the pediatric elbow and their average ages of appearance. CRITOE is the mnemonic to remember their order of appearance. The ages of appearance can also be effectively approximated by the numerical series 1,3,5,7,9,11. (Courtesy R. Dureseti.)

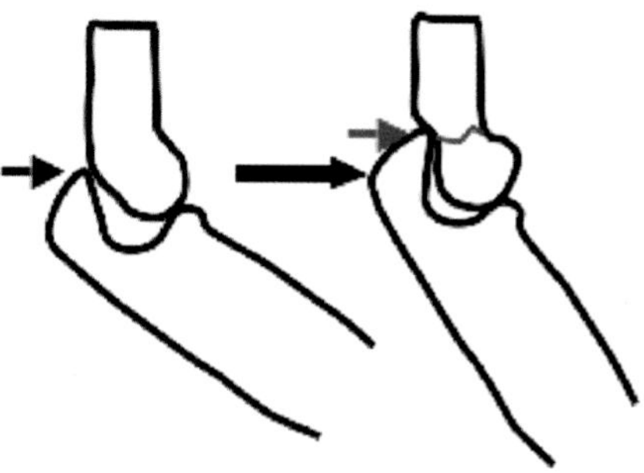

Figure 109.8 Mechanism of supracondylar fractures: With extreme extension and compression forces, the posterior supracondylar ridge fractures first. With even greater extension, the fracture displaces and the anterior supracondylar ridge fractures as well. (Courtesy R. Dureseti.)

Elbow fractures

The morbidity of elbow fractures is complicated by the challenging radiographic anatomy of the pediatric elbow. There are six major growth plates around the pediatric elbow. Each growth plate appears, on average, at a different age, and the mnemonic CRITOE (capitellum [C], radial head [R], internal [medial] epicondyle [I], trochlea [T], olecranon [O], and external [lateral] epicondyle (E]) is an effective way to remember the growth plates and their rough age of appearance (Fig. 109.7). In females, the growth plates appear 1–2 years earlier than they do in males.

Supracondylar fractures

Supracondylar fractures are more common in boys (3:1) and are most common in the 3–10-year-old age group with a mean age of incidence of roughly 7 years. Ninety-eight percent of supracondylar fractures are extension type injuries with a **f**all **o**n **o**ut-**s**tretched **h**and (FOOSH). The remaining few occur with the elbow in flexion (Fig. 109.8).

The most concerning element of supracondylar fractures is the propensity for significant functional morbidity. For supracondylar fractures that require operative repair, roughly 10% of patients will not have a satisfactory cosmetic or functional outcome. Neurovascular complications are the most dreaded outcomes with pediatric supracondylar fractures. Volkmann's contracture is a particularly morbid complication that is caused by a compartment syndrome secondary to limb ischemia from brachial artery injury. It occurs in only 0.5% of cases. Because of the significant morbidity associated with even properly treated supracondylar fractures, fewer general orthopedists are comfortable dealing with pediatric and even adult supracondylar fractures.

The Gartland classification for supracondylar fractures caused by extension injuries (98% of supracondylar fractures) is straightforward. Generally speaking, higher Gartland grades correlate with a more severe injury mechanism. Type I fractures are non-displaced supracondylar fractures. Type II fractures maintain an intact posterior humeral cortex while also maintaining contact between fragments (accounts for roughly 50% of displaced supracondylar fractures). Type III fractures are characterized by complete displacement of the fragments with no residual contact between the fragments. Both the anterior and posterior humeral cortex are involved. (Type III fractures represent the other 50% of displaced supracondylar fractures.). Intercondylar and transcondylar fractures are rare in children (they are more common in osteopenic elderly patients).

Diagnosis

Non-displaced supracondylar fractures can be a challenge to diagnose. Radiography of the uninjured limb has been recommended as a comparison. There are several radiographic clues that can facilitate diagnosis. The first and foremost is the presence of a non-physiologic "fat pad." When a joint effusion develops, the fat pads around the elbow joint are pushed outward. On a lateral view of the elbow, the anterior fat pad can be visible normally. When it is pushed out, it forms a characteristic "sail sign" because one can appreciate a triangular lucency anterior to the distal humerus just proximal to the capitellum. Normally, the posterior fat pad is not apparent. When an elbow joint effusion develops, the posterior fat pad becomes visible (Fig. 109.9). Additionally, the alignment

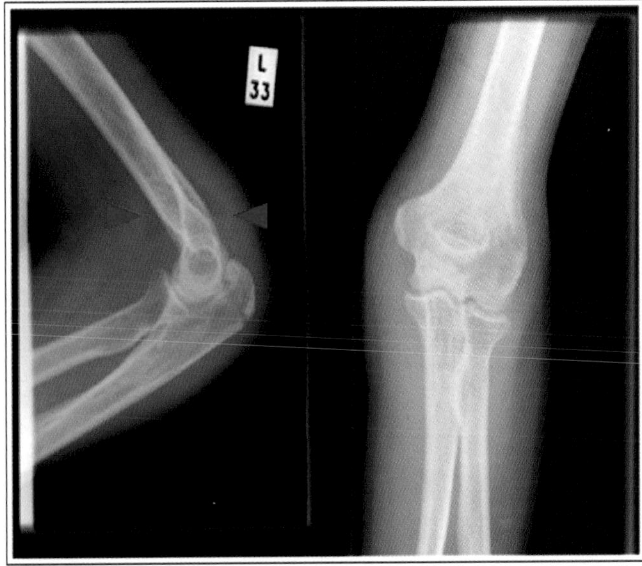

Figure 109.9 Anterior and posterior fat pads: notice the characteristic "sail" shape of the anterior fat pad in the presence of a joint effusion (arrowed). "Posterior fat pads are always pathologic." (Courtesy R. Duriseti.)

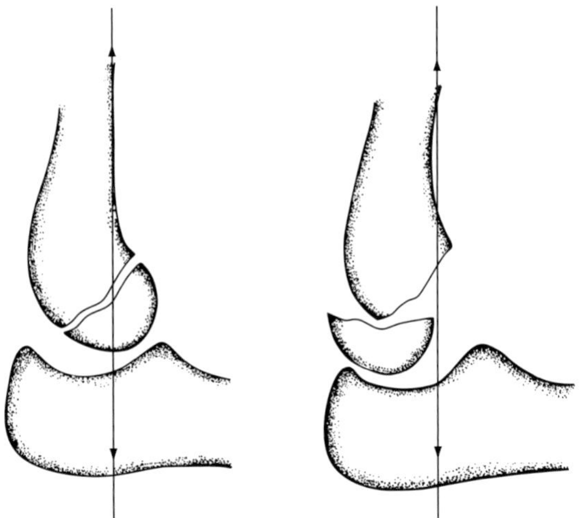

Figure 109.10 The anterior humeral line should intersect the posterior two-thirds of the capitellum. (Copyright N. Ewen Wang.)

between bones on a normal elbow is often disrupted in the setting of a fracture. The anterior humeral line is shown in Fig. 109.10.

Management

In the absence of neurovascular compromise or a fracture that is not oblique along the supracondylar ridge, an emergency orthopedic consultation in the ED is not required. However, these patients are often admitted for follow-up at a suitable time. Splinting is ideally performed with a posterior arm splint with the elbow flexed at 90 degrees and the hand in neutral position. Orthopedic follow-up within 24 h is appropriate in the absence of neurovascular injury or oblique fracture.

Table 109.3. Comparison of supracondylar and lateral condyle fractures

	Supracondylar fracture	Lateral condyle fracture
Age (years)	3–10	3–10
Mechanism	FOOSH	FOOSH
Frequency (%)	70	15
Diagnosis	Displacement obvious, usually initial injury is worst with no further displacement	Subtle, may displace late
Non-union, malunion	Rare and cosmetic	Common and functional injury
Neurovascular injury	10%	Rare
Non-surgical treatment	Anterior humeral line crosses capitellum	<2 mm displacement
Surgery	Can be done within week	Within 2–3 days

FOOSH, fall on out-stretched hand.

Lateral condyle fractures

Lateral condyle fractures are second to supracondylar fractures as the most common operative elbow fracture in children. They can be difficult to diagnose radiographically and are often misdiagnosed, leading to malunion.

The lateral condyle fracture results from a fall on outstretched hand in children 3–10 years old, similar to supracondylar fractures (Table 109.3). If the patient has <2 mm displacement, is neurovascularly intact, prompt orthopedic evaluation can be arranged. Otherwise, surgery is recommended within the first 48 h.

Forearm fractures

Along with clavicular fractures, forearm fractures are the most common pediatric fractures. Both types of fracture have fairly large degrees of post-reduction and preimmobilization deformity and, as a general rule, there is a high tolerance for initial or post-reduction deformity. The greater the period of time until growth plate maturation, the greater the allowable deformity without impacting cosmetic or functional outcome. For children <9 years, 15 degrees of angulation and up to 45 degrees of malrotation are acceptable. For children >9 years, 10 degrees of angulation and up to 30 degrees of malrotation are acceptable. With respect to bayoneting, complete bayonet apposition is acceptable as long as angulation does not exceed 20 degrees and at least 2 years of growth remain. Distal radial fractures are reduced in children in a manner similar to adults. Given the tough periosteum, they may sometimes be more difficult to reduce. "Both bone" forearm fractures are notoriously difficult to reduce.

The three main distal radius fracture types are similar to adults: Colles, Smith, and Barton's fractures. Colles fractures

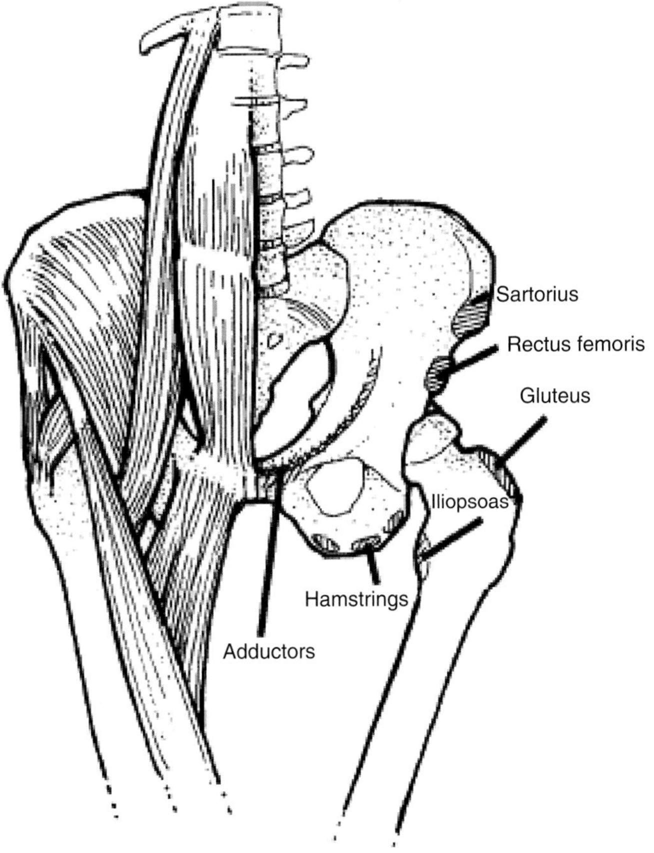

Figure 109.11 Locations of sites of major muscle origins and insertions of the pelvis and proximal femur. Avulsion injuries can occur at each of these sites. (Copyright N. Ewen Wang.)

result from a fall on an outstretched hand resulting in extension of the wrist with compression. Smith fractures are caused by flexion with compression and are, therefore, often referred to as reverse Colles fractures. Barton's fractures have significant radiocarpal dislocation associated with a fracture of the volar rim of the distal radius. These rarely do well without surgical fixation.

Avulsion fractures

Pelvic avulsion fractures can occur in active adolescents secondary to immaturity of the growth plates. They can occur at almost every site of muscle attachment in the pelvis.

The pelvic avulsion fracture is usually a consequence of a violent or sudden muscle contraction (Fig. 109.11). On examination, the patient will maintain a position that results in minimal stretching of the muscle. Point tenderness and swelling are evident on examination. These injuries can be suspected on history and usually diagnosed on radiography with comparison views of the uninjured side. Management depends on the site of injury, as well the degree and length of symptoms. Avulsion fractures will usually heal with rest, although sometimes surgical fixation is necessary. Patients should be made non-weight bearing and referred to an orthopedist for follow-up.

Toddler's and CAST fractures

Toddler's fractures are a subset of childhood accidental spiral tibial (CAST) fractures involving the distal half of the tibia. Toddler's and CAST fractures usually result from a low-energymechanism that twists the ankle or tibia in relation to the foot. Often presentation can be subtle with no history of trauma and refusal of the child to bear weight or walk. Radiological findings may initially be negative or may be subtle (see Ch. 106).

Box 109.2. Ottawa ankle and foot rules for pediatrics

Ankle films

- Pain in the ankle with inability to bear weight (four steps).
- Tenderness over the lateral or medial malleolus or the posterior tibia.

Foot films

- Pain in the mid-foot with inability to bear weight (four steps).
- Tenderness over the navicular bone.
- Tenderness at the base of the 5th metatarsal.

Ankle injuries

Next to forearm injuries, the ankles and feet are the most commonly injured musculoskeletal region. The Ottawa Ankle and Foot Rules are well validated and are accurate in children as well as in adults (Box 109.2, Fig. 109.12).

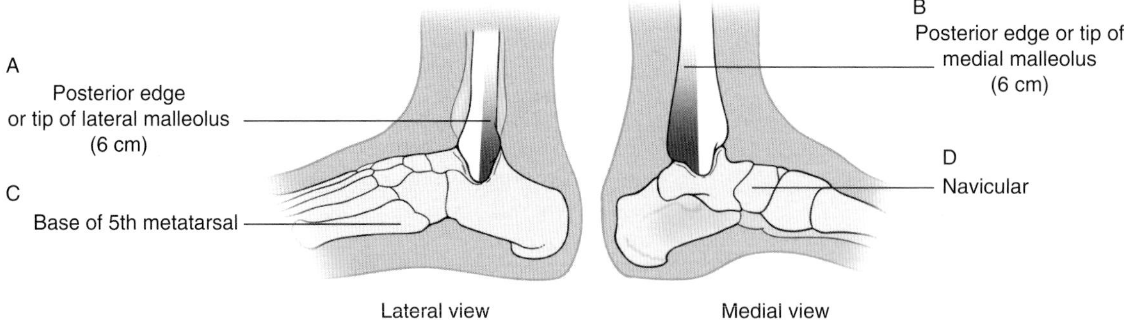

Figure 109.12 The Ottawa ankle rules. A radiograph to rule out fracture should be obtained if there is bony tenderness at posterior edge of distal 6 cm of lateral malleolus (A), posterior edge of distal 6 cm of medial malleolus (B), base of fifth metatarsal (C), or the navicular bone (D); or inability to bear weight immediately and in the ED. (Copyright Chris Gralapp.)

Pearls and pitfalls

Pearls

1. Always consider a growth plate injury when examining a child with an orthopedic injury.
2. A child with a suspected fracture should have it splinted even if initial studies are normal because of the high rate of occult fractures.
3. The mnemonic CRITOE (capitellum [C], radial head [R], internal [medial] epicondyle [I], trochlea [T], olecranon [O], and external [lateral] epicondyle (E]) can be used to remember the six pediatric elbow growth centers.

Pitfalls

1. Failure to systematically evaluate every joint of an affected extremity.
2. Failure to arrange close follow-up and give extensive return precautions to patients and caregivers.
3. Failure to distinguish between a nursemaid's elbow and an elbow fracture prior to attempting reduction.

Selected reference

Perron AD, Miller MD, Brady WJ. Orthopedic Pitfalls in the ED: pediatric growth plate injuries. *Am J Emerg Med* 2002;**20**:50–54.

Chapter

110 Tutorial: Splints

Betsy Encarnacion and Gregory H. Gilbert

Introduction

Typically, alignment of bone fragments is more important in children than it is in adults because of active growth and development of the bone. Immobilization via splints or casts is typically recommended for fracture or sprain injuries. If significant swelling or dressing changes are anticipated, splints tend to be the preferred modality of immobilization. Splinting is also associated with increased return of function to the child's daily activities, with less difficulty than casts. Of note, pediatric torus fractures of the wrist, radius, or ulna are not likely to refracture and can be safely managed with splinting in the ED and primary care follow-up. The basic technique for all splint application is similar (Fig. 110.1).

1. Position patient in the appropriate position.
2. Apply stockinette over the forearm and wrap a Webril roll over the stockinette.
3. Obtain the appropriate splint length and width.
4. Moisten the splint material with tepid water wring out excess water, and apply.
5. Roll an Ace bandage over the splint, molding it into shape.

Box 110.1 outlines the various types of splint used in children and specific lengths and widths of casting material used for each and Figs. 110.2 to 110.7 illustrates some of these.

All patients with splints should be assessed for capillary refill, pain and dysthesias.

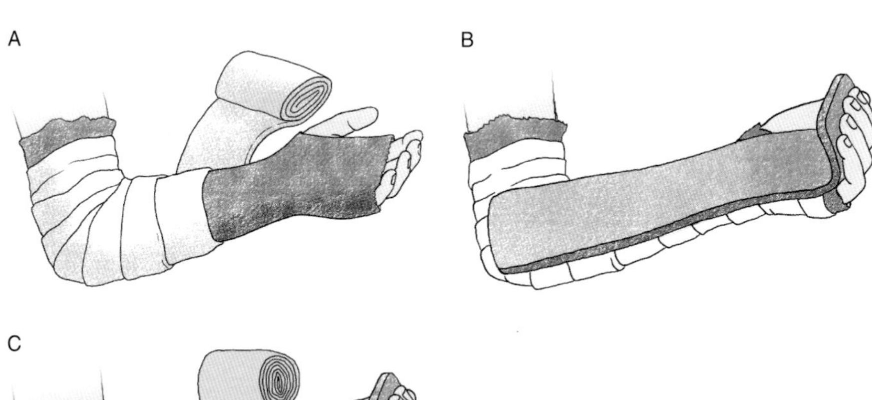

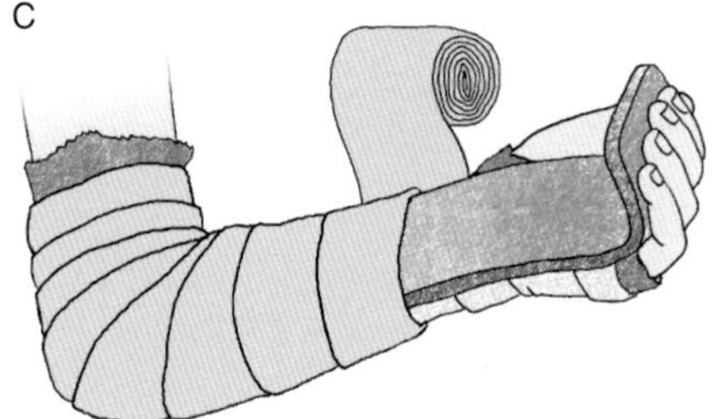

Figure 110.1 Process of placing a splint. (A) Webril roll is applied after stockinette. (B) The splinting material is positioned. (C) An ace bandage is rolled over splinting material and molded. A This Colles splint provides volar forearm support. The wrist is in neutral position and the digits are slightly flexed. (Copyright N. Ewen Wang.)

A Practical Guide to Pediatric Emergency Medicine: Caring for Children in the Emergency Department, ed. N. Ewen Amieva-Wang (associate eds. Jamie Shandro, Aparajita Sohoni, and Bernhard Fassl). Published by Cambridge University Press.

Box 110.1. Outline of splinting procedures

Colles splint (Fig. 110.1C)

Use

Distal forearm and wrist fractures; only provides volar support; used in older children instead of sugar tong splint.

Procedure specifics

1. Position the patient with arm placed as an "L."
2. Length should be from the proximal aspect of the fingers to the proximal forearm.
3. Width should fully cover the volar aspect of the forearm.
4. Place a piece of padding between fingers within the splint.

Gutter splint: radial or ulnar (Fig. 110.2)

Use

Metacarpal and or proximal phalangeal fractures.

Procedure specifics

1. Position the patient with forearm in vertical position.
2. Length should be from the base of the nail to the proximal forearm.
3. Width should be from the midline of the hand from the dorsal to the ulnar side.
4. If applying a radial gutter splint, cut a hole for the thumb to pass through.

Thumb spica (Fig. 110.3)

Use

First metacarpal, proximal phalangeal, or scaphoid fractures.

Procedure specifics

1. Position patient with forearm in vertical position.
2. Length should be from the base of the nail to the proximal forearm.
3. Width should be from the midline of the hand from the dorsal to the ulnar side.

Distal sugar tong (Fig. 110.4)

Use

Forearm and wrist fractures.

Procedure specifics

1. Position patient with arm placed as an "L."
2. Length should be from the dorsal aspect of the metacarpal–phalangeal joints, around the elbow, to the volar palmar flexion crease.
3. Width should overlap the radial and ulnar edges of arm.

Long arm (Fig. 110.5)

Use

Injuries at or near elbow without compromise of neurovascular or joint structures.

Procedure specifics

1. Position the patient prone with arm placed as an inverted "L."
2. Length should be from the mid-upper arm on the dorsal side, down the ulnar side to distal palmar flexion crease.
3. Width should cover half the arm circumference.

Long leg or knee immobilizer

Use

Knee immobilization, distal femur fractures, or fractures of proximal tibia or fibula.

Procedure specifics

1. Position the patient prone.
2. Length should be from the below the buttock to the heel of the foot.
3. If for knee immobilization only, length should be from mid-thigh to 7.5 cm (3 inches) above the malleolus.
4. Width should cover half the leg circumference.

Posterior short leg (Fig. 110.6)

Use

Fractures of distal tibia, fibula, ankle, and foot.

Procedure specifics

1. Position the patient prone, knee flexed 90 degrees.
2. Length should be from the fibular neck to base of toes; consider extending splint to cover toes in small children.
3. Width should cover half the leg circumference.
4. Ensure the patient flexes the foot 90 degrees.

Sugar tong short leg/stirrup (Fig. 110.7)

Use

Adds lateral support to posterior short leg splint.

Procedure specifics

1. Length should be from the fibular neck laterally, around the heel, to base of the knee medially.
2. Width should cover half the leg circumference.
3. Ensure the patient flexes the foot 90 degrees.

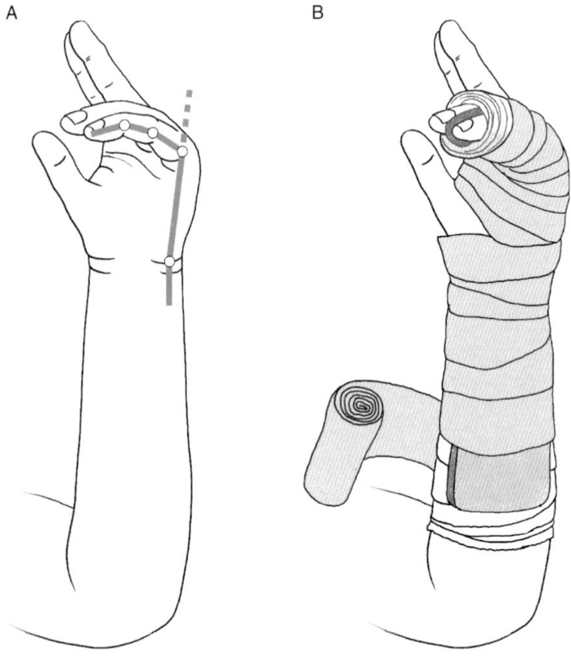

Figure 110.2 Ulnar gutter splint. (Copyright N. Ewen Wang.)

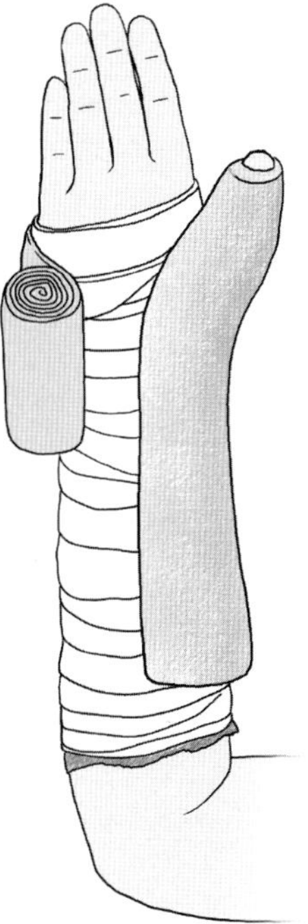

Figure 110.3 Thumb spica splint. (Copyright N. Ewen Wang.)

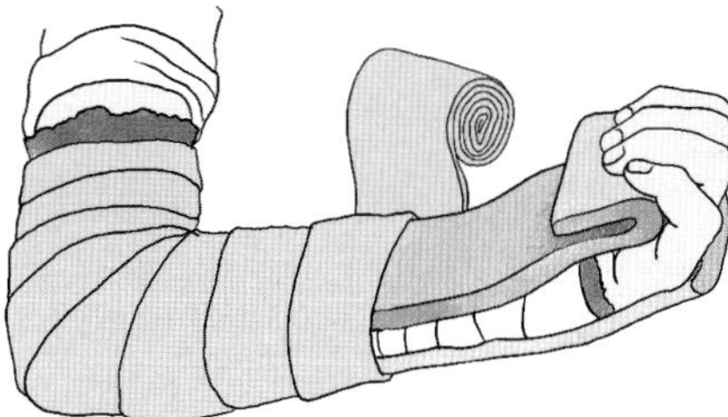

Figure 110.4 Distal sugar tong splint. This splint is recommended for young children for improved immobilization. (Copyright N. Ewen Wang.)

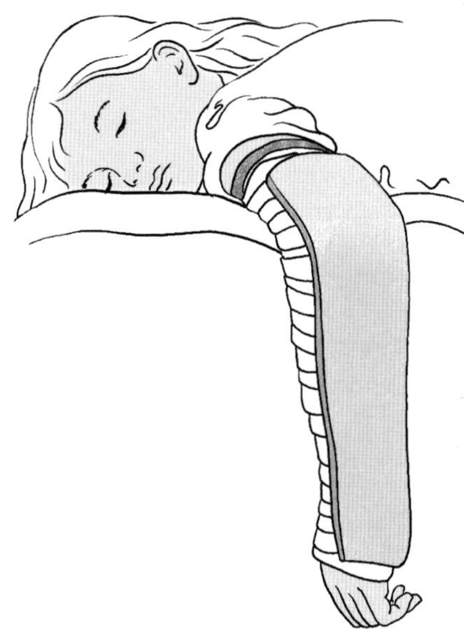

Figure 110.5 Long arm splint (Copyright N. Ewen Wang.)

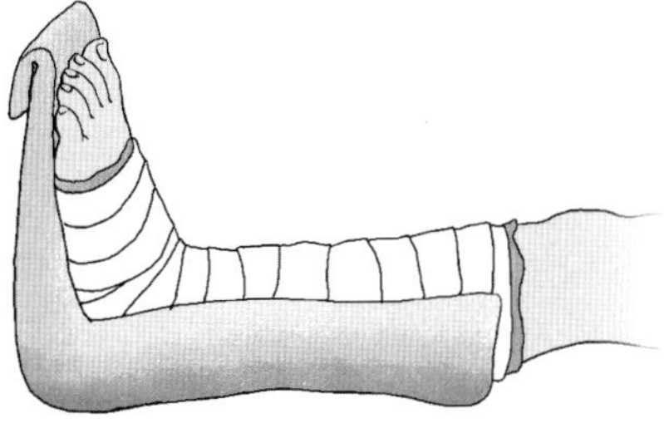

Figure 110.6 Posterior short leg splint. (Copyright N. Ewen Wang.)

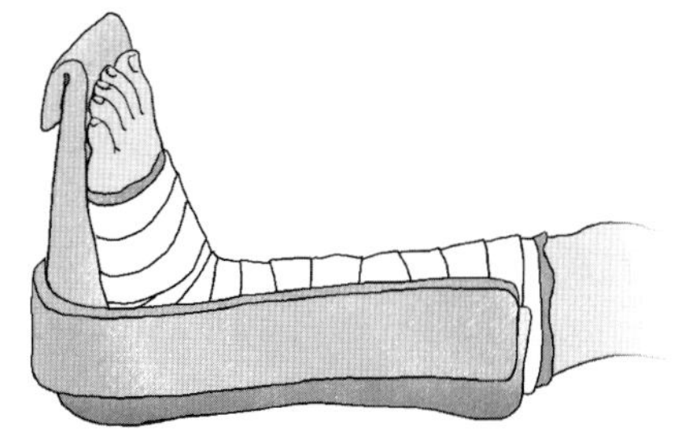

Figure 110.7 Sugar tong short leg/stirrup splint. This splint adds strength to the posterior short leg splint (Copyright N. Ewen Wang.)

Selected references

Klig JE. Splinting procedures. In King C, Henretig FM (eds.) *Textbook of Pediatric Emergency Procedures*, 2nd edn. Philadelphia, PA: Lippincott Williams & Wilkins, 2008, pp. 919–938.

Plint AC, Perry JJ, Tsang JL. Pediatric wrist buckle fractures. *CJEM* 2004;**6**:397–401.

Plint AC, Perry JJ, Correll R, Gaboury I, Lawton L. A randomized, controlled trial of removable splinting versus casting for wrist buckle fractures in children. *Pediatrics.* 2006;**117**:691–697.

Chapter

111 Emergency sports medicine

Daniel Garza, Tyler Johnston, and Gannon Sungar

Introduction

Nearly 30 million, or half of all children and adolescents in the USA, participate in organized sports. Not surprisingly, sports injuries are a common source of ED visits for children and adolescents, resulting in 23% of ED injury-related visits. Male sex, older age (6–18 years), and White race/ethnicity are associated with higher rates of visits related to sports injuries. Cycling, basketball, football, and playground injuries resulted in the largest numbers of ED sports injury-related visits. Leading diagnoses for sports injury-related visits included fractures and dislocations (24%), sprains and strains (20%), and open wounds (17%).

While physicians may be comfortable with the treatment of acute orthopedic trauma, there are multiple acute and overuse injuries that occur in the pediatric population. This chapter will address non-fracture sports injuries in children. These injuries tend to be secondary to overuse combined with rapid growth and/or to acute trauma.

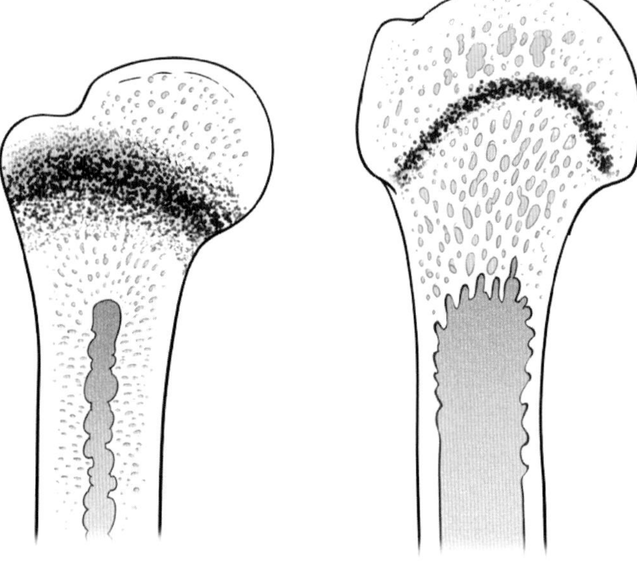

Figure 111.1 Anatomy of child bone. (Copyright Chris Gralapp.)

Pathophysiology

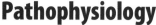

Because it is growing, pediatric bone is distinct from adult bone (Fig. 111.1 see also Fig. 109.1, p. 503). Bone components include:

- physis: growth plate
- epiphysis: secondary ossification site located at the ends of long bones
- apophysis: secondary ossification site at tendon insertions
- diaphysis: shaft of long bones
- metaphysis: bone adjacent to the physis.

Key differences between adults and children center around the nature of growing bone and the presence of ossification centers (physes and apophyses) in children. Pediatric bone is both more porous and more pliable than adult bone. This leads to bone that is more susceptible to fracture but is also able to undergo deformation without a traditional fracture pattern, as demonstrated by the greenstick fracture pattern. Growth plate cartilage is less resistant to stress than adult articular cartilage. It is also less resistant than adjacent bone to shear and tension forces. Therefore, when disruptive forces are applied to an extremity, failure may occur through the physis, which may be two to five times weaker than the surrounding fibrous tissue. For these reasons, injury mechanisms that may result in a complete ligament tear or a joint dislocation in an adult may produce a separation of the growth plate in a child. Similarly, a repetitive stress injury that would cause a soft tissue injury in an adult can be a potentially serious apophyseal injury in a child. The susceptibility of ossification centers to injury appears to be particularly pronounced during periods of rapid growth.

Common overuse injuries in children (Table 111.1) include

- apophysitis: inflammation of the tendon insertion site
- avulsion fractures: particularly at secondary ossification sites

A Practical Guide to Pediatric Emergency Medicine: Caring for Children in the Emergency Department, ed. N. Ewen Amieva-Wang (associate eds. Jamie Shandro, Aparajita Sohoni, and Bernhard Fassl). Published by Cambridge University Press.

Table 111.1. Different types of overuse injury

Area injured	Examples
Growth plate	Distal radial physis (gymnast's wrist), proximal humeral physis (little leaguer's shoulder), articular cartilage and subchondral bone, osteochondritis dissecans (medial condyle of femur, patella, talus, capitellum)
Apophysitis	Osgood–Schlatter disease (tibial tubercle), Sever's disease (posterior calcaneus), Iselin disease (fifth metatarsal), iliac crest apophysitis, little leaguer's elbow (medial epicondyle of humerus)
Bone stress fractures (low risk)	Medial tibia, fibula, ribs, radius, second and third metatarsals
Bone stress fractures (high risk)	Femoral neck, mid-anterior tibia, patella, medial malleolus, talus, tarsal navicular, pars interarticularis (spondylolysis)
Tendons	Rotator cuff tendonitis, de Quervain's tenosynovitis (extensor pollicis longus and abductor pollicis brevis), popliteus tendonitis, iliotibial band friction syndrome, patellar tendonitis, Achilles tendonitis
Bursa	Subacromial bursitis, olecranon bursitis, iliopectineal bursitis, trochanteric bursitis, prepatellar bursitis, pes anserine bursitis
Other	Lateral epicondylitis (tennis elbow), osteitis pubis (affecting symphysis pubis), Scheuermann's disease (vertebral end plates), idiopathic anterior knee pain, Sinding–Larsen–Johansson syndrome (distal pole of patella), Hoffa's fat pad syndrome (infrapatellar fat), medial tibial stress syndrome (shin splints), chronic exertional compartment syndromes of the leg, plantar fasciitis

Source: Adapted from Patel and Baker, 2006.

Table 111.2. Differential diagnosis based on location of chronic or recurrent shoulder pain in young athletes

Region	Causes
Shoulder joint region	Glenohumeral joint instability; arthritis of glenohumeral joint; glenoid labral tears; long head of biceps tendonitis; rotator cuff impingement, tendonitis, and tear; subacromial bursitis; stress fracture of proximal physis of the humerus
Acromioclavicular joint region	Arthritis of the acromioclavicular joint, acromioclavicular joint sprain, atraumatic osteolysis of the distal clavicle
Scapulothoracic region	Scapular dyskinesis, stress fracture of the scapula, suprascapular neuropathy, referred pain from the neck region, cervical spinal cord impingement, cervical spinal cord tumor, syringomyelia, cervical disk herniation, cervical nerve root impingement, brachial plexus injuries, thoracic outlet syndrome

Source: Adapted from Patel and Baker, 2006.

Table 111.3. Differential diagnosis based on location of elbow pain in young athletes

Location	Causes
Lateral	Lateral epicondylitis (tennis elbow), osteochondritis dissecans of the capitellum, posterior interosseous nerve entrapment
Medial	Flexor–pronator syndrome, medial collateral ligament sprain or insufficiency, ulnar neuritis or compressive neuropathy, medial epicondyle apophysitis, medial epicondylitis (golfer's elbow)
Posterior	Olecranon bursitis, triceps insertional tendonitis, stress fracture of the olecranon, intra-articular loose bodies
Anterior	Biceps strain, biceps tendonitis, flexor-pronator exertional compartment syndrome, anterior capsulitis

Source: Adapted from Patel and Baker, 2006.

- osteochondritis dissecans: injury of articular cartilage and subchondral bone
- physeal or epiphyseal injury: stress injuries and inflammation of the growth plate.

This chapter will emphasize the diagnosis and treatment of sports injuries as well as an approach to young athletes to support returning to participation in a safe and timely manner. Tables 111.2 to 111.5 outline the differential diagnosis of pain in different joints. Understanding the importance of gradual load bearing on skeletal and soft tissue after a period of recovery is essential for any sports physician.

Apophyseal injuries

The apophysis, or secondary ossification center, in pediatric bone is commonly an attachment site for the myotendinous unit, leading to a nidus for mechanical stress. Histologically, these injuries manifest as a series of microavulsions at the bone–cartilage interface. There are a variety of overuse injuries that occur as a result of traction placed on these "weak points" in the bones of children and adolescents.

Table 111.4. Causes of chronic low back pain in young athletes

Causes	Examples
Soft tissue injuries (most common cause)	Recurrent musculotendinous strains and ligamentous sprains
Disk conditions causing mechanical pain	Disk rupture, herniation, infection, degeneration, juvenile disk disease (lumbar Scheuermann's disease)
Acquired conditions of the spine	Spondylolysis and spondylolisthesis (most commonly detected specific cause), slipped vertebral apophysis, apophyseal ring fracture, facet joint syndrome, idiopathic juvenile osteoporosis, vertebral osteomyelitis
Developmental conditions of the spine	Adolescent idiopathic scoliosis, spina bifida occulta, lumbarization or sacralization
Chronic inflammatory disease of the spine	spondyloarthropathy, ankylosing spondylitis, juvenile rheumatoid arthritis, benign and malignant tumors of the spine
Conditions of the sacrum	Sacroiliac joint dysfunction, sacroliitis, stress fracture of the sacrum
Conditions of the spinal cord	Syringomyelia, tumors, tethered cord
Intra-abdominal conditions Mechanical low back pain	Inflammatory bowel disease, renal disease, urinary tract infection, gynecologic conditions, intra-abdominal neoplasms
Psychosomatic	Important consideration in all adolescents

Table 111.5. Causes of chronic and recurrent knee pain in young athletes

Area affected	Causes
Anterior	Idiopathic anterior knee pain (patellofemoral pain), patellar or quadriceps tendonitis, Hoffa's fat pad syndrome, prepatellar or infrapatellar bursitis, Osgood–Schlatter disease, multipartite patella, patellar stress fracture, juvenile osteochondritis dissecans of the patella, chondromalacia patellae, Sinding–Larsen–Johansson syndrome
Posterior	Baker's cyst (associated with meniscal tear), Fabella syndrome, gastrocnemius tendonitis, hamstring tendonitis or chronic strain
Medial	Medial meniscal tear, pathologic medial plica, pes anserine bursitis/tendonitis, semimembranosus bursitis/tendonitis, juvenile osteochondritis dissecans of the knee
Lateral	Iliotibial band friction syndrome, popliteus tendonitis, discoid lateral meniscus injury, proximal tibiofibular articulation pain, referred pain from the hip:, slipped capital femoral epiphysis, Legg–Calvé–Perthes disease, femoral neck stress fracture
Other	Benign and malignant tumors around the knee, acute lymphoblastic leukemia, sickle cell arthropathy, juvenile rheumatoid arthritis, septic knee and osteomyelitis, reflex sympathetic dystrophy

Source: Adapted from Patel and Baker, 2006.

Osgood–Schlatter disease

Osgood–Schlatter disease is perhaps the best-known apophysitis. Inflammation occurs at the tibial tubercle apophysis, which is the site of attachment for the patellar tendon, most frequently occurring in jumping sports such as basketball and volleyball, where forceful contraction of the quadriceps occurs repetitively. The presenting symptom is pain and edema at the tibial tubercle. Boys and girls develop Osgood–Schlatter disease most commonly between ages 10 and 15 years.

The diagnosis is clinical, but malignancy (osteogenic sarcoma) is in the differential and, if follow-up is not reliable, radiographs should be obtained. Radiographs may show calcification distally within the apophyseal-tendon junction. Resolution will occur in 90% of patients when ossification is complete, but this can take years to occur. The expected course of symptoms is typically 12–24 months.

Osgood–Schlatter disease represents a challenge to clinician, patient, and parent as mild to moderate pain is not an absolute contraindication to sport participation. In fact, pain is a reliable guide to what activity is allowable; persistent pain is the indication of the need for prolonged rest. The cornerstone of treatment is cryotherapy, compression with elastic wrap, and occasional anti-inflammatory drugs.

Sever's disease

A second common apophysitis, Sever's disease, occurs at the junction between the Achilles tendon and the calcaneal apophysis. It is frequently bilateral and presents in preteen athletes in field sports with tenderness at the insertion of the Achilles tendon, but not the calcaneal body. This helps to distinguish Sever's apophysitis from other conditions, including calcaneal stress fractures and osteomyelitis.

The treatment approach is similar to Osgood–Schlatter disease, with pain dictating activity level and the use of cryotherapy and anti-inflammatory medication. The use of heel cups or lifts and stretching to improve ankle dorsiflexion may be helpful.

Apophysitis of the medial epicondyle

Apophysitis of the medial epicondyle, "little leaguer's elbow," is most commonly found in throwing athletes. The mechanism is a repetitive distractive force occurring during the cocking and acceleration phases of throwing. Excessive number of pitches thrown and the use of a sidearm delivery are risk factors.

Examination reveals localized tenderness over the medial epicondyle, with or without swelling. Frequently there is pain with resisted forearm pronation. There should be no instability with valgus stress of the elbow, which would suggest an acute medial collateral injury.

If radiographs reveal an avulsion fracture, then referral should be made to an orthopedic surgeon. Displacement of <5 mm is generally treated conservatively, whereas >5 mm frequently requires repair.

As with all apophysites, treatment begins with rest, cryotherapy and a gradual return to activity. Once pain is resolved, a program of strengthening and stretching should be initiated. Pitching should be absolutely restricted for 4 weeks following presentation, with a gradual return thereafter. Pain is an absolute indication for reinstitution of rest.

Ligamentous injuries

While ligamentous injuries are not as common as physeal injuries in young children, they do occur with increasing frequency in older children and adolescents who participate in sports. It is important that the EP assesses the severity of the injury and counsels appropriate rehabilitation to allow for safe return to play or refers to a surgeon for possible operative repair.

Ankle sprains

Ankle sprains are common in sports and generally occur as a result of landing on a plantar flexed foot with inversion of the ankle. This can occur through an uneven field surface or through landing on another competitor's foot. The inversion ankle sprain most commonly results in injury to the anterior talofibular ligament. With increasing force, additional ligaments such as the calcaneofibular and posterior talofibular ligaments may be injured. Ankle sprains are most frequently graded on a scale of I to III for severity, loosely correlating with the number of ligaments injured.

Physical examination will reveal tenderness and edema over the affected ligament, ecchymosis, and pain with weight bearing. The anterior drawer test may be positive in significant injuries to the anterior talofibular ligament (Fig. 111.2).

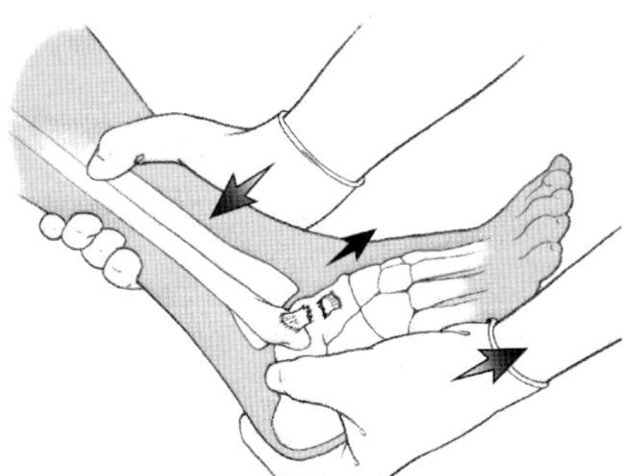

Figure 111.2 Positive anterior drawer (ankle) test. (Copyright Chris Gralapp; reproduced with permission from Mahadevan SV, Garmel GM. *An Introduction to Clinical Emergency Medicine.* Cambridge, UK: Cambridge University Press, 2005.)

The Ottawa rules can be used to determine if a radiograph is warrented (see Box 109.2 and Fig. 109.12, p. 510). The physician should inspect the radiograph for fractures, or a widened mortise, which may indicate instability.

Initial treatment consists of ice, compression, elevation, and crutches as needed to avoid painful weight bearing. Patients may benefit from the convenience of commercially available gel or air stirrup splints. Severe (grade III) sprains require immobilization in a plaster splint or orthopedic boot, no weight bearing, and referral to an orthopedic surgeon or sports medicine physician. When pain and edema improves, rehabilitation focuses first on range of motion and flexibility, and then progresses to gradual weight bearing and running, followed by multidirectional movements without pain. Physical therapy emphasizes strengthening and proprioception. Young athletes should not return to play until they demonstrate painless multidirectional movements at full speed (i.e., "cutting" and "backpedaling") as well as adequate strength and flexibility.

Eversion ankle sprains result in injury to the deltoid ligament along the medial aspect of the ankle. These injuries require significant force and the clinician should be suspicious for associated fracture (fibular, talar) and possible joint instability. Treatment and rehabilitation are similar to lateral ankle sprains.

A syndesmotic sprain (i.e., "high ankle sprain") generally occurs in the ankle that has associated external rotation with the injury mechanism. Physical examination findings include pain proximally, over the tibia–fibular syndesmosis, a positive squeeze test, pain with passive dorsiflexion and external rotation of the ankle, and generally less swelling than in sprains to the lateral or medial ligaments. These injuries frequently take longer to recover, although the principles of treatment and rehabilitation are the same.

Knee injuries

Similar to the ankle, knee ligament injuries are rare in children but occur more commonly in adolescents. Severity is graded as I (minimal laxity on exam), II (laxity with definite endpoint on examination), and III (laxity with no endpoint). A grade III tear is a complete disruption of the ligament. The most commonly injured knee ligaments are the medial collateral ligament and the anterior cruciate ligament.

Medial collateral ligament

The medial collateral ligament is confluent with the medial meniscus and is responsible for protecting the knee against valgus forces. It is typically injured when force is directed across the knee in a lateral to medial direction with contact (e.g., a football tackle) or without contact (e.g., a fall while skiing).

On examination there may be little or moderate effusion and pain/instability with application of valgus force.

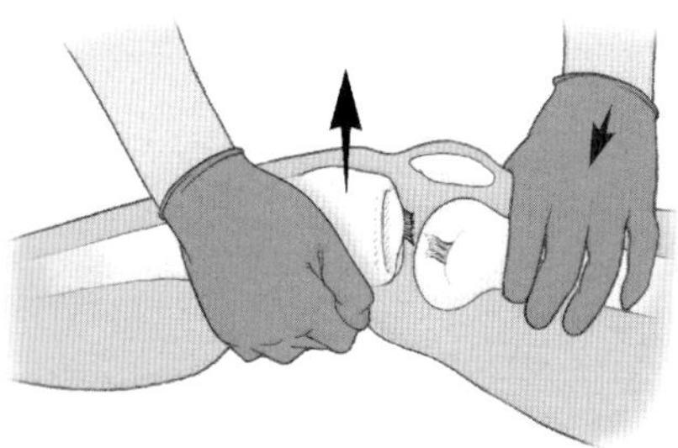

Figure 111.3 Positive Lachman test. (Copyright Chris Gralapp; reproduced with permission from Mahadevan SV, Garmel GM. *An Introduction to Clinical Emergency Medicine*. Cambridge, UK: Cambridge University Press, 2005.)

Treatment is non-operative with bracing for support, non-weight bearing as needed, cryotherapy, compression, and progression to rehabilitation for range of motion, strengthening, and proprioceptive training.

Anterior cruciate ligament

The anterior cruciate ligament helps to maintain the integrity of the knee in an anterior–posterior direction as well as limiting valgus and tibial external rotatory forces. The most common mechanism of injury is a non-contact flexion of the knee with external rotation of the tibia as the athlete plants and turns. A "pop" is often audible and there is normally a significant effusion.

Examination with either an anterior drawer or Lachman's test (Fig. 111.3) reveals laxity of the ligament. In complete disruption, there is noticeable anterior tibial translocation with no endpoint. Unlike in adults, surgery is often delayed as the procedure actually poses risk to the physes. Patients undergo bracing, activity modification, and rehabilitation until surgery can be performed.

Posterior cruciate ligament

Injuries to the posterior cruciate ligament are less common and often result from a direct force applied to the tibia in an anterior–posterior direction. On physical examination, an effusion is present and a posterior drawer test reveals laxity.

Treatment is non-surgical, with bracing and rehabilitation, unless there is extreme instability.

Management of knee ligament injuries

These ligament injuries may benefit from a knee immobilizer to reduce swelling and the pain associated with stress placed on the affected ligament, but they are not essential. Similarly, patients can carefully transition out of crutches if pain decreases and there is no frank instability. Follow-up within 1 week to a sports or orthopedic specialist allows for appropriate determination of the need for any functional bracing and/or rehabilitation.

Meniscal injuries

The menisci serve to transmit a more-uniform load to the underlying hyaline cartilage that they protect. Both the medial and lateral menisci are at risk from the shearing forces that occur when young athletes perform maneuvers that require the relative rotation of tibia and femur. If a meniscal tear is suspected, MRI is the imaging modality of choice to confirm and stage the location and extent of the tear.

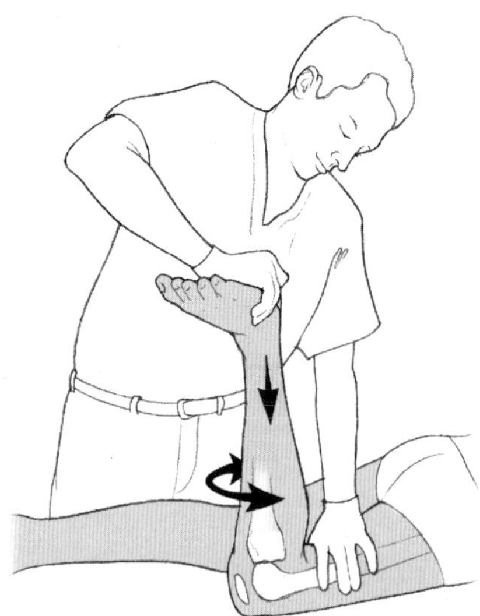

Figure 111.4 Positive Apley compression. (Copyright Chris Gralapp; reproduced with permission from Mahadevan SV, Garmel GM. *An Introduction to Clinical Emergency Medicine*. Cambridge, UK: Cambridge University Press, 2005.)

The onset of pain and swelling is generally less dramatic than with an acute ligamentous injury. Pain is along the joint line and patients may complain of a "locking" or "grinding" sensation. Physical examination reveals tenderness along the affected joint line as well as a mild to moderate effusion. A "bounce test," whereby the examiner applies intermittent force underneath a relaxed and fully extended knee with the patient supine, will frequently elicit pain. More specialized examination techniques, such as the McMurray's test and Apley Compression test (Fig. 111.4), will yield pain.

Initial treatment is cryotherapy, bracing and no weight bearing. Definitive treatment is surgical, with two options: (1) excision, if the tear is in a region with little or no vascular supply, or (2) repair, if the tear is within the better vascularized periphery. Referral to an orthopedic surgeon is essential, as patients who have few symptoms may opt to delay surgery to continue participating if the risks and benefits are clearly explained.

Osteochondritis dissecans

Osteochondritis dissecans results from the separation of a bone fragment and overlying articular cartilage in pediatric patients with open growth plates. This frequently leads to the free movement of the fragment within the joint, causing pain and accelerated damage. Although the exact etiology is unknown, most experts agree that repetitive stress is the primary cause. In the pediatric population, the most common site is the knee, and patients will present with generalized knee pain without prior trauma. Typical of bony lesions, pain is worse with activity. A small percentage of patients will be asymptomatic, and diagnosis will be made with incidental radiographs.

Importantly, the sensitivity of radiographs is improved by using a tunnel view. Initial diagnosis should be confirmed and delineated with MRI to fully evaluate the lesion.

Treatment is based on the goal of preservation of the articular cartilage. Immobilization of the extremity facilitates abstinence from sporting activity, with re-evaluation at 6–10 weeks. If reossification is demonstrated, then the patient may be progressed back to activity under the direction of a supervised rehabilitation program and the use of functional bracing. This process can take up to 1 year. Patients who are closer to skeletal maturity should be considered for surgical treatment with referral to an orthopedic surgeon.

Stress fractures

Stress fractures are properly viewed as overuse injuries of the skeletal tissue rather than acute fractures. Living bone responds to stress forces by remodeling to adapt, similar to muscle. However, if the load exceeds the limits of the tissue, a stress fracture can occur, resulting in inflammation, breakdown of the extracellular matrix, and pain.

The treatment is similar to that of soft tissue overuse injuries: rest followed by gradual return to activity, which allows the bone to actively remodel in a manner that will eventually support the offending activity in a reasonable manner. The use of immobilization for stress fractures is rare.

It is important for the physician to realize that stress fractures are ubiquitous: any region of the axial or appendicular skeleton subject to the force of tendon and muscle or repetitive impact can be susceptible. Often, these injuries occur in the weight-bearing bones of the body. Sites that are at high risk for fracture propagation or non-union include pars interarticularis of lumbar spine, anterior tibia, sesamoids of the great toe, base of the second metatarsal, and proximal fifth metatarsal. Shin splints (medial tibial stress syndrome) commonly causes anterior tibial pain as a result of increased exercise. These injuries represent a continuum with tibial stress fracture resulting after long-standing, repeated stresses.

The typical patient presents with weeks, rather than days, of slowly increasing pain that is worse with activity. Frequently, pain is present at night. Pain may often, but not always, be elicited with direct palpation and is usually more focal than diffuse.

Radiographs may show a small lucency or some periosteal scalloping, but are most often negative. This should encourage the EP to recommend weight bearing as tolerated initially. Definitive diagnosis is obtained by triple phase bone scan or MRI in most cases.

Treatment consists of rest from the offending activity followed by a supervised rehabilitation program that allows for gradually increasing loads to promote bone remodeling to the tolerance of the desired activity. This should also include a biomechanical assessment of factors that may be contributing to the development of the stress fracture. Clinicians should consider obtaining bone density results, particularly in adolescent females. Use of NSAIDs should be avoided as there is growing evidence in the literature that they may slow bone healing. Orthopedic or sports consultation is recommended for all stress fractures, and it is mandated for those with a high risk for non-union (navicular, femoral head/neck, anterior cortex of tibia, talus and base of second and fifth metatarsals).

Patellofemoral pain syndrome

Patellofemoral pain syndrome refers to chronic, yet vague anterior knee pain. The etiology is poorly understood. The mechanism likely involves overload, as well as abnormal tracking of the patella causing increased stresses at the lateral patellofemoral joint.

The symptoms typically occur with an increase in training and include pain associated with climbing or descending stairs, rising from a seated position, and/or other exercises requiring explosive quadriceps activity. Examination reveals tenderness around the patella and pain with compression of the patellofemoral joint.

Treatment focuses on avoidance of offending activities and patellar stabilization, accomplished through a variety of interventions including quadriceps strengthening (isometric training in full extension is recommended), hamstring stretching, patella-stabilizing braces, taping, ice, NSAIDs and orthotics.

Illiotibial band syndrome

Illiotibial band syndrome occurs most commonly in runners. Etiology involves repetitive rubbing of the illiotibial band over the lateral femoral condyle. It has been associated with excessive weekly running mileage, unidirectional running on a track, and downhill running.

Presentation is characterized by focal pain at the lateral femoral condyle with occasional radiation to the thigh. The Noble compression test is positive if pain is elicited with compression of the lateral femoral condyle at 30 degrees of flexion. History and physical examination (with possible use of local anesthetic injection) should be used to rule out intra-articular injuries, tendonitis, or peroneal nerve injury, or referred pain.

The goal of initial treatment is reduction of inflammation at the site of friction. To this end, oral NSAIDs, ice massage, phonophoresis, and iontophoresis may be used in conjunction with abstinence from the offending activities. Following inflammation management, conservative rehabilitation protocols designed to release myofascial restrictions and increase strength are recommended. The majority of patients may begin a ramped return to running protocol by 6 weeks, after demonstration of pain-free function. In rare unresolved cases, referral to an orthopedic surgeon may be indicated for surgical management, using a variety of techniques designed to decrease illiotibial band impingement.

Tendonitis

Tendonitis can occur with increased use of any muscle–tendon complex. Tendonitis of the patellar and quadriceps tendons (knee extensors) can commonly cause knee pain in athletes involved in running and jumping sports. Pain is worse after going up or down stairs and with prolonged sitting. Tenderness can occur in the patellar ligament, or the inferior and superior pole of the patella. In popliteal tendonitis, pain is localized to the posterior lateral knee after prolonged hiking up hill. Achilles tendonitis may also present in pediatric athletes, with excessive tightness of calf muscules.

Radiographs may demonstrate tendon calcifications. Treatment for patellar tendonitis includes quadriceps strengthening, increasing quadriceps and hamstring flexibility, rest, and ice. Treatment of Achilles tendonitis includes rest, ice, heel lifts, stretching, and may necessitate shoe inserts.

Spondylolysis and spondylolisthesis

Two common causes of chronic back pain in the pediatric and adolescent athlete are spondylolysis (pars interarticularis defect) and spondylolisthesis (anterior translation of one vertebral body relative to the segment inferior to it) (Fig. 107.1, p. 491).

Spondylolysis

Spondylolysis most frequently occurs at the L4 and L5 levels in athletes who experience repeated loads in hyperextension (e.g., gymnasts). Similar to stress injuries, spondylolysis may be seen as a continuum from stress reaction (no disruption of the cortex) to stress fracture (isthmic spondylolysis).

Presentation is usually insidious, and the pain is worse with extension. Unilateral pars defects may elicit a greater degree of pain with extension and rotation toward the affected side. There is generally no radiculopathy or neurological deficits.

The initial diagnostic test is a five-view lumbosacral series, with the oblique views offering the best chance of visualizing a cortical defect ("the Scotty dog sign") (Fig. 111.5). If the radiographs are negative and the history and physical suggest a stress reaction, the test of choice is a single photon emission computed tomography (SPECT). The stress reactions are visualized as increased tracer uptake in the affected region. Axial CT images may be used to delineate any fracture pattern not visualized by radiographs. The role of MRI is controversial in spondylolysis, with varied reports of sensitivity and specificity.

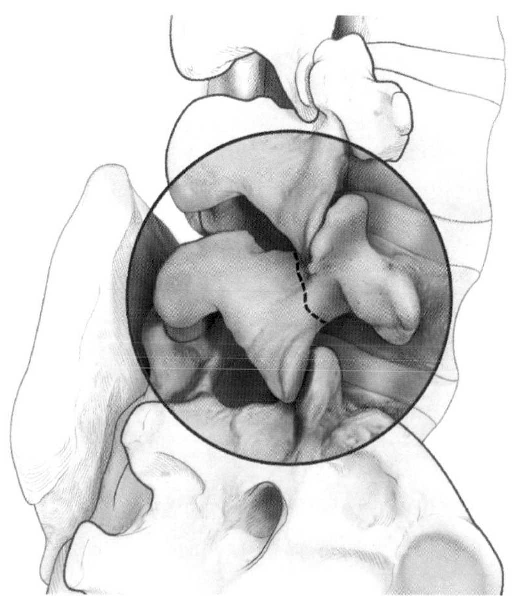

Figure 111.5 "Scotty dog" with a "collar appearance" seen on radiographs of patients with spondylolysis. (Copyright Scott Bodell, reproduced with permission from Cassas *et al.*, 2006.)

Treatment of spondylolysis depends on the presence of a cortical defect. A more conservative approach is taken with stress reactions to avoid progression to a cortical defect. Patients are placed in a thoracolumbar sacral orthosis brace for a period of 6–12 weeks until there is pain-free extension and rotation. The patient should progress in physical therapy to full activities once the brace has been removed. If a cortical defect is present, there is no likelihood of bony union and treatment is focused on alleviation of pain, increasing mobility, and gradual load bearing. Some studies have advocated the use of a soft corset to limit extension in the initial phase of treatment. Patients should be referred to physical therapy for a gradual return to play over 8–12 weeks. Treatment focuses on the strengthening of the deep ("core") abdominal muscles (internal obliques and transversus abdominis) and lumbar multifidus as well as increasing mobility in a controlled fashion.

Spondylolisthesis

Spondylolisthesis most often occurs at the L5–S1 level. In dysplastic spondylolisthesis, there is anterior translation of the L5 vertebra on the sacrum, resulting in lumbar stenosis and possibly L5 radiculopathy. Broadly, type I relates to congenital dysplasia, whereas type II refers to pars disruptions from either acute or overuse injuries.

Presentation is similar to spondylolysis; however, radiculopathy and/or bowel/ bladder incontinence may be reported by patients with high-grade spondylolisthesis. Therefore, physical examination should include a thorough neurologic evaluation of the lower extremities.

Lateral radiographs can be assessed via the Meyerding classification to quantify the amount of forward translation (slip) into four grades:

I: 0–25%
II: 26–50
III: 51–75%
IV: 76–99%.

Treatment options vary with the type and grade of spondylolisthesis as well as with response to initial conservative measures. Patients with low-grade (<50% slip) spondylolisthesis respond well to non-surgical measures, including activity restriction, bracing, and supervised physical therapy. Similar to spondylolysis, return to play is allowed when pain and spinal mobility have improved. In contrast, patients with symptomatic high-grade spondylolisthesis respond poorly to non-surgical measures and should be referred to a spinal surgeon. Patients with low-grade dysplastic spondylolisthesis are at greater risk for progression and should be followed with radiographs at intervals of 6–9 months through skeletal maturity. Any patients with any grade and neurologic symptoms should receive an MRI and referral to a spinal surgeon.

Pearls and pitfalls

Pearls

1. The growth plate is often the weak point of the pediatric skeleton and, therefore, an important site of injury
2. An increase in early participation in competitive sports has led to an increased incidence of ligamentous injuries as well as overuse injuries at earlier ages.
3. Most sports injuries respond well to rest followed by a gradual and supervised return to activity; those that do not warrant surgical consideration.

Pitfalls

1. Inappropriate return to play: a period of rest should never be followed by full activity; gradual return allows injured tissue to adapt to the load.
2. Failure to focus on the importance of growth plates or apophyses as the likely sites of injury.
3. Failure to refer to an orthopedic or sports specialist for follow-up.

Selected references

Caine D, DiFiori J, Maffuli N. Physeal injuries in children's and youth sports: reasons for concern. *Br J Sports Med* 2006;**40**:749–760.

Cassas KJ, Cassettari-Wayhs A. Childhood and adolescent sports-related overuse injuries. *Am Fam Physician* 2006;**73**:1014–1022.

Cavalier R, Herman MJ, Cheung EV, Pizzutillo PD. Spondylolysis and spondylolisthesis in children and adolescents: I. Diagnosis, natural history, and nonsurgical management. *J Am Acad Orthop Surg* 2006;**14**: 417–424.

Flachsmann R, Broom ND, Hardy AE, *et al.* Why is the adolescent joint particularly susceptible to osteochondral shear fracture? *Clin Orthop Rel Res* 2000;**381**:212–221.

Frederickson M, Wolf C. Iliotibial band syndrome in runners; innovations in treatment. *Sports Med* 2005;**35**:451–459.

Larson RL, McMahon RO. The epiphyses and the childhood athlete. *JAMA* 1966;**7**: 607–612.

Micheli LF. Pediatric and adolescent sports injury: recent trends. In Pandolf KB (ed.) *Exercise and Sport Science Reviews*. New York: Macmillan, 1986, pp. 359–374.

National Institutes of Health. *NIH Publication 93-3444: Conference on Sports Injuries in Youth – Surveillance Strategies, 1991*. Washington, DC: National Institutes of Health, 1992.

Patel DR, Baker RJ. Musculoskeletal injuries in sports. *Prim Care Clin Office Pract* 2006;**33**:545–579.

Saperstein AL, Nicholas SJ. Pediatric and adolescent sports medicine. *Pediatr Clin North Am* 1996;1014–1034.

Simon TD, Bublitz C, Hambridge SJ. Emergency department visits among pediatric patients for sports related injury. *Pediatr Emerg Care* 2006;**22**:309–315.

Wall E, Von Stein D. Juvenile osteochondritis dissecans. *Orthop Clin North Am* 2003;**34**:341–353.

Section 16

Neurology

Expert reviewer: Jin S. Hahn

Chapter 112 Approaches to the pediatric neurological examination

N. Ewen Amieva-Wang

Introduction

The pediatric neurologic examination can be difficult because children often cannot describe their symptoms, do not obey instructions, and develop different skills at different stages of development. While there are fundamental differences between children and adults, the same systematic approach should be used to examine children and adults. The neurologic examination should include mental status, cranial nerves, motor system, cerebellum and gait, sensory responses, and reflexes. Failure to meet developmental milestones (Table 112.1) as well as failure of primitive reflexes to disappear can denote pathology.

Table 112.1. Early developmental milestones

Task	Age range (months)
Sits with help or momentarily	4–8
Rolls	4–10
Sits without aid	5–9
Pulls to standing	6–12
Stands alone	9–16
Walks alone	9–17

Clinical presentation

History

In addition to specific details about onset of symptoms, duration, and associated factors, history should include:

- antenatal history (history of pregnancy, maternal history)
- perinatal events (labor and delivery, prolonged labor)
- developmental history (milestones)
- language development (compared with siblings)
- school information (attention span, grades, handedness)
- social history (abuse, toxin exposure)
- family history (neurodegenerative, genetic disease or epilepsy).

Physical examination

Upon entering the examination room, the child's general appearance, mental status, level of consciousness, attention, and cooperation should be assessed. Level of consciousness can be further characterized by the AVPU check (alert, responds to verbal stimulus, pain or unconscious.) The Glasgow Coma Scale also has a pediatric modification. Dysmorphic features, skin lesions (café au lait spots, depigmentation, hemangioma), and even unusual odors (metabolic disease) can give clues to underlying disorders. The neurologic examination should include assessment of normal growth, with an appropriate growth curve including head circumference.

Cranial nerve examination

The order of the neurologic examination should be tailored to the child's age. For younger children, starting with the cranial nerve examination is threatening. It is helpful to have the child sit in the parent's lap and then approach the examination systematically from "toe to head," starting with the lower extremities, and progressing to the upper extremities and lastly, the head (Table 112.2).

The cranial nerve examination in the infant and child is similar to that for an adult with the exception that smell, corneal reflex, and ability to locate sound are not present at birth.

Motor examination

Examination of the motor system involves observation, palpation, and assessment of tone, function, and strength (Table 112.3; see also Ch. 117). The first step in the examination of the motor system is to simply observe the patient. Observe the resting posture. Muscle strength in children, like adults, is assessed on a 5-point scale.

Pronator drift is a good method to elicit mild or moderate upper motor neuron weakness.

In school-aged children, one can assess individual muscle groups, but in younger children, it is reasonable to assess function of a group of muscles. For example, proximal lower

A Practical Guide to Pediatric Emergency Medicine: Caring for Children in the Emergency Department, ed. N. Ewen Amieva-Wang (associate eds. Jamie Shandro, Aparajita Sohoni, and Bernhard Fassl). Published by Cambridge University Press.

Table 112.2. Cranial nerve examination

Cranial nerve		How to test
I	Olfactory	Non-functional in newborns
II	Optic	Visual field acuity in Infants: introduce objects into visual field to grab; pupillary reflex
III	Oculomotor	Size of pupils, ability to fixate and follow object or light. Extraocular muscles and conjugate eye movements should be assessed
V	Trigeminal	Temporalis muscle (open and close mouth). Facial sensation with pinprick. Tickle. Nose with q-tip or tissue (might be less threatening for young children); in some circumstances, corneal reflex can be elicited with this method
VII	Facial	Smile, symmetry of facial movements
VIII	Vestibular	Hearing (watch child turn head towards noise)
IX	Glossopharyngeal	Test both afferent sensory, and efferent motor (gag), swallowing
XI	Spinal accessory	Shoulder shrug In younger children, palpate sternocleidomastoid muscle by extending head on the side of bed with infant in supine position
XII	Hypoglossal	Tongue movement (goes to side of lesion); if a patient can speak normally the hypoglossal should be intact

extremity and pelvic girdle muscle groups can be assessed by the child crawling, walking, or climbing stairs. Distal lower extremity function can be assessed by asking achild to walk on heels and toes. A child reaching for an object above his/her head can demonstrate upper extremity strength as a muscle group.

Tone

Tone is the baseline amount of muscle resistance to passive movement about a joint. The examiner must move each of the patient's limbs through full range of motion. Abnormalities include hypotonia or hypertonia. If hypertonia is suspected, the examiner should assess for increased spasticity or unidirectional resistance during flexion or extension (such as from an upper motor neuron lesion) or rigidity with increased resistance during both flexion and extension (such as from a basal ganglia lesion).

Cerebellum and gait

Coordination and cerebellar function can be difficult to assess in the young child. The central cerebellum controls balance while the cerebellar hemispheres control coordination. If a child can walk "normally" according to the parents this usually constitutes a normal cerebellar examination in the toddler. While finger to nose testing and heel–toe and tandem gait may be difficult for the young child, reaching for a toy, repeated high fives, or tapping a foot can also assess for cerebellar function.

Sensory system

Assessing the sensory system involves the examination of light touch, vibration, and proprioception. In newborns the examination is limited to touch and pinprick.

Reflexes

Abnormal reflexes may be the manifestation of electrolyte or endocrine pathology, or an anxious patient. Deep tendon

Table 112.3. Pediatric motor examination: specific tests

Test	Description	Pediatric adjustment	Pathology
Pronator drift	Test of upper motor strength	Extend upper arms with palms down. both eyes closed; after a few seconds, turn the palms up: elbow may pull down in upper motor neuron weakness; observe during hand extension for finger flexion, drift, or asymmetric pronation	Upper motor neuron lesion (trauma stroke)
Romberg	Stand with feet together and arms in front of body	None	If unable with eyes open, consider cerebellar lesion; If unable with eyes closed, indicates posterior column or peripheral nerve abnormality
Babinski	Stroke lateral aspect of foot and then move to big toe at metacarpophalangeal area: abnormal response is dorsiflexion of big toe and fanning of other toes	Positive response usually at birth until 1 year of age (can be positive without pathology to 2.5 years)	Pyramidal tract lesion
Clonus	Series of sustained rhythmic jerks following quick stretch of muscle	Sustained clonus is abnormal but a few jerks can be normal.	Upper motor neuron disease

Table 112.4. Primitive reflexes and age of disappearance

Reflex	Description	Age of disappearance	How to elicit reflex
Moro	Bilateral upper and lower extremity extension and abduction	Disappears by 3 months (persists in Tay–Sachs disease; is asymmetrical in Erb's palsy)	Elevate head 30 degrees above the body, then let head drop
Palmar grasp	Closure of fingers to grasp an object, when it is placed in the infant's hand or it strokes their palm	Disappears by 7 months	Stroke palm or place an object in the hand
Rooting reflex	Turns head towards cheek stimulation	Disappears by 4–6 months	Gently strok check

reflexes are considered normal if they are symmetrical and rate between 1+ and 3+. Asymmetrical reflexes or a substantial difference between the upper and lower extremities are indicative of abnormality and warrant further investigations.

Primitive reflexes are present at birth and assess the functional integrity of the brainstem and basal ganglia (Table 112.4). Disappearance is associated with normal maturation of the CNS.

Abnormal movements

If spontaneous abnormal movements are found, classify or characterize them based on type, age of patient at onset, mode of onset, and the clinical course of the movement. Abnormal hyperkinetic movements such as tremor, dystonia, chorea, ballismus, and myoclonus usually decrease in intensity and frequency during sleep (Table 112.5).

Table 112.5. Abnormal movements

Movement	Description	Possible cause/ pathology
Dystonia	Characterized by sustained muscle contraction that frequently causes twisting, repetitive and abnormal posture	*Primary*: inherited syndromes including mitochondrial and metabolic disease *Acquired*: perinatal injury, infections, drugs, toxins
Chorea	Involuntary, rapid and irregular jerky movement; it may affect one limb or all parts of the body and face	Primary inherited disorders Acquired disorder: Sydenham's chorea is one of acute manifestations of rheumatic fever; it occurs months after initial infection in children 5–13 years of age
Ballismus	Violent flinging movement of one or more limbs; can be intermittent or on a continuous basis; can involve one side (hemiballism) or both sides of the body	Strokes, tumors, medication
Myoclonus	Sudden, brief shock-like movement	Can occur with seizures

Conclusions

The pediatric neurologic examination tests similar function to the adult examination although in a developmentally appropriate fashion. Birth and family history, developmental milestones, and primitive reflexes are unique and integral to the systematic pediatric neurological examination.

Pearls and pitfalls

Pearls

1. Performing the neurological examination in a pediatric patient is challenging.
2. Age-appropriate adjustments must be made to perform a thorough neurological examination.

Pitfalls

1. Failure to assess developmental milestones in all pediatric patients.

Selected references

Mercuri E, Ricci D, Pane M, Baranello G. Neurological examination of the newborn baby. *Early Hum Devel* 2005;**81**:947–956.

Yang M. Newborn neurologic exam. *Neurology* 2004;**62**:15–17.

Chapter 113

Altered level of consciousness and coma

George Sternbach

Introduction

Assessment and management of the child with altered mental status parallels that of the adult in many respects. However, the relative frequency of the causes differs among the two groups. There are also some etiologies that are unique to the pediatric age group. Important causes of coma and altered mental status in children are:

- head trauma
- cerebral edema
- cerebral neoplasm
- CSF shunt malfunction
- seizure/post-ictal state
- meningitis/encephalitis
- toxic ingestion
- hypoxia
- hypoglycemia
- sepsis
- hypovolemia.

Various terms are applied to define deficits of consciousness. **Coma** has been defined as complete unresponsiveness and lack of awareness of self and environment. Other designations have been given to less pronounced alterations of consciousness. **Lethargy** describes reduced wakefulness with deficit of attention. **Obtundation** is mental blunting with slow responses to stimuli. **Stupor** is a state of diminished alertness from which a patient can be aroused only by vigorous stimulation. Because of the descriptive nature of these terms, a number of more objective scales have been developed to codify the clinical status of the patient with an abnormal level of consciousness (ALOC) and to allow for repeated assessment of such patients. The best-known of these is the Glasgow Coma Scale (GCS; Table 113.1) and the pediatric-modified GCS (Table 113.2).

This chapter will review common causes of ALOC, the approach to a patient with ALOC, and then special populations such as children with CSF shunts.

Table 113.1. The Glasgow Coma Scale

Sign	Finding	Score
Eye opening	Spontaneously	4
	To command	3
	To pain	2
	None	1
Verbal response	Oriented	5
	Confused, disoriented	4
	Inappropriate words	3
	Incomprehensible sounds	2
	None	1
Motor response	Obeys commands	6
	Localizes pain	5
	Withdraws from pain	4
	Flexion withdrawal (decorticate)	3
	Extension withdrawal (decerebrate)	2
	None	1
Total		3–15

Etiology

Altered level of consciousness involves a diffuse insult to the brain; for coma to occur, either the bilateral cerebral cortices or the ascending reticular activating system must be affected.

Such damage can occur from traumatic structural damage, which can cause global or focal symptoms, or infectious,

A Practical Guide to Pediatric Emergency Medicine: Caring for Children in the Emergency Department, ed. N. Ewen Amieva-Wang (associate eds. Jamie Shandro, Aparajita Sohoni, and Bernhard Fassl). Published by Cambridge University Press.

Table 113.2. The pediatric Glasgow Coma Scale

Sign	Finding	Score
Eye opening	Spontaneously	4
	To voice	3
	To pain	2
	None	
Verbal response	Coos, babbles	5
	Irritable, cries	4
	Cries to pain	3
	Moans to pain	2
	None	1
Motor response	Spontaneous movement	6
	Localizes pain	5
	Withdraws from pain	4
	Flexion withdrawal (decorticate)	3
	Extension withdrawal (decerebrate)	2
	None	1
Total		3–15

metabolic or toxic insults, which tend to cause more diffuse but symmetric findings. Lesions associated with trauma can usually be localized according to symptoms. Infratentorial lesions result in brainstem dysfunction, coma, cranial nerve disturbance, and pupillary findings.

The differential diagnosis of altered mental status changes with the age of the child (Table 113.3). In infants, infection, metabolic abnormalities, and inborn errors of metabolism are common causes. The last should especially be considered when vomiting, seizures, or metabolic acidosis is present. In the older child, infection, accidental ingestion of substances, and seizures are important considerations. In both these groups, trauma resulting from child abuse should be included in the differential. In the adolescent, the causes begin to more closely resemble those of adults. In this age group, head trauma and drug and alcohol ingestion are common etiologies.

Clinical presentation

History

The history taking should focus on the events preceding the ALOC but then should also include associated symptoms, past medical and family history.

Physical examination

The physical assessment begins, as with all emergency patients, with evaluation of the ABC status. Vital signs and oxygen

Table 113.3. Age-based differential diagnosis of altered level of consciousness

Diagnosis	Age	Associated findings	Comments
Trauma, child abuse	All ages; child abuse in infants and younger children	Focal and generalized findings depending on the lesion	EPs are mandatory reporters of child abuse; discuss with social worker and child protective services if suspected; consider admission of the child
Metabolic: inborn errors, hypo/ hyperglycemia, hypo/ hypernatremia	Young children are particularly susceptible to hypoglycemia given lack of glycogen stores	Neurovascular seizures	Disorders that can lead to gluconeogenesis include sepsis, dehydration, serious bacterial infection and alcohol intoxication
Infectious: herpes encephalitis	Infants, immunocompromised older children	Localized seizures, fever	Risk factors for neonatal herpes: maternal infection at the time of delivery, along with prolonged labor, placement of fetal scalp electrodes
Poisoning: alcohol, narcotics, sedatives, carbon monoxide, lead	Generally mobile children	Depends on substance ingested: tachypnea and odor of alcohol (alcohols), pinpoint pupils (narcotics), flushed face (carbon monoxide), sleepiness (sedatives)	In a child who is not ambulating or crawling, consider child abuse
Intussusception	Infants and young children	Abdominal pain, mass	Consider in the child with episodic abdominal pain and lethargy (Ch. 66)
Neoplasm	Any age, younger age generally portends a worse diagnosis	Hemorrhage; increased intracranial pressure, seizures or interruption of CSF flow	Acute hypdrocephalus caused by tumor growth classically produces a triad of headache, vomiting and lethargy

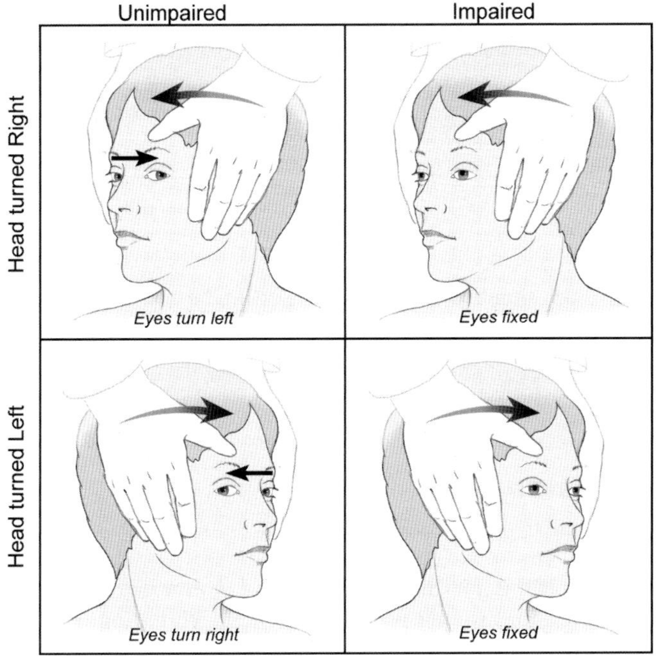

Figure 113.1 Oculocephalic reflex (doll's eyes). (Copyright Chris Gralapp; reproduced with permission from Mahadevan SV, Garmel GM. *An Introduction to Clinical Emergency Medicine.* Cambridge, UK: Cambridge University Press, 2005.)

saturation should be assessed and repeated frequently. A bedside serum glucose level should always be performed. A complete physical assessment should be performed, with particular attention applied to the respiratory pattern, eye and pupillary findings (Figs. 113.1 and 113.2), and neurologic examination. Fundoscopic examination should be attempted to assess for the presence of papilledema or retinal hemorrhages.

Identification of focal deficits or asymmetry is a priority in physical examination, as such findings suggest a structural intracranial lesion as a cause for coma. A positive Babinski reflex is indicative of an upper motor neuron lesion. Bilateral positive signs suggest bilateral CNS involvement.

In coma of metabolic cause, motor signs are usually symmetric and pupillary reaction to light is typically preserved.

A variety of respiratory patterns have been described in association with the unconscious state, and specific respirations identified as suggesting involvement of certain anatomic sites in the CNS. In practice, distinguishing between these patterns may be difficult in the emergency setting, and their identification may be of only limited practical value. In Cheyne–Stokes respirations, ventilatory effort cycles in a crescendo–decrescendo pattern between hyperventilation and apnea. This pattern may reflect bilateral cerebral hemispheric or upper brainstem lesions, but such breathing also occurs in metabolic

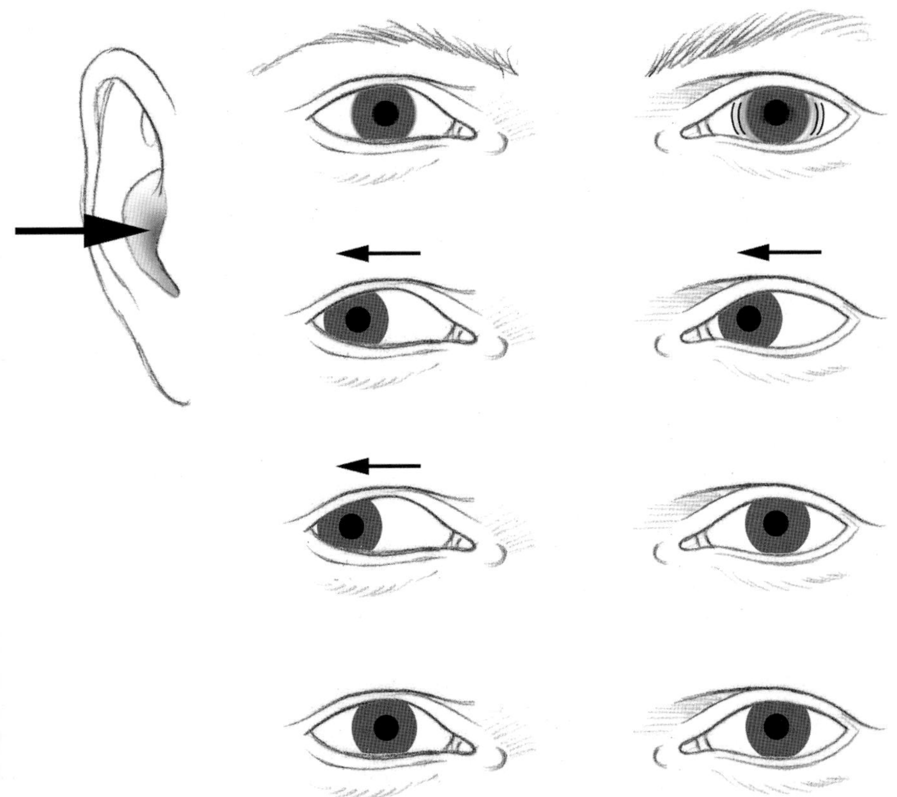

Figure 113.2 Oculovestibular testing (cold calorics). (Copyright Chris Gralapp; reproduced with permission from Mahadevan SV, Garmel GM. *An Introduction to Clinical Emergency Medicine.* Cambridge, UK: Cambridge University Press, 2005.)

encephalopathy and congestive heart failure. Sustained hyperventilation is seen in hypoxia, metabolic acidosis, and hepatic encephalopathy. Although a lesion of the upper brainstem may produce hyperventilation (central neurogenic hyperventilation), this is a much less common occurrence. Short-cycle Cheyne–Stokes respirations (cluster breathing), prolonged inspiratory pauses (apneustic breathing), and breathing that is irregular in rhythm and depth (ataxic breathing) have been linked to various brainstem and posterior fossa lesions.

A unilaterally dilated pupil in a patient with an altered mental status may be an indicator of transtentorial herniation of the temporal lobe against the third cranial nerve and brainstem.

The mass is usually on the same side as the dilated pupil. Bilateral pupillary dilation is usually caused by extracranial factors, such as prolonged hypoxia or drug intoxication. Bilateral pupillary constriction is seen in pontine hemorrhage and certain drug overdoses (e.g., opiates).

Testing of eye movements can differentiate brainstem and hemispheric lesions. In general, if both eyes cross the midline, the brainstem is intact. The oculocephalic (doll's eye) reflex involves moving the patient's head from side to side after the cervical spine is cleared (Fig. 113.1). If the eyes move in the opposite direction to the direction of movement, the brainstem is intact. The oculovestibular reflex (cold calorics) involves instilling 10–20 ml of cool water into the external auditory canal over approximately 10 s (Fig. 113.2). If the brainstem is normal, the eyes will turn toward the tested side ("slow" component). If the cerebral hemisphere is intact, the eyes will then move away from the side tested with a rapid, jerking motion ("fast" component). If there is no eye movement or only eye movement ipsilateral to the tested side then brainstem damage is probable.

Abnormal motor posturing may occur, either spontaneously or in response to stimulation. In decorticate posturing, the arms are flexed, adducted, and internally rotated, and the legs are extended. In decerebrate posturing, both the arms and legs are extended. Traditionally, decorticate posturing has been described as suggesting brain damage above the mid-brain, decerebrate posturing below this level. Such correlation between these postures and the anatomic location of CNS damage may, however, be inexact. Progression from decorticate to decerebrate posturing may indicate expansion of a structural lesion or herniation.

Diagnostic studies

Head computed tomography

Obtaining a CT of the head is an important priority in the child with persistent coma or with focal neurologic deficit. The diagnoses that can be made by CT include intracranial hemorrhage, subarachnoid hemorrhage, hydrocephalus, and cerebral tumor. The CT scan in HSV encephalitis may show frontal or temporal lobe changes, but it may be normal in many cases.

Box 113.1. Initial management of altered level of consciousness in the emergency department

1. Dextrose 25% 1 g/kg should be given as a bolus for hypoglycemia *or* glucagon 0.03 mg/kg SC (roughly 0.5 mg in a small child and 1 mg in larger child).
2. If narcotic overdose is suspected, give naloxone 0.1 mg/kg IV (max. 2 mg).

There are situations where MRI would be the first test of choice, such as in suspected encephalitis or encephalomyelitis. Since MRI is often more difficult to obtain than CT, these imaging arrangements can be made in conjunction with pediatric neurology.

Laboratory tests

Screening metabolic panel should be obtained to assess for common electrolyte abnormalities. Laboratory results and history suspicious for toxicological cause (anion gap, hypo- or hyperglycemia) should prompt more targeted testing (alcohol level, etc.). Lumbar puncture is necessary for suspected CNS infection.

Management

Initial management and stabilization should include glucose measurement and treatment (Box 113.1). Patients with suspected hypoglycemia should have glucose administered IV as soon as possible. If IV access cannot be established, glucagon should be administered SC.

If sepsis is considered, cultures of the blood, urine, and CSF should be obtained. In addition, cultures of nasal secretions, sputum, skin lesions, stool, and other sites should be sent to the laboratory, as indicated by the clinical picture. In children suspected of having HSV encephalitis, antiviral therapy with acyclovir should be initiated empirically. Note that acyclovir doses are higher than the recommended dosage for adults.

If meningitis is suspected and lumbar puncture must be delayed (by performance of head CT in appropriate cases, for example), a third-generation cephalosporin (cefotaxime, ceftazidime or ceftriaxone) should be started (see also Ch. 92). Some recommend the addition of vancomycin. In neonates under 3 weeks of age, the initial antibiotics of choice are ampicillin and gentamicin as well as acyclovir.

Special populations: cerebrospinal shunt malfunction

Children with hydrocephalus and surgically-placed CSF shunts may experience decreased level of consciousness. This can occur when shunt malfunction prevents adequate drainage of fluid from the ventricles, leading to increased intracranial

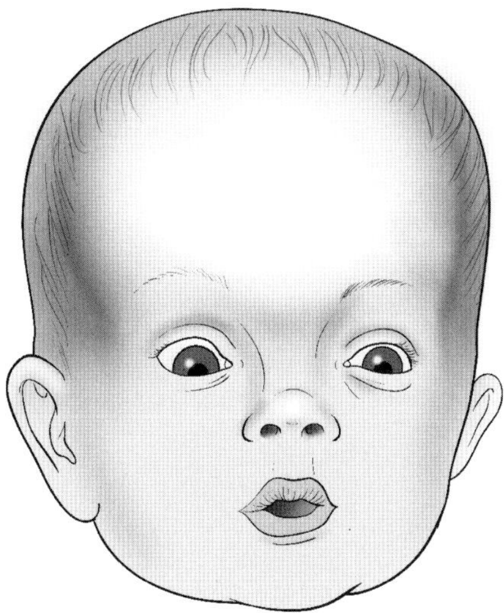

Figure 113.3 Sunsetting sign: forced downward deviation of the eyes so that the lower eyelid covers the inferior portion of the iris. (Copyright Chris Gralapp.)

pressure. Infants with hydrocephalus usually have macrocephaly, with a forehead that is disproportionately larger than the face and distended scalp veins over thin skin. Ocular findings include divergent gaze and decreased intraocular movement (specifically inability to look outward and up.) Severe hydrocephalus causes forced downward deviation of the eyes or the sunsetting sign (Fig. 113.3). Additional findings of acute intracranial pressure elevation include headache, nausea, vomiting, and papilledema. The most common shunt type is ventriculoperitoneal, with CSF drained from the lateral ventricles into the peritoneal cavity.

A CSF shunt consists of three components: a ventricular catheter; a valve and reservoir, which is palpable beneath the scalp; and a catheter leading to the site where the CSF is absorbed. The ventricular catheter traverses the skull through a burr hole and is joined to the valve that is seated beneath the scalp. Complications of shunts include infection and mechanical failure, and these are usually the result of contamination at the time of surgery. Mechanical failure occurs most commonly from tissue debris plugging the shunt's lumen. Separation or fracture of the shunt's components and migration of the catheter are additional causes of malfunction.

The time since the most recent shunt operation is an important item of historical information. Patients who are within 6 months of surgical shunt implantation or revision are more likely to experience failure than those who have been neurologically stable for more than 6 months. Infants with shunts who present for care are more likely to have shunt malfunction or failure than older children or adults.

It is often stated that assessment of the pump mechanism provides information regarding the shunt's function. If the reservoir is easily depressed and refills promptly, the implication is that the shunt is patent proximal to the reservoir. However, this is not a reliable maneuver, and it is not recommended that shunt failure be identified solely on the basis of such examination of the reservoir.

Diagnostic studies

Head computed tomography

When a brain CT is performed for purposes of assessing CSF shunt malfunction, it must be compared with a prior study. Without a comparison study, such imaging cannot be reliably interpreted. When a shunt malfunctions, ventricular volume usually increases over baseline, although this is not invariably the case. Plain radiographs (a "shunt series") can be obtained to demonstrate any discontinuity in the shunt's distal portion.

Summary

The workup of a patient with altered level of consciousness is complex and must be undertaken in a systematic fashion after thoroughly evaluating the patient and obtaining a detailed past medical history. When in doubt, the patient should be admitted for observation and further work-up. The EP should always check basic abnormalities such as electrolytes, glucose, and oxygen levels to screen for quickly correctable causes of ALOC. These signs, however, are often clues to the underlying disease process rather than the primary problem.

Pearls and pitfalls

Pearls

1. Apply age-related coma scales to preverbal children.
2. Administer appropriate antibiotics promptly in children with suspected meningitis even if lumbar puncture is delayed.
3. In suspected shunt malfunction, always compare head CT scans to prior imaging.

Pitfalls

1. Failure to consider child abuse in appropriate clinical settings with or without history of head trauma.
2. Failure to administer acyclovir in suspected viral encephalitis.
3. Failure to consider disease entities other than diabetes, such as sepsis or alcohol ingestion, in a patient with hypoglycemia.

Selected reference

Reilly PL, Simpson DA, Sprod R, *et al.* Assessing the conscious level in infants and young children: a pediatric version of the Glasgow Coma Scale. *Child Nerv Syst* 1988;**4**: 30–33.

Chapter 114

Dizziness and ataxia

Beau Briese, Millicent Marmer, and N. Ewen Amieva-Wang

Introduction

"Dizziness" is a patient complaint, which can be used to refer to vertigo, light-headedness, or ataxia. Ataxia is a movement disorder resulting in lack of coordination. Ataxia is rare in children. While in adults, acute cerebrovascular disease should be at the top of the differential diagnosis, with the exception of children with sickle cell disease or lupus, the incidence of thromboembolic events in the pediatric population is rare. Most causes of ataxia are benign and self-limited; however, it is an alarming symptom and can be a harbinger of serious disease such as brain tumor, encephalitis, and trauma.

Ataxia can reflect dysfunction of the cerebellum itself or of its afferent or efferent neuronal pathways.

Lesions to the central cerebellum cause truncal ataxia and a loss of balance. Lesions to the cerebellar hemispheres typically cause loss of coordination of fine movement.

Ataxia-like symptoms can be caused by a myriad of conditions, the major ones being vertigo, epilepsy, and weakness.

Vertigo. This is the sensation of movement while stationary. Peripheral vertigo is caused by pathology in the balance mechanism in the middle ear. Incidence of these syndromes (paroxysmal positional vertigo, vestibular neuronitis, labyrinthitis) in children is unknown. Symptoms are hard to communicate and describe. Examination should be benign for central deficits and patients should not have true ataxia. They often have horizontal nystagmus and the Dix–Hallpike test is positive. Of note, benign paroxysmal vertigo (BPV) is thought to be a migraine variant in infants and children (see below).

Epilepsy (pseudoataxia). Seizures, particularly partial and partial-complex seizures as well as their post-ictal states, may be confused with ataxia by parents. However, with epilepsy, the pseudoataxic symptoms are transient, lasting a matter of minutes and are generally associated with shaking, repetitive movements, or an ALOC.

Weakness. Weakness syndromes, such as botulism, tick paralysis, and Duchenne's muscular dystrophy, can easily manifest with an unsteady gate, particularly in toddlers and young children. Multiple sclerosis can present with ataxia in adolescents.

Middle ear pathology and muscular weakness are also known to cause ataxia.

In the ED, it is helpful to classify ataxia syndromes by age of onset and whether the ataxia is acute, episodic, or chronic (Table 114.1). Chronic etiologies of ataxia, congenital anomalies, hereditary ataxias, and degenerative CNS disease should present with a known diagnosis and will not be discussed here.

Differential diagnosis

Acute cerebellar ataxia is the most common cause of acute ataxia in young children and typically occurs in boys age 2 to 4 years of age.

Acute cerebellar ataxia. This syndrome is commonly preceded by a viral infection, most frequently varicella, days to weeks prior to the onset of ataxia. It is thought to be a post-infectious autoimmune process, although the pathophysiology is not well understood.

Traumatic head injury. A detailed history should raise suspicion for this process (Ch. 143). Non-accidental trauma must be on the differential diagnosis.

Infection. A careful past medical history, history of present illness, examination and directed diagnostics should offer clues that ataxia could be infectious in origin (Ch. 92).

Neoplasm. Medulloblastoma is the most common malignant pediatric tumor, comprising one-fifth of all pediatric primary CNS tumors (Ch. 80). The peak incidence is

A Practical Guide to Pediatric Emergency Medicine: Caring for Children in the Emergency Department, ed. N. Ewen Amieva-Wang (associate eds. Jamie Shandro, Aparajita Sohoni, and Bernhard Fassl). Published by Cambridge University Press.

Table 114.1. Causes of pediatric ataxia by age of onset, frequency, and acuity: most common diagnoses are listed first

	Infant/young child	School-age child/adolescent
Acute	Acute cerebellar ataxia 40%	Intoxication (alcohol, drugs of abuse)
	Intoxication (alcohol, medications) (30%)	Labyrinthitis
	Guillain–Barré	Guillain–Barré syndrome
	Trauma	Trauma
	Infection	Infection
	Malignancy (posterior fossa tumors and neuroblastoma)	Malignancy (posterior fossa tumors and neuroblastoma)
	Lead poisoning	Vertebrobasilar dissection (usually with a history of trauma)
		Psychologic
Intermittent	Benign paroxysmal vertigo	Migraine (basilar)
	Seizure	Seizure
	Inborn errors of metabolism	Benign paroxysmal vertigo
Chronic	Congenital	Congenital
	Hereditary ataxias	Hereditary ataxias
	Degenerative CNS disease Duchenne's dystrophy	Degenerative CNS disease (multiple sclerosis)

between 5 and 9 years. Since the tumors typically arise in the midline cerebellum, truncal ataxia, head bobbing (titubation), and unsteady gait commonly occur. The child usually also manifests with other symptoms and signs of increased intracranial pressure such as concerning headache, nausea, and vomiting.

Neuroblastomas. These occur in the peripheral nervous system, along the sympathetic chain (chest or abdomen). The presenting symptoms vary according to the location of the tumor. Neuroblastomas can present with an opsoclonus–myoclonus–ataxia complex (a paraneoplastic syndrome). Typically this consists of rapid, involuntary eye movements in all directions, rhythmic jerking, and ataxia.

Intoxication. Toddlers may ingest alcohol or other medications in the household as part of their exploratory actions. Adolescents may experiment with alcohol and drugs of abuse. Children medications such as anticonvulsant drugs may have elevated drug levels. A careful history should direct testing such as a urine toxicology screen, blood alcohol level, or specific drug level.

Migraine syndromes. These can manifest with disequilibrium. The history and recurrent nature of the disease should help with the diagnosis.

Benign paroxysmal vertigo. This is thought to be a migraine variant in infants and preschoolers. It is usually monosymptomatic, causing pure vertigo, which presents as ataxia (since the child may not be able to report the sensation of vertigo). This is not the same disease as paroxysmal positional vertigo, which occurs in adults as a result of displaced otoliths.

Basilar migraine. Incidence of basilar migraine peaks in adolescence and it may be more polysymptomatic than benign paroxysmal vertigo, with nausea, vomiting, headache, and other cranial nerve findings in addition to ataxia.

Clinical presentation

Ataxia although most easily confused with weakness, must be distinguished from other neuromuscular disorders such as spasticity, chorea, and myoclonus. Confirming the presence of these disorders and distinguishing them from one another requires knowledge of developmental milestones, a sense of the patient's baseline from the history, and a systematic and focused neurologic examination (See also Ch. 112).

Ataxia can manifest as an unsteady, wide-based gait. Normal infants learning to sit up and to walk can appear ataxic to a stranger, but parental history will help to distinguish abnormal movements from normal behavior. For children old enough to sit, truncal ataxia is often indicated by head titubation (bobbing or tremor) as well as by an inability to sustain a sitting position. For patients old enough to walk, a cerebellar hemispheric lesion will cause an ipsilateral veering gait.

A child who can walk to his caregiver with a gait that the caregiver claims is normal is normal.

By 4 to 7 months of age, an effective method of determining coordination is through playing with the infant and observing the infant's ability to transfer objects between hands. By 5 to 10 months, the infant's ability to perform raking movements towards toys and stickers should be intact. At this time, infants should also be able to finger feed, so a history of losing the capacity to do so may indicate dysmetria. Intention tremors (tremor is present when reaching out for objects but not at rest) are a sign of ataxia caused by ipsilateral hemispheric dysfunction. Infants aged 1 to 3 years should be able to perform basic coordination tests, including pointing to parents, colors, and named objects.

Ataxia and weakness can be differentiated by evaluation of muscle strength and deep tendon reflexes without movement. In ataxia, both are normal. Different tests to rule out weakness are appropriate at different ages. It is important to test axial, as well as upper and lower extremity strength. In infants aged 1 month to 6 months, clinicians should test the palmer and plantar grasp reflexes as well as the ability of a child to lift the head while prone. After 6 months, strength can be tested by assessing the infant's ability to roll. Children aged 18 months or older can have their strength and tone assessed through play as they grasp at and manipulate toys.

Spasticity is distinguished from ataxia by the presence of an unsteady but narrow gait as well as by hyperreflexia and increased muscle tone on passive movement. Chorea and myoclonus both continue to occur when a child is at rest, unlike ataxia, which presents only through voluntary movements or elicited reflexes.

Diagnosis and management

Acute cerebellar ataxia. Unless the history and presentation is classic and the ataxia is mild, workup includes neuroimaging and lumbar puncture. Although MRI is ideal because of better imaging of the posterior fossa and less radiation exposure, it is not available in all EDs. It is important to keep in mind that this is a diagnosis of exclusion. There is an 80–90% chance of complete recovery, often within days and generally within 6 weeks.

Infection. Bacterial and viral CNS infections cannot be reliably distinguished clinically. All patients with suspected CNS infection should undergo diagnostic testing including a lumbar puncture and receive prompt antibiotic treatment if there is a question of bacterial infection. Neuroimaging should be obtained in almost all cases before a lumbar puncture because of the concern about a posterior fossa tumor and risk of herniation with lumbar puncture.

Brain tumors. Brain tumors that either disrupt CSF flow or are located in the posterior fossa may cause ataxia. While ataxia may be the only presenting symptom of small tumors, ataxia-causing tumors usually present with other focal neurologic deficits such as nystagmus, head tilt, and aphasia. Nuchal rigidity, recurrent or chronic headaches, persistent vomiting, increased intracranial pressure signs, seizures, or altered mental status may also be present. Imaging with CT or MRI should be performed in those suspected of an intracranial malignancy. Up to 60% of all pediatric brain tumors occur on or near the cerebellum.

Neuroblastoma. Patients presenting with opsoclonus–myoclonus–ataxia should be assumed to have neuroblastoma until proven otherwise.

Toxins. Most cases are the result of accidental exposure in children 1 to 5 years old, although the physician should be aware of neglect and inappropriate exposure to substances of abuse. Adolescents may also present with experimental or suicidal exposure. Further laboratory testing depends upon the ingestion. Usually treatment requires supportive care except for specific ingestions such as lead.

Guillain–Barré syndrome. This post-infectious syndrome, usually characterized by ascending weakness, can also present with sensory ataxia. The Miller–Fisher variant can present with ataxia, areflexia, ophthalmoplegia, and relatively preserved strength.

Multiple sclerosis. This occurs in older children and adolescents and can initially present with episodes of ataxia. Bladder or bowel dysfunction, paresthesiae, visual changes secondary to optic neuritis, and an intention tremor may also be present. Demyelination lesions are seen on MRI. Neurological consult in the ED or close follow-up should be arranged depending on the severity of symptoms.

The constellation of presenting symptoms, combined with detailed history and physical examination, should guide ED testing and imaging.

Disposition

We recommend consultation with a pediatric neurologist in most cases for confirmation of the diagnosis as well as aid in management and follow-up. While some children with a clear diagnosis of acute cerebellar ataxia and full negative workup can be followed closely as an outpatient, most patients presenting to the ED with acute ataxia and continued inability to walk should be admitted to the hospital.

Pearls and pitfalls

Pearls

1. Parents are the best judge of whether their toddler has ataxia.
2. The most common causes of acute ataxia in children are ingestions or acute cerebellar ataxia.

Pitfalls

1. Failure to realize that children with chronic medical conditions, such as sickle cell disease or lupus, are at increased risk for thromboembolic events and stroke compared with the normal pediatric population.

Selected references

Casselbrant ML, Mandel EM. Balance disorders in children. *Neurol Clin* 2005;**23**:807–829, vii.

Davis DP, Marino A. Acute cerebellar ataxia in a toddler: case report and literature review. *J Emerg Med* 2003;**24**:281–284.

Dinolfo EA, Adam HM. Evaluation of ataxia. *Pediatr Rev* 2001;**22**:177.

Ryan MM, Engle EC. Acute ataxia in childhood. *J Child Neurol* 2003;**18**:309–316.

Wiener-Vacher SR. Vestibular disorders in children. *Int J Audiol* 2008;**47**:578–583.

Chapter 115

Headache

Sean Donahue

Introduction

Approximately 40–50% of elementary aged children have headaches, and this number increases to 60–80% by the time they are in high school. In addition, the prevalence of headaches varies by sex: prepubertal boys are more affected than girls, and conversely girls complain more of headaches after the onset of puberty. This chapter will review the approach to a pediatric patient with a headache, major categories of headaches in pediatric patients, and initial management.

Approach to the patient with a headache

There are several major differences in the approach to the child with a headache versus an adult. Not only do the the etiologies of headache differ within the pediatric population, but also the manner in which children respond to pain may not be as obvious. For instance, in younger non-verbal patients, headache pain may manifest as crying, hiding, or rocking back and forth. As the child becomes older, they will obviously be able to better describe and localize, as well as and remember, prior episodes. The extreme variability in presentation based on age makes the usual diagnosing scheme we use in adults (primary causes: migraines, tension type, or cluster headaches; secondary causes: trauma, intracranial anomalies, substance or metabolically related, etc.) not as feasible. In children we are often unable to easily illicit the "red flags" that may warn about underlying pathology of the headache, such as sudden onset, new headache in the setting of an underlying medical problem, or caused by trauma. An additional difference is that headaches, particularly migraines, may last longer in the pediatric population.

A careful and thorough history is paramount in making the proper diagnosis in a child with a headache. In particular, attention must be paid to the *temporal pattern* of the child's headache. Recognizing this pattern will greatly aid in both the differential diagnosis and the actual diagnosis. There are four main temporal patterns of headaches in children that are relevant to the EP (Table 115.1).

Table 115.1. The four temporal patterns of headaches in children relevant to the emergency department

Headache pattern	Definition	Miscellaneous
Acute	First-time episode of headache without a prior history of illness	May be traumatic or atraumatic; consider subarachnoid hemorrhage
Acute recurrent	Pattern of headaches with intervals in which the child is asymptomatic	Vast majority caused by migraines
Chronic progressive	A headache that increases in frequency and that gradually worsens over time	The most worrisome type of headache; neuroimaging is always warranted
Chronic non-progressive	A headache that occurs daily, or with constant frequency	Systemic, psychologic, or musculoskeletal

Source: adapted from Rothner, 1995.

A Practical Guide to Pediatric Emergency Medicine: Caring for Children in the Emergency Department, ed. N. Ewen Amieva-Wang (associate eds. Jamie Shandro, Aparajita Sohoni, and Bernhard Fassl). Published by Cambridge University Press.

These patterns can be elicited by asking if the headache is

- acute in onset
- acute and recurrent
- chronic and progressive
- chronic and non-progressive.

Classifying the onset of the headache and its temporal pattern, along with a thorough physical examination, will allow the clinician to understand when to worry about headaches in children, and how best to manage them.

Physical examination

The approach to the physical examination of a child with a headache requires a thorough neurologic evaluation and head-to-toe physical examination, starting with the vital signs head circumference, even in older children. Key features of the examination must focus on mental status, extraocular movements, the optic discs, motor and sensory symmetry, and coordination. The head should be thoroughly examined, carefully palpating the sutures and fontanelles in infants. The sinuses should be thoroughly examined, the temporomandibular joints palpated, and the auditory canals and tympanic membranes assessed. The mouth should be evaluated for dentition, throat, and neck as being possible sources of head pain in a child.

General management

Children with worrisome history and physical examination findings will require formal neuroimaging. Neuroimaging in young children must be undertaken judiciously because of the increased awareness of cancer-related illnesses from early radiation exposure. The risk of a child developing a neoplasm from radiation in a CT scan of the head is approximately 1/1500. As MRI is a safer, and often times, a more effective imaging modality, it should be used in select cases to evaluate worrisome headaches in a child. If this modality is not an option, or the headache is of an emergency nature, CT scans can be adjusted to lower radiation levels in the pediatric population.

The basic treatment regimens for children with headaches vary depending on the etiology (see below). Most will respond to traditional analgesic–antiemetic combinations. Specific migraine medications (triptans) should be reserved for the adolescent population. Refractory pain, or pain not responding to typical analgesia–antiemetic combinations, can be treated sparingly with narcotics. These treatment regimen is summarized in Table 115.2.

Table 115.2. Analgesic treatment regimens in the emergency department for children with headaches

Medications	Dosage	Forms available for children
First-line analgesia		
Acetaminophen	10–15 mg/kg q. 4–6 h	*Elixir*: 160 mg/5 ml *Chewable tablets*: 80 mg
Ibuprofen	10 mg/kg q. 6 h	*Elixir*: 160 mg/5 ml *Chewable tablets*: 50 or 100 mg
Naproxen	2.5–5 mg/kg q. 6–8 h	*Tablets* only: 220, 250, 500 mg
Second-line analgesia		
Sumatriptan (migraines only, >12 years only)	25 mg at onset of headache, may repeat q. 2 h to a total of 200 mg	*Tablets*: 15, 50 mg
Rizatriptan (migraines only, >12 years only)	1 tablet as needed	Tablets: 5, 10 mg
Third-line analgesia		*Narcotic analgesia*: reserved for refractory pain only
Codeine and acetaminophen (narcotic–analgesic combination)	*3–6 years*: 5 ml PO q. 6–8 h prn *7–12 years*: 10 ml PO q. 6–8 h prn *>12 years*: 15 ml PO q. 4 h prn	*Elixir*: 120 mg acetaminophen and 12 mg codeine in 5 ml
Morphine sulfate	0.1 mg/kg per dose IV/IM q. 2–4 h prn (max. dose 15 mg)	*Injection*: 0.5, 1, 2, 4, 5, 8 mg/ml
Codeine	0.5–1 mg/kg per dose IM/PO q. 4–6 h prn (max. dose 60 mg)	*Injection*: 30, 60 mg/ml *Elixir*: 15 mg/5 ml

prn, as needed.

Headache temporal patterns

Acute headaches

Traumatic injuries must be recognized.

Physicians must always be suspicious for occult trauma as a source of acute headaches in children.

Atraumatic headaches in children may result from a myriad of disease processes (Table 115.3). In most cases, acute, atraumatic headaches in children are the result of self-limited infectious causes such as fever, sinusitis, otitis media, dental disease, upper respiratory tract infections, or new-onset migraine. Streptococcal pharyngitis is notorious for associated symptoms of abdominal pain and headache. However, one must always consider more ominous causes of the acute-onset headache in a child in the setting of worrisome objective neurological findings.

Important subjective and objective findings may help the EP to identify the possibility of malignant intracranial or severe systemic pathology. Children with acute-onset headaches are at risk of serious pathology (meningitis, tumor, and hemorrhage) indicated by the following features in the history: absence of family history of migraine, vomiting, confusion, abnormal neurologic examination, or a headache awakening child from sleep. Other signs and symptoms suggestive of acute intracranial pathology would include nuchal rigidity, papilledema, and headache worsened with cough or defecation.

Any child with the above signs and symptoms should undergo formal neuroimaging. Treatment should be based on imaging results and final diagnosis. Pain should always be treated (Table 115.2).

Acute recurrent headaches

The most common cause of acute recurrent headaches in children is migraine, accounting for upwards of 95% of these types of headache. Most migraines have a strong genetic component; therefore, a family history is important. Approximately 3–5% of children have migraines before puberty. Girls after the age of 15 are more prone to having migraines (Table 115.4).

There are two main types of migraine in children: classic and common. The classic type includes a visual aura, is often unilateral, or bilateral, and is described as a throbbing pain that may last hours to days. The associated symptoms of migraine headaches include fatigue, hyperacusis, photophobia, and vomiting. Conversely, common type migraines include a throbbing headache without visual or auditory symptoms. Associated symptoms are also common. Several key differences are important to note in children with migraine headaches compared with adults. Typically, migraines in children can and will last longer (up to 48 h); they can be both unilateral and bilateral, and the child can have sensitivity to light and sound.

Table 115.3. Causes of acute-onset headaches in children

Diffuse/systemic etiologies	Focal etiologies
Upper respiratory tract infection/sinusitis	Migraine
Pharyngitis	Brain tumor
Meningitis	Hydrocephalus/ ventriculoperitoneal shunt malfunction
Hypertension	Subarachnoid hemorrhage
Substance abuse (stimulants), medications (methylphenidate, oral contraceptives)	Intracranial hemorrhage

Table 115.4. Prevalence of migraine headaches in children (both classic and common)

Features	3–6 years	6–15 years	≥15 years
Prevalence (%)	1–3	5–15	10–20
Male/female	M>F	M=F	F>M

In both types of migraine, a small percentage can be complicated by transient neurologic factors, such as visual disturbances, balance problems, or confusion. These symptoms may be attributable to basilar-type migraines. This rare disorder involves migraine with an aura and symptoms referable to the brainstem, usually without weakness. Girls and boys are equally affected, with age of onset between 7 and 17 years of age. The symptoms usually consist of a combination of vertigo, ataxia, dysarthria, tinnitus, diplopia, paresthesiae, and sometimes decreased level of consciousness. Brain MRI and MR angiography should be performed in conjunction with a pediatric neurology consultation if the diagnosis is suspected, in order to rule out vascular lesions, thrombosis, or aneurysms.

While the neurologist and not the EP should make the diagnosis, the diagnostic criteria for children with migraine consist of the following:

- five or more attacks which last 1–48 h
- two of the following features: bilateral or unilateral, pulsating, worsened with activity, and moderate to severe intensity
- accompanied with at least nausea and/or vomiting, plus hypersensitivity to light, and/or sound.

Therapeutic options in treating children diagnosed with migraine in the ED include both general measures and pharmacologic treatment. General measures include reassurance for parents as to the absence of serious problems, and further identifying triggers that may have precipitated the headache: caffeine overuse, sleep disturbances, feeding habits, and stress.

Table 115.5. Antiemetic treatment regimens in the emergency department for children (>2 years) with migraine headaches

Medication[a]	Dosage	Forms available for children
Promethazine	0.25–0.5 mg/kg q. 8 h prn	*Elixir*: 6.25, 25 mg/5 ml *Suppositories*: 12.5, 25, 50 mg
Prochlorperazine	0.25–0.5 mg/kg q. 4–6 h prn	*Elixir*: 5 mg/5 ml *Suppositories*: 2.5, 5 mg
Metoclopramide	1–3 mg/kg q. 4 h prn	*Elixir*: 5 mg/5 ml

prn, as needed.
[a] These medications have known extrapyramidal side effects, which can be dose related.

Children with the probable diagnosis of migraine should be referred to a neurologist for chronic care.

First-line pharmacologic measures should include single agent therapies such as acetaminophen and ibuprofen (Table 115.2). Narcotics should be avoided, and it is important to note that no ibuprofen agents have been approved for use in children, but they can be used safely in adolescents. In addition, if the diagnosis is certain and symptoms severe, antiemetic agents should be used in combination with the analgesic medications. Antiemetic agents can sometimes abate migraines on their own (Table 115.5).

Other less likely causes of acute recurrent headaches in children include tension-type headaches (headaches originating at the base of skull with radiation to the neck), tempormandibular joint dysfunction (an audible or palpable clicking or popping of the joint), and occipital neuralgia (shooting, sharp pain at the base of the skull and in the distribution of the occipital nerve). Pain originating from the occipital region of the scalp, or over the tempormandibular joint should alert the EP to these particular causes as the source of the headache.

Chronic progressive headaches

Chronic progressive headaches in children should always raise a red flag for the EP, and children with these types of headache should always be evaluated for intracranial pathology. The most common causes of these headaches in children are vascular malformations, tumors, abscess formation, slow-bleeding subdural hemorrhages, hydrocephalus, and idiopathic intracranial hypertension (pseudotumor cerebri).

Imaging will be based on the history of worsening headaches over time, and other red-flag symptoms such as awakening from sleep; morning headaches that improve in the afternoon; positional headaches, worsening with bearing down; gait disturbances; seizures; or vomiting. Always consider an arteriovenous malformation as a source of the child's headache, particularly if the headache occurs on the same side of the head and the child is not responding to conventional measures. Children with these types of headache should be evaluated with formal neuroimaging, particularly in the light of any focal deficits or a history of seizures.

Another cause of chronic progressive headaches in children is pseudotumor cerebri. This anomaly is caused by decreased CSF absorption as a result of arachnoid villi dysfunction. The signs and symptoms of this disorder are mostly from the elevated intracranial pressure: headache, vomiting, visual disturbances, and papilledema. The incidence in childhood is unknown, and the preferred imaging modality, if available, is MRI. A lumbar puncture can also lead to the diagnosis (after MRI to rule out herniation if this is a concern) by revealing an opening pressure of greater than 250 mmH_2O (approximately 20 mmHg). Therapy consists of acetazolamide, to decrease CSF production, serial lumbar punctures, or surgery in rare cases.

Other causes of chronic progressive headaches in children are depression, anxiety, and drug abuse; these can only be entertained as diagnoses of exclusion.

Chronic non-progressive headaches

The main causes of chronic non-progressive headaches in children include concussions, systemic inflammatory states (such as myositis), psychologic states (such as severe

Pearls and pitfalls

Pearls

1. Always remember the risks to children of early radiation exposure by using CT scans. Remember to include the parents as part of the treatment team, and remind them of the risks/benefits of such scans. MRI, if available, may be more useful if imaging is needed.
2. Migraines in children respond well to non-narcotic analgesia (single agents of Motrin and Tylenol are the mainstay), and antiemetics. Triptan drugs should only be used in the adolescent population.

Pitfalls

1. Failure to consider traumatic causes, including non-accidental trauma in acute-onset headaches in children.
2. Failure to consider elevated intracranial pressure in a child with headache and vomiting.
3. Failure to maintain a low threshold for diagnostic neuroimaging, as well as a formal neurological evaluation in a child presenting with a chronic progressive headache.

depression or conversion disorder), and musculoskeletal disorders (such as tempormandibular joint dysfunction, or cervical spine disease). These types of headache occur in <1% of the pediatric population and are classified as a headache that lasts for 4 or more hours per day, occurs at least 15 times per month, for a period of 4 or more months. Particulary in the adolescent population, depression must be considered as a source in chronic, stable headaches.

For these types of headache, particularly if another obvious source leading to the headaches has been identified, neuroimaging is not warranted. Treatment in the ED must be centered at localizing disease that may be contributing to the headache. Once any precipitating factors have been identified, first-line treatment is the use of analgesics.

Conclusions

While pediatric headaches are not uncommon and usually benign, the child with a headache warrants a careful and systematic workup. All children with acute recurrent and chronic non-progressive headaches should be evaluated by a neurologist; however, this can occur on an outpatient basis if the child is medically stable. Children with chronic progressive headaches should have imaging in conjunction with a pediatric neurologist. Management of acute headaches will be guided by the underlying cause. Headache pain should be treated expeditiously.

Selected references

Brenner DJ, Elliston CD, Hall EJ, Berdon WE. Estimated risks of radiation-induced fatal cancer from pediatric CT. *AJR Am J Roentgenol* 2001;**176**:289–296.

Evans, RW, Linder SL. Management of basilar migraine. *Headache* 2002;**42**:383.

Rothner AD. The evaluation of headaches in children and adolescents. *Semin Pediatric Neurol* 1995;**2**:109–118.

Winner P, Wasiewski W, Gladstein J, Linder S. Multicenter prospective evaluation of proposed pediatric migraine revisions to the HIS criteria. *Headache* 1997;**37**:545–548.

Chapter 116

Seizures

Claire Turchi

Introduction

Seizures are a common problem in childhood, with up to 6% of children experiencing at least one seizure sometime during childhood.

A seizure is defined as a transient, involuntary alteration of consciousness, behavior, motor activity, sensation, and/or autonomic function caused by excessive rate and hypersynchrony of discharges from a group of cerebral neurons. The following types of seizure are frequently encountered in the ED

Generalized seizure. There is involvement of both cerebral hemispheres. These seizures can be categorized as absence, myoclonic, tonic, clonic, atonic, and tonic–clonic.

Partial seizure. Involvement is limited to one cerebral hemisphere. Partial seizures may or may not cause ALOC and may evolve into a generalized seizure.

Status epilepticus. This is a state of prolonged seizure activity lasting more than 30 min or persistent repetitive seizure activity without recovery of consciousness between episodes. Status epilepticus occurs significantly more frequently in children and is typically divided into convulsive and non-convulsive types. The duration of seizures in both types can be underestimated because of failure to recognize subtle signs of seizure, including small-amplitude twitching or nystagmoid eye movements.

Non-convulsive status. There is altered mental status, with slow mentation, confusion, unresponsiveness, gross abnormal motor movements, twitches, lip smacking, mimicry, or automatisms. An EEG can confirm the diagnosis and should be obtained if non-convulsive status is suspected.

Epilepsy. This is a condition of susceptibility to recurrent seizures (commonly defined as two or more unprovoked seizures).

Post-ictal state. This is the period following a seizure, which may include confusion, lethargy, fatigue, irritability, headache, vomiting, or muscle soreness.

Seizures can also be classified as provoked or unprovoked, depending on whether there are clear inciting factors (such as fever, CNS infection, acute metabolic disturbances, and toxins). This chapter will review the differential diagnosis for seizures, common etiologies, the approach to the child who is seizing, and lastly will discuss special populations, such as children with febrile seizures and epileptic syndromes.

Pathophysiology

Pediatric patients are particularly vulnerable to seizures because in the young immature nervous system excitatory neurons tend to dominate the underdeveloped inhibitory system. During a seizure, the brain experiences increased blood flow, increased oxygen and glucose consumption, and increased carbon dioxide and lactic acid production. Prolonged seizures can lead to anoxic brain injury and ventilatory failure, causing hypoxia, hypercarbia, and respiratory acidosis, in addition to the risk of aspiration in patients with decreased level of consciousness. Prolonged skeletal muscle activity can lead to lactic acidosis, rhabdomyolysis, hyperkalemia, hyperthermia, and hypoglycemia.

Differential diagnosis

A seizure should not be viewed as a diagnosis, but rather as a symptom of an underlying pathologic process. Table 116.1 lists major secondary causes of seizures in children.

Many serious conditions may mimic seizures in their presentation. The following conditions comprise the differential diagnosis of seizures.

Psychogenic seizure. This is a movement disorder resembling seizures but with normal brain activity. Usually there is no associated biting, incontinence, or injury. This diagnosis is not commonly made in the ED setting – rather a neurologist will make this diagnosis after further workup usually including EEG monitoring.

A Practical Guide to Pediatric Emergency Medicine: Caring for Children in the Emergency Department, ed. N. Ewen Amieva-Wang (associate eds. Jamie Shandro, Aparajita Sohoni, and Bernhard Fassl). Published by Cambridge University Press.

Head trauma. Patients may experience a loss of consciousness following a head trauma with or without seizure activity (Ch. 143). Post-traumatic seizures should be considered in a patient with head trauma and a history consistent with a seizure. Impact seizures occur within 1 to 2 h of the trauma and are not an independent factor in predicting the severity of injury.

Syncope. Commonly confused for a seizure, syncope is a transient loss of consciousness resulting from inadequate cerebral perfusion or substrate delivery (Ch. 19). Some patients with true syncope will also exhibit convulsive activity, which can complicate the diagnosis. A prodrome of lightheadedness or diaphoresis should point the clinician towards a diagnosis of syncope. Patients with syncope do not exhibit post-ictal confusion.

Sleep disorders. Nightmares, night terrors, narcolepsy, sleep apne, hypersomnia, or somnambulism can be confused for seizures.

Atypical migraines. Migraines that are accompanied by an aura, motor dysfunction, clouding of consciousness, nausea, or vomiting can mimic seizures.

Movement disorders. Tics are rapid, repetitive, brief, involuntary movements that occur intermittently and in flurries. Patients do not lose consciousness. Shudder attacks usually occur in infants and are uncommon but can be mistaken for seizures and resemble a "sudden chill."

Psychiatric disorders. Day dreaming, attention-deficit hyperactivity disorder, or panic attacks all could be mistaken for seizures.

Gastrointestinal disorder. Sandifer syndrome is torticollis or dystonic posturing associated with gastroesophageal reflux disease. Infants will present with abnormal posturing, arching of the back, retrocollis, and torticollis.

Breath-holding spells. Up to 5% of children will have breath-holding episodes at some point in early childhood. These episodes typically present between ages 6 and 18 months and disappear by age 5 years. Episodes are triggered by pain or emotional upset that leads to crying. The child holds their breath during expiration and becomes either cyanotic or pallid. This can progress to loss of consciousness and could involve a brief period of clonic movements. The entire episode lasts less than a minute.

Apparent life-threatening event. This is any episode that frightens an infant's caregiver. Typically the events involve apnea, color change, marked change in muscle tone, or choking and gagging.

Arrhythmia. Abnormal heart rhythms can produce changes in respiratory pattern resulting in hypoxia and leading to seizure-like movements. If considered, obtain an ECG.

Table 116.1. Etiology of seizures in children

Etiology	Causes
Infections	Brain abscess, encephalitis, febrile seizure, meningitis, parasitic infection of CNS such as cysticercosis, syphilis
Toxicologic	Overdoses, including isoniazid, insulin, tricyclic antidepressants, others to (Chs. 138–140)
Hypoxic–ischemic injury	Drowning injuries, apparent life threatening events
Metabolic	Hypoglycemia, hyponatremia, other metabolic disorders
Oncologic	Primary brain tumor, metastatic disease
Endocrine	Addison's disease, hyperthyroidism, hypothyroidism
Obstetric	Eclampsia
Traumatic	Cerebral contusion, diffuse axonal injury, intracranial hemorrhage

Clinical presentation

History

Most seizures will have stopped prior to arrival in the ED, making the history and physical examination critical in determining diagnosis and management. Key aspects of the history include the events that led up to the seizure, the seizure itself, and the events directly afterwards.

Before the seizure. What was the patient doing preceding the possible seizure? Had the patient been ill recently? Any preceding trauma? Any potential toxin exposure? Any fever or systemic signs of illness? Any relevant medical history/developmental history/social history/travel history/family history of seizures? Was there an aura leading up to the convulsion? Did the patient complain of dizziness, an unusual odor, flashing lights? Did it start abruptly?

During the seizure. Was there loss of consciousness/awareness, tongue biting, or incontinence? Did the event involve the whole body or only part of the body? How long did the event last? Did the patient go stiff or limp? Did the patient shake? Were there different manifestations on one side of the body than the other? Did the eyes or head turn in one direction?

After the seizure. How did the patient behave after the event was over? Was the patient lethargic or confused? Did the patient complain of anything? Did the patient remember the event? Was there any focal or unilateral weakness (post-ictal Todd's paralysis).

The patient should be assessed for risk factors of epilepsy such as a history of meningitis, head injury, febrile seizures, congenital abnormalities, developmental delay, or a family history of epilepsy. Also any prior history of abnormal movements and/or seizure or epilepsy can be useful. Consider toxic ingestions and take a careful history from available caregivers to learn about possible accidental ingestions or toxin exposures.

Physical examination

As with any ED patient, it is important to obtain five vital signs. Examine the entire body, particularly the head for any evidence of trauma. Consider measuring head circumference in neonatal patients. Examine the skin for any rashes or congenital skin lesions, dysmorphic features sych as café au lait spots, or hypopigmented nevi. Examine the pupils, tympanic membranes (hemotympanum), and mouth for evidence of tongue biting. Examine the neck for evidence of meningeal irritation. Examine the chest, lungs, abdomen, and extremities. Complete neurologic examination should be performed. If the patient is post-ictal, neurologic examination should be performed frequently until the patient is back to baseline. Consider possible toxidromes while examining the patient.

The patient should also be examined for any injuries sustained during the seizure. This can be helpful both in addressing issues that may require additional medical attention (such as shoulder dislocation, wounds) and also in obtaining further evidence that the episode in question was a seizure.

Management

The ED approach to the actively seizing patient begins with management of the ABCs. Special considerations in the seizing patient include performing a focused neurologic examination prior to intubation, if possible. Paralytic and sedating agents should be short-acting, in order to avoid masking persistent seizure activity. The patient should, of course, be placed on a cardiac monitor with good IV access given the autonomic instability that can result from seizure activity. After securing the ABCs, the focus should shift to stopping the seizure and preventing neurologic damage. Anticonvulsant medications are recommended for any patient who has been seizing for more than 10 min. Benzodiazapines are standard medications to use initially with a seizing patient. If long-acting antiepileptics are needed, fosphenytoin or phenytoin are first line for pediatric seizures in the ED. Phenobarbital is used rarely, and usually only in newborns (Fig. 116.1).

MANAGEMENT OF SEIZURES

Lorazepam 0.05–0.1 mg/kg IM or IV, may repeat twice

If no IV access may also consider diazepam PR 0.5 mg/kg

(If the rectal preparation of diazepam is unavailable, the IV preparation can be inserted into the rectum through a lubricated feeding tube)

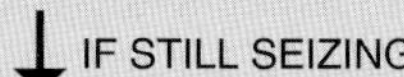

IF STILL SEIZING

Fosphenytoin 10–20 mg/kg at a rate of less than 1 mg/kg per min (can be given IM if no IV access, unlike phenytoin which can be given IV or PO). Cardiovascular monitoring must be maintained during phosphenytoin infusion. If hypotension occurs, the rate of infusion should be decreased

Consider IV valproate in patients in status epilepticus who are currently on valproate and have low levels: 10mg/kg IV can be given in subtherapeutic patients

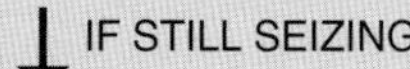

IF STILL SEIZING

Phenobarbital 10–20 mg/kg (causes respiratory depression, prepare to secure airway if patient not already intubated)

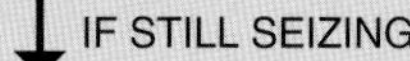

IF STILL SEIZING

- Consider other causes of seizure
- Consider pyridoxine deficiency in infant with refractory seizures
- Check glucose and electrolytes?
- Repeat history and physical – vital signs/toxidromes/rash/evidence of trauma/ history of ingestions

↓ ONCE SEIZURE HAS STOPPED

- Continue to re-evaluate for return of normal neurologic function
- If child fails to arouse after 30 min consider non-convulsive status epilepticus

Figure 116.1 Initial management of seizure.

Box 116.1. Assessment of patients with seizure

1. Check a glucose level in all seizing patients.
2. Seizure in setting of fever, consider meningitis/encephalitis/abscess as possible etiology. Follow guidelines regarding evaluation of fever and seizure in children.
3. Any patient with persistent abnormal mental status 30–60 min after the seizure requires a lumbar puncture to evaluate for meningitis, regardless of whether there is a fever:
   - in patients <12 months of age, clinical signs of meningitis can be subtle, so the threshold for performing a lumbar puncture should be low
   - antibiotics and antivirals (if appropriate) should not be delayed if lumbar puncture cannot be performed in timely fashion.
4. Check serum electrolytes in patients
   - with significant vomiting or diarrhea
   - with underlying renal, hepatic, neoplastic or endocrinologic disease
   - taking medications that may cause electrolyte disturbances
   - who are having refractory seizures: note that diluted formula can lead to hyponatremia and seizures in infants.
5. Consider checking magnesium level, hepatic transaminases, ammonia level, specific toxicology tests depending on history and physical examination.
6. Head CT should be obtained in following clinical scenarios
   - suspected increased intracranial pressure
   - focal seizure or secondarily generalized seizure
   - focal neurologic deficit
   - seizure following head trauma
   - persistent seizure activity
   - ill-appearing patient.
7. Check anticonvulsant levels if the patient is taking these medications. While these results are usually not available immediately, the results will aid in determining an etiology for the seizure, and guide further medication adjustments.
8. In a seizure following a traumatic event, in-line cervical spine stabilization should be maintained and Advanced Trauma Life Support guidelines should be followed.
9. In a patient with refractory seizures who is intubated and paralyzed, EEG monitoring should be obtained expeditiously to evaluate for continued seizure activity masked by the paralytic agent.

Once the patient is no longer seizing, use the guidelines in Box 116.1 to avoid missing a critical diagnosis, such as hypoglycemia, that may have caused the seizure.

Special situations

Febrile seizures

Febrile seizures are the most common convulsive disorder of children, occurring in 2–5% of the population. These seizures typically occur in children between 6 months and 5 years of age and are associated with a temperature >38°C without evidence of intracranial infection or other defined causes or neurologic disease. The seizures are most commonly tonic–clonic but could be any type:

- simple febrile seizures last <15 min and do not recur within a 24 h period
- complex febrile seizures are prolonged, recur within 24 h, or are focal.

There is a strong familial association of febrile seizures, and febrile seizures recur in a third of all patients; however, the risk of epilepsy in patients with a history of febrile seizures is <5%.

In patients with a history consistent with *simple* febrile seizure, no stigmata of CNS infection and a normal neurologic examination, no further evaluation for the cause of seizure is necessary. The evaluation should focus on the potential cause of the fever. A febrile seizure is *not* associated with an increased risk of occult bacteremia. No further treatment is recommended. Antipyretic drugs can be used to treat the fever but there is no evidence that they decrease the risk of febrile seizure. In complex febrile seizure (seizures may be focal, prolonged [>15 min], or recurrent during a single febrile illness), further neurological evaluations may be indicated.

The AAP recommends strong consideration of lumbar puncture in infants younger than 12 months with first-time febrile seizures, because the clinical signs of meningitis may be subtle. In a child >18 months old with no clinical evidence of meningitis, a lumbar puncture is generally not indicated. Clinicians should be aware that recent antibiotic treatment can mask the clinical signs and symptoms of meningitis and should have a lower threshold to perform a lumbar puncture on children who have a febrile seizure while taking antibiotics.

If a child recovers quickly from the febrile seizure (simple or complex), and CNS infections have been excluded, the child may be sent home. If the seizure was complex, further neurologic consultation and neurodiagnostic tests can be done as an outpatient.

Epileptic syndromes

Epilepsy is a disease characterized by recurrent unprovoked seizures. Table 116.2 reviews some of the epileptic syndromes that are common or noteworthy. Chapter 163 discusses children with neurological impairment on multiple seizure medications. Neonatal seizures are described in Ch. 157.

Table 116.2. Epilepsy syndromes

Syndrome	Age	Signs/symptoms	Prognosis
Infantile spasm	0–12 months	Rapid, jackknife flexor or extensor spasms that appear in clusters; infants draw legs up and cry; often mistaken for colic	Two-thirds of children with infantile spasms have underlying CNS disorder
Lennox–Gastaut syndrome	Any	Mental retardation, multiple seizure types (often difficult to control) and classic EEG pattern	Poor
Childhood and juvenile absence epilepsy	4–12 years	Frequently recurrent absence seizures manifested by staring spells or periods of inattention; spike and wave EEG pattern is classic.	Seizures typically stop by or during adolescence
Benign Rolandic epilepsy of childhood	3–13 years	Partial seizures that classically occur while sleeping and involve face; has potential to generalize	Seizures typically stop around 16 years of age

EEG, electroencephalography.

Disposition

In most cases of children presenting to the ED with a seizure, hospitalization is unnecessary. The further evaluation of a first-time seizure in a child who is now neurologically normal can be done as an outpatient. Children with febrile seizures can be discharged home with appropriate return precautions. Some children will be admitted if adequate follow-up cannot be arranged or for other psychosocial reasons.

Children who have had a prolonged seizure, have an underlying cause such as a possible infection, or who display an abnormal neurologic examination or persistently have an ALOC should be admitted. Pediatric neurology should be consulted to guide further workup and management, such as the decision to start antiepileptic therapy. In general, children with the first onset of unprovoked seizures are not treated with antiepileptic medications. Neurologists recommend waiting for a second unprovoked seizure (thus declaring the diagnosis of epilepsy) before starting antiepileptic medications. The decision to start treament depends on the child's neurodevelopmental status and other epileptic syndrome considerations.

Children who have a seizure and are discharged should be instructed not to engage in activities where they would be in danger if they had a sudden loss of consciousness until cleared by their physician. Specifically, teenagers should not drive a car until cleared, and swimming should be avoided.

Pearls and pitfalls

Pearls

1. A simple febrile seizure is a generalized tonic–clonic seizure lasting <15 min occurring once in a 24-h period in a febrile child between the ages of 6 months and 6 years.
2. An IV formulation of diazepam can be given per rectum in seizing patients with no IV access.
3. Consider the possibility of non-accidental trauma in pediatric patients with head injury.

Pitfalls

1. Failure to check a fingerstick glucose early in the workup.
2. Failure to realize that both seizures and altered mental status can be subtle in patients under 1 year of age.
3. Failure to exclude CNS infection by lumbar puncture in any child <12 months old with a febrile seizure.

Selected references

Chiang VW. Seizures. In Fleisher GR, Ludwig S, Henretig EM (eds.) *Textbook of Pediatric Emergency Medicine*, 5th edn. Philadelphia, PA: Lippincott, Williams & Wilkins 2006, pp. 629–636.

Friedman MJ, Sharieff GQ. Seizures in children. *Pediatric Clin North Am* 2006;**23**:275–277.

Gorelick MH, Blackwell CD. Neurologic emergencies In Fleisher GR, Ludwig S, Henretig EM (eds.) *Textbook of Pediatric Emergency Medicine*, 5th edn. Philadelphia, PA: Lippincott, Williams & Wilkins 2006, pp. 759–766.

Rubin DH, Kornblau DH, Conway EE Jr., Caplen SM. Neurologic disorders In Marx J, Hockberger R, Walls R (eds.) *Rosen's Emergency Medicine: Concepts and Clinical Practice*, 6th edn. St. Louis, MO: Mosby Elsevier, 2006, pp. 2665–2676.

Chapter 117

Weakness

Beau Briese, Millicent Marmer, and N. Ewen Amieva-Wang

Introduction

Weakness is a symptom that is rare in children and has many etiologies. Children may not complain of weakness, and weakness may first manifest as not moving an extremity or a limp particularly in a preverbal child (Ch. 106). Theoretically, weakness can stem from pathology anywhere from the motor cortex to the myocyte. Cerebral pathology such as a cerebrovascular accident or hemorrhage is relatively rare in children and would manifest with symptoms in addition to weakness. A cerebrovascular accident (stroke) in a child should cause a clinician to consider underlying hematologic or immunologic disease (e.g., sickle cell anemia or lupus) or cerebral spread of infectious disease (e.g., tuberculosis, malaria). Spinal cord trauma and infection also should manifest with other history and findings in addition to weakness (Chs. 107 and 111).

A systematic history and physical examination is imperative to evaluate weakness, particularly to differentiate perceived weakness from immobility secondary to pain or injury. Systemic signs and symptoms can give clues to the etiology of weakness.

Neuropathies

Pathophysiology

In general, upper motor neuron (UMN) disease will present with increased deep tendon reflexes and motor spasticity secondary to a lack of UMN inhibition, although flaccid paralysis may occur early in the course of disease. Lower motor neuron (LMN) disease refers to pathology anywhere from the anterior horn cells of the spinal cord, through the peripheral nerves to the neuromuscular junction (NMJ). Specific symptoms depend on the location of the lesion. In general, LMN disease causes hyporeflexia, fasciculations, atrophy, weakness, and hypotonia.

Differential diagnosis

Patients will most likely present to the ED for acute and subacute weakness rather than chronic progressive weakness disorders.

Transverse myelitis. This is an UMN disease, with acute demylination of the spinal cord. The etiology is thought to be immune or post-infectious. Patients can have fever and back pain at the affected level, followed by paresthesiae and weakness. On examination, patients have bilateral but not necessarily symmetric weakness, sensory loss (usually at the thoracic level), increased or decreased reflexes, and bowel and bladder incontinence. Workup must include MRI to rule out cord compression from tumor or epidural abscesses. In children, MRI with gadolinium often shows T_2 hyperintensities with variable enhancement over several spinal segments.

Anterior horn disease. This causes LMN symptoms. Sensation should be relatively unaffected. Reflexes are lost early. The patient develops muscle atrophy and fasciculations.

Polio. Poliovirus is a neurotropic enterovirus that lives in the GI tract. It destroys the motor neurons in the spinal cord and brainstem. Patients can have preceding "viral" gastroenteritis symptoms. Often they have pain prior to weakness and paralysis. Weakness can affect the muscles of respiration. In the extremities, weakness is often asymmetrical. Polio has been eradicated from the most of the world by vaccine.

Spinal muscular atrophy. This is an autosomal recessive disease of the LMNs located in the anterior horns. It causes muscle denervation, atrophy, and progressive weakness. Three phenotypes (types I–III) are recognized. Type III, the mildest form of disease, can present during childhood or adolescence.

A Practical Guide to Pediatric Emergency Medicine: Caring for Children in the Emergency Department, ed. N. Ewen Amieva-Wang (associate eds. Jamie Shandro, Aparajita Sohoni, and Bernhard Fassl). Published by Cambridge University Press.

Guillain–Barré syndrome. This acute demyelinating polyradiculoneuropathy is a post-infectious immune disorder. (Epstein–Barr virus, CMV, HIV and varicella have been associated with its development.) Patients can have preceding pain before weakness. Weakness begins in the lower extremities and progressively involves the trunk, upper limbs, and finally bulbar muscles (ascending paralysis). Respiratory insufficiency may occur. Deep tendon reflexes are lost, usually early in the course. Patients can have sensory symptoms including "pins and needles" and loss of sensation. Autonomic nerves may also be involved, resulting in blood pressure and cardiac rate instability. Classically, protein is elevated in CSF to more than 2× ULN, without elevated WBC. Motor nerve conduction velocities are greatly reduced and electromyography may show evidence of acute denervation. Because of potential rapid progression of weakness to respiratory failure, patients with suspected Guillain–Barré syndrome should be admitted for evaluation and treatment. Treatments include respiratory support, and plasma exchange or IV gammaglobulin. The Miller–Fisher variant presents classically with ataxia, areflexia, and opthalmoplegia.

Neuropathy. Heavy metals are neuropathic. Lead poisoning is the most common cause by far in children and can cause distal motor weakness with foot and wrist drop (Ch. 140).

Neuromuscular junction disease. This affects motor, including cranial nerves and autonomic function. Sensory nerves should not be affected.

Myasthenia gravis. This is an autoimmune disorder of the acetylecholine receptor that can affect children. Children may present with ophthalmoplegia (diplopia), bulbar weakness, and generalized weakness. The symptoms may fluctate and show signs of fatigability.

Infantile botulism. This can result in bulbar weakness (poor feeding), ptosis, and descending weakness into the trunk and limbs. Large, sluggishly reactive pupils may be present. Infantile botulism is caused by ingestion of botulinum spores, which then elaborate the botulinum neurotoxin in the GI tract of the infant. Diagnosis is made by clinical history and examination and is supported by toxin assay in stool. Infants suspected of having infantile botulism should be admitted due to potential for respiratory failure (Ch. 91).

Tick paralysis. Neurotoxins in the tick saliva act at the NMJ, mimicking the symptoms of Guillain–Barré syndrome. Recognition of the disorder and prompt removal of the tick is required for treatment.

Myopathies

The myopathies are disorders of muscle. Sensation should be normal and weakness usually starts in the larger muscle groups: usually lower extremities are affected before upper extremities and proximal muscles before distal.

In the muscular dystrophies, a group of inherited defects of muscle proteins, there is progressive skeletal muscle weakness and muscle cell death. In Duchenne's muscular dystrophy, patients present before 5 years of age with gait disturbances and history of falling. Becker's muscular dystrophy has a later onset with less morbidity.

In the ED, patients will largely present with subacute or acute myopathies such as inflammatory myositis, toxin-induced myopathy, and periodic paralysis.

Viral myositis. This is a more common cause of muscular pain and weakness in children. Symptoms follow a viral-like syndrome. On examination, muscles are painful and creatine phosphokinase can be elevated. Note that myositis often causes increased muscular pain rather than weakness. However, children may refuse to walk because of pain and will be presumed to be weak.

Toxin-induced myopathy. Steroids can cause a myopathy 3–14 days after medications are initiated.

Metabolic/endocrine causes. Pathology such as hyponatremia and inborn errors of metabolism can cause symmetric weakness in children.

Periodic paralysis. The periodic paralyses are a group of rare disorders with recurrent episodes of muscle weakness that resolve after hours to days. The hypokalemic periodic paralyses are the most common subset. These classically manifest as a flaccid paralysis occurring at night in young Asian males; the hypokalemia results from intracellular shifts of potassium into cells. Hypokalemic periodic paralysis is associated with hyperthyroid states.

Facial weakness. Specific facial weakness can be caused by central or peripheral disease of cranial nerve VII. Peripheral facial palsies can be caused by Lyme disease (Ch. 90) as well as Bell's palsy (as in adults). Central facial palsies are caused by contralateral CNS disease and are very uncommon in children. On examination, central lesions do not affect the forehead; peripheral facial nerve lesions affect the lower and upper face. Infant botulism must be considered in the infant with decreased facial movements or expression.

Management and disposition

Management in the ED should first focus on acute signs and symptoms. Decreased respiratory ability must be managed expediently. If neuromuscular pathology is considered, intubation should not be performed with succinylcholine. Basic electrolyte panel including calcium, and creatine phosphokinase should be obtained. Diagnostic tests should be based on clinical suspicion. If there is a suspected spinal cord lesion, MRI should be obtained.

A child should be admitted if she or he is likely to develop respiratory failure from progressive weakness.

Treatment is guided by the definitive diagnosis, which may be finally confirmed during the child's admission. Consultation with the pediatric neurologist can be invaluable in generating the differential, conducting the workup, recommending imaging, and disposition and follow-up in the unusual case of pediatric weakness. Patients unable to walk or with progressive symptoms should be admitted for monitoring and workup.

Pearls and pitfalls

Pearls

1. Weakness may manifest differently based on the child's age and developmental stage.
2. Weakness and pain may be confused. A child may not move a limb secondary to pain.
3. Reflex testing can help to localize the lesion. Reflexes are generally absent in lower motor neuron lesions, and increased in upper.

Pitfalls

1. Failure to anticipate respiratory distress in a child with acute weakness.
2. Failure to avoid succinylcholine (suxamethonium) if a child has respiratory failure and chronic neuromuscular disease.

Selected reference

Tsarouhas N, Decker JM. Weakness. In Fleisher GR, Ludwig S, Henretig FM (eds.) *Textbook of Pediatric Emergency Medicine*, 5th edn. Philadelphia, PA: Lippincott, Williams & Wilkins 2006 pp. 691–700.

Section

17

Ophthalmology

Chapter

118 Approach to the emergency pediatric eye examination

Douglas Fredrick

Introduction

The pediatric and adult ophthalmologic examinations are similar, with the pediatric examination often complicated by a child's inability to fully explain symptoms or cooperate with all aspects of the examination. As in all patients with eye complaints, the pediatric eye examination should systematically evaluate visual acuity/fields, the external eye, extraocular muscles, pupillary response, cornea, and anterior and posterior chambers. This chapter will review eye anatomy followed by a discussion of the standard physical examination of the eye, with age-appropriate tips and adjustments. The newborn eye examination is discussed in Ch. 155.

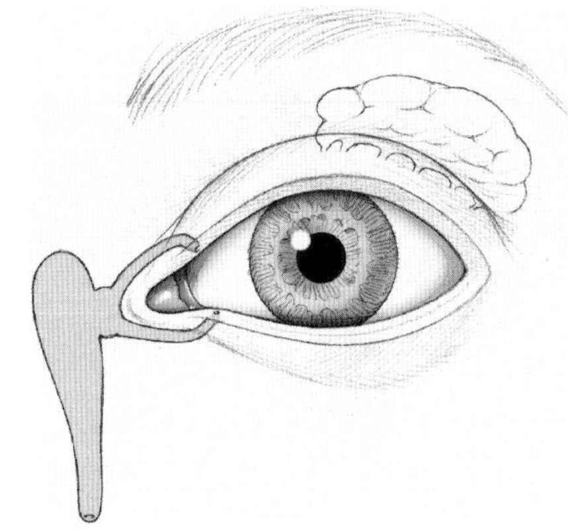

Figure 118.1 Anterior view of the eye and adnexal structures. The lacrimal gland is situated supertemporally. The superior and inferior puncta drain into the canalicular system, which eventually empties into the nasal cavity. (Copyright Chris Gralapp; reproduced with permission from Mahadevan SV, Garmel GM. *An Introduction to Clinical Emergency Medicine*. Cambridge, UK: Cambridge University Press, 2005.)

Anatomy of the eye

The orbit is composed of seven facial bones: the frontal, zygomatic, maxillary, ethmoid, lacrimal, sphenoid, and palatine bone. The eyeball is located in the orbit. The lacrimal gland is located on the superior temporal portion of the orbit. Accessory lacrimal glands are also located within the conjunctiva of the adnexal tissues. Tears are secreted and wash over the front of the eye, from where they drain through the puncta in the eyelid via the canalicular system to the nasolacrimal sac. The nasolacrimal duct drains the sac and passes through the nasal structures to empty underneath the inferior turbinate (Fig. 118.1).

The conjunctiva is the most superficial layer of the eye. It is an epithelium that contains mucus-secreting cells. The bulbar conjunctiva covers the eyeball; the palpebral conjunctiva covers the posterior aspect of the eyelids. Since the conjunctiva is a contiguous structure, foreign bodies cannot pass behind the eye unless there is a laceration or trauma to the conjunctival tissues. The cornea lies under the conjunctiva in the front of the eye, while the sclera, a dense tough collagenous membrane that is a derivative from dura mater, covers the posterior part of the eyeball. The iris is the colored part of the eye and separates the anterior and posterior chambers. Immediately behind the iris are the ciliary processes and ciliary body, an epithelial tissue that secretes aqueous humor. The aqueous humor passes through the pupil and is drained out of the eye at the trabecular meshwork (Fig. 118.2). The focus of the crystalline lens can be adjusted by constriction of the ciliary muscle to allow focus on near and far objects; this facility is gradually lost after around 40 years of age. Immediately behind the lens is the vitreous humor, which in young children is very viscous; it loses this viscosity with aging. The retina is the

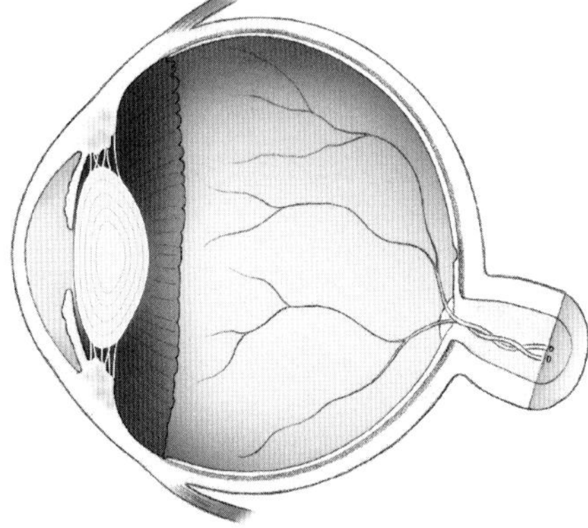

Figure 118.2 The globe in cross-section. The iris diaphragm outlines the margins of the pupil. The anterior surface of the lens abuts the posterior surface of the iris. Zonular suspensory fibers are seen emanating from the ciliary body adjacent to the iris root. (Copyright Chris Gralapp; reproduced with permission from Mahadevan SV, Garmel GM. *An Introduction to Clinical Emergency Medicine*. Cambridge, UK: Cambridge University Press, 2005.)

A Practical Guide to Pediatric Emergency Medicine: Caring for Children in the Emergency Department, ed. N. Ewen Amieva-Wang (associate eds. Jamie Shandro, Aparajita Sohoni, and Bernhard Fassl). Published by Cambridge University Press.

multilayered neural lining of the eye, which is responsible for converting light energy into electrical activity.

The cranial nerves as well as the sympathetic chain innervate the eye. While pathology can occur anywhere between the cortex and the eye structures themselves, the EP must be able to develop a pragmatic differential diagnosis of neuroocular findings in a child to guide the workup and treatment.

Clinical examination

Examination of the eye in the newborn is covered in Ch. 155.

Physical examination

If a child has pain and photophobia, and suspicion for a penetrating ocular injury is low, a drop of proparicaine or tetracaine will provide immediate relief of pain secondary to a corneal abrasion. This will facilitate a thorough ophthalmic examination and gain the child's confidence.

When dealing with children, the first look at the eye will be the best chance to obtain useful information.

Avoid multiple examinations and use distracting techniques such as videos or toys to allow an examination. Prying open the lids should only be done when all else fails, as this will make subsequent examinations very difficult.

Visual acuity

Visual acuity in children changes with growth (Table 118.1). Once a child becomes verbal and literate, the use of the standard Snellen chart is the gold standard in assessing visual acuity. However a variety of alternative symbols have been devised for the verbal but preliterate child. It is imperative to test both eyes together followed by each eye separately. Shy children who do not want to speak can use a response card placed in their lap to point to the object they see. Refractive errors such as myopia or near sightedness will present with decreased visual acuity at distance but normal visual acuity when using the pocket screening card or a pinhole. However children who have visual impediments such as cataracts or retinal abnormalities will show no improvement when a pinhole is placed in front of the affected eye.

Table 118.1. Age-based visual milestones

Age	Visual acuity
Birth/infancy	20/2000
6 months	20/80
4 years	20/40
6 years	20/20

Visual field assessment

Visual field testing is done to detect gross neurologic disorders such as hemianopia. The most important prerequisite for visual field assessment is that the child be able to maintain fixation for a brief period of time. For this reason, two examiners are often necessary to assess a child. One examiner will get the child's attention by making an entertaining noise or motion in front of the child. The second examiner will introduce a brightly colored toy or object with no audible cue from behind the patient into the child's peripheral vision. Eye movement on seeing the toy will indicate the extent of the peripheral visual field. This can be repeated in the four quadrants with both eyes and individually. In older children, visual fields can be tested in the standard fashion, covering each eye independently and presenting either one, two, or five fingers in each of the four visual quadrants. The extent of the peripheral visual field can be assessed by gradually moving a finger in from the peripheral field and asking the child to indicate when they see the object of regard.

External eye examination

In the absence of trauma, the two most commonly presenting signs of disease involving the external orbit are ptosis and proptosis.

Ptosis and proptosis are most often unilateral and the asymmetry will be apparent. Ptosis can be quantified by two simple techniques: First, as the child looks straight ahead, the distance between the upper eyelid and the lower eyelid (palpebral fissure) is measured with a ruler. The examiner should note whether there seems to be restriction or impediment of elevation of the eyelid as the patient goes from a down-gaze position to an up-gaze position.

Proptosis occurs when there is forward displacement of the globe as a result of inflammation, mass effect, or vascular congestion. The easiest way to assess for proptosis is to assess the amount of protrusion of the two eyes while standing behind and over the child. Proptosis of subtle degrees can easily be detected as the bulging eye will be more prominent as it clears the superior orbital rim.

Motility examination

Abnormalities of eye movement are common signs of underlying neurologic abnormality. The two components of the ocular motility examination are the assessment of eye movement and the assessment of the alignment of the eye. Movements are easily assessed by having the child fixate on an object of interest and testing them in all fields of gaze: elevation, depression, right gaze, left gaze, straight ahead, and near. The eye movements should be full and not restricted. Verbal children who have acute onset of restriction of eye movements may report double vision in certain fields of gaze, and it is important to specifically test the eye movements in these positions. Failure to move the eye into a desired field of gaze can indicate either paralysis or restriction.

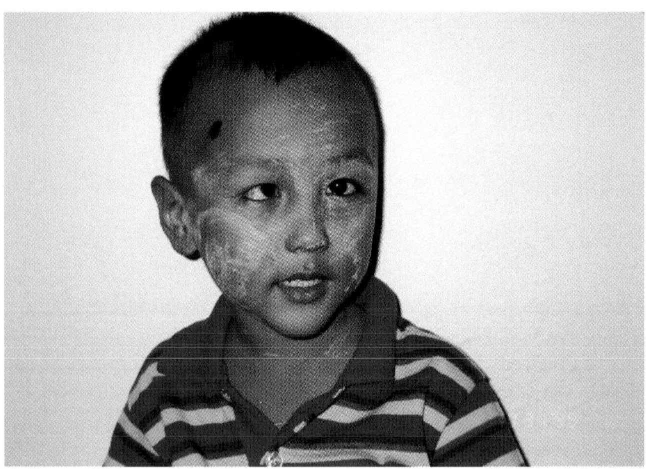

Figure 118.3 Esotropia of the right eye. (Courtesy of D. Fredrick.)

The second component, ocular alignment, is examined by an alternate cover test. Here again fixation is important. With a child fixating at an object of distance, an examiner occludes first the right eye and then the left eye in an alternating, repeating fashion. Children with aligned eyes show little movement of the eyes as the hand is alternated between the two eyes. Children who have an esotropia or inward deviation of the eyes will manifest an outward movement of the eyes as the hand is moved back and forth in front of the eyes (Fig. 118.3). In contrast, children with an exotropia or outward deviation of the eyes will manifest an inward movement of the eyes as the uncovered eye will move to pick up fixation. Finally, patients with a vertical deviation will elicit either downward or upward movement of the eyes as the eyes move back and forth. Simply by identifying whether the primary deviation is inward (esotropia), outward (exotropia), or vertical (hypertropia) will allow an appropriate differential diagnosis to be made.

Pupil examination

As with the visual field examination, the pupil examination requires the child to have steady fixation. Often a second examiner, a video monitor, or cooperative sibling can amuse the child as the examination light is used to look for both direct pupillary response to light and consensual response to light. To test for an afferent pupil defect, the swinging flashlight test is used. Fixation is maintained as the examiner swings the penlight back and forth rhythmically to alternately illuminate the two pupils (Fig. 118.4). A normal response is constriction to light on both sides. An abnormal result is when swinging the flashlight from the sound eye to the eye with suspected pathology yields a pupil that dilates rather than constricts. This indicates that the eye is receiving less visual input or afferant input than the fellow eye, which results in less pupillary constriction response. This finding is most commonly seen with injury to the optic nerve.

MARCUS GUNN PUPIL

To perform test:
Shine a bright light into each pupil for about 3–4 s. Alternate back and forth. Look for pupil to dilate, instead of constrict, with light

Left eye has decreased vision due to retinal lesion or optic nerve lesion

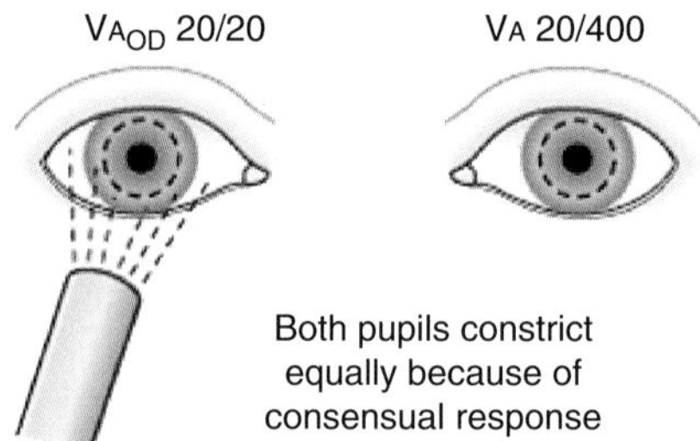

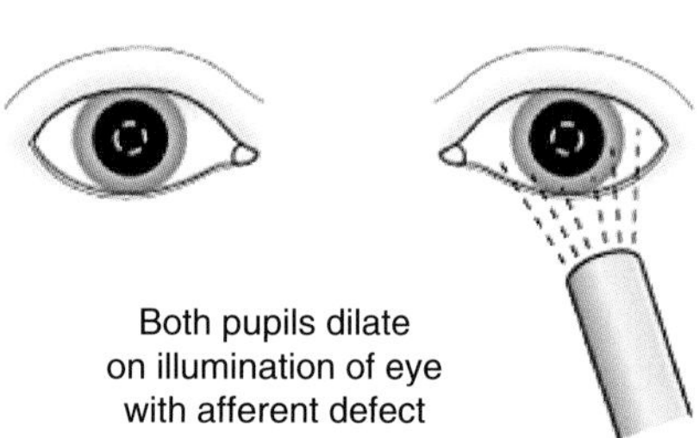

Both pupils dilate on illumination of eye with afferent defect

Figure 118.4 Afferent pupillary defect/Marcus Gunn pupil. (With permission from Zitelli BJ, Davis HW. *Atlas of Pediatric Physical Diagnosis,* 5th edn. Philadelphia, PA: Mosby Elsevier, 2007. © 2007 Mosby Inc., an affiliate of Elsevier Inc.)

Slit lamp examination

If a slit lamp is not available, a direct ophthalmoscope can be used in its place as the direct ophthalmoscope has a +20 diopter magnifying lens, which provides high magnification of the eye. When using a slit lamp on a young child, have the child sit on the parent's lap, then first demonstrate on the parent to allay the child's fears. A cellphone or gameplayer held next to the examiner's ear by an assistant will distract the child while you examine the eyes. Whether using a slit lamp or a direct ophthalmoscope, it is important to examine the surface of the eye systematically. Examine first the eyelids and eyelashes, looking for evidence of infection, laceration, or erythema. Both the bulbar and the palpebral conjunctival surface should be examined carefully. The cornea should be examined using a slit lamp to detect a corneal abrasion, corneal foreign body, or corneal laceration. The diagnosis of corneal abrasion can be facilitated by instilling fluorescein solution into the eye. An epithelial defect will illuminate brightly with a cobalt blue filter. With experience, it can also be used to identify inflammation within the aqueous humor, allowing a diagnosis of iritis. By narrowing the beam to a small spot, the floating white blood cells can be seen like specks of dust floating within the eye.

Direct ophthalmoscope

Once again, maintained fixation will greatly aid the examination of a child using a direct ophthalmoscope. Many EDs now keep a portable DVD player in the unit – this often distracts the child while the eye examination is conducted. For infants, the best time to examine them is when nursing or taking a bottle. Using an interesting fixation target, the examiner approaches the child from a 30 degree angle, placing the examiner's thumb on the child's brow and slowly moving in towards the child's face. If fixation is maintained, this will afford a view of the optic nerve and blood vessels.

If ophthalmic or neurologic consultation is not available and the presence of papilledema will change the course of therapy, then the child's eye can be dilated with tropicamide 1% ophthalmic solution. It should be kept in mind that the pupil will be dilated and unresponsive for 3 to 4 h; failure to notify other practitioners of pharmaceutical pupillary dilatation can lead to erroneous diagnoses.

Conclusions

To summarize, a few generalizations may be made in regard to the pediatric ophthalmic examination. It is important to note that the visual acuity is a subjective response. It can be greatly affected by anxiety, pain, parental expectations, and cognitive impairment. Therefore, the EP must feel comfortable about their ability to perform an eye examination on the young child. If a thorough examination of visual acuity, pupillary response, and cornea is performed, the chance of missing a serious diagnosis is low.

Chapter 119

Ophthalmic emergencies

Douglas Fredrick

Introduction

Pediatric ocular complaints presenting to the ED can be divided into three groups:

- acute disease processes affecting the eye
- ocular signs of underlying neurologic or systemic disease
- disorders of vision.

This chapter will discuss mainly acute disease processes affecting the eye, including red eye, inflammation about the eye, and eye trauma (Table 119.1). While disorders of vision will be discussed briefly, isolated acute loss of vision is rare in children. The most common causes of vision loss in children are refractive error and amblyopia, which occur in a chronic state but may present in an acute fashion.

Table 119.1. Summary of ophthalmic emergencies

Condition	What to do/rule out	How to treat
Conjunctivitis	R/o herpes and iritis, gonorrhea and chlamydia in neonates	Broad-spectrum topical antibiotics TID for 7 days
Corneal abrasion	R/o perforation or corneal ulcer	Antibiotic ointment, may use tight patch for large abrasion, recheck in 24 h
Hyphema	Sickle cell, glaucoma, ruptured globe	Cycloplegic (atropine), topical steroids, bed rest, eye shield
Blow-out fracture	Protect eye with eye shield; obtain orbital CT with 1.5 mm cuts; treat nausea	Ophthalmic referral, urgent if eye restriction
Chemical burn	Irrigate, check pH	Ophthalmic referral
Ocular perforation/ laceration	Nil by mouth; orbital CT to R/o intraocular foreign body; give eye shield, antibiotics	Prepare for surgery, ophthalmic referral
Vision loss	Eye examination, look for neurologic disease, visualize; the optic nerve obtain neuroimage for papilledema and optic atrophy	Close ophthalmic and neurologic follow-up

R/o, rule out.

Nasolacrimal duct obstruction

Tears are formed in the lacrimal gland, bathe the surface of the eye and are drained into the inferior and superior punctia of the eyelids. When there is obstruction of the distal end of the nasolacrimal duct, as occurs in 10% of all newborns, the infant will present with epiphora, a watery eye that is often accompanied by mucoid discharge. The discharge often seals the eye shut in the morning, and when cleared by cleansing, is replaced by tearing that persists for days and weeks. The conjunctiva will not be red, an important differentiating point that separates this condition from conjunctivitis. Oftentimes the skin around the lower eyelid will be red and macerated from the chronic moistness, but the lids will not be tender or swollen. Diagnosis will be confirmed by gently pressing on the lacrimal sac, which will cause mucoid or clear discharge to come from the lacrimal sac through the inferior puncta.

A rare but dangerous condition that can be mistaken with congenital nasolacrimal duct obstruction is **congenital glaucoma**. These infants also have epiphora but never have mucoid discharge, and they will frequently have enlarged corneas and symptoms of photophobia.

Treatment is symptomatic, as 50% of the obstructions will resolve spontaneously by 6 months of age, 90% by 1 year of age. Parents are instructed to instill erythromycin ophthalmic ointment into the eye before bedtime to control the discharge and help eyelid hygiene. Nasolacrimal sac massage (gently compressing the sac with the index finger stroking downward five strokes twice daily) will keep the sac decompressed and

A Practical Guide to Pediatric Emergency Medicine: Caring for Children in the Emergency Department, ed. N. Ewen Amieva-Wang (associate eds. Jamie Shandro, Aparajita Sohoni, and Bernhard Fassl). Published by Cambridge University Press.

Table 119.2. Differential diagnosis of red eye[a]

Diagnosis	Symptoms	Natural history	Recommended treatment
Viral Conjunctivitis	Watery discharge, concurrent upper respiratory tract infection, itching/preauricular adenopathy	Second eye less symptomatic than first, highly contagious, resolves in 5–7 days	Artificial tears, handwashing
Bacterial Conjunctivitis	Mucopurulent discharge	Resolves 5–7 days	Broad-spectrum topical antibiotic ointment or drops; erythromycin ointment (1.2 cm (½ inch) into affected eye twice a day for 7 days; polymyxin/trimethoprim ophthalmic solution 1 drop in affected eye QID for 7 days ; sulfacetamide 10% ophthalmic solution 1 drop in affected eye QID for 7 days
Herpetic conjunctivitis/ keratitis	Photophobia, watery discharge, foreign body sensation	Stain with fluorescein; if unrecognized lead to corneal scarring	Acyclovir 40–80 mg/kg daily in three divided doses; topical triflururidine 1 drop five times a day; ophthalmic referral
Allergic conjunctivitis	Allergic symptoms, chemosis, cobblestoning	Seasonal, will recur if trigger is repeated	Sodium cromolyn 4% 1 drop QID; olopatadine 1 drop each night for 2–3 weeks

[a]History of foreign body, trauma, contact lens should trigger suspicion of other disease processes.

help to prevent mucous from building up on the eyelids. Obstructions that fail to respond spontaneously can be treated by nasolacrimal duct probing performed using brief inhalation general anaesthesia at 1 year of age.

The red eye

Although a red eye in children is a common and usually benign eye condition, serious disease must be excluded (Table 119.2). Childcare facilities will often require proof of treatment before allowing a child with a red eye to return. All children with a red eye should have visual acuity checked as well as a thorough examination including fluorescein staining. While most therapy is outpatient and empiric with no need for cultures, ophthalmia neonatorum (Ch. 155) and herpetic conjunctivitis are notable exceptions.

Causes of red eye

Viral conjunctivitis

Viral conjunctivitis, also termed epidemic keratoconjunctivitis, is frequently caused by adenovirus. As adenovirus can survive on dry surfaces for hours, it is frequently associated with epidemics. Patients will complain of itchy eyes and present with a watery discharge and a mild amount of mucus. Often a concomitant upper respiratory tract infection is present. Viral conjunctivitis will often start in one eye and then spread to the other eye within a matter of days, with a far less severe course in the second eye. Multiple family members will often be infected at the same time.

On physical examination, a preauricular node ipsilateral to the affected eye may be palpated. Clinical examination is sufficient to make this diagnosis.

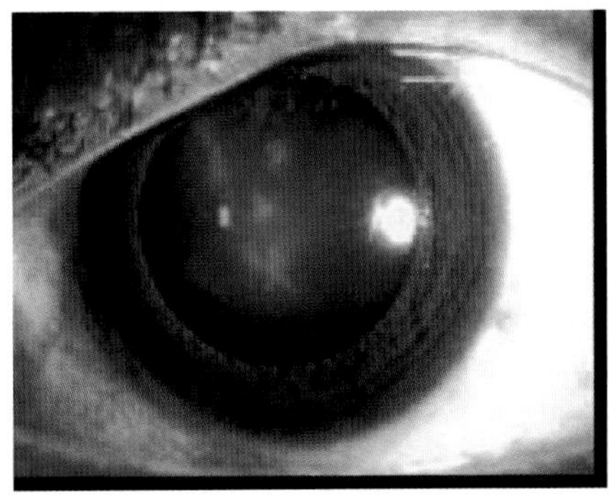

Figure 119.1 Herpetic keratitis with dendritic appearance of fluorescein stain. (Courtesy D. Fredrick.)

Treatment recommendations include careful hand washing, avoiding touching the eyes, and keeping the child away from other children while eye discharge is present. Artificial tears can provide symptomatic relief. Topical antibiotics are usually not indicated, but if there is concern for concurrent bacterial conjunctivitis, broad-spectrum antibiotics such as polymyxin/trimethoprim solution, sulfacetamide ophthalmic solution, or gentamicin ophthalmic solution may be used.

The preferred initial antibiotic eye solution is polymyxin/trimethoprim.

There is no evidence supporting the use of third-generation fluoroquinolones, as they are expensive and do not alter the course of the disease.

Herpetic keratoconjunctivitis

Patients often have presented to a primary care physician with a pink eye and will have completed a course of topical broad-spectrum antibiotics without resolution of their symptoms.

Table 119.3. Treatment of conjunctivitis

Antibiotic class	Antibiotic	Comments
Macrolides	Erythromycin effective against Gram-positive bacteria and atypical bacteria	Not toxic and well tolerated; penetration is poor and resistance increasing
Aminoglycosides: Gram-negative coverage with limited Gram-positive effect; increasing *Haemophilus influenzae* and pneumococcal resistance	Neomycin opthalmic drops	High incidence of allergic and hypersensitivity reactions
	Gentamicin	Can irritate conjunctiva and cornea
Sulfonamides	Sulfacetamide	Stings; requires frequent dosing; resistance increasing; associated with allergic reactions
Fluoroquinolones	Ciprofloxacin, ofloxacin	Second generation have good spectrum of activity but increasing resistance
Antibiotic combinations[a]	Trimethoprim sulfate and polymyxin B	Activity against Gram-positive and Gram-negative organisms

[a] Antibiotic corticosteroid combinations should not be used in the ED for presumptive bacterial conjunctivitis.

Herpetic keratoconjunctivitis is more common in children with atopy. Dendritic-appearance of fluorescein stain uptake can be readily diagnosed in the ED on macroscopic and the slit lamp examination (Fig. 119.1).

If diagnosed, prompt referral to an ophthalmologist is critical. Treatment involves the use of topical antiviral solution such as trifluoruridine or systemic antiviral agents such as oral acyclovir. Steroids should never be used in the ED. Complications of a delayed diagnosis result in corneal scarring and opacification.

Bacterial conjunctivitis

Bacterial conjunctivitis can result from infection with either Gram-positive (*Staphylococcus aureus* or *Streptococcus* spp.) or Gram-negative (*Haemophilus influenzae*) organisms. Common presenting complaints include a thick mucoid discharge, worse in the mornings, with an inability to open the eye upon awakening. Patients frequently deny concurrent upper respiratory tract complaints and are usually the only family member affected. However, epidemics of bacterial conjunctivitis have been reported.

Treatment is empiric and consists of broad-spectrum topical antibiotics, such as polymyxin/trimethoprim solution, erythromycin ointment, polymyxin bacitracin ophthalmic ointment, or sulfacetamide 10% applied four times daily for 7 days (Table 119.3). Children >1 year of age may not like blurred vision secondary to ointments. Decreased dosing frequency and number of drops increases compliance. While oral antibiotics can be used concurrently (e.g., to treat otitis media), topical antibiotics speed the resolution of symptoms secondary to a high concentration of drug at the site of infection.

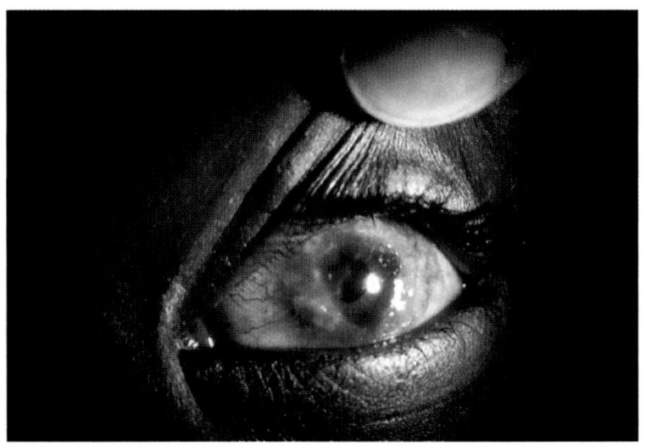

Figure 119.2 Limbal vernal conjunctivitis in atopic patient. (Courtesy D. Fredrick.)

Allergic conjunctivitis

Children with allergic conjunctivitis complain of itchy, watery eyes mainly during spring and fall months. These patients will often have a history of allergies as well as other allergic symptoms. On examination, the conjunctiva has limbal injection with gelatinous-appearing follicles near the corneal/sclera border, known as limbal vernal conjunctivitis (Fig. 119.2). The tarsal conjunctiva can have enlarged and erythematous papillae termed cobblestone papillae. The discharge from these folliciles is generally not sticky.

Treatment is symptomatic and consists of artificial tears and topical mast cell stabilizers. Topical NSAIDs have not been shown to improve symptoms and topical steroids should never be used in the ED.

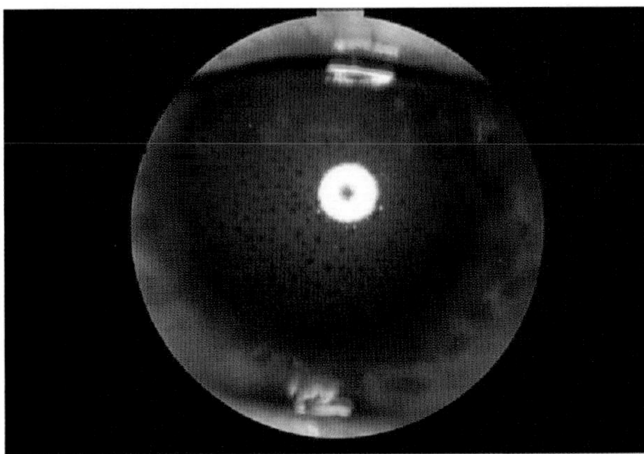

Figure 119.3 White blood cell aggregates called keratic precipitates in patient with iritis. (Courtesy D. Fredrick.)

Iritis

Iritis results from intraocular inflammation, which causes white blood cells to be liberated from vessels in the iris to circulate in the aqueous or vitreous humors (Fig. 119.3). This inflammation can lead to a red eye with symptoms of photophobia, pain, and tearing. The condition is frequently mistaken for allergic or viral conjunctivitis, and children are often treated empirically with antibiotics or anti-inflammatories until the correct diagnosis is made. Iritis should be considered in any child with a red eye without significant mucoid or purulent discharge and without symptoms of itching. Diagnosis is made by utilizing a slit lamp to see white blood cells in the aqueous humor in the anterior chamber.

Iritis in children is most often idiopathic or post-viral, but it can be seen in juvenile inflammatory arthritides or HLA-B 27 disorders, so a careful history for joint pain should be elicited.

Consider iritis in any child with a red eye who has failed to respond to topical antibiotics or anti-allergy regimens.

Management of red eye

Usually, the "red eye" can be treated as an outpatient. Patients are infectious for as long as they have discharge from the eye(s). Children should be kept out of school and daycare until their eyes are no longer watery and the discharge has resolved. The pink discoloration of the conjunctiva can persist for days after cessation of discharge. Redness alone should not be an indication for keeping the child at home.

Treatment of iritis involves use of topical corticosteroids to minimize inflammation and cycloplegics to prevent synechiae (adhesions) forming from the iris to the anterior lens surface. Use of corticosteroids should always be supervised by an ophthalmologist, as excess use can lead to glaucoma and cataract. Rheumatologic consultation should be initiated and follow-up arranged, as many children with juvenile inflammatory arthritides may develop iritis without any symptoms whatsoever, placing them at risk for vision loss if iritis is untreated.

Pearls and pitfalls: red eye

Pearls

1. All neonates with conjunctivitis should have a sample sent for Gram stain; if gonococcal conjunctivitis is suspected, the child should be admitted with topical, systemic antibiotic coverage and urgent ophthalmic consultation.
2. Conduct fluorescein examination in all cases of red eye.
3. Suspect herpetic keratitis in a conjunctivitis that does not resolve.

Pitfalls

1. Failure to exclude a retained foreign body, corneal abrasion, or corneal ulcer in a child with a red, watery eye, even though infectious conjunctivitis is the most likely cause.

Ocular trauma

In general, the management of ocular trauma in children does not differ vastly from management in adults (Fig. 119.4), except that the history may be more difficult to obtain, and the examination more difficult to perform. If pain, fear, or behavior prevents an adequate evaluation, oral sedation or an examination under anesthesia may be required. This should be coordinated with the ophthalmologist so that the examination does not need to be repeated.

Corneal abrasion

The sensation of a foreign body or irritation in the eye is a common ocular complaint seen in the ED. The history reveals mechanical trauma to the eye sustained during work or play. Seemingly benign mechanisms, such as scratching the eye with a finger, can result in a corneal abrasion. The classic presentation consists of pain in the eye with accompanying photophobia, tearing, and decreased vision.

Diagnostic studies

To confirm the diagnosis, a topical anesthetic should be applied to the eye to facilitate examination. Following application of fluorescein, a slit lamp examination, Wood's lamp, or direct examination of the eye should be performed. The fluorescein stain will illuminate bright green when examined with the blue filter on the slit lamp, direct ophthalmoscope, or Wood's lamp (Fig. 119.5). Care should be taken to rule out full-thickness laceration or penetration.

Whitening around an abrasion can indicate infected ulceration, which requires ophthalmic consultation.

A history of contact lens use should heighten suspicion for the possibility of corneal ulceration.

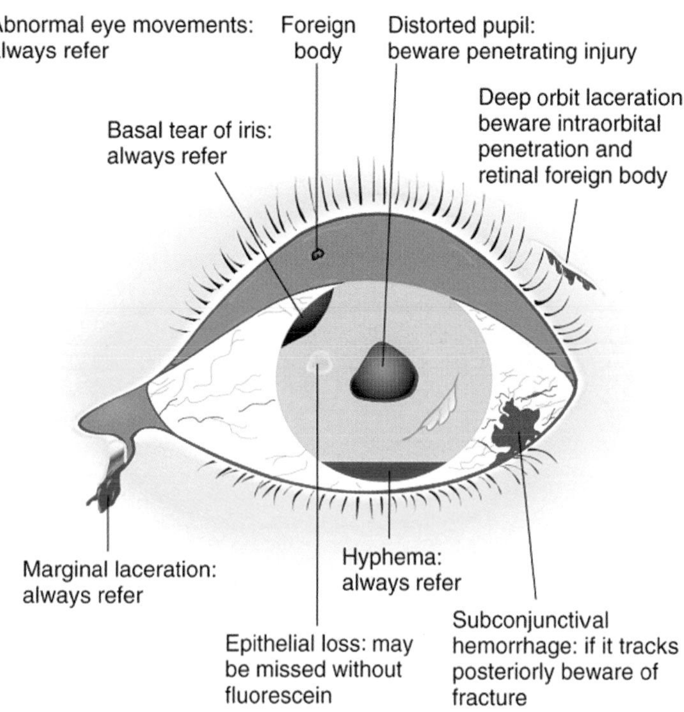

Figure 119.4 Overview of the injured eye. (Reproduced with permission from Khaw PT, Shah P, Elkington AR. Injury to the eye. *BMJ* 2004;328:36–38.)

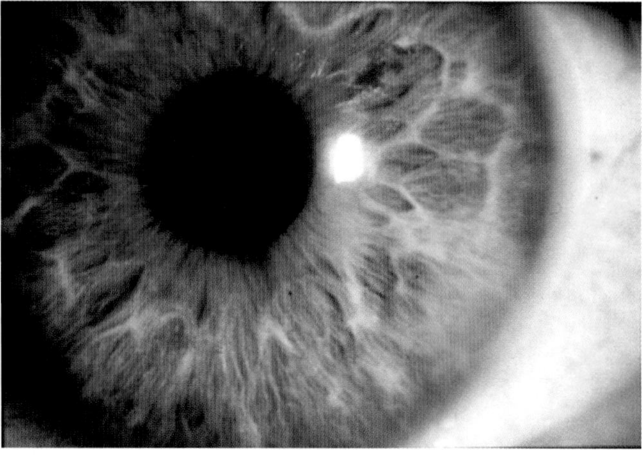

Figure 119.5 Corneal abrasion staining with fluorescein. (Courtesy D. Fredrick.)

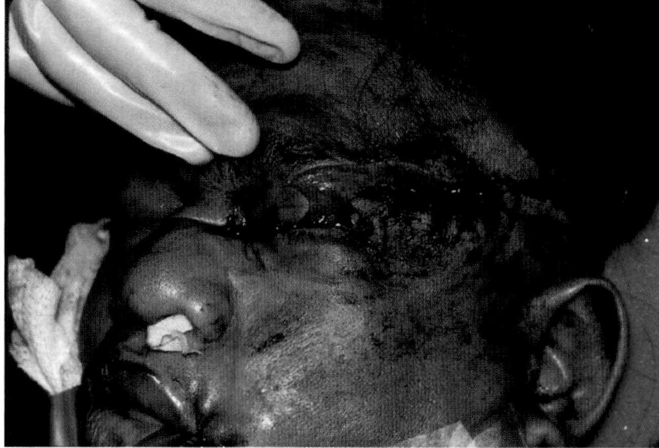

Figure 119.6 Full-thickness eyelid laceration involving the canaliculus that will require silicon intubation and microscopic repair. (Courtesy D. Fredrick.)

Management

A simple abrasion can be treated by instilling a topical antibiotic ointment. Patients may require oral analgesics. Topical anesthetics should never be prescribed, as these agents slow wound healing and can lead to further scarring. Topical NSAIDs have been used in adults, but because of expense and the occasional complication of corneal thinning, are not recommended for children. All patients should be seen again in 24 h, at which time most abrasions will be healed as evidenced by complete resolution of symptoms and lack of fluorescein staining on examination. Persistent epithelial defects warrant ophthalmic consultation.

Eyelid lacerations

Lacerations involving the eyelid must be carefully inspected to make certain that the eyeball itself is not injured. If globe trauma is ruled out, the laceration should be assessed to determine if it involves the eyelid margin or lacrimal structures (Fig. 119.6). If either structure is involved, surgical repair by ophthalmology is required within a few days.

Management

Any laceration that involves the lacrimal structures or the margin of the lid should be assessed and repaired by ophthalmology to prevent permanent drainage problems or lid notching, which can lead to further ocular pathology. If there is concern about need for ophthalmic repair, the wound can be treated with antibiotic ophthalmic ointment, patched and the patient placed on oral antibiotics until the patient is seen by ophthalmology within 48 h. If the laceration occurs medial to the upper or lower canaliculus, microsurgical repair will be needed to prevent chronic epiphora from scarring of the lacrimal drainage system.

Ruptured globe/corneal sclera laceration

The diagnostic workup is guided by the history and mechanism of injury. Any injury that involves high-velocity foreign bodies (i.e., machinery, pounding metal, or rock) should raise suspicion for penetrating ocular injury. Also, blunt trauma such as a high-velocity impact from a fist or a ball can cause the eye to rupture either at the corneal scleral limbus or directly behind the insertion of the extraocular muscles (which lie 5–7 mm posterior to the limbus). If there is any suspicion of globe rupture, the eye should be protected with a rigid Fox shield or with any other firm cover (i.e., top of a specimen cup).

Clinical presentation

Patients with a corneoscleral laceration will almost always complain of decreased vision, usually caused by disruption of corneal tissues, anterior or posterior chamber hemorrhage, or retinal detachment.

Penetrating trauma frequently presents with an irregular pupil, formed by the iris tissue being drawn toward the laceration. As aqueous humor escapes from the anterior chamber, the anterior chamber becomes shallow. When shining a penlight obliquely across the anterior chamber the temporal iris will be illuminated, but the nasal iris will be shadowed as the entire iris is vaulted forward, indicating a shallow anterior chamber. Finally, there will be an absent red reflex as an irregular cornea or hemorrhage in the anterior chamber or vitreous humor will prevent light from the ophthalmoscope from being reflected from the retina. An afferent pupillary defect may be present. The presence of bloody chemosis (hemorrhage underneath the conjunctiva) is an additional sign of ruptured globe.

Diagnosis and management

If there is any possibility of intraorbital or intraocular foreign body, a CT scan of the brain and orbits should be obtained.

For cases of intraocular foreign body, ophthalmic consultation should be obtained promptly, as emergency surgical repair within 24–48 h will be needed to prevent endophthalmitis, or infection of the globe. Tetanus toxoid should be given, if required. Antiemetics should be given to prevent vomiting, as any valsalva maneuvers can increase intraorbital pressure and potentially cause expulsion of the ocular contents. Broad-spectrum IV antibiotics (vancomycin 10–15 mg/kg twice a day and ceftazidime 50 mg/kg twice a day) should be given as soon as possible to minimize the risk of endophthalmitis. Risk factors for poor prognosis include length of time until surgical repair, length of laceration, and vitreous loss in the wound.

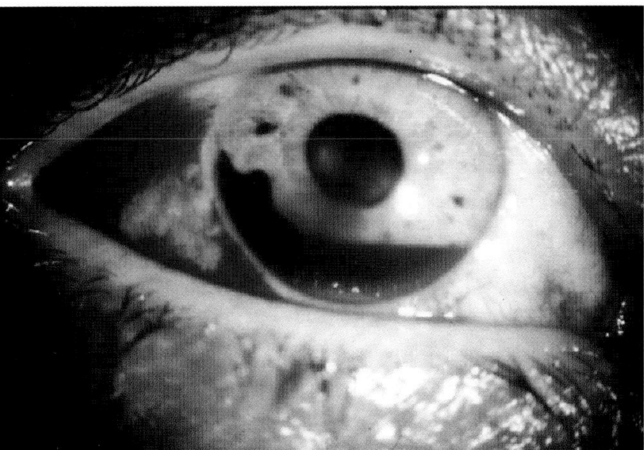

Figure 119.7 Layered red blood cells in anterior chamber in traumatic hyphema. (Courtesy D. Fredrick.)

Traumatic hyphema

A traumatic hyphema occurs when blood accumulates in the anterior chamber after blunt trauma (Fig. 119.7). As pressure rises rapidly within the anterior chamber, aqueous humor is forced into the trabecular meshwork, causing rupture of arterioles in the root of the iris. Blood enters the anterior chamber and coagulates to form a clot. Red blood cells in the anterior chamber can be caught in the trabecular meshwork and decrease outflow of aqueous humor, thereby increasing the intraocular pressure and precipitating glaucoma. The optic nerve can be damaged by the increased intraocular pressure and this causes permanently decreased visual acuity. Higher intraocular pressures can also force red blood cells into the cornea, a condition called cornea blood staining.

Clinical presentation

Patients with a hyphema generally complain of poor vision. On examination, they are found to have a poorly reactive, and sometimes unidentifiable, pupil. Diagnosis is made through a slit lamp examination where red blood cells can be seen both suspended and layering out in the anterior chamber.

Management

Ophthalmologic consultation is warranted to rule out concurrent ocular injuries, such as retinal detachment, vitreous hemorrhage, and damage to the intraocular lens. Treatment of the hyphema itself is aimed at speeding resolution of the bleeding and maintaining low/normal intraocular pressure. To protect the visual acuity, a cycloplegic such as atropine is used to dilate the pupil, thereby preventing the iris from moving and dislodging the clot. Topical prednisolone acetate should be prescribed. A rigid Fox shield should be placed over the eye at all times to prevent the child from rubbing the eye and further disrupting the clot. Attempts should be made to have the child rest for a few days to minimize this chance of rebleeding. When sleeping, the child's head should be elevated to allow the blood to layer in the inferior portion of the anterior portion of the chamber to improve visual acuity.

There is a higher risk of increased intraocular pressure from hyphema in those with sickle cell disease.

Patients with sickle cell disease often require treatment with topical eyedrops to lower intraocular pressure. The child should be seen daily to monitor the intraocular pressure. If a child cannot be kept calm at home, or if daily follow-up for the patient is difficult, inpatient hospitalization may be indicated. If intraocular pressure increases, topical and oral medications for glaucoma should be used.

Patients with a hyphema are at increased risk for chronic open angle glaucoma.

Long-term follow-up with an ophthalmologist is required to monitor their intraocular pressure. They are also at increased risk for retinal detachment and should be advised appropriately.

Orbital "blow-out" fracture

Blunt trauma to the globe can cause elevated intraorbital pressures that threaten the surrounding bony structures, or orbit. The weakest parts of the orbit are the ethmoid sinus and the orbital floor, formed by the roof of the maxillary sinus. The orbital floor can fracture, causing orbital contents to prolapse into the maxillary sinus and resulting in a blow-out fracture.

Clinical presentation

As the orbital contents are displaced from the orbit into the maxillary sinus, the eye will sink into the orbital socket, a condition called enophthalmos. The inferior rectus can become entrapped in the fracture site, preventing the eye from looking up or down. The orbital floor fracture can entrap the inferior rectus muscle and then snap backward, producing a "trapdoor" fracture. When the child looks up and down, the restriction of the muscle in the fracture can elicit a vagal response, causing significant nausea and vomiting. Commonly known as the "white eye blow-out", the child may appear relatively asymptomatic with minimal ecchymosis or swelling but will have significantly restricted eye movements with emesis. The patient will also complain of double vision on attempted up or down gaze.

Diagnostic studies

A CT scan with 1.5 mm orbital cuts should be obtained to confirm the diagnosis of an orbital blow-out fracture. Ophthalmic referral should be arranged.

Management

Urgent repair is indicated if there is entrapment of the extraocular muscles. If there is no entrapment of the muscles, surgical repair can be deferred until 7 to 10 days after the trauma to allow swelling to decrease. Patients should be placed on oral antibiotics to prevent secondary infection (cephalexin 50 mg/kg daily in three divided doses or trimethoprim–sulfamethoxazole 6–12 mg/kg daily in two divided doses for 10 days). The patient should be advised not to blow their nose as air from the sinus can go into the orbit, resulting in increased pressure from orbital emphysema.

Chemical burn

When assessing a patient with a chemical burn, it is imperative to determine whether the offending chemical is an acid or a base. Acidic burns cause rapid coagulation of the tissues of the eye. Alkali, or basic, burns cause saponification and necrosis of the blood supply to the eye, thereby leading to more significant long-term sequelae.

Clinical presentation

The history is key to identifying the source chemical, the time of the initial exposure, duration of exposure, and subsequent symptoms. Patients may complain of burning, sharp shooting pains, or a change in their visual acuity.

Management

The mainstay of therapy, regardless of acid or base, is immediate and continuous irrigation until the pH is neutralized as verified by pH paper. Ophthalmic consultation should be arranged, and topical antibiotics applied to prevent secondary infection. The ophthalmologist will begin a regimen of topical anti-inflammatories and anti-collagenases.

Pearls and pitfalls: ocular trauma

Pearls

1. If there is any question of penetrating trauma, obtain CT scan with 1.5 mm cuts through the orbit.
2. Carefully screen a patient with an eyelid laceration for ocular trauma.
3. A laceration in the medial one-third of the lower eye may involve the lacrimal system.

Pitfalls

1. Failure to check normal eye movement in all directions in patients with blunt trauma the globe.
2. Failure to recheck pH 20 min after discontinuing initial irrigation in cases of chemical burns to or near the eye.

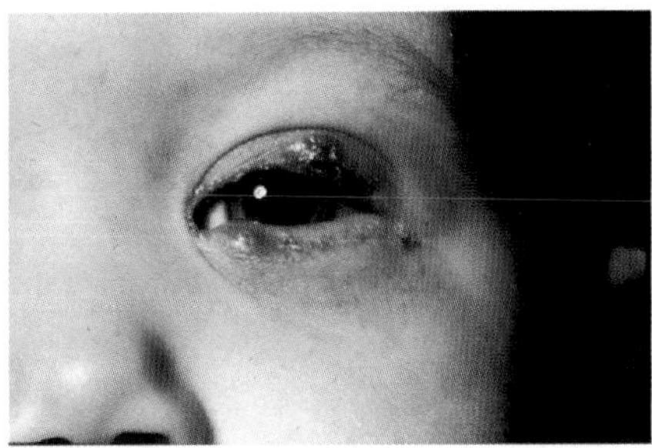

Figure 119.8 Infection of eyelashes leading to acute hordeola. (Courtesy D. Fredrick.)

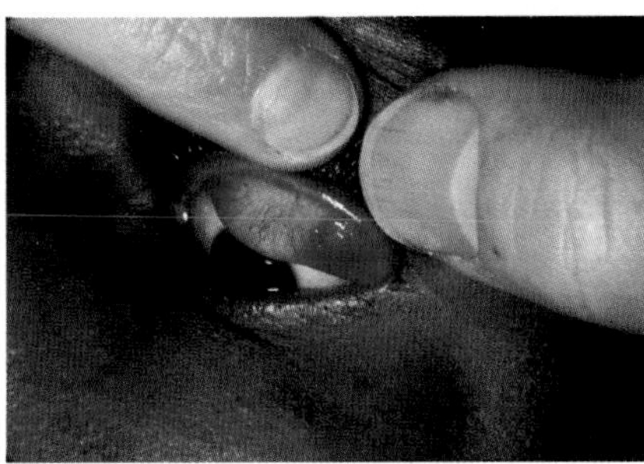

Figure 119.10 Chalazia should be drained with internal approach to avoid a scar on skin. (Courtesy D. Fredrick.)

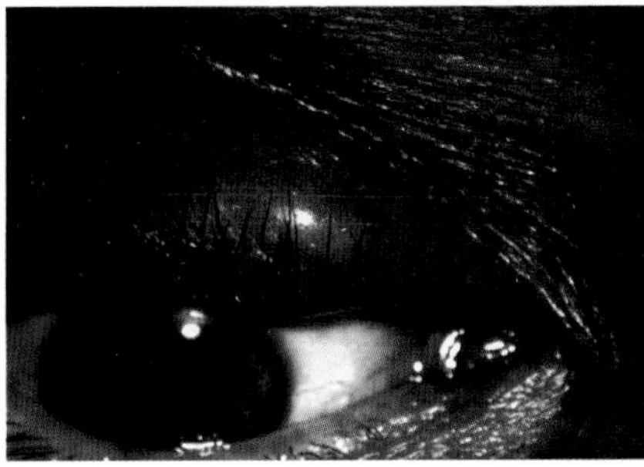

Figure 119.9 Chronic blepharitis causing recurrent hordeolum and chalazia. (Courtesy D. Fredrick.)

Ocular and periocular infection and inflammation

Swollen eyelids

The dermal structures surrounding the eye and orbit are particularly elastic and easily distended by inflammatory processes. Swelling of the eyelids can be sudden and dramatic. The patient is usually brought in with a caregiver complaining that the child can no longer see out of the affected eye. Once again, the history will usually provide clues to arrive at a proper diagnosis. Attention should be paid to any history of preceding upper respiratory or viral illness, any recent trauma involving the head and neck, or any history of atopy, allergies, or exposure to irritating substances that may have led to an allergic reaction.

Patients with atopy who manifest reactive airway disease or eczema are particularly prone to swelling of the eyelid structures. This swelling, or blepharochalasis, is usually painless. Blepharochalasis generally develops after extensive itching of the eyes has occurred. As children rub their eyes, the release of histamine causes further inflammation and swelling, and at times the eyelids can be swollen completely shut. When the eyelids are eventually forced open, the conjunctiva is often also edematous but without any notable discharge. The extraocular movements should be painless and without any restrictions. Often the condition is bilateral although it can be asymmetric.

Management

Antihistamines result in rapid resolution of the swelling. Cool compresses will often provide symptomatic relief as do chilled artificial tears.

Hordeolum (stye) and chalazia

An acute infection of the eyelash follicle or oil gland (meibomian gland) of the eyelids can lead to a hordeolum (Figs. 119.8 and 119.9). Hordeola are generally red, swollen, and painful. Treatment is warm compresses and erythromycin ophthalmic ointment. Patients will frequently have concomitant blepharitis, a chronic infection of the eyelids with *Staphylococcus* spp. leading to chronic itchy burning eyelids and recurrent symptoms.

Management

Treatment involves good eyelid hygiene, soaking the eyes with a warm compress at night, washing with baby shampoo, and using erythromycin ointment at night for 5 days. Periodic washing will minimize recurrent symptoms. Once the acute infection has resolved, the patient may be left with a sterile, painless lipogranuloma that is slow to resolve. These chalazia (Fig. 119.10) eventually resolve with warm compresses but occasionally require incision and curettage with local anesthesia if resolution is too slow.

Preseptal/periorbital cellulitis

Infection of the eyelid structures can sometimes spread from a localized source to diffuse cellulitis. In preseptal cellulitis, the infection is contained within the eyelid structures and does not involve the deeper orbital tissues.

Clinical presentation

The upper and lower eyelids can be edematous and tender to the touch. When the eyelids are opened gently, the eye has full motility, the pupils react briskly, there is minimal injection and swelling of the conjunctiva, and no vision loss. The initial source of the preseptal cellulitis is often a stye or hordeolum that spreads to the contiguous structures. They also may be a history of trauma with the introduction of Gram-positive organisms into the periorbital tissues.

Diagnosis

The diagnosis is usually clinical; however, any obvious purulent material should be sent for culture and sensitivities.

Management

Empiric treatment with broad-spectrum oral antibiotics is indicated. A first dose of IM ceftriaxone followed by oral medications with Gram-positive and Gram-negative organism coverage is appropriate (daily amoxicillin 90 mg/kg plus clavulanate 4–6 mg/kg, divided twice a day). With the increased prevalence of methicillin-resistant *S. aureus* (MRSA), the patient should be placed on sulfamethoxazole–trimethoprim or clindamycin in addition. Warm compresses will often aid the resolution of any external source of infection such as a hordeolum or chalazion. The patient should be followed closely to make sure that the preseptal cellulitis does not involve deeper tissues and progress to orbital cellulitis, which requires more aggressive diagnosis and management.

Orbital cellulitis

In orbital cellulitis, infection extends to the deeper tissues surrounding the eye, extraocular muscles, or optic nerve. Since the deeper orbital tissues are separated from the superficial tissues by an inelastic orbital septum, increased pressure from inflammation causes increased pressure on the optic nerve and subsequent ischemia. This sequence of events can cause irrevocable vision loss. For this reason, appropriate diagnostic and therapeutic maneuvers are necessary to preserve vision in patients with orbital cellulitis.

Clinical presentation

Patients with orbital cellulitis can present similarly to those with preseptal cellulitis. The eyelids may be erythematous, swollen, and painful. Most often patients with orbital cellulitis have an ill appearance. There is typically a history of upper respiratory tract infection or a history of sinusitis. The characteristic features of orbital cellulitis include:

- restriction of extraocular movements
- proptosis (forward displacement of the eyeball)
- poor pupil reaction as a result of ischemic pressure on the optic nerve
- decreased visual acuity.

Diagnostic studies

If orbital cellulitis is suspected, CT scan of the orbits using 1.5 mm cuts with coronal reformation should be obtained to confirm the diagnosis. Imaging may reveal the presence of a subperiostal or intraorbital abscess, contiguous sinusitis, and evidence of cavernous sinus involvement. Distention of the superior ophthalmic vein is concerning for involvement of the cavernous sinus, which can lead to more dire consequences such as cavernous sinus thrombosis, multiple cranial nerve involvement, or intracranial involvement.

Management

Patients with orbital cellulitis should be admitted to the hospital and placed on parenteral broad-spectrum antibiotics. Often vancomycin, clindamycin, and third-generation cephalosporins are used to cover resistant Gram-positive organisms (vancomycin 10–15 mg/kg q. 12 h and ceftriaxone 100 mg/kg daily divided BID). Ophthalmic consultation should be obtained to monitor for signs of optic nerve compression and retinal perfusion. An otorhinolaryngologic consultation is warranted as sinus infections often cause orbital cellulitis. Common routes of introduction of bacteria into the orbit include spread through the ethmoid sinus or maxillary frontal sinus. If the patient does not show rapid resolution of symptoms on parenteral antibiotics, surgical drainage through a sinus approach is indicated.

Pearls and pitfalls: ocular and periorbital cellulitis

Pearls

1. Significant periorbital (preseptal) cellulitis, and all cases of orbital cellulitis, require urgent ophthalmologic evaluation.
2. Orbital and periorbital cellulitis may appear similar clinically.
3. A careful eye examination to ensure preservation of visual acuity and visual fields is crucial in the workup for orbital or periorbital cellulitis.

Pitfalls

1. Failing to consider orbital cellulitis simply because there is evidence of concomitant periorbital cellulitis.

Vision loss

Poor vision in infancy

If a child has poor vision at birth as a result of structural or developmental anomalies of the eye, they will show signs of poor vision in the first few months of life. Poor vision in both eyes will lead to nystagmus, which begins at 2 month of age. If vision loss is in one eye, the affected eye may develop strabismus, with the eye turning inward (esotropia) or outward (exotropia). Family history of visual loss is important to elicit, as many forms of congenital blindness are hereditary. The pre- and perinatal history are likewise important, as a history of maternal fever or rashes may indicate congenital disease, while a traumatic birth can result in cortical visual impairment.

Poor vision in children

Poor vision may be unilateral or bilateral. Bilateral poor vision is most often caused by a refractive error. These children will have poor distance vision, but normal vision when tested with a near card. Visual acuity that improves with use of a pinhole occlusive device is also most commonly a refractive error. Bilateral poor vision that is unchanged with position and occlusive device warrants ophthalmic referral. Unilateral poor vision may be caused by a unilateral refractive error or amblyopia. Amblyopia is a cortically mediated process where an abnormal visual input to the striate cortex leads to anatomic and physiologic changes in the brain, causing poor visual acuity. If the condition is not detected and treated in the first decade of life, the vision loss can become permanent. The causes of amblyopia are misaligned eyes (strabismus), unequal refractive error between the eyes (anisometropia), or visual deprivation from a visual impediment (e.g., cataract).

Final diagnosis, including evaluating for a structural anomaly, should be made by an ophthalmologist. Treatment involves eliminating the cause (correcting the strabismus/giving glasses) and initiating occlusion therapy to the sound eye, thereby reversing the vision loss in the weak eye.

Sudden vision loss

When evaluating the child with the chief complaint of decreased vision, the most important questions are

- is the vision loss unilateral or bilateral?
- is the vision loss sudden or is there a sudden discovery of poor vision?

Children rarely complain of vision loss unless it is profound and sudden in onset. Longer-term poor vision will be noted by parents, caretakers, and teachers, and will seldom present to the ED.

True sudden loss of vision in children is most often neurologic in nature, so careful questioning looking for any neurologic signs and symptoms is important. The presence of headache, nausea, vertigo, paresthesiae, weakness, and tinnitus should be evaluated. A thorough infection history is important, as a multitude of infectious processes can lead to inflammatory conditions affecting the nerve and retina.

Differential diagnosis for vision loss

Refractive error. Vision will be poor at distance, better with a pinhole or with proximity.

Amblyopia. The patient may have strabismus, but otherwise normal eye examination.

Papilledema. This occurs with swollen optic nerves; vision loss occurs only when intracranial pressure elevation has been long standing or there is sudden onset of very high pressure (Fig. 119.11). Imaging with CT or MRI should be instituted and a lumbar puncture considered with opening pressure if neuroimaging shows no mass lesion and there is a concern for meningitis or pseudotumor cerebri.

Optic neuritis. This is a possible diagnosis if vision loss affects only one eye, and there is an afferent pupillary defect, poor visual acuity, and a swollen optic nerve. Use of MRI can evaluate for white matter disease.

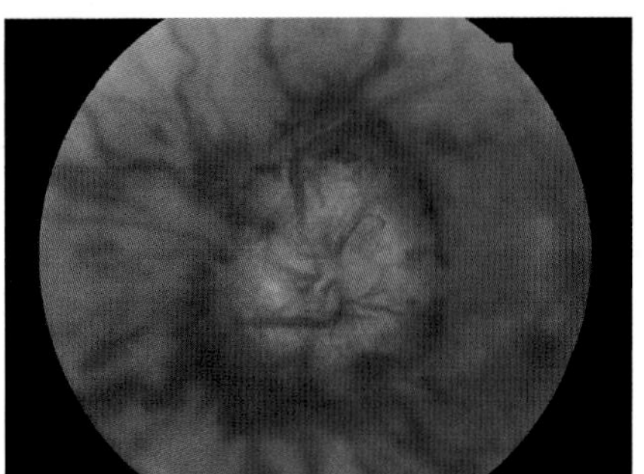

Figure 119.11 Papilledema with swollen nerve and peripapillary hemorrhage in a patient with high opening pressure during lumbar puncture. (Courtesy D. Fredrick.)

Retinal detachment. This presents as a sudden clouding of vision, "curtain falling down," and is painless. Assess with bedside ultrasound followed by urgent ophthalmology consultation. Retinal detachment can. occur with complaints of flashing lights or floating spots, previous history of ocular trauma, or high myopia.

Physical examination

A carefully conducted history and targeted physical examination will allow the EP to determine if ophthalmic or neurologic consultation is required. Visual acuity should be tested one eye at a time, both at a distance and with a near card. Pupils should be checked, looking for anisocoria, reaction to light, and for the presence of an afferent pupillary defect. The direct ophthalmoscope should be used to check for a red reflex, to examine the arterial structure of the eye, and to examine the optic discs. If the red reflex is absent and if the pupil looks white with direct illumination, the condition is called leukocoria. Leukocoria can be associated with vision- and life-threatening conditions and mandates urgent ophthalmic evaluation. Attempts should be made to examine the optic nerve to evaluate for swelling or atrophy. Pupillary dilatation can be accomplished using topicamide 1% ophthalmic solution.

Pearls and pitfalls: sudden vision loss

Pearls

1. Visual acuity is a subjective test; the EP must rely on objective findings (pupil reaction, motility, and appearance of optic nerve) to determine if neuroimaging or specialist consultation is necessary.
2. True sudden vision loss is rare in children and is most often neurologic in nature. Consultation with an ophthalmologist.

Section

18

Psychiatric emergencies

Expert reviewer: Shashank V. Joshi

Chapter

120 The agitated, anxious child

Robert Hilt

Introduction

Agitation in the ED can have many causes, including delirium, psychosis, family dysfunction, recent trauma, or simply patient frustration. Substance intoxication, as a cause of agitation, has a unique treatment need and is important to screen for early. Specific toxic syndromes are addressed elsewhere in this book. Agitated delirium requires treatment of any underlying medical cause, and possibly the short-term use of an antipsychotic drug to calm behaviors. Major medical emergencies such as severe trauma also require their own approach, such as rapidly moving toward physical restraint or occasionally using paralysis and intubation if necessary to facilitate safe medical care. If there is active violence of the child towards themselves or others, physical restraint may be needed for safety but only by staff educated in the use of safe physical restraint procedures.

Identifying the early stages of agitation helps the ED staff to initiate intervention with the child prior to needing restraints.

The early stages of agitation can be seen as a stepwise progression from verbal stage, to motor stage, to a property damage phase and then to an attack stage. If ED staff wait until they feel angry or frustrated with the child, then it is likely that the early warning stages have already passed and the intervention needed to calm the child will be more serious.

Stepwise approach to agitation

Generally, agitation care should start with everything except use of restraint or giving medications. Begin with altering the environment, such as bringing the child to a "safe room" in the ED where there is minimal breakable equipment and where staff containment, if needed, is more straightforward. A constructive interaction with the child and family starts by reminding oneself not to take a child or family's anger personally. Instead the EP needs to project a calm disposition, which works as an agitation treatment. A soft voice, slow movements, and calm demeanor pulls the child toward using verbal communication rather than agitated aggressive outbursts. Remember not to take their anger personally. Calming interventions include:

- clearly introducing yourself
- using simplified language, a soft voice, and slow movements
- explaining what will happen in the ED
- reducing the stimulation from the environment, if possible (less noise, light, or people)
- removing access to breakable objects/equipment
- allowing room for pacing, if possible
- offering food or drink, which is inherently calming
- reassuring the child that you are there to keep them safe, that this is your job
- listening and empathizing (a treatment cornerstone)
- telling the child how you plan to honor their reasonable requests
- clarifying the child's goal, and then trying to link his/her cooperation to that goal
- finding things for the child to control, like choice of drinks
- engaging available consultants (security, social work, psychiatry)
- offering distracting toys/sensory modalities
- keeping engaged as being perceived as ignored may encourage escalations.

Ask for the child's views and opinions without expressing judgement, and then help them to label and identify their feelings. Feeling understood is calming. For example one might observe aloud, "You feel really mad that Mom and Dad brought you in here." Separate arguing family members when appropriate and offer reassurance to the child that your job is to "make everyone safe." Stating this role explicitly can have a calming effect on both yourself and the child.

Food and drink can have anti-agitation effects in children that should not be underestimated. Food enhances relaxation and it delivers a clear non-verbal message to the child that the ED is a nurturing environment. Do not do this, however, if intubation or conscious sedation might reasonably be necessary for their care. Distraction, commonly used when performing painful procedures in children, can also have value in

A Practical Guide to Pediatric Emergency Medicine: Caring for Children in the Emergency Department, ed. N. Ewen Amieva-Wang (associate eds. Jamie Shandro, Aparajita Sohoni, and Bernhard Fassl). Published by Cambridge University Press.

reducing agitation. Movies, sensory toys (like Koosh balls), books, video games, art projects, and music are all potential distraction techniques.

To the extent that agitation is caused by a loss of control, a child's agitation can be reduced by giving the child forced choices in an ED. Examples of this are asking the child if they want their parents to wait outside during their interview, if they want their lights on or off, and so on. If a child is makes a particular demand that cannot be honored right away, then link care needs to the child's stated goal. For instance, "I heard you want to leave right now. To show us that you are safe to leave, can you [insert care need]?".

The calming interventions listed here should be the first-line approach; however, when that does not help, or when agitation is extreme, further interventions must be considered (Fig. 120.1). Using a chemical restraint, whose purpose is to halt a child's movements against their will, is controversial. Physical restraint or containment that follows state and federal guidelines may be the better short-term option, as chemical restraint agents can take up to 30 min to take effect while the reason for their use is often more immediate. However, one should consider a chemical restraint for a child who is continuing to struggle violently against a necessary physical restraint.

Besides chemical restraint, medications may also be used for symptom-focused treatment of agitation. Symptom-focused treatment is initiated with consent of the legal guardian and age-appropriate assent of the child, based on a measured plan of care to reduce the symptom of agitation. This is

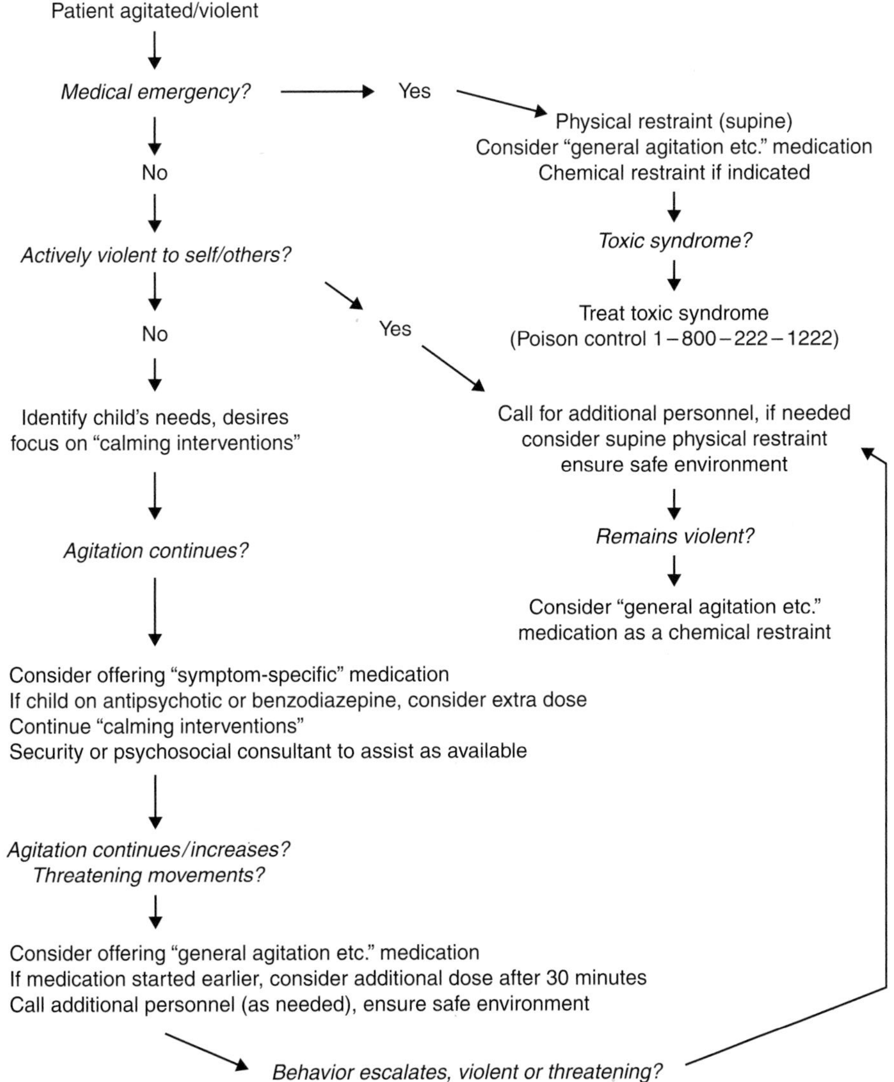

Figure 120.1 Algorithm for management of the agitated child. See Box 120.1 for "general agitation" and "symptom-specific" medication. (With permission from Hilt and Woodward, 2008.)

like treating other symptom-specific problems in medicine for which the underlying diagnosis may not be known, for example giving ibuprofen for headache or fever. The Centers for Medicare and Medicaid Services (CMS) and Department of Health and Human Services (DHHS) also make this distinction, in that if medication "is given as part of a plan of care to treat medical symptoms," then that medication is not a chemical restraint. Such "plans of care" are said to be created by a "brief assessment leading to determination of a general category of presentation," such as intoxication, anxiety, or psychosis, as the potential cause of observed agitation. If the child does not assent to use of medication (i.e., needing IM administration), it becomes difficult to argue that such administration is not, in fact, a "chemical restraint."

There are no randomized controlled trials on use of medication to treat agitated children in an ED. Ziprasidone IM shows benefit in open label reports with agitated child psychiatric inpatients. Haloperidol has had positive open label reports for agitated delirium in children, and positive randomized trial results treating aggression in child psychiatric inpatients. Risperidone improved maladaptive aggression in nine controlled trials in children across multiple diagnostic categories and settings. Benzodiazepines and antihistamines, despite their widespread usage, have no research reports on effectiveness for treating agitated children.

Despite the general lack of child data, most pediatric emergency medicine training directors note that medications are "regularly" used to treat agitation in their departments (e.g. Dorfman and Kastner reported use of benzodiazepines for 71%, haloperidol for 46%, and antihistamines for 25% of their cases when medicines are given).

Adult emergency medicine agitation research is more advanced, and should inform treatment choices with children. Adult agitation care guidelines based on both expert opinions and controlled trials support the use of the atypical antipsychotics risperidone or olanzapine (with or without a benzodiazepine added) if an oral agent is needed, and use of IM ziprasidone alone or IM haloperidol plus a benzodiazepine if IM agent is needed. Use of IM olanzapine is also supported for this indication but occasional potent sedation when combined with a benzodiazepine has limited its widespread use. Four different studies with agitated adults in EDs have shown that oral risperidone is as fast and as effective as IM haloperidol; consequently, oral administration is preferred over IM whenever patients will allow it.

Conclusions

A suggested medication use guideline for children appears in Boxes 120.1 and 120.2, and Fig. 120.1 gives an algorithm for decision making. It is preferred to have regional experts review these guidelines and tailor them to fit local best practices. When possible, medication treatments should match the suspected cause of agitation, such as using benzodiazepines for

Box 120.1. Chosing emergency psychopharmacology

Patient already on psychiatric medications

1. Give the patient's usual psychiatric medicines on schedule, unless toxicity suspected.
2. Consider giving one-quarter to one-half of their total daily amount of either antipsychotic or benzodiazepine as a single dose if between dose times.

If patient is not on psychiatric medications:

1. *Symptom-specific treatments* include:
   - anxiety: lorazepam, diazepam, or possibly diphenhydramine
   - psychosis, mania, maladaptive aggression, delirium: risperidone, olanzapine, ziprasidone IM, haloperidol IM.
2. *General agitation treatments* (PO preferred over IM):
   - PO options: risperidone, olanzapine, diazepam, lorazepam
   - IM options: lorazepam, diazepam, ziprasidone, haloperidol.

Note: Benzodiazepines and diphenhydramine may cause disinhibition, particularly in the very young or those with developmental delays. If there is muscle stiffness or movement problems from an antipsychotic drug, give diphenhydramine or benztropine.

Box 120.2. Suggested dosages for psychopharmacology

Diazepam: 0.04–0.2 mg/kg per dose PO/IM (max. 10 mg/dose).
Diphenhydramine: 1 mg/kg per dose PO/IM/IV (max. 50 mg).
Haloperidol: 0.025–0.075 mg/kg per dose IM (max. 5 mg).
Lorazepam: 0.05 mg/kg per dose PO/IM/IV (max. 2 mg/dose).
Olanzapine: 2.5 mg (school age) to10 mg (late adolescent) PO.
Risperidone: 0.25 mg (school age) to 2 mg (late adolescent) PO.
Ziprasidone: 10–20 mg IM (>15 years), 10 mg IM (12–16 years).
Adapted from Hilt and Woodward, 2008.

Pearls and pitfalls

Pearls

1. Use calming measures first.
2. Offer food/drink as appropriate.
3. Treatment is not equivalent to restraint.
4. Oral medication can work as effectively as IM.

Pitfalls

1. Failure to screen for acute medical conditions or substance intoxication, which could be the cause of agitation.

anxious agitation. Risks of benzodiazepines include potent sedation or paradoxic agitation or disinhibition, a particular problem in children. Risks of antipsychotic drugs include dystonia (treat with diphenhydramine or benztropine [benzatropine]), mild reduction of seizure threshold, lengthening of QT interval, and neuroleptic malignant syndrome.

Restraint use can be avoided in all but the most significant scenarios, but how often that is necessary is not well established. Institutions that provide staff education on restraint alternatives, and provide collaborative support and resources for staff (to manage agitated children), are predicted to have a lower need to use restraints.

Selected references

Allen MH, Currier GW, Carpenter D, Ross RW, Docherty JP. Introduction, methods, commentary and summary. *J Psychiatr Pract* 2005;**11**(Suppl. 1):5–25.

Dorfman D, Kastner B. The use of restraint for pediatric psychiatric patients in emergency departments. *Pediatr Emerg Care* 2004;**20**:151–156.

Heyneman EK. The aggressive child. *Child Adolesc Psychiatr Clin North Am* 2003;**12**:667–677.

Hilt RJ, Woodward TA. Agitation treatment for pediatric emergency patients. *J Am Acad Child Adolesc Psychiatry* 2008;**47**:132–138.

Pappadopulos E, Woolston S, Chait A, *et al.* Pharmacotherapy of aggression in children and adolescents: efficacy and effect size. *J Can Acad Child Adolesc Psychiatry* 2006;**15**:27–39.

Chapter

121 Psychiatric emergencies in children

Danielle M. McCarthy and Michael A. Gisondi

Introduction

It is estimated that one in every five children between ages 9 and 17 years in the USA has a diagnosable mental or addictive disorder resulting in some degree of impairment. The ED has become a frequent site for the care of patients with psychiatric and behavioral disorders. From 1993 to 1999, there were more than 3 million pediatric mental health visits to the ED, summing to an annual rate of 326 visits per 10 000 children. In these visits, the three most common diagnoses were depressive disorders, anxiety states, and other (non-specific) psychological issues. A systematic approach to this patient population will identify red flags necessitating more in-depth treatment. An awareness of available resources can help to reduce stress for the patient, family, and providers. This chapter will address issues common to psychiatric conditions and behavioral problems in children and teenagers.

Clinical presentation

General principles

Barriers to receiving psychiatric care for adults and children include lack of health insurance, a fragmented mental health care infrastructure, and the cultural stigma associated with mental health disorders. Mental healthcare access is also more difficult for children because of a shortage of pediatric mental health specialists. These barriers to consistent outpatient psychiatric services contribute to the use of the ED as a safety net for patients with both life-threatening and non-life-threatening mental health problems. While, in general, the ED team should be attuned to specific sociocultural aspects of the family when a child presents to the ED for any reason, this is particularly true with regard to psychiatric symptoms.

Differential diagnosis

While adult patients presenting to the ED often have an established psychiatric diagnosis, children more commonly present with undifferentiated psychiatric symptoms that can be confused with medical conditions. The *Diagnostic and Statistic Manual IV* (DSM IV) distinguishes between "mental disorders that are due to a general medical condition" and "primary mental disorders," rather than the terminology *organic* and *functional*.

Before assuming a primary psychiatric disease for a behavioral change, it is paramount to exclude a medical cause.

Several findings in the history and examination may be helpful in differentiating behavioral disturbances caused by primary psychiatric disorders from those stemming from medical disease. These include similar red flags to those identified in the adult population, such as a lack of previous psychiatric disease, ALOC or delirium, abnormal vital signs, or an abnormal neurological examination.

A thorough medical history is required for children with established psychiatric illness, as these patients may have co-existing medical conditions that can contribute to or exacerbate their mental illness. Toxicological causes of disease, including prescription drugs, illicit substances and over-the-counter medications, must always be considered in the differential diagnosis.

Patient age may help to differentiate undiagnosed psychiatric illness. Many disorders start in childhood but are not properly identified or treated until later in life (Table 121.1).

Acute depression and suicidal ideation

Children with depression and suicidality may initially present with a pervasive sense of sadness and hopelessness. The child may be preoccupied with death. The patient should be questioned carefully about suicidal intent. If a child has attempted suicide without success, the lethality of the attempt may have been miscalculated but the event should to taken seriously regardless of the result. These patients should be further evaluated in the ED setting with the help of the psychiatry team prior to disposition. If there is any doubt as to the safety of the patient, he or she should be placed on a hold according to hospital, county or state procedures. The acutely depressed

A Practical Guide to Pediatric Emergency Medicine: Caring for Children in the Emergency Department, ed. N. Ewen Amieva-Wang (associate eds. Jamie Shandro, Aparajita Sohoni, and Bernhard Fassl). Published by Cambridge University Press.

Table 121.1. Age of onset for psychiatric illnesses

Disorder	Median age of onset
Impulse control disorders	
Attention-deficit hyperactivity disorder	5–7 years
Oppositional-defiant disorder, conduct disorder, intermittent explosive disorder	7–12 years
Anxiety disorders	
Phobias and separation anxiety disorder	7–14 years
Generalized anxiety disorder, panic disorder and post-traumatic stress disorder	25–50 years, but may present in childhood
Mood disorders	29–43 years, but may present in childhood
Substance use disorders	14–29 years
Schizophrenia spectrum diagnoses	15–35 years
Eating disorders	14–18 years, but may present in late childhood

child without suicidal intent may be discharged home if the parents and primary care physician are in agreement. Prior to discharge, the psychiatric team should assist the family in creating a safety contract and give a specific psychiatrist for aftercare referral.

Be familiar with medications commonly used for the treatment of depression in pediatrics. Fluoxetine is currently the only FDA-approved psychotropic medication for depression in children and adolescents. Several other selective serotonin reuptake inhibitors (SSRIs) are commonly used, as is buproprion. The EP should not prescribe these medications as an acute intervention because the full clinical effect may take upwards of 1 month, and a prescription may decrease outpatient follow-up.

Psychosis, schizophrenia, and bipolar disease

Psychosis in children is broadly divided into two categories: medical psychosis and psychiatric psychosis. Medical psychosis may be caused by the exacerbation of an acute or chronic medical condition, or may be observed in the setting of alcohol or drug abuse. Certain psychiatric medications in overdose can lead to agitation and psychotic behavior (e.g., anticholinergic agents [benztropine, diphenhydramine] and prescription psychostimulants [methylphenidate, dextroamphetamine]). Psychiatric psychosis may result from schizophrenia, bipolar disorder, or an acute reaction to a traumatic event. Schizophrenic patients may present with a flat or withdrawn affect and, similar to the adult presentation, may have illogical thoughts and hallucinations.

Childhood bipolar disorder differs from the adult presentation in that mania more commonly manifests as an irritable mood rather than as euphoria.

Explosive outbursts and emotional lability are frequently seen. In the acute setting, particularly with an initial presentation, it may be difficult to differentiate bipolar mania and schizophrenia. Management of psychotic patients in the ED may require the use of physical or chemical restraints.

This subset of patients is particularly dangerous because impaired judgement and impulsive behavior can result in inadvertent physical harm to the child or others. If the child is not safe, he or she should be placed on a hold according to state or institutional protocol. If the psychotic behavior significantly improves with antipsychotic drugs, there are no other indications for admission, and the child has good supervision, the patient may be discharged home with close follow-up.

Attention-deficit hyperactivity disorder

Attention-deficit hyperactivity disorder (ADHD) is a syndrome with a prevalence of 3–7% in school-age children. Consequently, these patients will be seen frequently in the ED for both medical complaints and complaints related to their psychiatric condition. In adolescence, ADHD has been associated with learning disabilities, anxiety and mood disorders, and oppositional behavior. Typical features of the disorder include attention difficulty at home and at school, impulsivity, and hyperactivity. Although initiating treatment for ADHD is not recommended in the ED setting, the EP should be familiar with the most commonly used medications, including stimulants such as methylphenidate and dextroamphetamine. Children who are properly treated with stimulants and who receive regular follow-up care have been shown to require fewer subsequent ED visits. If there is a suspicion for ADHD, the patient should be given a referral to outpatient psychiatry.

Conduct disorders

A child or teenager with conduct disorder repeatedly engages in behavior that is socially unacceptable, both violent (e.g., assault, rape) and non-violent (e.g., lying, stealing, skipping school). On presentation to the ED, these patients may be cooperative or they may continue to act out. Maintaining the safety of the child and the staff is paramount and may require firm redirection as well as the presence of security staff. Those with severe problems or those with co-existent psychosis or depression may require hospitalization. Those with less severe problems may be followed as outpatients.

Autism

Autism is a type of pervasive developmental disorder. The approach to these children in the ED needs to be particularly sensitive, as they may become overwhelmed in new or high-stimulus environments. Children with autism have delayed or very abnormal communication and attachment patterns and generally play alone. They often have stereotyped behaviors. While this diagnosis will not often be made in the ED, the patient with autism may present for either medical conditions or behavioral issues. Many autistic children have seizure disorders. Agitation may ensue if any object in the child's environment has been changed. Most autistic children will have an outpatient psychiatrist to help to guide treatment for acute agitation. Hospitalization, although rarely necessary, requires careful forethought in order to find the best placement with staff who are appropriately skilled in working with these patients.

Eating disorders

Eating disorders often present during early to mid adolescence and may persist into adulthood. Approximately 0.5% of adolescent females in the USA have anorexia nervosa and 1–5% meet criteria for bulimia nervosa. These numbers likely underestimate the true prevalence of disease, as a large number of patients with disordered eating have physical and psychological sequelae but do not meet all of the requisite criteria of the DSM-IV.

Patients with the diagnosis, or possibility, of an eating disorder should have careful vital signs taken, a screening ECG, urinalysis, and electrolytes measured.

Emergencies related to eating disorders come from both caloric restriction and from purging. The most commonly seen emergencies include electrolyte abnormalities, which may precipitate unstable or fatal arrhythmias; GI abnormalities including dental caries, Mallory–Weiss tears; liver function abnormalities; and endocrinopathies, including amenorrhea, sick euthyroid syndrome, and osteopenia resulting in fractures. Irreversible myocardial damage may occur in patients using Ipecac to induce vomiting.

The AAP recommends the following criteria for hospital admission of children with eating disorders (Box 121.1).

Box 121.1. Criteria for hospital admission for children, adolescents, and young adults with eating disorders

Anorexia nervosa

- <75% ideal body weight, or ongoing weight loss despite intensive management.
- Refusal to eat.
- Body fat <10%.
- Heart rate <50 bpm daytime; <45 bpm nighttime.
- Systolic pressure <90 mmHg.
- Orthostatic changes in pulse (>20 bpm) or blood pressure (>10 mmHg).
- Temperature <35.5°C (96°F).
- Arrhythmia.

Bulimia nervosa

- Syncope.
- Serum potassium concentration <3.2 mmol/l.
- Serum chloride concentration <88 mmol/l.
- Esophageal tears.
- Cardiac arrhythmias including prolonged QTc.
- Hypothermia.
- Suicide risk.
- Intractable vomiting.
- Hematemesis.
- Failure to respond to outpatient therapy.

Drug abuse

Drug abuse is a problem which commonly begins in adolescence, although may not be recognized or treated until adulthood, thus resulting in increased morbidity and mortality. More than 50% of teenagers have smoked cigarettes, 75% have used alcohol, 40% have tried marijuana and 20% have used other illicit drugs. Substance use disorders have been associated with other mental disorders in adolescence including mood disorders, ADHD, and eating disorders. Substance abuse may be the first reason that a child presents for emergency psychiatric or medical services (see Ch. 161).

All children presenting with psychiatric complaints should be screened for substance use and abuse. The CAGE questions are often used in adults to identify alcohol problems, but other screening questions may be more age appropriate in younger patients. The CRAFFT mnemonic is one of the recommended screening tools for adolescents (Box 121.2). This tool has a high sensitivity for detecting children likely to benefit from treatment, if more than two questions are answered "Yes."

Box 121.2. Substance use screen for pediatric patients: CRAFFT

C: Have you ever ridden in a **car** driven by someone (including yourself) who was high or had been using alcohol or drugs?
R: Do you ever use alcohol or drugs to **relax**, feel better about yourself, or fit in?
A: Do you ever use alcohol or drugs while you are by yourself (**alone**)?
F: Do you ever **forget** things you do while using alcohol or drugs?
F: Do your family or **friends** ever tell you that you should cut down on your drinking or drug use?
T: Have you ever gotten into **trouble** while you were using alcohol or drugs?

Evaluation

A child may be referred for psychiatric evaluation by many sources. They may be brought to the ED by parents, teachers, baby sitters, the police, or shelters. The collateral information supplied by this broad spectrum of referrals is often indispensable in the evaluation of children as they sometimes do not provide an accurate history or explain the circumstances for their visit (e.g., suicide threat or escalating behavior at school).

A standard history should be obtained from the patient, including a careful review of their medications and family history. Take a moment to observe patient interactions with family or staff to help to determine both their developmental stage and their level of interaction and attention. These factors will influence how the interview is conducted and add information to the child's mental status examination. When appropriate, direct the questions to the guardian. Throughout the history and physical examination it is essential to pay attention to the privacy of the patient, which may include separating the patient from parents for portions of the evaluation. This attention to privacy is particularly important in gaining trust during the evaluation of an adolescent.

Several authors have recommended a structured psychosocial interview when evaluating adolescents. Use of these tools is not limited to the psychiatric setting and may be helpful in evaluating medical complaints in teenagers as well. One widely used tool in the ED setting is the HEADSS interview, which progresses from less-threatening issues to more sensitive topics:

home
education
activities
drug use and abuse
sexual behavior
suicidality/depression.

After a detailed history, a complete physical examination should be performed with close attention for signs of abuse or self-harm. Abuse is another sensitive issue often encountered in the care of pediatric mental health patients, and it may be the cause or the result of the presentation to the ED.

There are no mandated guidelines for a standard laboratory or imaging evaluation of the pediatric psychiatric patient. Laboratory evaluation should be directed at excluding medical diseases. Those patients with an established psychiatric diagnosis may be "medically cleared" by history and physical examination alone.

Management

Regardless of the specific psychiatric disease in question, initial care should be directed towards medical stabilization and patient safety. Once the patient is stable and medical etiologies have been excluded, child psychiatric consultation is required to guide individual management.

The need for physical restraint of the pediatric ED patient occurs almost daily in the setting of laceration repairs and IV placements; however, rarely does the need arise for the use of chemical or physical restraints in pediatric patients with psychiatric disease. When restraint is necessary, an attempt at verbal control should be made, with the help of the parent, before resorting to chemical or physical restraints (see Ch. 120). If verbal redirection is unsuccessful in controlling a violent or agitated patient, then chemical or physical restraints should be employed to protect both the patient and their caregivers. The use of restraints is not without risk, and as such, the Joint Commission for Accreditation of Health Care Organizations requires formal protocols for the use of restraints.

Chemical restraint is defined as "a medication used to control behavior or to restrict a patient's freedom of movement"; they are "not standard treatment for the patient's medical or psychiatric condition." The adverse effects of restraint medications should be weighed against the use of physical and/or chemical restraints. In a patient with mild agitation, careful use of an antihistamine alone may be sufficient. In all pediatric patients, but particularly those with autistic spectrum disorders, care should be taken regarding the dosing. While antihistamines can be helpful, they may also cause a paradoxical disinhibition. In moderate or severe agitation, benzodiazepines or antipsychotic drugs are more typically used. The medications most commonly used for chemical restraint in the treatment of pediatric psychiatric emergencies are summarized in Table 121.2.

Table 121.2. Medications for treating acute agitation/psychosis

Medication	Dose	Route of administration	Onset of action (min)	Side effects
Diphenhydramine	1 mg/kg	IV/IM/PO	5–15 (IV/IM) 20–30 (PO)	Sleepiness, possible disinhibition
Lorazepam	0.05–0.1 mg/kg	IV/IM/PO	5–10 (IV/IM) 20–30 (PO)	Sleepiness, respiratory depression
Haloperidol	0.025–0.075 mg/kg	IM/PO/IV[a]	20–30 (IM) 30–60 (PO)	Extrapyramidal symptoms, neuroleptic malignant syndrome,[b] QTc prolongation, possible restlessness
Olanzapine	*<12 years*: 2.5 mg *>12 years*: 5–10 mg	IM/PO (dissolvable tablet also available)	15–30 (IM) 45–60 (PO)	Sleepiness, bradycardia, headache, possible restlessness
Risperidone	*<12 years*: 0.25–1 mg *>12 years*: 0.5–1 mg	PO (dissolvable tablet also available)	30–60 (PO)	Sleepiness, abdominal pain, headache, hypotension, possible restlessness

[a] IV form not FDA approved.
[b] Management guidelines available at http://www.nmsis.org/services.shtml; 888-667-8367 (US; staffed 24/7 by MD); 315-464-4001 (outside US, also staffed 24/7).

Disposition

Disposition depends on both the clinical scenario as well as the medical and mental health resources available to the patient. If the child exhibits medical complications from a suicide attempt, or if medical causes of psychiatric illness have not been excluded, the patient should be admitted to an inpatient pediatric medical service; transfer to a psychiatric facility can be arranged at a later date. If the patient is a risk to themselves or others, precautions must be taken to ensure safety while completing the medical evaluation. For patients where all urgent medical issues have been addressed, the child should be admitted to an inpatient psychiatric service. The availability of these resources is limited and not all institutions will have such facilities readily available. Prearranged transfer agreements between hospitals should be established for this purpose.

Mental health consultation is recommended when available; however, this may not be an option at all institutions. For low-risk patients, discharge may be considered without immediate mental health consultation. The AAP recommends that if outpatient treatment is chosen, the provider must confirm that the patient has a comprehensive aftercare plan before discharge, that all firearms have been removed from the home, and that potentially lethal medications are not accessible to the child. Safety contracts alone have not been shown to be effective in preventing suicidal behavior.

The following resources can be given to families and patients:

- A 24-hour toll-free hotline for suicide prevention: 1–800-273-TALK, www.suicidepreventionlifeline.org
- American Association of Suicidology: www.suicidology.org
- National Depressive and Manic-Depressive Association: www.ndmda.org.

Pearls and pitfalls

Pearls

1. Always exclude a medical etiology for disturbed behavior. Many medical illnesses may mimic acute mental health symptoms.
2. Respect the privacy and confidentiality of the patient. Address this issue with both the patient and guardians prior to starting the interview process.
3. Use screening tools and have a list of resources for families and patients.

Pitfalls

1. Relying on triage to identify all psychiatric diagnoses. Multiple, non-specific complaints without a clear etiology may be the clue to a psychiatric diagnosis in a patient that is initially mistriaged.
2. Failure to realize that an inconsistent history, difficult examination, or parental interference in an assessment may be clues to trauma or abuse. Perform a violence screen (physical, emotional, and sexual) on all at-risk patients when they are separated from their guardians.

Selected references

Fournier ME, Levy S. Recent trends in adolescent substance use, primary care screening, and updates in treatment options. *Curr Opin Pediatr* 2006;**18**: 352–358.

Kessler RC, Amminger GP, Aguilar-Gaxiola S, *et al.* Age of onset of mental disorders: a review of recent literature. *Curr Opin Psychiatry* 2007;**20**:359–364.

Shain BN. Suicide and suicide attempts in adolescents. *Pediatrics* 2007;**120**: 669–676.

Section

19

Renal emergencies

Expert reviewers: Steven Alexander and Paul C. Grimm

Chapter

122 Kidney disease

Cynthia J. Wong and Steven Alexander

A Acute kidney injury

Introduction

Kidney disease can be categorized as prerenal, renal, or postrenal (Table 122.1). However, despite the etiology, the final outcome is the same, acute kidney injury (AKI). This is defined as a sudden decline in glomerular filtration rate (GFR) and inability of the kidneys to adequately regulate fluid, electrolyte, and acid–base homeostasis. The incidence of AKI in children is much lower than adults. Also, childhood AKI is often reversible if treated promptly. The most common causes of AKI in children are hypovolemic states, hemolytic uremic syndrome (Ch. 124), and acute glomerulonephritis (Ch. 123).

Prerenal insults are the most common causes of AKI in children.

Prerenal AKI occurs when there is inadequate kidney perfusion as a result of intravascular volume depletion and/or decreased cardiac output. Infants are particularly susceptible to excessive volume loss and prerenal AKI. The immature kidney is unable to maximally concentrate urine and appropriately conserve salt and water. A neonate has a relatively large body surface area compared with body mass and will have increased insensible water loss through the skin during illness and exposure.

Postrenal AKI occurs with bilateral urinary tract obstruction, which may result from anatomic abnormalities such as posterior urethral valves, bilateral ureteropelvic, or ureterovesicar junction obstruction. Functional bilateral obstruction from nephrolithiasis or mass can cause postrenal AKI, but this is rare.

Intrinsic renal disorders include renal vascular, glomerular, parenchymal, and/or tubulointerstitial pathologies.

- vascular: bilateral renal artery stenosis, renal vein thrombosis, hemolytic uremic syndrome (Ch. 124) and vasculitis
- glomerular: acute glomerulonephritis such as post-infectious glomerulonephritis, lupus nephritis, or Henoch–Schönlein purpura
- parenchymal: malignancies
- tubulointerstitial: interstitial nephritis and acute tubular necrosis (ATN) (most common form of intrinsic AKI).

Table 122.1. Age-based differential for common causes of acute renal injury

Age	Prerenal	Renal	Postrenal
Infant	Dehydration, sepsis, shock, hypoxic–ischemic insults, asphyxia and hyaline membrane disease, heart failure	ATN from nephrotoxic medications, congenital renal anomalies	Congenital malformations of urinary collecting systems, bladder outlet obstruction, neurogenic bladder
Children	Hypovolemia/dehydration from GI losses, congenital and acquired heart diseases resulting in decreased renal perfusion, sepsis	ATN secondary to medications, hypoxic–ischemic injury; hemolytic uremic syndrome, acute GN *2–12 years*: post-streptococcal GN, Henoch–Schönlein purpura	Bilateral urinary tract obstruction may be caused by anatomic abnormality, tumor, trauma, stones
Adolescents	Dehydration, sepsis	ATN secondary to medications; acute GN; rapidly progressive GN; sepsis, interstitial nephritis	Urinary tract obstruction may be caused by anatomic abnormality, tumor, trauma, stones

ATN, acute tubular necrosis; GN, glomerulonephritis.

A Practical Guide to Pediatric Emergency Medicine: Caring for Children in the Emergency Department, ed. N. Ewen Amieva-Wang (associate eds. Jamie Shandro, Aparajita Sohoni, and Bernhard Fassl). Published by Cambridge University Press.

Table 122.2. History for evaluation of causes of acute renal injury in children

History	Information
Clinical history	
Prerenal	Dehydration, vomiting, diarrhea, polyuria, fever, tachypnea, phototherapy, hemorrhage, nephrotic syndrome, liver failure, heart failure, sepsis
Acute tubular necrosis	Ischemia, hypoxia, toxins, sepsis, hemoglobinuria, myoglobinuria
Hemolytic uremic syndrome	Diarrhea, pallor
Henoch–Schönlein purpura	Palpable purpuric rash, abdominal pain, hematuria, arthralgias
Post-infectious glomerulonephritis	Gross hematuria, edema, hypertension, previous illness
Obstruction	Decreased urine output, abdominal mass, emesis
Past medical history	*Pregnancy and birth history*: previous renal insults, oligohydramnios, ischemic–hypoxic injury during pregnancy and/or delivery, complications after birth *Recurrent urinary tract infections*: history of past renal failure, neurogenic bladder, dysfunctional voiding *Other*: solitary kidney, hypertension
Family history	Kidney disease, dialysis, renal transplantation, kidney stones, recurrent urinary tract infections (vesicoureteral reflux), high-frequency hearing loss (Alport syndrome), hematuria/proteinuria

Acute tubular necrosis results from renal tubular injury in hypoxia, ischemia, or exposure to nephrotoxic agents, such as medications and radiographic contrast, and pigment nephropathy.

Clinical presentation

The diagnosis of AKI is often made by abnormal laboratory test results, which will spur a repeat history and re-examination to assess potential etiologies and extent of AKI.

The history and physical examination can often differentiate between prerenal, postrenal, and intrinsic renal failure (Table 122.2 and 122.3).

Physical examination

Vital signs should be assessed:

- **heart rate**: for a patient with tachycardia, evaluate for volume depletion and fever

Table 122.3. Physical examination findings and associated diseases

Organ system	Finding (clinical disease state)
General	Dry mucous membranes, no tears, and decreased skin turgor (volume depletion) Periorbital or generalized edema (volume overload, glomerulonephritis, nephrotic syndrome)
Head and mouth	Malar rash and oral ulcers (lupus) Uveitis (acute tubulointerstitial nephritis) Epistaxis (platelet dysfunction caused by uremia, hypertension) Sinus disease (Wegener's granulomatosis)
Heart	Hyperdynamic (fluid overload, anemia) Cardiac rub (pericarditis), gallop (fluid overload), muffled heart sounds (pericardial effusion)
Chest	Diminished breath sounds in bases (fluid overload and pleural effusion), pulmonary hemorrhage (microscopic polyangiitis and Wegener's granulomatosis)
Abdomen	Abdominal masses (polycystic kidneys, Wilms' tumor) Bruit (renal artery stenosis), bladder palpable (obstruction)
Skin	Palpable purpuric rash (Henoch–Schönlein purpura) petechiae (thrombocytopenia, hemolytic uremic syndrome), pallor (anemia, hemolytic uremic syndrome), skin turgor and capillary refill time

- **respiratory rate**: for a tachypneic patient, evaluate for fluid overload, pulmonary edema, metabolic acidosis, and/or infectious process; maintain renal perfusion and normal oxygen saturations to avoid hypoxic renal injury
- **blood pressure**: children with hypovolemia may be hypotensive; children with acute glomerulonephritis may be fluid overloaded and present with hypertensive urgency or emergency that needs to be recognized and treated promptly.

Physical examination findings may also suggest a specific etiology of renal disease.

Diagnostic studies

Laboratory tests

Immediate tests to guide treatment include a comprehensive metabolic panel, urinalysis, and CBC. Creatinine clearance should be calculated. The **Schwartz equation** for creatinine clearance (CrCl) is a standard age-based equation that is accessible on the web as well as in texts. It uses the patient's height (H), serum creatinine (Cr, mg/dl), and a proportionality constant (k), which varies with age:

$$\mathrm{CrCl} = k \times H(\mathrm{cm})/\mathrm{Cr}(\mathrm{mg/dl})$$

The values for k with age are:
infant (LBW <1 year): 0.33
infant (term <1 year): 0.45
child: 0.55
adolescent girl: 0.55
adolescent boy: 0.70.

There are a number of important caveats to using this approach.

- Normal serum creatinine varies by age (Table 122.4). While newborn infants have serum creatinine levels that reflect maternal levels for the first few days of life, as GFR increases, the infant's serum creatinine level decreases. Creatinine levels rise slowly in the first 10 to 15 years of life to adult parameters.

Table 122.4. Normal serum creatinine levels by age

Age	Creatinine (mg/dl)
Term infant >2 days	<0.4
2–8 years	0.5 to 0.7
9–18 years	0.6 to 0.9

Source: Avner, 2004.

- The BUN/creatinine ratio to evaluate for prerenal injury is not reliable in young pediatric patients as they have a lower muscle mass and creatinine levels.
- Azotemia is not a good indicator for acute renal injury in children since they may have low/normal BUN levels through decreased urea production, such as in severe liver disease or with protein malnutrition.

The fractional excretion (FE) of sodium is calculated using the following equation:

$$FE_{Na} = 100[U_{Na}P_{Cr}/P_{Na}U_{Cr}]$$

where U is urine, P is plasma, Na is sodium (mmol/l), and Cr is creatinine (mg/dl). It is important to remember that

- FE_{Na} not reliable after diuretic therapy
- low FE_{Na} can be seen in children who are not prerenal and who have normal tubular function but a low GFR, such as with acute glomerulonephritis, vasculitis, acute urinary tract obstruction, or ATN, superimposed upon a chronic sodium-retaining state.

Table 122.5 summarizes the laboratory and radiology results in different disease studies.

Imaging studies

In anuric children, and in children in whom there is a concern for urinary tract obstruction, a Doppler renal ultrasound and

Table 122.5. Laboratory and imaging studies

	Prerenal	ATN	HUS	HSP	PIGN	Obstruction
Urinalysis	Normal to minor changes	Granular casts, muddy brown casts	Hematuria, RBC casts, proteinuria	Hematuria, proteinuria	Hematuria, proteinuria, RBC casts	Normal
Urine osmolality	>400–500 mOsm (newborn >350 mOsm)	<350 mOsm (newborn <300 mOsm)	Variable	Variable	>400–500 mOsm	Variable
Urine sodium	<10 mEq/l (newborn <20–30 mEq/l)	>30–40 mEq/l	Variable	Variable	<10 mEq/l	Variable
Fractional excretion sodium[a]	<1% (newborn <2.5%)	>2% (newborn >2.5–3%)	Variable	Variable	<1%	Variable
BUN and creatinine	Increased BUN/ creatinine ratio					
Other laboratory tests			Anemia (hemolytic), uremia, thrombocytopenia		Post-streptococcal: low C3, + anti-streptolysin O titer + DNase B antibody	Variable, metabolic acidosis
Renal ultrasound	Normal	Normal or increased echogenicity with loss of CM differentiation	Normal or loss of CM differentiation	Normal	Nephromegaly and loss of CM differentiation	Dilated pelvis, ureter, and/or bladder depending on level of obstruction

ATN, acute tubular necrosis; BUN, blood urea nitrogen; CM, corticomedullary; HSP, Henoch–Schönlein purpura; HUS, hemolytic uremic syndrome; PIGN, post-infectious glomerulonephritis.
[a] Fractional excretion of sodium is not reliable after diuretics.

bladder ultrasound is useful. If there is a concern for nephrolithiasis, a helical CT scan may be indicated (Table 122.5).

Management

Initial management is to treat and avoid life-threatening complications including shock, hyperkalemia, hypertension, and cardiopulmonary compromise from fluid overload.

Fluid management

The goal is to establish an effective circulatory volume and maintain a normal intravascular volume. Children with volume depletion should be given IV fluids to restore intravascular volume and maintain renal perfusion. For oligouric/anuric renal failure, careful fluid resuscitation with close examination and re-evaluation after each fluid bolus is essential to avoid fluid overload and pulmonary edema.

Once the patient's intravascular volume is repleted, fluid management should be guided to replace insensible fluid losses, urine, and other output (see Ch. 53). Insensible fluid losses are estimated at approximately one-third maintenance. Insensible fluid losses will be higher in tachypneic and/or febrile children and in infants. In oliguric children, fluid should be restricted to insensible loss and volume of urine output, replaced milliliter for milliliter with fluids. Water losses from diarrhea should also be measured and replaced on these terms. Children in the recovery polyuric phase of ATN or the post-obstructive diuresis phase may have significant fluid and electrolyte losses that need to be monitored and replaced to avoid prerenal injury and dehydration.

Children with fluid overload need fluid restriction and, if indicated, a trial of diuretics. Significant fluid overload in an anuric child with pulmonary edema, respiratory distress, and/or heart failure who is not responsive to diuretics may need dialysis. Patients with hemolytic uremic syndrome and lupus can have severe anemia from hemolysis and may require transfusion. Packed red blood cell transfusions must be monitored closely in patients with AKI because of the potential for fluid and potassium overload. Patients with oliguric/anuric AKI who are fluid overloaded and resistant to diuretics may require dialysis for blood transfusions.

Electrolyte management

Hyperkalemia needs to be treated promptly because of concerns for cardiac arrhythmias (Ch. 17). If **hyponatremia** is caused by fluid overload, these children need to be fluid restricted. In contrast, children with hyponatremic dehydration as a result of large sodium and fluid losses require fluid and sodium replacement.

Metabolic acidosis

In children with AKI, acid excretion is impaired and acid production is frequently increased. Correction of acidosis should be limited to when arterial pH is <7.2 and/or the acidosis is contributing to hyperkalemia. Correction is limited by concerns for increase in intravascular volume, hypernatremia, hyperosmolarity, and lowering ionized calcium, leading to tetany or seizures when bicarbonate is given.

Hypertension

Consider using diuretics for a child with hypertension who is fluid overloaded and whose intravascular volume is replete. Calcium channel blockers, such as amlodipine 0.05 mg/kg (max. initial dose 5 mg), are also helpful to control blood pressure in children with normal cardiac and liver function.

Medications

Care must be taken to avoid further injury from nephrotoxic medications. Often dosage of medications that are cleared by the kidneys needs to be adjusted for the child's renal impairment, particularly when creatinine clearance falls to $<50\%$ of normal.

Dialysis

If the patient is not responding to medical management, dialysis may be necessary.

Indications for acute dialysis include severe fluid overload resistant to diuretics, leading to pulmonary edema, and heart failure, and/or hypertension; fluid overload that is refractory to medical therapy; severe electrolyte abnormalities that do not correct with medical management, such as hyperkalemia and severe metabolic acidosis; patients who are uremic and have symptoms such as mental status changes; uremic pericarditis; anuric or oligouric patients who need a significant amount of fluids, such as blood products, fluids needed to maintain hemodynamic stability, and/or nutritional needs; and/or drug/toxin accumulation.

Different modalities for dialysis include hemodialysis, peritoneal dialysis, and continuous renal replacement therapy (continuous venovenous hemodiafiltration). Peritoneal dialysis is continuous but slow. Intermittent hemodialysis can allow for rapid fluid removal but patients may have problems with hemodynamic instability. Continuous venovenous hemodiafiltration is continuous, slow, and patients may be hemodynamically more stable than with intermittent dialysis. This is a good approach for close fluid and electrolyte management in a critically ill patient.

Disposition

Children with AKI should be admitted to the hospital and a pediatric nephrologist should be consulted.

B Chronic kidney disease/dialysis and renal transplant

Introduction

It is important to differentiate acute from chronic renal failure since the causes and treatment may differ. The leading causes of end-stage renal disease in adults are diabetes, hypertension, and glomerulonephritis. In children, the leading causes are congenital abnormalities including hypoplastic/dysplastic kidneys, obstructive uropathy such as from posterior urethral valves, and focal segmental glomerulosclerosis.

Chronic kidney disease (CKD) is a progressive process and is usually not reversible. Initially, most patients are asymptomatic and different symptoms may be observed with gradual decline in renal function. Uremic patients may complain of anorexia, nausea, vomiting, peripheral neuropathy, and neurologic abnormalities, including seizures, difficulty concentrating, and lethargy.

In later stages of CKD when creatinine clearance declines, children may develop disorders of fluid, electrolyte, and acid–base balance and abnormalities in calcium and phosphorus metabolism, leading to hyperparathyroidism, hypertension, anemia, dyslipidemia, growth failure, and neurocognitive difficulties.

This section provides an overview of children on dialysis and renal transplantation; however, a nephrologist should be consulted whenever a child with CKD, particularly one with a renal transplant, is seen in the ED.

Hemodialysis

A child with CKD who is undergoing hemodialysis has unique physiologic needs and is exquisitely sensitive to alterations in blood pressure or electrolytes. With regard to blood pressure, both hyper- and hypotension can be dangerous. If hypertensive, with fluid overload, dialysis should be initiated. If there will be a delay to initiating dialysis, medications may be given to lower the blood pressure. Common antihypertensive medications include amlodipine if the child does not have depressed cardiac function. Hypotension can predispose the patient to developing thrombi in the arteriovenous fistula. Judicious use of fluids, as well as avoiding blood pressure measurements, tourniquets, and blood draws on the arm with the arteriovenous fistula, should be used to avoid thrombosing the fistula.

Children on dialysis are often on strict fluid and dietary sodium, potassium, and phosphorus restrictions. The exception are children with high-output (polyuric) renal failure. These children are encouraged to take in sufficient fluid to keep up with their urine output. Special caution should be used if prescribing any oral medication containing phosphorus or magnesium, or if prescribing a bowel preparation enema, to a child with CKD.

Lastly, children with a low estimated creatinine clearance should not receive gadolinium contrast because of concerns for systemic nephrogenic fibrosis, a debilitating and difficult-to-treat dermatologic disorder.

Management of the hemodialysis catheter

The majority of young children on hemodialysis will have a dialysis catheter versus an arteriovenous fistula or shunt for their dialysis access. Children with catheters or indwelling hardware are at the highest risk for blood-borne infection. If these children present with fever and/or chills during their evaluation, it is important to obtain blood cultures from each port of their hemodialysis catheter and start broad-spectrum empiric antibiotics. Doses of medications cleared by the kidney need to be adjusted in dialysis patients, since these children have significantly impaired ability to clear these medications.

Because of the limited lifelong vascular access in patients with end-stage renal disease, contamination of the catheter or thrombosis of the catheter from improper handling must be avoided. The hemodialysis catheter should only be accessed by a specialized nurse who is trained on the proper procedures needed to manage these catheters. Hemodialysis catheters tend to be locked with high concentrations of heparin (1000 U/ml) or alteplase and care must be taken not to flush these medications into the patient.

Peritoneal dialysis

Children on peritoneal dialysis are at increased risk for peritonitis because they have an indwelling catheter with a dextrose-containing fluid in their abdomen. In children who present with fever, abdominal pain, cloudy dialysate, and/or other symptoms concerning for peritonitis, a sample of the peritoneal dialysate needs to be obtained under proper sterile conditions and sent for Gram stain, cell count, and culture. A pediatric nephrologist should be consulted for further management and to guide use of empiric intraperitoneal antibiotics.

Children on peritoneal dialysis are also at increased risk for infection through hypogammaglobulinemia from IgG losses during dialysis.

Pearls and pitfalls

Pearls

1. Creatinine levels vary with age, what may be "normal" for an adult may be significantly elevated in a child.
2. The most common cause of acute kidney injury in children is a prerenal insult.
3. Most common cause of acute kidney injury in children are hypovolemia, hemolytic uremic syndrome, and acute glomerulonephritis.

Pitfalls

1. Failure to hydrate a child appropriately to prevent or reverse prerenal acute kidney injury.
2. Failure to avoid medications with phosphorus and magnesium in children on dialysis.

Renal transplant recipients

Proper fluid and blood pressure management is essential in a child with a renal transplant. Evaluation for rejection and infection is important in these immunosuppressed children.

Rejection may present as a rise in creatinine from the child's baseline. The child may have fever and flu-like symptoms with "rejection illness." They may experience pain over the graft and the graft may be firm and tender when palpated on examination.

Young children and toddlers who receive adult kidney transplants have high fluid requirements (1.5 or more liters a day) and higher blood pressures (systolic blood pressure >110–120 mmHg) in the first 6–12 months after transplant to maintain adequate blood flow to the graft. Therefore, dehydration and hypotension must be recognized and treated promptly to avoid a low flow state that could put the graft at risk for developing ATN and/or thrombosis, with permanent graft dysfunction.

Selected references

Andreoli S. Acute renal failure. *Curr Opin Pediatr* 2002;**14**:183–188.

Avner E. The fourth report on the diagnosis, evaluation, and treatment of high blood pressure in children and adolescents. *Pediatrics* 2004;**114**:555–576.

Corrigan Jr. JJ, Boineau FG. Hemolytic–uremic syndrome. *Pediatr Rev* 2001;**22**:365–369.

Noris M, Remuzzi G. Hemolytic uremic syndrome. *J Am Soc Nephrol* 2005;**16**:1035–1050.

Chapter 123

Glomerulonephritis and nephrotic syndrome

Cynthia J. Wong, Steven Alexander, and Ingrid T. Lim

A Glomerulonephritis

Cynthia J. Wong, Steven Alexander, and Ingrid T. Lim

Introduction

In the USA and Europe, glomerulonephritis is the third most common cause of end-stage renal disease. Acute glomerulonephritis is defined as inflammation of the glomeruli with gross or microscopic hematuria, proteinuria, and decreased renal function. Glomerulonephritis may occur as a primary renal disease or as a manifestation of a systemic disease process. Early detection of acute glomerulonephritis is important to provide appropriate management of the underlying disease. Children with acute glomerulonephritis may present with fluid overload and/or hypertension requiring emergency management. For children with glomerulonephritis, nephrology should be consulted for further management and follow-up. The differential diagnosis in a child who has acute glomerulonephritis should include post-infectious glomerulonephritis and primary glomerular diseases, including membranoproliferative glomerulonephritis, hereditary nephritis, Henoch–Schönlein purpura, IgA nephropathy, hemolytic uremic syndrome, and lupus. This chapter will review post-infectious glomerulonephritis and IgA nephropathy before moving on in Part B to nephrotic syndrome (NS).

Post-infectious glomerulonephritis

Post-infectious glomerulonephritis is the most common cause of glomerulonephritis in children. Nephrogenic strains of group A beta-hemolytic streptococci are most often involved. Poststreptococcal acute glomerulonephritis (PSGN) follows bacterial infection within 14–21 days. Most cases of PSGN occur between 4 and 15 years of age with a peak incidence at age 4 to 5 years.

Clinical presentation

The clinical presentation of PSGN is variable. Clinical features include hematuria, proteinuria, active urine sediment, fluid retention, hypertension, and reduced renal function: 30–50% of children with PSGN present with gross hematuria, described as coca cola or tea colored. Gross hematuria tends to clear within a few days but can last as long as 2 weeks. Microscopic hematuria may persist for years. Proteinuria is usually transient and not in the nephrotic range (i.e., $<40\ mg/m^2$ per h).

Hypertension is common and may be initially asymptomatic. Unmonitored and untreated, hypertension may lead to serious complications, including hypertensive encephalopathy and cardiac failure. Hypertension and fluid overload are related to sodium retention and increased intravascular volume. Blood pressures tend to improve with sodium and fluid restriction as well as diuretics. Aggressive antihypertensive therapy is needed for patients who present with hypertensive urgency or crisis.

Diagnostic studies

Laboratory studies to confirm recent streptococcal infection include elevated streptococcal antibodies. Anti-streptolysin O (ASO) titer is elevated in 50–80% of children with PSGN after a streptococcal pharyngitis. Titers should be present 2–3 weeks after infection, unless the antibody response was blunted by the use of antibiotics.

Management

Management of PSGN includes monitoring and treating hypertension, electrolyte abnormalities, and fluid overload. Antihypertensive therapy includes correcting hypervolemic state with diuretics, sodium and fluid restriction, and antihypertensive medications if necessary. Patients with oliguria should be evaluated for dehydration, euvolemia, or fluid overload and for intravascular volume status before restricting fluid. If urine output does not increase with diuretics, fluid intake should be restricted to insensible water loss and urine output. Children may have a variety of electrolyte imbalances including hyponatremia, which is usually caused by fluid overload; hyperkalemia from acute renal failure; hypocalcemia; and metabolic acidosis. Renal service should consult on all patients with acute glomerulonephritis. All patients should be strongly considered for admission.

A Practical Guide to Pediatric Emergency Medicine: Caring for Children in the Emergency Department, ed. N. Ewen Amieva-Wang (associate eds. Jamie Shandro, Aparajita Sohoni, and Bernhard Fassl). Published by Cambridge University Press.

Antibiotic therapy does not prevent or alter the course of PSGN, but streptococcal infections should be treated to prevent the complications of rheumatic heart disease. Repeat episodes of PSGN are rare since immunity is type specific and long lasting. Prognosis of PSGN is generally favorable with more than 95% of pediatric patients recovering spontaneously with return to baseline renal function within 3–4 weeks.

IgA nephropathy

IgA nephropathy is the most common cause of glomerulonephritis diagnosed in adolescents. Primary IgA nephropathy is an immune-complex-mediated glomerulonephritis with IgA deposits mainly in the mesangium of the glomeruli.

Clinical presentation

Classic presentation is asymptomatic gross hematuria at the time of a respiratory infection. Mild and transient reduction in renal function may occur during presentation and/or during episodes of gross hematuria.

Management

Treatment is not well defined and may include fish oil, ACE inhibitor, and/or immunosuppressant therapy with steroids, cyclophosphamide, and/or mycophenolate mofetil in more aggressive disease. Disposition should be decided in consult with renal service and follow-up should be arranged. These patients need long-term follow-up by nephrology.

Disposition in glomerulonephritis

All children with acute glomerulonephritis should have a detailed physical examination focusing on hypertension, fluid balance, and cardiorespiratory function. They also should have chemistry panel to determine the presence of uremia, acidosis, or hyperkalemia. Strong consideration for admission should include discussion with a pediatric nephrologist. Acute glomerulonephritis such as IgA nephropathy that presents with gross hematuria in the context of acute upper respiratory tract infection with normal blood pressure and normal chemistry can usually be treated as an outpatient unless there are extenuating social circumstances.

B Nephrotic syndrome

Ingrid T. Lim

Introduction

Nephrotic syndrome refers to a syndrome of increased permeability to protein across the glomerular filtration barrier. It is defined as the clinical manifestation of a variety of primary and secondary glomerular disorders characterized by the following findings:

- hypoproteinemia (serum albumin <3 g/dl)
- marked proteinuria (>40 mg/m^2 per h in a 24-h period)
- edema
- hyperlipidemia (predominantly triglycerides and cholesterol).

The most common cause of pediatric NS is idiopathic (also known as minimal change disease because of the minimal changes seen on renal biopsy). Idiopathic NS can be classified by its response to corticosteroids: steroid responsive (90%) and steroid non-responsive (10%). Lack of response to steroids portends a poor prognosis and a 50% risk of advancement to end-stage renal failure. Usually sporadic NS can be familial, with polygenic inheritance pattern. The typical age of presentation of primary NS is 18 months to 5 or 6 years. In adolescents, NS is most often associated with a primary or secondary form of an underlying nephritis.

Clinical presentation

The usual presenting sign in a child with NS is edema. The edema starts with early-morning periorbital swelling, often wrongly attributed to a cold or allergies. As the edema spreads to the abdomen, trunk, and extremities, children develop difficulty fitting into their pants and shoes, and parents often mistake it for weight gain. The child otherwise appears well, unless ascites, pleural effusion, or pulmonary edema is present. Ascites and edematous intestinal wall can manifest as abdominal pain, nausea, vomiting, and diarrhea. Scrotal or labial edema may also be present.

Complications

Acute renal failure can occur. Patients can also become hypovolemic. They can develop respiratory distress from pleural effusions, pulmonary edema and massive ascites.

Patients are also prone to infection because of their decreased serum immunoproteins. They are particularly susceptible to encapsulated bacteria such as *Escherichia coli, Haemophilus influenzae* and *Streptococcus pneumoniae*. The most common infection is peritonitis. Steroid therapy may mask the typical signs of infection. In fact, infections with these organisms are the main cause of death in children with NS.

Patients with NS are also prone to hypercoagulable states (seen in 3% of nephrotic patients). Hypoalbuminemia may enhance platelet aggregation. Thromboembolic events can involve both arteries and veins, but particularly the renal veins. Consequently, sudden onset of gross hematuria or renal failure should prompt investigation for renal vein thrombosis. Note that prednisone exerts an anti-heparin effect; deep venous punctures should not be attempted in nephrotic children unless no alternative exists.

Management

The goals for ED management are volume resuscitation and treatment of symptomatic edema. Shock is treated with isotonic hydration at 20 ml/kg bolus per hour until normotensive, even in the presence of edema. If the child is clinically dehydrated and hemoconcentrated but not in shock, a trial of sodium-deficient fluids orally at twice maintenance is preferable to IV hypotonic solutions. Frequent, small amounts of oral hydration should be given to avoid vomiting caused by an edematous gut.

If the patient is well hydrated and exhibits severe or symptomatic edema, diuretics can be started but should be used judiciously as these patients have decreased circulating volume and they are prone to thromboembolic events. Furosemide 1 to 2 mg/kg over 24 h PO or IV in divided BID doses can be used. Loop diuretics work best, but additional diuretics such as hydrochlorothiazide, metalozone, or spironolactone may be added to potentiate the effect of loop diuretics. Diuretics are not effective with albumin concentrations <1.5 g. Albumin infusions may be necessary prior to diuretic administration: 0.5 to 1 g/kg given as 25% salt-deficient albumin followed by 0.5 to 1 mg/kg furosemide. Diuretics are rarely if ever prescribed to outpatients because of the risk of aggravating hemoconcentration in patients who cannot defend their circulating blood volume owing to a low serum albumin.

The mainstay of treatment for NS is steroid therapy. Generally patients should be started on prednisone 2 mg/kg per 24 h (max. 60 mg/24 h) divided into two to three doses. Approximately 90% of patients with idiopathic NS will respond to steroid therapy by the end of a 4-week course, defined by trace or negative urine protein for 3 days. Failure to respond to steroid treatment increases the likelihood that the renal pathology is not caused by NS, and referral and renal biopsy are warranted.

Prophylactic antibiotics are not necessary unless infection is suspected and cultures collected. Any child with NS and an unexplained fever must be considered to have a bacterial infection until proven otherwise. Blood and urine cultures should be obtained, and coverage with broad-spectrum antibiotics is recommended while awaiting culture results. As patients on steroids may not demonstrate any abdominal pain or signs of peritonitis, a diagnostic paracentesis must be performed on children with fever and ascites, or signs of peritonitis without fever. Prophylactic aspirin may be considered for patients with hemoconcentration, history of thrombosis during a previous relapse, or elevated platelets.

Disposition

Admission is recommended for

- any infant with nephrotic syndrome
- any patient with respiratory distress or shock
- newly diagnosed patients in order to complete an evaluation and educate parents about management.

Pearls and pitfalls

Pearls

1. In patients with post-infectious glomerulonephritis, blood pressure monitoring is key.
2. Suspect IgA nephropathy in a child with asymptomatic gross hematuria at the time of a systemic infection, such as a respiratory infection.
3. Nephrotic syndrome is characterized by marked proteinuria, hypoalbuminemia, hyperlipidemia, and edema.

Pitfalls

1. Performing deep venous or arterial punctures in nephrotic children on chronic prednisone therapy. These patients are at increased risk for thromboembolic events.
2. Failure to admit a child with acute glomerulonephritis.
3. Failure to suspect a bacterial infection in a child with nephrotic syndrome and a fever.

Selected references

Andreoli S. Acute renal failure. *Curr Opin Pediatr* 2002;**14**:183–188.

Lau KK, Wyatt RJ. Glomerulonephritis. *Adolesc Med Clin* 2005;**16**: 67–85.

McCrory WW. Glomerulonephritis. *Pediatr Rev* 1983;**5**:19–25.

Chapter

124 Hemolytic uremic syndrome

Cynthia J. Wong and Steven Alexander

Introduction

Hemolytic uremic syndrome (HUS) is the most common primary renal disease that causes acute kidney injury (AKI) in children.

HUS is characterized by microangiopathic, non-immune hemolytic anemia, thrombocytopenia, and acute uremic renal failure.

The most common form of HUS is associated with diarrhea and has been associated with a Shiga toxin-producing strain of *Escherichia coli* O157:H7 or other Shiga toxin-producing organisms. Atypical, non-diarrhea-associated HUS is less common in children and has a worse prognosis. The annual incidence of diarrhea-associated HUS is estimated to be 2.1/100 000 persons. Peak incidence is in children <5 years of age.

Clinical presentation

The clinical picture of HUS is a previously healthy child who develops abdominal pain and diarrhea, which may progress to bloody diarrhea. The child has a normochromic, normocytic anemia with schistocytes and helmet cells seen on blood smear. Platelet counts may start off greater than 100 000/μl then decrease with thrombocytopenia, which may last for 7 to 20 days. Central nervous system symptoms, such as seizures (3–5% of patients), may also occur.

Renal involvement with HUS varies from isolated microscopic hematuria to anuric renal failure requiring dialysis; 55–70% of patients experience some degree of AKI. Within 4 to 7 days of onset of diarrhea, 60% of patients experience oligouria, which lasts an average of 1 week. Almost 50% of oliguric patients become anuric for an average of 3 days, but renal function recovers in the majority of patients.

Electrolyte and fluid imbalance is common. Patients may have a variety of electrolyte disturbances including hyponatremia from fluid overload, metabolic acidosis, hyperphosphatemia, hypocalcemia, and hyperkalemia from decreased glomerular filtration rate, hemolysis, and tissue catabolism. Almost 50% of children with HUS develop hypertension. Hypertension may be related to fluid overload or renin release in response to decreased renal perfusion.

Management

Management is primarily supportive. Careful control of fluid and electrolyte balance is essential. Volume expansion with isotonic saline during the diarrheal phase may be associated with less-severe renal involvement. Diuretics may be needed in patients with fluid overload.

Antimotility agents should also be avoided.

Hypertension must be recognized and treated. Diuretics are useful to help to control hypertension in patients with fluid overload who are not anuric. A calcium channel blocker, such as amlodipine or isradipine, is recommended as an initial choice for an antihypertensive agent.

Children with HUS may become profoundly anemic through the active hemolytic processes. Transfusion with packed red blood cells (RBCs) should be considered when the hemoglobin is <7 g/dl, or sooner in a patient with cardiac or pulmonary compromise. The target hemoglobin is between 8 and 9 mg/dl. A RBC transfusion should be volume and leukocyte reduced to avoid fluid overload and sensitization. For a child with anuric or oliguric AKI and fluid overload, packed RBCs may need to be given with dialysis to avoid cardiopulmonary compromise. Transfusions should be given slowly with monitoring for hyperkalemia, fluid overload, and hypertension. Platelet transfusions should be avoided in stable

A Practical Guide to Pediatric Emergency Medicine: Caring for Children in the Emergency Department, ed. N. Ewen Amieva-Wang (associate eds. Jamie Shandro, Aparajita Sohoni, and Bernhard Fassl). Published by Cambridge University Press.

patients who are not bleeding because of concerns for formation of new or expanding thrombi.

Although HUS is associated with *E. coli* O157:H7 infection, this infection generally should not be treated. Antimotility agents should also be avoided.

Antibiotics should be avoided in clinically stable patients who do not have sepsis or bacteremia because of concerns about toxin release and exacerbation of HUS.

Disposition

Children with HUS should be admitted. Nephrology should be consulted to aid in medical management as well as to provide long-term renal follow-up. For children with renal failure who are not responding to medical management for fluid and electrolyte balance, dialysis may be indicated.

Prognosis

The early mortality for diarrhea-associated HUS is <5%, with the exception of epidemics where the mortality is higher. For the first decade after HUS, up to 30% of survivors experienced adverse renal outcome such as persistent proteinuria, hypertension, or renal impairment, including end-stage renal disease in 5–10%. Long-term follow-up and monitoring for development of hypertension, proteinuria, and renal insufficiency is necessary as end-stage renal disease may increase by 60% in the second and third decades of life after HUS. Poor outcome is more likely if a patient has anuric AKI for greater than a week and/or requires more than 2 weeks of dialysis during the acute phase.

Pearls and pitfalls

Pearls

1. Hemolytic uremic syndrome (HUS) in children and thrombotic thrombocytopenic purpura in adults appear to have similar pathophysiology, but differ in terms of organ systems affected, with increased renal pathology in children and more prominent CNS, cardiac, GI, and some renal pathology in adults.
2. In children, HUS is the most common cause of acute kidney injury.
3. In HUS, there is microangiopathic hemolytic anemia, thrombocytopenia, and acute kidney injury.
4. Typical/diarrhea-associated HUS is the most common cause of HUS in children and is often associated with diarrhea caused by bacteria producing Shiga toxin, such as *Escherichia coli* 0157.

Pitfalls

1. Failure to consider/workup for HUS in a child with bloody diarrhea.
2. Failure to send stool culture.
3. Unnecessary treatment of bloody diarrhea with antibiotics.

Select references

Corrigan JJ Jr., Boineau FG. Hemolytic-uremic syndrome. *Pediatr Rev* 2001;**22**:365–369.

Noris M, Remuzzi G. Hemolytic uremic syndrome. *J Am Soc Nephrol* 2005;**16**:1035–1050.

Siegler RL, Pavia AT, Christofferson RD, Milligan MK. A 20-year population-based study of postdiarrheal hemolytic uremic syndrome in Utah. *Pediatrics* 1994;**94**: 35–40.

Chapter

125 Hypertension

Aparajita Sohoni

Introduction

Pediatric hypertension is an important and increasingly recognized phenomenon. In 2004, the National High Blood Pressure Education Program published guidelines regarding the diagnosis and management of pediatric hypertension. These guidelines define the following terms that are useful for the understanding of pediatric hypertension.

- hypertension is an average systolic blood pressure (SBP) and/or diastolic blood pressure (DBP) ≥95th percentile for gender/age/height on ≥3 occasions
- hypertension is further staged by severity:
  - "white coat hypertension": a child with SBP or DBP >95th percentile in a medical setting but who is normotensive outside the clinical setting
  - prehypertension: average SBP or DBP ≥90th percentile but <95th percentile (note: in adolescents, any blood pressure >120/80 mmHg should be considered prehypertension)
  - stage 1 hypertension: blood pressure measurements in the 95th–99th percentile plus 5 mmHg
  - stage 2 hypertension: blood pressure measurements in the 99th percentile plus 5 mmHg.

All pediatric patients >3 years of age should have their blood pressure measured once during an ED encounter. In patients <3 years, blood pressure should be measured if there is a history of congenital heart disease; prematurity or other neonatal complication; renal disease, recurrent urinary tract infections, hematuria, or proteinuria; a history of malignancy, bone marrow or organ transplantation; medication use thought to increase blood pressure; or other systemic illness associated with hypertension (e.g., tuberous sclerosis or neurofibromatosis).

While the overall prevalence of pediatric hypertension is approximated at 1–2%, with the current rise in childhood obesity the true prevalence of hypertension is thought to be much higher than current estimates suggest. Of equal concern is the contribution of obesity to the development of other cardiovascular risk factors, such as hyperlipidemia and hyperinsulinemia. The identification and appropriate management of pediatric hypertension is an important component of overall child health and prevention of future morbidity from cardiovascular disease.

Pediatric hypertension is divided into primary, or essential, hypertension and secondary hypertension. While in past decades the majority of pediatric hypertension was thought to be secondary, mainly from renal disease, surveys from the past few years have shown an increase in the prevalence of primary hypertension: from only 13% in studies from the late 1980s to as high as 50% in 2001. The most common etiologies of pediatric hypertension by age are shown in Table 125.1.

Clinical presentation

Pediatric patients with hypertension may present in a variety of manners. Most patients will have an incidentally high blood pressure noted on the ED visit for an unrelated issue. Some patients may be brought in because of an incidental elevated blood pressure reading noted at a supermarket or at a school screening-test. More uncommonly, a child may present with hypertension in the setting of a known associated medical condition. Hypertensive emergencies are rare in children. Hypertensive urgencies, where the elevated blood pressure is thought to imminently be able to cause end-organ damage but has not yet, are more common and often the cause of admission to the hospital.

The first step in evaluating a child with hypertension is to confirm that the blood pressure is indeed elevated. The inflatable bladders width is at least 40% of the arm circumference at a point midway between the olecranon and the acromion. The cuff bladder length should cover 80–100% of the circumference of the arm. Appropriate blood pressure cuff size is key to ensuring an accurate measurement, as is measuring the blood pressure when the child is calm, in a seated position, and with the arm at the level of the heart. In any child presenting with hypertension, coarctation of the aorta is a concern; therefore, blood pressure measurements in all four limbs should be obtained.

A Practical Guide to Pediatric Emergency Medicine: Caring for Children in the Emergency Department, ed. N. Ewen Amieva-Wang (associate eds. Jamie Shandro, Aparajita Sohoni, and Bernhard Fassl). Published by Cambridge University Press.

Table 125.1. Etiologies of pediatric hypertension

Newborn	1–12 months	1–6 years	6–12 years	12–18 years
Renovascular disease	Renovascular disease	Renovascular disease	Renovascular disease	Renovascular disease
Congenital renal disease	Renal parenchymal diseases	Renal parenchymal diseases	Renal parenchymal diseases	Renal parenchymal diseases
Coarctation of the aorta	Coarctation of the aorta	Coarctation of the aorta	Coarctation of the aorta	Coarctation of the aorta
Patent ductus arteriosus		Essential hypertension Endocrine disorders	Essential hypertension Endocrine disorders	Essential hypertension Endocrine disorders
Intraventricular hemorrhage			Iatrogenic (medications or postoperative)	
Bronchopulmonary dysplasia				

Source: Varda and Gregoric, 2005.

After confirmation of an elevated blood pressure, it is imperative to obtain a thorough history and conduct a careful physical examination. The review of systems should cover cardiac, renal, or endocrine diseases. A history of stimulant use should specifically be assessed. Past medical history, including urinary tract infections, surgeries, snoring, or patterns of sleep should be evaluated. All medications should be reviewed, and the family history of cardiovascular disease should also be obtained.

Diagnosis

Recently published guidelines have sought to unify the diagnosis and management of hypertension. A patient with an elevated blood pressure should be classified as clinically symptomatic or asymptomatic, as this will determine whether immediate blood pressure-lowering medication is warranted. Clinical symptoms vary with the age of the patient but include irritability, seizures, visual changes, headache, or cranial nerve palsies. All symptomatic children, and all children with stage 1 or 2 hypertension, should undergo laboratory testing for evidence of occult end-organ damage. End-organ damage is now thought to be more common in pediatric patients than formerly recognized, with some studies of patients with SBP or DBP measurements >90th percentile showing 36% having left ventricular hypertrophy and 50% having retinal vascular changes. Table 125.2 lists an appropriate diagnostic series for evaluating end-organ damage in a pediatric patient with either symptomatic hypertension or stage 1 or stage 2 hypertension.

Table 125.2. Diagnostic evaluation of hypertension

Test	Population		
	BP ≥95th percentile	BP ≥90th percentile plus co-morbid risk factors[a]	Family history of hypertension
BUN, creatinine, electrolytes	X		
Urine analysis, urine culture	X	X	X
Complete blood count	X		
Renal ultrasound	X		
Echocardiography	X	X	
Retinal examination	X	X	
Fasting lipid panel	X	X	X
Fasting blood glucose	X	X	X
Drug screen	If suggested by history	If suggested by history	If suggested by history

BP, blood pressure.
[a] Co-morbid risk factors include chronic kidney disease, diabetes mellitus, and obesity.

Management

The management of pediatric hypertension in the ED will depend on the stage of hypertension and the severity of symptoms, if present. For any patient with stage 1, stage 2, or symptomatic hypertension, diagnostic evaluations as well as oral antihypertensive medications should be initiated in close conjunction with the child's primary care physician and hypertension specialist. Ideally these patients will be admitted for gradual blood pressure lowering, workup, and to arrange optimal follow-up.

Pharmacologic therapy for the treatment of pediatric hypertension has advanced greatly. Oral antihypertensive medications are first-line treatment. Intravenous medications should only be used if severe, symptomatic hypertension with evidence of end-organ damage is present. Consultation with a specialist in selection of an antihypertensive medication is prudent, particularly if the etiology of the hypertension is known. If unknown, typically pediatric nephrology (or pediatric cardiology in some centers) can be consulted for hypertension management while the etiology is discovered.

For all patients with prehypertension who are asymptomatic, close follow-up should be arranged with their primary care doctor. Their primary care doctor will initiate the workup listed in Table 125.2 if they continue to have prehypertension at follow-up visits. All patients with prehypertension or hypertension should be counseled extensively regarding lifestyle modifications, such as weight loss and dietary changes. In general, pharmacologic therapy should be added only if end-organ damage is discovered, if the patient has diabetes mellitus, persistent hypertension despite lifestyle modifications, symptomatic hypertension, or secondary hypertension. For patients with suspected "white-coat hypertension", referral to the primary care clinician should be completed for outpatient ambulatory blood pressure monitoring.

The overall goal of blood pressure medications is to lower the blood pressure to <95th percentile or <90th percentile for children with co-morbidities or hypertension-induced end-organ damage.

Disposition

Any child with end-organ damage or symptomatic or severe hypertension should be admitted for close blood pressure management and workup to discover the etiology of the hypertension. Close follow-up for asymptomatic hypertensive patients should be arranged to recheck the blood pressure as well as the efficacy of pharmacologic or lifestyle modifications. Ideally, follow-up should be arranged with the primary care doctor. When not feasible, patients should return to the ED for a blood pressure recheck and evaluation. Return precautions should be provided to caregivers and the patient. Antihypertensive medications should only be started in conjunction with a specialist or the patient's primary care doctor.

Pearls and pitfalls

Pearls

1. In adolescents, any blood pressure (BP) >120/80 mmHg should be considered prehypertension.
2. The prevalence of end-organ damage is higher than initially recognized.
3. Close follow-up is key for outpatient management of hypertension.
4. An appropriate size BP cuff must be used.

Pitfalls

1. Failure to recognize hypertension in a pediatric patient.
2. Failure to give close follow-up for pediatric hypertension.
3. Failure to screen for stimulant use in adolescent patients with hypertension.

Selected references

Constantine E, Linakis J. The assessment and management of hypertensive emergencies and urgencies in children. *Pediatr Emerg Care* 2005;**21**:391–396; quiz 7.

National High Blood Pressure Education Program Working Group on High Blood Pressure in Children and Adolescents. The fourth report on the diagnosis, evaluation, and treatment of high blood pressure in children and adolescents. *Pediatrics* 2004;**114**:555–576.

Varda NM, Gregoric A A diagnostic approach for the child with hypertension. *Pediatr Nephrol* 2005;**20**:499–506.

Chapter 126

Tutorial: The abnormal urinalysis, hematuria, and proteinuria

Ingrid T. Lim

Hematuria

Hematuria can arise from the glomeruli, renal tubules and interstitium, or the urinary tract (including the collecting system, ureters, bladder, and urethra). In children, the more common cause is glomerular. Red blood cells (RBCs) cross the glomerular basement membrane through structural irregularities in the capillary wall.

Definitions

Hematuria can be macroscopic or microscopic:

- macroscopic hematuria: visible to the naked eye
- microscopic hematuria: usually detected on dipstick test and confirmed by microscopic examination of spun urine sediment.

Although there is no consensus on the definition of microscopic hematuria, RBC >5–10/high-power field is generally considered significant.

Clinical presentation

The etiology of hematuria can be further delineated by the history and associated symptoms.

Urine color

"Pink-tinged" urine denotes a much smaller amount of blood and is rarely a result of glomerular disease.

Patients with glomerular disease often have uniformly discolored urine, without clots; this can be brownish-red, tea colored, or coca cola colored. Patients with bright red or cherry-colored urine are likely to have vascular bleeding or lower urinary tract bleeding. Urine that is yellow with blood clots suggests a non-glomerular source, such as the lower urinary tract. If bleeding is severe, the urine may be opaque, dark burgundy. Urinary bleeding that occurs at the start versus the end of a void provide clues to either urethritis or cystitis, respectively. Discoloration of the urine is not necessarily from blood. Pink diaper syndrome in newborns, in which a red-brown spot of urine appears in the diaper, is caused by urate crystals. Many substances can cause discoloration of the urine, such as pigments (hemoglobin, myoglobin), food (e.g., blackberries and beets), drugs (e.g., rifampin, pyridium, nitrofurantoin, metronidazole), and organic biochemicals (e.g., porphyrins, methemoglobin).

Presence of pain

Painful macroscopic hematuria is usually caused by infection, calculi, or other urologic conditions. Glomerular diseases, such as post-streptococcal glomerulonephritis and IgA nephropathy, are usually painless. With microscopic hematuria, a history of dysuria, urgency, frequency, and hematuria suggests a diagnosis of a urinary tract infection or nephrolithiasis.

Associated symptoms

Patients with glomerular disease may complain of dyspnea, weight gain, and edema. A recent pharyngitis, skin infection, or other febrile illness suggests acute post-infectious glomerulonephritis. Abdominal pain, arthralgias, diarrhea, and rash would suggest systemic vasculitis, such as Henoch–Schönlein purpura (HSP). Recurrent hematuria, with concomitant upper respiratory illnesses, could be secondary to IgA nephropathy. Fevers, weight loss, alopecia, mouth ulcers, chest pain, fatigue, and arthritis suggest systemic lupus erythematosus (SLE). Hemoptysis or cough is seen in rare pulmonary–renal syndromes, such as Goodpasture syndrome or Wegener's granulomatosis.

Review of systems and history

In African-American patients, ask about a history of sickle cell hemoglobinopathy. Ask about medications that might cause interstitial nephritis (antibiotics, anticonvulsants, and NSAIDs). A history of menorrhagia, prolonged epistaxis, hemarthrosis, and prolonged bleeding may be from an undiagnosed bleeding disorder. Ask about recent travel history, particularly in areas where schisotosomiasis is endemic (e.g., Asia, Africa, South America), or exposure to tuberculosis. Think about foreign bodies, trauma, and sexual abuse. Transient hematuria could be from menstruation, strenuous exercise, or trauma.

Physical examination

The blood pressure is an important determinant for further evaluation. If the patient is normotensive, it is unlikely that the microscopic hematuria, whatever the cause, warrants immediate treatment. Presence of fever, suprapubic or costovertebral angle tenderness suggests a urinary tract infection or pyelonephritis. An abdominal mass could be secondary to a tumor, hydronephrosis, or polycystic kidney disease. The most common renal tumor seen in young children (aged 1–4 years) is Wilms' tumor, although other types do occur. Rashes and arthritis can occur with SLE and HSP. Edema is an important feature of nephrotic syndrome.

Perform a genital examination for foreign body, lacerations or tears caused by trauma or abuse.

Diagnostic studies

Laboratory studies

Macroscopic hematuria requires a urinalysis, looking for RBCs, RBC casts, and crystals; a urine culture should be ordered if infection is suspected. In patients with recent travel or immigration, *Schistosoma hematobium* can be diagnosed by finding ova in the urine.

Microscopic hematuria requires two tests: a test for proteinuria and a microscopic examination for RBC and RBC casts. Proteinuria may be present regardless of the cause of the bleeding, but it usually does not exceed 100 mg/dl (2+) if the only source of the protein is from the blood. Proteinuria greater than 2+ prompts further investigation for glomerulonephritis and nephrotic syndrome. Occurrence of RBC casts is a highly specific marker for glomerulonephritis, but their absence does not rule it out. Dysmorphic, misshapen red cells also suggest a glomerular cause of bleeding. Bacteria and significant pyuria indicate infection.

Isolated microhematuria in the absence of hypertension or significant proteinuria can be worked up as an outpatient. At least two of three urinalyses must show microhematuria over 2 to 3 weeks before further evaluation is needed.

Imaging

Macroscopic hematuria in the absence of significant proteinuria, hypertension, azotemia or RBC casts should be evaluated with renal and bladder ultrasound to look for hydronephrosis, nephrolithiasis, malignancy, or cystic renal disease; if abnormal, the patient should be referred to urology. Nephrology should otherwise be consulted.

Indications for prompt evaluation

Further evaluation should be performed in any child with hematuria and any of the following: hypertension, edema, oliguria, significant proteinuria, or RBC casts.

Additional studies include CBC (hemolytic uremic syndrome); throat culture, anti-streptolysin O (ASO) titer or streptozyme test, and serum C3 (post-streptococcal glomerulonephritis); serum creatinine and potassium (renal insufficiency). If the cause of hematuria still remains unclear after the above tests, consult nephrology.

Proteinuria

Normally, the glomerulus is virtually impenetrable to proteins of large molecular weight, such as albumin. The small amounts that are filtered are reabsorbed and degraded in the proximal tubule. Proteinuria occurs when either there is increased permeability of the glomeruli to serum proteins or there is decreased reabsorption of low-molecular-weight proteins in the tubules. Glomerular disease is marked by excretion of large-molecular-weight proteins, while tubular disease results in the excretion of low-molecular-weight proteins.

Proteinuria is often found on routine urinalysis. Most proteinuria is transient or intermittent and benign. In the absence of edema, hypertension, oliguria, or hematuria, a repeat urinalysis in 2 to 4 weeks is recommended.

Differential diagnosis

Proteinuria can be divided into conditions affecting the glomerulus or the tubule. Fortunately, benign conditions are the most common.

Transient proteinuria. This is unrelated to renal disease and resolves when the inciting factor, such as fever, stress, dehydration, or exercise, disappears; it is usually less than 2+ proteinuria (100 mg/dl).

Orthostatic proteinuria. This occurs only when the patient is in the upright position. It is thought to be caused by excessive glomerular filtration. Orthostatic proteinuria is the most common cause of proteinuria and accounts for over 60% of all the proteinuria in children. Incidence is higher in teenage girls.

Clinical presentation

History

Look for a history suggestive of renal disease. Questions should include short stature or growth failure (seen in chronic kidney failure), developmental delay, edema or swelling, weight gain, polydipsia, deafness, urinary tract infection, other recent infection, oliguria, and recent medications. Inquire about a family history of renal disease, diabetes, or hypertension.

Physical examination

The examination should check for:

- hypertension
- edema: cardinal finding in nephrotic syndrome, usually periorbital, but as the disease progresses, ascites or scrotal swelling may be present
- rash and arthritis: suggests SLE or HSP.

Diagnostic studies

Urinalysis and microscopic examination of urine is required. Protein is usually detected by a color change on the reagent dipstick. These strips detect primarily albumin, approximately 20 mg/dl albumin, so do not detect non-albumin proteinuria; low-molecular-weight proteins are mostly undetected. False-positive results can occur in highly concentrated urine, sodium bicarbonate ingestion, very alkaline urine, contaminating antiseptics (such as chlorhexidine and benzalkonium chloride), macroscopic hematuria, phenazopyridine, pyuria or bacteruria, or after radiographic contrast administration.

Proteinuria that is 3+ or 4+ requires further evaluation with urine culture, serum protein and albumin, serum electrolytes, BUN, and creatinine.

Selected references

Glassock RJ. Hematuria and proteinuria. In Greenberg A, Cheung AK, Coffman TM, editors. *Primer on Kidney Diseases*. 4th edn. Philadelphia, PA: Elsevier Saunders; 2005. p. 36–46.

Glick RD, Hicks MJ, Nuctem JG, Wesson DE, Olutoye OO, Cass DL. Renal tumors in infants <6 month of age. *J Pediatr Surg.* 2004;**39**:522–525.

Hogg RJ, Portman RJ, Milliner D, *et al.* Evaluation and Management of Proteinuria and Nephrotic Syndrome in Children: Recommendations from a Pediatric Nephrology Panel Established at the National Kidney Foundation Conference on Proteinuria, Albuminuria, Risk, Assessment, Detection, and Elimination (PARADE). *Pediatrics.* 2000;**105**:1242–1249.

Meyers KEC. Evaluation of hematuria in children. *Urol Clin North Am* 2001;**31**:559–573.

Pan CG. Evaluation of gross hematuria. *Pediatr Clin North Am* 2006;**53**:401–412.

Section 20

Respiratory emergencies

Chapter

127 Apparent life-threatening events

Stephen J. Liu

Introduction

An NIH Consensus Panel defined an apparent life-threatening event (ALTE) as "an episode that is frightening to the observer and that is characterized by some combination of apnea (central or occasionally obstructive), color change (usually cyanotic or pallid but occasionally erythematous or plethoric), marked change in muscle tone (usually marked limpness), choking or gagging. In some cases, the observer fears that the infant has died."

These episodes occur in infants <12 months of age. The incidence is estimated to range from 0.5 to 7.5% in the general population. Premature infants are at higher risk for ALTEs, particularly those who develop respiratory syncytial virus infection. The episodes have also been associated with children who feed rapidly, cough frequently, or choke during feeding. Usually, by the time the infant is examined by the EP, he or she is well appearing.

Despite a number of studies, it is controversial whether an ALTE is a predictor of subsequent death, sudden infant death syndrome (SIDS), or other serious disorder in an infant. The conflicting results of these various studies are at the heart of the controversy regarding the appropriate evaluation and disposition of patients who present to the ED with an ALTE. This chapter will review the approach to, and management of, a patient with an ALTE.

Background

It is important to note that an ALTE is not a diagnosis but rather a description of an event. The descriptions given by caregivers vary tremendously, and the potential diagnoses are myriad. Because there are many abnormalities that can lead to an ALTE, it is difficult to discuss any common pathophysiology. However, there are common events that are associated in the symptom complex of ALTEs. Four findings comprise the symptom complex of ALTEs as defined by the Consensus Panel:

- apnea
- cyanosis
- altered muscle tone
- choking, gagging or coughing.

Apnea is the most commonly associated symptom with an ALTE.

Apnea occurs in three forms, central, obstructive, and mixed.

Central apnea. This results from a failure of the respiratory centers of the brainstem and transmission of signals along the descending neuromuscular pathways. This type of apnea usually responds to positive pressure ventilation. Some causes include prematurity and head trauma.

Obstructive apnea. This is defined as breathing through an occluded airway, with normal neuromuscular physiology. It can result from tonsillar hypertrophy, laryngolmalacia, or vocal cord paralysis.

Mixed apnea. A combination of central and obstructive apnea can occur. For example, premature infants who suffer from central apnea can also have a respiratory infection that causes obstructive physiology. It is hypothesized in gastroesophageal reflux disease that apnea results from choking on regurgitated gastric contents, bronchospasm, and laryngeal chemoreceptor reflex central apnea.

Cyanosis can result from impaired oxygen exchange (apnea) or distribution (sepsis).

Plethora results from hyperemia and localized vasodilation while pallor results from vasoconstriction – both are mediated by autonomic activity.

Altered muscle tone may be manifested as limpness, tonic–clonic movements, or rigidity. This can be from the CNS, or secondary to a systemic process (vasovagal response).

Choking, coughing, or gagging is the normal response for airway protection. This reflex inhibits normal respiration by two processes. First, if the reflex is triggered by foreign material in the posterior pharynx, there is a mechanical obstruction by the foreign bodies. Second, the act of coughing and gagging blocks effective ventilation. This forceful reflex can

A Practical Guide to Pediatric Emergency Medicine: Caring for Children in the Emergency Department, ed. N. Ewen Amieva-Wang (associate eds. Jamie Shandro, Aparajita Sohoni, and Bernhard Fassl). Published by Cambridge University Press.

result in plethora and erythema of the head and face, and a sustained effort can result in a vasovagal response, leading to hypotonia.

Clinical presentation

The occurrence of ALTEs presents a diagnostic dilemma because the infants are usually well appearing by the time they are examined by the EP. If the patient arrives in extremis or pulseless/apneic, the usual acute resuscitation and life-support measures should be undertaken. Otherwise, a careful history and physical examination will usually provide some clues to the etiology. Judicious use of testing in combination with the history and physical can provide some answers:

- idiopathic: 50% of cases
- GI: 25% of cases with etiology determined
- neurologic: 15% of cases with etiology determined
- respiratory: 10% of cases with etiology determined
- cardiac: <2% of cases
- infection: <2% of cases
- metabolic: <2% of cases
- abuse: <2% of cases.

Even thorough testing can still result in a diagnosis of "idiopathic ALTE."

History

The evaluation begins with a careful history of the event (Table 127.1). Many ALTEs are associated with temporary airway obstruction owing to laryngospasm following gastroesophageal reflux or feeding, are self-resolving, and of benign nature. However because of the multitude of possible causes the clinician is obligated to have a high index of suspicion for other, potentially life-threatening etiologies.

Physical examination

The physical examination is focused on examination findings associated with common causes of ALTEs:

- general impression: arousal, irritability, somnolence, dysmorphic features
- vital signs: fever, oxygen saturation
- growth curves: height, weight, head circumference
- head, eyes, ears, nose, and throat: trauma, tympanic membranes, reactive of eyes and retinal hemorrhages, nasal

Table 127.1. History taking related to apparent life-threatening events

Question	Significance
What was the child doing during the event? (feeding, coughing, sleeping)	Association with feeding/regurgitation
What were the breathing efforts (none, shallow, increased, decreased)?	Airway obstruction vs. apnea vs. neurologic versus metabolic
What was the condition of the child (awake, asleep, position, pillows, blankets)?	Determine conditions surrounding event
What interventions were done (stimulation, blowing air in face, mouth-to-mouth breathing, cardiopulmonary resuscitation by medical personnel)?	Determine severity of event
What was the duration of the event?	Determine severity of event
How is the child now?	Determine severity of event
Any recent problems (recent illnesses, fever, poor feeding, rash, irritability, weight loss, sick contacts, new medications)?	Infectious exposure, upper respiratory tract infection symptoms, respiratory distress
What were the movements or tone? (tonic–clonic, limp, rigid, decreased, "seizure like")	Seizure
Was there any coughing (phlegm or dry), vomiting (milk, mucous or blood), or noise (silent, cough, stridor, crying, gagging)?	Respiratory syncytial virus, pertussis, gastroesophageal reflux disease, ENT causes
Is there any fever?	Presence of serious bacterial infection
What medications is the child taking (including maternal medications if breast feeding or immediately postpartum)?	Medication reaction (narcotics, dystonic reactions)
Is there any history of trauma (accidental, non-accidental)?	Traumatic brain injury
Is there a family history of apparent life-threatening events, sudden infant death syndrome, or unexpected sudden death?	Traumatic brain injury
Is there a history of prematurity, underlying medical conditions or neurologic impairment?	High-risk infant

congestion, nasal flaring, foreign bodies in throat, stridor, micrognathia, cleft lip/palate
- heart: rate, rhythm, capillary refill, murmurs, gallop
- lungs: breath sounds, rales, stridor, retractions
- abdomen: signs of trauma, acute infection, hepatomegaly, abdominal breathing
- musculoskeletal: range of motion, signs of trauma
- skin: rash, bruising
- neurologic: tone, movement, tracking, smile, posturing, developmental milestones for age.

Diagnostic studies

Laboratory tests

Laboratory testing and radiologic imaging will be guided by information obtained during the initial history and physical

Table 127.2. Overview of organ-specific causes,[a] common associated findings on history and suggested workup for apparent life-threatening events

Condition	Findings	Suggested workup
Cardiovascular		*ED*: ECG, chest X-ray *Other*: echocardiology
Arrythmias	Syncope	
Cardiomyopathy	Murmur, gallop, liver enlargement	
Respiratory		*ED*: chest X-ray, CBC
Breath-holding spell	Cyanosis	
Aspiration with reflex apnea	Respiratory distress	
Airway obstruction	Stridor	
Congenital airway anomaly	Cough	
Infection		*ED*: Sepsis workup
Sepsis, meningitis	Fever, ALOC	
Viral infection	Apnea, early symptoms of upper respiratory infection	Respiratory syncytial virus, influenza assay
Pertussis	Cyanosis, stacatto cough	Pertussis PCR/culture
Gastrointestinal		*ED*: history *Other*: swallow evaluation, pH probe
Gastroesophageal reflux	Association with feeding	
Swallowing abnormalities	Regurgitation/vomiting	
Metabolic		*ED*: blood glucose, lactate, ammonia, urine analysis *Other*: acylcarnitine profile, serum amino acids, urine organic acids
Inborn error of metabolism	Shock, seizures, change in mental status	
Neurologic		*ED*: Head CT scan, shunt series *Other*: MRI, EEG
Seizure, apnea, increased intracranial pressure (shunt malfunction)	History of shaking, ALOC, dysmorphic features, developmental delay	
Toxicology		
Ingestion, maternal drugs	ALOC, seizure, nausea and vomiting	*ED*: Drug screen
Carbon monoxide	Many members of household with same complaints	*ED*: CO_2 level
Social		
Non-accidental trauma	Inconsistent history and examination, changing history, repeated episodes	*ED*: Head CT; if non-accidental trauma suspected, do skeletal survey, fundal examination

ALOC, altered level of consciousness; EEG, electroencephalography.
[a]Note that with some diagnoses, depending on severity, the child will have continued symptoms and so would not fit fully under the classification of ALTE.

examination. Some experts recommend that, at minimum, the following tests should be obtained:

- fingerstick glucose
- ECG
- CBC
- basic metabolic panel (including magnesium and calcium), serum bicarbonate
- serum lactate, urinalysis
- chest radiograph.

Table 127.2 provides an overview of the most common causes, clues in history and examination and suggested workup. With some diagnoses, depending on severity, the child will have continued symptoms and so not fit fully under the classification of ALTE.

In the absence of a clear association with feeding, or emesis, a more detailed workup is warranted. Further testing will depend on positive and negative findings on history and physical examination. If there is a clear association with feeding, then the workup can be limited to GI causes (Table 127.2):

- most additional testing is not an emergency, but should be part of a thorough or directed workup, and can take place after admission
- if a clinician suspects an inborn error of metabolism, appropriate laboratiory testing should be attempted before reversal of metabolic derangement if patient is stable.

Disposition

Patients who present with an ALTE to the ED usually should be considered for admission. Hospitalization will allow for prolonged cardiovascular monitoring and further diagnostic testing can be quickly performed and interpreted. It also allows for further reassurance and education of caregivers regarding ALTEs and allows opportunity for specific training in cardiopulmonary resuscitation and modification of modifiable SIDS risk factors.

Special considerations

Respiratory syncytial virus

Apnea associated with respiratory syncytial virus infection occurs in 18–20% of young infants who are hospitalized with respiratory syncytial virus bronchiolitis. This frequency increases in premature infants (particularly those with a gestational age <32 weeks) and in those who have not yet reached 44 weeks from conception. The apnea occurs early in the disease, and may often be the presenting symptom. This non-obstructive central apnea occurs during quiet sleep. It rarely lasts more than a few days, but it is important to note that 10% of these infants will require intubation and mechanical ventilation. Bronchiolitis is discussed in Ch. 131.

Breath holding spell

A breath holding spell, while not described in children <12 months old as a disease entity, can be considered in toddlers with a classic description of circumstances and symptoms. A breath holding spell is a paroxysmal event in which a child stops breathing at the end of expiration after crying, typically because of pain or anger. These spells can be classified as simple, cyanotic, or pallid.

A simple spell is when the child becomes apneic (cyanotic or pale) but then takes a deep breath.

Cyanotic spells typically have an emotional precipitant (e.g., frustration or anger), and the child progresses from cyanotic to apneic with the breath holding. The child may then become limp and lose consciousness. Breath holding spells usually last <1 min. Sometimes seizures can occur during these episodes.

Pallid spells are usually a response to painful stimuli. The child quickly becomes apneic and pale. The etiology is postulated to be secondary to an enhanced vagal reaction and can be a precursor to bradycardia or asystole.

These breath holding spells are common and can occur in up to 4–5% of children younger than 8 years old. Peak incidence is at 2–3 years, with onset in infancy. Approximately 80–90% stop by 6 years of age. Associated injuries include traumatic injuries from the loss of consciousness and muscle tone. This behavior falls under the category of "habit disorders" and the particular etiology is not well established nor understood.

Sandifer syndrome

Sandifer syndrome involves a spasmodic arching of the back with opisthotonic posturing of the neck, back, and upper extremities. The head and neck will rotate to one side and the legs to the other side. The posture will typically last from

Pearls and pitfalls

Pearls

1. A thorough history and physical examination is key to guide the workup of an apparent life-threatening event (ALTE).
2. Most ALTE episodes are temporally related to feeding/reflux/emesis and represent reflex laryngospasm with subsequent changes in color and tone. Those not preceded by a GI event deserve a more thorough workup.
3. Consider admission for all patients to coordinate and complete further evaluation and treatment, and also for parental education.

Pitfalls

1. Failure to consider non-accidental trauma as an etiology for an ALTE.

1 to 3 min. It is associated with gastroesophageal reflux disease and hiatal hernias and often occurs after feeding. Sandifer syndrome is often mistaken for a seizure since an altered mental status is associated with the posturing; however, there is no clonic movement. While typically occurring in infancy and early childhood, Sandifer syndrome can occur in mentally impaired adolescents. This syndrome is not associated with mortality.

Selected references

Brooks JG. Apparent life-threatening events and apnea of infancy. *Clin Perinatol* 1992;**19**:809–838.

Burchfield DJ, Rawlings DJ. Sudden deaths and apparent life threatening events in hospitalized neonates presumed to be healthy. *Am J Dis Child* 1991;**145**:903–904.

Cousineau A, Savitsky E. Cardiac tamponade presenting as an apparent life threatening event. *Pediatr Emerg Care* 2005;**21**:104–108.

Davies F, Gupta R. Apparent life threatening events in infants presenting to an emergency department. *Emerg Med J* 2002;**19**:11–16.

DeWolfe CC. Apparent life threatening event: a review. *Pediatr Clin North Am* 2005;**52**:1127–1146.

Grey C, Davies F, Molyneux E. Apparent life-threatening events presenting to a pediatric emergency department. *Pediatr Emerg Care* 1999;**15**:195–199.

Hall KL, Zalman B. Evaluation and management of apparent life-threatening events in children. *Am Fam Physician* 2005;**71**:2301–2308.

Kahn A. Recommended clinical evaluation of infants with an apparent life-threatening event: consensus document of the European Society for the Study and Prevention of Infant Death, 2003. *Eur J Pediatr* 2004;**163**:108–115.

Kelly DH, Shannon DC, O'Connell K. Care of infants with near-miss sudden infant death syndrome. *Pediatrics* 1978;**61**:511–514.

Little GA, Ballard RA, Brooks JG, *et al.* National Institute of Health Consensus Development. Course on infantile apnea and home monitoring, Sept 1986. *Pediatrics* 1987;**79**:292–299.

McGovern MC, Smith MB. Causes of apparent life-threatening events in infants: a systemic review. *Arch Dis Child* 2004;**98**:1043–1048.

National Institutes of Health. Consensus statement: Consensus Development Conference on Infantile Apnea and Home Monitoring, 1986. *Pediatrics* 1987;**79**:292–299.

Pitetti RD, Maffei F, Chang K, *et al.* Prevalence of retinal hemorrhages and child abuse in children who present with an apparent life threatening event. *Pediatrics* 2002;**110**:557–562.

Ramanathan R, Corwin MJ, Hunt CE, *et al.* Cardiorespiratory events recorded on home monitors: comparison of healthy infants with those at increased risk for SIDS. *JAMA* 2001;**285**:2199–2207.

Rosenberg NM, Cruz MN, Chamberlain JM, *et al.* The least expensive diagnostic tool. *Pediatr Emerg Care* 1995;**11**:389–391.

Southall DP, Richards JM, Rhoden KJ, *et al.* Prolonged apnea and cardiac arrhythmias in infants discharged from neonatal intensive care units: failure to predict an increased risk for sudden infant death syndrome. *Pediatrics* 1982;**70**:844–851.

Steinschneider A. Prolonged apnea and the sudden infant death syndrome: clinical and laboratory observations. *Pediatrics* 1972;**50**:646–654.

Veereman-Wauters G, Bochner A, Van Caillie-Bertrand M. Gastroesophageal reflux in infants with a history of near-miss sudden infant death. *J Pediatr Gastroenterol Nutr* 1991;**12**:319–323.

Wennergren G, Milerad J, Westphall I, *et al.* Consensus statement on clinical management. *Acta Paediatr*1993;**82**(Suppl 389):S114–S116.

Chapter 128

Foreign body in the lower airways

Eric C. Walter

Introduction

Foreign body aspiration (FBA) occurs more commonly in children than adults and is a cause of unintentional death in children. Fortunately, deaths from FBA have dropped dramatically and are currently approximately 2%. The epidemiology of FBA has not changed. Approximately 75% of aspirated foreign bodies occur in children, most of whom are <4 years of age and male. Young children are at higher risk for aspiration because of the tendency to place items in their mouths. They also lack molars to adequately chew certain foods and swallowing control is less developed. This lack of oral control is important as food and other organic material are by far the most frequently aspirated products. In some series, up to 80–90% of aspirated material was reported to be organic. Frequently aspirated foods include peanuts, seeds or other nuts, and beans. Foreign bodies may lodge in either the upper or the lower airways. This chapter will focus on foreign bodies in the lower airways.

Clinical presentation

History

The strongest predictor of FBA is a witnessed choking event. Choking and cough are the most common symptoms. The positive predictive value approaches 90% if the event was witnessed. While a history of a witnessed choking event is a strong predictor for FBA, the absence of a witnessed event does not rule it out.

Physical examination

Foreign body aspiration can be life threatening. The initial physical examination should focus on the child's appearance on presentation and vital signs. Foreign bodies that obstruct the glottis or trachea can present with profound respiratory distress. Patients may appear in distress with tachypnea, little to no air movement, or cyanosis. Patients presenting in distress should be evaluated immediately according to the Pediatric Advanced Life Support (PALS) algorithm for upper airway obstruction.

Patients with foreign bodies in the lower airways may present with little or no signs of distress. However, most children have at least some abnormality on physical examination. Multiple studies have concluded that the presence of decreased breath sounds is the most common physical examination finding in children with FBA. Other abnormalities reported include localized wheezing, stridor, and cough. In some cases patients with proven FBA have a normal physical examination.

A normal physical examination should never be used to exclude foreign body aspiration, particularly if the history is suggestive of aspiration.

Location of the object

Most lower airway foreign bodies are located in the main stem bronchi.

In contrast to adults, where foreign bodies are more likely to be found in the right lung, in children foreign bodies are found equally in the right and left lungs; this is likely because in young children the right and left main stem bronchi bifurcate from the trachea at equal angles. Around 15 years of age the aortic knob reaches full development and increases the angle at which the left main bronchus branches from the trachea. After this age, foreign bodies are more likely to enter the right main stem bronchus. In addition, foreign bodies are more likely to be lodged in the proximal airways in children than in adults. This is likely because of the smaller diameter of children's airways.

Diagnostic studies

Imaging

Most aspirated foreign bodies will be radiolucent and chest radiography may be normal even in the presence of a foreign body.

A

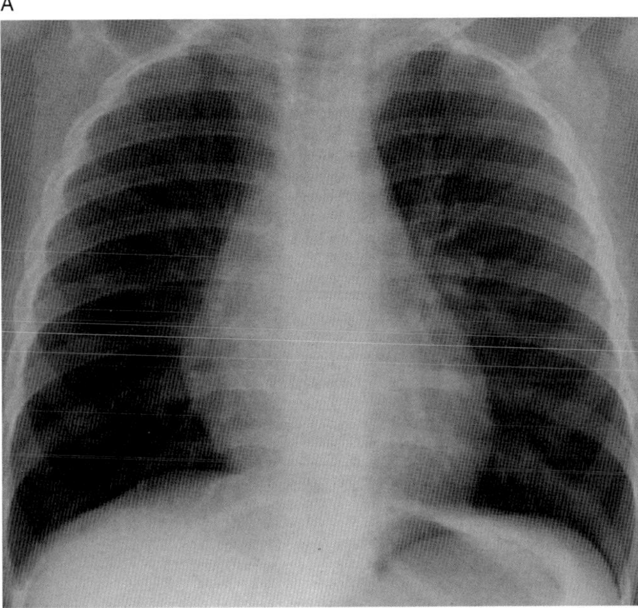

B

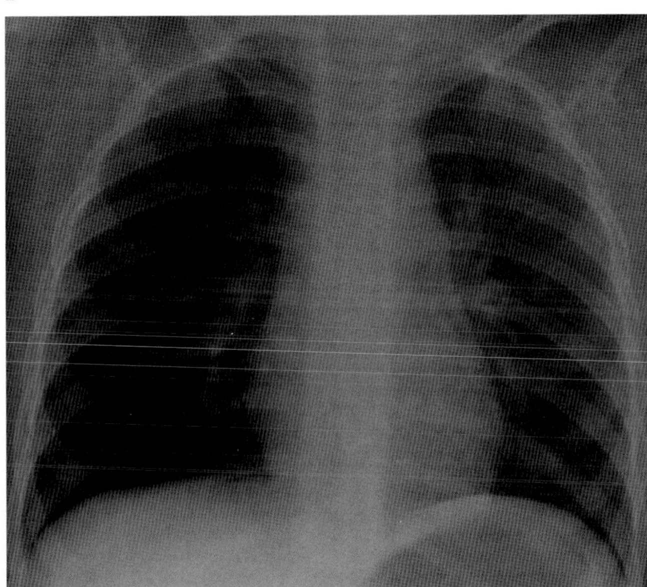

Figure 128.1 Right-sided bronchial foreign body in a 2-year-old girl presenting with wheezing. The inspiratory (A) and partially expiratory (B) chest radiographs show persistent hyperinflation and oligemia on the right side, indicative of partial right bronchial obstruction. Note the shift of heart towards the left on the expiratory view because of partial deflation of the left lung.

Nevertheless, a chest radiograph including the neck should be performed in all cases of suspected FBA, as an abnormality will be detected more than 50% of the time a foreign body is present. Chest radiograph findings differ between adults and children with aspiration. In adults, atelectasis is the most frequent finding. In contrast, air trapping or hyperinflation in the ipsilateral lung is the most frequent radiograph abnormality in children. Chest radiograph also has a higher likelihood of being abnormal 24 h or more after the aspiration.

Traditionally, inspiratory and expiratory films have been recommended to evaluate suspected FBA (Fig. 128.1). The side of the lung where the foreign body is located will appear hyperinflated as a result of air trapping. Unfortunately, young children frequently cannot cooperate with inspiratory and expiratory maneuvers. When this occurs, right and left lateral decubitus films have been recommended. The dependent lung should normally deflate. Theoretically, when a foreign body is present the air may be trapped and the dependent lung will not deflate as it normally should.

A normal chest radiograph should never be used to exclude the presence of FBA. Fluoroscopy and chest CT are additional imaging techniques that may be helpful. Fluoroscopy may show hyperinflation, mediastinal shift, and paradoxical movement of the diaphragm. Fluoroscopy has been reported to be more sensitive than chest radiographs but may still miss foreign bodies in up to 10% of cases. Use of CT may be recommended as a way of avoiding bronchoscopy when there is discordance between clinical and radiological findings. However, the risk–benefit of additional imaging studies must be considered, including radiation exposure. We would recommend further imaging in conjunction with ENT consultation.

Laboratory tests

Laboratory testing is unnecessary for the healthy child with suspected acute aspiration.

Pearls and pitfalls

Pearls

1. If a toddler has been exposed to chocolate or nuts and has any possible history of aspiration, ENT consult should be obtained for possible bronchoscopy regardless of imaging results or physical examination.
2. In contrast to adults where foreign bodies are more likely to be found in the right lung, in children foreign bodies are found equally in the right and left lungs.
3. Repeated or severe unilateral white out pneumonias in a toddler should raise suspicion for foreign body aspiration.

Pitfalls

1. A normal physical examination should *not* be used to rule out aspiration if the history is compelling.
2. Failure to realize that organic material may be radiolucent.

Management

If there is high suspicion for FBA the child should be admitted and a specialist in bronchoscopy consulted. Depending on the institution, bronchoscopy may be performed by pulmonary, otolaryngology, or pediatric surgery. In contrast to adults, most removals of foreign bodies in children require general anesthesia and rigid bronchoscopy. However, if the diagnosis of foreign body is questionable, particularly if the indication is for atelectasis or evaluation of recurrent pneumonia, diagnostic flexible bronchoscopy is useful and less invasive. If a foreign body is found, rigid bronchoscopy can be subsequently performed to remove the object.

Conclusions

The evaluation of children with possible foreign body aspiration should focus on a detailed history and physical examination. A history of choking and coughing, particularly if the onset was witnessed or acute, is the best predictor of FBA. Physical examination should be directed at the respiratory system, with particular attention to the symmetry of breath sounds. Chest radiographs and perhaps CT scan are useful adjuncts to history and physical examination. However, most foreign bodies are radiolucent and chest imaging may be normal even when a foreign body is present. The most common abnormality on chest radiograph is unilateral air trapping. If a foreign body is identified or is there is a high index of suspicion for FBA, bronchoscopy is recommended.

Selected references

Assefa D, Amin N, Stringel G, Dozor AJ. Use of decubitus radiographs in the diagnosis of foreign body aspiration in young children. *Pediatr Emerg Care* 2007;**23**:154–157.

Baharloo F, Veyckemans F, Francis C, Biettlot MP, Rodenstein DO. Tracheobronchial foreign bodies: presentation and management in children and adults. *Chest* 1999;**115**:1357–1362.

Even L, Heno N, Talmon Y, *et al.* Diagnostic evaluation of foreign body aspiration in children: a prospective study. *J Pediatr Surg* 2005;**40**:1122–1127.

Holinger LD, Baretto R. Foreign bodies of the airway and esophagus. In Cummings CW, Haughey BH, Thomas JR, Harker LA, Flint PW (eds.) *Cummings Otolarnygology: Head and Neck Surgery*, 4th edn. Philadelphia, PA: Saunders, 2005, pp. 4343–4353.

Rovin JD, Rodgers BM. Pediatric foreign body aspiration. *Pediatr Rev* 2000;**21**:86–90.

Chapter

129 Asthma

William Eidenmuller and Rebecca Smith-Coggins

Introduction

While asthma is a worldwide problem, it is 8–10 times more common in developed nations. The USA has one of the highest prevalences of asthma in the world. In the USA, asthma is the most common chronic illness of childhood and affects minority and socially disadvantaged children disproportionately; 17% of all pediatric ED visits are for asthma. Despite its prevalence, asthma is a disease that is both underdiagnosed and undertreated.

The diagnosis of asthma before puberty is three times higher in males than in females; however, this ratio equalizes during adolescence. Risk factors for asthma in children include allergies, parental asthma, male gender, low birth weight, and second-hand smoke. Puerto Rican and Black children have higher asthma prevalence rates than non-Hispanic White children. Rates of adverse outcomes, including death from asthma, are higher among Black children.

Because asthma has an increased prevalence in children with decreased healthcare access and poorer healthcare quality, EPs should understand how to grade asthma and initiate chronic treatment (Ch. 130), as well as treat acute exacerbations. While the treatment of an asthma exacerbation in a child is similar to the treatment of an adult exacerbation, there are important differences. For example, children's lungs continue to develop until around 8 years of age, making the prevention and controlling of asthma exacerbations in younger years significant for decreasing asthma morbidity in later years.

Pathophysiology

Transmitted upper airway sounds can be mistaken for wheezing. The differential diagnosis of upper airway stridor is listed in Table 134.1 (p. 622). Table 129.1 gives an aged-based differential diagnosis of wheezing in a child.

There are three criteria for the diagnosis of asthma in children: *recurrent*, *reversible* lower airway obstruction without an *alternative* diagnosis.

Airway inflammation contributes to and exacerbates bronchial reactivity. An asthma exacerbation is an acute worsening of the underlying disease manifested by "acute or subacute episodes of progressively worsening shortness of breath, cough, wheezing, and chest tightness – or some combination of these symptoms."

Clinical presentation

History

Asthma classically presents as a wheezing cough and difficulty breathing. Children commonly wheeze secondary to an allergic trigger such as a viral upper respiratory tract infection or antigen exposure. The adage "not all that wheezes is asthma" holds true (Table 129.1).

In cough-variant asthma, patients have a dry cough, usually worse at night. Patients often do not wheeze at all.

Treatment of cough-variant asthma is the same as classic asthma. The fact that the cough is responsive to bronchodilator therapy suggests a bronchial hyperreactivity component. Older children and adolescents can present with vague chest pain perhaps precipitated by activity or exposure.

Physical examination

Acute asthma exacerbation is a clinical diagnosis. The hallmark finding is auscultation of bilateral wheezes during the pulmonary examination; ideally, with a known history of asthma. Wheezing in a young child with no history of asthma should prompt a more thorough history and physical examination. Unilateral or focal wheezing in a toddler should raise the suspicion of an aspirated foreign body. At times, transmitted upper airway noises can be mistaken for wheezing; however, holding the stethoscope at the nares can usually elucidate the location of the sounds.

Evaluation of a patient with acute asthma should include:

- determination of exacerbation severity
- determination of chronic asthma symptom control (symptoms "in between" exacerbations).

A Practical Guide to Pediatric Emergency Medicine: Caring for Children in the Emergency Department, ed. N. Ewen Amieva-Wang (associate eds. Jamie Shandro, Aparajita Sohoni, and Bernhard Fassl). Published by Cambridge University Press.

Table 129.1. Aged-based differential diagnosis of wheezing in a child[a]

Disease	Age range	Diagnostic indications
Bronchiolitis	2–24 months	Usually with fever, upper respiratory tract infection symptoms
Foreign body aspiration	Toddler, young child	Wheezing is unilateral or focal; history of aspiration or exposure
Congestive heart failure	Any	Unusual in children; usually has been diagnosed previously
Cystic fibrosis, immunodeficiencies	Any	Association between poor weight gain and recurrent respiratory symptoms; frequent hospitalizations
Bronchopulmonary dysplasia	Any	History of prematurity and acute respiratory distress syndrome
Gastroesophageal reflux disease	Young child	Lack of response to standard asthma treatment, symptoms associated with positioning or feeds
Anaphylaxis	Any	Associated signs of anaphylaxis (e.g., urticaria, uvular edema)
Vocal cord dysfunction	Adolescence	Associated with chest or throat tightness, stridor and voice change
Aspiration events	Neurologically impaired children	Recurrent wheezing

[a]Transmitted upper airway sounds can be mistaken for wheezing.

Asthma severity assessment is based on clinical signs and symptoms and direct measurement of airflow obstruction. Table 129.2 provides an overview of assessing acute asthma severity.

The EP should be adept at gauging the severity of asthma based on history and physical examination. This is of particular importance in infants, who are unable to communicate verbally and with whom peak flow measurements are impossible. Clinicians should observe for overall respiratory distress, particularly the heart and respiratory rate (Table 129.3), as well as the more subtle indicators of respiratory distress such as accessory muscle use, retractions, nasal flaring, grunting, inability to feed, and active expiration. Head bobbing is a sign of severe respiratory distress in infants. Older children should have their position of comfort assessed. Patients without respiratory distress should be able to breathe comfortably in any position. The skin should also be inspected for eczema, which would support an asthma diagnosis, or urticaria, which would suggest an alternative reason for wheezing.

Peak flow measurement is useful in assessing the degree of airway obstruction in the older compliant child. The test can be diagnostic of a severe exacerbation (<40% of predicted or personal best). Additionally, it is a good tool to measure response to therapy and aids the clinician in deciding whether hospital admission is warranted. Peak expiratory flow is limited by the fact that it is effort/compliance dependent and is not useful in children under the age of 5 years.

Accessory muscles of respiration are the sternocleidomastoid and scalene muscles of the neck. During normal inspiration, these muscles do not contract. As airway resistance increases, the body recruits additional muscles to generate greater inspiratory force to overcome this increased resistance. In obese patients, it may be necessary to palpate these muscles during inspiration to determine if they are contracting. Expiration is normally a passive event, but in the setting of increased airway resistance, the body will recruit the abdominal muscles to assist with expiration. This so-called active expiration (abdominal breathing) is a sign of respiratory distress and should be specifically looked for in the physical examination.

In contrast to the accessory muscles, the external intercostal muscles are normal muscles of respiration. They provide a supportive role to the diaphragm to expand the thorax to produce active inspiration. As airway obstruction increases, the greater negative pressure generated in the chest cavity during inspiration draws these muscles inward, which is easily recognizable in an undressed child.

Grunting is an indication of self-generated positive end-expiratory pressure and is a subtle indicator of respiratory distress. Head bobbing refers to the action of the head lifting and tilting back during inspiration, moving forward with expiration. It is considered by many to be a late, ominous sign potentially signifying impending respiratory failure. Paradoxical respiration occurs when the diaphragm has become fatigued and accessory muscle use pulls the diaphragm (paradoxically) up during inspiration. Patients exhibiting paradoxical respiration should be considered critical.

Diagnostic studies

A chest radiograph is the first-line test for most patients in respiratory distress; however, it is not recommended for routine use in children with acute asthma. Its main utility is to exclude alternative diagnoses or co-morbidities, and so radiography would not be necessary in known asthmatics with a

Table 129.2. Gauging asthma exacerbation severity

	Mild	Moderate	Severe	Critical
Symptom				
Breathlessness	Only on exertion	At rest; infants have difficulty feeding	At rest; infants cannot feed	
Speech fluency	Normal	Phrases only	Few words only	
Alertness	Normal	May be agitated	Usually agitated	Drowsy or confused
Positioning	Any	Prefers sitting	Sits upright	
Signs				
Tachypnea	Mild	Moderate	Severe	May slow as patient fatigues
Tachycardia	Mild	Moderate	Severe	Bradycardia
Retraction/accessory muscle use	Usually not	Commonly	Usually	Paradoxical respiration
Wheeze	Moderate, often only end-expiratory	Loud, expiratory	Usually loud, both inspiratory and expiratory	Absent
Functional assessment				
Peak expiratory flow (PEF) compared with predicted or personal best (%)	≥70	40–69	<40	<25
Arterial oxygen saturation (Sao_2) with room air (at sea level) (%)	>95	90–95	<90	

Source: adapted from National Asthma Education and Prevention Program, 2007.

Table 129.3. Normal pediatric vital sign ranges

Age	Respiratory rate (breaths/min)	Heart rate (bpm)
Neonate	<60	<145
<2 months	<60	<160
2–12 months	<50	<160
1–2 years	<40	<120
3–5 years	<40	<110
6–8 years	<30	<110

presenting history and physical consistent with an asthma exacerbation.

Characteristic findings in chest radiography include peribronchial cuffing and flattened diaphragms. Laboratory studies are of limited utility in the ED management of asthma. Arterial/capillary blood gases should be considered in patients in severe distress to measure the PCO_2. Normal carbon dioxide levels in a tachypneic patient are a sign of respiratory failure as these patients would be expected to have a low PCO_2 secondary to their hyperventilation. Children taking theophylline should have its serum level measured to rule out theophylline toxicity.

Management

Treatment of critically ill children:

- ketamine and propofol are the preferred sedating agents in children with respiratory failure
- opioids should be avoided
- paralysis may be beneficial in patients who are difficult to ventilate
- beware of increased positive end-expiratory pressure in intubated/ventilated patients; they are at risk of dynamic hyperinflation owing to the highly increased expiratory airway resistance, leading to end expiratory gas trapping.

Bronchodilators

Bronchodilators can be given via nebulization or metered dose inhaler (MDI). Studies have shown that MDIs are equally efficacious as nebulization. The treatment requires a coordinated sequence of medicine administration and inhalation and so use of MDI can be difficult in children. Young children often object to the airtight face mask needed to deliver the aerosol. While spacers are known to help with medication administration, they can be expensive and are often lost.

Our institution commonly starts treatment with nebulized treatments and transitions to MDI treatment for children who are discharged. Nebulized treatments should routinely be given with oxygen as the gas vehicle as children are particularly susceptible to hypoxia. Beta-adrenergic agonists can lead to a transient fall in PO_2 secondary to worsening of ventilation–perfusion mismatching during treatment. While the concern of blunting a hypoxia-driven respiratory drive leads some practitioners to use air to deliver beta-2 agonists to their adult patients with chronic obstructive airway disease, there is no place for this practice in pediatric asthma management.

Beta-2 agonists: albuterol

The mainstay of asthma exacerbation treatment in children is inhaled beta-2 agonist. In the USA, the short acting beta-2 agonist albuterol (salbutamol) is by far the most commonly used agent. The (*R*)-enantiomer of albuterol (levalbuterol) has not been shown to be superior to the traditional racemic albuterol. There is no role for oral albuterol in the treatment of acute asthma exacerbations.

Albuterol is provided either as a continuous infusion or as separate doses. Nebulized albuterol is dosed at 0.15 mg/kg with a minimum dose of 2.5 mg. This dose is typically given every 20 min for three doses; dosage based on the child's weight is:

<20 kg: 2.5 mg
20–30 kg: 3.75 mg
>30 kg: 5 mg.

Alternatively, a 1 h long continuous treatment can be given at a dose of 0.5 mg/kg. For a continuous treatment, the medication needs to be diluted in a sufficient volume of saline.

Anticholinergic drugs: ipratropium

For adults, the standard of care for treatment of acute asthma exacerbation includes the addition of the inhaled anticholinergic ipratropium bromide. In children, ipratropium has been shown to decrease admission rates and there is some evidence that it may reduce the amount of beta agonist needed to treat an exacerbation. It is, therefore, recommended to add ipratropium to pediatric nebulizer treatments while the patient is in the ED.

Ipratropium dosage for children is 0.25 mg nebulized ipratropium every 20 min for three doses and then every 2–4 h. The adult dosage is 0.5 mg nebulized ipratropium every 20 min for three doses and then every 2–4 h.

Systemic beta agonists

The role of systemic beta agonists (terbutaline, epinephrine, and isoproterenol) in the management of asthma is controversial. Currently, there is not enough evidence to support their use in children or adults. Intravenous isoproterenol is specifically not recommended secondary to potential cardiac toxicity. Some clinicians will use epinephrine or terbutaline as second- or third-line drugs in patients not responding to conventional treatment. Their systemic side effects result from β_1-adrenoceptor stimulation and are generally well tolerated in children.

Systemic beta agonist dosing is controversial and should not be used in children with cardiac disease. The recommended dosages are:

- **terbutaline**: 0.01 mg/kg SC up to 0.3 mg q. 20 min, three doses maximum *or* 10 μg/kg IV load over 10 min followed by 0.4 μg/kg per min
- **epinephrine**: 0.01 mg/kg up to 0.3 mg/dose SC (use 1:1000 solution).

Systemic steroids

Recognition that inflammation is the underlying pathology in asthma has led to increasing usage of both systemic and inhaled steroids. In addition to their anti-inflammatory properties, steroids are believed to potentiate the effects of beta-2 agonists on airway smooth muscle. Children may display an even greater responsiveness to steroids than adults. The efficacy of oral versus parenteral steroids seems to be equivalent in adults and children, and the decision as to which route to use should be based more on the child's condition and ability to tolerate oral medication. Current guidelines are to give systemic corticosteroids for moderate to severe exacerbations or to any patient who does not respond "promptly and completely" to short-acting beta agonists. Steroids take time to work and should not be counted on to have an effect during the initial stabilization of an acute exacerbation. Inhaled corticosteroids do not have a role in acute exacerbation but are a mainstay of long-term management.

In order to prevent early relapse, patients discharged from the ED should complete a 3–5 day treatment course of systemic corticosteroids after discharge.

Systemic steroid dosing is 1 mg/kg daily divided BID (max. 60 mg daily) either orally or parenterally.

Magnesium sulfate

Guidelines for asthma treatment recommend consideration of IV magnesium sulfate in life-threatening exacerbations or in those patients whose exacerbations remain severe after 1 h of intensive conventional therapy. Magnesium sulfate probably is of no added benefit in less severe exacerbations.

Magnesium sulfate dosing is with 25–75 mg/kg (2 g max.) in children. Commonly used doses are 25 mg/kg and 40 mg/kg.

Heliox

Heliox is a commercially available gas mixture containing atmospheric oxygen (21%) mixed with 79% helium. The concept behind heliox therapy is that by replacing the nitrogen in air with the less-dense helium, airway resistance is lowered, which leads to decreased work of breathing. When nebulized medications are given using heliox as the delivery gas, pulmonary aerosol delivery is likely increased. Outcome data are controversial; however, the safety profile for heliox seems to be good, with increased tachycardia being the most commonly reported side effect. It seems reasonable to try heliox in children with severe attacks.

Theophylline

Theophylline and aminophylline are methylxanthines, which have long been known to produce bronchodilatation. However, these agents are associated with significant toxicity. The National Asthma Education and Prevention Program Expert Panel Report 3 *Guidelines for the Diagnosis and Management of Asthma* (EPR-3) specifically recommends against the use of theophylline/aminophylline in the treatment of asthma.

Fluids

In theory, the increased respiratory rates of patients suffering from acute asthma exacerbations will lead to increased fluid losses, which could potentially lead to dehydration. In small children and infants, there is a potential for significant fluid loss. The EPR-3 recommends fluid hydration either orally or IV. Furthermore, the inhaled beta-2 agonists will temporarily shift extracellular potassium to the intracellular compartment, leading some to recommend adding potassium chloride to the IV fluids of patients receiving albuterol therapy.

Intubation

Unlike upper airway problems, where intubation is the definitive treatment, asthma requires continued (even increased) medical management of the airway.

The last resort in the management of a pediatric asthma exacerbation is intubation. The decision to intubate is based on clinical judgement. In-line nebulizers should be aggressively used, and the second- and third-line medical treatments such as magnesium, heliox, and terbutaline/epinephrine should be considered.

Ventilator management of severe asthmatics is complicated. Efforts must be taken to minimize barotrauma from the high airway pressure while still maintaining adequate oxygenation. The basic recommendation is referred to as "controlled hypoventilation." Maximum fraction of inhaled oxygen (FIO_2) is used with decreased tidal volumes to limit barotrauma secondary to hyperinflation. Additionally, decreased respiratory rates and longer expiratory phases are used to prevent "stacking" of breaths. Because a longer time is needed for the asthmatic lung to exhale its air, should the next inspiration come before the lung has fully deflated, hyperinflation and resultant barotrauma can occur.

Ketamine

There are several anecdotal reports in the literature describing improvement of pediatric asthma patients after administration of ketamine (usually as an induction agent prior to intubation). Currently there is neither an FDA approval nor enough data to support the use of ketamine in the treatment of pediatric asthma. Further studies are needed to see if there is a role for ketamine as a "last resort" treatment in status asthmaticus.

Disposition

As with adults, the subjective clinical picture is the primary guiding factor in the decision to discharge or admit a pediatric patient suffering from an acute asthma exacerbation (Table 129.4). For children, clinicians have the added complexity of needing to consider the reliability of the parents in deciding whether it is safe for a child to go home. Clues in the history suggesting a child may need to be admitted include either an abrupt onset severe attack, or a prolonged duration attack. Prior ICU admissions or intubations suggest severe disease and should lower the threshold for admission. Frequent ED visits and frequent hospitalizations are also concerning, and these details should be specifically sought during history taking.

There is evidence that repeat pulse oximetry after 1 h of treatment may be a predictor of a need for admission, particularly in infants. Children at sea level with a pulse oximetry of <92% after 1 h of treatment should be considered for admission.

Discharge goal should be a peak expiratory flow of 70% or greater of the child's "personal best" peak flow.

Tachycardia on presentation may be an indicator of a more severe exacerbation. Arterial blood gas measurements for patients with severe exacerbations can help to guide the level of care a patient will need. Clinicians should keep in mind that

Table 129.4. Indications for admission for asthma exacerbation

Clinical parameter	Comments
Clinical judgement	Always first and foremost
History	Prior intubations or ICU admissions; abrupt or prolonged attack
Physical examination	Persistent wheezing or signs of respiratory distress despite aggressive ED therapy; tachycardia on presentation prior to beta-2 agonist administration
Pulse oximetry	<92% on arrival, or perhaps more importantly after 1 h of treatment
Peak flow	<70% of personal best likely needs admission
Parental reliability	Most importantly, must be able to accurately gauge severity of child's asthma attack
Severe exacerbation in a high-risk patient	Admit

tachypneic patients are expected to have a decreased PCO_2. Therefore a normocapnic patient in respiratory distress is at high risk for respiratory failure.

Components of the asthma history associated with fatal or near-fatal asthma include:

- previous severe exacerbation requiring intubation or ICU admission
- two or more hospitalizations for asthma in the past year
- three or more ED visits for asthma in the past year
- hospitalization or ED visit for asthma in the past month
- increasing beta-2 agonist usage, and utilizing greater than 2 canisters/month of short acting beta agonist.

Difficulty perceiving asthma symptoms or severity of exacerbations is a risk factor for death from asthma. The provider must also assess the parents' comfort level with perceiving their child's symptoms or severity of attack, particularly for younger patients. Other risk factors for death from asthma include a lack of a written asthma action plan, documented sensitivity to the mold *Alternaria*, and low socioeconomic status or inner city residence.

The disposition of infants requires special consideration because they are at greater risk for respiratory failure. As peak flow measurements have no use in the assessment of infants, the physical examination becomes paramount. Use of accessory muscles, paradoxical breathing, cyanosis, and respiratory rate >60 breaths/min are all signs of distress that should prompt consideration for admission. An oxygen saturation of <90% in an infant indicates serious distress as well.

Patients improved enough for discharge should have a follow-up appointment with the doctor who manages their asthma. They should also receive counseling from the EP regarding trigger control. Specific recommendations include avoiding known allergic triggers, strict no smoking in house rules, plastic seals on bedding to avoid dust mite exposure, consideration of removal of carpet from household, cockroach control, and avoidance of wood-burning stoves. All patients should have a *written* asthma action plan as well. At a minimum, this plan should detail daily management of the patient's asthma as well as give detailed instruction on how to manage exacerbations. The more severe a patient's asthma, the more important a written action plan is. Highlighting the importance of a written action plan, it is now a Joint Commision requirement that all children admitted for an asthma exacerbation be discharged with a written action plan.

Acknowledgement

The authors would like to thank Cristina Zeretzke, for comments and suggestions on this chapter.

Pearls and pitfalls

Pearls

1. Management should focus on treating the acute exacerbation *and* the chronic asthma symptoms.
2. The "personal best" peak flow can be a more sensitive detector of severe exacerbation than history and physical alone.
3. Routine chest radiographs and antibiotic treatment are not indicated if the clinical presentation is consistent with asthma.
4. In infants, fever accompanying acute wheezing episodes is usually secondary to viral infection.

Pitfalls

1. Failure to completely undress infants to assess their respiratory status.
2. Failure to consider other diagnoses, such as foreign body aspiration or croup.
3. Failure to address the need for preventive medications, trigger avoidance, and ongoing follow-up with caregivers.
4. Failure to realize that the normocapnic patient in respiratory distress is at high risk for respiratory failure.

Selected references

Akinbami, L. *Advance Data From Vital and Health Statistics 381: The State of Childhood Asthma, United States 1980–2005.* Atlanta, GA: Centers for Disease Control and Prevention, 2006.

MoormanJE, Rudd RA, Johnson, CA, et al. National surveillance for asthma: United States, 1980–2004. *MMWR Surveill Summ* 2007;**56**;1–54.

National Asthma Education and Prevention Program. *Expert Panel Report III: Guidelines for the Management of Asthma.* Bethesda, MD: National Heart, Lung, and Blood Institute, National Institutes of Health, 2007.

National Asthma Education and Prevention Program. *Expert Panel Report II: Guidelines for the Diagnosis and Management of Asthma.* Bethesda, MD: National Heart, Lung, and Blood Institute, National Institutes of Health, 1997, pp. 1–50.

Chapter 130

Tutorial: Management of outpatient asthma from the emergency department

Bernhard Fassl, William Eidenmuller, and Rebecca Smith-Coggins

Introduction

Treatment of pediatric asthma needs to focus on the long-term management of the disease. This responsibility used to be handed to the primary pediatrician; however, evidence shows that preventive care measures initiated in the ED setting are associated with better patient outcomes. Because of access to care issues, increasing numbers of patients utilize EDs as their sole access point to the healthcare system. It is common to encounter patients with poorly controlled asthma who are well enough to be discharged home but who do not have access to immediate outpatient follow-up. These patients may need to be started on control medications, or have them increased, by the ED provider (Table 130.1). Box 130.1 offers a simple approach for the algorithm to help the EP start this appropriate care.

Inhaled corticosteroids

The effectiveness of inhaled corticosteroids (ICSs) is attributed to their anti-inflammatory properties. Inhaled steroids have substantially less systemic absorption than oral steroids and, therefore, have a much better side-effect profile.

ICS sare the most important long-term control medications for asthma.

Commonly used ICS include budesonide, fluticasone, and triamcinolone. Data comparing the inhaled corticosteroids against each other are, at best, difficult to interpret. Clearly, these drugs have very different potencies. The reality is that the drug most asthmatics end up on is the one covered by their insurance carrier. Tables exist giving the low, medium, and high dosages for each of the ICS. Current consensus is that most of the effectiveness of ICS is achieved with the "low" (standard) dose, but that with more severe cases of asthma, increased dosing may be of benefit. It should be kept in mind that with increased doses come increased side effects. The best approach is to use the lowest dose possible that gives adequate control.

Long-acting beta agonists

Long-acting beta agonists (LABAs) such as formoterol and salmeterol are not recommended for the management of acute asthma exacerbations. However, clinicians will encounter many children who utilize these medications as part of their

Table 130.1. Summary of drugs for management of chronic asthma

Drug class	Drugs	Comments
Inhaled corticosteroids	Beclomethasone, budesonide, flunisolide, fluticasone, mometasone, triamcinolone	First-line drugs for all poorly controlled asthmatics; for children <5 years of age, increasing their dosage is preferable to adding adjunct medication
Long-acting beta agonists	Formoterol or salmeterol	Preferred adjunct to ICS in children ≥12 years; for children 5–12 years can either add one of these or increase ICS dose Good for exercise-induced asthma Never prescribe as monotherapy
Mast cell stabilizers	Cromolyn/nedocromil	Second-line treatment for mild persistent asthma
Anti IgE antibodies	Omalizumab	Use only in children ≥12 years; use as adjunct for severe persistent asthma in patients with allergies

A Practical Guide to Pediatric Emergency Medicine: Caring for Children in the Emergency Department, ed. N. Ewen Amieva-Wang (associate eds. Jamie Shandro, Aparajita Sohoni, and Bernhard Fassl). Published by Cambridge University Press.

Box 130.1. Management of asthma exacerbations presenting to the emergency department

Treat the acute exacerbation (Ch. 129).
Treat underlying chronic asthma symptoms.

Chronic symptoms

Inquire about presence of chronic asthma symptoms:

- nighttime cough/awakening because of asthma once or more per month
- daytime asthma symptoms more than twice a week
- activity limitations
- rescue inhaler use more than twice per week
- one or more exacerbations in previous 12 months.

1. If one or more of these questions above was answered Yes *and* the patient is *not* taking preventive medication regularly, then start preventive medication.
2. If any of these questions above was answered Yes *and* the patient *is* taking preventive medications, check usage of these medications and then step up treatment.

Usage of preventive medications

Inquire about use of preventive medications:

- type and dosage
- frequency of use.
- ability to take inhaler.

Treatment

In *treatment-naive patients* start inhaled steroid at low dose: fluticasone 44 μg/puff BID.

Step-up algorithm

Step-up treatment when the patient has had an asthma exacerbation when already taking preventive medication appropriately:

- leukotriene modifier → low-dose inhaled corticosteroids (ICS)
- low-dose ICS → medium-dose ICS
- medium-dose ICS → high-dose ICS or medium-dose ICS plus long-acting beta agonist
- high-dose ICS or medium-dose ICS + long acting beta agonist → referral to specialist after steroid burst to treat the exacerbation.

General rules

1. Always educate the patient and caregivers about how to take recommended medications.
2. Always refer the patient for follow-up to have asthma symptoms reassessed within 2 weeks.

long-term asthma management. Moreover, EPs may need to consider prescribing these medications to patients who present to ED with poor asthma control. A LABA is the preferred therapy to combine with ICS in those 12 years of age or older. Additionally, the National Asthma Education and Prevention Program Expert Panel Report 3 *Guidelines for the Diagnosis and Management of Asthma* (EPR-3) recommends "giving equal weight" to the options of increasing the dose of low-dose ICS versus adding a LABA in patients <5 years with poorly controlled asthma. It is worth mentioning that inhaled LABA are particularly effective when used before exercise to control exercise-induced bronchospasm. However, LABAs should *never* be prescribed as monotherapy for long-term asthma control. Consideration should be given to the fact that the subset of patients who showed increased morbidity/mortality while taking LABAs were predominantly African-American.

Other anti-inflammatory drugs

Given that asthma is a chronic inflammatory disease, it makes sense that other anti-inflammatory medicines could benefit asthmatic patients. The challenge to pediatric providers is that these medicines are often only tested on adults as they are developed.

Anti-IgE antibodies

The anti-IgE monoclonal antibody omalizumab, available under the commercial name Xolair, is now approved for children 12 years of age or older only. It works by blocking inflammatory cells from binding IgE. Its recommended use is as an adjunct to treatment of patients who have allergies and severe persistent asthma.

Leukotriene receptor antagonists

The family of medications known as leukotriene receptor antagonists (LTRAs) work by blocking leukotriene-mediated inflammatory pathways. Promising data have emerged for the use of IV montelukast in acute asthma exacerbations (in adults), showing improved pulmonary function in as little as 10 min. However, the IV form is currently not commercially available, pending FDA approval. Oral montelukast (Singulair)

Pearls and pitfalls

Pearls

1. In patients who are new to inhaled steroids, start with a low dose, such as fluticasone 44 μg/puff BID.
2. Long-acting beta agonists should never be used as the sole medication for a patient with asthma.

Pitfalls

1. Failure to recommend or arrange follow-up with a pediatrician for long-term management of asthma.

and zafirlukast (Accolate) are currently the only LTRAs approved for use in pediatrics. Zafirlukast can be used in children >7 years of age; montelukast is approved for children as young as 1 year. Delayed onset of action may limit their usefulness in an acute exacerbation. For chronic asthma management, they are considered alternative but not preferred treatments for mild persistent asthma.

Selected reference

National Asthma Education and Prevention Program. *Expert Panel Report II: Guidelines for the Diagnosis and Management of Asthma.* Bethesda, MD: National Heart, Lung, and Blood Institute, National Institutes of Health, 1997, pp. 1–50.

Mast cell stabilizers

Cromolyn and nedocromil make up a family of drugs known as mast cell stabilizers. They block the release of inflammatory mediators from mast cells. They are a second-line medication for the treatment of mild persistent asthma. They can also be used prior to exercise as a preventive medication.

Chapter 131

Bronchiolitis

Yi-Mei Chng and Laura Edgerley-Gibb

Introduction

Bronchiolitis is a viral lower respiratory tract infection that occurs mostly in children between the ages of 1 month and 2 years. It is the most common lower respiratory tract infection in children of these ages. It is characterized by acute inflammation and edema of the small airways, small-airway epithelial cell necrosis, increased mucus production, and bronchospasm. Children with history of premature birth, immunocompromise, pulmonary problems, or cardiac disease are at the highest risk for severe disease.

Bronchiolitis is a seasonal disease, occurring from November to March in the northern hemisphere. There are regional variations in the onset and length of season. While known causative viral agents include parainfluenza, influenza A and B, rhinovirus, and adenovirus, respiratory syncytial virus (RSV) is the most common etiologic agent, infecting up to 90% of children by 2 years of age. Unfortunately, infection with RSV does not confer permanent immunity. Children may have multiple bronchiolitis episodes from different viruses, or be reinfected with the same virus. Severe bronchiolitis infection requiring hospital admission in infancy has been linked with asthma and increased frequency of respiratory infection in older children. Patients who have received prophylaxis against RSV with palivizumab (a monoclonal antibody) in the past may still develop RSV infection. These patients are also likely to have risk factors for developing severe bronchiolitis because palivizumab is only given to infants with prematurity, lung disease, congenital heart disease, and other serious illnesses. Affected children may be symptomatic anywhere from a few days to 3–4 weeks, with the median duration of symptoms being 12 days.

Clinical presentation

History

The typical patient's history consists of a viral prodrome with rhinorrhea, fever, and cough followed by increased respiratory effort and wheezing.

Physical examination

Increased respiratory effort can be signaled by the patient's use of accessory muscles during inspiration, paradoxical abdominal wall motion, as well as grunting or nasal flaring. Tachypnea is frequently present and its absence is highly correlated with lack of lower respiratory infection in this age group.

Apnea may also be the presenting symptom of RSV infection in up to 20% of children who are early in the course of disease.

Very young infants (<3 months old) or infants with a history of premature birth at risk for RSV apnea.

On physical examination, children can have fever, copious rhinorrhea as well as respiratory distress with wheezing, rhonchi, and fine crackles on auscultation. The respiratory sounds of bronchiolitis have been likened to a washing machine.

Diagnostic studies

Radiography and laboratory studies should be done only to disprove other diagnoses in the differential or to assess a patient with worsening clinical course. While chest radiograph may reveal hyperinflation, bronchial cuffing, atelectasis, or consolidation (Fig. 131.1), there is no correlation between these abnormalities and the severity of disease. Routine radiography is discouraged.

Although routine testing for RSV or influenza virus also has little value in the ED diagnosis or treatment, testing is widely utilized in the inpatient setting to place patients in cohorts and to prevent the spread of disease.

Differential diagnosis

Respiratory distress and crackles on lung auscultation can be seen in a variety of other illnesses (Table 131.1). The clinician must maintain a high index of suspicion for other diagnoses particularly in the absence of a typical history of prodromal findings or lack of exposure.

A Practical Guide to Pediatric Emergency Medicine: Caring for Children in the Emergency Department, ed. N. Ewen Amieva-Wang (associate eds. Jamie Shandro, Aparajita Sohoni, and Bernhard Fassl). Published by Cambridge University Press.

A

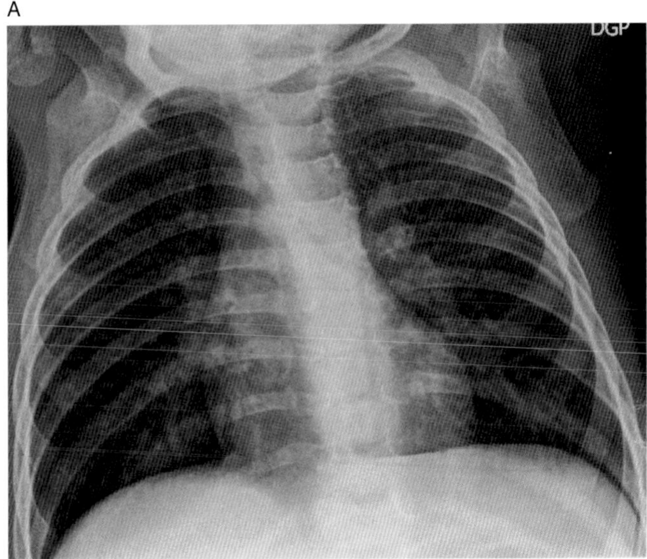

B

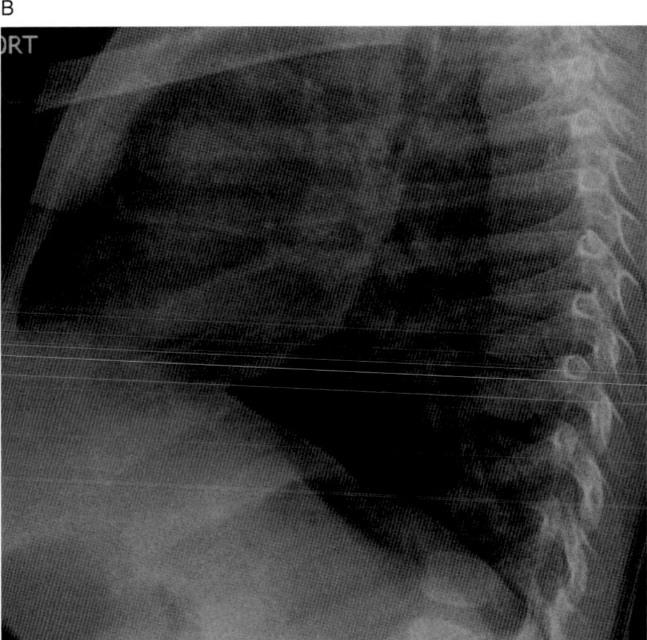

Figure 131.1 Viral bronchiolitis presenting with cough in an 11-month-old girl. (A,B) Chest radiographs demonstrate diffuse peribronchial thickening and mild hyperinflation seen as flattening of the diaphragm and air seen anterior to the heart (B), better appreciated on the lateral view.

Management

Immediate treatment is guided by examination and vital signs and is primarily supportive. Supplemental oxygen should be provided to infants with oxygen saturation <90%. Patients may require endotracheal intubation in the setting of respiratory fatigue or inability to maintain oxygenation. Infants with clinical evidence of dehydration or inability to feed because of severe tachypnea or nasal secretions may require IV fluids.

The pharmacologic treatment of bronchiolitis has been a subject of much study and debate. While bronchiolitis shares the common findings of wheezing with asthma, the routine use of bronchodilators has shown no improvement in outcomes. As some patients may improve in the short term, a trial of bronchodilators, either albuterol or racemic epinephrine, is sometimes warranted. These treatments should be discontinued if the patient exhibits no clinical response. Racemic epinephrine has shown slightly more promising results in terms of oxygen saturation and respiratory rate than albuterol. As such, it is the preferred agent in the ED and inpatient settings. Anticholinergics, such as ipratropium, have not been shown to have any short- or long-term benefit and should not be used. The use of systemic or inhaled corticosteroids in bronchiolitis has shown no benefit over placebo and is not recommended.

Rates of bacteremia in patients <3 months of age with documented RSV infection are quite low (<1%); therefore, workup for sepsis should be based on clinical suspicion. Antibiotics should be used only where there is co-existing bacterial infection. At this time, the AAP recommends the use of ribavirin only for infants with severe disease or infants with cardiac disease, pulmonary disease or who are immunocompromised.

Disposition

The decision whether to admit a patient with bronchiolitis from the ED depends on a number of factors:

- stability of the patient
  - pulse
  - oximetry: hypoxemia Sa_{O_2} <94% after treatment
  - oxygen requirement
  - respiratory distress (retractions, elevated respiratory rate)
  - dehydration or poor oral intake
  - degree of tachypnea
- underlying co-morbid illness, e.g., pulmonary, cardiac, metabolic or immunologic conditions
- history of apnea
- age <3 months or history of prematurity
- poor follow-up/social factors.

Children with positive viral testing should be placed on droplet precautions if admitted.

Table 131.1. Age-based differential diagnosis of lower lung findings and respiratory distress

Differential diagnosis	Common age of onset	Clues in history
Congestive heart failure secondary to congenital heart disease	Neonate	History of poor weight gain, sweating with feeds, cardiomegaly
Cystic fibrosis	Neonate	History of recurrent wheezing, failure to thrive
Aspiration	Neonate	Neurologically impaired children, ex-premature infants
Immunodeficiency syndromes	Any	Recurrent sinopulmonary infections
Bacterial pneumonia	Any	Lack of upper respiratory tract infection symptoms in history
Reactive airway disease/asthma	Any	History of past respiratory syncytial virus infection, presence/history of eczema, family history
Pertussis	Any	Leukocytosis, severe cough, apnea as presenting sign
Croup	3 months to 6 years	Inspiratory stridor
Foreign body aspiration	Toddler	Age, lack of prodrome

Pearls and pitfalls

Pearls

1. Bronchiolitis is a clinical diagnosis. The routine use of laboratory analyses and chest radiography is only indicated when other causes are suspected for patient symptoms.
2. Saline drops and nasal suctioning can greatly improve congestion in infants and young children with bronchiolitis.
3. Consider oxygenation, hydration status, ability to feed, and work of breathing when deciding whether to admit patients with bronchiolitis.
4. Infants <3 months or with a history of prematurity are at risk for respiratory syncytial virus apnea.

Pitfalls

1. Apnea, rather than respiratory distress, is the presenting sign in up to 20% of young infants with early respiratory syncytial virus infection.
2. Recurrent wheezing in infants can also be a presenting sign for congenital heart failure or cystic fibrosis.

Selected references

American Academy of Pediatrics Subcommittee on Diagnosis and Management of Bronchiolitis. Diagnosis and management of bronchiolitis. *Pediatrics* 2006;**118**:1774–1793.

Corneli HM, Zork JJ, Majahan P, for the Bronchiolitis Study Group of the Pediatric Emergency Care Applied Research Network (PECARN). A multicenter, randomized, controlled trial of dexamethasone for bronchiolitis. *N Engl J Med* 2007;**357**:331–339.

Wainwright C, Altamirano L, Cheney M, *et al.* A multicenter, randomized, double-blind, controlled trial of nebulized epinephrine in infants with acute bronchiolitis. *N Engl J Med* 2003;**349**:27–35.

Chapter

132 Cough

N. Ewen Amieva-Wang

Introduction

Cough is a symptom caused by airway reflexes that are essential to protect and clear the airway. It is a common complaint of children presenting to the ED. The cough can be acute and alarming, such as the barking cough of croup, or it can be more chronic and bothersome, such as a dry cough that occurs at night when the child is trying to sleep. Cough in the infant during the first 2 months of life is concerning and has an increased incidence of serious pathology, including congenital and infectious etiologies:

- congenital/anatomic
  - pulmonary: tracheoesophageal fistula, laryngeal web, pulmonary edema
  - congenital heart disease
  - neurologic abnormalities: aspiration
- infectious
  - pertussis
  - chlamydial infection
- gastroesophageal reflux disease: cough associated with feeding.

The clinician should also consider foreign body aspiration in a toddler with a new cough without associated infectious symptoms. Cough-induced asthma should be suspected in a child with nighttime cough responsive to beta adrenergic drugs.

Clinical presentation

History

Past medical history should include birth history including prematurity (bronchopulmonary dysplasia) or past pneumonia (immunodeficiency, cystic fibrosis). Family history of asthma, atopy (bronchospasm), or cystic fibrosis is important. Social history should include familial smoking as well as child experimentation with smoking or recreational inhalants.

The history (onset, quality of cough, timing, associated symptoms) offers clues to the etiology of the cough (Box 132.1). While sputum quality may offer clues to etiology for adults, children usually swallow their sputum; clues to sputum production are wet/dry cough. Acute onset is concerning for infection or foreign body aspiration while chronic onset suggests a more insidious process.

Associated symptoms can give clues to the severity of disease and etiology of cough. History of dyspnea, cyanosis, and hemoptysis are concerning for serious lung disease. Acute onset of fever, congestion, or headache suggests infection, including upper respiratory tract infection, sinusitis and pneumonia. Choking in association with cough suggests aspiration.

Box 132.1. Historical clues to etiology of cough

Onset

- *Acute*: foreign body, infection (pertussis, pneumonia, laryngotracheitis, bronchiolitis, upper respiratory tract infection, sinusitis).
- *Chronic*: gastroesophageal reflux, asthma, congenital anomalies, cystic fibrosis, neoplasm, congestive heart failure, otic foreign body.

Quality

- *Bark*: croup (often associated upper respiratory tract infection symptoms and fever).
- *Staccato cough*: chlanydial or mycoplasma pneumonia; can be afebrile pneumonia.
- *Paroxysmal*: series of coughs without intervening respirations: pertussis (characteristic whoop may be absent in infants and children).
- *Honking*: psychogenic (often follows an upper respiratory tract infection).

Timing

- *Morning*: asthma, sinusitis, postnasal drip, gastroesophageal reflux, croup.
- *Night*: asthma, gastroesophageal reflux disease and sinusitis.
- *Related to feeds*: gastroesophageal reflux, mechanical/neurologic abnormality suggestive of aspiration.
- *Seasonal*: reactive airway disease, allergic rhinitis.
- *Associated with exercise/cold*: suggests asthma.

Sputum

- *Productive*: lower airway infection (sinusitis, pneumonia).
- *Hemoptysis*: tuberculosis, abscess, foreign body aspiration, cystic fibrosis.

A Practical Guide to Pediatric Emergency Medicine: Caring for Children in the Emergency Department, ed. N. Ewen Amieva-Wang (associate eds. Jamie Shandro, Aparajita Sohoni, and Bernhard Fassl). Published by Cambridge University Press.

Physical examination

General appearance can indicate whether the child may have a chronic illness such as cystic fibrosis. Allergic signs include "shiners," nasal salute, and edematous nasal turbinates. Sinusitis can be suspected in a patient with halitosis and facial tenderness. Stridor indicates upper airway disease. Wheezes, rhonchi, or rales indicate lower airway disease, such as asthma, bronchiolitis or pneumonia.

Differential diagnosis

Probably the most common cause of acute cough is upper respiratory infection with or without bronchospasm. This should be considered after other causes have been ruled out.

Chlamydial pneumonia. This usually manifests within 2 weeks of birth; it may or may not be associated with conjunctivitis. The cough is typically stacatto in nature, and the children are afebrile.

Pertussis. Infants can contract pertussis from adults who are unimmunized or in whom immunization has worn off. Infants are usually not capable of generating enough force to emit the characteristic whoop. Cough may be associated with cyanosis and or apnea. While infants can look surprisingly well when not coughing, they are at risk for death with pertussis.

Congenital disease or anomaly. Undiagnosed laryngeal webs or tracheoesophageal fistulae can cause cough in the neonate. A young infant should never be diagnosed with croup without a workup for underlying causes of cough or stridor.

Cystic fibrosis. Chronic cough, poor weight gain, and recurrent infections are suspicious for cystic fibrosis.

Tuberculosis. Children with tuberculosis have increased incidence of systemic disease spread (versus primary lung disease). A child with exposure, hemoptysis, or other systemic signs should have workup to exclude tuberculosis (Ch. 99).

Gastroesophageal reflux/aspiration. If cough is associated with feeds in an infant, or in a child with seizure or neurologic impairment, think of aspiration.

Reactive airway disease. Bronchospasm can cause cough even in the absence of wheezing. Patients with a history of atopy, allergic rhinitis, and nighttime cough should have a trial of bronchodilator treatment (Chs. 129 and 130).

Diagnostic studies

Laboratory tests

Laboratory investigation should be done according to associated symptoms (suspected pneumonia might warrant a CBC).

Imaging

Patients with mild symptoms and a probable etiology, known asthma, or suspected bronchiolitis and pneumonia with a classic examination do not need radiographic evaluation. History of recurrent right middle lobe "pneumonia" is common in children with asthma secondary to poor collateral ventilation in the right middle lobe.

Severe presentations may warrant a radiograph to rule out other pathology. Suspected pulmonary foreign body warrants a radiograph (Ch. 128). Although organic matter will not be visible, indirect signs may be apparent. Recurrent pneumonia in one lobe of the lung can be caused by obstruction.

Management

Children with cough should be stabilized and treated for the underlying cause of their symptoms.

Antitussives have been shown to be ineffective and even harmful to young children, and should not be recommended or prescribed.

Sometimes a trial of bronchodilator in a child with possible bronchospasm in association with a virus is effective. Elevation of head and cool mist are also innocuous treatments that can help a viral cough.

Disposition

Most children with cough can be discharged home with treatment for the cause of the cough and follow-up with their primary care physician.

Young infants with possible pertussis, cystic fibrosis, or tuberculosis should be admitted for observation, definitive diagnosis, and treatment.

Children with suspected congenital anomaly must be assessed carefully. If they are stable to go home, good follow-up must be arranged for definitive workup. Toddlers with probable foreign body aspiration should undergo bronchoscopy. As always, good return precautions and follow-up with the primary care doctor should be provided.

Pearls and pitfalls

Pearls

1. The main causes of chronic cough in children are bronchospasm, gastroesophageal reflux, and postnasal drip/allergic rhinitis.
2. Cough during the first 2 months of life is more likely to be more serious than cough in older children.
3. Pertussis in an infant can cause death. Suspected disease in an infant up to 4–6 months of age warrants admission.

Pitfalls

1. Failure to consider congenital causes of cough in an infant.
2. Failure to consider foreign body aspiration in a toddler.

Chapter 133

Pneumonia

Yi-Mei Chng and Laura Edgerley-Gibb

Introduction

The WHO estimates that pneumonia is the number one cause of death in children <5 years of age. In Europe and North America, the incidence is thought to be approximately 34–40/1000 in children <5 years of age, who have a higher attack rate than older children. Some of the current recommendations continue to be based on data acquired prior to the initiation of widespread pneumococcal heptavalent conjugated vaccine (Prevnar) use, and may change as more is known about community-acquired pneumonia in the post-Prevnar epoch.

There are many pathogens associated with community-acquired pneumonia in the pediatric population. Viral infections are the most common cause of pneumonia in the pediatric age group, particularly in older infants and toddlers. Common viral pathogens include respiratory syncytial virus, influenza, parainfluenza, adenovirus, and rhinovirus. Fungal agents are uncommon but require a high level of suspicion for proper treatment, particularly in children with chronic diseases or immune deficiencies. Aspiration pneumonia should also be considered in children with chronic aspiration or other deficiencies in their protective airway reflexes.

The pathogens causing pneumonia vary with age in children (Table 133.1). The most common bacteria causing pneumonia in neonates include group B beta-hemolytic streptococci, Gram-negative enteric bacteria, *Listeria monocytogenes*, and *Chlamydia trachomatis*. In infants 1–3 months, *C. trachomatis* continues to be an important cause along with multiple viruses and *Streptococcus pneumoniae*. Toddlers are commonly infected with the common upper respiratory pathogens such as *S. pneumoniae* although viruses are the most common pathogen in this age group. As children transition into the school-age population, "atypical" pathogens become more prevalent. *Bordetella pertussis* can cause pneumonia even in vaccinated children, since immunization is only 80% effective in providing immunity after three doses, although the illness may be milder in vaccinated children. Pneumonia from pertussis is most common in infants <6 months old but can occur in older children and adults. It begins with 1–2 weeks of upper respiratory tract symptoms before progressing to the classic paroxysmal cough. Infants <6 months of age may have apnea rather than the classic "whoop."

Clinical presentation

Children with pneumonia may have a variety of complaints including difficulty breathing, fever, lethargy, cough, chest or abdominal pain. Presenting symptoms are often most vague in infants, with parents noting difficulty feeding, changes in breathing, irritability, and sometimes hypothermia.

The clinical signs of pneumonia include increased work of breathing, manifested by grunting, nasal flaring, intercostal and sternal retractions, and paradoxical abdominal motion, as well as tachypnea.

Tachypnea has been suggested as the best indicator of lower respiratory tract infection in children.

Other signs include low oxygen saturation, so pulse oximetry should always be included in the measured vital signs. Lung auscultation findings can range from diffuse rales to areas of absent breath sounds. It can be difficult to ascertain the etiologic agent from the presenting symptoms even in older children, although typical presentations for various pathogens are shown in Table 133.2. The lung examination may be particularly difficult in young children who are crying or uncooperative.

Diagnostic studies

Laboratory tests

Laboratory studies such as CBC, CRP, and ESR may signal infection, but are non-specific.

Sputum samples are difficult to collect in children and blood cultures are often low yield (2–10%). Nasopharyngeal swabs for viral testing are available for agents such as respiratory syncytial virus, parainfluenza and influenza. Up to 40% of children will have mixed viral and bacterial infection; consequently, even in the presence of positive viral testing, bacterial

A Practical Guide to Pediatric Emergency Medicine: Caring for Children in the Emergency Department, ed. N. Ewen Amieva-Wang (associate eds. Jamie Shandro, Aparajita Sohoni, and Bernhard Fassl). Published by Cambridge University Press.

Table 133.1. Common pathogens in pneumonia by age-range and suggested treatment[a]

Age	Most common infectious agents	Outpatient treatment	Inpatient treatment
0–1 month	Group B streptococci, Gram-negative enterics, cytomegalovirus, *Listeria monocytogenes*	Admit	Ampicillin + gentamicin ± cefotaxime
1–3 months	*Chlamydia trachomatis, Streptococcus pneumoniae*	Erythromycin or azithromycin	Ampicillin + cefotaxime (or ceftriaxone if >5weeks old) Erythromycin for *C. trachomatis*
	Viruses (respiratory syncytial virus, parainfluenza)	Supportive care	Supportive care
4 months to 4 years	Viruses		
	S. pneumoniae, Haemophilus influenzae; less prevalent, *Mycoplasma pneumoniae*, or *Chlamydia pneumoniae*	Amoxicillin or amoxicillin + clavulanic acid or cefuroxime or azithromycin (for chlamydia) or clarithromycin; supportive care	Ampicillin or cefuroxime or cefotaxime or clindamycin; supportive care
	Resistant *S. pneumoniae*/methicillin-resistant *Staphylococcus aureus* (MRSA)	Add macrolide	Add macrolide, vancomycin
5–18 years	*M. pneumoniae, C. pneumoniae, S. pneumoniae*	Macrolide or doxycycline if >8 years	Macrolide + cefuroxime or cefotaxime or ceftriaxone or clindamycin
	Resistant *S. pneumoniae*/MRSA	Macrolide or doxycycline if >8 years	Add vancomycin
	Viruses	Supportive care	Supportive care

[a] Consult antibiotic dosing guides for dosages.

infection cannot be excluded. Serum and serological testing lack specificity and are not currently recommended for routine use. Empiric treatment is probably sufficient in children with an uncomplicated medical history, mild symptoms, and on initial presentation.

Imaging

Although chest radiographs remain the gold standard in the diagnosis of pneumonia, findings are variable and range from areas of consolidation and air bronchograms to streaky or diffuse infiltrates or hilar adenopathy (Figs. 133.1 and 133.2).

British Thoracic Society Guidelines recommend against routine radiographic study in children with suspected pneumonia eligible for outpatient treatment.

However, chest radiograph is warranted in children and infants with respiratory complaints and uncertain diagnosis and in patients with severe illness.

Differential diagnosis

Differential diagnosis for pneumonia includes:

- bronchiolitis
- sepsis
- foreign body aspiration
- asthma
- viral upper respiratory infection.

Children with recurrent pneumonias or evidence of chronic lung disease on chest radiograph deserve special attention. The main differentials include:

- *cystic fibrosis*: recurrent respiratory infections, sinus infections, failure to thrive, bronchiectasis on chest radiograph
- *immunodeficiency syndromes*: recurrent sinopulmonary infections
- *aspiration pneumonia*: recurrent pneumonias in neurologically impaired children
- *occult foreign body aspiration*: repeated unilateral "white out" pneumonias in previously healthy toddlers.

Management

Patients should be stabilized in the ED with respiratory support as needed. Oxygen should be administered to maintain oxygen saturation >95%. Children with severe respiratory distress may require intubation and mechanical ventilation. Patients with signs of dehydration and inability to take oral liquids may require IV hydration.

Treatment for pneumonia is based on the patient's age and most likely etiologic agent (Table 133.1). Infants and children aged 4 months to 5 years with mild symptoms, appropriate short-term follow-up, and caregivers who will be able to assess

Table 133.2. Pneumonia syndromes and common presentations

Etiologic agent	Onset	Characteristics
Bacterial	Sudden onset, often associated with high fever and toxic appearance	High WBC more common; radiography findings variable; more likely to be associated with pleural effusions, abscesses, or lobar infiltrates than other causes of pneumonia
Viral	More gradual onset; often seasonal depending on the virus (most occur during the winter)	Fever more low grade; WBC lower than in bacterial pneumonia; associated with lymphocytosis
Mycoplasma	Tends to occur between ages 5 and 18 years; less toxic appearance; gradual onset May be associated with prodrome of headache, fever, and malaise before onset of cough with rash, sore throat, or chest pain	Bullous myringitis is not common, but classic for this infection
Chlamydia		
C. trachomatis	Pneumonia occurs in infants 3–19 weeks after colonization at birth	Associated conjunctivitis can occur in about half the children; may be associated with eosinophilia; often mild but can be associated with apnea
C. pneumoniae	Older children	Associated with flu-like symptoms and a stacatto cough
Pertussis	First stage can last 1–2 weeks and resembles catarrhal upper respiratory infection and is already contagious Second stage progresses to paroxysmal staccato cough, although this may not be present in infants <6 months old, who may have apnea instead; contagious	Can be associated with high WBC and lymphocytosis; exposure to an adult with a chronic cough should increase suspicion for pertussis
Tuberculosis	Longer-standing symptoms	Can progress to severe disease; exposure to an infected person is the biggest risk factor

for worsening illness may not require antibiotics given the high rates of viral infection in this group. Otherwise, treatment should proceed with appropriate antibiotic coverage for the patient's age group. Most patients should be treated with a course of oral antibiotics. Children with severe illness or the inability to tolerate oral antibiotics because of vomiting should be treated with IV antibiotics. For children with known exposure to or diagnosis of tuberculosis, management is covered in Ch. 99.

For outpatients, the British Thoracic Society guidelines recommend 7–14 days of treatment based on clinical response for most antibiotics including amoxicillin ± clavulanic acid, clarithromycin, cefaclor, and erythromycin. If treating with azithromycin, 5 days is recommended. *S. pneumoniae* resistant to penicillin has emerged in recent years but can still be treated effectively with the use of high-dose beta-lactam antibiotics. For the outpatient, high-dose amoxicillin (80–100 mg/kg daily) is preferred; the addition of beta-lactamase inhibitors does not help, as the mechanism of resistance in *S. pneumoniae* does not rely on that enzyme. If there is high suspicion for pertussis (exposure to an adult with known pertussis or symptoms consistent with pertussis), treat with azithromycin for 5 days or erythromycin for 14 days.

Disposition

Infants <1 month of age and any child who is immunocompromised or with intrinsic lung disease such as cystic fibrosis should be admitted for IV antibiotics.

Infants 1–3 months should strongly be considered for admission.

Some experts also recommend admission in all infants <6 months of age. In older, otherwise healthy infants and children, the decision to admit is based on their respiratory status, ability to take oral feedings, ability of parents to care for the child at home with proper precautions, and availability of follow-up.

Hospitalization should be considered for infants with

- arterial oxygen saturation ($SaO_2 \leq 92\%$)
- cyanosis
- respiratory rate >70 breaths/min
- difficulty breathing
- intermittent apnea
- grunting
- inability to feed
- family incapable of assessing the patient for indicators for admission at home.

A

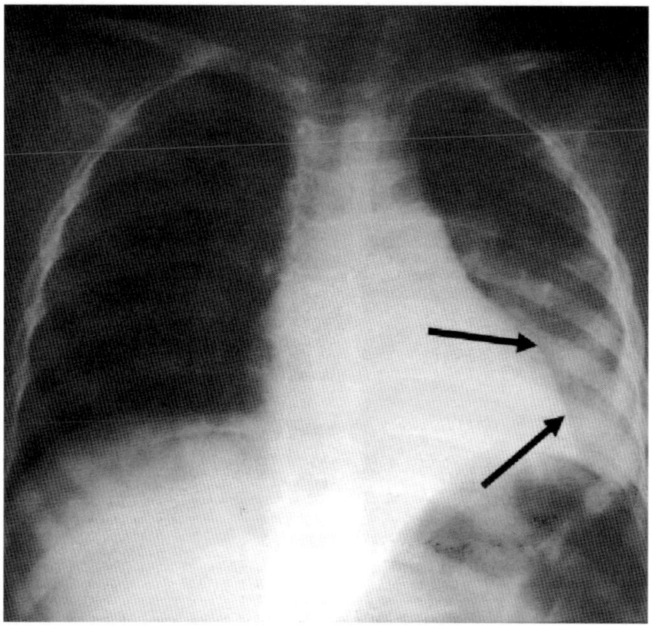

B

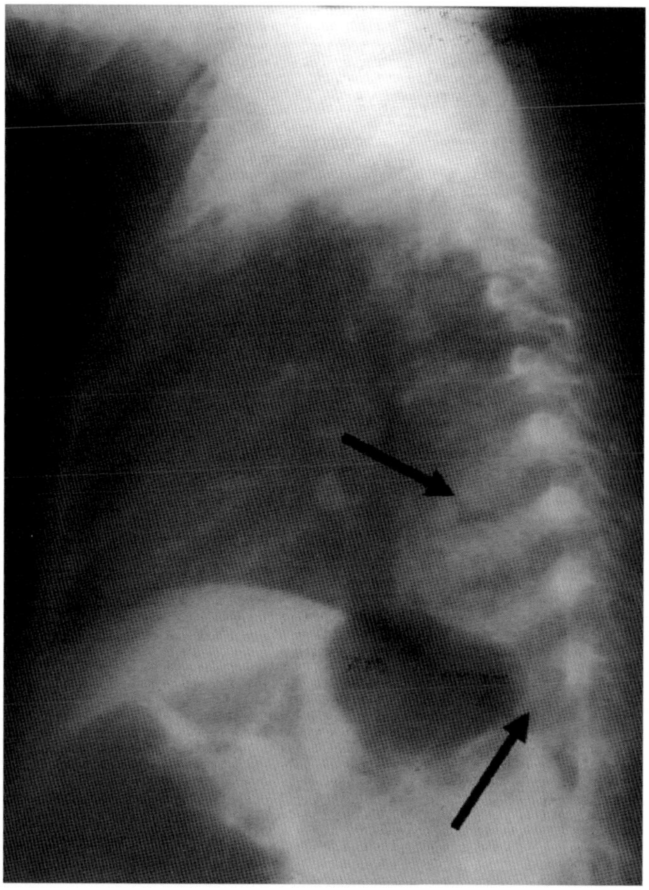

Figure 133.1 Pneumococcal pneumonia in a 5-year-old child. (A) Frontal chest radiograph demonstrates air space consolidation in the left lower lobe with preservation of the left heart border (arrows). (B) Opacity overlying the spine on the lateral view (arrows).

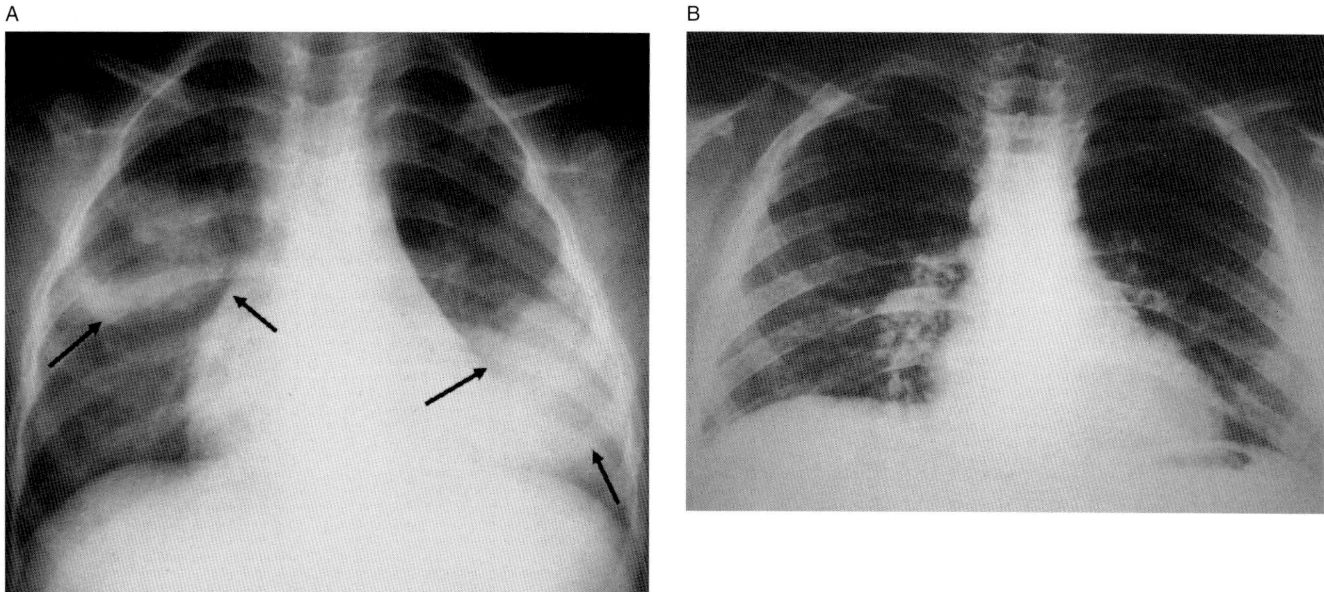

Figure 133.2 Variable pattern of *Mycoplasma* pneumonia. (A) Frontal chest radiograph in a 7-year-old child shows patchy air space consolidation in both lungs (arrows). (B) Frontal chest radiograph in a 4-year-old child shows reticulonodular infiltrates in bilateral perihilar and lower lobes.

For older children, admission should be considered for SaO_2 $\leq$92%, cyanosis, respiratory rate >50 breaths/min, difficulty breathing, grunting, signs of dehydration, or family incapable of assessing the patient for indicators for admission at home. Hospitalization should also be considered for children who have any of the following: a toxic appearance even without meeting the criteria above, pleural effusions, or an immunocompromised state.

In children with no signs of increased work of breathing who have a caregiver who can adequately assess warning signs for bringing the child back to the hospital, discharge home with an oral antibiotic regimen may be warranted. Patients with pneumonia should always have a follow-up visit within 24 h to assess response to medications.

Pearls and pitfalls

Pearls

1. Pneumonia in pediatric patients is frequently caused by a viral infection.
2. Tachypnea is considered one of the most reliable signs of lower respiratory infection in children.
3. Sputum cultures are of low yield, and difficult to obtain, in pediatric patients.

Pitfalls

1. Failure to consider atypical pathogens in children not improving on their current antibiotic regimen.
2. Failure to consider pertussis in the differential diagnosis of pneumonia.
3. Failure to consider aspiration of a foreign body in a child with repeated pneumonia.

Selected references

McIntosh K. Community acquired pneumonia in children. *N Engl J Med* 2002;**346**:429–437.

Michelow I, Olsen K, Lozano J, *et al.* Epidemiology and clinical characteristics of community-acquired pneumonia in hospitalized children. *Pediatrics.* 2004;**113**:701–707.

Chapter 134

Upper airway emergencies

Sangeeta Kaur Gill Schroeder

Introduction

Pediatric upper airway obstruction affects different age groups and can be caused by congenital/anatomic anomalies, infection, and foreign bodies (Fig. 134.1 and Table 134.1). The epidemiology of upper airway emergencies in the USA has changed dramatically since the institution of immunization for *Haemophilus influenzae* type b (Hib) and the use of steroids in viral croup. While croup is still the most common infectious reason for pediatric airway obstruction, bacterial tracheitis has become the most common infectious etiology of the true pediatric airway emergency.

Children are more prone to upper airway obstruction than adults because of airway size as well as a tendency to put things into their mouths. With a smaller airway diameter, children are at increased risk for respiratory compromise with even a small amount of airway blockage from mucous production, inflammation, congenital anomalies, or a foreign body. Once airway obstruction has occurred, a child can decompensate quickly.

Anatomy

A good way to differentiate the causes of upper airway obstruction in children is to separate them by location: extrathoracic/supraglottic, glottic/subglottic, and intrathoracic. The anatomic location of the obstruction also directly informs the clinical presentation.

Extrathoracic/supraglottic. The supraglottic airway lacks cartilaginous support and is composed primarily of soft

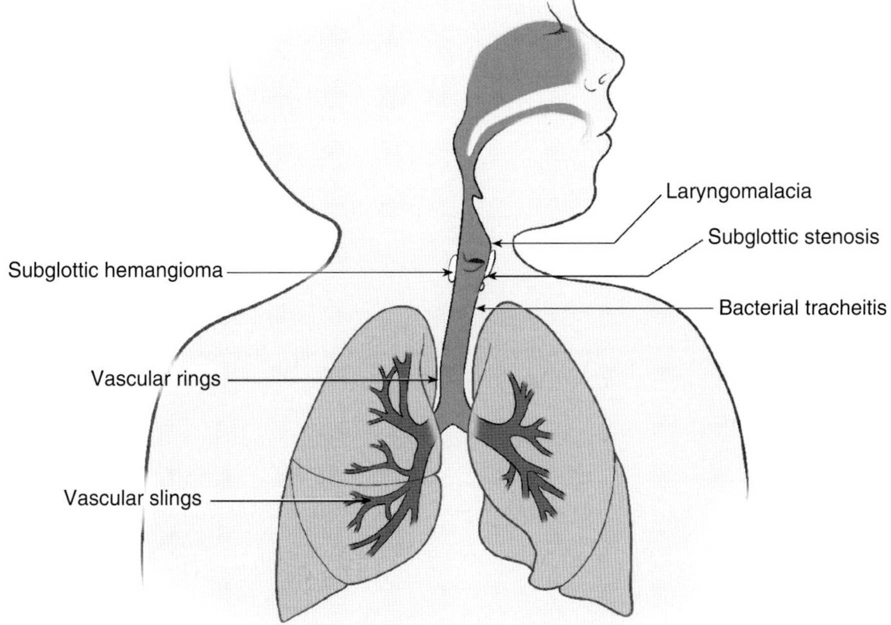

Figure 134.1 Pathology of upper airway.

A Practical Guide to Pediatric Emergency Medicine: Caring for Children in the Emergency Department, ed. N. Ewen Amieva-Wang (associate eds. Jamie Shandro, Aparajita Sohoni, and Bernhard Fassl). Published by Cambridge University Press.

Table 134.1. Age-based differential of upper airway obstruction and symptoms

Age	Diagnosis	Presentation	Risk factors	Signs/symptoms
3 months to 6 years	Croup	Gradual onset	Underlying anatomic narrowing of the airway	Varying degrees of stridor associated with upper respiratory tract infection symptoms
Any age	Bacterial tracheitis	Gradual onset with sudden progression; can also present suddenly without prodrome	Underlying croup infection; immunocompromised	Often starts as croup with sudden worsening of stridor and coughing; child is anxious and toxic appearing; diagnosis often confirmed on bronchoscopy
Unvaccinated child (peaks at 3 years), vaccinated child (peaks at 6–7 years)	Epiglottitis	Sudden onset of sore throat, fever, inability to control secretions and inspiratory distress	Incomplete or absent Hib vaccination; complication of varicella infection, immunocompromised	Child sits forward and often unable to control secretions; anxious and toxic appearing; usually without signs of retractions, stridor, or coughing; diagnosis often confirmed via airway endoscopy or direct laryngoscopy
6 weeks to 1 year	Laryngomalacia	Intermittent episodes of stridor without fever	Male infants, associated with gastroesophageal reflux disease	Stridor worsens with activity or infections
Any age (most prominent in infancy)	Tracheomalacia, bronchomalacia	Appears insidiously after the first few weeks of life; symptoms are more persistent in nature than with laryngomalacia	Underlying neuromuscular or genetic disorder	Stridor and wheezing worsen with minor activity (coughing, feeding) or infections; can cause significant cyanotic spells
Infants	Vascular rings/ slings	Incomplete rings often present after a child has been introduced to solid foods (usually between 4–8 months of life)	Congenital heart disease (most commonly tetralogy of Fallot)	Complete rings present with stridor and wheezing in early infancy; incomplete rings present with dysphagia (if compressing the esophagus) or with intermittent stridor/wheezing (if compressing the trachea)
Neonates (complete webs), infants and toddlers (incomplete webs)	Laryngeal webs	Different degrees of respiratory distress	DiGeorge syndrome and other congenital cardiac abnormalities	Stridor, weak cry in infants; complete webbing is found at birth with significant respiratory distress requiring surgical intervention
Infant (congenital), any age (acquired)	Subglottic stenosis	Chronic stridor	History of prolonged intubation, gastroesophageal reflux	Varying degrees of respiratory distress depending on the degree of stenosis, considered congenital if there is no history of airway instrumentation
Infants and toddlers	Subglottic hemangioma	Insidious presentation of stridor that worsens as the lesion enlarges	Face and neck hemangiomas	Progressively loud biphasic stridor and respiratory distress associated with an enlarging hemangioma
Peritonsillar abscess (>10 years old)	Peritonsillar abscess	Dysphagia, hot potato voice, trismus	Recent viral upper respiratory tract infection	Displaced uvula, fluctuance

Table 134.1. *(cont.)*

Age	Diagnosis	Presentation	Risk factors	Signs/symptoms
Retropharyngeal abscess (4 years old)	Retropharyngeal abscess, etc.	High fever, dysphagia; in infants can simulate nuchal rigidity	Immunocompromised, trauma	Child can be anxious with difficulty controlling secretions
Any	Anaphylaxis (see also Ch. 10)	Many times this will be the first presentation of reaction to an unknown offending agent	History of food or medication allergy	Airway and facial swelling. Often both stridor and wheezing is appreciated
Toddlers	Foreign body obstruction (see also Ch. 128)	History of aspiration or choking	Unattended child	Cough and stridor or wheezing, depending on the location of the foreign body

tissue and muscles including the epiglottis. Epiglottitis is often caused by an invasive bacterial infection of the epiglottis but can also infect the arytenoid cartilages, aryepiglottic folds, and false vocal cords.

Glottic/subglottic. The glottis and subglottic larynx make up the lower extrathoracic airway. While this area is composed of some cartilaginous support (cricoid cartilage and incomplete tracheal rings), the subglottic area is the smallest point in the pediatric airway. This is a common location for both infectious causes of stridor (croup and bacterial tracheitis) and non-infectious causes; 75% of laryngeal webs (webbing caused by residual embryonic tissue that did not normally regress) also occur in the glottic area.

Intrathoracic. The intrathoracic airway is synonymous with the tracheobronchial tree. Usually, obstruction at this level is secondary to congenital etiologies such as vascular rings/slings and bronchomalacia. Vascular rings/slings arise from an abnormal persistence or regression of the embryonic tissue that made up the aortic arch. The most common reasons for airway compression secondary to vascular anomalies are a double aortic arch (50–60%), a right aortic arch with an aberrant left subclavian artery (12–25%), and a pulmonary artery sling. Bronchomalacia, like tracheomalacia, is a result of inadequate cartilaginous and muscle fiber support.

Clinical presentation

After determining whether emergency airway management is needed, it is important to differentiate whether the upper airway obstruction is infectious or not and then where the obstruction is. Fever and upper respiratory tract infection symptoms suggest an infectious process. If the child is toxic or the symptoms rapidly progress, a bacterial etiology must be considered. If the symptoms are insidious and/or intermittent, a congenital etiology is likely.

Anatomical abnormalities that cause airway obstruction are also often worsened by an upper respiratory infection.

History

Obtaining a good past medical history is also key to the diagnosis. Acquired subglottic stenosis is a known sequela of prolonged intubation. Congenital subglottic stenosis is seen more frequently in children with trisomy 21. Other genetic defects increase the risk of having laryngeal webs. A diagnosis of hypotonia points to tracheo- or bronchomalacia.

A history of hemangiomas indicates a possible subglottic hemangioma.

While most hemangiomas require no intervention and decrease in size by the age of 2, they usually increase in size first. If the hemangioma is within the airway, this increase in size can be the cause of sudden upper airway obstruction in a young child.

Physical examination

On physical examination, neck mass or edema are suggestive of an underlying abscess. Edematous nasal turbinates with nasal secretions suggest viral croup. Intermittent cyanotic spells with nasal congestion could represent an underlying congenital abnormality aggravated by a viral infection.

When auscultating, make sure to listen to the mouth, neck and lungs. If a child has snoring that is audible without a stethoscope, the child likely has a nasal or oropharyngeal obstruction. Referred upper airway sounds or “gurgling” without definitive stridor or wheezing in an anxious-appearing child should provoke the EP to rule out epiglottitis. Inspiratory stridor indicates a glottic or subglottic obstruction, while expiratory stridor indicates a lesion lower in the trachea. Skin findings, such as café au lait spots (suggestive of neurofibromas of the airway) or hemangiomas (give rise to the possibility of a subglottic hemangioma) can also help the EP to determine an etiology to the child’s illness.

A change in the tone and quality of the voice can also help in determining the etiology of the patient's stridor. A muffled, "hot potato" voice usually is a sign that the patient has a supraglottic obstruction such as epiglottitis. A subglottic obstruction, such as croup, usually presents with a "barky" cough, while a "weak" cry and hoarseness is often the presentation of an incomplete laryngeal web.

Differential diagnosis

Epiglottitis, bacterial tracheitis, and croup all cause upper airway obstruction.

Epiglottitis

Epiglottitis involves the acute onset of edema and inflammation of the area from the epiglottis to the false vocal cords and can often present with significant inspiratory distress and "gurgling" sounds without concurrent stridor or retractions. This is a key distinguishing factor between epiglottitis and bacterial tracheitis or severe laryngotracheitis (croup). In the USA, with the advent of the Hib vaccine, *S. pneumoniae* and group A beta-hemolytic streptococci have become the major bacterial causes of epiglottitis, transforming epiglottitis from a disease of infancy to one of older children.

Classically, epiglottitis presents with a sudden onset of fever and toxic appearance in a child who has not received Hib vaccine. The child is often anxious and toxic-appearing out of proportion to their signs of respiratory distress. The child will often sit forward with the hands extended in front of the body (tripod positioning), the jaw thrust forward with an open mouth and copious drooling present. While the child will have inspiratory "gurgling" sounds, they will not cough or produce much stridor as this would produce motion of the epiglottis and intensify the pain.

Laryngotracheitis/croup

In viral laryngotracheitis (croup), the obstruction is inflammation and mucous production at the subglottic area, secondary to viral invasion. The most common viruses to cause croup are parainfluenza virus types 1, 2 and 3, influenza virus types A and B, respiratory synctial virus, and adenoviruses.

Children classically present with a history of mild upper respiratory tract infection symptoms and sudden onset of barking cough and/or stridor. Determining whether the child has mild, moderate, or severe croup is important. Mild croup is defined as a child without stridor or significant chest wall retractions at rest, who may have some stridor with activity. Moderate croup consists of stridor and chest wall retractions at rest. Severe croup is characterized by stridor and substernal retractions associated with agitation or lethargy.

Bacterial tracheitis

The hallmark of bacterial tracheitis is the formation of a pseudomembrane composed of mucous, bacteria, and inflammatory products. The most common causes of bacterial tracheitis are *Staphylococcus aureus* and *Streptococcus pyogenes*. It is usually a superinfection of a viral upper respiratory infection (most commonly parainfluenza and influenza) but can also be caused by direct invasion of the bacteria into the subglottic area without a prodromal viral infection. Children with bacterial tracheitis will present with stridor and cough but appear more toxic and infectious than children with croup.

Differentiating epiglottitis, bacterial tracheitis, and severe croup

A key feature to differentiating epiglottitis from bacterial tracheitis and severe croup is the absence of retractions or other signs of increased work of breathing (Table 134.2). Severe viral croup and bacterial tracheitis, by comparison, will almost always produce stridor and cough as they do not produce pain while epiglottitis causes pain. These children will also often demonstrate suprasternal retractions and would not produce the muffled, "hot potato" voice that is characteristic of epiglottitis.

Anatomic abnormalities

Congenital obstruction must be excluded in any child who presents with intermittent stridor within the first 3 months of life or has been diagnosed with croup multiple times in the past.

Patients with laryngeal webs often present with a weak cry, hoarseness, and varying degrees of respiratory distress depending on the degree of webbing.

Patients are classified as type I ($\leq$35% webbing) through to type IV (>75% webbing). Type IV webs are usually diagnosed at birth and require urgent airway stabilization.

Vascular ring presentation also depends on the degree of compression of the trachea and/or esophagus. The most common clinical findings are stridor and wheezing, although these children can also present with cyanotic or apneic episodes. While wheezing is the direct result of the vascular ring itself, stridor can also be heard secondary to laryngeal inflammation from the associated gastroesophageal reflux that many of these children have. Secondary to the mixture of pulmonary sounds heard in these children, they are commonly misdiagnosed as having bronchiolitis. Children can also present with difficulty feeding on introduction of solid foods if there is a component of esophageal compression. Often children do not present until they develop a mild upper respiratory tract infection, which causes symptomatic obstruction of an already narrowed airway.

Diagnosis

Diagnosis of upper airway obstruction is mainly clinical. While neck radiographs have historically been used for diagnosis they are not recommended for toxic children and are not particularly sensitive or specific.

Table 134.2. Differentiation of croup, bacterial tracheitis, and epiglottitis

	Croup	Bacterial tracheitis	Epiglottitis
Age	<6 years	<6 years	Median 6–7 years in vaccinated children
Risk factors	Sick contacts	Often starts as croup, rarely starts without prodrome; intubated children are more at risk	Immunizations not complete (<6 months of age, born in non-vaccinating country, parents refused immunizations, etc.)
Fever	Low grade	High or low	High
Onset	Gradual	Gradual with sudden progression	Sudden
Airway examination	Not significant	Purulent with pseudomembrane formation; often seen by bronchoscopy, which is needed for definitive diagnosis and treatment (suctioning of secretions)	Swollen cherry-red epiglottis, *but* if the child fits the clinical picture, evaluation of the airway should only be done by someone experienced in managing a tenuous airway
Lung examination	Stridor with or without retractions	Stridor with retractions	Normal, usually no signs of retractions
Toxic appearing	Rarely	Almost always	Almost always
Viral symptoms of congestion/ runny nose	Almost always present	Often starts with these symptoms prior to progression	Can be seen with these associated symptoms as a secondary infection, but it usually is a primary infection
Treatment	Dexamethasone ± racemic epinephrine	Antibiotics and careful airway management, with need for constant suctioning	Antibiotics and careful airway management
Disposition	Home or observation unit; rarely severe enough for ICU admission	Admit to ICU	Admit to ICU

Radiography is not recommended unless a foreign body is suspected. Use of CT is indicated for possible neck abscess. Inpatient studies to further identify malacia, vascular rings, or laryngeal webs utilize laryngoscopy, bronchoscopy, barium swallow or MRI.

Management

If the child is toxic appearing, emergency airway management should be initiated. With suspected epiglottitis and bacterial tracheitis, ideally intubation should be conducted in the operating room. The practitioner should be prepared to use an endotracheal tube that is smaller than indicated because of the likelihood of significant airway edema.

Epiglottitis

In most cases of epiglottitis, the child should be taken to a controlled environment and an artificial airway should be placed by an experienced practitioner. In the current age of post-Hib immunization, the question of automatic intubation in all patients with epiglottitis is being posed. Once the airway is stabilized, antibiotics should be started without delay. Appropriate antibiotic choices would be ceftriaxone or cefotaxime with vancomycin if concerned for methicillin-resistant *S. aureus* (MRSA). All children with epiglottitis should be admitted to a pediatric ICU.

Croup

While humidified air and cool mist are age-old treatments, their efficacy has yet to be proven. All children presenting to the ED with symptoms of viral croup, regardless of their severity, should be given a dose of 0.6 mg/kg dexamethasone IM/PO (max. 10 mg). In moderate to severe croup, airway edema is decreased with racemic epinephrine 2.25% nebulized treatment along with corticosteroids. Once the treatment with racemic epinephrine is given, the child should be observed for at least 2 h. While the rebound effect is controversial, it is imperative to observe the severity of a child's obstructive symptoms after the medication effects have worn off. A second treatment is sometimes needed after 1 to 2 h, and in severe stridor, continuous nebulized racemic epinephrine treatments are warranted. A child requiring more than two nebulized treatments should be admitted. If continuous nebulized treatment is needed, the child should be admitted to a pediatric ICU. Other indications for admission would be dehydration secondary to poor oral intake or moderate respiratory distress with a lack of adequate follow-up. In children who do not respond to continuous racemic epinephrine nebulized treatments, bacterial tracheitis should be put back at the top of the differential.

Bacterial tracheitis

Treatment of bacterial tracheitis is with airway management and antibiotics. Often these children will require urgent airway stabilization and bronchoscopy to suction purulent and necrotic debris from within the airways. Even after an artificial airway is placed, these children require constant observation in a pediatric ICU for continued suctioning of secretions. Initial antibiotic coverage should be broad, and include coverage of Gram-positive cocci, usually vancomycin, along with a third-generation cephalosporin.

Anatomic abnormalities

The responsibility of the EP is to suspect possible underlying anatomic disorders and refer for definitive diagnosis in the very young patient or child with recurrent symptoms. If there is a viral infection and worsening symptoms of any known or suspected anatomic disorder, treatment should be directed at decreasing airway inflammation. Most cases of laryngomalacia and tracheomalacia resolve once the child's airway grows in size, usually around 1 year of age, and require no other therapy.

Treatment for laryngeal webs and vascular rings is surgical. Often webbing of the larynx is observed until the child is 3–4 years of age before surgical intervention is required. Vascular rings, however, are often corrected early.

Subglottic hemangiomas also require surgical intervention if the obstruction is causing significant respiratory distress. Indications for admission would be hypoxia, significant respiratory distress, dehydration from decreased feeding, and poor follow-up.

Pearls and pitfalls

Pearls

1. Croup should not be diagnosed in the first month of life; instead, suspect a congenital anomaly.
2. In a child with a hemangioma and stridor, consider subglottic hemangioma.
3. Dexamethasone 0.6 mg/kg IM or PO has become the mainstay of treatment for croup, regardless of severity.
4. Bacterial tracheitis, frequently caused by *Staphylococcus aureus* or *Streptococcus pyogenes*, is now the most common infectious cause of pediatric upper respiratory emergencies.

Pitfalls

1. Failure to consider laryngomalacia in the differential diagnosis for intermittent respiratory distress.

Selected references

Bjornson C, Johnson D. Croup. *Lancet* 2008;**317**:329–339.

Hartnick CJ, Cotton RT. Congenital laryngeal anomalies. Laryngeal atresia, stenosis, webs and clefts. *Otolaryngol Clin North Am* 2000;**33**: 1293–1308.

Hopkins A, Lahiri T, Salerno R, Heath B. Changing epidemiology of life-threatening upper airway infections: the reemergence of bacterial tracheitis. *Pediatrics* 2006;**118**: 1418–1421.

Kussman BD, Geva R, McGowan F. Cardiovascular causes of airway compression. *Paediatr Anaesth* 2004;**14**:60–74.

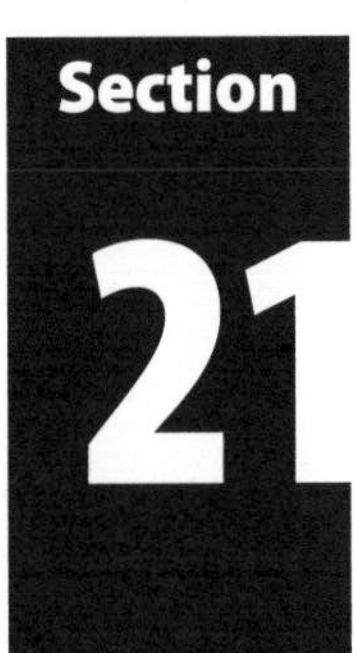

Social and emotional emergencies

Expert reviewer: Tonya Chaffee

Chapter 135

Child abuse and maltreatment

Bryce Inman and Jamie Shandro

Introduction

Child maltreatment is defined as intentional harm or threat of harm to a child by a person who is acting in the role of caretaker. The exact incidence of child maltreatment in the USA is unknown, but according to the US Department of Health and Human and Services approximately 3.6 million cases of child abuse were investigated by child protective services (CPS) in 2006. Of those, 900 000 were classified as victims by CPS and close to three quarters of them had no prior history of abuse.

Four types of maltreatment are commonly described: physical abuse, sexual abuse, emotional abuse, and neglect. The large majority of affected children are maltreated in the setting of neglect (64%), but there is a still-significant portion of this population exposed to physical (16%) or sexual (9%) abuse. Certain populations are more vulnerable, with infants and children with chronic disease or disabilities more likely to suffer from abuse. Those under the age of 4 years make up 78% or more of the deaths resulting from child abuse.

There are mandatory reporting laws for suspected child abuse in all 50 states (http://www.childwelfare.gov/). The specific reporting requirements and definition of abuse and maltreatment may vary, but all affirm that healthcare professionals are mandated to report suspected child abuse. Reportable cases include discrepancies between physical findings and the suggested mechanism of injury, inconsistent histories, unusual fractures, delays in seeking care, multiple fractures/injuries in varying degrees of healing, and sexual trauma. Failure to report cases may result in civil and/or criminal liabilities, including fines or imprisonment.

The goal of this chapter is to provide a concise guide to the EP who is faced with a possible case of child maltreatment. Child maltreatment is often seen first in the setting of an ED, and it is, therefore, imperative that healthcare professionals in these settings are able to identify and manage suspected abuse. This chapter provides guidelines for management as well as disposition and notification issues in the case of suspected child maltreatment, as well as a guide to the various presentations of non-accidental trauma and how to distinguish non-accidental from accidental trauma.

Clinical presentation and differential diagnosis

Maltreatment may manifest in many different ways and involve any body system. Maintain a high index of suspicion for abuse in the setting of an acutely injured child in order to accurately diagnose the trauma as well as institute actions that prevent future injury or death. A careful history and physical examination is the best tool for the initial investigation of abuse.

History

History may provide the initial clues to child abuse:

- delayed presentation
- contradictory/vague/untenable history
- <3 years of age
- behavioral problems
- poor growth.

If the reported history is vague, conflicting, or repeatedly changing then include abuse as part of the differential diagnosis. The same is true if injuries are out of proportion to the history. Other suggestive histories include a caregiver who blames another caregiver who is not present, unwitnessed accidents, multiple prior injuries, and delays in seeking treatment. Behavior of the caregiver may raise suspicion as well, as they may be detached and unconcerned regarding the injury or, conversely, extremely concerned over seemingly minor injuries.

When evaluating for possible sexual abuse, the history is highly valuable, as the most common manifestation of sexual abuse is a positive history. Those children who have been sexually maltreated may present with vague abdominal pains, hematuria, dysuria, enuresis, and/or vaginal discharge. Children who can relate a history of sexual abuse must be taken seriously as it is extremely unlikely they could make up such an

A Practical Guide to Pediatric Emergency Medicine: Caring for Children in the Emergency Department, ed. N. Ewen Amieva-Wang (associate eds. Jamie Shandro, Aparajita Sohoni, and Bernhard Fassl). Published by Cambridge University Press.

Table 135.1. Physical examination findings and injury patterns suggestive of abuse by body system

System	Examination findings suggestive of abuse	Injury patterns suggestive of abuse
Skin	Bites, burns, abrasions, or diffuse bruising at different stages of healing	Injuries on cheeks, ears, thighs, buttocks, abdomen, and flank Deep burns or immersion burns
Neurologic	Retinal hemorrhages, lethargy, focal neurological deficits	Skull fractures, intracranial bleeds such as a subdural or epidural hematoma
Musculoskeletal	Point tenderness, swelling, joint deformities, or bony step-offs Multiple injured extremities; rib or sternal fractures	Metaphyseal–epiphyseal and spiral fractures; fractures of ribs, sternum, pelvis Multiple fractures in various stages of healing: long bone fracture <2 years old (tibia/humerus/femur most common)
Gastrointestinal	Rebound, guarding, ecchymoses of abdomen/flank	Solid organ rupture, elevated pancreatic/liver enzymes
Genitourinal	Brusing, tearing, scarring around the genitals or anus, genital discharge	Aside from zipper injuries, almost all injuries in this area are suspicious of abuse

allegation. The EP's history should focus on understanding the etiology of the symptoms (trauma, infection, abuse.) If the suspicion for sexual abuse is high, after assuring there are no acute injuries, a thorough history should be obtained by professionals trained in pediatric sexual assault evaluation. Referral to a team or professional specifically trained in pediatric sexual assault is vital for several reasons: (1) history may be the most important evidence since often physical examination is negative in cases of abuse, (2) the examiner will likely be called to testify in court, and (3) relegating the history to the definitive forensic examiner will obviate the need for the child to repeat painful or distressing history to multiple caregivers.

Psychological/emotional abuse is deliberately conveying to a child that he or she is worthless, flawed, unloved, endangered, or unwanted. Examples of caregiver behavior productive of this abuse include intimidating, blaming, ridiculing, exploiting, and terrorizing. Long-standing abuse leads to impaired social and psychological growth and development. Although one of the most common forms of child abuse, it represents only 7% CPS reports. The history will often include emotional disturbances such as depression, agitation, and social withdrawal, as well as problems outside the home such as drug/alcohol problems and difficulty in school.

Neglect occurs in four forms; physical, emotional, educational, and medical. A careful history can yield useful information and guide further evaluations. If there is evidence of physical neglect then ask the caregiver about resources and their ability to care for the child. If there is suspicion of emotional neglect, ask the caregiver about how he or she feels towards the child, and how each conveys affection towards the other. Failure to enroll a child in school or maintain their attendance, or failure to provide intellectual stimulation are suggestive of educational neglect. If a child has a medical condition and the caregiver is consistently lax in following recommended care, managing treatment (e.g., medications), or the child has experienced harm through lack of care, then medical neglect is likely. In all cases of neglect, assess the caregiver's attitudes and their understanding of the problem as some cases of neglect may result from inadequate education, insufficient resources, or cultural differences.

Physical examination

A complete physical examination is necessary to evaluate for potential maltreatment. Certain injuries are much more likely to result from abuse than from accidental trauma, and this may suggest the diagnosis of abuse is likely (Table 135.1). Furthermore, injuries that do not correspond to the reported mechanism of injury may be indicative of abuse.

The skin is the most often involved organ system and will provide important diagnostic clues. Bruises, bites, abrasions, and burns are often easy to find and may be suggestive of more serious lesions. Important characteristics in assessing these lesions include location, chronology, and appearance. "Normal" bruising (i.e., accidental bruising) often occurs in children on extensor surfaces such as shins, forearms, and even the forehead and need not necessarily raise alarm unless the child is still too young to ambulate. The presence of bruising on more centrally located and softer areas including buttocks, genitalia, inner/anterior thighs, abdomen, lower back, chest, and upper arms are much more suggestive of abuse. Bruising of the cheeks, ears, and neck should also arouse suspicion of abuse.

Injury appearance may provide clues as to mechanism. Parallel linear marks on cheeks or elsewhere are typically indicative of a slap from either a closed or open hand. These may also appear as oval-shaped bruises, similar to pinch marks. Teeth marks are easily identifiable and should be measured and documented carefully to later match the wound marks against a probable perpetrator. While, historically, dating of bruises by color has been described, it may be not be accurate.

Young ambulatory children are at risk for acquiring slight contact burns as a result of grasping hot objects such as curling irons. This should produce a single, superficial burn because of the quick response by the parent. Burns that involve multiple sites, immersion burns, or deep burns are indicative of abuse. Immersion burns are specific for abuse and manifest as well-demarcated lesions on the buttocks, hips, or hands and feet in a stocking and glove pattern. Burn marks resulting from cigarettes appear as round lesions, typically 10 mm in diameter, and the abused child may have multiple burn marks particularly on the hands, arms, and feet.

Head injuries are the most frequent cause of childhood morbidity and mortality related to abuse.

The initial manifestations of head injuries in children are typically non-specific, including listlessness, lethargy, irritability, poor feeding habits, and vomiting; they are, therefore, easy to miss. If the injury is severe enough, the child may present with seizures or coma. The mechanisms needed to produce such symptoms are often divided into two categories of force: direct or indirect. Direct injuries are caused by an impact of the child's head against a solid surface, either from a caregiver striking the child with a solid object or throwing the child against a wall or other fixed surface. These injuries more commonly present with external injuries such as contusions of the scalp or face, although many will present without any external signs of trauma. Indirect trauma is typically the result of being shaken violently, leading to a whiplash injury commonly known as the "shaken baby syndrome." This type of injury causes significant intracranial shearing forces affecting the brain and vascular supply. They are almost always devoid of external signs of trauma, and the EP must, therefore, carefully screen for injuries in these children. A household fall is often the stated history, but these accidents are unlikely to produce neurological trauma. In such cases an ophthalmologic examination should be conducted to screen for retinal hemorrhages as these are highly associated with abuse. Order a non-contrast head CT and skeletal survey if retinal hemorrhages are present or if there is suspicion of abuse.

Fractures are the second most common injury seen after skin lesions in abused children. Young children commonly sustain fractures; therefore, it is important to carefully assess the fracture in light of the history to determine if it was an accidental injury or the result of abuse. The differential diagnosis includes true accidental fractures, osteogenesis imperfecta, and metabolic bone disorders (i.e., rickets). Mild cases of osteogenesis imperfecta may be difficult to diagnose clinically. However, metaphyseal corner, skull, and rib fractures are rare in osteogenesis imperfecta.

Some injuries are highly specific for abuse, such as metaphyseal-epiphyseal fractures and fractures of the scapulae, posterior ribs, sternum, and pelvis.

Metaphyseal fractures, described as corner or "bucket handle" fractures depending on the radiographic image, result from a strong force pulling on the affected limb and are considered diagnostic of abuse as these are not likely to be produced by direct blows or falls onto the outstretched limb. The most common fractures, however, are diaphyseal fractures of the femur or humerus. These are less specific for abuse but should still raise a red flag if the child is young, the mechanism of injury unlikely, or other fractures in various stages of healing are found on plain films. A spiral fracture of the diaphysis results from excessive twisting forces and is also unlikely to result from a fall. Falling out of a bed or off a dresser is a commonly reported history but is unlikely to produce such a fracture.

The radiographic appearance of extremity fractures can be used to help date the injury. As with bruising, however, fracture appearance is highly variable, depending on many factors including age, nutritional status, and the force that produced the fracture. Imaging can only provide a rough estimate of dates. Of more importance is accurately distinguishing new and old fractures so as to identify long-standing abuse. On radiographs, an acute injury will manifest soft tissue swelling and the fracture if it is extensive. Soft tissue swelling should be visible up to 5 days after the injury has occurred. Callus and new periosteal bone may appear between 1 and 2 weeks. From 2 to 8 weeks, callus formation and bone resorption increases, enhancing the fracture appearance. After 8 weeks the fracture begins to take on a more "normal" appearance as the calluses smooth and fragments are incorporated into the healing bone.

Abdominal injuries may also present with non-specific symptoms such as poor feeding and listlessness/irritability. These account for a smaller subset of injuries but are the second most common cause of childhood deaths related to abuse. They typically result from blunt trauma to the abdomen which may rupture solid organs, particularly spleen and liver. A history of a short fall is often given, once again from a bed or down a set of stairs. These mechanisms have been shown to be highly unlikely to produce serious abdominal injuries and suggest abuse if the injury is out of proportion to the history. Examination of the child's abdomen, inguinal region, and flank should be performed to assess for signs of bruising or tenderness, although these are not always immediately evident. Intra-abdominal rupture may present with an acute abdomen or shock. Elevated serum liver enzymes or amylase provide evidence of intra-abdominal injury, and plain films may show evidence of free air in the abdomen in cases of perforation.

While genitourinary trauma is suggestive of sexual abuse and should be evaluated carefully, sexual abuse may be quite subtle in children, and physical signs can be absent even after anal penetration.

The main object of the initial genitourinary examination is to ensure medical stability; forensic examination should be deferred to regional sexual abuse teams if possible.

Inspection of the genitals and anus should be performed in both males and females with special attention to abrasions, bleeding, bruising, fissures, and scarring. Genital examination should form part of a "regular examination." Inspection is best carried out in the knee–chest position (Fig. 74.3, p. 325). Examine the oral cavity for tears of the frenulum and injuries to the soft and hard palates. Internal pelvic examinations on prepubescent girls are unnecessary unless there is concern for acute penetrating injuries and/or there is vaginal bleeding. These girls should be referred to a pediatrician or gynecologist.

Although the manifestations of physical abuse may be dramatic, the majority of child abuse occurs in the form of neglect. Neglect is oftentimes unapparent and may go unrecognized for long periods of time, but most commonly manifests as abandonment, failure to thrive, and medical neglect in the ED setting. The initial evaluation should include an assessment of the child's nutritional and hydration status as well as a full physical examination. Physical neglect is suspected based on inadequate clothing, hygiene, or nutrition. In cases of medical neglect, consider if harm has occurred through medical non-compliance by the parent or caregiver. Failure to thrive is reviewed in Ch. 61. Neglect takes many forms, although not all manifest somatically (e.g., emotional neglect). Observation of the caregiver–child interactions may demonstrate a lack of affection or caring, or even deleterious behaviors such as threatening, name-calling, or pressuring. If abandonment is suspected, consider how long a child was left alone and if any adverse consequences resulted.

Management

The first step in the management of child maltreatment is the immediate identification and correction of life-threatening injuries. If a child is stable, conduct a careful history regarding the present illness or injury as well as past medical problems and previous hospitalizations or past ED visits. If verbal, attempt to ascertain a history from the child. Conduct a meticulous physical examination and identify lesions not included in the chief complaint. Document all external abnormalities, using diagrams or photographs if necessary. The first step in identifying abuse is suspecting abuse; therefore, assess the history in light of the injuries and decide if there is enough suspicion to warrant further investigation.

In cases of suspected abuse, it is important to understand the role of the different providers involved. The role of the EP is generally to suspect abuse and initiate the involvement of police, CPS, and social services. If a child is brought to the ED with suspected abuse, it is important to notify the police in the county where the abuse occurred, as they are usually in charge of investigating the crime. In many areas, police are in charge of activating the forensic medical examination (such as a dedicated sexual abuse team); the CPS is charged with making sure the child is safe if it is suspected the maltreatment occurred in the house or in the school. Hospital social services can often facilitate the interaction of the different providers.

Box 135.1. Current recommendations on radiographic skeletal survey from the American Academy of Pediatrics

Mandatory survey if child is 2 years old or younger, with individualized use in those aged 2–5 years, and limited, if any, use in those over 5 years. Yield of survey is low for children 3 years of age and older. Survey includes antero–posterior (AP) and lateral radiographic films:

- bilateral AP arms/forearms/hands
- bilateral AP thighs/legs/feet
- AP and lateral skull
- AP and lateral axial skeleton and trunk.

It is imperative in abuse, particularly sexual abuse, to avoid repeating the initial trauma during the medical examination.

Three techniques to complete an initial screening examination are (1) to emphasize that adults undergo these examinations also, (2) to explain that the examination is to see that their entire body is "OK" and healthy, and (3) to give the child as much choice as possible (does the child want to wear this gown or that one, have the ears or the nose examined first). Screening examination is usually appropriate in the ED. If a child will be treated with antibiotics, cultures must be taken. Urgent evaluation is necessary if abuse occurred within 72 h or there are genital and anal injuries requiring treatment. If there is possibility that the abuse occurred within 72 h and the child will be discharged to complete the detailed examination with a specially trained sexual abuse team, it should be emphasized that the child should not shower. The scheduled or urgent sexual assault examination should ideally be performed by professionals trained to conduct a non-traumatizing examination, gather evidence and to testify in court.

Laboratory studies and imaging can be obtained to assess various injuries. A CBC with smear, platelet count, and PT/PTT should be drawn for evaluation of "easy bruising" and bleeding tendencies. Serum osmolality and electrolytes may be abnormal in dehydration or drowning. If abdominal trauma is suspected, then serum liver and pancreatic enzymes should be assessed for elevations, and imaging should be obtained. A urinalysis and urine toxicology screen should be ordered if renal injury or forced intoxication is suspected.

If the child presents with a fracture and a questionable history, then a radiographic skeletal survey should be performed to assess for evidence of other injuries. The AAP survey guidelines are given in Box 135.1. Serum calcium, phosphorus, and alkaline phosphatase, if normal, can help to exclude bone disorders such as rickets and osteogenesis imperfecta. Radionuclide bone scans are sometimes used to further evaluate for abuse if the skeletal survey is negative but the suspicion for abuse remains high, because this technique has higher sensitivity for acute fractures. If there is any concern for head injury, then an ophthalmologic examination and non-contrast head CT scan should be performed. If sexual abuse is suspected than a sexual assault kit can be used to collect specimens for identification of the perpetrator as well as detection of sexually transmitted diseases. Serology studies for HIV, syphilis, hepatitis B and C, and a pregnancy test are recommended for any sexual abuse victim who is at risk.

Disposition

The evaluation of child abuse is a multidisciplinary pursuit and should involve help from a social worker or other appropriate authorities. Consultations from physicians with more experience in child abuse are also warranted. A report should be made to the the appropriate child welfare authorities when child abuse is suspected; a report does not need to rely on proven abuse. The failure to report suspected abuse may result in penalties for mandated reporters including physicians. Those who report abuse are commonly given protection from legal action if a suspected abuse turns out to be negative. Reports are most commonly made to CPS but may also involve police departments or other authorities.

An important and challenging step is notifying the parents that child abuse is being considered and a report is being filed. This can be quite difficult and may lead to a variety of reactions from the parents. Inform the parents that your primary concern is for the safety and well-being of their child, and let them know in a non-accusatory and empathetic manner that an investigation is legally required whenever concern for possible abuse or neglect arises and/or the injuries are inconsistent with the described mechanism.

Hospitalization may be necessary if you feel the child may be unsafe upon returning home. This is often difficult as some parents are reluctant to admit their child and may become defiant when notified, but the priority remains the child's safety and well-being. Often social workers, CPS workers, and/or police officers can be helpful in explaining the process of a CPS investigation and can help to answer parents' questions and concerns.

Pearls and pitfalls

Pearls

1. Injuries must be considered within the developmental context of the child. "Those who don't cruise, don't bruise."
2. Examine the child–parent interactions carefully as this may be the initial clue to abuse
3. Delays in seeking treatment are worrisome.
4. Obtain help in dealing with suspected child maltreatment.
5. Know your local resources and reporting procedures (http://www.childwelfare.gov/).

Pitfalls

1. Reliance on a "classic" presentation of abuse: any unusual history or physical finding should prompt consideraton of this diagnosis.
2. Failure to identify the cutaneous manifestations that can mimic inflicted trauma, such as Mongolian spots and birthmarks, but are benign.
3. "Traumatizing the traumatized." Have the most trained person available sensitively perform a sexual assault evaluation.

Selected references

Duhaime AC, Christian CW, Rorke LB, Zimmerman RA. Nonaccidental head injury in infants: the "shaken-baby syndrome." *N Engl J Med* 1998;**338**:1822–1829.

Hymel KP, Jenny C. Child sexual abuse. *Pediatr Rev* 1996;**17**:236–249.

Kocher MS, Kasser JR. Orthopaedic aspects of child abuse. *J Am Acad Orthoped Surg* 2000;**8**:10–20.

Sugar NF, Taylor JA, Feldman KW. Bruises in infants and toddlers; those who don't cruise don't bruise. *Arch Pediatr Adolesc Med* 1999;**153**:399–403.

Chapter 136

Delivering difficult news about a child

Chere Taylor and Colleen O'Connor

Introduction

Delivering difficult news to parents about their child is one of the most challenging experiences EPs face. This chapter covers aspects of parental presence during codes and procedures, delivering the diagnosis of a life-changing illness, and delivering the most difficult news of all – the death of a child.

Parental presence during codes and procedures

Surveys of parents suggest that parents overwhelmingly report they would want to be present when invasive procedures are performed on their children. As procedures become more invasive, this desire to be present is diminished, but most parents report they would want to be present if their child were likely to die, and nearly all parents wanted to participate in the decision about their presence. Medical providers often feel more discomfort with parental presence during codes than do families, yet families report afterwards that being present helped them to understand and process the experience. The following suggestions will help to manage these situations.

- Offer parents a choice to stay in the room with their child or step outside. If parents choose to stay in the room explain that they can leave at any time.
- Assign a member of the ED team to stay with parents to answer questions, explain procedures, and/or update parents.
- Include parents in decision making about the patient's care.
- If a parent begins to interfere with the medical care of the child, explain to the parent they must stay back and let the medical team continue with treatment of their child or the parent will have to leave the room.
- Assist parents in calling family/friends to come to the ED for support.
- After the medical team is finished treating the child, one of the physicians should approach the parents regarding outcome and/or plan of care for their child before leaving the room.

Parental involvement in a new diagnosis of life-changing illness

Delivering a new diagnosis of a life-changing illness to parents is also challenging. Keep in mind that parents will need time to absorb this information and will likely have many questions. The way in which the information is delivered significantly affects the process for the family.

1. State to parents that you have the test results back and your child appears to have some type of ... (cancer, diabetes, brain tumor, etc.).
2. Explain to parents that, because this is very serious, you would like to admit their child or recommend that they take their child to see a specialist in this field as soon as possible. Present the parents with some names and phone numbers of a few specialists in their area or, if possible or indicated, call the specialists prior to discussing with the family so you have more information for them.
3. Explain to parents that you are not a specialist in this field and you would like to defer any specific questions to the specialist but if they have any general questions you would be more than happy to answer them.
4. Offer the parents some paper/notebook with a pen so they can write down the questions that come to mind for the specialist.
5. Assist parents in calling family/friends to offer support; offer social work assistance if available.

Death in the emergency department

An estimated 8000 children <14 years of age are pronounced dead in an ED each year. While pediatric deaths are rare when compared with adults, the infrequency leads to further discomfort for EPs. Recent surveys showed that 70% of EPs indicated that the most stressful aspect of their job was managing a pediatric death, while 40% reported prolonged resuscitative efforts they knew to be futile because of a reluctance to tell the parents the child had died. Another factor leading to physician's

A Practical Guide to Pediatric Emergency Medicine: Caring for Children in the Emergency Department, ed. N. Ewen Amieva-Wang (associate eds. Jamie Shandro, Aparajita Sohoni, and Bernhard Fassl). Published by Cambridge University Press.

discomfort with pediatric death and notification stems from the lack of grief training.

The sudden and unexpected death of a child is an unfathomable loss that leaves no opportunity for psychological preparation for the surviving support system.

Members of staff are entrusted with the care of not only the patient but also the family members.

The words and actions of the medical team have a significant impact on the grief process of the family system. The family gives tremendous value to the words they hear and often remember them for the rest of their lives. From the time that the family enters the ED, a designated staff person should be present to communicate and be with the parents/family throughout the ED experience. This person should ideally be trained in risk assessment and have a strong clinical background in working with death and dying (social worker, resource nurse).

Creating a systematic and consistent approach to the situation of death and grief in the ED is helpful to the practitioner and the family. A few basic concepts can be adapted to fit the personal style and preferences of each caregiver. An important way to communicate to the family that the care of their loved one was taken seriously and that everything possible was done to change the outcome is to have the physician responsible for the care of the patient be the one to provide notification to the family.

If you remember nothing else, remember that the manner in which you deliver the news is critical. The medical facts are less important than compassion. Be your authentic, present, caring self. Before meeting with the family:

1. Take time to review the events that have transpired leading to the eventual death, including information about the causing trauma and the procedures and care administered during the resuscitative measures and to put your thoughts into chronological order.
2. Be prepared to discuss coroner/autopsy process and organ/tissue donation.
3. If there is a language barrier, secure an interpreter before meeting with the family.
4. Prepare to have a calm, caring, compassionate, professional demeanor.
5. Avoid giving a cold clinical impression by making the transition from managing a crisis to responding to a family's emotional trauma.
6. Gather information about whom in the family is present.
7. Have the designated staff identified above and other pertinent team members be present when giving notification to share the emotional demands of the interaction.
8. During disclosure/discussion of child's death:
   - introduce yourself and other team members that are present
   - have family members identify themselves
   - refer to the patient by their name
   - ask them what they know and share what they observed.
9. Briefly, in chronological order, tell in layman terms what you know about the event leading to the trauma, problems that occurred, actions taken, the patient's response to each intervention. The gentle, gradual delivery of factual information facilitates an intellectual acknowledgement of death. Deciding how detailed to be in the delivery is a delicate balance.
10. Emphasize that everything medically possible was done.
11. Reassure the family that their loved one did not suffer.
12. Confirm that they have died. Wait silently for around a minute, allowing time for the family to absorb the information and then address any questions they have.
13. Tell them how sorry you are.
14. Tell them that you are making arrangements for them to be with their loved one.
15. Confirm that their questions have been answered and make yourself available should more questions arise.

While you may not have an active role in the tasks that follow the notification interview, it is critical to be aware and mindful of the importance and significance of the necessary tasks that might occur. Providing an understanding of what happens next: viewing of the body, grief support and education for siblings and other family members, completion of paperwork, the medical examiner process, and "goodbyes" all take place in the busy ER setting. Please be supportive of the process and the time parents and families may need despite all the other responsibilities that continue to exist within the ED.

Conclusions

Physicians have identified pediatric death and serious illness as the most stressful events within their role. Additional support, education, and training can help EPs and staff to deal with feelings of loss, suffering, and death in a more professionally and personally satisfying way. Use these tips to help to deliver this news as humanely as possible. Remember to include families in decision making, and be supportive of the process and the time parents and families may need despite all the other responsibilities that continue to exist within the ED.

Pearls and pitfalls

Pearls

1. For a critically ill patient, designate a staff person to be with the family and to communicate with the parents/family throughout the ED experience.
2. Include parents and/or guardians in decision making about their child.
3. Be supportive of the process and the time parents and families may need after receiving difficult news.

Pitfalls

1. Failure to make a transition mentally from the clinical to the human when going to meet the family and deliver difficult news.
2. Failure to remember that the manner in which news is delivered is critical. Medical facts are less important than compassion. Be your authentic, present, caring self.

Selected references

Ahrens WR, Hart RG. Pediatric death: Managing the aftermath in the Emergency Department. *Am J Emerg Med* 1997;**15**:601–605.

Ahrens WR, Hart RG. Emergency physicians' experience with the death of pediatric patients. *Am J Emerg Med* 1997;**15**: 642–643.

Boie ET, Moore GP, Brummett C, Nelson DR. Do parents want to be present during invasive procedures performed on their children in the emergency department? A survey of 400 parents. *Ann Emerg Med* 1999;**34**:70–74.

Isaacs E, D'souza P. Grief Support in the ED. *eMedicine* **14** January, 2008 http://emedicine.medscape.com/article/806280-overview (accessed 27 April 2010).

Knapp J, Mulligan-Smith D and the Committee on Pediatric Emergency Medicine. Death of a child in the emergency department. *Pediatrics* 2005;**115**:1432–1437.

Section 22

Toxicology

Chapter 137

Toxidromes and general management

William T. Hurley and Donald H. Schreiber

Introduction

Pediatric poisoning occurs in a bimodal distribution. Ingestions by children aged 1 to 5 years are commonly accidental and result from oral exploration. Such ingestions seldom produce severe symptoms. Only a few substances have the potential to significantly harm or kill a toddler with just a single dose (Ch. 139). Ingestions by adolescents are commonly recreational or the result of attempted suicide. These usually follow an adult pattern, involving potentially toxic substances, but commonly in small amounts. Ingestions outside of these ages are uncommon. Children younger than 6 months of age are often incapable of acquiring substances to ingest. Children aged 5 years to adolescence rarely present with ingestions.

Most children presenting with significant intoxication manifest altered mental status, but there can be a number of different causes:

- poisoning
- drugs, common causes include opiates, benzodiazepines, ethanol, anticholinergics, salicylates
- environmental toxins, including carbon monoxide, lead, mercury (Ch. 140)
- hypoglycemia
- infection
- intracranial pathology.

Providers must maintain skepticism concerning the diagnosis of poisoning, as altered mental status may be caused by hypoglycemia, infection, or intracranial pathology.

Toxicological syndromes

The diagnosis of poisoning is often clinical.

Toxicological screening seldom leads to a change in patient management.

An exception to this rule is testing for acetaminophen. Blood acetaminophen should be checked in every substantial overdose, particularly when the agent is unknown. The key to diagnosis and management of poisoning is identification of a toxicological syndrome or toxidrome. A toxidrome is a constellation of symptoms and signs that represent the effects of a particular drug, toxin, or class of agent. Characteristic vital sign abnormalities and physical findings point to common classes of chemical intoxication. Key areas of examination include vital signs, pupils, mucus membranes, lungs, abdomen, and the skin (Table 137.1). It is important to know a few representative drugs of each class and recognize the typical clinical presentation of these drugs, understand the pharmacokinetics and reversal agents where applicable, and anticipate the most common ominous complications.

Anticholinergic toxidrome

The anticholinergic syndrome is precipitated by exposure to anticholinergic agents such as diphenhydramine, scopolamine (hyoscine) and other medications with significant anticholinergic effects. The clinical syndrome is characterized by agitation, confusion, or psychosis associated with elevated heart rate, dry skin, flushing and mydriasis.

The mnemonic "mad as a hatter, blind as a bat, and dry as a bone" characterizes the anticholinergic syndrome.

Table 137.1. Findings in common toxicological syndromes

Toxicological syndrome	Common physical findings
Stimulant or sympathomimetic	Hypertension, tachycardia, hyperthemia, dilated pupils, CNS stimulation, diaphoresis
Anticholinergic	Tachycardia, hyperthermia, dilated pupils, CNS depression, dry skin/mucus membranes
Cholinergic	Bradycardia, small pupils, seizures, paralysis, hypersecretions, bronchospasm, diaphoresis
Opiate or opioid	Hypothermia, small pupils, CNS depression, respiratory depression
Cardiotoxic	Hypotension, bradycardia, CNS depression, respiratory depression

A Practical Guide to Pediatric Emergency Medicine: Caring for Children in the Emergency Department, ed. N. Ewen Amieva-Wang (associate eds. Jamie Shandro, Aparajita Sohoni, and Bernhard Fassl). Published by Cambridge University Press.

Treatment is primarily supportive, but physostigmine has been used as a reversal agent. It should be used with caution for patients taking tricyclic antidepressants and other drugs with significant anticholinergic effects because it may precipitate seizures. Other complications are rhabdomyolysis, severe hyperthermia, and tachyarrhythmias.

Cardiotoxic toxidrome

A cardiotoxic syndrome presents after ingestion of cardiac agents including beta-blockers, calcium channel blockers, and/or digoxin. Signs and symptoms may include profound hypotension, bradycardia with conduction delay, CNS depression, and respiratory failure.

Cholinergic toxidrome

The cholinergic toxidrome is most commonly seen as an occupational hazard in farmworkers exposed to organophosphate or carbamate pesticides. In the USA, these toxic insecticides are rapidly being replaced by the much less toxic pyrethrins and pyrethroids. Cholinergic agents are still available in many homes and toxicity is occasionally seen in children.

Carbamates do not produce CNS toxicity because of poor penetration into the CNS.

The cholinergic toxidrome consists of generalized muscle weakness, fasciculations, miosis, bradycardia, depressed respiratory rate, and excessive secretions manifesting as bronchorrhea, diarrhea, and excessive salivation. Reversal agents include atropine, pralidoxime (2-PAM), and benadryl. Ventilatory support may be required. The most serious complications are seizures, acute respiratory failure, and paralysis.

Opioid toxidrome

The opioid toxidrome (typified by morphine) clinically presents with depressed respiration, miosis, hypotension, and relative bradycardia. A decreased level of consciousness associated with hypothermia, dry skin, and decreased bowel sounds is typical. Assisted ventilation with oxygen may be required and naloxone is the reversal agent. The most serious complications are respiratory arrest and non-cardiogenic pulmonary edema.

Sedative and alcohol toxidrome

Hypnotic sedatives and alcohol are common ingestions. The clinical toxidrome is characterized by an ALOC leading to coma and respiratory depression. Mixed ingestions are frequently encountered when alcohol is combined with other sedative agents. Treatment is primarily supportive. Flumazenil is a reversal agent for acute benzodiazepine ingestions. It may induce withdrawal seizures in patients who are chronically taking benzodiazepines, or lead to intractable seizures with cyclic antidepressants, limiting its use. Because of this risk, the routine use of flumazenil is not recommended in a "coma cocktail" for general toxicological emergencies.

Serotonin syndrome

The serotonin syndrome is a particularly ominous toxidrome precipitated by an overdose of selective serotonin reuptake inhibitors (SSRIs), simultaneous ingestion of two or more SSRIs, ingestion of MDMA (ecstasy), or the combination of monoamine oxidase inhibitors (MAOIs) with other agents such as SSRIs, cocaine, methamphetamines, dextromethorphan, and tricyclic antidepressants. The patient develops acute hyperthermia, increased muscle tone, fasciculations, hyperereflexia, altered mental status, and diaphoresis. This toxicological emergency should be urgently treated with IV fluids, benzodiazepines, cooling, and occasionally cyproheptadine. Serious complications include cardiac arrest, disseminated intravascular coagulation, and severe hyperthermia.

Sympathomimetic toxidrome

Cocaine and amphetamines are representative drugs causing the sympathomimetic toxidrome. The typical clinical presentation is characterized by psychomotor agitation, elevated heart rate and blood pressure, mydriasis, and diaphoresis. There are no specific reversal agents, but cooling agents, benzodiazepines, and hydration are cornerstones of therapy. Cardiovascular effects include chest pain, myocardial ischemia, myocardial infarction, hypertension, congestive heart failure, arrhythmias, and aortic dissection. Other severe complications include cardiac arrest, seizures, intracranial hemorrhage, and rhabdomyolysis.

Hypoglycemia

Hypoglycemic reactions are common from accidental exposure to oral hypoglycemic agents or excessive doses of insulin. Clinical manifestations include ALOC, progressing to coma or seizures, in the setting of mildly elevated blood pressure and pulse. Diaphoresis and pale, cool skin are often seen. Focal neurological signs may occur and hypoglycemia is a known stroke mimic. Therefore, fingerstick evaluation of serum blood glucose should be performed on all patients with an altered mental status, confusion, coma, or seizures. The antidote is glucose administered either orally or IV. Major complications include intractable seizures and aspiration pneumonia.

General management

General management of poisonings in children focuses on the ABCs (Box 137.1). The most common cause of death from poisoning is loss of airway protection and inadequate ventilation. Control of the airway, prevention of aspiration, adequate ventilation, and oxygenation are imperative for the patient suffering from significant poisoning. This should be followed by assessment of cardiac rhythm and circulation. Several drugs and toxins produce sodium channel blockade and widening of the QRS complex. Cardiac monitoring and ECG should be performed.

Box 137.1. General management in toxicology

ABC protocol

Follow the ABC protocol:

- control the airway
- provide ventilation or breathing
- support circulation with fluid and pressors.

D: decontamination

In poisonings, D stands for decontamination; provide appropriate eye, skin, and gut decontamination:

- activated charcoal is the standard for gut decontamination; the appropriate oral dose is 10 times the ingestion, with a starting dose of 1–2 g/kg.
- gastric lavage or whole bowel irrigation may be useful for specific ingestions but is not routinely indicated.

Further steps

Assessment and treatment includes:

- ECG
- serum glucose
- obtain a history
- focused physical examination
- specific agents have available antidotes
- naloxone, oxygen, and glucose should be available and used when indicated
- consult the regional Poison Center (1-800-222-1222) to aid selection of the most appropriate method of decontamination.

If QRS interval is >0.12 s in the limb leads, poisoning by a tricyclic antidepressant, antiarrhythmic, or other sodium channel blocking agent should be suspected

This is managed with sodium bicarbonate bolus infusion of 1–2 mEq/kg. Intravenous fluid administration (20 ml/kg) and pressors should be used to maintain systemic perfusion.

Decontamination appropriate to the specific agent and route of exposure should be performed. Corrosive agents should be quickly and rapidly flushed from the skin and eyes. Hydrocarbons should be washed off. Gastric decontamination is a controversial topic. Studies have shown little benefit in emptying the stomach, so recommendations have moved to providing the least dangerous option; oral activated charcoal. A more aggressive approach using gastric lavage may be indicated in recent (within 1 h) ingestions of large amounts (aspirin) or highly toxic substances (calcium antagonists, cyclic antidepressants, antimalarials). The use of syrup of ipecac has fallen out of favor because of the occurrence of prolonged emesis and the inability to effectively administer activated charcoal. Syrup of ipecac may still be indicated in recent ingestions of potentially toxic agents with a prolonged anticipated delay in healthcare. Vomiting should be avoided with agents expected to produce burns, aspiration, rapid loss of airway protective reflexes, or seizures.

Activated charcoal is effective in preventing the absorption of most compounds from the GI tract. The recommended dose of charcoal is 10 times the estimated ingested dose of compound. Charcoal is ineffective in binding small molecules (metals, hydrocarbons) and is contraindicated with suspected perforation (caustics) or ileus. Charcoal is available mixed with water or sorbitol. Sorbitol has been shown to increase vomiting and to cause dehydration and hypernatremia in young children. Young children should not be given a second dose of charcoal with sorbitol. Also, charcoal can be damaging if aspirated, so it should be given only to alert patients who can safely drink it or else by nasogastric tube. Stomach volume limits the initial dose of charcoal to 1–2 g/kg. In large overdoses, repeat doses each 1–2 h may be needed to achieve a charcoal dose 10 times the estimated ingestion.

Whole bowel irrigation has been shown useful to be in selected ingestions. The technique uses non-absorbable bowel-preparation solution (polyethylene glycol) to move compounds through the GI tract before they can be absorbed. Case reports describe its use with iron, lithium, valproic acid, theophylline, verapamil, diltiazem, and enteric-coated aspirin. The recommended dose is 35 ml/kg per h (max. 2 l/h) until the rectal effluent is clear or until 200 ml/kg has been given.

Laboratory evaluation

The routine ordering of comprehensive urine or serum drug screens has not been shown to impact clinical management of most patients. Measuring specific drug levels can be useful in the clinical management of certain situations. Acetaminophen overdose may be clinically silent after a significant ingestion. The blood acetaminophen level at 4 h predicts hepatotoxicity and the need for antidote use. Salicylate levels may correlate with toxicity and the need for enhanced elimination with bicarbonate or dialysis. Anticonvulsant drug levels are helpful in the evaluation of patients who present with possible toxicity and CNS effects such as seizures, ataxia, or altered mental status.

Rapid qualitative urine drug screen tests identify classes of drug and may help to establish a diagnosis in confusing cases. These tests identify drugs by class and not by specific agents. The most commonly used urine drug screen can detect benzodiazepines, barbiturates, opioids, cannabinoids, cocaine, amphetamines, tricyclic antidepressants, and phencyclidine. Some drugs can be missed as the concentrations fail to reach the detection limit of the test. Urine drug screens often do not detect fentanyl unless it is present in extremely high doses. Certain agents are commonly mis-identified through cross-reactivity. Decongestants and psychotropic medications such as amphetamine plus dextroamphetamine (Adderall) will cross-react with the amphetamine assay and give a positive result.

Routine evaluation of the CBC, basic chemistry panel and LFTs may be required to assess the toxic effects of common ingestions. Certain metabolic "gaps" are utilized in the evaluation of patients. The anion gap is useful in the evaluation of metabolic acidosis; a normal anion gap is <14 meq/l. An elevated anion gap may be seen in certain settings. Agents that commonly cause an elevated anion gap are given in Box 137.2.

Box 137.2. Substances that may cause elevated anion gap acidosis

Acetaminophen (high dose)	Ethylene glycol	Niacin
Amiloride	Formaldehyde	Nitroprusside
Ascorbic acid	Hydrogen sulfide	NSAIDs
Carbon monoxide	Iron	Papaverine
Chloramphenicol	Isoniazid	Paraldehyde
Colchicine	Ketamine	Propofol
Cyanide	Metformin	Salicylates
Dapsone	Methanol	Terbutaline
Ethanol	Ethylene glycol	Toluene

The anion gap may help to identify the poison, assess its severity, and guide treatment.

The osmol gap is helpful in the evaluation of patients with suspected ethanol (alcohol), methanol, or ethylene glycol ingestions. These small molecules elevate the serum osmolarity. The serum osmolality may be calculated by doubling the serum sodium concentration and adding to that the BUN concentration divided by 2.8 and the glucose concentration divided by 18.

Calculated serum osmolality

$$= 2[Na^+] + [BUN(mg\%)/2.8] + [Glucose(mg\%)/18]$$

The serum osmolality is measured in the laboratory by the freezing point depression method. The difference between the calculated osmolarity and measured serum osmolality is the osmol gap. If the osmol gap exceeds 10 mOsm, there is an excessive amount of small molecules contributing to osmolality present in the serum. The most common cause of an elevated serum osmolality and osmol gap is ethanol ingestion. Ethanol contributes to serum osmolality. This contribution can be calculated by:

$$\text{Osmolality of ethanol} = [\text{Ethanol}(mg\%)/4.6]$$

In the absence of ethanol ingestion, an increase in serum osmolality and the osmol gap can result from methanol or ethylene glycol ingestion. Measurement of methanol and ethylene glycol is not commonly available in the hospital laboratory, but measuring the serum osmolality and calculating the osmol gap can be used to diagnose life-threatening ingestions of methanol and ethylene glycol. In patients who present with coma or ALOC where the history is often unreliable or unobtainable, a serum osmolality is a useful laboratory screening test.

Table 137.2. Antidotes for selected toxins

Toxin	Recommended antidote
Sodium channel antagonists (cyclic antidepressants, antimalarials, local anesthetics)	Sodium bicarbonate bolus 1–2 mEq/kg for QRS widening greater than 0.12 s
Antidiabetic agents, ethanol	25% dextrose 2–4 ml/kg, 10% dextrose infusion Octreotide 1 μg/kg (for refractory hypoglycemia)
Calcium channel antagonists	Calcium gluconate 0.2–0.3 ml/kg or calcium chloride 0.1–0.2 ml/kg Atropine 0.02 mg/kg Epinephrine 1 μg/min (titrated) Insulin 1 U/kg bolus, then 0.5–1 U/kg per h infusion + 25% dextrose 1–2 ml/kg and 10% dextrose infusion (keep glucose 100–200 mg/dl)
Acetaminophen (paracetamol)	Acetylcysteine 140 mg/kg, then 70 mg/kg q. 4 h or 150 mg/kg bolus slowly IV, then 50 mg/kg over 4 h and 100 mg/kg over 16 h (use reduced dilution in children)
Ethylene glycol or methanol	4-Methylpyrazole 15 mg/kg (up to 1 g) slowly IV, then 10 mg/kg IV every 12 h
Opioids or clonidine	Naloxone 0.4–2 mg IV/IM/nebulized/by ET tube; 0.05 mg carefully titrated up in opiate-dependent patients
Iron	Deferoxamine (desferrioxamine) 15 mg/kg per h IV

Antidotes

Specific agents respond to key antidotes (Table 137.2). Only those more commonly used will be mentioned.

- Sodium bicarbonate overcomes sodium channel blocking compounds (cyclic antidepressants, antimalarials, local anesthetics); it is also effective in reversing acidosis and manipulating pH in salicylate intoxication.
- Glucose monitoring and supplementation is required for intoxication with alcohols and oral hyperglycemic agents, which produce hypoglycemia. Calcium, atropine, pressors, and high-dose insulin euglycemic therapy are used in escalating treatment to manage calcium channel blocker poisoning.
- Intralipid has been shown to reverse the severe toxic effects of calcium channel blockers, beta blockers, or IV anesthetic poisoning, as well as for that with other highly lipophilic agents.

- Acetylcysteine is highly effective as an antidote for acetaminophen poisoning.
- Chelators are available for iron, lead, mercury, arsenic, and other metals.
- Antibodies to digoxin have proven effective.
- Fomepizole and ethanol inhibit the metabolism of methanol and ethylene glycol to toxic metabolites.
- Hydroxocobalamine is recommended for cyanide poisoning.
- Naloxone is commonly used in opioid and clonidine overdose.
- Methylene blue reverses methemoglobinemia.
- Pyridoxine helps to halt seizures caused by isoniazid.

Certain poisonings respond to enhanced renal elimination. Salicylates, lithium, ethylene glycol, methanol, and theophylline respond well to dialysis. Alkaline diuresis is recommended for salicylates.

Poison prevention

Exposure of a child to a toxin provides an opportunity for the provider and family to prevent future similar events. Analysis of the cause of the incident should be performed. Concerning circumstances or multiple incidents should prompt a referral to child protective services or other appropriate agency. Children are at greatest risk of exposure during disruptions in social circumstances, such as vacations, moving, or visiting relatives (especially grandparents). Adults should be encouraged to store medications and chemicals in appropriate child-resistant containers and away from food items. Toxic liquids should never be kept in beverage or drinking bottles.

Child abuse and neglect can present as poisoning. Inconsistencies in the story, inappropriate behaviors for age, physical signs of abuse or neglect, repeat incidents, or suspected intentional sedation should arouse suspicion and prompt referral to the appropriate agency.

Special populations: neonates

Neonates present a unique risk of intoxication. Metabolic pathways are incompletely developed, allowing for the accumulation of certain agents (acetaminophen, caffeine, morphine, phenytoin, and theophylline) and progressive development of toxicity over time. Toxicity from cutaneous absorption of hexachlorophene, boric acid, and alcohols has been described in neonates. Placental transfer of agents produces toxicity and withdrawal in the newborn. Opioid withdrawal in the neonate can present with hypertonia, hyperreflexia, seizures, poor feeding, dehydration, and acidosis. It is critical to differentiate intoxication or withdrawal from sepsis, hypoglycemia, or intracranial hemorrhage. Supportive care includes a quiet room, hydration, glucose support, and sedation with benzodiazepines.

Disposition

The decision to admit the poisoned patient is usually dictated by the patient's clinical condition. Those with obvious clinical manifestations of their ingestion require admission. Patients who require assisted ventilation or circulatory support or those who are obtunded or comatose will require admission to the ICU. The difficult disposition involves the patient with a potential serious ingestion who is asymptomatic. Most consultants recommend a minimum period of observation of 6 h after the ingestion for all potentially poisoned patients. Certain agents require significantly longer periods of observation. After consultation with the regional Poison Center, the asymptomatic patient may be safely discharged, keeping in mind that if a patient is a danger to him or herself, a psychiatric consultation and admission are warranted.

Conclusions

Pediatric poisoning provides unique challenges. Most pediatric ingestions produce no significant toxicity. Key toxins can produce significant poisoning with ingestion of only a few milliliters or one to two tablets. Involvement of the regional Poison Center (1–800–222–1222) can provide advice and consultation on a 24/7 basis.

Pearls and pitfalls

Pearls

1. Children commonly ingest non-toxic substances or non-toxic doses of toxic substances.
2. Control of the ABCs plus decontamination are the mainstays of treatment for the majority of poisonings.
3. With the exception of hypoglycemia, focal neurological signs are inconsistent with poisoning.
4. Poison Centers in the USA are available through a national toll-free number 1–800–222–1222.

Pitfalls

1. Avoid premature diagnosis. Remember infections and intracranial pathology may mimic poisoning.
2. Failure to suspect abuse or neglect in ingestions by school-age children.
3. Failure to check a blood glucose level in all patients with altered mental status, confusion, coma, or seizures.

Selected references

Agency for Toxic Substances and Disease Registry. http://www.atsdr.cdc.gov/ (accessed 28 April 2010).

American Association of Poison Control Centers. http://www.aapcc.org (accessed 28 April 2010).

Boyer EW, Duic PA, Evans A. Hyperinsulinemia/euglycemia therapy for calcium channel blocker poisoning. *Pediatr Emerg Care* 2002;**18**:36–37.

Erickson TB. The approach to the patient with an unknown overdose. *Emerg Med Clin North Am* 2007;**25**:249–281.

Erickson TB, Ahrens WR, Aks SE, Baum C, Ling L. *Pediatric Toxicology: Diagnosis and Management of the Poisoned Child*. New York: McGraw-Hill, 2005.

Ford M, Delaney KA, Ling L, Erickson T. *Clinical Toxicology*. Philadelphia, PA: Saunders, 2001.

Megarbane B, Borron SW, Baud FJ. Current recommendations for treatment of severe toxic alcohol poisonings. *Intensive Care Med* 2005;**31**:189–195.

Mycyk MB, Szyszko AL, Aks SE. Nebulized naloxone gently and effectively reverses methadone intoxication. *J Emerg Med* 2003;**24**:185–187.

Olson KR (ed.). *Poisoning and Drug Overdose*, 5th edn. New York: McGraw-Hill, 2007.

TOXNET Toxicology Data Network. http://toxnet.nlm.nih.gov/ (accessed 28 April 2010).

Chapter 138

Common poisonings

William T. Hurley, Donald H. Schreiber, and Jamie Shandro

Introduction

Understanding the nuances of management of common and dangerous agents provides insight into the management of poisonings in children. The majority of substances ingested by children under 6 years of age are household products (cosmetics, cleaning agents) and plants. The vast majority of these ingestions are non-toxic and can be managed at home or in the ED in consultation with a poison control center. It is helpful to know which plants are potentially toxic (Table 138.1), as well as commonly ingested plants that are non-toxic (Box 138.1). This chapter focuses on the management of potentially more lethal ingestions such as acetaminophen, salicylates, iron, opiates, and methanol/ethylene glycol.

Acetaminophen

Acetaminophen ingestion and toxicity are very common. Acetaminophen is the single most common drug causing acute fulminant liver failure necessitating liver transplantation in the USA. Its clinical toxidrome is manifested initially by a relative paucity of symptoms. The onset of liver necrosis is often delayed for 18 to 72 h, after which it may progress to acute fulminant liver failure with coagulopathy and encephalopathy. Such a time course demonstrates the importance of early identification of the child with a toxic acetaminophen exposure.

Children are more tolerant of acetaminophen overdose than adults because they have higher levels of hepatic sulfate stores and less production of the toxic metabolite NAPQI. The Rumack-Matthews nomogram (Fig. 138.1, below) is useful to predict toxicity after a single acute ingestion. Ingestions of greater than 200 mg/kg are often toxic. A plasma acetaminophen level of greater than 200 μg/ml at 4 h after ingestion predicts potential toxicity and guides antidote therapy.

Acetaminophen is metabolized in the liver by two pathways: 90–95% is metabolized by conjugation with sulfation and then glucuronidation in the liver, which is a non-toxic pathway and does not lead to liver necrosis; the remainder is metabolized through the P450 cytochrome system and produces a toxic metabolite (NAPQI) that leads to liver necrosis. NAPQI can be removed by interaction with glutathione to give a non-toxic metabolite. Fortunately, children <10 years of age are at lower risk of hepatotoxicity because acetaminophen is primarily detoxified by the sulfation pathway and less by the cytochrome P450 system. Approximately 4% of children will develop hepatotoxicity after acetaminophen overdose, but <2% will progress to acute fulminant liver failure.

An effective antidote (*N*-acetylcysteine [NAC]) is available but is most effective if used before significant hepatic injury develops. *N*-Acetylcysteine removes acetaminophen in two ways: it is a precursor of glutathione and so increases the sulfation of acetaminophen to a non-toxic metabolite, and it also binds to NAPQI.

The identification of acetaminophen poisoning relies on the history and the interpretation of specific acetaminophen drug levels using the Rumack–Matthews nomogram (Fig. 138.1). A toxic dose should be strongly suspected if the amount ingested is greater than 200 mg/kg body weight. In a 10 kg toddler, this amounts to approximately 2000 mg or only four extra strength 500 mg acetaminophen tablets. Absorption is rapid and occurs in approximately 30 to 120 min. A blood sample drawn 4 h after ingestion will allow for assessment of acetaminophen distribution and the potential for hepatotoxicity. The Rumack–Matthews nomogram compares drug levels with the time of ingestion. If the acetaminophen level falls above the potential hepatotoxicity range, then antidotal therapy with NAC is indicated. If the level falls within the potential hepatotoxicity range but below the probable hepatotoxicity range, consult with a toxicologist. If a hepatotoxic dose is strongly suspected clinically prior to the 4 h level, then treatment with NAC should be initiated empirically. This therapy can be easily aborted without serious adverse effects if the drug measurement ultimately confirms a non-hepatotoxic ingestion. It is far better to initiate early therapy when strongly suspected than to wait for a drug measurement at the 4 h timepoint. Also obtain baseline CBC, electrolytes, BUN, creatinine, LFTs, and coagulation studies.

N-Acetylcysteine has been commonly administered orally in the USA but has recently been approved for IV use. As it has a foul smell and taste, it can be difficult to administer orally.

A Practical Guide to Pediatric Emergency Medicine: Caring for Children in the Emergency Department, ed. N. Ewen Amieva-Wang (associate eds. Jamie Shandro, Aparajita Sohoni, and Bernhard Fassl). Published by Cambridge University Press.

Table 138.1. Potentially toxic plants and symptoms

Name	Symptoms
Typically do not require treatment	
Capsicum (pepper)	Skin and mucous membrane irritation
Narcissus, amaryllis, daffodil	Vomiting and diarrhea
Philodendron, peace lily, devil's ivy	Mucous membrane irritation
Poinsettia	Mild mucous membrane and GI irritation
Chrysanthemum	Contact dermatitis
Rhododendron azalea	Local and GI irritation, vomiting; rare respiratory depression
English holly, mistletoe	Vomiting, diarrhea
Potato (foliage), tomato (foliage)	GI irritation, headache, dermatitis
May require specific therapy	
Pokeweed, inkberry	Vomiting, abdominal pain, CNS depression
Monkshood, larkspur	Salivation, tachycardia, restlessness.
Poison hemlock	Salivation, vomiting, diarrhea, seizures, coma
White snakeroot	Weakness, debilitation, vomiting, death
Lily of the valley, foxglove, oleander	Mucous membrane irritation, cardiac toxicity
Poison ivy, poison oak	Contact dermatitis
Jimson weed, horse nettle	Anticholinergic syndrome
Rhubarb (leaves)	Mucous membrane irritation, rarely hypocalcemia and renal failure
Castor bean	GI irritation, CNS depression, seizures, hepatic and renal failure
Cherry, apple, peach trees (pits and leaves)	Potential cyanide toxicity in large doses
Toxic mushrooms, *Amanita phalloides, Gyromitra*	Hepatic or renal failure

Box 138.1. Commonly ingested non-toxic plants

African violet	Geranium	Prayer plant
Aluminum plant	Grape hyacinth	Rose
Asparagus fern	Grape ivy	Rubber tree
Begonia	Hens and chicks	Snake plant
Christmas cactus	Hibiscus	Snapdragon
Coleus	Honesuckle	Spider plant
Corn plant	Jade plant	Swedish ivy
Crocus	Lady's slipper	Violets
Dandelion	Lilac	Wax plant
Dwarf cactus	Palm	Weeping fig
Gardenia	Piggyback plant	Zebra plant

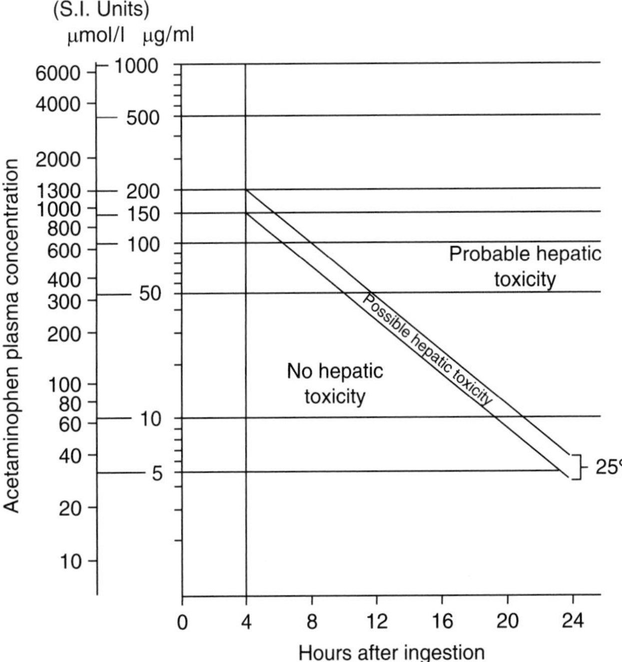

Figure 138.1 The Rumack–Matthews nomogram shows the relationship of time after ingestion (h) and serum acetaminophen concentration (μg/ml). Values under the line indicate no hepatic toxicity, values over the line indicate probable hepatic toxicity. Serum concentrations within the lines indicate possible toxicity. All values above the upper line indicate treatment with *N*-acetylcysteine (NAC) should occur.

The oral NAC regimen uses an initial dose of 140 mg/kg followed by 17 doses of 70 mg/kg each 4 h.

If oral administration is not tolerated, a 150 mg/kg IV load is administered over 1 h followed by 50 mg/kg IV over a 4 h period and then 100 mg/kg IV over a 16 h period.

Take care to concentrate IV NAC and avoid excessive fluid administration in small children, as hyponatremia has occurred.

Salicylates

Salicylate poisoning may present after acute or chronic ingestion. The incidence of salicylate poisoning has decreased as the use of aspirin has declined because of its potential association with Reyes syndrome. Symptoms of salicylate poisoning include confusion, tachycardia, tachypnea, tinnitus, and nausea or vomiting.

The toxic dose of aspirin ranges from 150 to 200 mg/kg or approximately five to seven regular strength 325 mg aspirin tablets for a 10 kg toddler.

Salicylates are rapidly absorbed from the stomach and small intestine. Aspirin in therapeutic concentrations is primarily metabolized by the liver, but renal excretion predominates in overdose. The half-life is normally 2.5–4 h, but it can be prolonged to 18–36 h in overdose.

Multisystem toxicity characterizes the salicylate toxidrome. Salicylates uncouple oxidative phosphorylation, ultimately leading to intracellular toxicity, an anion gap, and metabolic acidosis. Stimulation of the respiratory center in the CNS leads to an initial respiratory alkalosis. Neurotoxicity manifests as seizures, coma, or severe hyperthermia. Ototoxicity presents as tinnitus, which may be an early clue to the diagnosis. Gastrointestinal symptoms include nausea and vomiting. Upper GI bleeding may occur, particularly if coagulopathy develops. Other possible findings include platelet function abnormality, electrolyte disturbances, renal insufficiency, and hypoglycemia.

Specific measurement of blood salicylate is an essential component of management. Values on blood drawn prior to 6 h following ingestion are inaccurate in assessing toxicity. If measurement of salicylates has a long turnaround time from the laboratory, venous or arterial blood gas results can be used to rapidly assess toxicity. Early mild toxicity presents as an isolated respiratory alkalosis. In intermediate toxicity, a mixed respiratory alkalosis and metabolic acidosis develop. Severe toxicity produces metabolic acidosis and an increased anion gap. Acid–base status can be used to assess the severity of toxicity and guide treatment.

Decontamination of the GI tract with activated charcoal to limit absorption is indicated. In large ingestions and with enteric-coated salicylate compounds, activated charcoal can be repeated every 2 to 6 h. Since salicylate is primarily excreted by the kidney, IV fluid hydration and urine alkalinization are useful. Baseline laboratory investigations should include electrolytes, renal function, glucose, and salicylate drug levels. Acetaminophen should also be measured to detect a possible co-ingestion.

Urinary alkalinization increases the excretion of salicylates via ion trapping, which occurs as urine pH is raised. Intravenous sodium bicarbonate is used as a bolus (1–2 mEq/kg) to raise the urine pH to 7.4 or higher. An infusion of 3–4 mEq/kg per h is given to maintain urinary alkalosis. Sodium bicarbonate (2–3 ampules or 100–150 mEq) can be added to 1 liter of 5% dextrose for the infusion. Successful urinary alkalinization and prevention of hypokalemia often require supplementation with potassium (20 mEq/l KCl) as well. Urinary pH can be checked each hour using dipsticks. Electrolytes, glucose, and renal function must be regularly monitored.

Indications for dialysis for severe salicylate toxicity are:

- hemodynamic instability
- acute respiratory failure with endotracheal intubation
- severe acidosis
- acute renal failure
- seizures
- rhabdomyolysis
- serum salicylate levels >80 mg/dl (800 μg/ml)
- chronic salicylate ingestion, with significant toxicity, independent of drug level.

Narcotics and opioid poisoning

Opioid poisoning is rapidly becoming one of the most common causes of accidental death in the USA. The hallmarks of the opioid toxidrome are respiratory depression, CNS depression, and pupillary miosis. The diagnosis is usually established from the history and physical examination. Diagnostic laboratory testing is of little value other than to perhaps identify the specific agent for forensic purposes. The clinical response to naloxone, a narcotic antagonist, often helps to confirm the clinical impression. Because aspirin and acetaminophen are frequently combined with opioids, these should also be measured.

Other drugs that mimic opioid toxicity include clonidine, tramadol, gamma-hydroxybutyrate (GHB), valproic acid, and some selective serotonin reuptake inhibitors (SSRIs). The combination of CNS depression with respiratory depression and miosis narrows the differential diagnosis. Clonidine requires special consideration because it is often prescribed for narcotic withdrawal and also produces pupillary miosis.

In the setting of miosis, CNS depression, hypotension, and failure to respond to naloxone therapy, clonidine should be considered as the etiologic agent.

Management of opioid toxicity is supportive and based on the correction of hypoxia and hypoventilation.

Naloxone is the primary antidote, at a dose of 0.01–0.1 mg/kg IV, to a maximum of 2 mg.

In patients with known or suspected narcotic dependency, smaller doses of naloxone titrated to relief of respiratory depression are recommended (0.1–0.2 mg every 1–2 min) to prevent acute opioid withdrawal. Naloxone can be administered IV, IM, intranasally, intraosseously, by nebulizer, by sublingual injection, and through an endotracheal tube.

The usual 1 h duration of action of naloxone is often significantly shorter than the duration of action of the opioid. Close monitoring for recurrent respiratory depression and hypoxia is critical. Repeat bolus dosing is commonly required. A naloxone infusion may be necessary to maintain respiratory drive in the setting of longer-acting opiate ingestion.

Acute lung injury is not uncommon after respiratory depression from opioids and is more common after the use of naloxone. Aspiration syndrome is a well-recognized complication of narcotic overdose. Patients must be observed closely until their respiratory status is stable without naloxone. Consultation with psychiatry or childhood protective services may be necessary.

Iron

Iron has historically Iron has historically been associated with fatal intoxication in children, causing GI bleeding followed by hepatic injury. Toxic iron ingestions by toddlers have involved iron supplements in coated tablets resembling candy, particularly prenatal iron supplements. Recently there has been a dramatic decline in significant poisonings, thought to be achieved through packaging in smaller quantities.

Iron toxicity is dose dependent, and different formulations of iron supplements contain different amounts of elemental iron. Ferrous gluconate contains 12% elemental iron, ferrous sulfate contains 20% elemental iron, and ferrous fumarate contains 33% elemental iron. Prenatal vitamins typically contain 60–65 mg elemental iron, while most other multivitamins contain 15–20 mg elemental iron. Enteric-coated iron tablets may have delayed release of iron.

The exact toxic dose has not been established, but generally <20 mg/kg produces no significant symptoms, 20–60 mg/kg may or may not produce toxic symptoms, and >60 mg/kg will likely produce significant toxicity. By determining the type of iron formulation ingested, the total amount of elemental iron can be calculated and the toxic dose in milligrams per kilogram body weight can be ascertained.

Symptoms of iron intoxication are classically divided into phases (Table 138.2). The GI phase is characterized by abdominal pain with vomiting, diarrhea, and occasionally GI bleeding. Death during this phase is usually caused by hypovolemic shock. These symptoms typically occur within 6 h of ingestion unless the ingestion was enteric-coated or extended release preparation. Generally, a patient who is asymptomatic 6 h after ingestion is unlikely to develop iron toxicity. The latent phase is a period of symptomatic improvement. Patients who progress beyond this phase progress into a phase of shock and metabolic acidosis, followed by hepatotoxicity. If the patient survives these phases, they may present 2–4 weeks later with gastric outlet obstruction secondary to gastric scarring.

When considering iron ingestion, obtain serum iron levels on all patients with systemic symptoms, those who have ingested greater than 40 mg/kg elemental iron, and those who have ingested an unknown quantity. Obtain a serum iron concentration (ideally at least 6 h after ingestion of non-extended release tablets), a CBC, chemistry panel including creatinine, LFTs, coagulation studies, and an arterial or venous pH if the patient is symptomatic. An abdominal radiograph can be helpful to look for radiopaque pills.

Table 138.2. Clinical phases and symptoms of iron toxicity

Clinical phases	Timing	Signs/symptoms
Gastrointestinal phase	30 min to 6 h	Abdominal pain, vomiting, diarrhea, hematemesis, melena, lethargy, hypotension
Latent phase	6–24 h	Improved GI symptoms; may have poor perfusion, tachypnea, tachycardia
Shock and acidosis phase		
Shock and metabolic acidosis	4 h to 4 days	Shock with significant metabolic acidosis, coagulopathy, renal failure, respiratory failure, CNS dysfunction
Hepatotoxic phase	Within 2 days	Hepatic dysfunction with jaundice, coagulopathy, encephalopathy, acidosis
Late sequela: bowel obstruction	2–4 weeks	Abdominal pain, distention, vomiting, dehydration

Serum iron concentrations of <350 μg/dl are associated with minimal toxicity, while those between 350 and 500 μg/dl generally produce mild to moderate GI symptoms. Peak serum iron concentrations >500 μg/dl are associated with serious systemic toxicity, and those >1000 μg/dl are potentially lethal.

Initial management of iron toxicity consists of ABCs, managing volume depletion with aggressive fluid boluses, and supportive care. Consider whole bowel irrigation for patients with a significant number of pills on abdominal radiograph. Activated charcoal does not effectively bind iron. For severe ingestions, chelation therapy with deferoxamine (desferrioxamine) is the antidote of choice. As deferoxamine can cause hypotension and possibly acute respiratory distress syndrome, it should be used only for significant ingestions. Indications for chelation therapy with deferoxamine include altered mental status from iron toxicity, shock, significant anion gap acidosis, a serum iron concentration >500 μg/dl, persistent vomiting and diarrhea, and a large number of iron pills visualized on abdominal radiograph.

Hydrocarbons

Hydrocarbons are available as petroleum distillates and plant oils. Oral ingestion often produces little toxicity, but aspiration of even small amounts can be fatal from severe pneumonitis. Most hydrocarbons are aliphatic compounds that should be left in the GI tract if ingested. Some halogenated and aromatic hydrocarbons produce more systemic toxicity. The risk of their removal by gastric lavage should be weighed against the risk of aspiration. Activated charcoal does not adsorb hydrocarbons and is not recommended. Hydrocarbon compounds, particularly gasoline, can produce burns if left on the skin, so patients with hydrocarbon exposure may require external decontamination.

Methanol and ethylene glycol

Methanol and ethylene glycol are commonly available as solvents, starter fluids, and antifreeze. Even a small ingestion, such as a swallow, can produce significant toxicity. The parent compounds are relatively non-toxic, but toxic metabolites produce acidosis, altered mental status, retinal injury, and renal failure. Calculation of an anion gap and osmol gap are important in establishing this diagnosis. Competitive blockade of metabolism using fomepizole or ethanol followed by dialysis improves outcome.

Conclusions

Identifying the ingested agent is the key to developing an appropriate management plan for the poisoned patient. Know the common ingestions and indications for therapy, and use symptoms and laboratory investigations to guide management.

Pearls and pitfalls

Pearls

1. The majority of plant and household substance ingestions are non-toxic.
2. There is little risk but great potential benefit in administering *N*-acetylcysteine if significant acetaminophen ingestion is suspected.
3. Consider deferoxamine therapy in significant iron ingestion.
4. Calculate an osmol gap to look for possible methanol or ethylene glycol ingestion in the setting of metabolic anion gap acidosis.

Pitfalls

1. Failure to consider serial salicylate levels.
2. Failure to initiate urine alkalinization or dialysis with significant salicylate toxicity.
3. Failure to consider the short half-life of naloxone and observe for full recovery after naloxone administration in the setting of opiate ingestion.

Selected references

Alber, IA, Alber, DM. *Baby-safe Houseplants and Cut Flowers: A Guide to Keeping Children and Plants Safely under the Same Roof.* Highland, IL: Genus Books, 1990.

American Academy of Pediatrics, Committee on Injury and Poison Prevention. *Handbook of Common Poisonings in Children*, 3rd edn. Elk Grove Village, IL: American Academy of Pediatrics, 1994.

Chyka PA, Butler AY, Holley JE. Serum iron concentrations and symptoms of acute iron poisoning in children. *Pharmacotherapy* 1996; **16**:1053–1058.

Erickson TB, Ahrens WR, Aks SE, Baum C, Ling L. *Pediatric Toxicology: Diagnosis and Management of the Poisoned Child.* New York: McGraw-Hill, 2005.

Fine JS. Iron poisoning. *Curr Probl Pediatr* 2000; **30**:71–90.

Ford M, Delaney KA, Ling L, Erickson T. *Clinical Toxicology*. Philadelphia, PA: Saunders, 2001.

Hartington K, Hartley J, Clancy M. Measuring plasma paracetamol concentrations in all patients with drug overdoses; development of a clinical decision rule and clinicians willingness to use it. *Emerg Med J* 2002;**19**:408–411.

Kunkel, DB. Plant poisoning in children. *Pediatr Ann* 1987; **16**:927–932.

Lawrence, RA. Poisonous plants: when they are a threat to children. *Pediatr Rev* 1997; **18**:162–168.

Mills KC, Curry SC. Acute iron poisoning. *Emerg Med Clin North Am* 1994; **12**:397–413.

Olson KR (ed.). *Poisoning and Drug Overdose*, 5th edn. New York: McGraw-Hill, 2007.

Sporer KA, Khayam-Bashi H. Acetaminophen and salicylate serum levels in patients with suicidal ingestion or altered mental status. *Am J Emerg Med* 1996;**14**:443–446.

Chapter 139

Drugs that kill in small doses

Donald H. Schreiber

Introduction

Although most pediatric poisonings have good outcomes, it is important to recognize those ingestions that in small doses are potentially lethal. This chapter will focus on medications that with a single dose have the potential to kill a 10-kg child (Table 139.1). Rapid recognition and prompt treatment are essential to prevent a fatal event.

Chloroquine and hydroxychloroquine

Chloroquine is an antiparasitic agent indicated for the treatment and prophylaxis of malaria. Hydroxychloroquine is increasingly being used as an anti-inflammatory agent for systemic lupus erythematosus, rheumatoid arthritis, and other autoimmune disorders. Both agents have a narrow therapeutic index.

Acute overdose presents with the onset of nausea and vomiting followed by rapid deterioration to coma, cardiac arrhythmias, and cardiac arrest. The toxicity is thought to be related to a direct cellular effect. The cardiac arrhythmias have been attributed to its structural quinidine ring, which produces similar cardiotoxic effects. Hypokalemia is common and is thought to be precipitated by increased activity of the Na^+-K^+-ATPase pump.

Treatment is primarily supportive but optimal outcomes are achieved with early intubation, mechanical ventilation, and high-dose epinephrine (0.1–1.0 µg/kg per min) for hypotension. Although this regimen has not been well studied in children, there are no contraindications to its use in the pediatric population.

Most deaths from chloroquine occur within 1–3 h of ingestion. Its rapid onset and high mortality rate is well recognized. The Hemlock Society recommends chloroquine as the ideal agent for patient assisted suicide.

Camphor

Camphor is commonly found in many over-the-counter topical products for supportive care of upper respiratory tract symptoms and musculoskeletal complaints. The list of products include Vicks VapoRub, Ben Gay, Adsorbine, and Tiger Balm. Since 1983, federal regulations limit the concentration of camphor to <11.1% (1.1 g/10 ml) but foreign products may still contain higher concentrations. The potential lethal dose is 100 mg/kg or only 10 ml in a 10-kg toddler. Vicks Vaporub contains 4.8% camphor (480 mg/10 ml) and a potentially lethal dose would be approximately 20 ml. Some products such as Ben Gay contain other toxic substances such as methyl salicylate in concentrations of 30%.

Camphor has a distinct aromatic odor and pungent taste. It is rapidly absorbed through skin, mucous membranes, and the GI tract. Common symptoms include sore throat, nausea and vomiting, and sinus tachycardia. Worrisome neurological effects include agitation, delirium, and seizures. Both CNS depression and respiratory failure can ensue.

Treatment focuses on limiting absorption by washing the substance, and administering activated charcoal.

Benzodiazepines are recommended to control CNS agitation and seizures.

Airway protection and mechanical ventilation may be required. There are no antidotes available for camphor toxicity. Treatment is essentially supportive.

Clonidine and other imidazolines

Clonidine is approved for the treatment of hypertension in the USA but off-label uses include treatment for narcotic withdrawal, attention-deficit hyperactivity disorder, and Tourette syndrome. Other imidazolines are naphzoline, oxymetazoline, and tetrahydrozoline, all marketed as nasal decongestants, and apraclonidine for glaucoma. All the imidazolines have similar toxicological profiles.

A Practical Guide to Pediatric Emergency Medicine: Caring for Children in the Emergency Department, ed. N. Ewen Amieva-Wang (associate eds. Jamie Shandro, Aparajita Sohoni, and Bernhard Fassl). Published by Cambridge University Press.

Table 139.1. Medications with lethal potential as a single dose for a 10 kg child

Drug	Potential lethal dose (mg/kg)	Drug formulation	No. unit doses
Antimalarials			
Chloroquine	50	500 mg tablet	1 tablet
Hydroxychloroquine	20	200 mg tablet	1 tablet
Sulfonylureas	0.1		
Glipizide	0.1	5 mg	1 tablet
Glyburide	0.1	10 mg	1 tablet
Calcium channel blockers			
Diltiazem	15	360	1 tablet
Nifedipine	15	90	1 tablet
Verapamil	15	360	1 tablet
Narcotic analgesics			
Codeine	7–14	60	1–2 tablets
Methadone	1–2	40	1 tablet
Antipsychotics			
Chlorpromazine	25	200	1–2 tablets
Thioridazine	15	200	1 tablet
Tricyclic antidepressants			
Amitriptyline	15	100	1–2 tablets
Desipramine	15	75	1–2 tablets
Imipramine	15	150	1 tablet
Other			
Camphor	100	1.1 g/10 ml	2 tsp
Clonidine	0.01	0.3 mg tablet	1 tab
Methyl salicylate	200	1.4 g/ml	1.5 ml
Theophylline	8.4	500 mg tablet	1 tablet

Clonidine is available as 0.1, 0.2, and 0.3 mg tablets and in a variety of transdermal patches for weekly application with total dosages of 2.5, 5, and 7.5 mg, respectively. The potentially lethal dose is 0.01 mg/kg or 0.1 mg for a 10 kg toddler. Used patches may contain as much as 75% of the total dose even after 1 week.

The setting of CNS depression, hypotension, miosis, and failure to respond to naloxone, a clonidine overdose should be suspected.

Clinical manifestations of toxicity include CNS depression and hypotension. The presence of miotic pupils can mislead the clinician to consider an opioid toxidrome. Failure to respond to naloxone suggests a clonidine exposure. Hypotension and relative bradycardia are caused by its α_2-adrenoceptor agonist effects. Treatment is generally supportive including fluid resuscitation and inotropic support with norepinephrine.

Methyl salicylates

The incidence of salicylate poisoning in children has fallen dramatically as the use of aspirin has decreased in the pediatric age group because of its association with Reyes syndrome. However, salicylates are still a common ingredient in a number of over-the-counter preparations such as Oil of Wintergreen and Peptobismol. It is not widely appreciated that these products contain large amounts of salicylates and are potentially lethal in small doses. Oil of Wintergreen contains 5 g methyl salicylate in 5 ml (one teaspoon). A potentially lethal dose is 200 mg/kg, representing only 2 ml in a 10 kg toddler. Peptobismol contains 236 mg salicylates per 15 ml (tablespoon); a lethal dose is 120 ml.

Sulfonylureas

Oral hypoglycemic agents are frequently prescribed in the adult populations. The incidence of toxic exposures in children under the age of 6 years is relatively high.

The most common agents reported are glipizide and glyburide. The primary clinical manifestations are related to hypoglycemia. The sulfonylureas stimulate insulin release from the pancreas and inhibit compensatory gluconeogenesis and glycogenolysis in the liver. Sulfonylureas are metabolized primarily in the liver to active metabolites, which are ultimately excreted renally.

Hypoglycemia typically occurs within 8 h of ingestion, but there are many reports of delayed onset. Severe hypoglycemia may present with coma and seizures. Treatment is primarily supportive, focusing on the close monitoring of blood glucose every 2 h using fingerstick glucose monitoring. Conscious patients are encouraged to eat. Supplemental IV glucose is not recommended for asymptomatic children as it will mask hypoglycemia. Symptomatic patients with hypoglycemia may be treated with boluses of 25% dextrose in water (D25W) or as a continuous IV solution of 5–10% dextrose and water.

Octreotide, a synthetic somastatin analogue, inhibits the secretion of glucagon and insulin. Studies have shown that giving octreotide produces a statistically significant decrease in the number of ampules of 50% dextrose (D50) required to maintain euglycemia in patients poisoned with sulfonlyureas. The drug is administered as 1–2 μg/kg IV every 8 h.

All symptomatic patients must be admitted to hospital for close glucose monitoring and treatment because of the prolonged duration of action of these drugs. All children suspected of having ingested a sulfonylurea should also be admitted for observation.

Calcium channel blockers

The incidence of calcium channel blocker poisoning has increased in parallel with the frequency of prescriptions for these drugs. The three classes of calcium channel blockers are based on their molecular structure. The phenylalkylamines (verapamil) and the benzothiaprines (diltiazem) act primarily on cardiac tissue. The dihydropyridines (nifedipine, nimodipine) act predominately on vascular smooth muscle. Pediatric deaths have been reported with single tablet ingestions of verapamil and nifedipine in toddlers.

The clinical manifestations of toxicity are related to cardiac effects, primarily hypotension and bradyarrhythmias. Hypotension may persist for more than 24 h despite therapy, and cardiac conduction abnormalities may persist for 7 days. Except for nimodipine, the calcium channel blockers do not penetrate the CNS effectively. Therefore, adverse CNS effects such as drowsiness, confusion, and seizures in the absence of hemodynamic compromise are unusual and a co-ingestion must be considered. Hyperglycemia is common. Delayed onset of symptoms will occur with extended- or sustained-release formulations.

Treatment is primarily supportive. Activated charcoal is indicated to limit absorption if it can be administered within 1 h of ingestion. Hypotension should initially be treated with fluid boluses of saline. Vasopressors may be required. An adrenergic agent such as norepinephrine or phenylephrine may be preferred, although in the setting of co-existent bradycardia, epinephrine has both alpha- and beta-adrenergic agonist activity.

Calcium would seem to be the rational choice as an antidote for calcium blocker toxicity but its efficacy has been mixed. It seems to be most effective in mild toxicity but has had little effect in severe toxicity. Calcium may be administered as 10% calcium chloride (0.10–0.25 ml/kg, max. 1 g) or 10% calcium gluconate (0.3–0.75 ml/kg, max. 3 g). It may be repeated every 20 min up to 3 or 4 doses.

Glucagon has inotropic activity and has been recommended in severe beta-blocker toxicity. Anecdotal case reports have been published on its use in severe calcium channel blocker toxicity refractory to traditional vasopressors. The successful use of a glucose–insulin infusion as an inotropic agent has also been published in a small case series. Glucose–insulin infusions have also been utilized in patients with acute myocardial infarction and in cardiogenic shock after coronary artery bypass surgery. Recently, intravascular lipid emulsion has been reported to reverse the cardiotoxicity in a number of patients. A bolus dose of 1.5 ml/kg of 20% intralipid followed by an infusion of 0.25 ml/kg per min has been used.

All symptomatic children with calcium channel blocker toxicity should be admitted to the ICU. Asymptomatic patients with a suspected ingestion should be observed for at least 6 h and up to 24 h in the case of suspected ingestion of sustained-release agents.

Beta-blockers

In 2006, there were 9041 single beta-blocker exposures reported to poison centers in the USA. Of these, 613 had moderate or major adverse outcomes and there were four deaths (2007 *Poison Control Report*). The primary clinical effects of beta-blockers are on the β_1- and β_2-adrenoceptors. Howevers beta-blockers also have a membrane-stabilizing activity that accounts for their antiarrhythmic effects. Lipophilic beta-blockers with high lipid solubility rapidly cross the blood–brain barrier and may cause CNS toxicity, such as delirium and seizures (e.g., propranolol). Selective beta-blockers have intrinsic sympathomimetic activity, which accounts for their use in heart failure (e.g., metoprolol, carvedilol). However this intrinsic sympathomimetic activity does not mitigate severe cardiovascular toxicity. Bronchoconstriction and hypoglycemia are common clinical findings associated with beta-blocker toxicity. It is critically important to rapidly identify and treat the hypoglycemia precipitated by beta-blocker toxicity.

The pharmacokinetics of beta-blockers depend on their formulation (e.g., sustained release) and their clearance. Some are cleared by the liver and others by the kidney (sotalol, atenolol, labetalol).

The initial management focuses on correcting the cardiovascular effects.

Intravenous crystalloid and atropine (0.5 to 1.0 mg doses up to a maximum of 0.03–0.04 mg/kg) are the first-line therapies for hypotension and bradycardia.

Hypoglycemia is corrected with 2.5 ml/kg of 10% dextrose in water (D10W). Glucagon has inotropic effects and has been effective in case reports although no clinical trial has been conducted. The initial dose is 50 µg/kg followed by an infusion of 70 µg/kg per h titrated to a mean arterial blood pressure of 60 mmHg.

As with calcium channel blocker toxicity, IV calcium has also been successfully used in severe beta-blocker toxicity. Pressor support with epinephrine has been associated with poor outcomes in animal models and isolated case reports but it may be tried if the above are unsuccessful.

Preliminary studies on insulin–glucose infusions have also recently been reported. A bolus of 2.5 ml/kg D10W is given IV followed by regular insulin 2 U/kg IV. An insulin infusion of 0.5–2.0 U/kg per h is initiated simultaneously with an infusion of 2.5 ml/kg D10W. Serial blood samples are carefully monitored for glucose and potassium.

The hydrophilic, minimally protein-bound beta-blockers are amenable to removal by dialysis. Hemodialysis has been successfully used with acebutolol, atenolol, and sotalol but is not effective with metoprolol or propranolol. All symptomatic children must be admitted for cardiac monitoring. Asymptomatic children should be observed for a minimum of 6 h for any evidence of cardiovascular toxicity and may then be discharged. However, observation for 24 h is warranted in the setting of co-ingestions with other agents with cardiovascular toxicity, with long-acting or extended-release formulations, and, specifically, with sotalol ingestions because of its unique antiarrhythmic activity.

Tricyclic antidepressants

Antidepressants are the second most common cause of death from poisoning in the adult population. Amitriptyline is still prescribed for childhood enuresis. A potentially lethal dose is only 15 mg/kg and a single 150 mg tablet can be deadly in a 10 kg toddler.

The clinical toxicity is related to a combination of CNS and cardiac effects. Anticholinergic effects, alpha adrenergic blockade, and quinidine-like activity all contribute to the clinical manifestations. Clinical manifestations include the classic triad of the three Cs: coma, convulsions, and conduction abnormalities. Onset of toxicity is rapid and the EP should anticipate rapid progression of symptoms. Prolongation of the QRS interval >100 ms is a marker of severe toxicity. Early intervention to support the airway with ventilatory support is strongly recommended. Acidosis increases the uptake of the drug into the CNS and potentiates the cardiotoxicty. Once seizures develop, toxicity exponentially worsens, associated with the resultant metabolic acidosis.

A serum or urine qualitative drug screen may help to establish the diagnosis but serum drug levels are of no benefit. Rapid uptake into the CNS and body fat stores as well as protein binding render serum drug measurements an inaccurate assessment of toxicity.

Sodium bicarbonate therapy is currently recommended to treat the cardiotoxic effects.

Boluses of 1–2 mEq/kg IV sodium bicarbonate are given for patients with signs of clinical toxicity, including sinus tachycardia, supraventricular tachyarrhythmias, ventricular arrhythmias, and widening of the QRS interval. The benefits of sodium bicarbonate therapy have been observed even in the setting of a normal pH. Doses of sodium bicarbonate may be repeated to elevate the arterial pH to 7.5. Benzodiazepines are recommended as first-line treatment for seizures.

Asymptomatic children with a suspected ingestion should be observed for at least 6 h. Children with signs of clinical toxicity must be admitted to the ICU.

Conclusions

The potential gravity of small ingestions of selected drugs that are associated with severe adverse outcomes must be clearly understood by the EP. A potential toxic ingestion should be included in the differential diagnosis of common clinical problems. A careful history is of paramount importance to avoid potential catastrophes.

Pearls and pitfalls

Pearls

1. Staff in ED must be familiar with the medications that can be lethal in a single dose.
2. A poison control center must be consulted for any pediatric exposure or ingestion.
3. All children with ingestion of beta-blocker, hypoglycemic agents, or calcium-channel blockers should be admitted for close observation and management because of the delayed onset of symptoms.

Pitfalls

1. Failure to ask about combination medications (i.e., Vicks Vaporub) when attempting to determine possible toxic exposures.
2. Failure to document a likely time of ingestion on which to base further management and observation.
3. Failure to educate parents regarding the toxicity of certain medications present in the home.

Selected references

Bailey B. Glucagon in beta blocker and calcium channel blocker overdoses: a systematic review. *J Toxicol Clin Toxicol* 2003;**41**:595–602.

Harrigan RA. Oral agents for the treatment of type 2 diabetes mellitus: pharmacology, toxicity and treatment. *Ann Emerg Med* 2001;**38**:68–78.

Holger JS, Engebretsen KM, Fritzlar SJ, *et al.* Insulin versus vasopressin and epinephrine to treat beta-blocker toxicity. *Clin Toxicol (Phila)* 2007;**45**:396–401.

Holger JS, Engebretsen KM, Obetz CL, *et al.* A comparison of vasopressin and glucagon in beta-blocker induced toxicity. *Clin Toxicol (Phila)* 2006;**44**:45–51.

Ling Ngan Wong A, Tsz Fung Cheung J, Graham C. Hydroxychloroquine overdose: case report and recommendations for management. *Eur J Emerg Med* 2008;**15**:16–18.

Michael JB, Sztajnkrycer MD. Deadly pediatric poisons: nine common agents that kill at low doses. *Emerg Med Clin North Am* 2004;**22**: 1019–1050.

Seger DL. Clonidine toxicity revisited. *J Toxicol Clin Toxicol* 2002;**40**: 145–155.

White NT. Cardiotoxicity of Antimalarial Drugs. *Lancet Infect Dis* 2007;**7**:549–558.

Chapter 140

Environmental toxins: common environmental exposures

Richard N. Bradley

Introduction

Many environmental toxins pose significant health risks to children. Priorities in the emergency treatment of pediatric patients exposed to toxic environmental substances are:

- termination of the exposure
- supportive care
- specific therapy, if indicated.

The most common environmental toxic substances that cause acute morbidity in North American children under 6 years of age are plants and pesticides. While mortality from environmental toxic exposures in children is rare, carbon monoxide (CO) exposure is the most common cause of death from toxic environmental exposure.

Children are more susceptible than adults to toxic environments because they breathe more air, drink more water, and eat more food per unit of body mass. An infant's respiratory rate is twice that of adults. Since infants and toddlers are frequently on the floor, carpet, or grass, they incur more exposure to chemicals present in these surroundings. If unable to walk or crawl, children may sustain exposure to noxious agents because they cannot remove themselves from hazardous environments. Adolescents are also at higher risk because they may misjudge or ignore risks.

This chapter will review the approach to, diagnosis, and management of some of the most common environmental exposures in the pediatric population (Table 140.1).

Common environmental toxins

Lead

There has been a resurgence in concern about childhood lead poisoning, particularly from lead contamination in toys. Abdominal pain, arthralgia, and constipation are common early complaints. While the time course may range from weeks to months, the child may also display signs of early encephalopathy such as clumsiness, staggering, headache, and behavioral changes. While extremely rare, symptoms may progress to diminished level of consciousness, stupor, and convulsions.

The primary test for evaluation of lead poisoning is the whole blood lead concentration; however, it may not be available on an emergency basis. Alternative tests include an erythrocyte protoporphyrin concentration, radiographs for lead paint chips or other ingested lead objects, and radiographs looking for lead lines in long bones.

Emergency treatment depends on the severity of the symptoms. Admit patients with symptomatic lead toxicity or transfer them to a hospital with expertise in caring for children.

Treat patients with more severe symptoms using parenteral chelation therapy with high-dose British Anti-Lewisite (BAL).

The first dose of BAL for patients of any age with encephalopathy is 4 mg/kg administered IM. The next dose is given 4 h later and then an IV infusion of calcium disodium ethylenediaminetetraacetic acid (EDTA) is immediately started. Continuing treatment and management of patients with mild lead poisoning may be carried out with oral succimer. Benzodiazepines and phenytoin are useful for seizures. Consider whole bowel irrigation if there is major contamination of the digestive tract.

Carbon monoxide and smoke

The affinity of hemoglobin for CO is approximately 200 times greater than its affinity for oxygen. A leftward shift in the oxyhemoglobin dissociation curve occurs when CO binds to hemoglobin and forms the carboxyhemoglobin molecule, which is incapable of delivering oxygen to the cells. Within cells, CO acts as an intracellular toxin and interferes with mitochondrial oxidative phosphorylation. Thus, CO poisoning reduces the oxygen-carrying capacity of blood, the amount of oxygen delivered to the tissues, and subsequent energy production.

Symptoms of CO poisoning include non-specific signs such as headache, nausea, vomiting, dizziness, and fatigue.

Patients with serious CO poisoning present with lethargy, coma, seizures, metabolic acidosis, hypotension, or cardiac arrest. It is important to note that the severity of CO poisoning

Table 140.1. Pediatric presentation of common environmental exposures

	Symptoms	Investigations
Lead	Encephalopathy, ataxia, constipation, abdominal pain, arthralgia, or seizures	*History*: possible exposure (older house) *Analyses*: blood lead, erythrocyte protoporphyrin concentration *Imaging*: radiographs for lead lines in long bones or ingested lead paint chips or objects
Carbon monoxide	Headache, nausea, lethargy, unconsciousness, or seizures	*Analyses*: CO oximetry; however, the breakdown of protoporphyrin to bilirubin also produces CO, so CO–hemoglobin may be elevated in children with jaundice and many oximeters give falsely elevated carboxyhemoglobin in proportion to the amount of fetal hemoglobin present
Organophosphates	Unlike adults, children are less likely to present with bradycardia, and may show tachycardia; they are also more likely to have mental status changes and seizures	*History*: exposure to pesticides *Analyses*: none relevant to the acute phase of presentation and management

may not correlate with carboxyhemoglobin levels. Many patients who survive significant exposures have delayed neurological sequelae, which may manifest as focal motor deficits, seizures, or as cognitive deficits that may only be detectable with neuropsychological testing. Prevention of these sequelae is the primary goal of current therapy.

Routine blood gases are not appropriate because they do not measure carboxyhemoglobin levels. The oxygen saturation from routine arterial or venous blood gas measurements is actually a calculated value based on a normal oxygen–hemoglobin dissociation curve. Pulse oximetry measures only the calculated oxygen saturation value and may be normal even in the setting of severe toxicity. Therefore, the diagnosis of CO poisoning is confirmed by Co-oximetry performed on an arterial or venous blood gas sample in the laboratory. The co-oximeter will accurately measure the true oxygen saturation and the carboxyhemoglobin level.

The first step in the treatment of CO poisoning is to administer high-flow oxygen.

The half-life of CO is inversely related to the fraction of inspired oxygen (FIO_2). On room air, the half-life is approximately 250 min; on 100% oxygen by non-rebreathing mask the halflife falls to 90–120 min. Hyperbaric oxygen provided at a pressure of 3 atm reduces the half-life to 40 min. For most patients, 100% oxygen administered via a properly fitting non-rebreathing mask is recommended as initial therapy.

The rationale for hyperbaric therapy in CO poisoning is to prevent the delayed neurologic sequelae and not as acute life-saving therapy. Because the degree of toxicity does not necessarily correlate with the CO level and because pre-hospital oxygen therapy further reduces the CO level, any patient with neurological deficits (altered mental status, syncope, severe headache) or cardiac effects (arrhythmias, myocardial ischemia) should undergo hyperbaric therapy. Similarly, patients with high levels of carboxyhemoglobin (>25%) without significant symptoms should also be considered for hyperbaric therapy. Consultation with the regional poison control center and local hyperbaric therapy facility is recommended.

Indications for hyperbaric oxygen therapy after carbon monoxide poisoning are:

- syncope
- coma
- seizure
- altered mental status or confusion
- carboxyhemoglobin >25%
- abnormal cerebellar examination
- fetal distress in pregnancy.

Patients with smoke inhalation often have co-existent cyanide toxicity. The symptoms and clinical manifestations of cyanide poisoning are often identical to CO poisoning; therefore, consideration should be given to initiate empiric therapy with hydroxocobalamin or the cyanide antidote kit after consultation with the regional poison control center. Usually therapy must be provided before confirmatory cyanide levels can be returned from the laboratory.

Pesticides (organophosphates)

Several types of pesticide, such as rodenticides and pyrethrins, are of toxicological concern in children, but the ones most likely to cause significant illness or death in children are organophosphates. Organophosphate insecticides are neurotoxins that inhibit acetylcholinesterase. The resulting accumulation of acetylcholine at the neuromuscular junction causes cholinergic overstimulation. Symptoms of toxicity include:

- strange or confused behavior
- severe difficulty breathing
- severe secretions
- severe muscular twitching and general muscle weakness
- involuntary urination and defecation (in toilet trained children)

- lacrimation
- bronchorrhea
- bradycardia
- miosis
- convulsions, seizures
- unconsciousness.

Chapter 141 has more information on the organophosphate toxidrome.

Ensure that decontamination is complete before a patient exposed to organophosphates enters the treatment area. This limits the total dose that the patient will receive as well as protects healthcare workers.

Atropine, an anticholinergic medication, is the primary treatment for organophosphate insecticide poisonings.

The dosage is 0.05 mg/kg atropine, repeated every 10–30 min until symptoms resolve. Pralidoxime hydrochloride (2-PAM) enhances the regeneration of acetylcholinesterase. It is administered immediately to patients with severe symptoms and repeated every 6–12 h, as needed. The dose is 20–40 mg/kg (max. 2 g) diluted to 5% and infused over 10–15 min. Benzodiazepines are given to patients with severe symptoms to treat or reduce the occurrence of seizures.

AtroPen is a prefilled autoinjector that is available for self-use or use by bystanders when a patient is symptomatic after an exposure. In patients with mild symptoms, the appropriate dose is one AtroPen. When a patient has severe symptoms, the clinician or rescuer may need to administer two or three auto-injectors in order to achieve atropinization (flushing, mydriasis, tachycardia, dryness of the mouth and nose) (Table 140.2). The user should hold the autoinjector perpendicular to the skin and administer it into the muscles of the thigh.

Air pollutants

The major components of air pollution come from combustion of fossil fuels. These include nitrogen dioxide, ozone, and suspended solid or liquid particles. Environmental tobacco smoke is also a concern. The primary effect of environmental pollutants in children is asthma exacerbations. Traditional treatment with bronchodilators and steroids is appropriate in these patients.

Table 140.2. AtroPen strengths

Age group	Strength (color code)
Adults and children weighing <41 kg (90 lbs) (generally <10 years of age)	2 mg (green)
Children 18–41 kg (40–90 lbs) (generally 4–10 years of age)	1 mg (dark red)
Children 7–18 kg (15–40 lbs) (generally 6 months to 4 years of age)	0.5 mg (blue)
Infants weighing <7 kg (15 lbs) (generally <6 months of age)	0.25 mg (yellow)

Paints and solvents/inhalant abuse

Inhalant abuse is most common among young teenagers. Abused substances include glues, paints, lacquers, correction fluid, butane, and gasoline. Methods of abuse include "sniffing" (inhalation of vapors directly from an open container or a heated pan), "bagging" (inhalation of vapors from a plastic or paper bag), and "huffing" (oral inhalation of vapors from a soaked piece of cloth against the face). Symptoms of intoxication include euphoria, hallucinations, nystagmus, seizures, and coma. Damage occurs in the CNS and the peripheral nervous systems. Some agents, particularly hydrocarbons, may produce vasodilatation and decreased cardiac output, leading to hypotension. Cardiac arrhythmias are the most common cause of sudden sniffing death syndrome.

The focus of treatment is to decontaminate clothing and skin, to provide supportive care, and to maintain hydration.

Disposition

Children with any degree of symptoms after lead poisoning or with blood lead >70 µg/dl should be admitted for parenteral chelation therapy. Asymptomatic children with blood lead levels of 45–70 µg/dl may be treated as outpatients with oral chelation alone, as long as the physician can ensure that the child will not return to a residence with ongoing lead exposure.

For CO exposure, children are admitted if they meet the indications for hyperbaric oxygen or are still symptomatic after oxygen administration in the ED.

Any child with organophosphate poisoning or probable exposure to chemical or biological weapons should be admitted for management and/or monitoring for clinical deterioration.

Pearls and pitfalls

Pearls

1. Decontamination is one of the highest priorities to consider in toxicological emergencies.
2. Symptoms and signs of environmental toxins may present differently in children to adults.

Pitfalls

1. Failure to consider environmental exposures when children present with unusual symptoms or altered mental status.
2. Failure to alert the hospital administration, emergency response team, and other potential victims when treating one individual exposed to an environmental toxin.

Selected references

Clark RF. Insecticides: organic phosphorus compounds and carbamates. In Flomenbaum NE, Goldfrank LR, Hoffman RS, *et al.* (eds.) *Goldfrank's Toxicologic Emergencies*, 8th edn. New York: McGraw-Hill, 2006, pp. 1689–1704.

Henretig FM. Lead. In Flomenbaum NE, Goldfrank LR, Hoffman RS, *et al.* (eds.) *Goldfrank's Toxicologic Emergencies*, 8th edn. New York: McGraw-Hill, 2006, pp. 1308–1324.

Reigart JR, Roberts JR. Pesticides in children. *Pediatr Clin North Am* 2001;**48**: 1185–1198, ix.

Chapter

141 Environmental toxins: biological, chemical, and radiological terrorism

Richard N. Bradley

Introduction

This chapter will review radiation, chemical, and biological environmental toxins, as well as discuss the general principles of management and specific pediatric treatments.

Radiation

Children may be injured either by direct exposure to ionizing radiation or by coming into contact with contaminated radioactive materials. One of the primary differences between the routes of exposure is that ionizing radiation will not make patients radioactive, whereas patients who are contaminated by radioactive material (e.g., after exposure to a dirty bomb) receive ongoing injury and pose a risk to others until decontaminated.

Radiation injuries generally do not produce immediate physical effects. If patients are symptomatic shortly after a radiation injury, this is indicative of a very high exposure dosage and, therefore, the prognosis is usually poor.

Chemical warfare agents

Chemical warfare agents may be divided into four categories: nerve agents, blister agents, cyanides, and choking agents (Table 141.1).

- *Nerve agents* block acetylcholinesterase, leading to both nicotinic and muscarinic effects. Some nerve agents are volatile liquids, while others produce less vapors but are more persistent. Symptoms are similar to organophosphate pesticide toxicity.
- *Blister agents* produce cutaneous bullae and may produce leukopenia or pancytopenia several days after the exposure.
- *Cyanide* interferes with cellular respiration by inhibiting cytochrome oxidase at the cytochrome a_3 portion of the electron transport chain.
- *Choking agents* produce pulmonary edema and include substances such as chlorine and phosgene.

Table 141.1. Chemical warfare agents, symptoms and treatment

Agent class	Symptoms	Treatment
Nerve agents	Seizures, miosis, organophosphate poisoning symptoms	Atropine, pralidoxime hydrochloride (2-PAM)
Blister agents	Blisters; presentation delayed several hours after exposure	Supportive care
Cyanides	Oxygen utilization prevented at the cellular level, resulting in cellular asphyxia with a normal arterial oxygen content	Hydroxocobalamin, 70 mg/kg IV over 30 min (or rapid push in cardiac arrest) (max. 5 g)
Choking agents	Dyspnea or pulmonary edema	Supportive care

Bioterrorism

There are a large number of potential bioterrorism agents. The agents posing the greatest threats are the "Category A" agents/diseases as defined by the CDC (Table 141.2). These include agents that are easily disseminated or transmitted; those that result in high mortality or have potential major public health impact; those that might cause panic, and those that require special public health preparedness. Examples of Category A diseases that show person-to-person transmission are smallpox, plague, and viral hemorrhagic fevers. There are also three Category A diseases that are not transmitted person to person: anthrax, tularemia, and botulism.

Some diseases caused by bioterrorism agents can be difficult to diagnose because their symptoms appear as a generic flu-like illness. Exposed patients often present with fever, chills, and upper respiratory symptoms. The Category A diseases that

A Practical Guide to Pediatric Emergency Medicine: Caring for Children in the Emergency Department, ed. N. Ewen Amieva-Wang (associate eds. Jamie Shandro, Aparajita Sohoni, and Bernhard Fassl). Published by Cambridge University Press.

Table 141.2. Class A bioterrorism agents[a]

Agents	Symptoms	Person-to-person transmission	Treatment
Smallpox	Pustular rash (centripetal, not sparing palms or soles), fever, ill-appearing	Yes	Supportive care (cidofovir if approved by CDC)
Plague	Flu-like symptoms; bubos are less likely in a terrorism scenario	Yes	Gentamicin 2.5 mg/kg IM/IV, TID
Tularemia	Flu-like symptoms	No	Gentamicin 2.5 mg/kg IM/IV TID
Anthrax	Flu-like symptoms *or* skin lesion with black eschar	No	Ciprofloxacin 10–15 mg/kg q. 12 h (max. 1 g/day) or doxycycline Add two additional antimicrobials, such as rifampin, vancomycin, penicillin, clindamycin, or clarithromycin
Botulism	Afebrile, descending, flaccid paralysis	No	Supportive care; antitoxin from the CDC
Viral hemorrhagic fevers	Fever and hemorrhagic rash	Yes	Supportive care

[a]Category A agents/diseases as defined by the US Centers for Disease Control and Prevention (CDC).

present with influenza-like illness include pulmonary anthrax, pneumonic plague, and tularemia.

Other Category A agents present with skin findings. The papulopustular rash is characteristic of smallpox. Clinicians can differentiate this rash from chickenpox because the lesions tend to be peripheral and usually do not spare the palms and soles. Unlike chickenpox, which will have "crops" of lesions in various stages of development, all of the lesions in smallpox will be at the same stage of development on the spectrum from macule to papule to vesicle to pustule. The CDC has produced an online risk evaluation algorithm for evaluating rashes potentially caused by smallpox (http://emergency.cdc.gov/agent/smallpox/diagnosis/riskalgorithm/).

Additional Category A agents with skin findings are the viral hemorrhagic fevers. Patients with these conditions have fever and some cutaneous manifestations of hemorrhage, such as a hemorrhagic conjunctivitis or petechiae. There is a wide variety of these viral hemorrhagic fevers, including Ebola and Marburg virus.

The final Category A agent is botulism. This presents as an afebrile, descending, flaccid paralysis.

Management

Biological warfare agents

Anthrax

Bacillus anthracis is the causative agent for anthrax, a disease that is challenging to treat in children. It may produce a cephalosporinase or contain an inducible beta-lactamase, which may decrease the effectiveness of penicillins.

The treatment of choice for anthrax is ciprofloxacin or doxycycline.

The dosage for ciprofloxacin is 10–15 mg/kg every 12 h (not to exceed 1 g per day) and for doxycycline is

$\leq$8 years: 2.2 mg/kg every 12 h
>8 years and $\leq$45 kg: 2.2 mg/kg every 12 h
>8 years and >45 kg: 100 mg every 12 h.

In addition to the ciprofloxacin or doxycycline, one or two additional antimicrobial drugs, such as rifampin, vancomycin, penicillin, clindamycin or clarithromycin, should be administered to patients with inhalational anthrax and to those with cutaneous anthrax and signs of systemic involvement, extensive edema, or lesions on the head and neck. These drugs may have adverse effects in children. After a week or more of treatment is completed, physicians may change the therapy to amoxicillin if the strain is penicillin-sensitive, in order to reduce the likelihood of adverse effects from the ciprofloxacin or doxycycline. Amoxicillin may also be appropriate for post-exposure prophylaxis in asymptomatic children.

Plague and tularemia

The preferred therapy for both plague and tularemia in children is gentamicin at a dose of 2.5 mg/kg IM or IV, three times per day.

Smallpox

There is no proven treatment for smallpox; however, in an outbreak, the CDC would likely make cidofovir (Vistide) available as a potential therapy.

Box 141.1. Age-based treatment for nerve agent intoxication

Atropine

Infant (0–2 years)

- Mild/moderate symptoms: 0.05 mg/kg IM or 0.02 mg/kg IV.
- Severe symptoms: 0.1 mg/kg IM or 0.02 mg/kg IV.

Child (2–10 years)

- Mild/moderate symptoms: 1 mg IM.
- Severe symptoms: 2 mg IM.

Adolescent (>10 years)

- Mild/moderate symptoms: 2 mg IM
- Severe symptoms: 4 mg IM

Repeat atropine (2 mg IM or 1 mg IM for infants) at 5–10-min intervals until secretions have diminished and breathing is comfortable or airway resistance has returned to near normal.

Pralidoxime hydrochloride (2-PAM)

Give 15 mg/kg IV slowly.

Other treatment

- Assisted ventilation as needed.
- Phentolamine for 2-PAM-induced hypertension (1 mg IV for children).
- Diazepam for convulsions:
  - 0.2 to 0.5 mg IV for infants to 5 years
  - 1 mg IV for children >5 years.

Botulism

Supportive care, along with passive immunization with equine antitoxin, is appropriate for children with botulism. Botulinum antitoxin should be administered as soon as possible after the clinical diagnosis, unless the patient's paralysis is definitely improving. In the USA, botulinum antitoxin is available from the CDC via state and local health departments.

Chemical warfare agents

Patients with symptomatic nerve agent intoxication should be treated with atropine (Ch. 140). Box 141.1 gives the treatment for nerve agent intoxication.

Cyanide

If the patient has been poisoned by cyanide, the first step, as with other chemical contamination scenarios, is to decontaminate the patient. If the child ingested cyanide, aspirate the stomach contents and then administer charcoal. The antidotes for cyanides are sodium thiosulfate (25% solution; 1.65 ml/kg IV) or hydroxocobalamin (70 mg/kg IV).

If hydroxocobalamin, the preferred agent, is not available, then sodium nitrite and sodium thiosulfate are used. Sodium nitrite dosage is 0.12–0.3 ml/kg (up to 10 ml) given IV over no shorter a time than 5 min. Blood pressure should be monitored closely and the infusion discontinued if the patient develops hypotension. The sodium nitrite is followed by IV 25% sodium thiosulfate, 1.65 ml/kg. One-half of the initial dose can be repeated in 30 min if needed. It is important to note that young children are particularly susceptible to excessive methemoglobinemia, which is an expected effect of nitrite administration.

Blister agents

There is no known antidote to most blister agents; treatment is primarily supportive. Topical mydriatic–cycloplegic solution, antibiotics, and corticosteroids may be useful in injuries to the eyes. Petroleum jelly may reduce the likelihood of lid adhesion. Silver sulfadiazine or bacitracin zinc may reduce the incidence of secondary skin infections. Analgesics including narcotics, are given as necessary for pain control. Early intubation should be considered if the airways are involved.

Disposition

Any child with organophosphate poisoning or probable exposure to chemical or biological weapons should be admitted for management and/or monitoring for clinical deterioration, as should any patient with a potentially significant radiation exposure. Anyone exposed to the agent (i.e., parents or caregivers) must also be treated appropriately.

It is wise to assess your hospital's mass casualty or mass exposure triage and treatment protocol.

Pearls and pitfalls

Pearls

1. While the threat of biological, chemical, and radiological terrorism is concerning, terroristic attacks are much more likely to involve conventional weapons such as explosives and firearms.
2. Atropine antidote kits are available with pediatric dosages.

Pitfalls

1. Failure to decontaminate patients and those accompanying them before allowing access to the ED.
2. Failure to triage effectively in a multiple casualty event involving weapons of mass destruction. There may be a tendency to treat the patients who scream or complain the loudest, but the quietest patients, such as some children, may be the sickest and most in need of immediate care.

Selected references

Centers for Disease Control and Prevention. Notice to readers: update. Interim recommendations for antimicrobial prophylaxis for children and breastfeeding mothers and treatment of children with anthrax. *MMWR Morb Mort Wkly Rep* 2001;**50**:1014–1016.

Centers for Disease Control and Prevention. *Smallpox Response Plan and Guidelines*. Atlanta, GA: Centers for Disease Control and Prevention, 2002.

Geller RJ, Barthold C, Saiers JA, Hall AH. Pediatric cyanide poisoning: causes, manifestations, management, and unmet needs. *Pediatrics* 2006;**118**: 2146–2158.

Section

23

Trauma

Expert reviewers: James Holmes Jr., Michael S. B. Edwards, and William A. Kennedy II

Chapter 142

Trauma overview and injury prevention

Jamie Shandro

Introduction

Injuries are the leading cause of death for children aged 1 to 18 years. There are biphasic peaks of incidence and case fatality, with higher rates for children <3 years of age and those aged 13–18 years. The leading mechanism of injuries among all children is motor vehicle crashes. For younger children, falls are a significant source of morbidity and mortality, whereas for adolescents, violent injuries increase in numbers. It is vital to remember that in trauma, as in medical emergencies, hypoxia, resulting from airway compromise or respiratory failure, is the most common cause of cardiac arrest in children.

The goals of this section are to outline general management for pediatric trauma care, highlighting differences in pediatric anatomy and physiology that lead to important clinical considerations. This chapter will also emphasize the importance of injury prevention. Subsequent chapters will address details of head, spinal, chest and abdominal, genitourinary, and non-accidental trauma. Wound care is covered in Section 25 and sprain and fracture care is covered in detail in Section 15.

Children experience unique patterns of injury secondary to their size and developmental stage.

Waddell's triad. This is femur fracture, abdominal/pelvic injury, and head injury and results from a school-age child being hit by a car while running across the street.

Chance fractures (flexion injury of the spine). These are also known as seatbelt injuries. They occur secondary to the sudden flexion of the spine that can occur in a head-on collision. They are linear fractures through a lumbar vertebral body, pedicles, and spinous process. While their incidence has decreased with the adoption of lap/shoulder harnesses, 50% of these fractures are associated with intra-abdominal injuries.

Poorly fitting seatbelts and airbags cause pediatric morbidity in motor vehicle accidents. There are also more head injuries among young children because of their large heads relative to their short immature neck musculature. While cervical spine injuries are relatively rare in children, injuries tend to occur at higher levels (C2–C3) in young children and lower levels (C5–C6) in adolescents. Handle bar injuries causing duodenal and pancreatic injuries occur in bicycle accidents. Because of the increased elasticity of pediatric bones, they can experience significant trauma unmarked by overlying fracture.

In young children, the liver, spleen, kidneys, and bladder are less protected by overlying ribs or abdominal musculature than in adults; remember that the bladder is an intra-abdominal organ.

Clinical presentation

History

Injured children are often unable to recount the events of their trauma, so the EP must rely on information obtained from secondary sources including parents, family members, school teachers, and emergency medical services (EMS) personnel. Despite the need to take the history in a timely manner, the focus of care should be on proper resuscitation and management of the child's injuries. The history should be taken concurrently with the primary survey or by an additional EP who is not directly contributing to the primary survey.

Obtain the history of the mechanism of injury from available sources. Certain mechanisms of injury elicited in the history will give clues as to the anatomic structures at greatest risk. For motor vehicle crashes, EMS personnel provide information about the child's location in a motorized vehicle, type of restraints used, extent of intrusion into the passenger cabin, and the approximate speed of the vehicle. Other types of information may include a report on injuries to other victims at the scene, if a child had significant blood loss or was ambulatory prior to EMS arrival, the height of a reported fall, or the type of weapon used.

The primary survey and therapeutic adjuncts

The 'primary survey' is a methodological approach to the initial trauma evaluation and resuscitation presented by the American College of Surgeons in the Advanced Trauma Life Support (ATLS) course. The primary survey is composed of five ordered steps, referred to by the acronym ABCDE for

A Practical Guide to Pediatric Emergency Medicine: Caring for Children in the Emergency Department, ed. N. Ewen Amieva-Wang (associate eds. Jamie Shandro, Aparajita Sohoni, and Bernhard Fassl). Published by Cambridge University Press.

airway, breathing, circulation, disability, and exposure. If a problem with one of these functions is identified, it should be promptly addressed. These priorities are the same for adults and children although pediatric pathology can manifest differently.

When the ED receives a prehospital call regarding a pediatric patient, there is often a short period of time to anticipate the equipment and procedures that will be needed. If major trauma is anticipated, precalculating age- and weight-based equipment sizes and airway medication doses (in addition to one size larger and smaller) will expedite care. Since the majority of trauma resuscitation is carried out in the presence of a team of providers, many parts of the primary survey and its adjuncts can be done simultaneously.

Obtaining IV access, interpreting age-appropriate vital signs, and using the Broselow Pediatric Emergency Tape to confirm appropriate equipment size and drug dosing for the child's weight should all be initiated while the primary survey is ongoing.

Airway

The first component of the primary survey is airway assessment. The goals are to find evidence that the child has the appropriate mental status required to protect his or her airway from obstruction and to look for signs of injury to the neck, trachea or oropharynx that may compromise the patency of the airway. The airway must be maintained in conjunction with cervical spine stabilization. This evaluation can be carried out rapidly by listening for adequate crying or asking a child to speak. Examine the oropharynx and neck for signs of significant wounds or hematoma formation. Decreased level of consciousness indicates not only a need to protect the airway but may also result in obstruction of the airway by the tongue.

Supplemental oxygen should be given to all children with significant trauma. Airway adjuncts such as jaw thrust and/or the placement of nasopharyngeal and oropharyngeal airways can maintain the airway when obstructed. Patients unable to protect their airway should be endotracheally intubated.

Breathing

The second part of the primary survey is assessment of the child's breathing. The goals are to identify respiratory distress or other signs of tension pneumothorax, hemothorax, or flail chest, which significantly compromise ventilation and oxygenation. Pulse oximetry and continuous capnography should be obtained with vital signs to assess oxygenation and ventilation.

Children can have significant lung injury without manifesting outward signs of trauma. Lung sounds can be misleading because they are often transmitted throughout the thorax.

Gastric distention in the child from crying can add to respiratory distress. Bag-valve mask can usually be performed indefinitely on a child, although after intubation a nasogastric tube should be placed to decrease gastric distention and prevent emesis and aspiration.

Circulation

The third step in the primary survey is assessment of the child's circulatory status. The goal is to look for evidence of life-threatening hemorrhage. First, assess for strong and symmetric pulses: palpate the brachial arteries in infants; and the carotid, radial, or femoral arteries in older children. Globally diminished pulses, tachycardia, and mottled or poorly perfused skin are suggestive of hemorrhagic shock. Focal, asymmetric loss of a pulse suggests an arterial laceration or compromise caused by compartment syndrome. After examination of pulses and skin perfusion, quickly search for bleeding wounds and establish control of bleeding by applying a dressing and holding direct pressure. This maneuver will control external blood loss until the wounds can be cleaned and repaired.

During this portion of the primary survey, evaluate the abdomen for signs of tenderness, rebound, guarding, or distention, all of which may be suggestive of intra-abdominal injury as a cause of hemorrhagic shock. Assess the stability of the child's pelvis at this time, as open-book or other pelvic fractures may also be a cause of significant intra-abdominal bleeding. Open-book pelvic fractures should be stabilized as well as possible with the use of a wrapped bed sheet to keep the fracture components aligned until external fixation or surgical repair can be done.

Tachycardia or signs of hemorrhagic shock should prompt aggressive fluid resuscitation beginning with two boluses of 20 ml/kg warmed lactated Ringer's solution or normal saline. Remember that children will often not become hypotensive until they are very decompensated. If shock continues despite crystalloid fluid resuscitation, packed red blood cell transfusion should be administered at 10 ml/kg. Initially, O^- blood can be used in females and O^+ blood in males until type-specific blood is available from the blood bank. In the setting of massive hemorrhage when significant blood transfusion is required, coagulation factors should also be repleted by transfusing fresh frozen plasma, cryoprecipitate, and platelets.

Disability and exposure

Evaluation of neurological disability and exposure are the last two portions of the primary survey. A rapid assessment of gross motor and sensory function in all extremities should be completed and a Glasgow Coma Scale calculated according to the child's age.

Remove the child's clothing but take care to maintain appropriate body temperature with blankets, heating lamps, or warmed IV fluids. After clothing is removed, log-roll the child while maintaining in-line spinal immobilization, and look for easily missed injuries to the back of the head, thorax, buttocks, axillae, perineum, or thighs.

The secondary survey

After completion of the primary survey, a more thorough secondary survey should be performed. This is similar in adults and children and entails a complete head to toe physical examination of all body areas. Of importance in the secondary survey is evaluation of the child's ears, nose, mouth, face, heart, abdomen, pelvis, back, and extremities. If the primary survey produces clear indication for exploratory thoracotomy or laparotomy in the operating room, the secondary survey should not delay these procedures or transport to the operating theater.

Differential diagnosis

Generating a list of differential diagnoses when dealing with a trauma patient depends largely on the history (mechanism of injury and complaints) as well as the physical examination findings encountered during the primary survey. During the primary survey, the key goal is to address life-threatening issues at each step. The specific injury patterns will be discussed by system in subsequent chapters of this section.

Diagnostic studies

Radiographic studies

During the primary survey, easily obtainable portable radiographs include chest and pelvis radiographs. Further details of these studies as well as radiology studies carried out after the secondary survey in stable patients are discussed by system in subsequent chapters of this section.

Laboratory tests

In most cases of significant trauma, early ordering of a blood type and cross-match is crucial to starting type-specific blood transfusion. It may also be important to send samples for hemoglobin, basic chemistries, amylase, and liver enzymes, as these values help to establish a baseline that can then be followed during the child's hospital stay. Blood for INR and PTT should be sent for severely injured children, particularly those with traumatic brain injury. An arterial blood gas aids in measuring the respiratory and ventilatory status of a patient. Urinalysis is useful in screening for abdominal and genitourinary trauma. All female patients of menstruating age should also have a pregnancy test.

Management

Management will depend on the type and extent of injury and is covered for specific trauma in the subsequent chapters.

Tetanus booster. Most children have been immunized against tetanus. Administration of booster should be discussed with the guardians of injured children who have sustained open wounds and have not been properly vaccinated.

Pain control. Traumatic injuries can be very painful, and it can be easy to overlook the need for analgesia in small children. In a stable patient in pain, provide analgesia (IV in the case of potential operative injuries requiring nil by mouth status).

Disposition

Consider resources when determining the disposition for pediatric trauma patients. If the facility lacks a trauma surgeon able to care for patients in ED, begin to arrange transfer to a facility with a higher level of care as early as possible during resuscitation and evaluation. Transfer of care to designated pediatric trauma centers does improve outcomes for seriously injured children.

In the setting of pediatric trauma, it is important to consider non-accidental trauma in the differential diagnosis, particularly where the mechanism of injury is not clearly congruent with the observed injuries or there has been a delay in seeking medical care. Data evaluated from the National Pediatric Trauma Registry has shown the incidence of non-accidental trauma to be approximately 10% of all trauma cases leading to hospitalization, with non-accidental trauma more common in infants under 1 year of age. When concerned for non-accidental trauma, it is important to involve social work, the department of child and family services (DCFS), hospital security services, or local police as needed.

Pearls and pitfalls

Pearls

1. Remember the protocol ABCDE (ABC plus disability and exposure): assess, intervene as needed, and reassess frequently for changes.
2. Use the length-based resuscitation tape as a quick reference to find appropriate dosing of medications and correct equipment sizes when a child's weight is not known.
3. Do not delay transfer; it is better to transfer early than to delay necessary treatment while obtaining additional studies.

Pitfalls

1. Failure to rewarm, or maintain, a normal body temperature during resuscitation.
2. Failure to realize that hypotension is a *late* sign of blood loss in children.
3. Failure to suspect non-accidental trauma in children with an unusual mechanism of injury or delayed presentation.

Table 142.1. Common mechanisms of injury by age, and prevention messages for parents

Age group	Injury mechanism	Prevention message
Infants (<1 year)	Unintentional suffocation, non-accidental head injury	Infants sleep on back, screen for child maltreatment
Toddlers (1–3 years)	Motor vehicle crashes, drowning falls	Reinforce car-seat safety; pools isolated with fencing, swimming skills; window screens or secure latches, stair gates
Children (4–11 years)	Motor vehicle crashes, drowning, pedestrian hit by vehicle, closed head injury	Booster seats for 4–8 years, children in back seat, swimming skills, pedestrian safety, helmet use on bikes and skateboards
Adolescents (12–18 years)	Motor vehicle crashes, homicide, suicide, sports-related injuries	Driver's safety (no drinking and driving), violence prevention, suicidality screen, safety in sports (e.g., helmets)

Injury prevention

Injuries are the most common cause of death for ages 1–18 years, and they are often preventable. The ED visit should be used to educate or remind parents and patients about safe practices to decrease the risk of recurrent injury. Table 142.1 lists common mechanisms of injury by age and anticipatory guidance/prevention messages.

Selected references

American College of Surgeons. *Advanced Trauma Life Support for Doctors*, 7th edn. Chicago, IL: American College of Surgeons, 2004.

National Center for Injury Prevention and Control, Centers for Disease Control and Prevention. *Injury Prevention and Control: Data and Statistics*. Atlanta, GA: Centers for Disease Control and Prevention http://www.cdc.gov/injury/wisqars/index.html (accessed 28 April 2010).

Chapter 143

Traumatic brain injury

Pichaya Waitayawinyu, Pimwan Sookplung, and Monica S. Vavilala

Introduction

Traumatic brain injury (TBI) is a leading cause of injury-related morbidity and mortality in the USA. Children <4 years of age have a higher incidence of TBI. Approximately 75% of children with multiple injuries have TBI and almost 80% of all trauma deaths are associated with TBI. However, 90% of pediatric TBI cases are mild and these patients can often be discharged home after an ED visit.

Mechanism of injury

The mechanisms of injury leading to TBI differ by age. Among children <4 years of age, falls account for 41%. In comparison, motor vehicle accidents cause 43% of TBI among adolescents. Inflicted TBI (abuse) should be suspected in children <2 years of age if they have an unclear mechanism of injury, or the physical examination reveals injuries inconsistent with history.

Acceleration or deceleration forces can produce diffuse brain injury, which is the most common type of severe TBI in children. Focal injur patterns include subdural hematoma, epidural hematoma, brain contusions, intracerebral hemorrhage, and subarachnoid hemorrhage. Subarachnoid hemorrhages and subdural hematomas are usually associated with more severe TBI.

Pathophysiology

The pathophysiology of severe TBI involves two insults. The primary event involves direct injury to brain parenchyma. Subsequently, a cascade of biochemical, cellular, and metabolic responses causes secondary damage. Secondary injury also occurs as the result of exogenous insults such as hypoxia and hypotension. Cerebral blood flow may be decreased in children immediately after TBI, but cerebral metabolic rate may be normal, decreased, or increased. Cerebral swelling can develop between 24 and 72 h after TBI, resulting in intracranial hypertension (intracranial pressure (ICP) >20 mmHg). Cerebral perfusion depends on blood pressure since cerebral autoregulation is commonly impaired after pediatric TBI. Interventions to improve cerebral perfusion may involve preventing and treating hypotension and/or the use of temporary hyperventilation ($PaCO_2$ <35 mmHg) to treat increased ICP. However, excessive and/or sustained hyperventilation may lead to cerebral ischemia, while marked increases in blood pressure may lead to cerebral hyperemia.

Injury types

Combined injuries are common.

Epidural hematoma. An epidural hematoma results from an arterial or venous tear and is usually found with a concomitant skull fracture. These are biconvex and most often require neurosurgical intervention. If expediently evacuated, they have an excellent prognosis as the underlying brain is usually unaffected.

Subdural hematoma. A subdural hematoma usually results from tearing of the bridging veins between the dura and cerebral cortex. On CT, these lesions conform to the shape of the brain and cross suture lines. This shear injury to the brain results in higher morbidity and mortality than epidural hematomas. Subdural hematomas may develop with minimal trauma and are not necessarily linked to underlying skull fractures. In an infant, a subdural hematoma can be indicative of inflicted TBI.

Subarachnoid hematoma. Subarachnoid hemorrhage (SAH) results in blood collecting beneath the arachnoid, within the potential space, and spreading along the subarachnoid CSF space to adjacent sulci and gyri. This injury can have severe neurological consequences through irritation, vasospasm, or mass effect of the underlying parenchyma.

Diffuse axonal injury. Shearing forces can cause disruption of the white matter of the brain. External trauma may not be evident. Diffuse brain swelling develops over the course of 24–48 h. Diffuse axonal injury is usually seen in infants <36 months.

A Practical Guide to Pediatric Emergency Medicine: Caring for Children in the Emergency Department, ed. N. Ewen Amieva-Wang (associate eds. Jamie Shandro, Aparajita Sohoni, and Bernhard Fassl). Published by Cambridge University Press.

Contusion. An area of focal brain injury can be seen on the CT scan. Neurologic deficits may be present.

Concussion. Traumatic brain injury associated with or without loss of consciousness, confusion, and other non-specific signs; CT is usually negative. Concussions are graded.

grade I: transient confusion, <15 min of mental confusion, no LOC

grade II: transient confusion, more than 15 min, no LOC.

grade III: any LOC.

Concussion is the most common type of injury in pediatric TBI.

Clinical presentation

History

The history should elicit mechanism of injury, loss or deterioration of consciousness, vomiting, or persistent headache.

Physical examination

Initial trauma management priorities, as always, should start with assessment and stabilization of the ABCs. Subsequently, a brief neurological examination assigns a Glasgow Coma Scale (GCS) score as an early indicator of the severity of the traumatic brain injury. Severity of TBI is classified based on the GCS score:

14, 15: mild

9 to 13: moderate

≤8: severe.

(Table 143.1). A more focused neurological examination should pay specific attention to the following features to more fully understand the level of brain injury: level of consciousness, pupillary examination, fundoscopic examination, cranial nerve evaluation, sensory and motor testing, deep tendon reflexes, and signs of herniation (Cushing's reflex: hypertension, bradycardia and irregular respirations).

Cervical spine immobilization should be maintained throughout the evaluation particularly in severe TBI and in children incapable of verbal communication. Methods of immobilization have been modified for use in children based on their stage of development.

Initial management should avoid causing secondary insults that could lead to secondary brain damage:

- hypoxia may lead to brain ischemia
- hypocarbia may lead to brain ischemia through low cerebral blood flow
- hypercarbia may increase cerebral blood flow and worsen intracranial hypertension
- hypotension may lead to brain ischemia through low cerebral perfusion pressure
- hyperglycemia has been associated with poor outcomes for children and adults with TBI
- pyrexia may lead to brain ischemia through increased cerebral metabolic rate, particularly with limited cerebral oxygen supply.

Table 143.1. Glasgow Coma Scale assessment in adults and children

Assessment	Adults	Children <3 years	Score
Eye opening	Spontaneous	Spontaneous	4
	To verbal command	To speech	3
	To pain	To pain	2
	None	None	1
Verbal response	Oriented	Smile, orients to sound, follows objects, interacts	5
	Confused	Crys but consolable, interacts but inappropriately	4
	Inappropriate	Crys inconsistently consolable; interacts with moaning	3
	Incomprehensible	Inconsolable, interacts with irritability, restless	2
	None	None	1
Motor response	Obeys command	Spontaneous (obeys command)	6
	Localizes pain	Localizes pain	5
	Withdraws to pain	Withdraws from touch	4
	Abnormal flexion to pain	Abnormal flexion to pain	3
	Extensor response to pain	Extensor response to pain	2
	None	None	1

Diagnostic studies

Laboratory studies

In patients arriving in the ED with moderate or severe TBI, hematocrit, glucose, electrolytes, and coagulation values should be obtained. Extracranial injuries may necessitate other tests during the primary and secondary surveys.

Imaging

Children with moderate and severe TBI should have a head CT following initial evaluation and stabilization.

Management

Moderate and severe brain injury

Rapid identification and stabilization of children with moderate and severe TBI is essential. Identify injuries that require immediate neurosurgical intervention and associated injuries that impact management during the systematic primary and secondary survey.

Children with severe TBI require endotracheal intubation to maximize oxygenation and ventilation, to protect the airway from aspiration, and to decrease ICP. Special considerations for tracheal intubation include cervical spine immobilization and avoiding nasotracheal intubation in patients with mid-face trauma or signs of basilar skull fracture (raccoon's eyes, battle's sign, CSF otorrhea or rhinorrhea, hemotympanum). Propofol or thiopental can be used as induction agents for intubation. If there is hypotension, etomidate is the preferable agent. Although succinylcholine can increase ICP, this increase is transient and succinylcholine is commonly used in TBI. Pretreatment with lidocaine may minimize the increase in ICP that can occur with intubation.

The use of hyperventilation is controversial. While decreased PaCO2 from hyperventilation will decrease ICP, hyperventilation may lead to hypocapnia and cause cerebral ischemia. In general, normocapnia (PaCO2 35–40 mmHg) should be maintained. Aggressive hyperventilation (PaCO2 <30 mmHg) is not recommended except in the setting of refractory intracranial hypertension (ICP >20 mmHg), acute neurologic deterioration, or signs of pending herniation

Hypovolemia should be prevented and aggressively treated. Recent recommendations suggest that systolic blood pressure should be maintained above the 5th percentile for age and gender, which may be estimated by the formula:

$$70\,\text{mmHg} + 2(\text{Age in years})$$

When ICP monitors are used, cerebral perfusion pressure (mean arterial pressure minus ICP) should be maintained between 40 and 65 mmHg, depending on age.

The head should be slightly elevated at 15 to 30 degrees in order to decrease ICP; if the child is not hypotensive, hyperosmolar therapy with mannitol or 3% hypertonic saline can be used to decrease ICP and increase cerebral perfusion pressure. Hyperosmolar therapy should be used in patients with increased ICP or brain herniation. While hypothermia may theoretically be benefical, it is not routinely used. However, hyperthermia should be aggressively prevented and treated. Glucose control to <200 mg/dl is associated with better outcome. Early prophylactic anticonvulsant therapy within the first week after TBI to prevent late onset of seizures is controversial.

Mild brain injury

Approximately 90% of childhood TBI is mild. The decision to obtain neuroimaging is mediated by patient age, mechanism, symptoms, and social situation (Tables 143.2 and 143.3). There is some controversy as to whether GCS score of 13 constitutes mild or moderate TBI.

Imaging

The clinical usefulness of skull radiograph is debatable because it cannot reveal underlying TBI or hemorrhage. However, if

Table 143.2. Summary of recommendations for imaging in head trauma for children based on level of risk

Features	Minimal risk	Low risk	Moderate/high risk
Examination	Normal	Normal	<2 years
Loss of consciousness	None	<1 min	>1 min
Mental state	No symptoms	Lethargy	Depressed
Neurologic	None	Amnesia, headache	Seizures, abnormal examination
Vomiting	None	Yes	Persistent
Degree trauma	–	–	Facial injury, multiple trauma
Observation/CT	Yes	Yes or head CT	CT scan

Sources: Committee on Quality Improvement, American Academy of Pediatrics and Commission on Clinical Policies and Research, American Academy of Family Physicians, 1999; Schutzman, 2001.

Table 143.3. Summary of recommendations for obtaining head CT imaging in patients with mild head injury, GCS ≥14, and no localizing signs by age

	<3 months	3 months to 2 years	2–20 years
Past medical history		No pre-existing neurologic disorder or significant medical condition	No pre-existing neurologic disorder or significant medical condition
Social history		Reliable family; no red flags	Reliable family; no alcohol or drugs
History		Low energy fall (<1 m [<3 feet]), no symptoms, injury >2 h previous	No loss of consciousness, no multiple trauma
Physical examination		No scalp hematoma	No sign of skull fracture, non-focal examination, ocular signs
Disposition	CT for any non-trivial mechanism despite normal examination	Can be safely discharged with close follow-up and no head CT	Can be safely discharged with close follow-up and no head CT

Sources: Committee on Quality Improvement, American Academy of Pediatrics and Commission on Clinical Policies and Research, American Academy of Family Physicians, 1999; Schutzman, 2001.

CT is not readily available, skull radiographs can provide screening information. If a fracture is detected, CT imaging is indicated to assess for associated TBI.

The indications for CT scanning in children with minor TBI are controversial particularly in those who have had a loss of consciousness but who upon admission to the ED have no abnormal neurological findings. While symptoms of headache, vomiting, drowsiness, irritability, amnesia, visual disturbance, focal neurologic signs, dizziness, or ALOC suggest increased ICP or worsening TBI, there are no reliable negative predictors of TBI. Even normal GCS score does not preclude TBI because approximately 30% of children with mild TBI are neurologically intact.

Historical features that suggest an increased risk of TBI, include high-risk mechanisms (fall from significant height, motor vehicle accident, penetrating injury, inflicted injury), seizure, convulsion, headache, persistent vomiting, loss of consciousness and/or pre-existing neurologic conditions or a bleeding disorder that might increase risk of TBI. Findings on physical examination such as scalp anomalies or signs of basilar skull fracture suggest the possibility of having TBI.

Young children are at higher risk for TBI despite normal ED presentation. Risk factors for delayed complications from TBI are age 0–6 months, since they may lose a significant amount of blood into large scalp hematomas; large scalp swelling; high-energy mechanisms in particular locations (e.g., fall >1 m (3 ft) or more than three times the height of the child); or fractures crossing a suture or dural venous sinus, vascular groove, or extending into the posterior fossa.

Since the use of CT scans is associated with increased cost and risk of radiation exposure in children, clinical decision rules have been developed to decrease unnecessary CT scan exposure. While controversy exists, most decision rules suggest head CT scans for injured children with the following (Tables 143.2 and 143.3):

- age <2 years
- GCS score <15
- loss of consciousness >1 min
- depressed mental status
- presence of scalp bruising, swelling, or laceration (>5 cm) on the head
- open or depressed skull injury or signs of basilar skull fracture
- focal neurological deficits, vomiting, seizures
- dangerous mechanism of injury.

A recent prospective cohort study by the Pediatric Emergency Care Applied Research Network of 42 412 children in North America is the largest trial to date attempting to identify children at very low risk of clinically important brain injury after head trauma. The authors derived and validated decision rules to identify children above and below 2 years of age at very low risk of clinically important brain injury. The severity of the mechanism of injury was one factor in the analysis. Severe mechanisms were defined as:

- motor vehicle crash with patient ejection, death of another passenger, or rollover
- pedestrian or bicyclist without helmet struck by a motorized vehicle
- falls of >1.5 m (5 ft) for patients aged ≥2 years or >0.9 m (3 ft) for those <2 years
- head struck by a high impact object.

Mild mechanisms included ground-level falls or running into stationary objects; moderate covered any other mechanism.

The study listed six predictors for children >2 years of age for risk of brain injury:

- GCS score of 14, or other signs of altered mental status
- signs of basilar skull fracture

- history of loss of consciousness
- history of vomiting
- severe headache
- severe mechanism of injury (listed above).

Without any of the six predictors, the risk of brain injury was <0.05% with a negative predictive value of 99.95% and CT was not recommended. Patients with GCS score of 14 or any loss of consciousness and those with signs of basilar skull fracture had a 4.3% risk of traumatic brain injury and CT was recommended. Children with the other four predictors had a 0.9% risk and observation versus CT should be decided on the basis of other clinical factors (physician experience, worsening symptoms or signs after observation, and parental preference).

In children <2 years of age, an alternative set of six predictors were outlined:

- GCS score of 14 or other signs of altered mental status
- palpable skull fracture
- occipital or parietal or temporal scalp hematoma
- history of loss of consciousness ≥5 s
- severe mechanism of injury (listed above)
- not acting normally according to parent.

The risk of clinically important brain injury in those without these six predictors was <0.02%, with a negative predictive value of 99.9–100.0% and CT was not recommended. Patients with GCS score of 14 or ALOC and those with palpable skull fracture had a 4.4% risk of traumatic brain injury and CT was recommended. Those with the other four predictors had a 0.9% risk and observation versus CT should be decided on the basis of other clinical factors (those listed above plus age <3 months).

Disposition

Children with moderate and severe TBI should be admitted to the hospital. Children with remote injury, normal CT scan (if obtained), a normal examination in the ED, and reliable social situation may be safely discharged home with at least telephone follow-up within 24 h since they are at low risk for subsequent intracranial bleeding and neurologic sequelae. Indications for returning to hospital are persistent headache, increased drowsiness or confusion, vomiting, abnormal breathing, lethargy, or weakness. Some children may require observation in the ED. Hospital admission should be considered in some situations if there are concerns for associated injuries or an unsafe home environment, or simply concern for families residing far from the medical center with limited access to care.

Children with concussions secondary to sports injuries deserve special mention since this is an emerging area of investigation in TBI research. We believe even children with grade 1 concussions should not participate in sports until cleared by a sports or family physician who documents that they are asymptomatic, and the child can follow a stepwise symptom-limited program before return to play. The 2004 Prague sports concussion assessment tool offers a stepwise symptom-limited activity plan that ranges from no activity and mild rest to full game play after assessing the patient's signs, memory, symptom score, cognition, and conducting neurological screen. Although most children who suffer from mild TBI return to school, the long-term disability may be significant; this has not been fully characterized and is underappreciated.

Pearls and pitfalls

Pearls

1. Use the pediatric Glasgow Coma Scale score to evaluate severity of traumatic brain injury in children.
2. In children with mild TBI, the risks of unnecessary CT must be balanced against the need for imaging, particularly when the mechanism is unknown. Obtain head CT if severe mechanism, skull fracture, ALOC, and/or altered mental status.
3. Maintain systolic blood pressure higher than 5th percentile for age.

Pitfalls

1. Failure to stabilize the cervical spine.
2. Failure to prevent secondary insults, such as hypoxia or hypotension.
3. Failure to transfer a patient with moderate-to-severe traumatic brain injury to a pediatric trauma center.

Selected references

Adelson PD, Clyde B, Kochanek PM, *et al.* Cerebrovascular response in infants and young children following severe traumatic brain injury: a preliminary report. *Pediatr Neurosurg* 1997;**26**:200–207.

Adelson PD, Bratton SL, Carney NA, *et al.* Guidelines for the acute medical management of severe traumatic brain injury in infants, children, and adolescents. Ch. 4. Resuscitation of blood pressure and oxygenation and prehospital brain-specific therapies for the severe pediatric traumatic brain injury patient. *Pediatr Crit Care Med* 2003;**4**:S12–S18.

Adelson PD, Bratton SL, Carney NA, *et al.* Guidelines for the acute medical management of severe traumatic brain injury in infants, children, and adolescents. Ch. 12. Use of hyperventilation in the acute management of severe pediatric traumatic brain injury. *Pediatr Crit Care Med* 2003;**4**:S45.

Committee on Quality Improvement, American Academy of Pediatrics and Commission on Clinical Policies and Research, American Academy of Family Physicians. The management of minor closed head injury in children. *Pediatrics* 1999;**104**:1407–1415.

Keenan HT, Runyan DK, Marshall SW, *et al.* A population-based study of inflicted traumatic brain injury in young children. *JAMA* 2003;**290**:621–626.

Kuppermann N, Holmes JF, Dayan PS, for the Pediatric Emergency Care Applied Research Network (PECARN). Identification of children at very low risk of clinically important brain injuries after head trauma: a prospective cohort study. *Lancet* 2009;**374**:1160–1170.

Myburgh J, Cooper DJ, Finfer S, *et al.* Saline or albumin for fluid resuscitation in patients with traumatic brain injury. *N Engl J Med* 2007;**357**:874–884.

National Institute for Health and Clinical Excellence. *NICE Clinical Guideline No 56. Head Injury: Triage, Assessment, Investigation and Early Management of Head Injury in Infants, Children and Adults.* London: National Institute for Health and Clinical Excellence, 2007 www.Nice.org.uk/CG056 (accessed 28 April 2010).

Rutland-Brown W, Langlois JA, Thomas KE. *Traumatic Brain Injury in the United States: Emergency Department Visits, Hospitalizations, and Deaths*. Atlanta, GA: National Center for Injury Prevention and Control, Centers for Disease Control and Prevention, 2004.

Schutzman SA, Barnes P, Duhaime AC, *et al.* Evaluation and management of children younger than two years old with apparently minor head trauma: proposed guidelines. *Pediatrics* 2001;**107**:983–993.

Vavilala MS, Bowen A, Lam AM, *et al.* Blood pressure and outcome after severe pediatric traumatic brain injury. *J Trauma* 2003;**55**:1039–1044.

Chapter 144

Cervical spine injuries

Kirsten E. Mewaldt and Swaminatha V. Mahadevan

Introduction

Pediatric cervical spine injuries are quite rare. Of the 11 000 new cases of spinal cord injury each year, fewer than 16% occur in individuals ≤18 years of age (Spinal Cord Injury Information Network). Spinal cord injuries may be caused by various mechanisms. Motor vehicle collisions (47%) are the leading cause, followed by falls, acts of violence (e.g., gunshot wounds), and recreational sports. Although pediatric cervical spine injuries are uncommon, a missed or delayed diagnosis may have devastating consequences for both the patient and the parents. The challenge is to correctly identify these injured patients while minimizing their radiation exposure from diagnostic imaging. This chapter will review the evaluation and management of children at risk for cervical spine injury.

Anatomy

Anatomic differences between the cervical spines of adults and children influence the types of injury sustained by these two populations. The spine of a growing child does not take on adult characteristics until preadolescence (about 8 years of age). Distinguishing characteristics of preadolescent cervical spines include:

- anatomic fulcrum between C2 and C3
- relative ligamentous laxity
- comparatively large head with underdeveloped neck musculature
- incomplete ossification
- horizontal orientation of the shallow facet joints
- anterior wedging of the vertebral bodies.

Preadolescent children (≤8 years) tend to sustain upper cervical spine (C1–C3) injuries secondary to an anatomic fulcrum at C2–C3, while adolescents and adults are predisposed to lower cervical spine injuries (C5–C7) as the anatomic fulcrum is at C5–C6. Children are prone to hyperextension and hyperflexion injuries (because of the greater elasticity of their cervical spine), subluxation (made more likely by the horizontal orientation of articular facets), and fractures (secondary to the weakness of cartilaginous structures compared with ligaments).

Clinical presentation

History

Children with cervical spine injuries may complain of neck pain, spasm, or pain with movement. Patients with a cervical spine injury and an accompanying painful, distracting injury (e.g., femur fracture) may not experience neck pain. Always suspect occult cervical spine injury in patients who are unconscious, have ALOC, or are intoxicated. The spectrum of symptoms associated with spinal cord injuries ranges from subtle neurologic deficits to clear paralysis. Patients may describe numbness, tingling, paresthesiae, or focal weakness. Symptoms may be transient or complete. Complaints of either urinary or fecal retention or incontinence are concerning.

Physical examination

Patients with cervical spine injury may exhibit tenderness of the cervical spine upon palpation. Signs of spinal cord injury include impaired motor/sensory function and abnormal deep tendon reflexes. Other concerning signs include diaphragmatic breathing, neurogenic shock (hypotension and bradycardia), priapism, ileus, abnormal rectal tone, temperature instability, Horner syndrome, and clonus without rigidity.

Patients with spinal cord injury without radiologic abnormality (SCIWORA) may present with profound or progressive paralysis; however, these symptoms may be delayed up to 48 h following injury. Transient symptoms such paresthesiae in the hands and legs, subjective feelings of generalized weakness, and L'ermitte phenomenon (shock-like sensation shooting down the spine with the neck movement) should raise suspicion for a spinal cord injury. Admission and serial examinations may be necessary.

Patients with occult cervical spine injuries (e.g., subtle fractures, ligamentous disruption) may not experience neck

A Practical Guide to Pediatric Emergency Medicine: Caring for Children in the Emergency Department, ed. N. Ewen Amieva-Wang (associate eds. Jamie Shandro, Aparajita Sohoni, and Bernhard Fassl). Published by Cambridge University Press.

pain until they attempt to range (flex, extend or rotate) their neck. Patients who are awake and alert will typically stop any neck movement when they experience pain. Physicians should never manipulate (e.g., passively range) a patient's neck, as a serious injury can occur in the absence of this protective mechanism.

A child's inability to perceive pain, as a result of a spinal cord injury, may mask other potentially serious injuries elsewhere in the body. Look for occult injuries in high-risk regions, such as the abdomen, and other areas of the body that exhibit swelling or bruising.

Identifying signs of cervical spine injury is particularly challenging in young children (particularly preverbal), who may not be able to describe their pain or response to palpation of their spine. Neck injuries are more likely to go undiagnosed in such children. A child with inconsolable crying following trauma should also raise suspicion for a cervical spine injury.

Differential diagnosis

Until the diagnosis of cervical spine injury can be excluded, physicians should assume the worst and take the necessary precautions.

Specific cervical spine injuries occurring in children include:

- occipitoatlantal dislocation
- atlas fractures
- atlantoaxial injuries
- os odontoideum
- hangman's fracture
- atlantoaxial rotary subluxation.

However, the differential diagnosis for neck pain in a trauma patient is not limited to just vertebral, ligamentous, and spinal cord injuries; a broader differential should also be considered.

Burner or stinger. A cervical root or brachial plexus injury resulting from stretching or compression of the nerves usually in the C5–C6 distribution. The injury is typically associated with immediate pain followed by burning along the affected arm. Patients may also have a transient paresis with an ill-defined area of decreased sensation. The radicular symptoms usually resolve within 5–10 min but the local tenderness remains. Unlike a spinal cord injury, which affects multiple limbs, a "burner" affects just one extremity.

Carotid artery dissection. Stretching of the carotid artery over the cervical vertebrae leads to a tear following high-impact trauma or rapid deceleration. Patients are at risk for stroke from thromboembolism or stenosis. Patients typically present with neck pain. Focal neurologic symptoms, such as hemiparesis or cranial nerve deficits, are usually delayed. Despite hemiparesis, patients may be awake and alert. Seat belt injury (ecchymosis of the neck from the shoulder strap) is a risk factor. Angiography using CT or MRI is diagnostic.

Cervical strain (whiplash). An abrupt force to the neck (as experienced in rapid deceleration injury) leads to strain of the neck musculature and/or sprain of cervical ligamentous structures. Patients present with pain on movement of the neck, typically worsening in the hours following the trauma. On examination, patients typically have reproducible paraspinal or midline tenderness spanning multiple vertebral levels.

Intravertebral disc herniation. The disc may impinge on a spinal nerve root leading to focal spinal or radicular pain. Some disc herniations may exert pressure on the spinal cord (i.e., SCIWORA).

Ligamentous disruption. An unstable spinal column may result without associated injury to the vertebrae or spinal cord. Conventional imaging (radiograph, CT) may reveal abnormal subluxation, angulation, or uncovering of facet joints, but may also appear completely normal despite the injury. Awake patients will typically complain of focal neck pain and restricted motion. Obtunded, impaired, or distracted patients should remain in their cervical collar until the diagnosis can be excluded.

Spinal cord injury. Typically, spinal cord injury presents with neck pain and neurologic deficits; however, symptoms may be transient or subjective, and signs may be delayed. Patients with complete spinal cord injury have no demonstrable motor or sensory function below the level of injury whereas patients with incomplete injury have motor function, sensation, or both, partially present below the level of the injury.

SCIWORA. Children, particularly preadolescent patients, are at risk for SCIWORA, condition first described in the pediatric population. It results from flexion, extension, or distraction forces that produce hypermobility of the spinal column, leading to injury to the spinal cord without vertebral fracture or subluxation. Patients experience immediate or delayed (up to 48 h) neurological symptoms such as paresthesiae or weakness. These injuries, while not visible on CT or plain film, are visible on MRI.

Vertebral fracture. Typically, the fracture presents with neck pain associated with significant midline spinal tenderness on palpation. Associated findings include spinal soft tissue swelling, ecchymosis, or step-off misalignment of the spine.

Diagnostic studies

Imaging

While deciding whether to image the cervical spine or the "clinically clear" patient, it must always be ensured that the patient's spine is protected until injuries can be identified or excluded. The National Emergency X-Radiography Utilization

Study (NEXUS) derived a set of five clinical criteria that can be used to identify low-risk patients who do not need cervical spine imaging; patients meeting all five criteria do not require diagnostic imaging:

- absence of a focal neurologic deficit
- no midline cervical spine tenderness
- normal level of alertness
- no evidence of intoxication with alcohol or drugs
- absence of a clinically apparent injury that could distract the patient from the pain of a cervical spine injury.

Care should exercised when applying the NEXUS criteria to young children, particularly those <2 years of age.

Imaging studies (i.e., plain films, CT) are frequently utilized to identify the presence of vertebral column fractures or spinal instability. Advantages of plain film radiography are wide availability, reduced radiation risk and low cost. Cervical spine plain films should include three views: antero-posterior, lateral (with visualization of the C7–T1 junction), and open-mouth (or odontoid). The open mouth (odontoid) view is difficult to obtain in uncooperative children and can be replaced with CT of C1 and C2. A systematic approach to evaluating cervical spine plain films is crucial to identifying subtle abnormalities (see Ch. 148). Advantages of CT compared with plain films include improved accuracy (sensitivity 98% versus 53%) and rapid diagnosis; the disadvantages are greater expense and higher radiation doses (14× the radiation to the thyroid). The prudent approach is to utilize CT for patients at high risk for cervical spine injury. Any of the following factors increases risk:

- high-risk mechanisms of injury
- suspected head injury or ALOC
- significant head or neck trauma
- multisystem trauma (including pelvic or extremity fractures)
- neck pain, focal neck tenderness or physical signs of neck trauma
- neurologic symptoms (even transient) or abnormal neurologic examination
- unreliable examination because of intoxication or substance abuse
- preverbal children or those too young to express pain
- inconsolable children.

While CT is the preferred adjunct to plain films for the identification of bony injuries, MRI can visualize soft tissue structures including the intervertebral discs, ligaments, and spinal cord. Indications for MRI include complete or incomplete neurologic deficits associated with fracture or subluxation, neurologic deficits not explained by CT or plain films (e.g., SCIWORA), deterioration of neurologic function, and suspicion of ligamentous injury.

In pediatric patients with suspected ligamentous injury and normal imaging, flexion–extension plain films can evaluate vertebral column stability. The patient must be awake, alert, without neurologic deficits, and able to actively flex and extend the neck 30 degrees. Vertebral body subluxation, angulation or focal widening between the posterior elements suggests an unstable ligamentous injury. No serious adverse outcomes have resulted from voluntary neck movement by an awake, alert, cooperative pediatric patient without neurologic deficits. However, the inability to adequately flex and extend (from muscle spasm) could lead to false negative results.

Management

The first priority in managing acute cervical spine injury is protecting the spine and spinal cord from further injury. Placement of a rigid cervical collar and immobilization (in the supine, neutral position) on a long spinal board are the first steps. The standard adult backboard is not appropriate for young children as it allows flexion of the cervical spine secondary to the child's large head and small chest. This potentially harmful flexion can be avoided by using a modified backboard with a cutout beneath the occiput or a standard pediatric backboard with a thickened mattress pad under the body. In infants <6 months, using a spine board with tape across the forehead and blankets or towels around the neck is appropriate. In infants ≥6 months of age, the head can be immobilized in the manner described above or by using a small rigid pediatric cervical collar. Children >8 years of age require a medium-sized cervical collar. It should be noted that many children come in from the field with the cervical spine inadequately protected. Appropriate cervical spine immobilization should be maintained or attained during the initial ABCs.

The logroll maneuver may be employed to prevent aspiration in the vomiting child, to allow examination of the back, and to facilitate patient removal from the spinal board. For patients who require endotracheal intubation, in-line cervical immobilization (not traction) can prevent extension of the head during laryngoscopy.

Children able to cooperate with the examination (usually >3 years of age) who also conform to the NEXUS criteria are candidates for clinical clearance of the cervical spine. Unfasten the cervical collar and carefully palpate the patient's cervical spine without flexing the neck. In the absence of significant midline tenderness, ask the patient to actively lift the head off the gurney and range the neck by looking right, left, caudad, and cephalad. In a younger child, release the collar and watch if the patient will spontaneously move the neck or look around. If the patient is able to do so without significant pain or the development of neurological symptoms, the patient's neck is considered "clinically cleared." The collar may be removed and no imaging is required.

A patient with persistent neck pain, a normal neurologic examination, and normal CT might still have unstable cervical ligamentous injury. The diagnosis may be established by MRI or flexion–extension plain films. Alternatively, cooperative patients can be discharged with a semi-rigid cervical collar (e.g., Aspen or Philadelphia collar) and asked to return in 7–10 days for delayed flexion–extension radiographs.

All confirmed or suspected cervical spinal cord injuries mandate immediate spine subspecialty consultation. Serial neurologic examinations can identify neurologic improvement or deterioration. Early endotracheal intubation should be considered for patients with cervical spinal cord injury, as paralysis of the respiratory muscles and respiratory failure can rapidly ensue. Neurogenic shock (hypotension, relative bradycardia) may be treated with vasopressors and atropine. Surgical reduction of the displaced spinal column and decompression of the spinal cord has been associated with recovery from otherwise devastating spinal cord injuries. The optimal timing of surgery following a spinal injury remains controversial. The sole absolute indication for immediate surgery is a progressively worsening neurologic status in patients with spinal fracture/dislocations who initially present with incomplete or absent neurologic deficits

The use of corticosteroid therapy for children with acute spinal cord injury has been extrapolated from the National Acute Spinal Cord Injury Study (NASCIS), which did not include any patients <14 years. Unfortunately, no studies have evaluated utility of steroids in pediatric spinal cord injury. The dosage of methylprednisolone sodium succinate recommended is:

loading dose: 30 mg/kg over 15 min
infusion following this: 5.4 mg/kg per h; continued for 23 h (in patients treated within 3 h of injury) or 48 h (for patients treated 3–8 h after injury).

There is no benefit from steroids administered more than 8 h after injury, and steroid therapy is not indicated for penetrating injuries. Given the limited potential benefits and possibility for adverse affects (GI bleeding, wound infections, sepsis, pneumonia), the use of steroids for blunt traumatic spinal cord injury should not be initiated without subspecialist consultation and approval.

All diagnoses of cervical ligamentous injuries and vertebral fractures warrant spine subspecialty consultation. Management depends on the type of injury and stability of the vertebral column. In general, partial ligamentous injuries and stable fractures (e.g., spinous process, transverse process) do not lead to spinal column instability. If the spine is stable, treatment is largely supportive (i.e., pain control and physical therapy). In contrast, unstable fractures and/or complete ligamentous injury may require surgery, placement of a halo, or another form of extended spinal immobilization.

Most patients with traumatic neck pain are diagnosed with cervical strain, a benign diagnosis with an excellent prognosis. Neck pain typically worsens over the first day or two secondary to muscle spasm and can last up to a month. A combination of NSAIDs, narcotic analgesics, and muscle relaxants is typically prescribed. Gentle range of motion exercises (as tolerated) should be encouraged. Soft cervical collars do not hasten recovery and may promote stiffness.

Disposition

Children with traumatic cervical spine fractures require spine subspecialty consultation (neurosurgeon or orthopedist) and admission to the hospital if they have intractable pain, an unstable fracture pattern, or potential for development of a spinal cord injury. Any child with a significant mechanism of injury and neurologic symptoms (transient or complete) requires early spine subspecialty consultation and admission. This may require patient transfer to a spine specialty center. The level of spinal cord injury, associated deficits, and other injuries will determine the patient level of care (ICU, neurosurgical observation unit, or general ward). All obtunded, impaired, or otherwise critically ill trauma patients should be admitted to the hospital and remain in their cervical collar.

Patients with stable cervical spine injuries (fractures, ligamentous sprain) may be discharged home after consultation with a spine subspecialist. Awake, alert, neurologically intact patients with negative imaging and persistent neck pain may still harbor an unstable ligamentous injury; these patients should be discharged home in a semi-rigid cervical collar until definitive imaging can exclude an injury. All discharged patients should be warned about signs and symptoms of spinal cord injury, and reasons to return to the ED.

Pearls and pitfalls

Pearls

1. Significant anatomic differences between pediatric and adult cervical spines predispose children to unique patterns of injury.
2. Often, a high-risk mechanism identified by history is the first suggestion of a possible cervical spine injury.
3. The differential for neck pain in a trauma patient is not limited to spinal injury; however, cervical spine precautions should be maintained while the workup is completed.

Pitfalls

1. Failure to pay special attention to preverbal children as there are higher rates of missed injuries in this difficult to examine population.
2. Failure to consider that normal variants in cervical spines of preadolescent children can take on the appearance of injuries.
3. Failure to consider that neurologic symptoms may be delayed in spinal cord injury without radiologic abnormality (SCIWORA).

Selected references

Bonadio WA. Cervical spine trauma in children: part I. General concepts, normal anatomy, radiographic evaluation. *Am J Emerg Med* 1993;**11**:158–165.

Bonadio WA. Cervical spine trauma in children: part II. Mechanisms and manifestations of injury, therapeutic considerations. *Am J Emerg Med* 1993;**11**:256–278.

Bracken MB. Steroids for acute spinal cord injury. *Cochrane Database Systemat Rev* 2002;(3):CD001046.

Bracken MB, Shepard MJ, Collins, WF, *et al.* A randomized, controlled trial of methylprednisolone or nalaxone in the treatment of acute spinal-cord injury. Results of the Second National Acute Spinal Cord Injury Study. *N Engl J Med* 1990;**322**:1405–1411.

Bracken MB, Shepard MJ, Collins, WF, *et al.* Administration of methylprednisolone for 24 or 48 hours or tirilazad mesylate for 48 hours in the treatment of acute spinal cord injury. Results of the Third National Acute Spinal Cord Injury Randomized Controlled Trial. *JAMA* 1997;**277**:1597–1604.

Buhs C, Cullen M, Klein M, Farmer D. The pediatric trauma C-spine: is the "odontoid" view necessary? *J Pediatr Surg* 2000;**35**:994–997.

Congress of Neurological Surgeons. Management of pediatric cervical spine and spinal cord injuries. *Neurosurgery* 2002;**50** (Suppl.):S85–S99.

Dormans JP. Evaluation of children with suspected cervical spine injury. *J Bone Joint Surg* 2002;**84A**:123–132.

Eleraky MA, Theodore N, Adams M, Rekate HL, Sonntag VK. Pediatric cervical spine injuries: report of 102 cases and review of the literature. *J Neurosurg Spine* 2000;**92**:12–17.

Eubanks JD, Gilmore A, Bess S, Cooperman DR. Clearing the pediatric cervical spine following injury. *J Am Acad Orthoped Surg* 2006;**14**:552–564.

Herzenberg, RN, Hensinger RN, Dedrick DK, Phillips WA. Emergency transport and positioning of young children who have an injury of the cervical spine. The standard Backboard may be hazardous. *J Bone Joint Surg* 1989;**71**:15–22.

Hoffman JR, Mower W, Wolfson AB, Todd KH, Zucker MI, *et al.* Validity of a set of clinical criteria to rule out injury to the cervical spine in patients with blunt trauma. *N Engl J Med* 2000;**343**:94–99.

Lin M, Mahadevan SV. Spine trauma and spinal cord injury: In Adams J (ed.) *Emergency Medicine: Expert Consult.* Philadelphia, PA: Saunders, 2008, pp. 765–781.

Mahadevan SV, Navarro M. Evaluation and clearance of the cervical spine in adult trauma patients: clinical concepts, controversies and advances: part 1. *Trauma Rep* 2004;**5**:1–10.

Mahadevan SV, Navarro M. Evaluation and clearance of the cervical spine in adult trauma patients: clinical concepts, controversies and advances: part 2. *Trauma Rep* 2004;**5**:11–12.

Norman C, Lopez BL. Pediatric C-spine injury. *Crit Decision Emerg Med* 2007;**21**:2–8.

Pang D, Pollack IF. Spinal cord injury without radiographic abnormality in children: the SCIWORA syndrome. *J Trauma* 1989;**29**:654–664.

Ralston M, Chung K, Barnes PD, Emans JB, Schutzman SA. Role of flexion–extension radiographs in blunt pediatric cervical spine injury. *Acad Emerg Med* 2001;**8**:237–245.

Spinal Cord Injury Information Network. *Facts and Stats: 2006 NSCISC Statistical Annual Report.* Birmingham, AL: University of Alabama, 2007 www.spinalcord.uab.edu (accessed December 15, 2007).

Viccellio P, Simon H, Pressman BD, for the NEXUS Group. A prospective multicenter study of cervical spine injury in children. *Pediatrics* 2001;**108**:e20.

Woods WA. Pediatric cervical spine injuries: avoiding potential diaster. *Trauma Rep.* 2003:**4**:1–17.

Chapter

145 Chest and abdominal trauma

Katrina Leone and Michael A. Gisondi

Introduction

According to the National Trauma Data Bank *Pediatric Report 2007*, 16.4% of pediatric traumatic incidents result in injury to the chest or abdomen, with >85% of these injuries caused by blunt mechanisms. The injuries sustained can be exceptionally variable and are dependent upon the mechanism of injury, the amount of force applied, and the size of the patient. The goal of this chapter is to provide a thorough differential diagnosis for chest and abdominal injuries based upon the mechanism of injury. It will also review data for diagnostic testing utilized in the evaluation of traumatized children and discuss management considerations for commonly encountered injuries.

Differential diagnosis

Because of the multitude of injuries that may be sustained as a consequence of trauma to the chest or abdomen, it is helpful to have a framework of possible injuries to utilize when creating a differential diagnosis. Often, patients are initially categorized by the mechanism of their injury, because blunt and penetrating mechanisms typically create different patterns of trauma. With blunt injuries, force is distributed over a wider area of the child's body, resulting in multiple or widespread injuries. Pediatric patients are more vulnerable to injuries from blunt abdominal trauma than adults, because the immature pediatric axial skeleton and abdominal musculature cause the liver, spleen, and bladder to be less protected (Table 145.1).

Diagnostic studies

Studies regularly performed in the course of an evaluation for trauma include chest and pelvis radiographs and a focused abdominal sonography in trauma (FAST) examination. Secondary studies include CT of the chest, abdomen and pelvis; laboratory testing; and organ-specific evaluations. Where there is a significant mechanism of injury or concerning physical examination findings, the algorithm for imaging is quite standard: chest and/or pelvis plain film, followed by FAST examination, then CT. The utilization of other secondary studies should be based upon the suspicion for specific injuries, as described in Table 145.1. Diagnostic testing is only indicated when the child is hemodynamically stable and should not delay prompt operative exploration when indicated.

Chest radiography

Chest radiography is a commonly utilized diagnostic test in pediatric chest trauma. Indications for chest radiograph include both blunt and penetrating chest trauma, particularly in the setting of abnormal vital signs, complaints of chest pain or shortness of breath, and abnormal chest examination findings. When evaluating a pediatric chest radiograph, it is

Table 145.1. Differential diagnosis of blunt thoracic and abdominal injuries

Mechanism of injury	Structures at risk	Diagnostic studies
Deceleration	Thoracic aorta, mesenteric attachments	Chest radiograph, FAST, CT chest and abdomen, echocardiogram
Direct blow to chest	Ribs, sternum, lung parenchyma, heart	Chest radiograph, FAST, ECG, CT chest
Direct blow to abdomen	Liver, spleen, pancreas, kidneys, small and large bowel, pelvis, bladder, urethra	Pelvic radiograph, FAST, CT abdomen and pelvis, urinalysis, laboratory testing
Seatbelt sign	Lumbar spine (Chance fractures), small and large bowel	CT abdomen, pelvis, spine; lumbar spine radiographs, CT

FAST, focused abdominal sonography in trauma.

A Practical Guide to Pediatric Emergency Medicine: Caring for Children in the Emergency Department, ed. N. Ewen Amieva-Wang (associate eds. Jamie Shandro, Aparajita Sohoni, and Bernhard Fassl). Published by Cambridge University Press.

important to remember the differences between the pediatric and adult skeleton.

The pediatric chest wall is highly flexible, so it is possible for lung parenchymal injury to occur in blunt chest trauma without evidence of overlying bony fractures.

Rib or sternal fractures seen on radiography are then suggestive of a significant blunt force applied to the chest wall.

Pelvis radiography

Pelvis radiography is used routinely in the evaluation of adult trauma but is less commonly used in the evaluation of pediatric trauma.

Traumatic fractures of the pelvis occur with less frequency in the setting of blunt trauma in children than in adults because ossification is incomplete and the pediatric pelvis is more flexible.

Pelvic radiographs are reserved for significant blunt trauma with concerns for fracture based upon the mechanism of injury, findings of pelvic instability or tenderness on examination. When interpreting pediatric pelvic radiographs, it is important to look for symmetry and compare any sites of abnormal lucency with the contralateral side to avoid mistaking incomplete ossification for fracture.

Focused abdominal sonography in trauma

A FAST examination has become an important tool in early evaluation of trauma to the abdomen since its conception in the 1970s. It was initially utilized for adult trauma, but it is slowly being utilized for pediatric trauma as well. The goal of FAST is to search for evidence of free peritoneal or pericardial fluid, presumed to be blood, in the setting of trauma. The indications for performing FAST include blunt or penetrating injury to the abdomen and penetrating injury to the chest with concern for pericardial effusion. Studies in children have shown that FAST is helpful for the identification of significant intraperitoneal fluid requiring exploratory laparotomy in hemodynamically unstable patients. The utility of FAST is more uncertain in hemodynamically stable children. With parenchymal injuries to the liver, spleen, and kidneys often managed conservatively in hemodynamically stable children, a positive FAST examination in this setting may not alter management or alleviate the need for further diagnostic evaluation with CT of the abdomen and pelvis. Also, for patients with significant abdominal tenderness, a negative FAST examination does not alleviate the need for further evaluation. The examination is performed similarly in adults and children (Ch. 147).

Computed tomography

The regular utilization of CT began in the early 1980s and it has become an integral diagnostic test for evaluation of children and adults with traumatic injuries to the chest and abdomen. In many studies of trauma, CT is now used as the gold standard for comparison of other diagnostic tests. Chest CT is indicated for any hemodynamically stable child with significant blunt or penetrating injury to the chest that is not adequately evaluated with chest radiography. Likewise, CT of the abdomen and pelvis is indicated for hemodynamically stable children with blunt or low velocity penetrating abdominal trauma in the setting of a concerning mechanism of injury or abdominal tenderness on examination. It is particularly reliable for identifying injuries to solid abdominal organs, lung parenchyma, and bony structures. It is limited in its ability to identify diaphragmatic or mesenteric injuries.

In light of increasing awareness that pediatric radiation exposure has the potential to cause future malignancy, the question of whether or not to image with CT is less clear. Figure 145.1 illustrates a sample algorithm for imaging in blunt abdominal trauma. Children with stable vital signs and a reassuring physical examination following minor abdominal trauma may be observed or discharged with close follow-up without performing CT.

Diagnostic peritoneal lavage

Diagnostic peritoneal lavage is a test historically used to assess for free peritoneal fluid in the setting of blunt and penetrating abdominal trauma:

- red blood cell count >100 000 cells/ml: positive for blunt abdominal trauma/stab wound to anterior abdomen
- red blood cell count >10 000 cells/ml: positive for gunshot wounds to the abdomen/stab wound to back or flank
- frank bowel contents or fluid significantly positive for amylase or lipase: positive regardless of mechanism of injury.

This technique has been supplanted by FAST, which provides similar information about free abdominal fluid but is non-invasive.

Laboratory testing

Routine use of a panel of laboratory tests is rarely helpful for diagnosing traumatic injuries in the acute setting because of the slow turn around time and low sensitivity and specificity. In the critically injured child, it is important to quickly obtain a blood type and cross-match in order to start type-specific blood transfusion. It is also helpful to send samples for hemoglobin and hematocrit levels, as these values help to establish a baseline that can then be followed during the course of non-operative management for blunt abdominal organ injuries. In blunt liver injury, elevation of AST or ALT >400 IU/l on initial laboratory assessment has been shown to correlate with significant injury, although smaller elevations of these laboratory values are neither sensitive nor specific for significant liver lacerations. Elevation of amylase or lipase is not sensitive for the identification of pancreatic injury immediately after blunt abdominal trauma but is highly specific. The low sensitivity causes these tests to have little utility to assist physicians with the decision to perform CT imaging of the abdomen. Performing a urinalysis to assess for hematuria is an important component of the evaluation of genitourinary trauma.

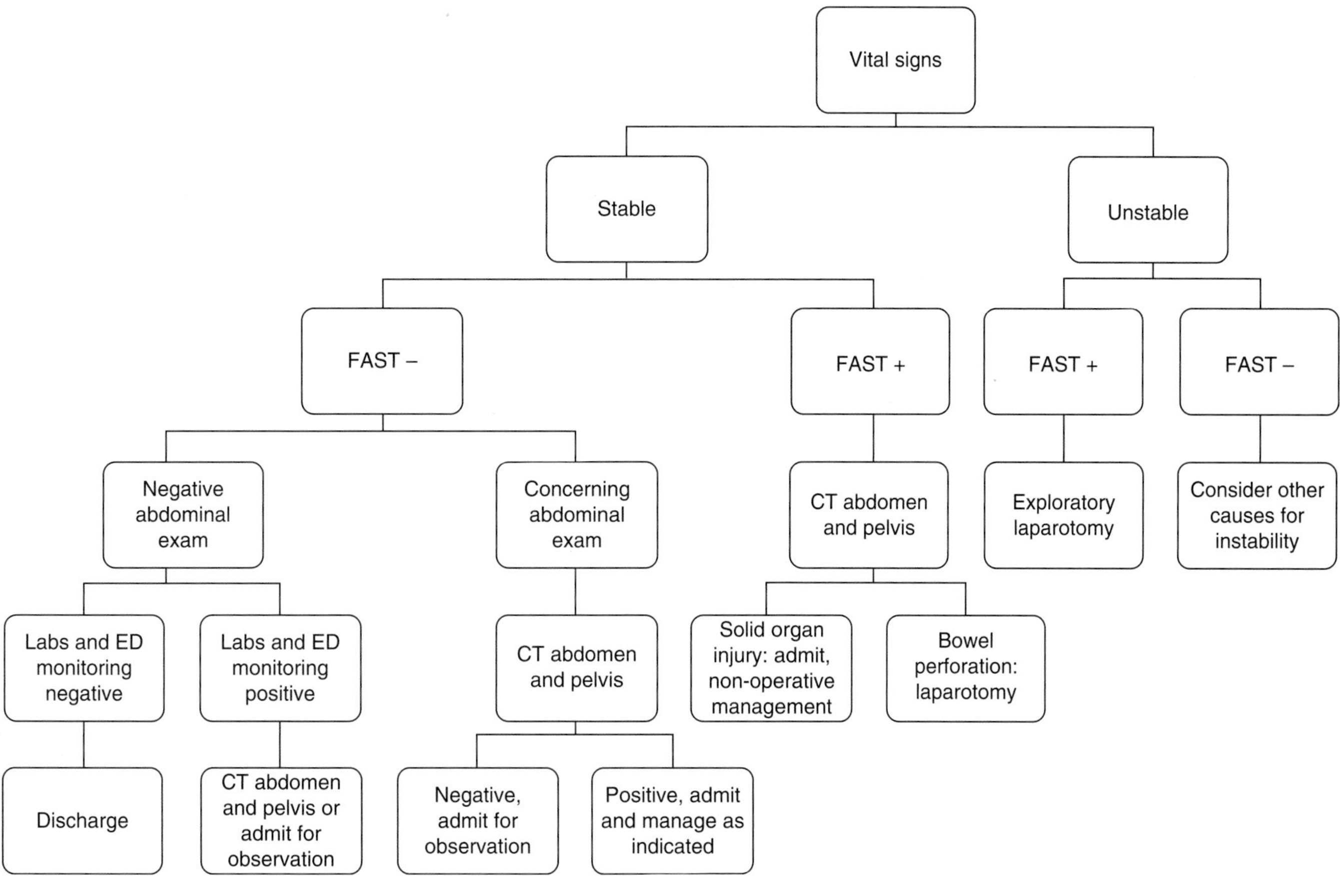

Figure 145.1 Algorithm for imaging and disposition in blunt abdominal trauma. Imaging and disposition decisions hinge upon whether vital signs are stable or unstable, if the FAST (focused abdominal sonography in trauma) is positive or negative, and the abdominal examination. Unstable vital signs with positive FAST indicate exploratory laparotomy; unstable vital signs with negative FAST warrant consideration of other causes of instability such as retroperitoneal bleeding or intrathoracic injury. Stable vital signs and positive FAST indicate further imaging with CT of the abdomen and pelvis; Stable vital signs, negative FAST and concerning abdominal examination indicate further imaging with CT of abdomen and pelvis; Stable vital signs, negative FAST, and negative abdominal exam indicate further assessment and disposition based upon these results.

Management of chest injuries

Rib fractures

Rib fractures are uncommon, but because of the flexibility of the pediatric skeleton, fractures of the ribs, clavicles, or sternum suggest that significant force was applied to the chest wall. Rib fractures are managed similarly in children and adults. Analgesia and deep breathing maneuvers or incentive spirometry (to discourage atelectasis and pneumonia) are the hallmarks of management.

Hemothorax and pneumothorax

Hemothorax results from both blunt and penetrating injury to the lung parenchyma or to intrathoracic vessels. Possible causes of copious thoracic bleeding include laceration of an intercostal or internal mammary artery, or a pulmonary hilum injury. On chest radiography, a hemothorax has the appearance of a densely radiopaque pleural effusion. Pneumothorax is a commonly encountered complication of chest trauma that results from the puncture or rupture of the lung parenchyma. Small or anterior pneumothoraces can be missed on physical examination but are often identified on chest radiography, ultrasonography, or CT.

Needle thoracostomy to decompress a possible tension pneumothorax is indicated in patients with diminished breath sounds in the setting of hemodynamic instability. The procedure is similar to that in adults. Drainage of a hemothorax is with a 14- or 16-gauge angiocatheter inserted into the second intercostal space in the mid-clavicular line.

Tube thoracostomy procedure

Placement of a chest tube, also known as tube thoracostomy, is indicated for a significant pneumothorax or hemothorax in the setting of chest trauma. Any traumatic pneumothorax associated with respiratory failure requiring mechanical ventilation should be managed with the placement of a chest tube because of the risk for transformation into a tension

Table 145.2. Chest tube size by weight[a]

Patient weight (kg)	Chest tube size (F)
3–9	10–12
10–11	16–20
12–18	20–24
19–22	24–32
24–28	28–32
>30	32–38

[a]Weight-based sizes can also be found on the equipment section of a pediatric emergency tape.

pneumothorax after the application of positive pressure ventilation. In the non-intubated patient, chest tube placement depends upon the size of the pneumothorax and the hemodynamic stability of the patient. A chest tube should be placed for moderate to large pneumothoraces and in any hemodynamically unstable patient with a known pneumothorax or hemothorax. An open pneumothorax (sucking chest wound) requires placement of a chest tube in a site separate from the open wound and a dressing placed over the open wound itself.

Tube thoracostomy in children is more challenging than in adults because procedural sedation, rather than just local anesthesia, may be required. Table 145.2 lists suggested tube sizes based upon a child's weight. Although a smaller sized tube can be used for a simple pneumothorax, in the setting of trauma, a larger tube size should be used to ensure adequate drainage of a hemothorax without tube clogging. Just as in adults, chest tubes in the setting of trauma are placed at the anterior axillary line at the level of the 4th intercostal space.

Indication for operative thoracic exploration is immediate return of >20% of the child's estimated blood volume through the chest tube or more than 2 ml/kg per h of persistent bleeding. In a 10 kg child, with an estimated blood volume of 700–800 ml, loss of 140–160 ml indicates need for surgical intervention.

Tracheobronchial tree injuries

Tracheal and bronchial injuries have the potential for significant morbidity and mortality. These injuries result in pneumothoraces with air leak refractory to chest tube placement, pneumomediastinum, or subcutaneous emphysema. Minor tracheobronchial tears can occasionally be treated conservatively, but successfully, with chest tube, IV antibiotics, and placement of an endotrachial tube distal to the injury to preserve ventilation. Successful conservative management is rare, limited to case reports in the literature. Bronchoscopy can be used for evaluation of suspected tracheobronchial injuries.

Pulmonary contusion

Patients with pulmonary contusion can present with a broad spectrum of symptoms, ranging from asymptomatic to severe respiratory distress. A pulmonary contusion is defined as a focal infiltrate in a defined lung area, consistent with blood and edema filling the alveolar spaces. Radiographic evidence of contusion often lags behind the clinical symptoms and may take 24 to 48 h to become fully defined. Significant contusions seen on initial chest radiograph often result in tachypnea, hypoxia, or respiratory distress; these should be managed supportively. Small contusions, not visible by X-ray but found on CT, do not significantly increase mortality in patients who are without signs of respiratory distress.

Blunt cardiac injury

Chest trauma has the potential to cause a variety of pediatric cardiac and aortic injuries. Pediatric blunt cardiac injury ranges in severity from arrhythmia to valvular insufficiency to severe pump failure. The diagnostic criteria for blunt cardiac injury are not well defined but have been described in the literature to include clinical or radiographic evidence of heart failure, new heart murmur, new ECG conduction abnormality or arrhythmia, abnormal echocardiographic findings, or elevated cardiac enzyme levels in the setting of a blunt traumatic mechanism. For children who present in normal sinus rhythm with normal vital signs after blunt cardiac injury, the risk of decompensation is low. If significant cardiac injury has occurred, unstable vital signs or physical examination findings are apparent on initial presentation.

Blunt cardiac injury is managed supportively. Supraventricular and ventricular arrhythmias should be managed as described by the American Heart Association's Pediatric Advanced Life Support (PALS) protocol. Telemetry monitoring to observe for recurrence of arrhythmia is recommended for children initially presenting with a rhythm disturbance. The ECG should be used to identify new conduction abnormalities when suspected. Echocardiography is useful for identifying new valve dysfunction or quantifying the extent of new pump failure.

In addition to cardiac injuries, blunt chest trauma can result in traumatic injury to the thoracic aorta. This injury most often results from motor vehicle collisions with a rapid deceleration mechanism, but it is much more commonly seen in adults. Confirmatory diagnostic testing includes CT chest or transesophageal echocardiography. Initial management includes fluid resuscitation to lower heart rate and prevent expansion of the injury. The majority of children with aortic injuries will require endovascular graft or surgical repair.

Penetrating cardiac injury

Penetrating chest trauma may result in laceration or puncture of the myocardium, which has the potential to induce tamponade physiology or massive hemothorax. If the FAST examination is positive for pericardial effusion in the setting of chest trauma, the fluid should be assumed to be blood until proven otherwise, even in a hemodynamically stable patient. If tamponade physiology is present, an emergency pericardiocentesis is performed. The procedure for pericardiocentisis is similar in adults and children. All patients with positive cardiac FAST or need for pericardiocentisis should have operative exploration of the heart and pericardium to assess for injuries.

Management of abdominal injuries

Solid organ injury

The spleen and liver are the most commonly injured abdominal organs after blunt abdominal trauma.

Non-operative management of blunt solid organ injury has become the standard of care for hemodynamically stable children.

Non-operative management decreases hospital length of stay and avoids the risk of overwhelming post-splenectomy infection. A typical protocol for non-operative management includes bed rest, serial abdominal examinations for signs of peritonitis, and serial hematocrit and vital sign monitoring for evidence of hemorrhage. These children should then have followed by delayed return to activities and contact sports. Transfer to a designated pediatric trauma center increases the success rate of non-operative management after solid organ injury. Failure of non-operative management for blunt solid organ injury is approximately 5% at designated level 1 pediatric trauma centers. Failure of non-operative management increases with increasing grades of organ injury and with multiple solid organ injuries. The majority of patients failing non-operative management do so quickly, with a peak time to failure at 4 h post-admission. Spleen and liver lacerations are radiographically graded I–IV, and as the grade of laceration increases, so does the length of healing time and the longer the recommended delay in return to contact activities. The mortality associated with isolated liver injury is higher than that for isolated spleen injury, and injury to multiple intra-abdominal organs further increases mortality. The American Pediatric Surgical Association Committee on Trauma recommends activity restriction for up to 6 weeks in children with grade IV lacerations to the liver or spleen.

Unlike blunt spleen and liver injuries, non-operative management of blunt trauma to the pancreas remains controversial. Some pediatric trauma centers recommend aggressive surgical intervention, while other centers have had success with non-operative management. One retrospective study of data from seven level 1 pediatric trauma centers demonstrated that blunt pancreatic injuries were associated with a nine-fold increase in need for operative management relative to other solid organ injuries. Chapter 146 discusses traumatic renal injuries.

Bowel injury

Blunt or penetrating perforation to a hollow viscus requires surgical repair to prevent the development of peritonitis. Because of the rising trend in non-surgical management of blunt solid organ injury, it has become increasingly important to observe for clinical signs of peritonitis in the post-injury period, because hollow viscus injuries may rarely be missed on CT scan. Clinical outcome after bowel injury is dependent upon the amount of bowel injured and the extent of surgical repair required.

Duodenal perforation or hematoma, resulting from a direct blow to the abdomen or a fall onto bicycle handle bars, is seen more commonly in children than in adults. Frank duodenal perforation requires surgical repair, but hematoma without radiographic or clinical suspicion for perforation may be managed non-operatively with hospital admission, nasogastric tube decompression of the stomach to relieve gastric outlet obstruction, total parenteral nutrition, and slow return to enteral feeding.

Bowel injuries are associated with lumbar fractures in children restrained with improperly fitting lap belts during motor vehicle collisions. A seatbelt sign (horizontal bruising to the abdominal wall) is a physical examination finding that should prompt evaluation for bowel and lumbar bony injuries. Chance fractures are defined as linear fractures through a lumbar vertebral body, pedicles, and spinous process. These fractures are seen at the mid-lumbar levels in young children and at the higher lumber levels in adults or larger children. Plain radiographs or CT of the lumbar spine can be used to identify these injuries. The incidence of bowel, pancreatic, liver, or spleen injuries approaches 50% in children with Chance fractures, so CT imaging of the abdomen is indicated in patients with this injury. Chance fractures are generally managed with immobilization in a thoracolumbosacral orthosis, but occasional operative fixation may be required.

Pelvic fractures

Pelvic fractures are rare in children and are a result of significant blunt force applied to the body. Assessment of the stability of the child's pelvis should be performed during the secondary survey and a suspected open-book pelvic fracture should be supported with the use of a wrapped bed sheet or pelvic binder. Pelvic radiographs or CT should be performed when fractures are suspected. Differing from adults, pelvic fractures in children rarely result in hemodynamic compromise or require transfusion. Major sacral or acetabular fractures may require surgical repair or fixation, but other fractures are generally treated with bed rest for 4–6 weeks and slow return to activities.

Disposition

When determining the disposition for pediatric patients who have suffered trauma to the chest or abdomen, consider the resources available at the hospital where resuscitation is taking place. Trauma surgeons with pediatric expertise should be involved in management decisions early in the evaluation process. Transfer of care to designated pediatric trauma centers improves success rates for non-operative management of blunt abdominal organ injuries. Children with a benign examination and normal radiographic imaging may be discharged with a reliable family member after explicit return precautions are given and understood.

Pearls and pitfalls

Pearls

1. Pediatric patients are more vulnerable to injuries from blunt abdominal trauma than adults because of their relatively compact torso and smaller area for distribution of traumatic forces.
2. Transfer to a designated pediatric trauma center improves success rates for non-operative management of blunt liver and spleen injuries.
3. Involve a pediatric trauma surgeon early in the evaluation of significant chest and abdominal trauma.

Pitfalls

1. Failure to recognize that significant contusion to the lungs can occur without evidence of rib fractures.
2. Failure to assess for intra-abdominal injuries associated with lumbar spine fractures (Chance fractures) in children inappropriately restrained with lap belts during motor vehicle collision.

Selected references

American College of Surgeons. *National Trauma Data Bank Pediatric Report 2007, version 7.0*. Chicago, IL: American College of Surgeons http://www.facs.org/trauma/ntdb/ntdbpediatricreport2007.pdf (accessed 28 April 2010).]

Dowd MD, Krug S. Pediatric blunt cardiac injury: epidemiology, clinical features, and diagnosis. Pediatric Emergency Medicine Collaborative Research Committee: Working Group on Blunt Cardiac Injury. *J Trauma* 1996;**40**: 61–67.

Hall JR, Reyes HM, Meller JL, Loeff DS, Dembek R. The outcome for children with blunt trauma is best at a pediatric trauma center. *J Pediatr Surg* 1996;**31**:72–76.

Holmes JF, Gladman A, Chang CH. Performance of abdominal ultrasonography in pediatric blunt trauma patients: a meta-analysis. *J Ped Surg* 2007;**42**:1588–1594.

Paddock HN, Tepas III JJ, Ramenofsky ML, Vane DW, Discala C. Management of blunt pediatric hepatic and splenic injury: similar process, different outcome. *American Surgeon* 2004;**70**:1068–1072.

Rice H. Review of radiation risks for computed tomography: essentials for the pediatric surgeon. *J Ped Surg* 2004;**42**:603–607.

Chapter

146 Genitourinary trauma

Ingrid T. Lim

Introduction

Approximately 10% of pediatric patients with trauma have urogenital trauma. Most injuries (90%) are a result of blunt trauma involving crush or acceleration/deceleration forces. Other mechanisms include falls and sports-related injuries. Penetrating genitourinary injuries are much less common in children than in adults. Genitourinary and renal injuries and their treatment are summarized in Table 146.1.

Diagnosis

The general diagnostic approach to evaluate the genitourinary tract in pediatric trauma is similar to that in adults, and should include the following four factors.

Hemodynamic stability. If a patient is hemodynamically unstable, gross hematuria should be noted. Further evaluation of the kidneys, ureters, and bladder can be assessed intraoperatively. Unlike adults, children maintain normal blood pressures despite large volumes of blood loss, which makes the absence of hypotension an unreliable indicator of significant injury. The stable patient can undergo diagnostic imaging.

Hematuria (microscopic versus gross). The presence of gross hematuria is a sign of urologic injury, necessitating further evaluation. Gross hematuria is defined as bloody or blood-tinged urine. Microscopic hematuria is defined as red blood cell count >5/high-power field, although significant injury is usually associated with >50 cells/high-power field. Microscopic hematuria associated with hypotension must be evaluated. Renovascular pedicle injuries or penetrating ureteral injury may not produce any hematuria.

Mechanism of injury. In blunt trauma, obtain imaging on all patients with microscopic hematuria and shock or with gross hematuria. Penetrating injury is clinically more subtle and may exist even when hematuria is absent. Therefore, consider evaluation of all patients with penetrating injuries in proximity to the urinary tract (e.g., flank, back, abdomen, or groin), regardless of the presence or degree of hematuria.

Anatomic site of injury (upper versus lower tract). The kidneys and ureters are considered the upper urinary tract, while the external genitalia, urethra, and bladder constitute the lower urinary tract. In general, urologic injuries should always be assessed in a retrograde fashion: lower tract injury should be excluded before evaluation of the upper tract. When lower tract injury is suspected (e.g., pelvic fracture and hematuria), the urethra should be evaluated before the bladder. When upper tract injury is suspected (e.g., rapid deceleration; direct blow to the back, flank, or abdomen; penetrating torso injury), a targeted radiologic evaluation of the ureters and kidneys with abdominal CT and delayed imaging of the kidneys should be performed.

Urethral trauma

Although urethral trauma in children is far less common than injuries to the kidney or bladder, it is potentially the most debilitating of all urologic injuries because of the high incidence of complications (e.g., strictures, impotence, incontinence).

Clinical presentation

Most urethral injuries in childhood result from motor vehicle accidents, straddle injuries, and instrumentation. Urethral injuries occur more commonly in boys; they are exceedingly rare in girls because of the shorter more mobile urethra. Consider urethral injuries in the female patient if there is blood at the introitus or rectal injury. Female urethral injuries are usually associated with unstable pelvic fractures, in which a bony fragment lacerates the urethra.

In males, the urogenital diaphragm divides the urethra into anterior and posterior segments (Fig. 146.1). The **anterior urethra**, located below the urogenital diaphragm, includes both the bulbous and penile urethra. Injuries to the anterior urethra occur with straddle injuries or direct blows to the perineum. The major sign of acute anterior injury is blood at

A Practical Guide to Pediatric Emergency Medicine: Caring for Children in the Emergency Department, ed. N. Ewen Amieva-Wang (associate eds. Jamie Shandro, Aparajita Sohoni, and Bernhard Fassl). Published by Cambridge University Press.

Table 146.1. Summary of guidelines for diagnosis and treatment of genitourinal trauma

Injuries	Clinical presentation	Imaging modality of choice	Treatment
Urethra			
Anterior (bulbous and penile urethra)	Blood at the meatus, hematuria, inability or difficulty voiding, periurethral or perineal edema and ecchymosis	Retrograde urethrogram; CT scan is not adequate for diagnosing urethral injuries	7–10 days of urinary catheterization and antibiotics; more severe injuries require suprapubic cystostomy
Posterior (membranous and prostatic urethra)	95% of patients have a pelvic fracture, particularly any disruption of the anterior pelvic ring Dysuria, perineal pain, inability to void; late findings, perineal or scrotal discoloration	Retrograde urethrogram; CT scan is not adequate for diagnosing urethral injuries	Controversial; immediate laparotomy with primary repair versus suprapubic catheter with delayed urethroplasty; all penetrating wounds require early surgical exploration
Bladder: extraperitoneal (80%), intraperitoneal (15%), combined (5%)	80% associated with pelvic fractures and penetration of bladder by bony fragment Gross hematuria (in 90%); dysuria, lower abdominal pain, palpable fluid wave or peritoneal signs if extravasation into the peritoneal cavity	Initial assessment with pelvic radiograph to assess for fractures; CT cystography is superior to retrograde cystogram (sensitivity 95% and specificity 100%), contrast must be instilled to distend the bladder	*Bladder contusion*: treat conservatively with or without catheter drainage *Extraperitoneal bladder rupture*: urinary catheter for 7–10 days *Intraperitoneal bladder rupture*: exploratory laparotomy and suprapubic cystostomy tube *Combined or penetrating injuries*: surgical exploration
Ureteral	80–90% have microscopic hematuria, symptoms develop later when extravasated urine causes local inflammation or obstruction Right-sided injury three times more common; usually associated with penetrating injuries; suspect if transverse process fracture of lumbar vertebra, pelvic fracture, splenic or liver laceration	Intravenous pyelogram; CT urography (images obtained in the excretory phase) is the modality of choice now if the patient is already going for CT scan	*Discovered within 5–10 days of injury*: prompt surgical repair *Discovered >10 days*: urinary diversion above the lesion and definitive repair 4–6 months later
Renal	Most common GU tract injury; usually associated with blunt trauma Associated abdominal and head injuries are common; localized flank tenderness, hematomas or mass Associated findings: rib fractures, fractured transverse processes, macroscopic and microscopic hematuria	*Urgent imaging*: gross hematuria, hypotension, or severe mechanism of injury *Imaging*: microscopic hematuria because of the large number of undetected congenital anomalies *Preferred imaging*: contrast-enhanced CT with delayed renal images	*Grades I–III*: conservative management *Grades IV–V* hemodynamically stable: conservative management with serial hematocrits and broad-spectrum antibiotics. *Grades IV–V* hemodynamically unstable: vascular injuries, urine extravasation: surgery
Renovascular	Left-sided injuries are more common. Most common injury is thrombosis of the renal artery from an intimal tear Hematuria can be lacking in one-third	Contrast-enhanced CT	Controversial; conservative management if hemodynamically stable without associated injuries

the meatus, seen in 90% of patients. Other findings include hematuria, inability or difficulty voiding, periurethral or perineal edema, and ecchymosis.

The **posterior urethra** consists of the membranous and prostatic urethra. The posterior urethra firmly attaches to the pubis by the puboprostatic ligaments. A posterior urethral injury should be suspected in any patient with a disruption of the anterior pelvic ring, particularly in pubic rami fractures or symphyseal disruptions. Between 5 and 25% of patients with pelvic fractures have an associated urethral injury. Conversely, a pelvic fracture is present in >95% of patients with an injury to the posterior urethra. Patients typically complain of dysuria,

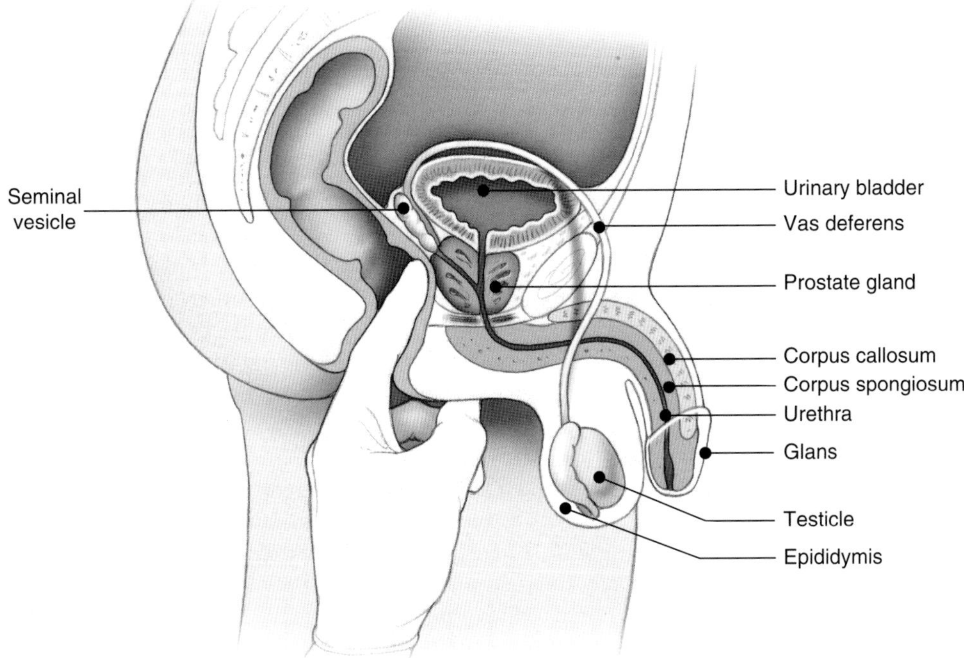

Figure 146.1 Male urinary tract. (Copyright Chris Gralapp; reproduced with permission from Mahadevan SV, Garmel GM. *An Introduction to Clinical Emergency Medicine*. Cambridge, UK: Cambridge University Press, 2005.)

perineal pain, or inability to void. Attempts at micturition can cause penile or perineal swelling. Blood at the urethral meatus is not always present. Perineal and scrotal discoloration is usually a late finding. Rectal examination may demonstrate a "high-riding" prostate, resulting from pelvic hematoma or transection of the puboprostatic ligaments.

Diagnostic studies

No attempt should be made to insert a urethral catheter if urethral injury is suspected. There is an increased risk of infection, stricture formation, or conversion of a partial tear into a complete one. A retrograde urethrogram must be performed under sterile conditions. To perform a urethrogram, a size-appropriate Foley catheter is inserted into the penile urethra without inflating the balloon. Water-soluble contrast is injected and antero–posterior and oblique views taken. Gross extravasation of the contrast without visualization of proximal structures suggests complete rupture of the urethra. Partial injury shows localized extravasation and contrast passing to the proximal urethra and bladder. If no extravasation is noted, the Foley catheter can be gently advanced into the bladder. A CT scan is not adequate for diagnosing urethral injuries; it only provides presumptive evidence of disruption if extravasation is detected at the bladder neck or urethra.

Management

Anterior urethral injuries can be managed with 7 to 10 days of urinary catheterization and antimicrobial therapy. More severe injuries may require a suprapubic cystostomy.

Posterior urethral injuries usually occur with severe trauma, associated most commonly with pelvic fractures. Initial management remains controversial, varying from immediate laparotomy with primary repair to placement of a suprapubic tube with delayed urethroplasty. Penetrating wounds of the urethra demand surgical exploration.

Bladder trauma

Bladder injuries most often occur after blunt injury secondary to motor vehicle collisions or crush injuries to the pelvis. Approximately 80% of bladder injuries are associated with pelvic fractures and penetration of bladder by a bony fragment. However, only 10% of pelvic fractures have associated lower tract injury. The probability of bladder injury increases proportionally with the number of fractured pubic rami.

In childhood, the bladder has a higher abdominal location, rendering it more susceptible to injury than in adults. In addition, a full bladder is more prone to injury. Bladder injuries can range from contusions, in which there is an incomplete, non-perforating tear in the mucosa, to complete rupture. Bladder ruptures are classified as extraperitoneal, intraperitoneal, or combined. Extraperitoneal bladder rupture accounts for 80% of all bladder injuries and frequently occurs with pelvic fractures or penetrating trauma. Intraperitoneal injuries usually arise from blunt trauma to a distended bladder, causing a rupture of the dome. The least common bladder rupture – combined – is usually seen with gunshot wounds or multiple pelvic fractures. Differentiation of the injury type dictates management.

Clinical presentation

Hematuria, dysuria, and lower abdominal pain are the common presenting symptoms. Most patients with bladder rupture have gross hematuria. Microscopic hematuria may be seen in bladder contusions. Clear urine and the absence of a pelvic fracture virtually eliminate the possibility of bladder rupture. A palpable fluid wave and peritoneal signs on abdominal examination may occur if urine extravasates into the peritoneal cavity.

Diagnostic studies

Absolute indications for bladder imaging after blunt trauma are gross hematuria with a pelvic fracture and the inability to void.

Pelvic radiograph. This is the initial study to exclude a pelvic fracture.

Retrograde cystogram. Prior to the advent of CT imaging, retrograde cystograms were the standard of care in detailing bladder injuries. However, it is time consuming and does not provide information about surrounding structures.

Cystography with CT. Conventional cystography has largely been replaced by CT cystography. It is the ideal study in the patient with polytrauma already undergoing abdomino-pelvic CT. It is quicker, more convenient, and involves less radiation dose to the patient if performed as part of the initial CT than conventional cystography. Contrast enhancement of the bladder is necessary because extravasated urine can mimic ascites or hematoma. Although bladder contents can be enhanced by performing delayed scanning after the administration of IV contrast, the bladder distention is often suboptimal compared with that in CT cystography, in which dilute contrast is directly infused into the bladder, allowing a dramatic increase in the sensitivity and specificity for diagnosing bladder injuries. The standard rule of thumb for contrast administration in pediatric cystograms is to instill half of the estimated bladder capacity (calculated using the equation: 30(Age [years] + 2) (max. 300 ml). If the patient does not require CT for any other reason, a traditional cystogram is still preferred.

Management

Bladder contusions. Treat conservatively with or without urethral catheter drainage.

Extraperitoneal vesicle rupture. Urethral catheter or suprapubic catheterization for 7 to 10 days.

Intraperitoneal vesicle rupture (and large extraperitoneal tears). Exploratory laparotomy and placement of a suprapubic cystostomy tube.

Combined or penetrating injuries. Surgical exploration and direct closure.

Ureteral trauma

Ureteral trauma accounts for <1% of all urologic trauma; children have a predilection for ureteral injury while adults account for only one-third of cases. The mechanism of injury can be penetrating, blunt, or iatrogenic. More than 90% of ureteral injuries are associated with other intra-abdominal injuries. Suspicion should be heightened if patients have fractures of the transverse processes of lumbar vertebrae, pelvic fractures, splenic or liver lacerations, or diaphragmatic rupture.

Clinical presentation

Transection of the ureter does not cause any specific signs or symptoms, often leading to a delayed diagnosis. Hematuria, usually microscopic, is present in 80–90%. Symptoms usually do not develop until the extravasated urine produces local inflammation, or there is obstruction to urine flow from the ipsilateral kidney. Ureteral injury may manifest as fever, chills, lethargy, leukocytosis, pyuria, bacteriuria, flank mass or pain, ileus, urinoma or abscess formation, fistulae, or strictures.

Diagnostic studies

Urography with CT is the modality of choice for evaluation of ureteral trauma, as the other abdominal organs can be assessed simultaneously. The images must be obtained in the excretory phase for contrast in order to visualize the collecting system and the ureter. Retrograde pyelography remains the gold standard (sensitivity >90%).

Management

Prompt urologic consultation is indicated when ureteral trauma is identified. The prevalence of nephrectomy is approximately 5% when the injury is detected early, and as high as 32% when diagnosis is delayed.

Renal trauma

The most common urinary tract injury encountered in the pediatric population is injury to the kidney. Blunt trauma accounts for up to 90% of renal injuries, usually sustained in motor vehicle collisions. Children are more susceptible to renal injuries for several reasons:

- the paucity of surrounding fat and fascia
- the less-developed abdominal musculature
- the kidney's proportionally larger size compared with the surrounding abdominal organs
- the immature thoracic cage providing less protection
- remnants of fetal lobations being prone to parenchymal shearing.

The Organ Injury Scaling Committee of the American Association for the Surgery of Trauma grades renal injuries on a scale of I to V.

Clinical presentation

Renal injuries may manifest as localized signs of flank tenderness, flank hematomas, lower abdominal pain, and inability to void. Associated findings include ipsilateral rib fractures and fractured transverse processes of vertebral bodies. Hematuria is the marker for renal injury. Generally, increased blood in the urine is associated with increased grade of injury although some high-grade injuries can have minimal hematuria. Hematuria can be absent in up to 50% of patients with vascular pedicle injuries and in 29% of patients with penetrating injuries. Other intra-abdominal injuries should be suspected in patients with hematuria – some series suggest that clinically significant liver and spleen lacerations are more common in children with hematuria than are renal injuries.

Diagnostic studies

In adults, patients with gross hematuria or microscopic hematuria with shock require emergency imaging. In children, hypotension is not a reliable marker of significant renal injuries because they can have significant blood loss but remain normotensive. Regardless of the degree of hematuria, children with other major associated injuries or a significant mechanism should have radiographic evaluation.

Traditionally, IV pyelogram was the cornerstone of evaluation of the integrity and function of both kidneys. However, it cannot reliably identify and stage renal trauma. Delayed contrast-enhanced CT imaging is the preferred study for evaluation of intra-abdominal injury, including renal injury. The use of CT can delineate the degree of parenchymal injury, the presence of non-viable tissue, the integrity of the vasculature and renal parenchyma, and the presence of perirenal collections. The only role for IV pyelography is if the child is unstable and goes directly to the operating theater. Ultrasonography is not generally recommended because of its low sensitivity (70%).

In blunt trauma, minor renal injuries (contusions and lacerations without urine extravasation) can be managed conservatively with rest, analgesics, and antibiotics. Management of grades IV and V is controversial. Current opinion is that stable patients can be managed conservatively with urologic consultation, close monitoring, serial hematocrits, and broad-spectrum antibiotics. Penetrating renal injuries have traditionally been treated with surgical intervention. Patients with hemodynamic instability, vascular injuries, or urine extravasation almost always need surgical repair.

Renovascular injuries

Renovascular injuries are relatively uncommon in adults; the prevalence in children is nearly twice that seen in adults. Associated injuries are common, with more than half of children with renovascular injury sustaining another abdominal injury. Left-sided injuries outnumber right-sided injuries in blunt trauma, probably because the left renal artery is shorter and at a more acute angle that the right renal artery. The most common injury is thrombosis of the renal artery from an intimal tear and dissection.

Clinical presentation

Hematuria may not be seen in patients with major renovascular trauma. Renal artery pseudoaneurysms and arteriovenous fistulae can also develop, usually in penetrating injuries, and should be suspected if there is recurrent gross hematuria approximately 14 days after the injury.

Diagnostic studies

The study of choice is CT, which will diagnose most arterial injuries; venous injuries can be diagnosed indirectly by the presence of a large hematoma.

Management

Management of major renovascular injuries in children continues to spark debate between, historically, operative management versus non-operative observation when considering the hemodynamically stable patient without associated injuries. Prompt urologic and/or vascular consultation is indicated.

Scrotal trauma

Because of the small size and mobility of the testes in the prepubertal child, testicular injuries are exceedingly rare. Injuries are usually secondary to a direct blow, straddle injury, bicycle accidents, or sports activities. Potential injuries include skin or dartos ecchymosis, lacerations, and minor testicular hematomas, which can be managed conservatively with ice packs and scrotal support. More serious problems such as testicular dislocation, testicular rupture, large intrascrotal hematomas, or degloving injuries, may require operative treatment. The imaging modality of choice is ultrasound.

Penile trauma

See Ch. 149.

Perineal injury

Perineal injury typically occurs in female patients who experience a blunt straddle-type injury, but it can happen with penetrating injury, sexual assault, or sexual intercourse.

A meticulous examination of the urethra, vagina, and rectum should be carried out and it should be ensured that the patient can urinate. Patients may have vulvar hematomas, superficial lacerations, or urinary retention because of discomfort when voiding. Typically, treatment consists of ice packs to the perineum and sitz baths for superficial lacerations. Urination can be facilitated by having the child urinate in a warm bath. More severe injuries to the urethra, vagina, or rectum may occur. Urethral disruption may require suprapubic cystostomy or primary repair. Vaginal lacerations must be suspected in patients with severe trauma or penetration by a foreign object. These patients need a careful examination under anesthesia and laceration repair with absorbable sutures. Rectal penetration or perforation may warrant surgical intervention.

Pearls and pitfalls

Pearls

1. Genitourinary imaging is required in any child with *penetrating* abdominal trauma, and in any child with *blunt* trauma and microscopic hematuria, hypotension, fractures of the spine or pelvis, or significant deceleration mechanism.
2. In patients with pelic fractures, 5–25% have concomitant urethral or bladder injuries.
3. Although hematuria is present in 95% of significant genitourinary injuries, it may be absent, particularly with penetrating injuries.

Pitfalls

1. Failure to suspect urogenital trauma in a patient with blunt abdominal trauma.
2. Failure to perform a retrograde urethrogram prior to inserting a Foley catheter into a bloody urethral meatus.
3. Failure to suspect other intra-abdominal injuries in patients with hematuria; clinically significant liver and spleen lacerations may be more common than renal injuries in children with hematuria.

Selected references

Perez-Brayfield MR, Gatti JM, Smith EA, *et al.* Blunt traumatic hematuria in children. Is a simplified algorithm justified? *J Urol* 2002;**167**:2543–2547.

Santucci RA, Wessells H, Bartsch G, *et al.* Consensus on genitourinary trauma. Evaluation and management of renal injuries: consensus statement of the renal trauma subcommittee. *BJU Int* 2004;**93**:937–954.

Srinivasa RN, Akbar SA, Jafri SZ, Howells GA. Genitourinary trauma: a pictorial essay. *Emerg Radiol* 2009;**16**:21–33.

Chapter 147

Tutorial: The pediatric FAST and EFAST examination

Teresa S. Wu

Introduction

Rapid, accurate diagnosis and treatment is of utmost importance in the management of critical pediatric trauma patients. Computed tomography and ultrasound have become the two most popular modalities for assessing abdominal trauma and predicting the need for imminent laparotomy. Ultrasound enables physicians to rapidly assess for the presence of intrathoracic and intra-abdominal free fluid in a quick, simple, and non-invasive manner, without exposing the patient to the risks and dangers of ionizing radiation. First introduced in 1971, the use of ultrasound to assess thoraco-abdominal trauma has since gained worldwide acceptance, and in 1995 Rozycki and colleagues coined the term "focused assessment with sonography for trauma" (FAST) to encompass the goal-directed scans used in trauma management today. Bedside ultrasound has quickly become a mainstay in the management of pediatric trauma patients, and in 2004, the extended FAST (EFAST) examination was introduced. With the EFAST examination, practitioners can evaluate for the presence of a pneumothorax by interpreting just a few simple sonographic findings. Although bedside ultrasound is not the imaging modality of choice for detecting solid organ injury, its ability to detect free fluid and diagnose pneumothoraces with a sensitivity and specificity of nearly 100% makes it an excellent diagnostic adjunct in the assessment of unstable pediatric trauma patients.

Ultrasound

In order to master the FAST examination, three fundamental principles will need to be remembered:

- echogenicity: blood collections appear *hypoechoic*, or darker than the surrounding tissues on the ultrasound screen
- transducer probe: the lower-frequency 3.5 MHz probe is used
- spatial directionality and orientation: the dot on the probe correlates with the dot on the screen.

Echogenicity

To better understand echogenicity, it is important to remember that ultrasonography is founded upon the principles of sound and energy. During a scan, sound is transmitted as energy through mediums such as air, liquid, and solid at a frequency ranging between 2.5 and 10 MHz. As sound waves travel through a medium, they cause periodic changes in the pressure of the medium. The subsequent oscillation of molecules within the medium is detected by the ultrasound transducer and generates the images displayed on the ultrasound monitor. With collections of blood, most of the sound waves are absorbed and are minimally reflected back to the transducer. Thus, the low-amplitude signal from blood correlates with a darker, *hypoechoic* image on the screen.

In contrast, *hyperechoic* structures, such as the diaphragm, appear brighter and whiter on the monitor because of the increased amplitude of their sound echoes. Structures that are *isoechoic*, or similar in brightness to the surrounding tissues, will be difficult to distinguish because they share the same echogenicity. Finally, fluid-filled structures, such as cysts, do not reflect any sound waves and are, therefore, considered *anechoic*, or black in color on the monitor.

Transducer probe

Although many types of ultrasound probe are available, in most pediatric patients, the FAST examination should be performed using the 3.5 MHz curvilinear probe, which can penetrate deeper tissue depths. In contrast, the higher-frequency 7.5 MHz vascular probe allows for more detailed tissue resolution at the expense of more shallow tissue imaging (Fig. 147.1).

Spatial directionality and orientation

It is important to ensure that the directionality of the images obtained remains consistent and that orientation interpretation is not reversed. Most transducers have an external identification mark or dot located on one side. This marker

A Practical Guide to Pediatric Emergency Medicine: Caring for Children in the Emergency Department, ed. N. Ewen Amieva-Wang (associate eds. Jamie Shandro, Aparajita Sohoni, and Bernhard Fassl). Published by Cambridge University Press.

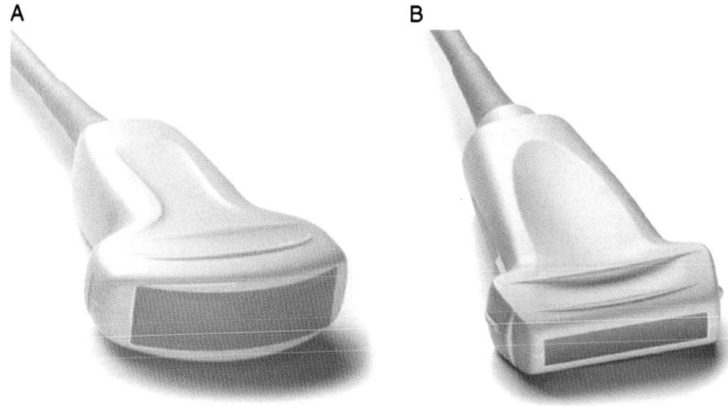

Figure 147.1 Probes. (A) A 3.5 MHz curvilinear probe for scanning deeper structures. (B) A 7.5 MHz linear probe for scanning superficial structures.

should be oriented to the corresponding identification mark or dot located on the ultrasound monitor. Then, if the probe is pointing towards the patient's head, the dot on the left-hand side of the screen corresponds to a cephalad direction.

The FAST examination

There are four basic ultrasound views utilized during trauma resuscitations. These four views (perihepatic, perisplenic, pelvic, and pericardial) are the foundation by which ultrasound has revolutionized the approach to trauma management in pediatric patients. These views are utilized for the rapid detection of hemoperitoneum, pericardial effusions, and pleural effusions.

The FAST examination operates on the premise that intraperitoneal free fluid will collect in anatomically defined pockets. In a supine patient, fluid in the abdomen usually flows to the most dependent supramesocolic location. This location is the right hepatorenal fossa, otherwise known as Morrison's pouch. Fluid will also localize in the pelvis. In males, it will rest in the rectovesicular space; in females, it will flow into the pouch of Douglas just anterior to the uterus.

Anatomy and technique

Most pediatric patients with trauma will present in a supine position, immobilized on a backboard, in cervical-spine precautions. In order to optimize the amount of free fluid accumulating in the most dependent anatomical pockets, the patient is placed in a slight Trendelenburg posture. The 3.5 MHz curvilinear transducer is used.

Many ultrasound machines will have preset windows for abdominal views, cardiac views, or gynecological studies. If the ultrasound machine has that option, begin with the machine cued to view the abdomen. Because Morrison's pouch is the most dependent position when the patient is lying supine, most experts advocate beginning the FAST examination with a view of the RUQ, unless there is concern for blunt or penetrating thoracic trauma. If such thoracic trauma is evident, cue the machine for cardiac windows and begin with a pericardial view to rule out pericardial effusion and tamponade.

Utilizing four primary views, the FAST examination aims to rapidly identify free fluid in the four most dependent locations:

Perihepatic view of the right upper quadrant

The area visualized:

- is otherwise known as Morrison's pouch or the hepatorenal space
- encompasses the interface between the liver and Gerota's fascia of the right kidney
- has the interface residing at the vertebral level between T12 and L3
- has the long access of the interface running almost parallel to the body.

The RUQ is evaluated by looking for the presence of free fluid in Morrison's pouch (Fig. 147.2), a right pleural effusion above the diaphragm, and free fluid below the diaphragm in the right pericolic gutter. During these perihepatic views, the ultrasound probe is placed at an oblique angle in the mid-axillary line between the 8th and 11th ribs. The probe indicator is angled towards the patient's right axilla, and the probe is swept back and forth in an attempt to obtain the best possible image. Placing the probe at an oblique angle between the ribs will minimize the amount of rib shadowing obstructing the view of the hepatorenal space. In order to evaluate the structures adjacent to the hyperechoic right diaphragm, the ultrasound beam is directed more cephalad. Free fluid above or below the diaphragm or in Morrison's pouch will be seen as an anechoic stripe.

Perisplenic view of the left upper quadrant

The area visualized:

- is otherwise known as the splenorenal space
- encompasses the interface between the spleen and Gerota's fascia of the left kidney
- has the interface residing at the vertebral level between T11 and L2
- has the long access of the interface running almost parallel to the body.

The steps used in scanning the RUQ are repeated to carefully evaluate the patient's left upper quadrant (LUQ), looking for the presence of free fluid in the splenorenal space (Fig. 147.3), a left pleural effusion above the diaphragm, and free fluid below the diaphragm in the left subphrenic recess. The ultrasound probe is placed at an oblique angle at the left posterior axillary line between the 7th and 10th ribs. The probe is angled towards the patient's left axilla and swept to maintain an image with minimal rib shadowing. The probe is placed almost flush against the backboard or gurney and the posteriorly located spleen is used as an acoustic window to maximize picture quality in this view. The angle of the probe is directed cephalad to examine for pleural fluid above and below the hyperechoic left diaphragm. Free fluid around the

A

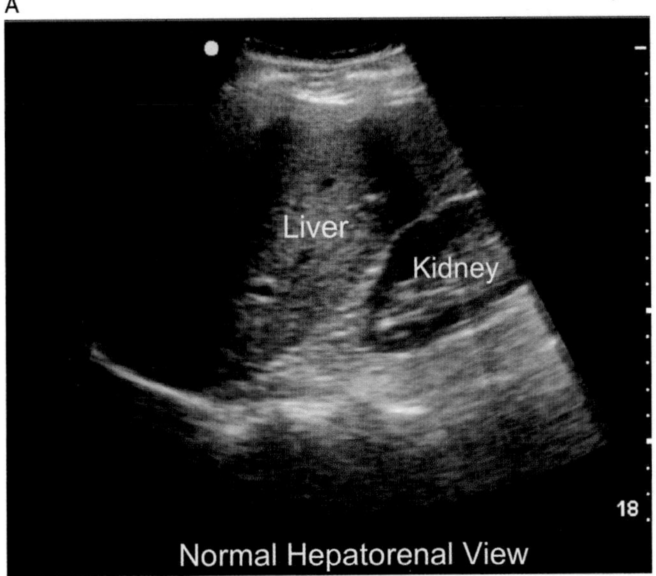

B

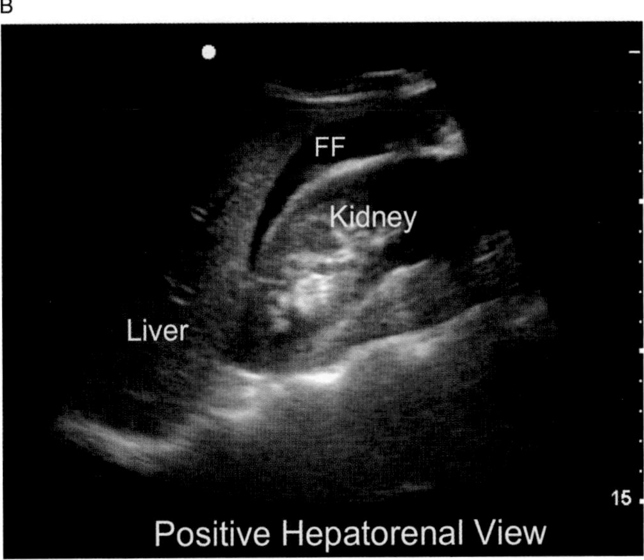

Figure 147.2 Hepatorenal images. (A) normal hepatorenal recess. (B) Free fluid (FF) in the hepatorenal recess.

A

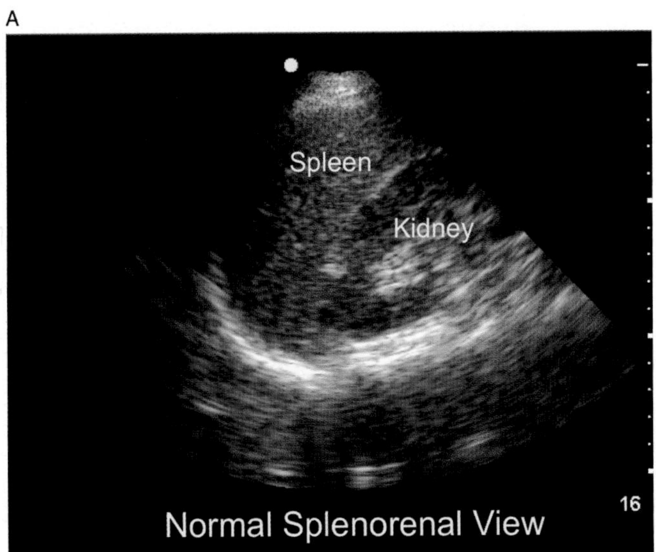

B

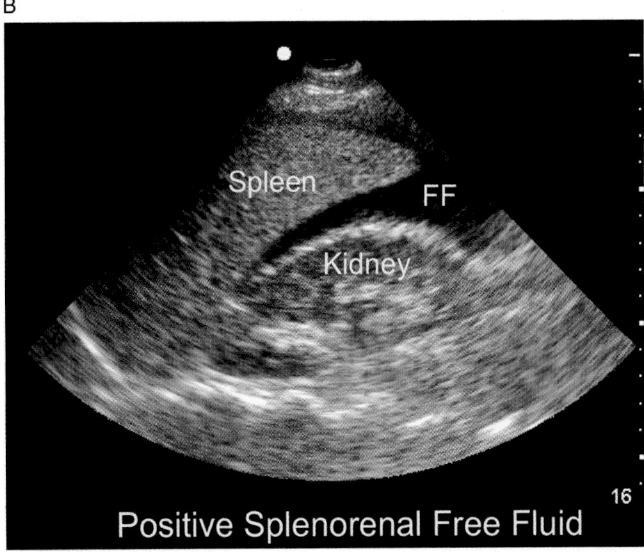

Figure 147.3 Splenorenal images. (A) Normal splenorenal recess. (B) Free fluid (FF) visible in surrounding the spleen and in the splenorenal recess.

diaphragm or in the splenorenal recess will be seen as an anechoic stripe.

Pericardial view

The pericardium has:

- two parts, making up a double-walled conical fibroserous sac: a tough fibrous pericardium externally, and the double-layered sac of transparent membrane called the serous pericardium internally
- a parietal surface of the serous pericardium fused with the fibrous pericardium, and the deeper visceral serous pericardium reflected on the heart where it forms the epicardium
- a potential space between the parietal and visceral layers of the serous pericardium, the pericardial cavity
- a location in the middle mediastinum, posterior to the body of the sternum and the 2nd to 6th costal cartilages, and anterior to the 5th through 8th thoracic vertebrae.

Both blunt and penetrating trauma can cause bleeding to occur into the pericardial cavity between the double-layered serous pericardium.

Examination of the heart uses either the subxiphoid view (using the liver as a window; Fig. 147.4), or the intercostal view. To obtain a view of the pericardium, the ultrasound probe is placed just below the xiphoid process and the beam is angled

A

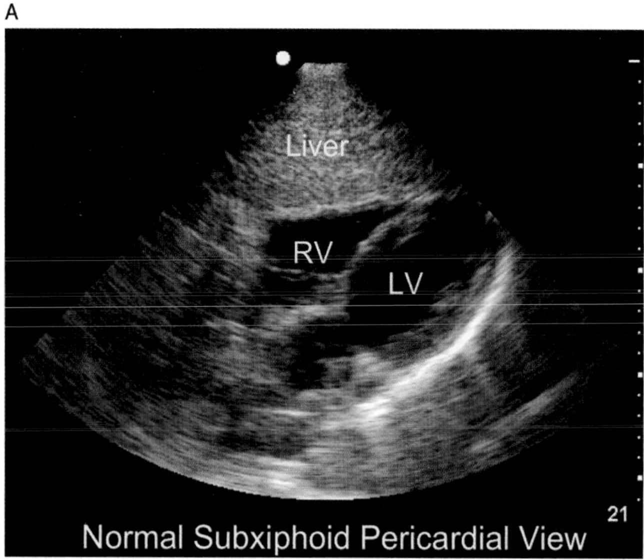

B

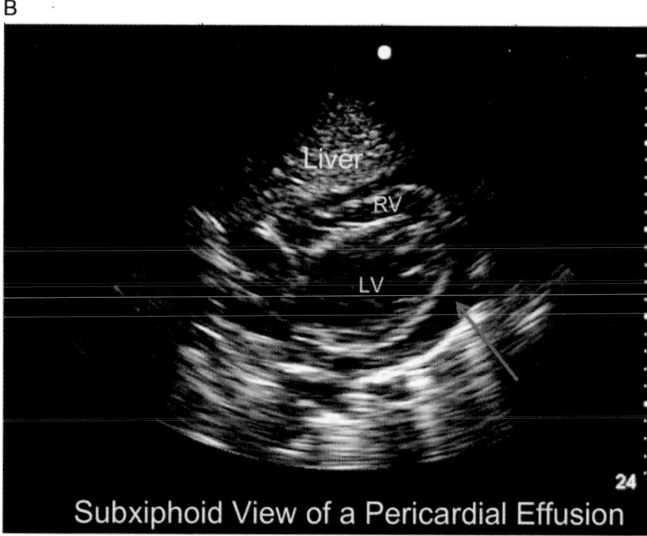

Figure 147.4 Pericardial images. (A) Subxiphoid view of a normal pericardial sac. (B) Hypoechoic pericardial effusion (arrowed) noted on subxiphoid view of the heart. RV, right ventricle; LV, left ventricle.

towards the patient's left shoulder. The body of the probe is placed flush against the patient and a small amount of pressure is exerted at the transducer head to direct the beam superoposteriorly. A coronal section of the heart will provide an adequate four-chamber view in this position. Global cardiac function and chamber size can be observed through a few cardiac and respiratory cycles. Normal pericardium will be seen as a hyperechoic line surrounding the heart. Pericardial free fluid will appear as a hypoechoic stripe internal to the pericardium.

Suprapubic view

The area visualized:

- is otherwise known as the pouch of Douglas in females, and the rectovesicular space in males
- will have an empty bladder lying almost entirely in the pelvis minor, inferior to the pelvic floor and posterior to the pubic symphysis
- with a full bladder, its sonographic window may rise as high as the umbilicus.

This final view of the basic FAST examination involves examination for free fluid in the anterior pelvis or rectovesicular space. A full bladder will provide an excellent acoustic window, so it is better to try to get these views before a Foley catheter is placed. If the patient has been placed in the Trendelenburg position for the previous views, they should now be positioned in a slight reverse Trendelenburg to maximize the final pelvic view. The ultrasound probe is placed longitudinally 2 cm superior to the pubic symphysis along the midline of the abdomen. The uterus or prostate, the lateral walls of the bladder, and the rectovesicular space can be inspected. Directing the ultrasound beam posteriorly and sweeping cephalad will allow anechoic free fluid lying posterior to the bladder in the rectovesicular recess to be visualized (Fig. 147.5). Often, a prominent rectum may appear as a hypoechoic stripe posterior to the bladder. Rotating the probe 90 degrees to a sagittal plane allows assessment for layering of the hypoechoic stripe. True free fluid will appear as an anechoic stripe layering in the most dependent/inferior portion of the image.

Limitations

It is important to understand the basic limitations of the FAST examination in order to avoid common pitfalls in patient management. First, certain serious traumatic injuries cannot be detected with ultrasound limited to the four basic views. These injuries include, but are not limited to, renal pedicle injury, viscus perforation, bowel wall contusion, pancreatic trauma, diaphragmatic injury, or retroperitoneal trauma.

Second, the amount of time lapsed between the inciting trauma and the FAST examination must be taken into account. Over time, older blood becomes less anechoic and may appear as a dark gray stripe on ultrasound. Once the blood begins to clot, it may adhere to the surrounding tissue and will not layer out as well as fresh blood.

Finally, intraperitoneal fat can often appear relatively hypoechoic on ultrasound and can be mistaken for free fluid or a hematoma. Its identity can be verified by evaluating its variation with respiration or movement, analyzing its density on multiple views, and correlating its presence with the entire clinical scenario. Box 147.1 gives some useful hints for the FAST examination.

The EFAST examination

The EFAST examination calls for additional views of the thorax to be obtained during the initial trauma scan. Bedside

A

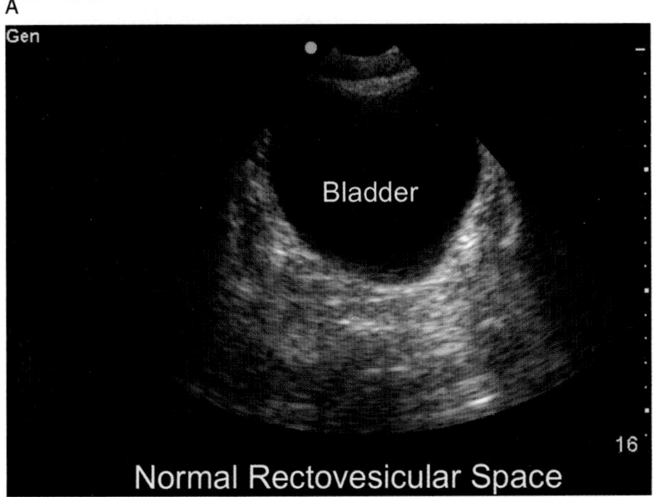

B

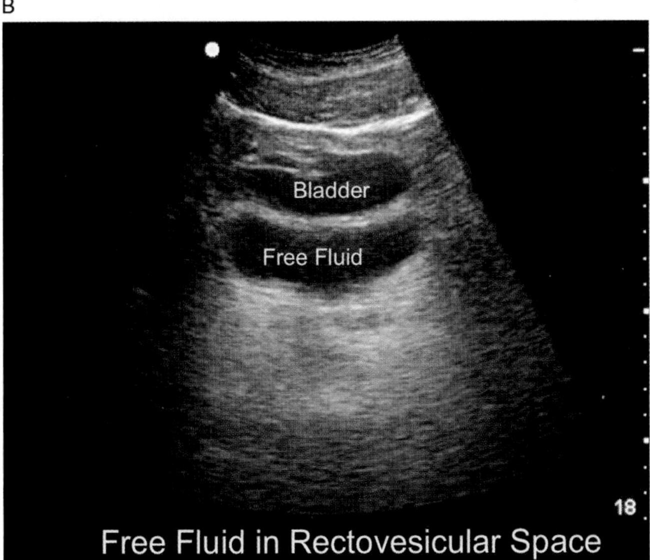

Figure 147.5 Rectovesicular space. (A) Transverse view of a normal rectovesicular space. (B) Free fluid visible behind the bladder in the rectovesicular space.

ultrasound is particularly useful in clinical scenarios where auscultation of breath sounds is limited by ambient noise or patient body habitus, and it can also provide valuable information when supine radiographs are equivocal. Its portability and ability to provide time-sensitive information has prompted many practitioners to incorporate bedside thoracic scanning into their initial patient evaluation.

Diagnosis of a pneumothorax

In the reassessment of hypoxic or dyspneic patients, bedside ultrasound can determine if the patient has a pneumothorax in a matter of seconds.

1. Use the highest resolution probe available (7–10 MHz); in most clinical situations, use the linear/vascular probe.
2. If a scan for a pneumothorax is to occur as a continuation of the FAST examination and a curvilinear or phased array probe is being used, adjust and decrease the depth settings on the machine.

Box 147.1. Helpful hints for the FAST examination

Unable to visualize the left upper quadrant (LUQ)/ splenorenal junction because of rib shadowing or bowel
Move the transducer probe more posteriorly and superiorly. A common pitfall is to position the probe too anteroinferiorly. The probe should lie parallel and virtually flat against the patient's gurney.

Only the bottom half of the heart is visible on a subxiphoid view
Try to increase the depth of the scan first. Then have the patient take in a deep breath and hold it. This will bring the entire pericardium into view.

A small sliver of hypoechoic fluid can be seen in the RUQ or LUQ view but it is not certain that it is free fluid
Take a moment and re-evaluate the entire clinical scenario. If the patient is stable, try placing the patient in steeper Trendelenberg position. This will cause free fluid to flow towards the most dependent supramesocolic location (Morrison's pouch). If repositioning does not improve the view of the suspicious area, consider completing serial ultrasound examinations until a definitive diagnosis can be made.

What if a Foley catheter has already been placed to decompress the bladder before the suprapubic scan could be performed
Most pelvic scans should be performed before catheter placement because the full bladder makes a great acoustic window. If the bladder is empty and a Foley catheter is in place, it may be helpful to instill 250 ml of warm normal saline into the bladder to improve the sensitivity of the suprapubic scan. Clamp the catheter during the scan, and then unclamp the catheter to allow normal output after the scan is completed.

The LUQ is the most difficult quadrant to scan; how to ensure that the entire splenorenal junction has been evaluated adequately
Remember that the spleen lies more posteriorly than the liver. Place the probe flush against the patient's gurney and use the spleen as the acoustic window to visualize the splenorenal recess. Sweep the probe inferiorly until the inferior tip of the spleen is visualized. Also sweep the probe superiorly until the infradiaphragmatic region just above the spleen is fully observed. Often times, free fluid will accumulate in the supraslenic recess before it flows into the splenorenal junction.

What is the large hypoechoic structure that can sometimes obstruct a scan of the splenorenal space?
An enlarged stomach can confuse a scan or obstruct the view of the LUQ. Lying just medial to the splenic hilum, the stomach will appear anechoic with a bright hyperechoic lining. When filled with liquid contents, the enlarged stomach may impede a clear view of the splenorenal space. The anechoic stomach should not be mistaken for free fluid.

3. The patient can be sitting upright or lying supine.
4. Place the linear probe in the 2nd or 3rd intercostal space along the mid-clavicular line.
5. The scan can be completed in either a longitudinal or transverse plane.
6. Find the bright, white, hyperechoic pleural line and look for lung sliding across the screen (to and fro movement of the parietal pleura gliding against the visceral pleura).
7. If a pneumothorax is present, it will not be possible to visualize the parietal pleura gliding against the visceral pleura. The sonographic sign of lung sliding will be absent.
8. Next, observe for comet tails (bright white, echogenic streaks that shoot farfield off the pleura from apposition of the parietal–visceral pleural interface; Fig. 147.6). If air is separating the parietal pleura from the visceral pleura, the parietal–visceral interface is interrupted and comet tails will be absent.

Tricks of the trade in evaluation of a pneumothorax

- Augment findings by also scanning in M-mode (M, motion).
- Split the screen to show both B-mode and M-mode images.
- On M-mode, the parietal–visceral pleural interface will appear again as a bright, white, hyperechoic line traversing horizontally across the screen (Fig. 147.7).

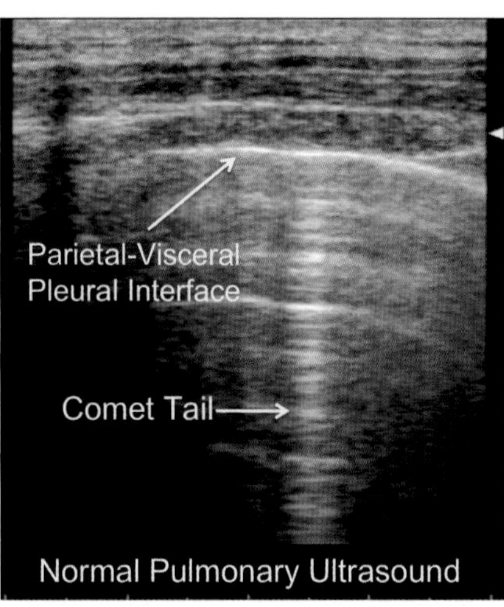

Figure 147.6 Normal pulmonary ultrasound demonstrating a hyperechoic comet tail coming off from the parietal–visceral pleural interface.

- Normal lung parenchyma will demonstrate the "seashore sign." Transmission of ultrasound signals to the lung parenchyma farfield to the pleural line produces a pattern that appears like the sea crashing along the shore.
- If the patient has a pneumothorax, air trapped in between the parietal and visceral pleura will impede ultrasound signals from reaching the parenchyma farfield to the pleural line. The resulting artifact transmitted on the screen looks like a barcode running across the monitor and is, therefore, called the "barcode sign" of a pneumothorax.

Summary of sonographic findings in a pneumothorax

- There is no pneumothorax if there is:
  - lung sliding
  - comet tails (Fig. 147.6)
  - the "seashore sign" on M-mode.
- A pneumothorax is present if there is:
  - absence of lung sliding
  - absence of comet tails
  - the "barcode sign" on M-mode.

Conclusions

Since the late 1970s, the use of goal-directed bedside ultrasound has become widely accepted as a mainstay of trauma management. With the introduction of new technology comes the recognition of its current limitations. Understanding and accepting these limitations will allow EPs in pediatric and adult medicine to take full advantage of the FAST and EFAST examinations, while avoiding pitfalls in their application.

Like most operator-dependent procedures, the more practice EPs have, the more comfortable they will be with the results obtained. As skills evolve, so too will technology and the role of bedside ultrasound in the management of pediatric trauma patients. The simple technology that once revolutionized the approach to ectopic pregnancies, gallbladder disease, and cardiovascular medicine will inevitably continue to change the way we approach pediatric trauma management in the future.

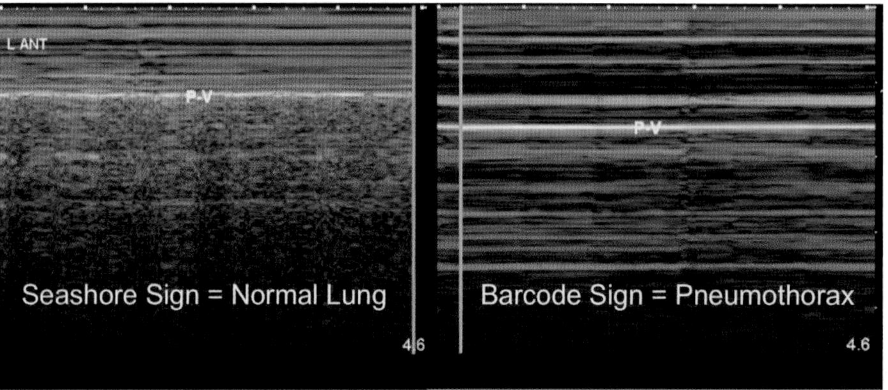

Figure 147.7 M-mode ultrasound of a normal lung ("seashore sign") and ultrasound of a pneumothorax ("barcode sign").

Selected references

Kirkpatrick AW, Sirois M, Laupland KB, *et al.* Handheld thoracic sonography for detecting post-traumatic pneumothoraces: the extended focused assessment with sonography for trauma (EFAST). *J Trauma* 2004;**57**:288–295.

Kristensen JK, Buemann B, Keuhl E. Ultrasonic scanning in the diagnosis of splenic hematomas. *Acta Chir Scand* 1971;**137**:653–657.

Rozycki GS, Ochsner MG, Schmidt JA, *et al.* A prospective study of surgeon-performed ultrasound as the primary adjuvant modality for injured patient assessment. *J Trauma* 1995;**39**:492–498.

Chapter 148

Tutorial: Pediatric cervical spine radiology

Swaminatha V. Mahadevan

A systematic approach to evaluating cervical spine plain films is crucial to identifying subtle abnormalities. Several common variations of the pediatric cervical spine may simulate injury.

1. Pseudosubluxation of either C2 on C3 (up to 4 mm), or C3 on C4 (Fig. 148.1).
2. Increased (anteroposterior) predental space (up to 5 mm) (Fig. 148.2).
3. Anterior wedging (up to 3 mm) of the vertebral bodies.
4. Overriding of up to two-thirds of the anterior arch of C1 above the odontoid tip.
5. Absence of normal cervical lordosis.
6. Delayed fusion of the anterior arch of the atlas with the neural arches.
7. Asymmetric positioning of the odontoid between the lateral arches of C1.
8. Lucent apical odontoid epiphysis.
9. Persistent basilar odontoid synchondrosis.
10. Secondary ossification centers of spinous processes and unfused ring apophyses of the vertebral bodies.
11. Widening of the prevertebral soft tissues secondary to expiration.

Figure 148.3 gives an overview of the approach to evaluating cervical spine radiographs. When abnormalities are identified on plain films, a CT should be performed.

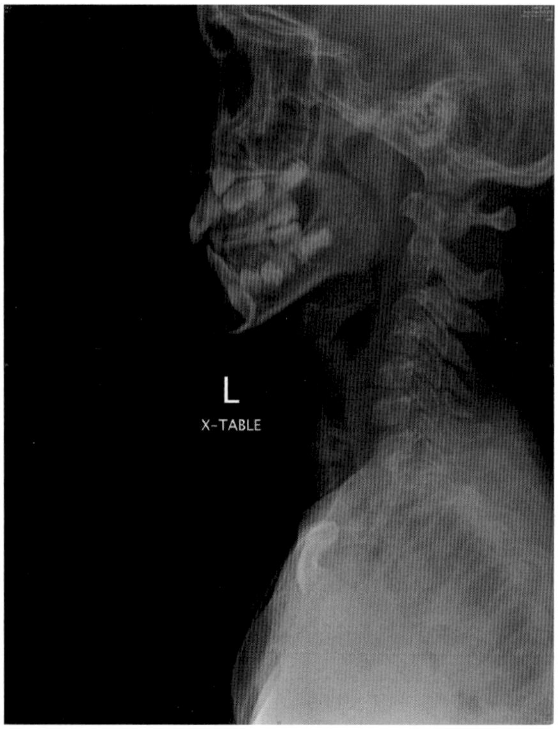

Figure 148.1 Pseudosubluxation. Anterior displacement of C2 on C3; the posterior cervical line is normal. (Courtesy S. V. Mahadevan.)

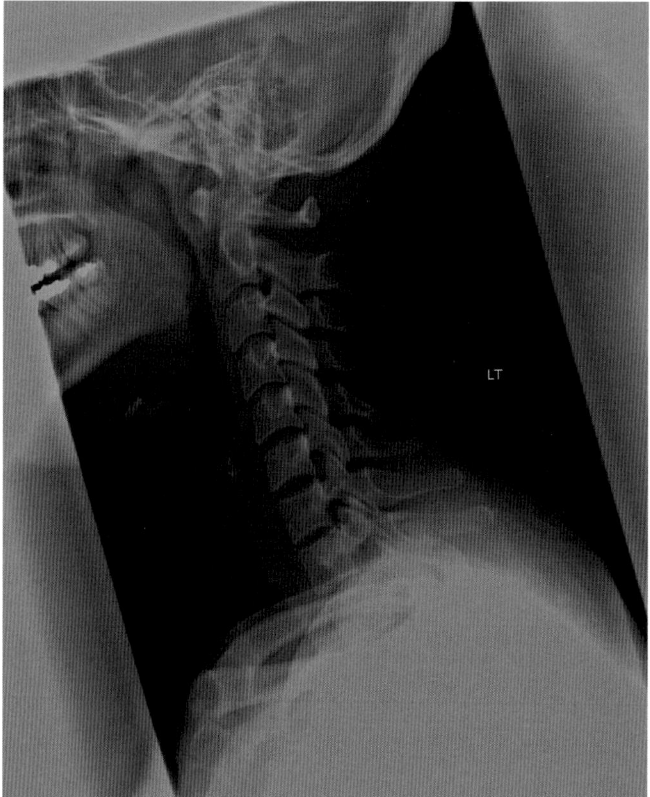

Figure 148.2 Increased predental space. (Courtesy S. V. Mahadevan.)

A Practical Guide to Pediatric Emergency Medicine: Caring for Children in the Emergency Department, ed. N. Ewen Amieva-Wang (associate eds. Jamie Shandro, Aparajita Sohoni, and Bernhard Fassl). Published by Cambridge University Press. Copyright © N. E. Amieva-Wang, J. Shandro, A. Sohoni, and B. Fassl 2011.

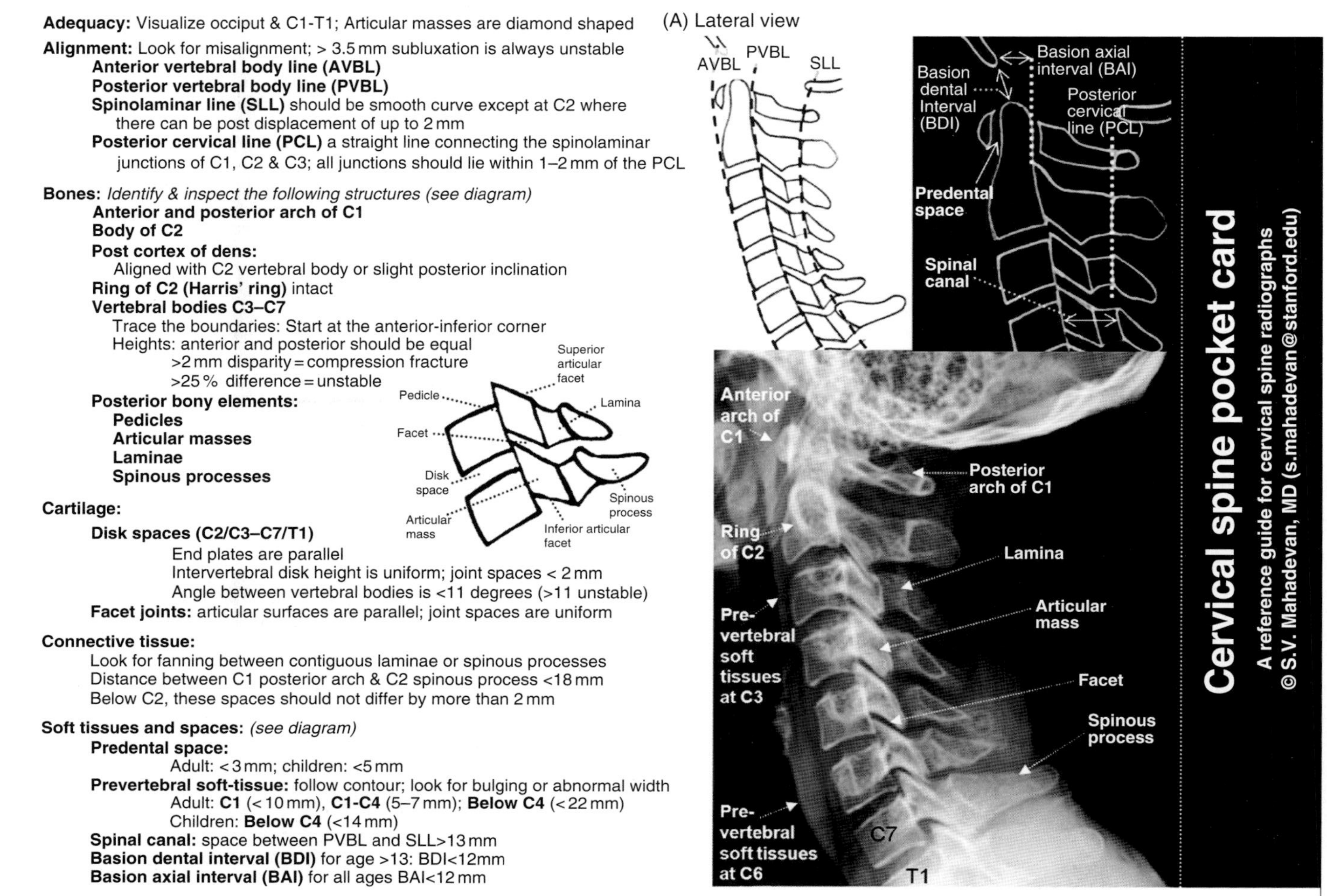

Adequacy: Visualize occiput & C1-T1; Articular masses are diamond shaped
Alignment: Look for misalignment; > 3.5 mm subluxation is always unstable
Anterior vertebral body line (AVBL)
Posterior vertebral body line (PVBL)
Spinolaminar line (SLL) should be smooth curve except at C2 where there can be post displacement of up to 2 mm
Posterior cervical line (PCL) a straight line connecting the spinolaminar junctions of C1, C2 & C3; all junctions should lie within 1–2 mm of the PCL
Bones: Identify & inspect the following structures (see diagram)
Anterior and posterior arch of C1
Body of C2
Post cortex of dens:
Aligned with C2 vertebral body or slight posterior inclination
Ring of C2 (Harris' ring) intact
Vertebral bodies C3–C7
Trace the boundaries: Start at the anterior-inferior corner
Heights: anterior and posterior should be equal
>2 mm disparity = compression fracture
>25 % difference = unstable
Posterior bony elements:
Pedicles
Articular masses
Laminae
Spinous processes
Cartilage:
Disk spaces (C2/C3–C7/T1)
End plates are parallel
Intervertebral disk height is uniform; joint spaces < 2 mm
Angle between vertebral bodies is <11 degrees (>11 unstable)
Facet joints: articular surfaces are parallel; joint spaces are uniform
Connective tissue:
Look for fanning between contiguous laminae or spinous processes
Distance between C1 posterior arch & C2 spinous process <18 mm
Below C2, these spaces should not differ by more than 2 mm
Soft tissues and spaces: (see diagram)
Predental space:
Adult: < 3 mm; children: <5 mm
Prevertebral soft-tissue: follow contour; look for bulging or abnormal width
Adult: C1 (< 10 mm), C1-C4 (5–7 mm); Below C4 (< 22 mm)
Children: Below C4 (<14 mm)
Spinal canal: space between PVBL and SLL>13 mm
Basion dental interval (BDI) for age >13: BDI<12mm
Basion axial interval (BAI) for all ages BAI<12 mm
Superior articular facet
Pedicle
Lamina
Facet
Disk space
Spinous process
Articular mass
Inferior articular facet
(A) Lateral view
AVBL
PVBL
SLL
Basion dental Interval (BDI)
Basion axial interval (BAI)
Posterior cervical line (PCL)
Predental space
Spinal canal
Cervical spine pocket card
A reference guide for cervical spine radiographs
© S.V. Mahadevan, MD (s.mahadevan@stanford.edu)
Anterior arch of C1
Posterior arch of C1
Ring of C2
Lamina
Pre-vertebral soft tissues at C3
Articular mass
Facet
Spinous process
Pre-vertebral soft tissues at C6
C7
T1

Figure 148.3 Approach to evaluating cervical spine plain films: the ABCs of assessment. (A) Lateral view; (B) open–mouth view; (C) anterior–posterior view. (Copyright S. V. Mahadevan.)

(B) Open mouth

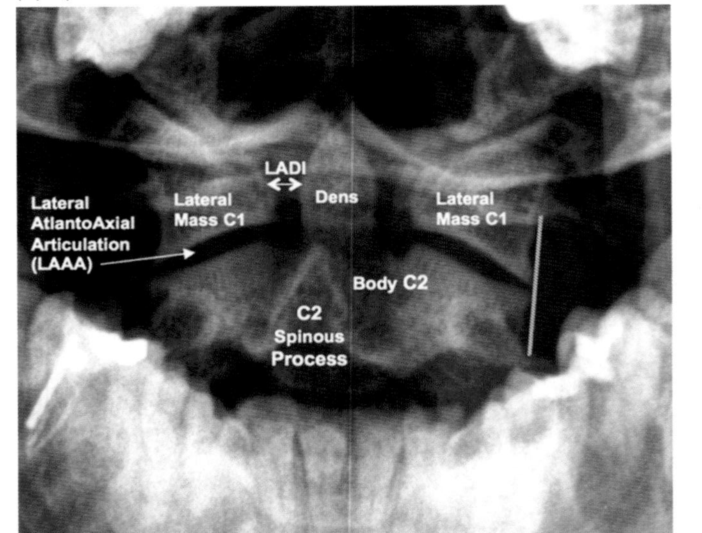

Adequacy: The dens and lateral masses (C1 and C2) are visible including the entire **lateral atlantoaxial articulation (LAAA)**
Rotation is minimized: Dens and C2 spinous process are in the midline

Alignment: Lateral margins of the articular surfaces of C1-C2 are aligned (═══)
About 1–2 mm symmetric overriding is allowable medially or laterally

Bones: *Identify & inspect the following structures (see diagram above)*
Lateral masses of C1
Spinous process of C2
Peg and base of the dens
Body of C2

Cartilage: The **lateral atlantoaxial articulation** of C1–C2 form parallel joint surfaces

Spaces: **Lateral atlantodental intervals (LADI)** are similar but not necessarily equal

Figure 148.3 *(cont.)*

(C) Anterior–posterior

Adequacy: No tilt or rotation
The vertebral bodies of C3-T1 are visible

Alignment: The spinous processes are aligned in the midline
The articular masses form a smooth, undulating and continuous lateral margin

Bones: *Identify & inspect the following structures (diagram above)*
Vertebral bodies: Are rectangular and of uniform height/width
Uncinate processes
Lateral masses
Spinous processes

Cartilage: Disk spaces are of uniform height
articular surfaces are parallel

Spaces: Spinous processes are equidistant

Section

24

Urologic emergencies

Expert reviewer: William A. Kennedy II

Chapter 149 Penile complaints

Jonathan E. Davis

Introduction

Emergency penile conditions include priapism and paraphimosis. Sexually transmitted diseases (STDs) will also be discussed in this chapter.

Anatomy

The penis consists of the corpora cavernosa (erectile bodies) and the corpus spongiosum, which surrounds the urethra (Fig. 149.1). In uncircumcised males, the retractile penile foreskin is a sleeve that covers the head of the penis (glans penis). Each corpus cavernosum is surrounded by a dense connective tissue layer, the tunica albuginea.

History

Practitioners should inquire specifically about any history of prior surgery or procedures (including circumcision), medication use, as well as underlying medical problems. In addition, history regarding sexual habits, including number and gender of sexual contacts as well as condom use, is important for peri- and post-pubescent males.

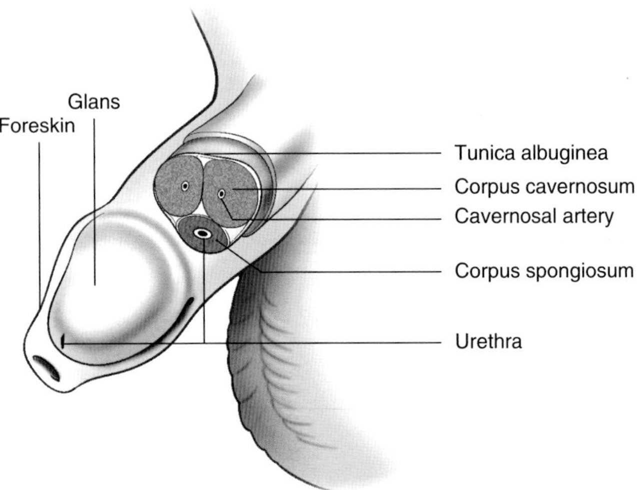

Figure 149.1 Anatomy of the penis. (copyright C. Gralappe.)

Differential diagnosis

Patients with penile complaints often present with nonspecific complaints such as a "painful" or "swollen" penis (Table 149.1). It is imperative to distinguish localized processes (such as constriction [i.e., paraphimosis, entrapment injury], inflammation [i.e., balanoposthitis], infection [i.e., "bite" injury], or other trauma [i.e., abrasion, contusion]) from edema resulting from a systemic derangement.

Priapism

Priapism is a pathologic condition defined as the presence of a persistent erection lasting longer than 4 h. It most frequently results from engorgement of the corpora cavernosa with stagnant blood flow (termed low-flow priapism). Patients with low-flow priapism often complain of an exquisitely painful and prolonged erection. Stagnant, oxygen-poor, acidic blood accumulates in the corpora, resulting in "ischemic" pain. Ischemia resulting from prolonged duration of the pathologic erection may lead to irreversible cellular damage, permanent fibrosis, and impotence. The more prevalent etiologies of low-flow priapism in the pediatric population include medications or hematologic disorders (such as sickle cell disease and leukemia).

Although rare, high-flow priapism results from the development of traumatic arterial–cavernosal fistulae, resulting in the accumulation of oxygen-rich blood in the corpora. These patients complain of a persistent, yet painless, erection as there is continuous inflow of oxygen-rich blood through the traumatic arterial–cavernosal fistulae. High- and low-flow priapism are definitively differentiated by a penile blood gas.

Paraphimosis

Paraphimosis classically develops in uncircumcised males of any age when the proximally retracted foreskin acts as a constricting band on the distal portion of the penile shaft (Fig. 149.2). Initial disruption of venous drainage by the constricting foreskin leads to a cycle of progressive glans edema.

A Practical Guide to Pediatric Emergency Medicine: Caring for Children in the Emergency Department, ed. N. Ewen Amieva-Wang (associate eds. Jamie Shandro, Aparajita Sohoni, and Bernhard Fassl). Published by Cambridge University Press.

Table 149.1 Aged-based differential diagnoses for penile complaints

	Common age	Symptoms	Signs
Most threatening			
Priapism	Any (sickle cell disease)	Persistent erection	Persistent erection
Paraphimosis	Any	Swelling and pain of head of the penis, uncircumcised male	Edema of retracted penile foreskin; glans edema, with possibility of distal penile vascular compromise
Entrapment injury (hair tourniquet)	Infant, adolescent	Swelling and pain of head of the penis, circumcised or uncircumcised male	Glans edema, with possibility of distal penile vascular compromise; may see constricting object proximal to glans
Penile fracture	Postpubescent	Sudden "snapping" sound, followed by immediate loss of erectile function	Edema, tenderness, ecchymoses, flaccidity of penile shaft
Genitourinal trauma	Any	History of blunt or penetrating mechanism of injury	Variable depending on mechanism
Other etiologies			
Balanitis	Any, typically school-age male	Pain, itching, swelling of glans penis	Tenderness, excoriation, rash
Posthitis	Any, typically school-age male	Pain, itching, swelling of penile foreskin	Tenderness, excoriation, rash
Phimosis	Any, physiologic common in uncircumcised <4 years	Foreskin "stuck" in position, covering head of penis; may present with entrapment of urine under foreskin with poor/no drainage	Inability to retract foreskin
Sexually transmitted disease	Postpubescent; consider abuse if prepubescent	Variable depending on cause	Genital ulceration(s); penile discharge

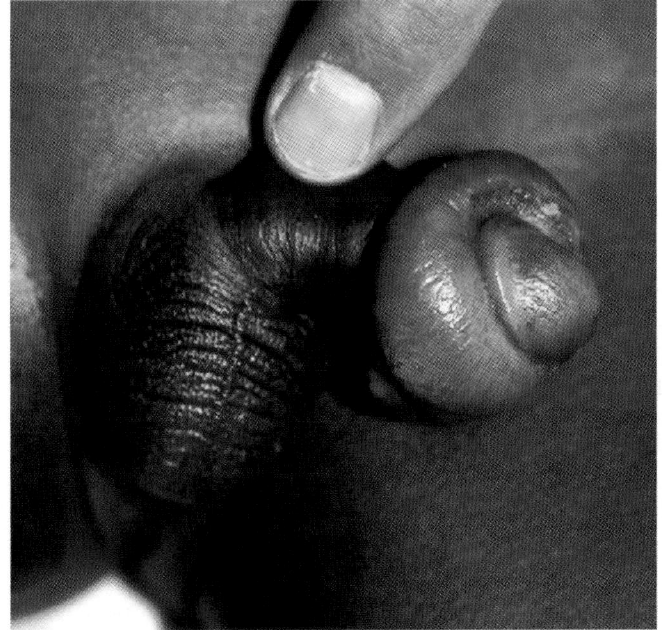

Figure 149.2 Paraphimosis in the uncircumcised male results from entrapment of the foreskin proximal to the glans. In this image, the foreskin has been retracted proximal to the glans penis and has become markedly swollen secondary to venous congestion. (Reproduced with permission from Kliegman RM, Behrman RE, Jenson HB, Stanton BF (eds.) *Nelson Textbook of Pediatrics*, 17th edn. Philadelphia, PA: Saunders, 2007, p. 2256. © Saunders Inc., an affiliate of Elsevier Inc.)

Progressive glans edema may eventually lead to arterial compromise and subsequent glans necrosis and gangrene. The penile foreskin should always be replaced after retraction for examination or urethral catheter placement to avoid development of an iatrogenic paraphimosis.

Glans edema mimicking a paraphimosis can occur in circumcised or uncircumcised males in the case of penile entrapment injuries. In these instances, external objects may constrict the mid to distal shaft, leading to the same pathophysiologic derangements seen with paraphimosis. These objects may either be placed intentionally for sexual stimulation (i.e., string, metal rings, or rubber rings), or may occur sporadically, as in the case of a hair tourniquet in male infants. Hair tourniquets may be particularly difficult to diagnose, as the offending hair may be nearly invisible within an edematous coronal sulcus of the glans penis. An occult hair tourniquet should be considered in the infant with inconsolable crying.

Phimosis

Phimosis is the inability to retract the penile foreskin proximally. A pathologic phimosis exists when the failure to retract results from distal scarring of the prepuce. This is typically a subacute condition that may present acutely to the ED when a patient develops entrapment of urine beneath the foreskin with poor to no drainage.

A non-retractile foreskin is common among boys in the first few years of life (physiologic phimosis).

In contrast to a pathologic variety, a physiologic phimosis consists of a pliant, unscarred preputial orifice as seen on physical examination. The foreskin gradually becomes retractile over time as a result of intermittent erections and keratinization of the inner preputial epithelium. By 3 years of age, fewer than 10% of foreskins remain non-retractile, with nearly all becoming retractile by late adolescence.

Balanitis and posthitis

Balanitis and posthitis are defined as inflammation of the glans penis or penile foreskin, respectively, and they typically result from inflammation (i.e., local irritation) with or without co-existing bacterial (i.e., typically *Streptococcus* or *Staphylococcus* spp.) or fungal (i.e., *Candida* sp.) infection. Balanoposthitis refers to these two conditions occurring together. It may occur as a result of poor hygiene and is commonly seen in boys who wear diapers. Recurrent episodes of balanoposthitis may lead to scarring or, in extreme cases, a pathologic phimosis.

Trauma

The most common causes of penile trauma in children are circumcision and zipper trauma. The most common complication of circumcision is hemorrhage, although usually it is minimal.

Tourniquet injuries of the penis can result from any object that can constrict penile blood flow, such as bands, rings, or human hair. Hair tourniquet should be included in the differential diagnosis for inconsolable crying of an infant. The glans becomes swollen and painful. Often misdiagnosed as paraphimosis or balanitis, hair tourniquets may require local anesthesia or procedural sedation to remove.

A penile fracture is an acute tear or rupture of the tunica albuginea of the corpus cavernosum. Patients often report a history of a sudden "snapping" sound during intercourse or other sexual activity, or as a result of blunt trauma in the setting of an erect penis. Physical examination reveals a swollen, ecchymotic, detumescent (limp) penis, which is tender to palpation. A penile contusion results from less-severe direct blunt force to a typically detumescent penis. In a penile contusion, the tunica albuginea remains intact, and the patient presents with localized ecchymoses and tenderness at the site of trauma. This may result from a toilet seat injury sustained while "potty-training" in the toddler/preschool-age groups, or as a result of a "straddle" mechanism in any age group. Penile injuries from penetrating trauma are rare and, similar to blunt trauma, can be associated with urethral injury. Blood at the meatus or inability to void are highly suspicious for urethral injury. In cases of genitourinary trauma, it is prudent to remain particularly vigilant to the possibility of child abuse.

Sexually transmitted diseases

Genital infections that are likely to cause acute symptoms can be divided into diseases characterized by genital ulceration and diseases causing penile discharge (i.e., urethritis). Among the many infections that can cause genital ulceration, genital herpes, syphilis, and chancroid are most commonly seen in the USA, with genital herpes most prevalent. In addition, human papillomavirus may present in males as raised, verrucous penile lesions. Urethritis is typically characterized by discharge of mucopurulent or purulent material, with or without accompanying dysuria or urethral pruritis. The principal bacterial pathogens of proven clinical importance in men with urethritis are *Neisseria gonorrhoeae* and *Chlamydia trachomatis.*

Sexually transmitted disease is common among adolescents. Younger adolescents (<15 years old) who are sexually active are at particular risk for STDs. In prepubertal males, the confirmed presence of an STD is either diagnostic (gonorrhea, chlamydia, syphillis) or suspicious (trichomonas, genital herpes, anogenital warts, new HIV infection) for sexual abuse.

Urethritis

Any patient presenting to the ED with penile discharge should be assumed to have urethritis. Testing to determine the specific etiology is recommended. The distinction between urethritis with or without accompanying epididymitis is critical as it has important therapy implications.

Diagnostic studies

The diagnosis of priapism and paraphimosis are made on clinical grounds, with the physical examination providing confirmatory evidence. In genitourinary trauma, a sonogram can be very useful in delineating the extent of injury and for assessing distal penile vascular integrity. The STDs may require additional confirmatory microbiologic laboratory testing, including direct culture or other automated techniques such as PCR.

Management

Priapism

It may be necessary for the EP to initiate treatment for low-flow priapism prior to availability of a urologist. Oral (or SC) terbutaline has long been proposed as the initial treatment for low-flow priapism, regardless of inciting etiology. It is thought that terbutaline, a β_2-adrenergic agonist, serves to increase venous outflow from the engorged corpora by way of relaxing venous sinusoidal smooth muscle. Although consensus expert opinion questions the utility of this intervention, an initial trial of terbutaline is reasonable, as it is the least invasive therapeutic option. Other treatments include corporal blood aspiration, saline irrigation (to break-up the clots), and direct corporal injection of an α-adrenergic receptor agonist (such as phenylephrine or epinephrine). The goal of treatment in the patient with sickle cell disease and priapism is reduction of red cell sickling, thereby reducing vascular sludging and vaso-occlusion. Optimal treatments in this setting include oxygen, IV hydration, and possibly simple or exchange transfusions. As they can cause permanent impotence, surgical shunt procedures are used as a last resort in patients with low-flow priapism unresponsive to the aforementioned treatments.

Paraphimosis

Paraphimosis is relatively unique among the genitourinary emergencies, as it can frequently be managed in the ED without the need for emergency specialty consultation. There are many reported methods of successful paraphimosis reduction. The most commonly employed initial maneuver involves manual compression of the distal glans penis to decrease edema, followed by reduction of the glans penis back through the proximal constricting band of foreskin. A variant of this procedure entails wrapping the penis with a self-adherent wrap to apply steady pressure to decrease edema before manual reduction. Application of an iced glove to the distal penis for 5 min is reported to work. We do not recommend applying granulated sugar or placement of multiple puncture wounds in the swollen glans, although this has been reported in the literature as an approach.

Phimosis

Prudent treatment of physiologic phimosis is "tincture of time." Alternatively, a trial of topical corticosteroids applied to the preputial outlet may be initiated to help to expedite the process, although this treatment needs to be continued for 6–8 weeks and its overall utility is debated in the literature. With a pathologic phimosis, ensure the ability to void spontaneously, and refer to urology for timely follow-up.

Balanoposthitis

Treatment of balanoposthitis typically consists of local cleansing and application of antibacterial or antifungal ointment, depending on the appearance of the skin lesion. On occasion, a course of oral antimicrobial drug may be needed.

Trauma

Post-circumcision bleeding is usually controlled with direct pressure, silver nitrate application, or an absorbable suture. With zipper entrapment, a bone or wire cutter can be used to cut the median bar of zipper. Simply applying anesthetic gel can allow the foreskin to slip out. Edema can be subsequently treated with warm soaks.

Hair tourniquets may require local anesthesia or procedural sedation to remove. Over-the-counter hair removal products, such as Nair, have been used successfully for the removal of digital (finger, toe) hair tourniquets, leading some to suggest its utility for penile hair tourniquets as well. These products however, are very caustic and should not be used near mucous membranes such as the urethral meatus or inner preputial tissue.

Penile fractures and penetrating penile injuries necessitate specialty consultation in all cases.

Sexually transmitted diseases

Treatment for presumptive STD should be initiated empirically based on historical and examination findings. Patients found to have one STD are at risk for others as well. As such, the use of additional confirmatory tests should be considered. Alternatively, empiric treatment for all likely pathogens should be initiated before the patient leaves the ED, particularly if the adequacy of follow-up care remains a concern.

A key treatment decision rests in distinguishing urethritis from epididymitis. When accompanying epididymal pain or tenderness is present, both the dosage and the duration of antimicrobial treatment increase, as epididymitis represents a more advanced stage of reproductive tract disease. For instance, a typical treatment regimen for isolated urethritis is a single dose of ceftriaxone 125 mg (IM) plus azithromycin 1 g (PO), whereas typical treatment for epididymitis is ceftriaxone 250 mg (IM) plus doxycycline 100 mg (PO) twice daily for 10 days (CDC Sexually transmitted diseases treatment guidelines).

Disposition

Emergency conditions that require discussion with an appropriate specialist in the ED include priapism, paraphimosis and genitourinary trauma. Patients with acute penile pain who have been ruled out for conditions necessitating emergency

Pearls and pitfalls

Pearls

1. There are three true penile emergencies: priapism, paraphimosis, and any form of genitourinary trauma until proven non-operative.
2. Differentiating true genitourinary emergencies (requiring prompt action) from urgent conditions (safe for outpatient management) takes precedence over definitive diagnosis in the majority of patients.
3. Successful reduction of paraphimosis can often be performed in the ED.

Pitfalls

1. Failure to perform a genitourinary examination in an infant with inconsolable crying, or in a non-communicative male patient.
2. Failure to replace penile foreskin following examination or urethral catheter placement in an uncircumcised male.
3. Failure to consider abuse in genitourinary complaints with an inconsistent history.

consultation can be referred for specialty or primary care follow-up. Whenever in doubt, appropriate consultation should be obtained while the patient remains in the ED. When evaluating pediatric genitourinary complaints, the EP must always remain vigilant to the possibility of child abuse and always address pain by providing adequate analgesia.

Selected references

Centers for Disease Control and Prevention. Sexually transmitted diseases treatment guidelines, 2006. *MMWR Morb Mortal Wkly Rep* 2006;**55**(RR-11):49–56.

Kellogg N for the American Academy of Pediatrics Committee on Child Abuse and Neglect. The evaluation of sexual abuse in children. *Pediatrics* 2005;**116**:506–512.

Lowe JC, Jarow JP. Placebo-controlled study of oral terbutaline and pseudoephedrine in management of prostaglandin E_1-induced prolonged erections. *Urology* 1993;**42**:51–54.

McGregor TB, Pike KJG, Leonard MP. Pathologic and physiologic phimosis: approach to the phimotic foreskin. *Can Fam Physician* 2007;**53**:445–448.

Priyadarshi S. Oral terbutaline in the management of pharmacologically induced prolonged erection. *Int J Impotence Res* 2004;**16**:424–426.

Chapter 150

Scrotal complaints

Jonathan E. Davis

Introduction

When a child presents with scrotal pain, the most important conditions to consider, correctly diagnose, and treat expediently are testicular torsion, a strangulated inguinal hernia, and necrotizing fasciitis of the perineum (Fournier's disease or Fournier's gangrene).

Anatomy

The scrotal wall consists of several layers. Each testis is encapsulated within a dense connective tissue layer termed the tunica albuginea (Fig. 150.1). External to the tunica albuginea is the tunica vaginalis, which envelops each testicle and fastens it to the posterior scrotal wall. The scrotal ligament (gubernaculum) anchors each testicle inferiorly. A lack of firm attachment of the testicle to the posterior scrotal wall makes each testis prone to rotation in a horizontal plane about the spermatic cord within the tunica vaginalis, a condition termed testicular torsion (Fig. 150.2). The spermatic cord contains the testicular blood supply (via the gonadal vessels) as well as the vas deferens. Interruption of testicular blood flow by twisting of the spermatic cord can rapidly lead to ischemia and subsequent infarction. The appendix testes are embryologic remnants with no known physiologic function. These appendages may torse as well, leading to localized, self-limited necrosis. This results in pain which can be confused with pain from torsion of the testicle.

An inguinal hernia may occur when there is a defect in the anterior abdominal wall musculature (direct inguinal hernia) (Fig. 150.3). Alternatively, a persistent embryologic communication (patent processus vaginalis) between the peritoneal cavity and the tunica vaginalis may result in an indirect

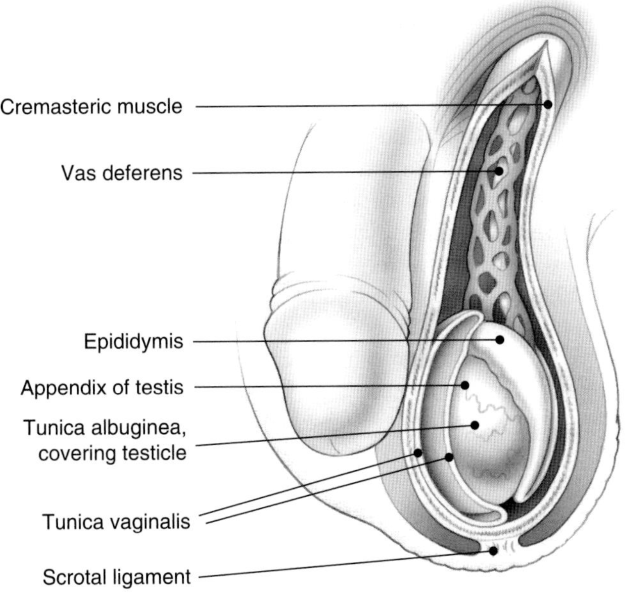

Figure 150.1 Anatomy of the scrotum (Copyright Chris Gralapp; reproduced with permission from Mahadevan SV, Garmel GM. *An Introduction to Clinical Emergency Medicine*. Cambridge, UK: Cambridge University Press, 2005.)

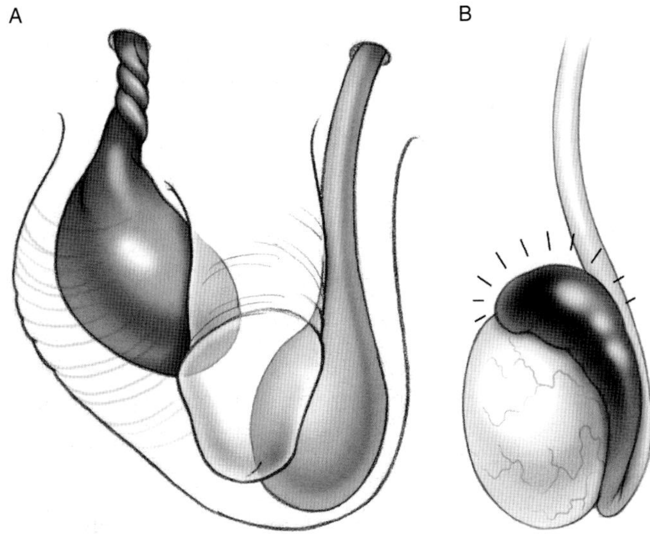

Figure 150.2 (A) Testicular torsion and (B) epididymitis. (Copyright Chris Gralapp; reproduced with permission from Mahadevan SV, Garmel GM. *An Introduction to Clinical Emergency Medicine*. Cambridge, UK: Cambridge University Press, 2005.)

A Practical Guide to Pediatric Emergency Medicine: Caring for Children in the Emergency Department, ed. N. Ewen Amieva-Wang (associate eds. Jamie Shandro, Aparajita Sohoni, and Bernhard Fassl). Published by Cambridge University Press.

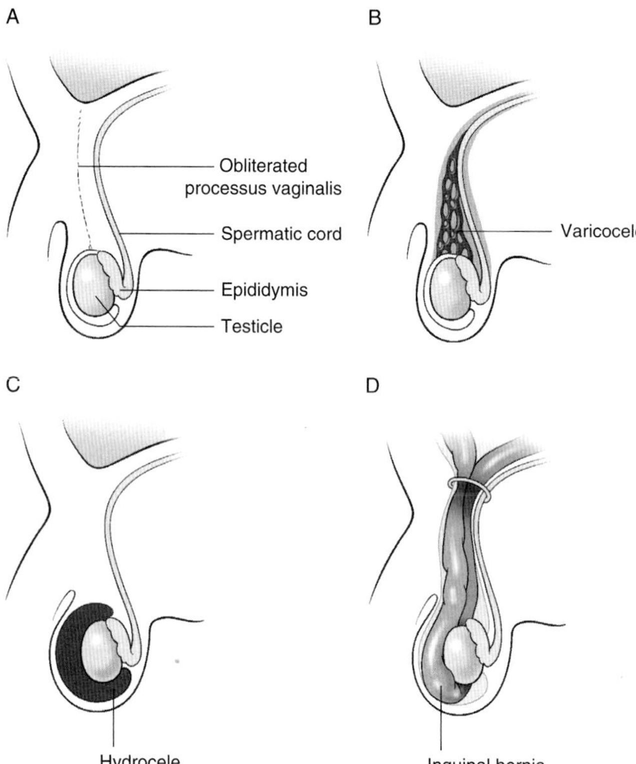

Figure 150.3 (A) Normal anatomy. (B) Varicocele. (C) Hydrocele. (D) Inguinal hernia. (Copyright Chris Gralapp.)

inguinal hernia. Fluid accumulation in the tunica vaginalis occurs through a similar mechanism (congenital hydrocele). A reducible hernia occurs when abdominal contents can freely (or with simple manipulation) move between the abdomen and the hernia sac. An irreducible (or incarcerated) hernia cannot return to its normal site spontaneously or by simple manipulation. An irreducible hernia may become strangulated, where pressure on the hernial contents compromises blood supply. Both direct and indirect herniae present when incarcerated or strangulated. Inguinal hernias are identified usually in the first year of life; there is a 10:1 male:female predominance. Femoral herniae are rare in pediatric patients.

Differential diagnoses

The majority of patients with the complaint of acute scrotal pain will have a problem isolated to the genitalia. However, it is also important to consider that genitourinary pain may be referred from other anatomic regions (e.g., intra-abdominal or retroperitoneal). Likewise, it is important to consider acute genitourinary pathology in the differential for any male patient presenting with seemingly isolated pain to the abdomen, thigh, or flank.

A wide variety of clinical conditions may all present in an identical fashion: with a male patient complaining of acute, unilateral (or bilateral) scrotal pain and swelling (the "acute scrotum") (Table 150.1). In the vast majority of pediatric patients, acute scrotal pain can be attributed to one of three diagnostic entities (Table 150.2):

- testicular torsion
- epididymitis
- appendage torsion.

Clinical presentation

A diligent and focused history and physical examination of the patient complaining of acute scrotal symptoms is the cornerstone of providing appropriate care. Patients and also their parents may be uncomfortable in discussing the symptoms. Take care to respect and address privacy issues, particularly in the adolescent and prepubescent age groups.

History

Pain that begins abruptly and severely is concerning for testicular torsion. The sudden twisting of the spermatic cord characteristic of testicular torsion leads to rapid diminution of blood supply to the affected testicle, causing "ischemic" pain. Pain may occur intermittently, as the spermatic cord may spontaneously torse and detorse. Whereas the pain of testicular or appendage torsion often develops over seconds or minutes, the pain associated with epididymitis frequently develops over the course of days. Epididymitis is a gradually progressive inflammatory process that is characterized by a more indolent and smoldering pain (Fig. 150.2). Patients may exhibit pain with ambulation or movement as a result of the inflammation.

As a general rule, males with testicular torsion appear more ill, with associated systemic signs and symptoms such as nausea and emesis, than patients with appendage torsion or uncomplicated epididymitis. While patients with epididymitis may present with nausea, malaise, or low-grade fever, it is typically those with more advanced degrees of infection (epididymo-orchitis) who exhibit more "systemic" involvement.

The EP should always inquire about changes in urination, including urgency, frequency, dysuria, hesitancy, and hematuria. Urinary symptoms may accompany many causes of acute scrotal pain. Classically, epididymitis may be accompanied by urinary complaints such as dysuria and urgency.

Physical examination

Patients with intermittent colicky pain (i.e., testicular torsion or renal colic) tend to writhe on the gurney as they cannot find a position of comfort. In contrast, patients with progressive inflammatory conditions (such as epididymitis or epididymo-orchitis) tend to minimize activity, as the slightest degree of movement may exacerbate their pain.

A complete abdominal examination is crucial in any patient presenting with an acute scrotum, as many intra-abdominal conditions may present with a component of genitourinary

Table 150.1. Aged-based differential diagnoses of scrotal pain

	Peak incidence	Symptoms	Signs
Most threatening			
Testicular torsion	Any age, high-risk in neonates, adolescents	Sudden and severe onset of pain; often associated with nausea and emesis ("systemic" symptoms)	High-riding testicle with transverse lie; intact ipsilateral cremasteric reflex decreases the probability of testicular torsion
Fournier's disease	Any age, high-risk in immunosuppressed, diabetic	Perineal pain, swelling, redness, bruising; fever, vomiting, lethargy, weakness ("systemic" signs of illness)	Paucity of local findings in early stages ("pain out of proportion to physical findings"); may rapidly progress to fulminant sepsis and shock
Genitourinal trauma	Any age	History of blunt or penetrating mechanism of injury	Highly variable depending on mechanism
Other genitourinal etiologies			
Appendage torsion	Prepubescent	More indolent onset of symptoms compared with testicular torsion; rarely "systemic" symptoms such as nausea and vomiting	Tender nodule at head of testicle or epididymis; "blue dot sign" pathognomonic
Epididymitis	2 years and adolescent	More indolent onset of symptoms compared with testicular torsion	*Early*: tenderness isolated to epididymis *Late*: with progression, inflammation becomes contiguous with testicle (epididymo-orchitis)
Epididymo-orchitis	2 years and adolescent	Often more "systemic" findings compared with isolated epididymitis	Large, swollen scrotal mass; indistinct border between testicle and epididymis
Hematocele	Any age	Painful scrotal mass; often antecedent history of trauma	Ecchymoses of scrotal skin; testicular/scrotal tenderness
Hydrocele	Any (most commonly found first year of life)	Gradual or sudden onset of swelling, secondary to fluid accumulation	Transillumination can be helpful in differential diagnosis
Idiopathic scrotal edema	Primarily in children <10 years	Typically unilateral scrotal swelling and edema	Scrotal, perineal, inguinal erythema and edema
Orchitis	Any age	Gradual onset of unilateral (or bilateral) testicular swelling and pain	Swelling and tenderness isolated to testicle (or testes); no epididymal involvement
Scrotal skin disorders	Any age	Variable depending on cause	Must distinguish between lesions localized to scrotal wall and those contiguous with deeper structures
Tumor	More common in children <5 years and those postpubertal	Gradually progressive testicular mass; often painless	May appreciate mass, firmness, or induration
Varicocele	Adolescents, rare in prepubertal males	Gradual onset of unilateral swelling; often painless	Abnormally enlarged spermatic cord venous plexus (described as a "bag of worms" on palpation)
Vasculitis (HSP)	School age	Testicular swelling and pain	Associated vasculitis findings (such as buttock/lower extremity purpura and renal involvement in HSP)

Table 150.1. *(cont.)*

	Peak incidence	Symptoms	Signs
Other pathology			
Acute appendicitis	Any age	Fever, nausea, vomiting, anorexia, RLQ pain	RLQ tenderness classic; may have associated abdominal rebound/guarding
Inguinal hernia	More common in first year of life	Unilateral inguinal/scrotal swelling and pain	Reducible, incarcerated and strangulated forms; last two often more tender on examination
Renal colic	Adolescents	Sudden, severe, "colicky" pain, may be referred to ipsilateral groin/testicle mimicking testicular torsion; often associated flank pain or urinary symptoms, and systemic findings such as nausea, vomiting, diaphoresis	CVA tenderness, low abdominal tenderness
Pyelonephritis	Any	Constant and progressive flank pain, may be referred to ipsilateral groin/testicle; often associated urinary symptoms, and systemic findings such as nausea, vomiting, fever	CVA tenderness, low abdominal tenderness, fever

CVA, costovertebral angle HSP, Henoch–Schönlein purpura; LRQ, lower right quadrant.

Table 150.2. Differentiating testicular torsion, epididymitis, and appendage torsion

	Testicular torsion	Epididymitis	Appendage torsion
History			
Age	Incidence peaks in neonatal and adolescent groups, but may occur at any age	<2 years and adolescents Its	Prepubescent
Risk factors	Undescended testicle (neonate), rapid increase in testicular size (adolescent), failure of prior torsion surgical repair	Voiding dysfunction in young children (chemical epididymitis), sexual activity, GU anomalies, GU instrumentation	Predisposing anatomy
Pain onset	Sudden	Gradual	Sudden or gradual
Prior episodes of similar pain	Possible (spontaneous detorsion)	Unlikely (unless recurrent)	Occasional (torsion/ detorsion of appendage or multiple appendages)
History of trauma	Possible	Possible	Possible
Nausea/ vomiting	Common	Rare	Rare
Dysuria	Rare	Common	Rare
Physical findings			
Fever	Rare (except late presentation with possible necrosis)	Seen in advanced disease (epididymo-orchitis)	Rare
Location of swelling/ tenderness	Testicle, progressing to diffuse hemiscrotal involvement	Epididymis, progressing to diffuse hemiscrotal involvement	Localized to head of affected testicle or epididymis
Cremasteric reflex	Typically absent	Typically present	Typically present
Testicle position	High riding testicle with transverse alignment	Normal position with vertical alignment	Normal position with vertical alignment
Pyuria	Rare	More common	Rare

pain. It is important to examine the male genitalia both while the patient is standing and when lying supine. Exercise caution when examining a standing patient as some males may experience a strong vagal response to scrotal stimulation, leading to presyncope or syncope. Also, examination of the testicle and epididymis may cause significant discomfort even in the absence of pathology. The unaffected side is examined first. Key visual features of testicular torsion include a high-riding testicle with a transverse lie resulting from twisting of the spermatic cord. Unfortunately, such "textbook" presentations are rare. More commonly, patients with acute scrotal pain, regardless of underlying etiology, present with acute unilateral (or bilateral) scrotal swelling and testicular enlargement, with blurring of the distinction between the testicle and epididymis.

If isolated swelling and tenderness of the epididymis (adjacent to the posterolateral aspect of each testis) is present, epididymitis is the likely diagnosis. The natural progression of this infection is first to affect only the epididymis and then to progress to affect the ipsilateral testicle as well (epididymo-orchitis). Isolated nodularity at the superior pole of either the testicle or the epididymis is often the result of appendage torsion, given the anatomic location of these vestigial structures. In the case of hydrocele (or hematocele), the ability to distinguish the ipsilateral testis from the adjacent fluid-filled (or blood-filled) mass is variable. Hydroceles may be congenital or acquired, the latter resulting from local inflammation and associated fluid accumulation. Hematoceles typically develop following direct trauma. A varicocele is frequently described as a "bag of worms," which results from engorgement of the spermatic cord (pampiniform) venous plexus (Fig. 150.3). It can be felt superior to the testicle along the spermatic cord. A varicocele is more prominent in the standing position and decreases in size when supine. A mass or bulge in the vicinity of the inguinal canal may be indicative of an inguinal hernia. Ability to reduce a hernia is crucial, as an incarcerated (or strangulated) hernia necessitates immediate surgical intervention.

Idiopathic scrotal edema typically occurs in males <10 years old and presents with unilateral erythema and edema of the perineal/scrotal/inguinal skin, which may be very difficult to differentiate from an acute bacterial skin infection. It is a self-limited process with an unclear etiology, although allergic mechanisms have been proposed.

Additional techniques

The presence of an intact ipsilateral cremasteric reflex is reportedly highly sensitive for excluding the diagnosis of testicular torsion. This reflex is elicited by stroking the inner thigh with a tongue depressor or gloved hand, resulting in a reflexive elevation of the ipsilateral testicle through contraction of the cremasteric muscle (Fig. 150.4). Although the presence of an intact cremasteric reflex is useful in excluding torsion, the absence of this reflex is non-specific, as some healthy individuals lack the reflex altogether (particularly males in their first few years of life). Prehn's sign, or relief of pain with scrotal elevation, was previously thought to help in differentiating epididymitis (pain relieved with scrotal elevation) from testicular torsion (no change in symptoms with elevation). However, this sign is generally considered unreliable and its use is not recommended.

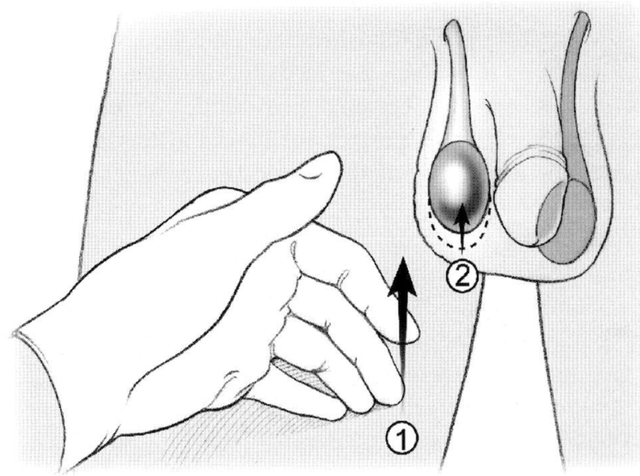

Figure 150.4 Cremasteric reflex. (Copyright Chris Gralapp; reproduced with permission Mahadevan SV, Garmel GM. *An Introduction to Clinical Emergency Medicine*. Cambridge, UK: Cambridge University Press, 2005.)

Appendage torsion is most common in the prepubescent age group, where the infarcted appendage (the "blue dot") may be seen through thin, non-hormonally stimulated prepubertal skin. The pathognomonic blue dot, however, is usually only seen prior to development of secondary skin changes. Scrotal transillumination may be performed in suspected hydrocele. The scrotal contents should, in theory, transilluminate when the tunica vaginalis is filled with light-transmitting fluid. However, practitioners tend to "overcall" positive test results (i.e., every scrotum transilluminates), so many experienced practitioners do not derive any additional diagnostic information by performing this test.

Fournier's gangrene may occur in diabetic or other immunocompromised children of any age. Key features of early Fournier's gangrene include pain out of proportion to findings on physical examination. Overt and progressive skin necrosis may be evident in advanced Fournier's disease.

Diagnostic studies

Routine blood work and urinalysis adds little to distinguish among the common etiologies of acute scrotal pain. These tests in fact only cause delays in diagnosis.

When utilized in the appropriate clinical setting, ultrasound remains the most useful diagnostic modality in the evaluation of genitourinary complaints. A color flow duplex Doppler ultrasound may be helpful in indeterminate cases of acute scrotal pain. The classic sonographic finding suggestive of testicular torsion is diminished intratesticular arterial blood flow. However, if a testicle has recently "detorsed," the blood flow may actually be increased (hyperemic) on ultrasound. This underscores the importance of clinical history and physical examination in making the diagnosis of testicular torsion. In epididymitis, perfusion will be normal (or increased) because of the effects of inflammatory mediators on local vascular beds. An infarcted appendage (resulting from appendage torsion) may also be visualized on ultrasound. Ultrasonography may also identify hydroceles, hematoceles, varicoceles, hernias, tumors, abscesses, or gonadal vasculitis.

Computed tomography may be helpful in assessing the degree of extension in genitourinary abscess or Fournier's disease.

Management

The key to managing acute genitourinary problems is the timely recognition of fertility- or life-threatening conditions. As testicular torsion produces end-organ ischemia, rapid detorsion (often accomplished in the operating room) must occur in order to prevent testicular infarction and necrosis.

If the history and examination suggests the diagnosis of testicular torsion, urology (or pediatric surgery) consultation and plans for immediate surgical exploration should be initiated without delay.

A patient of appropriate age (neonate, adolescent) with a classic history (sudden onset of scrotal pain with associated nausea/vomiting) and examination (high-riding gonad with transverse lie) findings of testicular torsion will not require any diagnostic tests. However, in less-distinct circumstances, a confirmatory diagnostic study (typically ultrasound) is indicated. In addition, the EP should always err on the side of caution and obtain specialty consultation sooner rather than later in indeterminate situations. If testicular torsion is strongly suspected, manual detorsion may be attempted; although the genitourinary consult should be called simultaneously, as the examination may be compromised. Pain medications should be given before attempting detorsion. As the testes most frequently torse in a lateral to medial fashion, detorsion is often accomplished by rotation of the affected testicle from medial to lateral (frequently described as "opening a book"). The end-point of the detorsion procedure is relief of pain.

In Fournier's disease, delays in recognition and definitive surgical debridement can be life threatening. Early consultation and administration of broad-spectrum antibiotics is indicated in all suspected cases; surgical debridement remains the definitive treatment. Interestingly, in contrast to adults, children with Fournier's disease may appear relatively non-toxic despite marked tissue inflammation and necrosis.

The question remains regarding the prudent management of patients presenting with an acute scrotum who have a "negative" ultrasound examination for testicular torsion. Sonography for the diagnosis of testicular torsion has its limitations; false negatives have been reported in up to 25% of cases in some series. As such, maintaining a high level of clinical suspicion based on historical and examination features is paramount, and diagnostic results need to be interpreted cautiously within the context of the overall clinical picture. If torsion is highly suspected, delay for diagnostic ultrasound is inappropriate if in-house surgical expertise to explore it is available, as time is of the essence.

Treatment

The primary goals of treatment in the ED setting are physiologic stabilization, symptom relief, administration of antibiotics when indicated, prompt referral, and, in some cases, preparation for immediate surgical intervention.

Pain relief

Acute scrotal problems encountered in the ED commonly present with significant pain. Initial pain medications should, in many cases, be administered parenterally. Analgesia should not be withheld pending consultation. If the likelihood of surgical intervention is low, or if the pain is mild on presentation, a trial of oral medications can be offered. Agents used most frequently are narcotic analgesics, NSAIDs, or acetaminophen. Scrotal elevation may be beneficial in patients with inflammatory conditions such as epididymitis. This is

Pearls and pitfalls

Pearls

1. There are four true "scrotal/testicular" emergencies that require immediate evaluation by an appropriate specialist in the ED: testicular torsion, an incarcerated or strangulated inguinal hernia, Fournier's disease, and genitourinary tra.
2. In suspected testicular torsion, emergency specialty consultation is imperative: "time is testicle."
3. Ultrasound examination is extremely useful for differentiating among the etiologies of acute scrotal pain.
4. When examining the testes, always examine the unaffected side first.

Pitfalls

1. Failure to perform a genitourinary examination in a male infant with inconsolable crying, a male patient with "abdominal" pain, or a non-communicative male patient.
2. Failure to consider sexual abuse with a genitourinary complaint and inconsistent history.
3. Although Prehn's sign is frequently taught as a historical method of differentiating testicular torsion from epididymitis, it is unreliable and should not be used in clinical decision making.

easily accomplished by use of a towel roll or supportive undergarment (such as a "jock strap"). Ice may reduce edema and provide a mild degree of analgesia.

Antibiotics

Antimicrobial agents are indicated in suspected or proven infection. Early broad-spectrum antibiotic therapy (covering Gram-positive, Gram-negative, and anaerobic species) is imperative in suspected Fournier's disease.

Epididymitis in prepubescent males is often caused by reflux of sterile urine, often as a result of congenital genitourinary anomalies. Recommendations regarding treatment of the resulting "chemical" inflammation vary from treating all boys with antibiotics to limiting their use to patients with documented urinary findings (pyuria, bacteriuria, positive urine culture). If utilized, prophylactic antibiotics should cover the common urinary pathogens.

Disposition

There are four urologic emergencies that require immediate evaluation by an appropriate specialist in the ED: testicular torsion, Fournier's disease, incarcerated or strangulated hernia, and genitourinary trauma. Whenever in doubt, the EP should err on the side of caution and obtain appropriate consultation while the patient remains in the ED. When evaluating pediatric genitourinary complaints, the EP should always remain vigilant to the possibility of child abuse.

When patients leave the ED, they should be provided with adequate home analgesia, whether prescription medications, recommendations for over-the-counter analgesics, or a combination. Patients with unclear diagnoses, intractable pain, vomiting, unreliable follow-up, or an unstable home/social situation may require inpatient management by an appropriate specialist or a primary care provider.

Selected references

Adams JR, Mata JA, Venable DD, *et al.* Fournier's disease in children. *Urology* 1990;**35**:439–441.

Caldamome AA, Valvo JR, Altebarmakian VK, *et al.* Acute scrotal swelling in children. *J Pediatr Surg* 1984;**19**:581–584.

Ciftci AO, Senocak ME, Tanyel FC, *et al.* Clinical predictors for differential diagnosis of acute scrotum. *Eur J Pediatr Surg* 2004;**14**:5:333–338.

Klin B, Lotan G, Efrati Y, *et al.* Acute idiopathic scrotal edema in children: revisited. *J Pediatr Surg* 2002;**37**:1200–1202.

Melekos MD, Asbach HW, Markou SA. Etiology of acute scrotum in 100 boys with regard to age distribution. *J Urol* 1988;**139**:1023–1025.

Rabinowitz R. The importance of the cremasteric reflex in acute scrotal swelling in children. *J Urol* 1984;**132**:89–90.

Section

25 Wound management

Chapter

151 Selected procedures in pediatric emergency medicine

Betsy Encarnacion and Gregory H. Gilbert

Introduction

Children commonly visit the emergency room for cuts, scrapes, and lacerations that may need treatment. Efforts to address the needs of children, particularly their fear of pain and sharp instruments, have led to advancements in laceration repair and resulted in new non-invasive approaches to wound management. This section reviews newer non-invasive techniques in wound repair and approaches to specific procedures. Techniques that are similar for adults and children, such as suturing techniques, will not be covered.

Laceration repairs and wound closure

Wound assessment is the same as with adults, although it may be more difficult in a frightened child. A general approach to different lacerations by site is given in Table 151.1. As with adults, all wounds need to be irrigated and explored. In young children, a thorough examination and repair may require the use of procedural sedation. Alternatives include maximizing parental cooperation to distract or to manipulate injuries.

Wound repair techniques

Tissue adhesives

Tissue adhesives such as Dermabond (octylcyanoacrylate, OCA), Indermil and Histoacryl (*n*-butyl-2 cyanoacrylate) have grown in popularity since their development. They can be used in a variety of settings, including superficial scalp wounds, facial lacerations, and selected extremity and torso lacerations. Tissue adhesives are intended for use on non-contaminated, non-mucosal wounds under minimal tension or as a superficial adhesive over deep suture placement. Tissue adhesives are not a good option if there is concern for too much wound tension. However, splinting an extremity or joint can lead to the immobility required to use a tissue adhesive.

The advantages of tissue adhesives are many, including that they allow for painless, quick closure with a similar short- and long-term cosmetic outcome as standard suture closure. Infection and dehiscence rates between lacerations repaired by tissue adhesives and suturing appear to be comparable, and tissue adhesives have the added benefit of providing a microbial barrier. Tissue adhesives thus essentially eliminate the use of sharp instruments as well as the need for a return visit for suture removal, features that are particularly important and appealing to children, parents, and physicians.

Table 151.1. Approach to specific wounds by site

Wound site	Site features	Methods of repair
Scalp	Good blood supply, so lacerations tend to heal well	Staples, non-absorbable sutures, hair apposition technique
Forehead	Relaxed skin tension lines run horizontally across forehead; horizontal lacerations heal better than vertical ones	Consider sutures for vertical lacerations and wound closure tapes to provide additional support
Lip	Approximate vermillion border to preserve cosmetic outcome	Close in layers with absorbable sutures
Chin	Common site for blunt trauma in children	Wound tape or tissue adhesive

A Practical Guide to Pediatric Emergency Medicine: Caring for Children in the Emergency Department, ed. N. Ewen Amieva-Wang (associate eds. Jamie Shandro, Aparajita Sohoni, and Bernhard Fassl). Published by Cambridge University Press.

Tissue adhesives, however, should not be used in or near eyes, over joints, in the wound itself, in areas of dense hair, or on wounds under tension. Their use is also contraindicated on infected wounds and those on mucous membranes or mucocutaneous junctions, such as the perioral rim. All tissue adhesives work through an exothermic reaction, which may cause children discomfort if applied in large droplets and not evenly spread over the wound edges. No reports were found regarding how well children tolerated the use of particular tissue adhesives.

Run-off of the adhesive into an unintended area and subsequent unintentional adhesion is another disadvantage. Fortunately, tissue adhesives can be removed with acetone or petroleum-based jellies such as bacitracin or vasoline. In fact, pretreating areas such as the eyelid with bacitracin can help to prevent adhesion if run-off did occur. Two formulations of Dermabond are on the market: a low-viscosity formulation that has a consistency similar to water, and a high-viscosity syrup-like formulation. Although both forms are still sold, the high-viscosity version has become the more popular choice as it reduces the occurrence of run-off onto unintended sites.

A wound should be clean and dry, with no active bleeding, before the tissue adhesive is applied.

Even a slow ooze of blood can lead to a less than desirable closure as the adhesive tends to bond with the blood and bubble, making it difficult to visualize the actual wound closure itself. This can be best controlled with direct pressure or lidocaine with epinephrine; however, after the injection of a local anesthetic, suturing may indeed be the better option. Often, one practitioner holding the wound together while the other applies the tissue adhesive has good results.

A major limitation for use in children, particularly in the summertime, is that tissue adhesives are not resistant to excessive moisture and must be used with caution in patients who will be soaking in water, such as with swimming or water sports. Showering is allowed, although children and parents should be advised to keep the wound as dry as possible and not to soak the wound until the adhesive has worn off.

Box 151.1 describes the technique used when applying a tissue adhesive.

Wound closure tapes

Wound closure tapes such as Steri-strips are easy to apply and they eliminate the need for suture removal at a return visit. These filamented tapes are painless to apply and are commonly used in young children with minor, low-tension wounds. As with tissue adhesives, wound closure tapes cannot be used on moist areas, the palms or soles, or hair-bearing areas. Wound closure tapes have similar rates of wound complications and cosmetic outcomes compared with wound adhesives and are more cost-effective. For longer cuts, wound closure tapes can be placed first to get good approximation and glue can be applied over them. Another more difficult practice is to

Box 151.1. Use of tissue adhesives

Method

1. Clean, irrigate, and debride wound as necessary. Obtain hemostasis and close deeper layers, if necessary.
2. Make sure the wound is dry.
3. Position the wound so that the edges are well opposed (may require another set of hands).
4. Crush glass vial or twist off cap to plastic container, depending on type of tissue adhesive used.
5. Allow the adhesive to soak through to the tip of the applicator until a drop is almost ready to fall off.
6. Apply tissue adhesive to wound immediately.
7. Allow the adhesive drop and not the applicator to touch the wound.
8. Pull the drop across the wound with the applicator.
9. For Dermabond, apply in at least two layers, waiting 10–15 s between layers and extending 5–10 mm beyond wound edges. For Indermil, apply one layer or sparingly in small drops along wound edges.
10. Full polymerization may take 2–5 min.

Tricks of the trade

Gloves sticking to the wound site. Latex gloves often stick to the wound site during attempts to approximate wound edges. Vinyl gloves seem to stick less than latex gloves.

Unwanted gauze adhesion. The tissue adhesive can run off onto adjacent skin and dry gauze can glue to this area. Using dampened or vasoline soaked gauze will reduce the adhesion to the wound area.

Unwanted spread of the tissue adhesive. Tissue adhesive can run off onto adjacent sensitive areas, such as mouth and eyes, or to uneven surfaces that cannot be positioned horizontally. Applying ointment or petroleum jelly to the adjacent site(s) before tissue adhesive application will reduce this.

Adhesion of tissue adhesive to plastic forceps. Forceps are needed to hold the wound together and metal forceps are prefered as tissue adhesive tends to adhere to metal objects only if held still for a period of time.

Seepage of tissue adhesive into the wound. This can create a gap or a wound that is "frozen apart". The wound must be held firmly closed and Steri-strips can aid in this. Gluing over the strips or removing them after polymerization are both viable options.

Words of wisdom

1. Although local anesthesia may not be necessary for wound closure with tissue adhesive, do not shy away from copious and aggressive wound irrigation and debridement before closure with tissue adhesive.
2. Do not use tissue adhesive in areas under tension. They will be at risk for dehiscence.
3. Tissue adhesive does not facilitate hemostasis as sutures do. Be sure complete hemostasis is achieved prior to application of the tissue adhesive.
4. Avoid use of tissue adhesive over skin sutures; it will be difficult to remove the sutures until the tissue adhesive has broken down.

Box 151.1. *(cont.)*

5. Use tissue adhesive only in situations where the laceration edges can be approximated; avoid use on wounds too deep for skin closure alone.
6. Be aware that chin lacerations often have fat nodules that protrude from the edges of the wound. Try to push the fat nodules below the skin surface or remove them prior to the application of tissue adhesive.
7. Avoid using tissue adhesive on the thumb or finger as the child has a tendency to suck; alternatively place a non-adherent covering over tissue adhesive.
8. Spread tissue adhesive evenly over wound edges to avoid discomfort when applying.
9. Tissue adhesive should breakdown and slough off in 5–10 days. In cases of delayed breakdown of more than 2 weeks, advise parents and patients to soak, the area and apply petroleum jelly or acetone to the area.

Box 151.2. **Use of wound closure tape**

1. Clean, irrigate, and debride the wound as necessary.
2. Obtain hemostasis and close deeper layers, if necessary.
3. Make sure the wound is dry.
4. Apply adhesive adjunct (i.e., tincture of benzoin) and let dry.
5. Apply skin tapes perpendicularly across wound. One method is to apply one end of the Steri-strip and then use the tape to pull the wound closed before adhering the other side.

glue between the tape, allow the glue to set, and then remove the tape before glueing the rest of the laceration.

Pitfalls of wound closure tape use include decreased adherence with improper coating of the entire skin surface with adjunctive adhesive, such as benzoin. Overlapping tape strips and placing strips parallel to the wound (tacking strips) are also known to decrease wound tape adhesion.

Box 151.2 outlines the technique for using wound closure tape.

Hair tying and hair apposition techniques

Scalp lacerations are not uncommon in the pediatric population. Hair tying and hair apposition are commonly used as a non-invasive means of repairing small, superficial scalp lacerations, particularly in children. Hair tying involves separating the hair on each side of laceration and twisting it to form ropes of hair. The ropes of hair are tied together across the wound, tightly opposing the skin edges. As the wound heals, the knot grows away from the wound edge. Parents can then cut the knot of hair in 2–4 weeks as it grows away from the wound site. Another method for repairing scalp injuries is the hair apposition technique, where hair on either side of the laceration is twisted together along the wound and tissue adhesive is used to secure the laceration together (Fig. 151.1). Compared with standard sutures, hair apposition is faster, has fewer complications, is less painful, and has less scarring. Both hair apposition and hair tying have the added benefit of no return visit for stitch or staple removal and are cheaper than conventional suturing or stapling of scalp lacerations.

A

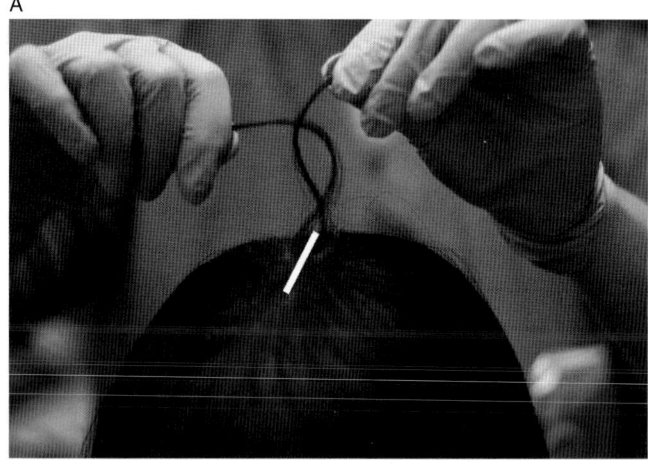

B

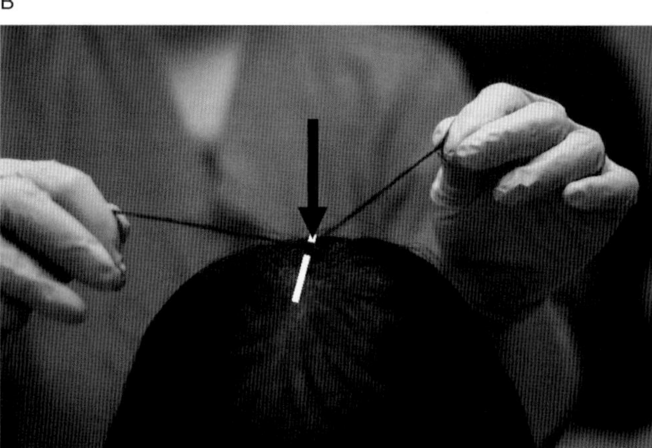

Figure 151.1 Hair apposition technique. The white line represents the laceration site. (Courtesy of Michele Lin.)

Invasive techniques

Although the trend in pediatric emergency medicine has been to use non-invasive techniques of wound repair, deep lacerations or wounds under high tension warrent use of stronger, more traditional methods of wound closure, such as sutures or staples.

Sutures

Deep lacerations or those that are under high tension require consideration of standard invasive wound closure techniques with appropriate procedural sedation (Ch. 152). The choice between non-absorbable and absorbable sutures in children has long been a source of controversy, because non-absorbable sutures were believed to provide the best cosmetic effect, less wound infection, and less dehiscence. Suture removal in a child, however, may be as difficult as the placement of the suture itself.

Absorbable sutures have been found to provide a similar cosmetic outcome and no difference in dehiscence or infection compared with non-absorbable sutures.

Comparisons of non-absorbable sutures, absorbable sutures, and tissue adhesives found no difference in cosmetic outcome of facial lacerations amongst all three groups, emphasizing the use of absorbable sutures or tissue adhesives in children. Choice among the different types of rapidly absorbing suture should be based on physician experience.

Staples

Stainless steel staples are commonly used for scalp lacerations not involving galea in the ED. Their use is as fast and cosmetically acceptable as suturing for simple scalp lacerations. However, staples must be removed with a specific surgical staple remover, which may cause an obstacle for patients seen in the ED. Furthermore, case reports have documented scalp staples to have rotated 90–180 degrees in pediatric patients, posing an obstacle to staple removal. Staples were removed in these circumstances with use of a hemostat to clamp and open the visible leg, and then the staple was worked out the rest of the way.

Management of specific wounds

Common facial wounds

Since the head is disproportionately larger in children than adults, and many table tops are at toddler eye level, children frequently lacerate their face and scalp. Depending on the location, repair can be done with glue, sutures, or, in some instances, hair. One common location of pediatric lacerations is under the chin. While typically closed with sutures in the past, many EPs are finding these injuries to be extremely amenable to glue. This is in large part because a slightly larger scar is less likely to be seen in the area under the chin, while patient and parent comfort is maximized.

It is always important to check the mouth for lacerations, bites, and loose teeth. A lacerated frenulum does not need to be repaired. Most intraoral lesions can be left open as well. However, intraoral lesions that gape open should be loosely approximated to avoid food particles becoming trapped in them. Lacerations through the vermillion border will require sutures to ensure proper repair. The same is true with lacerations that involve the eye. If there is suspicion of the tear duct system or tarsal plate involvement, opthalmology consultation should be obtained. Pre-marking the vermillion border or lines of the eye before anesthesia can be extremely helpful during the repair.

Forehead lacerations that run with the lines of Langer are amendable to glue. Those that run against them may require sutures. For longer cuts, Steri-strips can be placed first to get good approximation and glue can be applied over them. The only problem with leaving Steri-strips on the wound is that children will tend to pick at it more.

Animal and human bites

Bites can be either provoked or unprovoked. The most common provocation is when a child disturbs the family pet while it eats. Unprovoked bites should raise the concern for rabies. Dog bites are the most common type of animal injury presenting to the ED, and they frequently involve children and young adults. Dog bites tend to occur on the face and extremities and be more lacerating in nature. Cat bites tend to be puncture wounds mostly occurring on the hand. Human bites tend to involve the hand and are most commonly seen in young children bitten by a sibling, or adolescents and young adults after having been in a fight, also known as the "fight bite."

In general, dog bites tend to have a lower rate of infection than cat or human bites. Most dog bites, therefore, can actually be closed primarily after copious irrigation and debridement. Cat bites are not closed primarily because of the nature of the puncture wound and the difficulty it poses in adequate cleaning and irrigation. Human bites have a higher rate of infection and should not be closed primarily but rather should be copiously irrigated and closed with skin closure tapes. Relative contraindications to primary wound closure, therefore, include:

- deep puncture wounds (such as cat bites)
- human bites
- wounds more than 24 h old at presentation
- wounds in immunocompromised hosts
- hand wounds, as these have relatively poor vascularity and are at higher risk of infection.

Antibiotics are important in situations where the patient presents with an infected bite wound. However, the role of prophylactic antibiotics in cat, dog, and human bites is less clear. Cat bites are notorious for deep puncture bites and subsequent wound infection.

There is a higher rate of wound infection and a shorter interval between bite and presentation for cat bites than for dog bites, suggesting a faster onset of symptoms.

The use of prophylactic antibiotics in dog and human bites is dependent on the location and depth of the bite, and the patient's own risk factors for infection. Antibiotics should be considered in deep wounds; those involving the hands, feet, or skin overlying joints or cartilaginous structures; and bites affecting immunosuppressed patients.

Prophylactic antibiotics such as augmentin 10–15 mg/kg TID is recommended to cover for *Pasturella* infection in the setting of cat bites.

Fingertip and hand injuries

Fingertip and hand injuries are common in children and adolescents. Infants and young children tend to suffer fingertip crush injuries while older children and teenagers tend to have hand lacerations and sports-related fractures. Crush injuries frequently result from getting a finger trapped in a door or window. This injury often produces either a subungal hematoma or partial to complete amputation of the distal tip of the affected digit. Traditionally, formal nail removal and nail bed repair was recommended for an injury involving the nail bed or a subungal hematoma greater than 50% of the nail bed.

Subungal hematomas should be drained by nail trephination rather than nail bed repair regardless of size, as long as there is an intact nail bed.

This approach avoids additional trauma to the injured finger. Damage and laceration of the nail bed itself still requires fingernail removal. For partial to complete amputations, repair typically has a good prognosis, particularly in younger patients. As a meticulous repair is required, a hand surgery consult is always prudent and conscious sedation is usually required to allow for the best results. Use of antibiotic prophylaxis is controversial in fingertip injuries.

Penile injuries

Zipper injuries, although uncommon, do occur and present to the pediatric ED. These injuries are most common in young school-aged boys and tend to involve uncircumcised penile foreskin. Techniques to release penile skin have been well described and include unzipping the zipper, cutting the median bar, or using mineral oil to extract entrapped skin:

1. Apply mineral oil liberally to entrapped skin
2. Let mineral oil sit for several minutes
3. Apply gentle traction to the zipper.

Another technique involves cutting the zipper teeth themselves to unzip the remaining zipper. However, the technique chosen is dependent on the location of the entrapped skin in relation to the median bar and zipper teeth. Swelling often complicates zipper injuries, and in some situations, procedural sedation, local anesthesia, or a penile block may be necessary.

Pain control

Decisions need to be made between use of topical, local, or regional anesthetics. Procedures are often anxiety provoking for children in the ED. The field of pediatric emergency medicine has aimed to create an "ouchless ED," where non-invasive techniques are often favored over the traditional, often more painful, approaches. Parents particularly prefer painless procedures for their children, and they have been found to be willing to wait longer and/or pay to provide a painless procedure for their child. Topical anesthetics can often eliminate pain from procedures, such as IV cannulation and laceration repair, yet certain situations require the use of local or regional techniques. This section outlines the various types of topical anesthetic, their uses and limitations, as well as local and regional anesthetics and the situations in which they must ultimately be used. Procedural sedation is discussed in Ch. 152.

Table 151.2. Comparison of topical anesthetics

	Eutectic mixture of lidocaine and prilocaine (EMLA)	Lidocaine 4% (ElaMax)
Time to maximal effect	45–60 min	30 min
Occlusive dressing needed	Yes	No
Age restrictions	Not recommended for use in infants <3 months of age	None

Topical anesthetics

Topical anesthetics have several advantages that have led to their increased use in the pediatric ED. They are easy to apply and do not distort wound edges upon application as local injected anesthetics tend to do. Unfortunately, topical anesthetics are costly and tend to have a slow onset of action, limiting their use in many emergency situations. Options for topical anesthesia on intact skin include an eutectic mixture of lidocaine and prilocaine (EMLA), and 4% lidocaine (ElaMax). Both are often used in the pediatric ED prior to venipuncture or IV cannulation and EMLA has also been described to aid in analgesia during suprapubic catheterization and lumbar punctures. Studies comparing EMLA and ElaMax have shown them to be equivalent in efficacy. Both EMLA and ElaMax have a delay in onset of maximal effect; therefore, it is best to apply the agent to the desired site as soon as the child arrives to the ED. Differences in use of the two products are listed in Table 151.2.

Ongoing efforts aim to find a topical anesthetic that has a faster onset and similar efficacy as these. Ethyl chloride is a topical cooling spray, used for quick, minor procedures on intact skin, such as venipuncture, IV access, arthrocentesis, and incision and drainage of a superficial abscess. Ethyl chloride, while as efficacious as topical anesthetics, is flammable and must not be used near heat sources or electrocautery. Iontophoresis has also emerged as another means of fast topical anesthesia on intact skin. It works by transdermal administration of lidocaine using an electric current from two externally placed electrodes. It is non-invasive, provides similar pain relief to EMLA for insertion of IV catheters, and only takes 10 min for onset of maximal anesthesia. Use of iontophoresis requires the appropriate equipment and may cause a sensation of flowing electrical current through the application site, erythema, and blanching.

Table 151.3. Comparison of local anesthetics lidocaine and bupivacaine

Agent	Onset	Duration	Maximum dosage Without epinephrine	With epinephrine
Lidocaine	Seconds	1 h	5 mg/kg	7 mg/kg
Bupivacaine	Seconds +	>6 h	2 mg/kg	3 mg/kg

Non-intact skin requires use of different topical anesthetics. A mixture of tetracaine, epinephrine, and cocaine (TAC) has many side effects and potential complications, such as agitation and seizures. For the most part, TAC has been largely replaced by different forms of topical anesthetic, including a lidocaine, epinephrine (adrenaline) plus tetracaine mixture (LET or LAT), which has been found to be as effective as TAC for topical anesthesia during suturing of uncomplicated lacerations on the face and scalp in children. It comes in a gel or solution that can be used on non-mucosal, lacerated skin, and seems to work best on highly vascular skin such as the face, but less well in the extremities. The gel formulation is highly viscous and stays in the wound, which makes it at least as effective as the solution, which tends to drain out of the laceration. Furthermore, the lack of drainage of the gel formulation leads to less contamination of mucous membranes and ocular surfaces. A comparison of LET with EMLA indicated similar pain relief and analgesia with both. Because LET contains epinephrine, it should not be used on distal extremities, such as fingers and toes, the ear, nose, or penis.

Local anesthetics

Despite the advances in topical anesthetics, local injection of anesthetic must be performed in certain deeper procedures, such as some laceration repairs, foreign body removal, and abscess drainage. Lidocaine and procaine are the most commonly used local anesthetics in children. Bupivacaine is also commonly used; however, because of its high potency, long duration of action, and known cardiac toxicity, caution must be used in children younger than 12 years of age (Table 151.3). Two newer local anesthetics with characteristics similar to bupivacaine, ropivacaine and levobupivacaine, have been shown to provide similar anesthesia to bupivacaine but with decreased systemic toxicity.

The techniques of direct infiltration and parallel margin infiltration are similar amongst children and adults. It is important, however, to minimize the pain a child may feel with direct infiltration or parallel margin infiltration of a local anesthetic by applying LET to the open wound prior to the injection of lidocaine. Lidocaine injection itself can burn and be painful on application. To minimize pain with injection, it is advised to inject the anesthetic slowly, use a small needle, warm the anesthetic to 40°C, and use a sodium bicarbonate buffer in a 1:10 ratio to buffer the anesthetic. As with adults, CNS and cardiovascular toxicity is a concern with the use of local anesthetics.

Box 151.3. Hematoma block technique

1. Clean skin around fracture site well.
2. Insert needle into the area of the fracture, aspirate, and look for flash of blood to confirm placement into hematoma.
3. Inject local anesthetic into site: 10 ml of 0.5% bupivacaine into the hematoma and 5 ml around the site.
4. Allow 10–15 min prior to attempting manipulation.

Regional anesthesia

Regional anesthesia provides analgesia over large anatomical areas without distortion of wound edges. This is particularly significant for cosmetically important areas, when local anesthetic would cause extreme pain, such as the fingertip, nail bed, or palms and soles, or when laceration repair requires potentially toxic doses of local anesthetic. Regional anesthesia is also important for larger procedures, such as fracture reductions, because it provides sensory block with use of less anesthetic agent. Although IV procedural sedation is commonly used for fracture reductions, there is a large role for regional anesthesia with hematoma blocks in reducing fractures. Sedation techniques take more time for administration, more personnel, and a longer recovery period when compared with local or regional anesthetics, and tend to have significant side effects.

Amongst orthopedic surgeons and pediatric EPs performing forearm fracture reduction in children, hematoma blocks were the most common form of regional anesthetic technique used, mostly on older children and adolescents. Hematoma blocks have also been found to be as effective and safe for fracture reductions as procedural sedation. While no guidelines currently exist regarding the use of regional anesthesia versus procedural sedation in fracture reduction in children, there is an evolving and potentially central role for regional anesthesia with hematoma blocks. Box 151.3 describes the hematoma block technique.

Pearls and pitfalls

Pearls

1. Consider using one of many non-invasive methods (hair-tying techniques, tissue adhesives) for wound closure for a pediatric patient.
2. Dry the wound surface prior to applying tissue adhesive.
3. Think of hair-tying techniques for scalp lacerations
4. Apply topical analgesia to an open wound prior to injecting lidocaine.

Pitfalls

1. Failure to provide adequate sedation and analgesia for wound repair in children

Selected references

Constantine E, Steele DW, Eberson C, Boutis K, Amanullah S, Linakis JG. The use of local anesthetic techniques for closed forearm fracture reduction in children: a survey of academic pediatric emergency departments. *Pediatr Emerg Care* 2007;**23**:209–211.

McCreight A, Stephan M. Local and regional anesthesia. In King C, Henretig FM (eds.) *Textbook of Pediatric Emergency Procedures*, 2nd edn. Philadelphia, PA: Lippincott Williams & Wilkins, 2008, pp.439–467.

McNamara R, DeAngelis M. Laceration repair with sutures, staples, and wound closure tapes. In King C, Henretig FM (eds.) *Textbook of Pediatric Emergency Procedures*, 2nd edn. Philadelphia, PA: Lippincott Williams & Wilkins, 2008, pp.1018–1044.

Roser SE, Gellman H. Comparison of nail bed repair versus nail trephination for subungual hematomas in children. *J Hand Surg* 1999;**24**:1166–1170.

Zempsky WT, Parrotti D, Grem C, Nichols J. Randomized controlled comparison of cosmetic outcomes of simple facial lacerations closed with Steri Strip skin closures or Dermabond tissue adhesive. *Pediatr Emerg Care* 2004;**20**:519–524.

Chapter 152

Procedural sedation and analgesia

Judith R. Klein

Introduction

Procedural sedation is an underutilized tool in the armamentarium of most physicians caring for children. Several million children undergo procedural sedation each year, the vast majority not experiencing any significant complications. This chapter will discuss, in detail, how to provide safe and effective procedural sedation and analgesia for children.

Procedural sedation is defined as "the technique of administering sedatives or dissociative agents with or without analgesics to induce a state that allows the patient to tolerate unpleasant procedures while maintaining cardiorespiratory function." The implied goal is to depress level of consciousness while allowing for maintenance of airway control. The benefits of providing procedural sedation include pain relief, anxiety reduction, amnesia, immobility, and muscle relaxation. Often, without such sedation, procedures such as dislocation or fracture reductions would be nearly impossible. Along with these benefits, however, there are some risks, most notably respiratory compromise (depression and obstruction), cardiovascular depression, vomiting/aspiration, allergic reactions, and some adverse reactions unique to particular drugs such as myoclonus or laryngospasm. Of these effects, respiratory depression or vomiting are the most common.

Pre-procedure planning

Monitoring/equipment

Proper monitoring and preparation for possible adverse events is essential. Monitoring for procedural sedation includes cardiac rhythm, blood pressure, respiratory rate, and continuous pulse oximetry. Increasingly, end-tidal carbon dioxide monitoring is being added to this list in EDs across the USA. End-tidal carbon dioxide monitoring, typically through a slipstream in a nasal cannula, allows for early detection of hypoventilation through either a rise in the carbon dioxide or a loss of the waveform.

In addition to the use of proper monitoring devices, preparation for procedural sedation includes organizing potential airway interventions if hypoxia, hypoventilation, or airway obstruction occurs. Essential equipment includes:

- oxygen
- suction
- appropriately sized bag-valve mask and tubing
- nasopharyngeal and oropharyngeal airways (appropriate sizes)
- intubation equipment (rarely needed).

In addition to airway equipment, rescue medications should be readily available, including:

- naloxone (opiate reversal)
- flumazenil (benzodiazepine reversal)
- epinephrine and diphenhydramine (anaphylactic/allergic reactions).

These items and other essential equipment (IV equipment, nasogastric tubes, etc.) can all be stored in a specially designated "pediatric crash cart" that can be wheeled in wherever procedures are being performed. Finally, a standardized sedation record should be available for nursing to record vital signs, pain scores, and adverse events.

Nil by mouth

Another important consideration is a child's nil by mouth (NPO) status. According to the official recommendations of the American Society of Anesthesiologists, children should be kept NPO of liquids for 2 h and NPO of solids for 4 to 8 h prior to procedural sedation. This recommendation is difficult to follow in the ED because of the urgency of procedures, parental demands, and concerns regarding patient flow. Several studies involving children fasted for different lengths of time have demonstrated that there is no association between pre-procedural fasting and the incidence of adverse events during procedural sedation. Physicians should, therefore, perform emergency procedures without delay and without concern for fasting state. If the procedure is not an emergency, physicians

A Practical Guide to Pediatric Emergency Medicine: Caring for Children in the Emergency Department, ed. N. Ewen Amieva-Wang (associate eds. Jamie Shandro, Aparajita Sohoni, and Bernhard Fassl). Published by Cambridge University Press.

Table 152.1. Contraindications to the use of particular agents in procedural sedation

Medical problem/symptom	Medications to avoid
Asthma/respiratory distress	Morphine because of histamine release Propofol because of sulfites Narcotics because of respiratory depression
Hypotension	Benzodiazepines, barbiturates, narcotics
Elevated intracranial pressure	Ketamine, nitrous oxide; use propofol with caution
Elevated intraocular pressure	Ketamine
Seizure disorder	Ketamine, methohexital, meperidine
Severe hypertension	Ketamine
Psychosis/psychiatric disease	Ketamine
Air in closed space (e.g., pneumothorax, small bowel obstruction)	Nitrous oxide
Severe allergies/anaphylaxis	Morphine because of histamine release
Abundant respiratory secretions	Use ketamine with caution; use atropine or glycopyrolate as adjunct
Porphyria	All barbiturates
Hepatic disease	Caution with morphine, codeine, midazolam because of active hepatic metabolites
Renal disease	Many drugs dependent on kidneys for excretion; beware of repeat dosing and prolonged effects

should consider some delay in children who have had a recent large meal.

Choosing an agent

Choosing an appropriate agent for procedural sedation involves consideration of both patient and procedural characteristics. The patient's age and stage of development strongly influence the choice of an agent. While 2 to 3 ml of 30% oral sucrose water and local anesthetic may be adequate for a lumbar puncture in a neonate, a toddler will likely require much more extensive sedation and analgesia. A child's medical history and active health issues also dictate drug choice. The presence of a chronic cardiac, respiratory, metabolic/excretory, or neuropsychiatric problem is a contraindication to the use of certain medications (Table 152.1) Similarly, if a child is experiencing certain active symptoms – wheezing, upper respiratory congestion, vomiting, seizures, psychosis, head/eye injury – certain agents should also be avoided. Based on their chronic and active medical issues, children should be classified according the American Society of Anesthesiologist (ASA) classification system.

I Healthy
II Mild systemic disease
III Severe systemic disease
IV Severe systemic disease with constant life threat
V Moribund, requiring procedure
E Emergency procedure.

Procedures in children with an ASA class III or IV may best be carried out in an operating room (OR) setting, not in the ED.

The second part of choosing an agent for procedural sedation involves consideration of procedural characteristics. Specifically, the practitioner should answer the following questions:

- Is the procedure painful?
- Is complete immobility required?
- Will the procedure last <15 min or longer?

The answers to these questions coupled with the patient assessment noted above will allow for selection of the most appropriate agent(s) for sedation and analgesia.

Pre-procedure examination

Physical examination of children prior to performing procedural sedation is also essential, both for choosing an agent and for choosing an appropriate locale for performing the procedure (OR or ED). Physical examination considerations include:

- general appearance: morbid obesity
- head and neck: craniofacial abnormalities, limited mouth opening, receding chin, large tongue, short neck
- pulmonary: respiratory distress, stridor, wheezing
- cardiovascular: hypotension, signs of hypovolemia.

As part of this physical examination, children should also be given a Mallampati score by asking or enticing them to open their mouths maximally and peering in (Fig. 152.1).

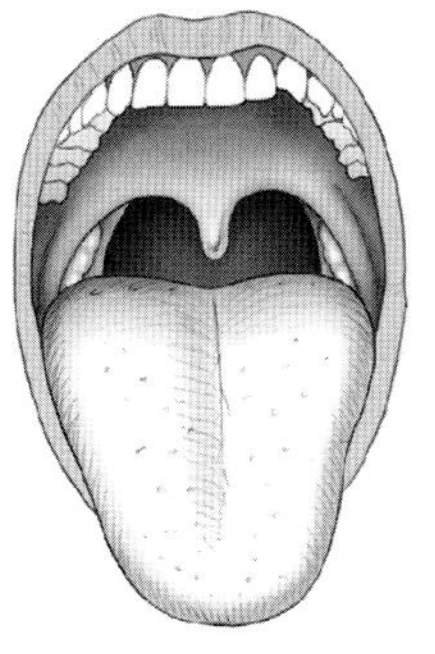

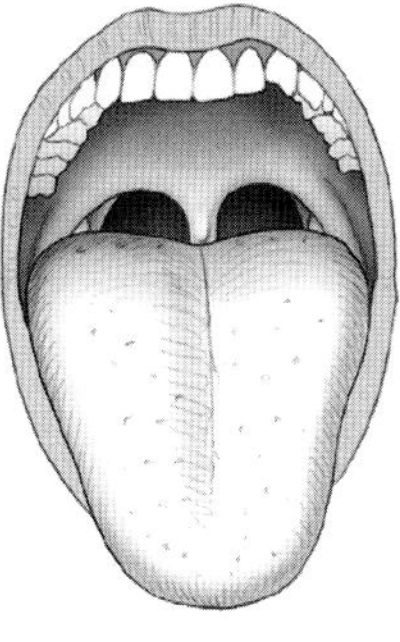

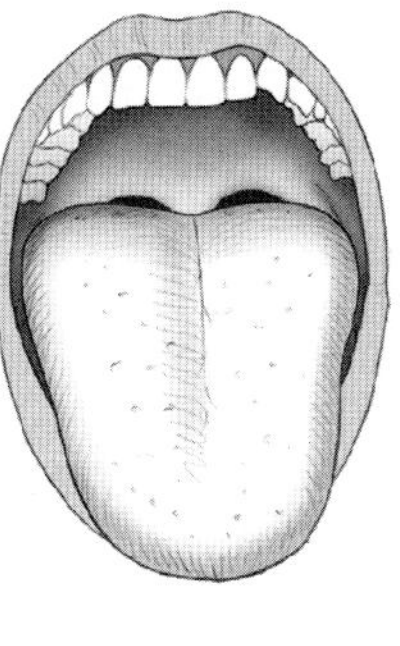

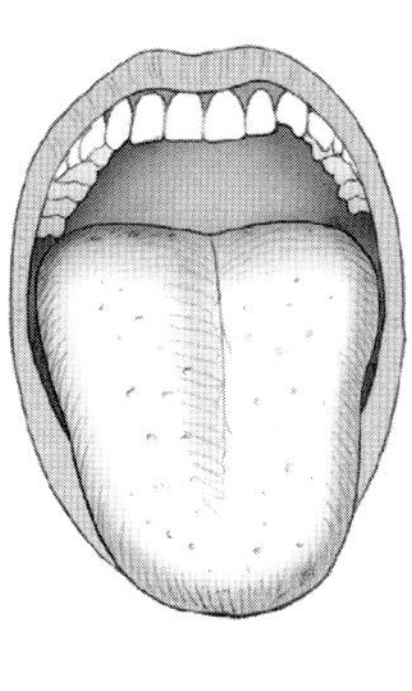

Figure 152.1 Mallampati classification. The classification of tongue size relative to the size of the oral cavity. Class I: faucial pillars, soft palate, and uvula visualized. Class II: faucial pillars and soft palate visualized but the uvula is masked by the base of the tongue. Class III: only the base of the uvula can be visualized. Class IV: none of the three structures can be visualized. (Copyright Chris Gralapp; reproduced with permission from Mahadevan SV, Garmel GM. *An Introduction to Clinical Emergency Medicine.* Cambridge, UK: Cambridge University Press, 2005.)

Mallampati scores correlate with ease of assisted ventilation and intubation should a child require it. Procedures in children with Mallampati scores of class III or IV may be most safely performed in the OR. Similarly, the presence of one or more of the physical examination characteristics noted above increases the risk of adverse events during sedation and should be considered when choosing medications and sedation locales.

Pre-procedure preparation of the child

Preparing a child for procedural sedation and creating a calming setting is equally important as the selection of the appropriate drug. Be calm and confident in explaining procedures to children and use language that is suitable for their stage of development. Avoid high anxiety words such as cut, shot, and pain. Give children realistic expectations and address their concerns. Consider demonstrating procedures on a doll or use an illustrated book or video. When preparing the setting for sedation, choose a calm, quiet environment without beeping monitors and children crying nearby. Allow children to hold comfort items – a blanket or stuffed animal – or listen to music to soothe them. When possible, let children help and give them a choice (e.g., holding gauze with the left or right hand). Encourage parents to help to comfort children through distraction, guided imagery, and praise. Discourage parents from criticizing children, apologizing to them, or giving them too much control. Finally, do not let parents assist with restraining a child, even for brief periods. This is not their role and they will not be as effective as trained medical professionals.

Types of agent

Medications used in procedural sedation can be administered in a variety of ways: orally, transmucosally (sublingual, intranasal, rectal), topically, SC, IM, and IV. Those agents that can be administered with minimal or no pain (e.g., topical medications) should be included in a sedation plan as often as possible.

Specific agents that are available for procedural sedation and analgesia in children can be categorized as follows (Table 152.2):

- pure analgesics
- pure sedatives
- mixed sedative/analgesics
- dissociative agent
- adjunctive/alternative techniques.

Pure analgesics

The pure analgesics provide pain relief only and can be administered orally (e.g., acetaminophen, ibuprofen), topically (e.g., liposomal lidocaine, an eutectic mixture of lidocaine and prilocaine [EMLA], lidocaine, epinephrine plus tetracaine [LET]), or SC (e.g., lidocaine with or without epinephrine, bupivacaine). The use of topical analgesics, EMLA and liposomal lidocaine on intact skin, and LET for lacerated or abraded skin, can significantly reduce the pain of IV placement, lumbar punctures, and laceration repair. Application of these agents at triage for children with lacerations will provide the added benefit of reduced total treatment time. Practitioners should keep in mind that EMLA and liposomal lidocaine require 45–60 min of application time for efficacy, while LET requires approximately 10–15 min. This is covered in Ch. 151.

Pure sedatives

The pure sedatives are CNS depressants that act principally by enhancing gamma-aminobutyrate (GABA) neurotransmission. They frequently provide anxiolysis and amnesia, in addition to sedation, but do not provide any analgesia. This category of agents consists primarily of the barbiturates, benzodiazepines, etomidate, propofol, and nitrous oxide (N_2O).

Barbiturates

The most commonly used barbiturates are pentobarbital and methohexital. Pentobarbital (2.5 mg/kg IV, repeat 1.25 mg/kg

Table 152.2. Medications for procedural sedation and analgesia

Medication	Route (dosing [mg/kg])	Maximum recommended single dose	Onset (duration)
Pure analgesia			
Lidocaine	SC	4 mg/kg	5–10 min (60–90 min)
Lidocaine/epinephine	SC	7 mg/kg	5–10 min (90–120 min)
Bupivacaine	SC	3 mg/kg	10 min (3–6 h)
Lidocaine, epinephrine (adrenaline) plus tetracaine (LET)	Topical	1.5 ml/10 kg	10–15 min (60–90 min)
Eutectic mixture of lidocaine and prilocaine (EMLA)	Topical	–	45–60 min
Liposomal lidocaine	Topical	–	60–90 min
Acetaminophen	PO (15–20)	1000 mg	20–30 min (4 h)
Ibuprofen	PO (10)	800 mg	20–30 min (6–8 h)
Pure sedation			
Midazolam	IV (0.1)	5 mg	5 min (45–90 min)
	IN/PR (0.3–0.7)	5 mg	10–15 min (variable)
Lorazepam	IV (0.05)	2 mg	5 min (8–12 h)
Pentobarbital	IV (2.5; repeat 1.25 q. 5 min as needed)	200 mg	3–5 min (30–90 min)
Methohexital	IV (0.5–1)	100 mg	0.5–1 min (5–10 min)
	PR (25)		8–10 min (45–80 min)
Etomidate	IV (0.15; repeat 0.05 q. 2–3 min)	20 mg	0.5–1.0 min (10–15 min)
Propofol	IV (1–2 bolus then 0.5 q 1–2 min *or* 1–2 bolus then 0.05–0.1 mg/kg per min drip)	100 mg	1–2 min (6–10 min)
Nitrous oxide	Inhaled N_2O:O_2 50:50 to 70:30		Minutes
Mixed agents			
Codeine	PO (1)	60 mg	20–30 min (4 h)
Morphine	IV (0.1)	10 mg	10–15 min (2–4 h)
Hydromorphone	IV (0.01–0.02)	2 mg	20–30 min (3–4 h)
Fentanyl	IV (1–3 μg/kg)	50 μg	5–10 min (30–60)
Dissociative agent			
Ketamine	IV (1.5)		1 min (15–20 min)
	IM (4)		5–10 min (30–45 min)

IN, intranasal.

in 5 min) is a short-acting barbiturate that acts as a GABA receptor agonist. It is particularly effective in young children for diagnostic procedure sedation (CT or MRI), much more so than etomidate or midazolam. Induction times are short (3–5 min) and the medication effects typically last 30–90 min. The most common side effects are transient respiratory depression (1–7%) and hypotension. Methohexital is another short-acting barbiturate than can be administered both parenterally and rectally. It should be avoided in children under 1 month of age or those with a history of seizures. Administered IV (1 mg/kg), it has a very rapid time of onset (30–60 s) and lasts only 5–10 min. Parenteral administration is, therefore, only useful for very short procedures such as fracture/dislocation reductions or simple foreign body removals from the ear or nose. In contrast, with rectal administration (25 mg/kg), induction time is longer (8–10 min) but the effects will last 45–80 min. Rectal administration is, therefore, more appropriate for diagnostic imaging or complex laceration repairs. Transient respiratory depression and hypotension can occur with either route of administration but is much less common with the rectal route, likely because of the slower absorption of medication.

Benzodiazepines

The benzodiazepines, principally midazolam (0.1 mg/kg) and lorazepam (0.05 mg/kg), are also used to provide immobility and anxiolysis for various procedures. While these agents are effective for some children, others experience paradoxical excitation in response to this class of medications. In addition, children who do respond appropriately to the benzodiazepines often require large doses (up to 0.6 mg/kg or more of midazolam) for effective sedation. In studies evaluating the efficacy of midazolam for diagnostic imaging sedation, the agent failed to provide adequate conditions nearly 50% of the time. Side effects such as respiratory depression and hypotension occur more commonly with midazolam than with other medications used for procedural sedation, such as ketamine.

Etomidate

Etomidate (0.15 mg/kg IV, repeat 0.05 mg/kg q. 2–3 min), an imidazole derivative, is another short-acting sedative that functions through enhancement of GABA neurotransmission. It is highly effective for brief procedures such as fracture/dislocation reduction, more so than midazolam. Some of the advantages of using etomidate are that it has minimal cardiovascular effects and lowers intracranial pressure. It is, therefore, an ideal agent for use in children who are hypovolemic or have traumatic brain injuries. Its time of onset is rapid, typically 30–60 s, and effects typically last 10–15 min. It is generally a very safe agent, whose side effects include brief respiratory depression, self-resolving myoclonus (up to 20%), and nausea. Cortisol depression noted in response to etomidate is transient and more typically associated with long-term use in an ICU setting.

Propofol

Propofol is a highly lipid-soluble, alkyl phenol sedative that prolongs the duration of contact of GABA and its receptor. The advantages of propofol include rapid onset, short duration, rapid recovery, and antiemetic properties. The medication is administered IV either as repetitive boluses for shorter procedures (1–2 mg/kg over 1–2 min then 0.5 mg/kg every 1–2 min) or as a bolus followed by a continuous infusion for longer procedures (1–2 mg/kg over 1–2 min, then 0.05–0.1 mg/kg per min drip). Patients receiving propofol have complained of pain at the injection site; this can be minimized through the administration of 1% lidocaine (0.5 mg/kg) through the vein prior to propofol infusion. Propofol rapidly distributes to the brain after administration, is metabolized by the liver, and excreted by the kidney. It is an excellent agent for brief, painful procedures such as fracture/dislocation reduction. Rapid administration of the drug increases the risk of its most common side effects: respiratory depression and hypotension. Both side effects are common enough – 40% respiratory depression and up to 92% transient hypotension – that children should be provided supplemental oxygen prior to the procedure. Practitioners should also be prepared to reposition the airway, provide brief bag-valve mask ventilation, and administer IV fluid. Propofol should be used carefully in children with asthma or sulfite allergies and those with suspected increased intracranial pressure.

Nitrous oxide

Finally, nitrous oxide (N_2O) is a unique sedative in that it is inhaled and administration requires a special delivery device that scavenges unused gas. Nitrous oxide is typically provided premixed in a N_2O to oxygen ratio of 50:50 to 70:30. Studies of N_2O use in the ED are limited; its use in children has primarily been studied in the OR. There are several advantages of N_2O: no IV is required for administration and it is very safe and effective, with recovery times of just a few minutes. It can be combined with local or regional analgesia for painful procedures that require immobility and anxiolysis. It is recommended for use in children >4 years of age because most safety/efficacy studies have only included children older than 4 years. The most common side effects are nausea and vomiting, which occur in up to 10% of patients. Nitrous oxide is contraindicated in patients with elevated intracranial pressure, altered mental status, pneumothorax or any disease where gas has accumulated in a closed space (e.g., bowel obstruction). The biggest concern with N_2O use in the ED is control of its use and diversion/abuse.

Mixed agents: sedatives and analgesics

The category of mixed agents consists of medications that have both sedative and analgesic properties. This group consists primarily of the opiates (e.g., codeine, morphine, fentanyl, and hydromorphone). In smaller doses, analgesic qualities predominate; at larger doses, CNS depression will also occur. Opiates are available as either oral or parenteral preparations and are often used along with the pure sedatives to provide analgesia for painful procedures. If high doses of opiates are used with sedatives, side effects of both medications, notably respiratory and cardiovascular depression, will become synergistic. While an oral lozenge of fentanyl exists, it is not ideal for procedural sedation. Studies have shown a high rate of respiratory depression and vomiting, or the child becomes sleepy after initially licking the lozenge but not sedated enough to perform the procedure. Its use is not recommended.

Dissociative agents

The dissociative category only contains one drug: ketamine. Ketamine is an *N*-methyl-D-aspartate (NMDA) glutamate receptor antagonist that produces a trance-like state characterized by profound sedation, analgesia, and amnesia, with retention of protective airway reflexes, spontaneous respirations, and cardiovascular stability. In one study of procedural sedation in community ED settings, ketamine was the most commonly used agent. This is primarily because ketamine is very effective and has a long proven safety record in tens of thousands of patients undergoing procedural sedation. Unless particular contraindications exist (see below and Table 152.1), ketamine should be considered the first-line agent for procedural sedation in children. It can be administered IV (1.5 mg/kg) or IM (4 mg/kg). Given IV, its time of onset is typically 1 min and duration of efficacy is approximately 15–20 min. Administered IM, time of onset is a little more variable (5–10 min), and duration of efficacy is 30–45 min. In studies comparing IV and IM administration, ketamine given IM was more effective in sedating children but had a significantly longer recovery time (129 versus 80 min) and a slightly higher incidence of vomiting. Decisions regarding route of administration should be made based on ease of IV placement, need for IV for other reasons, and parental preference.

The most common side effect of ketamine is vomiting, occurring in 8–10% of all children receiving the drug. Children waking up from ketamine sedation can also experience nightmares (emergence reactions). While some have suggested using midazolam to decrease the incidence of these reactions, studies have shown that midazolam is ineffective in this regard and increases the risk of respiratory depression. Emergence reactions can be minimized by allowing children to recover in a quiet, minimally stimulating environment in their parent's arms. Ketamine can also increase the production of secretions in the upper respiratory tract. This rarely poses a problem except in children <1 year old (smaller airways), children starting the procedure with heavy secretions, or with procedures in the oropharyngeal area where secretions could pose challenges. In these settings, glycopyrolate (5 μg/kg) or atropine (0.02 mg/kg) can be considered to minimize secretions. Ketamine can, rarely, cause laryngospasm (1% incidence). This side effect typically resolves spontaneously, or with brief supplemental oxygen or bag-valve mask ventilation. Contraindications to ketamine use are age <3 months (higher rate of airway complications), severe hypertension, elevated intraocular pressure, history of psychosis, or excessive secretions. Historically, elevated intracranial pressure has been a contraindication to ketamine use; however, recent studies have demonstrated that this is probably not clinically significant.

Preventing adverse outcomes

Adverse outcomes during procedural sedation in children do occur (up to 17% of the time in one study) but can be minimized by following some basic guidelines. Most adverse events (90%) occur during the procedure or in the immediate post-procedure period, but they may occur up to 40 min after the procedure is completed. In most cases, these delayed events are repeat occurrences in children who experienced the same event during the procedure. Box 152.1 contains guidelines that should assist the practitioner in minimizing adverse outcomes during sedation.

Box 152.1. Guidelines to minimize adverse outcomes during sedation

1. Adverse events occur less often because of the drug itself, and more commonly because of drug administration practices. Avoid rapid administration ("pushing") or too frequent dosing ("stacking") of medications.
2. Administer medications in appropriate settings with appropriate monitoring and trained personnel. Outside the ED, take necessary equipment with you.
3. Be familiar with the medications you are using: patient contraindications, pharmacokinetics and dynamics, and dosing (particularly when someone other than the physician [i.e., nursing staff] has drawn up medications in different dilutions).
4. Be careful with transcription when writing orders for medications.
5. Avoid combining more than two medications. The rate of adverse outcomes rises dramatically.
6. Beware of drugs with long half-lives and those administered IM (depot effect).
7. Beware of drug overdoses (doses exceeding adult maximum), particularly in obese children. Beware of local anesthetic overdoses in children with multiple lacerations
8. Have a comprehensive recovery plan in place including established discharge criteria and discharge instructions. Children who were able to walk and eat prior to the procedure should demonstrate that they are able to do so before they are discharged.

Procedural sedation in specific settings

As discussed above, choosing an agent for procedural sedation is based on patient characteristics (age, symptoms, chronic medical problems, physical examination) and procedure characteristics (pain, immobility requirements, duration). Some contraindications to the use of certain medications based on patient characteristics are discussed earlier in the chapter and are listed in Table 152. 1.

To guide the practitioner in the selection of agents, Table 152.3 suggests possible agent(s) for use in sedation/analgesia for some of the most common procedures performed in children in the ED. These are options only, not an exhaustive list of acceptable medications.

Table 152.3. Agents to consider for specific procedures

Procedure	Agents to consider
Laceration repair	Ketamine Etomidate + local anesthetic ± fentanyl Propofol + local anesthetic ± fentanyl Nitrous oxide + local anesthetic
Complex/multiple laceration repair	Ketamine Propofol + local anesthetic ± fentanyl Rectal methohexital + local anesthetic
Fracture/ dislocation reduction	Ketamine Etomidate + fentanyl Propofol + fentanyl Midazolam + fentanyl
Lumbar puncture	Etomidate + local anesthetic Propofol + local anesthetic Rectal methohexital + local anesthetic Sucrose water 30% + local anesthetic (neonates)
Foreign body removal: nose/ear	Ketamine, etomidate, propofol, nitrous oxide (ear foreign body)
CT	Rectal methohexital, pentobarbital, propofol, etomidate
MRI	Pentobarbital, rectal methohexital

Pearls and pitfalls

Pearls

1. Procedural sedation, if properly conducted, can be a very safe method of providing sedation and analgesia to child undergoing a painful procedure.
2. Children who meet the criteria for American Society of Anesthesiologist class III or IV should have sedation peformed in the operating room rather than the ER.
3. Providers should be thoroughly familiar with one or two agents in each of the analgesic, sedative, mixed, and dissociative categories.

Pitfalls

1. Failure to consider the child's chronic medical conditions when selecting an appropriate anesthetic or sedative agent.
2. Failure to perform an emergency procedural sedation because of nil by mouth status.
3. Failure to have a pediatric crash cart, along with antidotes to the various medications, available at the bedside.

Conclusions

Procedural sedation is an essential tool of the ED physician caring for children. In addition to allowing greater patient and parent satisfaction, it also provides a better environment in which to successfully perform painful and/or anxiety-provoking procedures. The recipe for successful sedation includes through patient evaluation, a proper sedation setting, appropriate monitoring and resuscitation equipment, careful medication selection and administration, and, finally, a well-defined recovery plan. Appropriate and clear parental consent and proper documentation are also vital, particularly in the event of an adverse outcome.

Selected references

Bar-Joseph G, Guilburd Y, Tamir A, Guilburd JN. Effectiveness of ketamine in decreasing intracranial pressure in children with intracranial hypertension. *J Neurosurg Pediatr* 2009;**4**:37–39.

Cote CJ, Karl HW, Notterman DA, *et al.* Adverse sedation events in pediatrics: analysis of medications used for sedation. *Pediatrics* 2000;**106**:633–644.

Hoffman GM, Nowakowski R, Troshynski TJ, *et al.* Risk reduction in pediatric procedural sedation by application of an American Academy of Pediatrics/ American Society of Anesthesiologists process model. *Pediatrics* 2002;**109**:236–243.

Mace SE, Barata IA, Cravero JP, *et al.* Clinical policy: evidence-based approach to pharmacologic agents used in pediatric sedation and analgesia in the emergency department. *Ann Emerg Med* 2004;**44**:342–377.

Roback MG, Wathen JE, Bajaj L, *et al.* Adverse events associated with procedural sedation and analgesia in a pediatric emergency department: a comparison of common parenteral drugs. *Acad Emerg Med* 2005;**12**:508–513.

Chapter

153 Tutorial: Ultrasound-guided procedures

Teresa S. Wu

A Abscess drainage

Care of the pediatric patient in the ED can be greatly enhanced when bedside ultrasound is utilized to augment clinical practice. Ultrasound's ability to provide additional data in a rapid, non-invasive manner has made it an appealing tool for practitioners to have in their armamentarium. Because children, in general, have less body fat to interfere with sonographic imaging, ultrasound images are usually very easy to obtain. The information provided by a quick bedside ultrasound can aid in the management of a multitude of common ailments encountered in the ED. In pediatric practice, bedside ultrasound has been used in clinical scenarios ranging from the detection of subcutaneous abscesses for incision and drainage to the use of ultrasound to guide procurement of central venous access during a resuscitation. This chapter covers historically, elevated intracranial pressure has been a contraindication to ketamine use; however, recent studies have demonstrated that this is probably not clinically significant.

Evaluation of a subcutaneous abscess

Bedside ultrasound can be utilized to determine if a patient has a simple cellulitis or an underlying abscess that requires incision and drainage. A quick scan of the area will not only establish whether or not an occult abscess is present but will also help to delineate the size and depth of the fluid collection requiring drainage. The following steps are used when performing a bedside ultrasound for abscess evaluation.

1. Use a higher frequency probe. Superficial structures are seen best with higher frequency transducers. In general, soft tissue applications should be performed with a 7.5-to 10-MHz linear array transducer (Fig. 153.1).
2. Apply a large amount of ultrasound gel to improve the acoustic interface. If the patient is thin and has little subcutaneous fat, use an acoustic standoff pad to improve the sonographic window.
3. If acoustic standoff pads are not available, an acoustic window can be easily created with a small bag of normal saline or a fluid-filled glove sandwiched between two layers of ultrasound gel (Fig. 153.2).

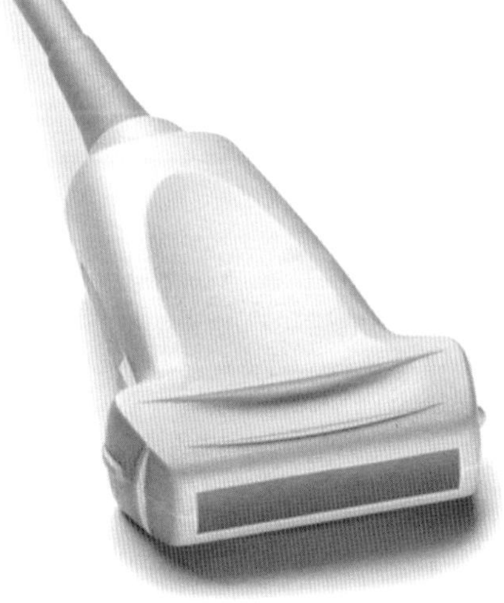

Figure 153.1 Linear array transducer. (Image courtesy of SonoSite, Inc.)

4. Begin by scanning normal tissue margins surrounding the area of interest. Note that normal subcutaneous tissue will have dark, hypoechoic regions of fat mixed in with hyperechoic (white) striations of muscle, brightly hyperechoic facial planes, and brightly hyperechoic fibrillar tendon planes (Fig. 153.3).
5. As the scan moves towards the area of interest, look for a spherical or elliptical collection of hypoechoic (dark) material indicating abscess formation. The hypoechoic (dark) or anechoic (black) fluid collection may have ring enhancement indicated by a rim of hyperechoic (white) surrounding tissue (Fig. 153.4).
6. Abscesses may appear hypoechoic (dark) or anechoic (black) during the initial stages of formation. As the inflammatory process progresses, the pus may begin to appear more heterogeneous with a mix of hypoechoic (dark) and hyperechoic (white) material swirled together.
7. Differentiating between cellulitis and small abscess pockets may be difficult. Cellulitis will typically have a

A Practical Guide to Pediatric Emergency Medicine: Caring for Children in the Emergency Department, ed. N. Ewen Amieva-Wang (associate eds. Jamie Shandro, Aparajita Sohoni, and Bernhard Fassl). Published by Cambridge University Press.

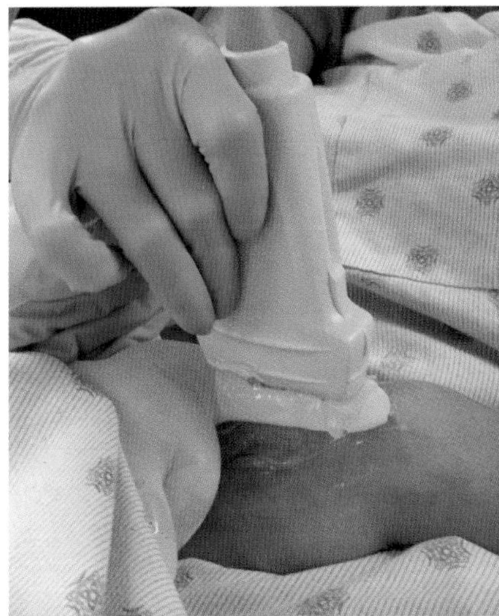

Figure 153.2 Enhancing the acoustic window with a water-filled glove. Scanning through a water-filled glove sandwiched between two layers of gel will provide an excellent acoustic window and allow better visualization of superficial structures.

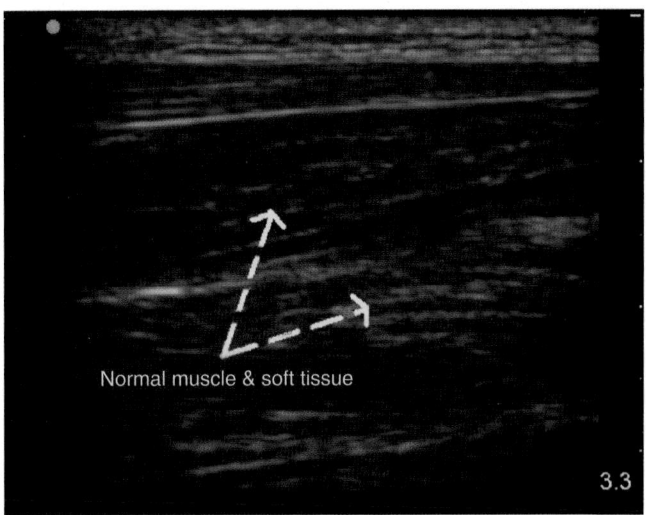

Figure 153.3 Ultrasound of normal soft tissue. Note the hypoechoic (dark) fat mixed in with hyperechoic (bright) muscle striations and brightly hyperechoic fascial planes.

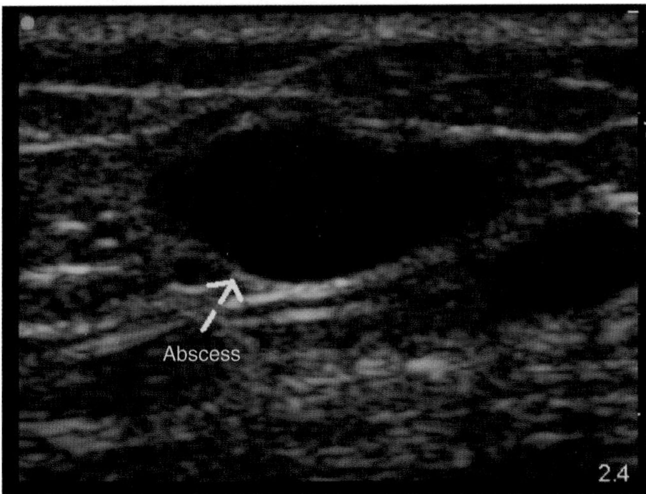

Figure 153.4 Ultrasound image of a hypoechoic (dark) soft tissue abscess.

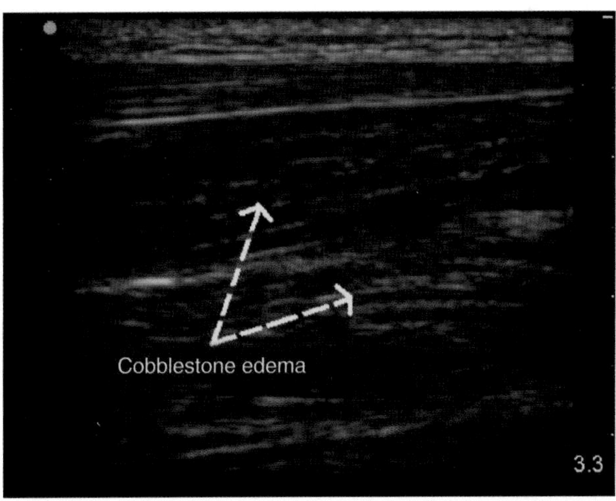

Figure 153.5 Ultrasound image of cellulitis. Note the "cobblestone" appearance and absence of a loculated fluid collection.

"cobblestone" appearance on ultrasound (Fig. 153.5). This appearance is created by the presence of fluid associated with cellulitis. The absence of a discrete fluid collection differentiates it from an abscess.

8. If a small hypoechoice (dark) fluid collection is visualized within a cellulitic area, apply a small amount of pressure over the fluid collection. Small fluid collections secondary to cellulitis will redistribute with pressure; abscess pockets will not.
9. Always obtain images in multiple planes (longitudinal, transverse, oblique) to help to define the borders of the abscess.
10. Utilize the electronic calipers available on the ultrasound system to make measurements of the abscess depth, width, and length.
11. Identify surrounding nerves, lymphatic channels, and vessels to help to prevent accidental puncture during incision and drainage.
12. Remember that pseudoaneurysms and large vessels may look like a fluid-filled abscess on ultrasound. When in doubt, apply color Doppler to the area of interest (Fig. 153.6). If there is flow on the color Doppler setting, the structure is likely a vessel.
13. Scan contralateral limbs and adjacent areas of normal appearing tissue for comparison.
14. Incision and drainage can be performed in a dynamic fashion under ultrasound guidance or in a static manner after the target area has been scanned and marked.

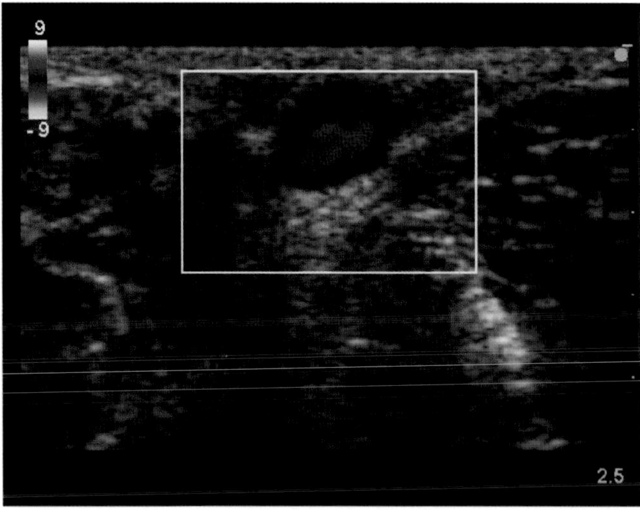

Figure 153.6 A large vessel can be mistaken for a small fluid collection. Apply color-Doppler to help to differentiate between the two.

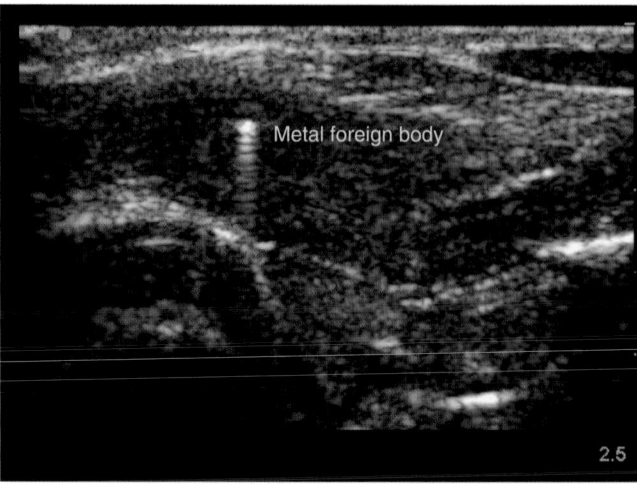

Figure 153.7 Ultrasound of a metal foreign body. Note the ring-down artifact cast deep (farfield) to the object.

B Foreign body removal

Soft tissue foreign bodies are often very difficult to detect clinically and, if left untreated, can lead to scar tissue formation, increased patient discomfort, infection, or delayed operative intervention. Although plain radiography is used frequently in the management of suspected soft tissue foreign bodies, it can only detect radiopaque substances such as gravel, metal, and certain types of leaded glass. Radiolucent substances such as wood, plastic, organic matter, and most types of glass are usually missed on plain radiographs. Although CT scan and MRI are more sensitive and specific, obtaining a CT scan or MRI in all cases of a suspected foreign body is not only expensive but also impractical. When a soft tissue foreign body is clinically suspected, bedside ultrasound can be used to aid in detection and localization.

Evaluation of a soft tissue foreign body

The following steps are performed using a bedside ultrasound for evaluation of a soft tissue foreign body.

1. Use a higher frequency probe to scan superficial structures, and a lower frequency probe when searching for deeper foreign bodies.
2. Most soft tissue applications should be performed with a 7.5 to 10 MHz linear array transducer (Fig. 153.1).
3. Apply a large amount of ultrasound gel to improve the acoustic interface. If the patient is thin and devoid of much subcutaneous fat, use an acoustic standoff pad to improve your sonographic window.
4. If acoustic standoff pads are not available, an acoustic window can be easily created with a small bag of normal saline or a fluid-filled glove sandwiched between two layers of ultrasound gel (Fig. 153.2).

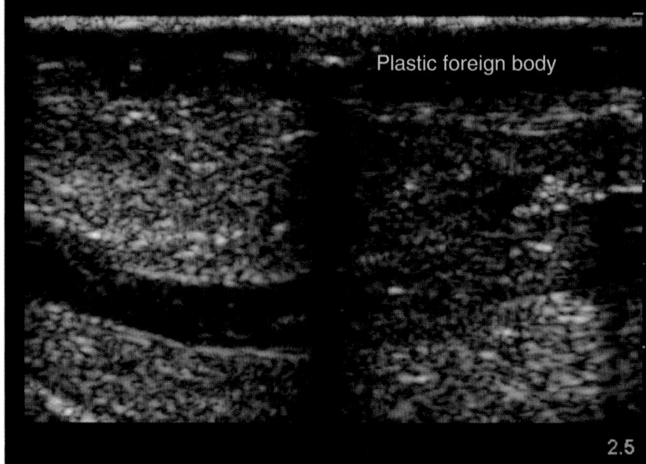

Figure 153.8 Ultrasound of plastic foreign body. Note the dark acoustic shadow cast deep (farfield) to the object.

5. Use sterile gel and scan with a transducer covered with a sterile sheath or glove to prevent contamination of the open wound. Remember that you must put gel between the transducer and the sterile sheath, and also between the sterile sheath and the object being scanned.
6. Begin by scanning normal tissue margins surrounding the area of interest. Note that normal subcutaneous tissue will have dark, hypoechoic regions of fat mixed in with hyperechoic (white) striations of muscle, brightly hyperechoic facial planes, and brightly hyperechoic fibrillar tendon planes (Fig. 153.3).
7. Foreign bodies will have different sonographic appearances depending on their density and constituents. Dense substances such as metal and gravel will be easier to detect

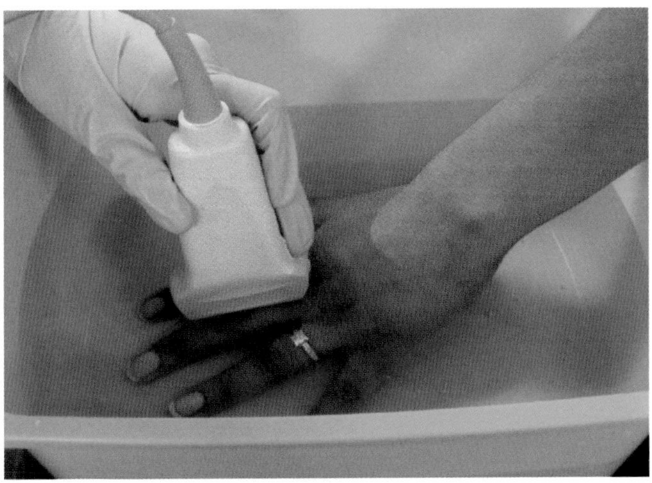

Figure 153.9 Water immersion to enhance the acoustic window. Immerse the target area in water and obtain sonographic images by floating the ultrasound probe a few centimeters above the area of interest.

than substances that are filled with more air, such as plastic and wood (Figs. 153.7 and 153.8).

8. Evaluation of a foreign body deep to a large, gaping wound can be difficult because imaging will be distorted by tissue damage and air. Imaging through an open wound can be enhanced with water immersion of the target area. Water serves as an excellent acoustic medium for ultrasound. Place the area of interest under water and direct the ultrasound beam at the target area through the water (Fig. 153.9).
9. Soft tissue foreign bodies can be removed in a static or dynamic fashion after ultrasound localization.

Section

26

Special populations: neonates

Expert reviewers: Janice Lowe, Arun Gupta, and Anand Rajani

Chapter

154 The normal neonate and common problems

J. Grace Park and N. Ewen Amieva-Wang

Introduction

The evaluation of neonates in the ED requires an understanding of normal behaviors for this age group. This chapter will describe the normal behaviors for neonates, followed by a discussion of common presenting complaints as well as an accompanying differential diagnosis. Emergency conditions in the neonatal age will be covered in Ch. 157.

The normal neonate

Birth history

While the past medical history for a neonate is seldom long, it is important to elicit specific information about the prenatal and peripartum course. A thorough prenatal history should include prenatal care, complications such as vaginal bleeding, and the presence of maternal diseases such as diabetes or hyperthyroidism. The number of weeks of gestation, length of labor with possible complications such as fever, mode of delivery, and hospital course including length of stay for mother and baby are also important. Normal term newborns weigh on average 3.4 kg (7.5 lb) with a range between 2.8 kg (6 lb 2 oz) and 4.2 kg (9 lb 2 oz). Babies who are small or large for gestational age (typically <10th and >90th percentile for gestational age) are at risk for congenital syndromes and complications.

Feeding, weight gain and stool patterns

During the first few days of life, a normal infant can lose up to 10% of the birth weight. Infants should regain their birth weight by 7–10 days of life. The average weight gain during the first 3 months of life is 20–30 g (approximately 1 oz) per day.

Bottle-fed infants usually feed between six and nine times every 24 h. Breast-fed infants tend to feed more frequently – as many as 12 times a day. A broad rule of thumb for appropriate feeding volumes is 2 oz every 2 h for neonates and 5–6 oz five to six times a day for babies up to 3 months of age. At older ages, babies will take 6–8 oz at a feeding.

Overfeeding can occur when parents try to feed a baby every time he or she cries. Overfeeding can also occur when parents use formula to supplement breast-feeding. Spitting up partially digested milk is not uncommon. However, if parents or caregivers describe true vomiting, a workup is warranted. A newborn should pass the first stool, or meconium, within the first 48 h of life. Constipation in neonates is not common. Straining up to 10 min before defecation of soft stools is caused by inability to relax the pelvic floor muscles (infant dyschezia) and is normal in infants. If there is a delay in passing of the first stool, a history of constipation, or failure to thrive, an organic cause must be ruled out. The differential diagnosis for constipation in a neonate includes

- cow's milk intolerance
- intestinal stenosis or atresia
- Hirschsprung disease
- hypothyroidism
- megacolon: meconium ilius or plug (associated with cystic fibrosis).

After the first passing of meconium, infants may stool one or two times a day or with every feed. Breast-fed infants tend to stool more frequently, averaging 27 stools in 7 days. Breast-fed infants also have looser, less-voluminous stools than bottle-fed babies since they absorb most of breast milk. If parents complain of "loose stool," it is important to differentiate this from regular breast-feeding stools. Reasons for loose stools include overfeeding, maternal use of laxatives, use of a formula that is too concentrated or high in sugar content, or infection.

Breathing

Neonates are obligate nasal breathers. Nasal congestion or choanal atresia can present with significant symptoms in the neonate. Choanal atresia can result in respiratory distress or cyanosis during feeding, which resolves with crying.

Breathing patterns

Beyond the postnatal adaptation period, the normal respiratory rate in infants is between 30 and 60 breaths/min.

A Practical Guide to Pediatric Emergency Medicine: Caring for Children in the Emergency Department, ed. N. Ewen Amieva-Wang (associate eds. Jamie Shandro, Aparajita Sohoni, and Bernhard Fassl). Published by Cambridge University Press.

Premature infants may have even higher respiratory rates. A periodic breathing pattern consists of alternating periods of normal breathing with respiratory pauses for 3 s or longer that last through three cycles of breathing. Periodic breathing usually occurs in premature infants, but full-term infants can also exhibit periodic breathing. Apnea longer than 20 s, or apnea of a shorter duration associated with cyanosis or bradycardia (heart rate $<$100 bpm), is not a normal breathing pattern and should be investigated for pathologic causes.

Sleeping patterns

Neonates usually sleep 18–20 h per day. Usually infants sleep for 2–4 h at a time and wake to be fed. During the first days of life, an infant should be awakened to be fed, if sleeping for more than 4 h at a time. Most full-term infants should be able to sleep through the night at around 3–6 months of age. Neonates with persistently increased sleep should be evaluated for possible pathologic causes of lethargy, such as sepsis or metabolic disorders.

Common complaints

While the majority of neonates brought to the ED for these complaints will be healthy, each patient deserves a careful history and physical examination to rule out a neonatal emergency or congenital disease process. Any toxic, irritable, or inconsolable patient should undergo a full workup to exclude sepsis as well as a workup of focal signs and symptoms.

Crying

Infants who presents with increased crying should be observed closely for an underlying cause. A careful history, asking about onset and pattern of crying, trauma, fever, and medication use, and a through physical examination are most important in determining the cause of crying. Laboratory tests are often not required.

A differential diagnosis of inconsolable crying includes:

- localized pain
- corneal abrasion or foreign body
- anal fissure
- improper feeding practices
  - overfeeding without adequate burping during feeding
  - underfeeding
  - milk protein allergy
- infections
  - meningitis
  - sepsis
  - otitis media
  - urinary tract
  - gastroenteritis
  - necrotizing enterocolitis
- requiring surgery
  - incarcerated hernia
  - anal fissure
  - intestinal malrotation/volvulus
- colic: diagnosis of exclusion in young neonate.

Localized pain, such as a corneal abrasion or a hair tourniquet (around fingers, toes or penis) can cause excessive crying in an infant. Infants can scratch their eyes with their fingernail, resulting in conjunctival inflammation and eye discharge. Fluorescein examination should be considered in infants with crying. All digits and penis should be examined for any signs of strangulation such as edema or erythema.

Infants should be examined carefully for signs of infection or anatomic reasons for discomfort. Examination should include ophthalmoscopic examination looking for retinal hemorrhage, otoscopic examination, palpation of the fontanel, and documentation of vital signs. Rarely, supraventricular tachycardia and congenital heart disease have been documented to cause neonatal crying. The remainder of the physical examination should include evaluation of the abdomen for distention, checking the groin for hernias, and surveying the skin for any bruising or petechiae that could signify either trauma or underlying bleeding tendency. If crying is truly inconsolable and no other etiology for crying can be found, a workup for sepsis should be performed.

"Colic", or excessive crying with no organic cause, is a diagnosis of exclusion. Colic is defined as daily paroxysmal crying, sometimes lasting for a few hours. Colic can start as early as the second to third week of life, and peaks at 6 to 8 weeks of age. Colic may last as late as 6 months of age. The crying is louder than usual, paroxysmal, clusters in the evenings, and is not related with any activity. The baby is usually inconsolable. Additional features such as burping, a reddened face, or drawing up the legs to the stomach can be present.

Most important to the diagnosis of colic is that the infant is completely normal between episodes, feeding well, and is otherwise healthy and gaining weight.

The crying pattern of a "colicky" infant is described by the wessel criteria or "rule of threes." Colic is crying that

starts during the third week of life
lasts more than 3 h per day
occurs more than 3 times a week
lasts longer than 3 weeks.

Proposed causes of colic include excessive intake of air, insufficient intake of fluid, milk allergy, parental anxiety, and "silent reflux." No single treatment has been shown to be effective for colic. However, some suggested interventions include decreasing external stimulation, sucking on a pacifier, listening to white noise, and rocking the infant. Use of medications rarely is beneficial or indicated. However, a trial of hypoallergenic or hydrolyzed formula may be useful. Reassuring the parents that colic is a common, self-limited problem in young infants and encouraging them to share care-giving responsibilities during this time can be helpful.

Rapid breathing

A neonate's breathing patterns can, at times, be alarming to the parent or caregiver. The adage "sleep like a baby" is misleading, as often caregivers will note respiratory pauses or an accelerated respiratory rate. The most common reason for true tachypnea in a neonate is infection, although abdominal, cardiac, and metabolic pathology are also in the differential diagnosis. Again, careful examination should be able to detect abdominal distention, rales, or heart murmur associated with tachypnea. If the patient is truly tachypneic, a chest radiograph as well as CBC and electrolytes are warranted. The practitioner should count the respiratory rate for a full minute as well as examine the neonate for signs of increased work of breathing. Differential diagnosis of rapid breathing includes:

- Infection
  - pneumonia
  - septicemia
  - meningitis
- abdominal distention
- metabolic derangement (acidosis)
- congenital diseases
  - diaphragmatic hernia
  - heart diease
  - tracheoesophageal fistula.

Vomiting

Vomiting should be differentiated from regurgitation in the neonate. While regurgitation is normal in a neonate, vomiting can be a serious symptom of an underlying neonatal emergency (Ch. 157). Differential diagnosis includes:

- malrotation: bilious vomiting
- hungry infant
- pyloric stenosis: vomiting of undigested feed in healthy with no history.
- milk allergy
- gastrointestinal reflux (GER)
- necrotizing enterocolitis
- infectious colitis.

A small amount of spitting with feeding is common in neonates and is caused by the reduced lower esophageal sphincter pressure and the relatively increased intragastric pressure. These infants do not have forceful vomiting, are not irritable, are growing normally, and have at least four to six wet diapers a day. Approximately 40–65% of newborns have some degree of reflux (see also Ch. 62), while only 3 to 5% of all infants have serious GER. These infants may exhibit signs of respiratory distress, failure to thrive, vomiting, or increased irritability. Infants may exhibit inconsolable crying, irritability with feeding, choking with feeding, refusal to feed, or frequent nighttime feeding. Infants with what appears to be severe GER should be investigated for anatomic causes of regurgitation or chronic aspiration.

Treatment of GER is initially conservative using non-pharmacologic intervention. Some of the proposed treatments include avoiding positions that can increase intra-abdominal pressure. Prone positioning is not recommended because of the increased risk of sudden infant death syndrome. Infants with GER also should avoid swings, slings, umbrella strollers, chairs, carriers, and any other device that increases intra-abdominal pressure. Smaller amounts of formula/breastmilk administered at higher frequencies may decrease the GER episodes. Some infants with GER are managed with hypoallergenic formula and thickening of feedings (1 tablespoon of dry rice cereal per ounce of formula). Also, formula with high calories may be used for those with weight loss or poor weight gain. Efficacy of pharmacologic interventions with histamine H_2 receptor antagonists, proton pump inhibitors, or prokinetic agents are controversial.

Blood in the diaper

Causes of blood in the diaper in a neonate include:

- swallowed maternal blood
- coagulopathies
- necrotizing enterocolitis
- infectious colitis
- congenital defects
- anal fissure
- milk allergy
- vaginal bleed from maternal estrogen withdraw
- urate crystals.

The emergency diagnoses to consider include coagulopathies, necrotizing enterocolitis, colitis, and congenital defects. If the neonate does not appear toxic and has no abdominal distension, then non-emergency diagnoses can be considered. There are a number of reassuring causes of blood or blood-like substances seen in the diaper: orange or brick-red urate crystals are often mistaken for blood but usually result from a chemical reaction of the urine with diaper fibers. Urate crystals can indicate dehydration. Breakthrough vaginal bleeding can occur in an estrogenized female.

Blood in the diaper or stool during the first 2 to 3 days of life is most commonly caused by swallowed maternal blood during birth. The Kleihauer–Betke or Apt–Downey test historically has been reported to confirm the diagnosis by differentiating fetal from maternal hemoglobin in the stool. However, these tests usually require fresh blood, which is not available from a diaper. Other possibilities include swallowed maternal blood during breast-feeding, which can be confirmed by examining the mother's breasts. Anal fissures are another common cause of bloody stools and can be seen with careful examination of the anus. Cow's milk allergy can also cause bloody stools. The incidence of cow's milk allergy worldwide is up to 7.5%. The diagnosis is made by

- resolution of symptoms after elimination of cow's milk and cow's milk products
- recurrence of identical symptoms after reintroduction of milk or milk products.

For unresponsive or severe allergy, biopsy may be needed to make a diagnosis. Infants usually start having symptoms within 1 week of exposure to cow's milk. The symptoms can start within a few minutes, an hour, or several days after ingestion.

Table 154.1. Indications for treatment of jaundice by age and bilirubin level

Age (h)	Treatment at bilirubin concentration (mg/dl)[a]		
	Follow-up[b]	Phototherapy	Exchange transfusion
>24	>5 (6–8)	>10	>20 (>18)
24–48	>9 (11–13)	>12 (>10)	>20 (>20)
48–72	>11 (13–15)	>15 (>12)	>25 (>20)

Source: adapted from the Provisional Committee on Quality Improvement and Subcommittee on Hyperbilirubinemia.
[a]Value in parentheses is the trigger level for those infants with risk factors including (1) family history of jaundice or hemolysis, (2) born at 34–38 weeks of gestation, (3) polycythemia, (4) bleeding internally or externally, (5) postnatal hemolysis, (6) increased rate of bilirubin rise (>0.5 mg/dl per h), (7) increased bilirubin production (high ETCOc [end-tidal carbon monoxide concentration]), (8) hypoxemia, acidosis, sepsis, or hypoalbuminemia.
[b]Follow-up is with a physician and with a repeat bilirubin measurement in 48 h.

Rash

The majority of rashes in the newborn are benign (Ch. 156). One of the exceptions is the seemingly innocuous group of vesicles found on a neonate. Localized HSV infection can occur on a neonate on days 7–14 of life. While a maternal history of herpes lesions is diagnostic, the absence of this history should not dissuade the EP from considering this disease. If a child presents with localized signs suggestive of HSV infection, the child should be admitted regardless of how well-appearing the child is (Fig. 156.10, p. xx). The lesions should be sampled for HSV direct fluorescent antibody test and viral culture. Empiric systemic acyclovir should be started.

Other rashes not unique to the newborn period and suggestive of potentially life-threatening conditions include

- maculopapular rash in erythema multiforme and rubeola
- petechial rash in meningococcemia
- staphylococcal pustulosis.

Often these rashes will be accompanied by systemic signs including irritability and fever.

Jaundice (hyperbilirubinemia)

The most common causes of jaundice seen in neonates are:

- hemolysis caused by ABO isogroup incompatibility, Rh incompatibility
- physiologic: sepsis or breast-milk jaundice
- excessive bruising from birth trauma (cephalohematoma or intramuscular hematoma)
- sepsis
- congenital infections (e.g., rubella, toxoplasmosis, CMV infection)
- congenital atresia of bile ducts, serum hepatitis
- congenital hemolytic anemias (sickle cell anemia, spherocytosis)
- hemolytic anemia caused by drugs (e.g., in glucose-6-phosphate dehydrogenase deficiency)
- hypothyroidism.

This section will focus on the common reasons for a well-appearing neonate to be jaundiced.

Physiologic jaundice occurs in up to 60% of full-term and 80% of preterm infants. This form of jaundice is caused by hemolysis of fetal red blood cells at a time when there is still a deficiency in the ability to conjugate bilirubin. The bilirubin level peaks between 3 and 5 days and requires no treatment. Well-appearing infants are most likely to have physiologic jaundice. A CBC, total bilirubin, direct and indirect bilirubin should be obtained. In a well-appearing, afebrile infant with unconjugated or indirect hyperbilirubinemia and a normal hemoglobin, no further tests are needed.

Jaundice associated with breast-feeding is mainly a result of suboptimal breast-feeding practices, resulting in dehydration. There may also be substances that inhibit glucuronyl transferase in the breast milk. Breast-feeding jaundice may start as early as days 3–4 of life. Initial management consists of supplementation with formula or other acceptable fluid such as pedialyte. Breast-feeding jaundice is unlikely to cause kernicterus and can be treated with phototherapy when necessary.

The AAP recommends initiation of phototherapy based on age and gestational age and neurotoxicity factors (Table 154.1). All infants requiring phototherapy or IV hydration from the ED require hospitalization. The Bilitool™ (http://bilitool.org/ [accessed July 2010]) carries treatment plans for jaundice according to age and level of bilirubin.

Eye discharge, redness, and conjunctivitis

In infants, nasolacrimal duct obstruction or dacryostenosis can be confused with conjunctivitis. However, these infants rarely have conjunctival injection but usually have eye discharge and crusts on lashes. Initially, lacrimal massage is recommended. Obstruction usually spontaneously resolves within 12 to 18 months of life (Ch. 119).

Neonatal conjunctivitis is the most common infection in neonates, occurring in 1.6–12% of newborns during the first month of life. Hyperemia with a thick mucopurulent discharge and pseudomembrane formation or eyelid edema should raise suspicion for infectious conjunctivitis. Red eye in a neonate is presumed an eye-threatening emergency until proven otherwise (Ch. 155).

Timing of the onset of conjunctivitis is an important consideration in evaluation of neonatal conjunctivitis. Conjunctivitis within the first 24 h of life is most frequently a chemical conjunctivitis caused by antimicrobial prophylaxis. Conjunctivitis occurring after the first few days of life, in association with facial rash or purulent discharge, warrants workup for conjunctivitis neonatorum (Ch. 155) secondary to gonococcal and chlamydial infection, as well as herpetic conjunctivitis. The peak time of onset for gonococcal conjunctivitis is between 3 and 5 days after birth. Chlamydial infection becomes the most frequent cause of conjunctivitis by the end of the first week of life and throughout the first month of life.

Acute glaucoma also can also cause a red eye in neonates. On examination, a stained or cloudy cornea with large pupils is usually seen. Slit lamp examination may show a shallow anterior chamber. The intraocular pressure should be also measured. An ophthalmologist should be consulted for suspected opthalmalgia neonatorum, glaucoma, or ocular HSV infection.

Pearls and pitfalls

Pearls

1. Neonates may lose up to 10% of their birth weight in the first week of life.
2. The majority of well-appearing jaundiced neonates have physiologic jaundice that will resolve without intervention.
3. Colic is a diagnosis of exclusion in the neonate.

Pitfalls

1. Failure to workup bilious vomiting in a neonate.
2. Failure to workup constipation in a neonate.
3. Failure to consider gonorrhea in a neonate with purulent eye discharge during the first week of life.

Selected references

Colletti JE, Kothari S, Jackson DM, Kilgore KP, Barringer K. An emergency medicine approach to neonatal hyperbilirubinemia. *Emerg Med Clin North Am* 2007;**25**:1117–1135, vii.

Henry SM. Discerning differences: gastroesophageal reflux and gastroesophageal reflux disease in infants. *Adv Neonatal Care* 2004;**4**: 235–247.

Martorell A, Plaza AM, Boné J, *et al.* Cow's milk protein allergy. A multi-centre study: clinical and epidemiological aspects. *Allergol Immunopathol (Madr)* 2006;**34**:46–53.

Provisional Committee on Quality Improvement and Subcommittee on Hyperbilirubinemia. Practice parameter: management of hyperbilirubinemia in the healthy term newborn. *Pediatrics* 1994;**94**:558–565.

Savino F. Focus on infantile colic. *Acta Paediatr* 2007;**96**:1259–1264.

Subcommittee on Hyperbilirubinemia. Management of hyperbilirubinemia in the newborn infant 35 or more weeks of gestation. *Pediatrics* 2004;**114**: 297–316.

Teoh DL, Reynolds S. Diagnosis and management of pediatric conjunctivitis. *Pediatr Emerg Care* 2003;**19**:48–55.

Chapter

155 Newborn ophthalmology

Douglas Fredrick

Introduction

Normal visual development depends not only on the eye anatomy but also on the absence of visual impediments (i.e., a droopy eyelid, cataract, or vitreous hemorrhage), having well aligned eyes, and an equal refractive error between the two eyes. Routine ED examination of a newborn should include a quick assessment of the red reflex (Fig. 155.1) and lack of leukocoria (Fig. 155.2), using the direct ophthalmoscope to make certain that light is reflected through the pupil in a symmetric pattern signifying absence of cataracts.

Assessment of vision in newborns

Assessing visual function in a newborn is difficult. A method to facilitate the eye examination in a newborn is to gently rock the patient from side to side, and then up and down. These maneuvers generally lead to natural eye opening in the newborn.

Newborns will not fix or follow, respond to visual threat, and often have an immature corneal sensation reflex. The best response is wincing to light, indicating that the child has light perception vision. By 2 months of age, a child should fix and follow the parent's or caretaker's face with the help of visual and auditory cues, such as making a clucking sound or a whistling sound while moving the face back and forth in front of the child. The child will then fix and follow. The examiner should stop making the auditory cues to see whether or not the child continues to follow the examiner's moving face. Fixation and following should be assessed first in both eyes and then in each eye separately by occluding the opposite eye. It is important to avoid physical contact when occluding an eye, as children will object to having either eye covered. A thumb or a small occluder can be used to occlude the visual axis without touching the child. A child who has poor vision in one eye will often violently object to covering the better eye and will become inconsolable if the sound eye is patched. When the eye with poor vision is patched, the child will stop fussing. This is indicative of visual asymmetry between the two eyes.

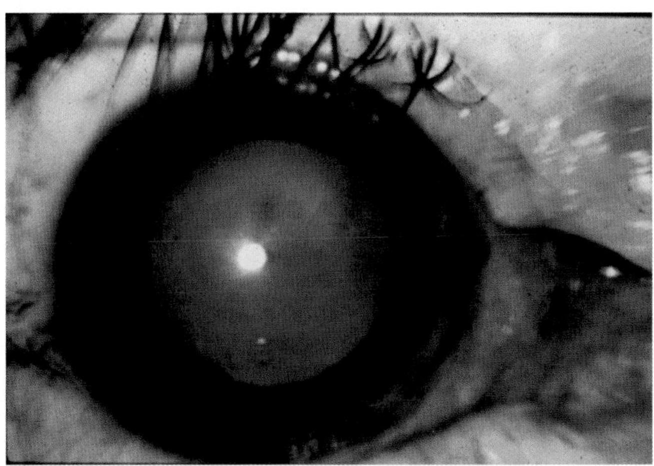

Figure 155.1 Normal appearance of red reflex. (Courtesy D. Fredrick.)

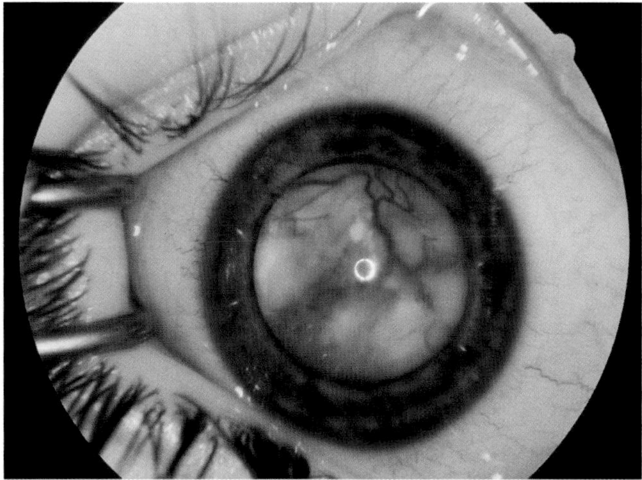

Figure 155.2 Leukocoria caused by a retinoblastoma. (Courtesy D. Fredrick.)

A Practical Guide to Pediatric Emergency Medicine: Caring for Children in the Emergency Department, ed. N. Ewen Amieva-Wang (associate eds. Jamie Shandro, Aparajita Sohoni, and Bernhard Fassl). Published by Cambridge University Press.

Table 155.1. Differential diagnosis of neonatal conjunctivitis

Diagnosis	Symptoms	Natural history	Time course of symptoms	Diagnosis and treatment
Chemical conjunctivitis	Watery discharge	1–3 days after birth	1–3 days after birth	Symptomatic and observation
Chlamydial conjunctivitis	Bilateral inflamed conjuntiva and initial watery discharge	Conjunctival scarring and pneumonitis if systemic treatment not initiated	5–14 days after birth	Topical tetracycline or erythromycin ophthalmic ointment (0.5–1 cm ribbon of ointment to affected conjunctival sac once daily) Oral erythromycin for chlamydial pneumonitis (50 mg/kg daily divided every 6 h)
Gonorrheal conjunctivitis	Red eye, purulent discharge	Corneal perforation if untreated	2–5 days after birth	Gram stain, culture and sensitivity Systemic ceftriaxone (50 mg/kg IV) Screening child for other sexually transmitted diseases, ophthalmic consultation
Herpetic conjunctivitis/ keratitis	Photophobia, watery discharge, foreign body sensation	Stains with fluorescein; if unrecognized leds to corneal scarring	Part of neonatal herpes simplex virus syndrome; 7–14 days after birth	Acyclovir IV (20 mg/kg per dose q. 8 h), topical trifluridine, ophthalmic referral, consult ophthalmology and infectious diseases specialist, with possible lumbar puncture to rule out CNS involvement

Newborn eye emergencies

Ophthalmia neonatorum refers to conjunctivitis caused by gonorrhea or chlamydial infection in the newborn period (Table 155.1). Every neonate who presents to the ED with a red eye should be evaluated for ophthalmia neonatorum given the potential for severe morbidity. Gonococcal conjunctivitis presents as hyperacute conjunctivitis with massive amounts of purulent discharge from both eyes. Patients with suspected gonococcal conjunctivitis require immediate swabbing of the exudates for Gram stain and culture. The presence of Gram-negative diplococci will confirm the diagnosis and guide treatment. Treatment includes hospital admission, ophthalmology consult, systemic third-generation cephalosporin, hourly saline irrigation to remove the mucoid material from the eye, and use of a topical broad-spectrum antibiotic, such as polysporin ophthalmic ointment. *Neisseria gonorrhoeae* can liberate collagenases that will lead to corneal perforation within days if untreated. If there is any swelling of the lids, erythema, or other signs of celluitis, a sepsis workup should be initiated.

Chlamydial conjunctivitis is more gradual in onset than gonorrheal conjunctivitis and usually presents in the second week of life. The child presents with bilateral inflamed conjunctiva and initially a watery discharge, which becomes mucopurulent or bloody if untreated. While rapid bedside tests can be used to initiate treatment (direct fluorescent antibody [DFA], enzyme-linked immunosorbent assay [ELISA] and PCR), sensitivity and specificity studies are lacking in infants and the gold standard for diagnosis is culture of epithelial cells from the palpebral conjunctiva (everted eyelid) as well as from the nasopharynx. (Culture of the exudate is not sufficient since *Chlamydia trachomatis* is an obligate intracellular pathogen.)

Treatment includes topical tetracycline or erythromycin ophthalmic ointment. In addition, oral erythromycin base should be administered since more than 50% of patients with chlamydial conjunctivitis have concomitant nasopharyngeal infection and are at risk of chlamydial pneumonitis. Complications include the development of a pseudomembrane formed by exudates adhering to conjunctiva or, in severe cases, the deposition of a layer of granulation tissue. These complications can develop as early as 2 weeks from onset of symptoms, making the early diagnosis and treatment of this condition imperative.

Neonates with either gonorrhea or chlamydia conjunctivitis require further evaluation for other sexually transmitted diseases. In addition, the mothers and their sexual partners should be screened for sexually transmitted diseases. Cases of gonorrhea or chlamydia must be reported to the state public health agencies.

Chapter 156

Neonatal dermatology

Theresa M. van der Vlugt

Introduction

This chapter includes benign neonatal skin findings, and a brief discussion of vesicular and pustular diseases of the newborn (Table 156.1).

Benign neonatal rash

Milia

Milia are whitish round 1–2 mm papules seen on the forehead, cheeks, and nose of 40–89% of newborns, more common in Caucasians (Fig. 156.1). They can occur in the oral cavity, where they are called Epstein's pearls. They are superficial epithelial cysts filled with keratin. They are frequently grouped and can also be found on the upper trunk, limbs, or penis. They usually resolve spontaneously by 2–3 months. The main differential diagnosis is sebaceous hyperplasia, discussed below. Acne are inflammatory lesions and do not appear until after 2 weeks of age.

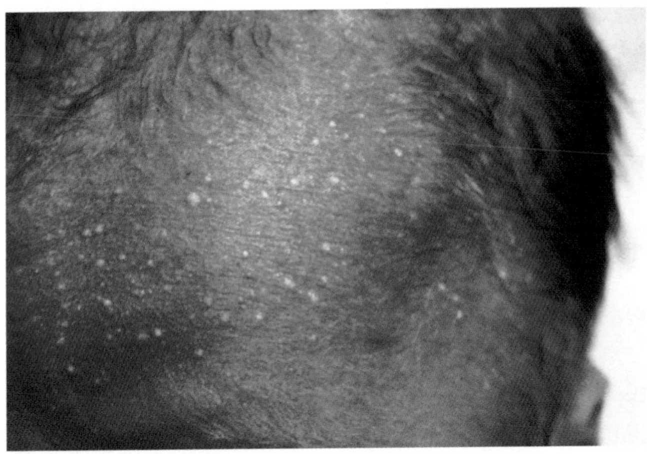

Figure 156.1 Milia: multiple white papules on the forehead of a neonate. (Reproduced with permission from Weston WL, Lane AT, Morelli JG. *Color Textbook of Pediatric Dermatology*, 4th edn. Philadelphia, PA: Mosby Elsevier, 2007. © 2007 Elsevier Inc.)

Table 156.1. Benign neonatal rash by distribution

Distribution	Rash
Face	Milia, sebaceous hyperplasia, neonatal acne, stork bite, infantile hemangioma
Head and neck	Cephalohematoma, caput succedaneum, stork bite, miliaria rubra, miliaria crystallina, infantile hemangioma
Trunk, back, extremities	Miliaria rubra, miliaria crystallina, subcutaneous fat necrosis, Mongolian spot, infantile hemangioma
Diffuse	Erythema toxicum neonatorum, transient neonatal pustular melanosis, congenital cutaneous candidiasis

Sebaceous hyperplasia

Sebaceous hyperplasia causes small, follicular, regularly spaced yellowish or flesh-colored papules clustered on the nose and upper lip, where sebaceous glands are most dense (Fig. 156.2). These lesions are yellower than milia. They occur in half of term infants. They are a function of intrauterine androgen stimulation, and involute completely over weeks to months.

Miliaria rubra

Miliaria rubra or "prickly heat" causes erythematous 1–3 mm pinpoint papules or papulopustules on the trunk, head and scalp, and flexural areas (Fig. 156.3). These papules are not follicularly based but are caused by obstruction of eccrine sweat glands, and they can be brought on by overheating and bundling with thick, non-breathable clothing. It is common on the back of young infants from supine sleep positioning, and the incidence is high in the first weeks of life because of the

A Practical Guide to Pediatric Emergency Medicine: Caring for Children in the Emergency Department, ed. N. Ewen Amieva-Wang (associate eds. Jamie Shandro, Aparajita Sohoni, and Bernhard Fassl). Published by Cambridge University Press.

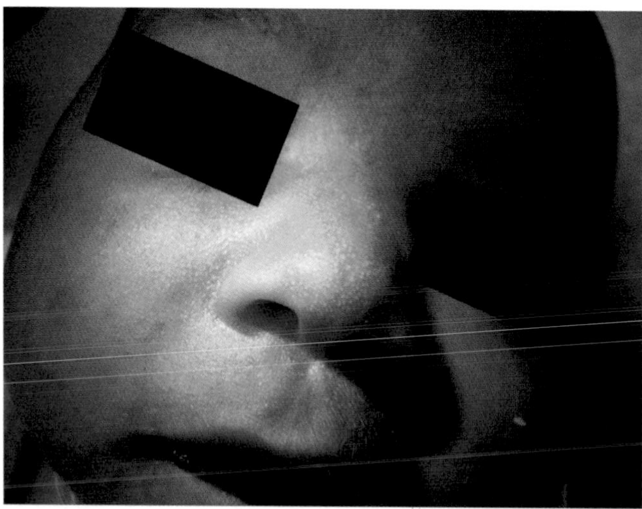

Figure 156.2 Sebacious hyperplasia on the nose and upper lip of an infant. (Courtesy Dr. Paul Matz.)

Figure 156.3 Miliaria rubra occurs with obstruction of sweat glands deeper in the epidermis or dermis, resulting in the reddened papulopustular lesions of "prickly heat." Papulopustular lesions dot the skin of this infant's face, neck, and upper trunk. (Courtesy of Logical Images, Inc.)

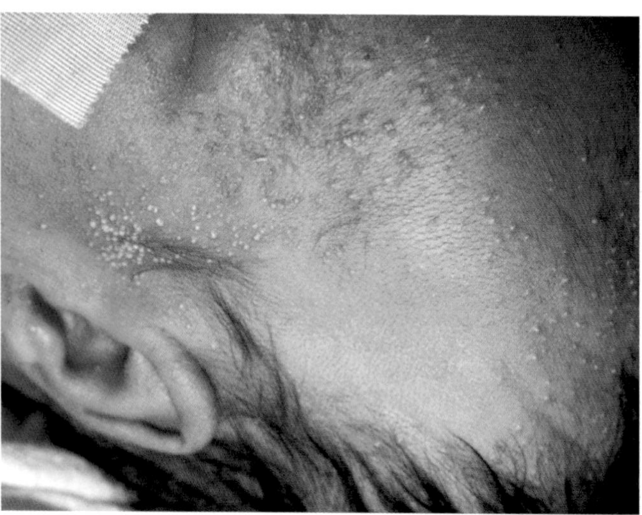

Figure 156.4 Miliaria occur with blockage of the sweat glands. Miliaria crystallina results from blockage of superficial eccrine sweat glands and leads to tiny thin-walled sweat-retention vesicles, which rupture then desquamate, typically on the head, neck, and upper trunk. (Courtesy of Logical Images, Inc.)

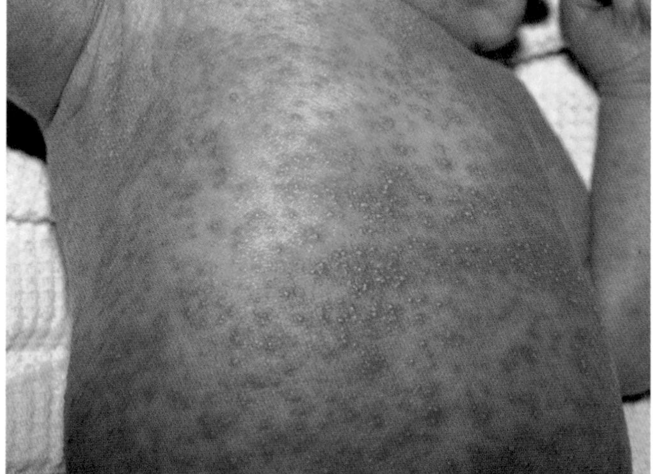

Figure 156.5 Erythema Toxicum Neonatorum. Blotchy erythematous macules with tiny central pustules that come and go over hours or days. (Courtesy of Logical images).

immaturity of epidermal appendages. Treatment centers on avoiding excessive heat, humidity, and occlusive non-breathable clothing.

Miliaria crystallina

Miliaria crystallina (Fig. 156.4) are clear pinpoint vesicles without inflammatory or erythematous background, seen in 3–15% of infants. They are caused by eccrine sweat duct obstruction at a more superficial level than miliaria rubra. These tiny vesicles are fragile and can be wiped away. They occur most commonly in the first few days of life and are encouraged by fever or environmental heating and occlusion. They are not often confused with other vesicular disorders because of their size, superficiality, and particular precipitating conditions.

Erythema toxicum neonatorum

Erythema toxicum neonatorum, despite its ominous name, is a well-known benign eruption in the newborn period, usually having onset in the first 48 h of life and seen in 21–72% of term infants (Fig. 156.5). Incidence increases with gestational age and weight of the infant. Lesions start as a blotchy macular erythema with many macules developing barely elevated central 1–3 mm yellowish papules or pustules. Lesions are evanescent and may last hours or days, and they can occur anywhere on the body, sparing the palms and soles. The eruption has

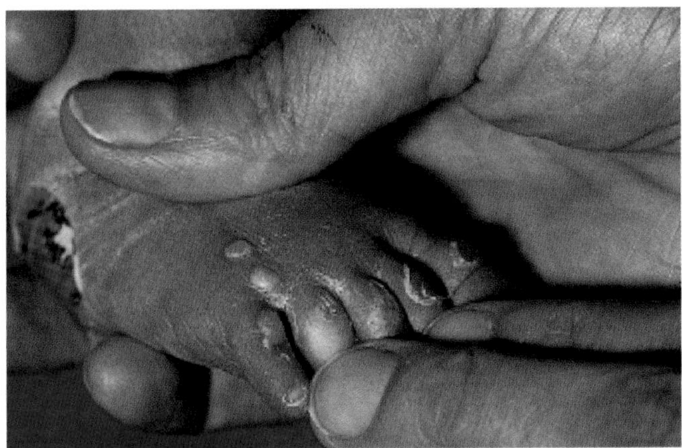

Figure 156.6 Transient neonatal pustular melanosis. Tense pustules and collarettes of scale at sites of older lesions. (Reprinted with permission from Paller, AS, Manicini AJ (eds.) *Hurwitz Clinical Pediatric Dermatology: A Textbook of Skin Disorders of Childhood and Adolescence* 3rd edn. Philadelphia, PA: Elsevier Saunders, 2006. © 2006 Saunders Inc., an affiliate of Elsevier Inc.)

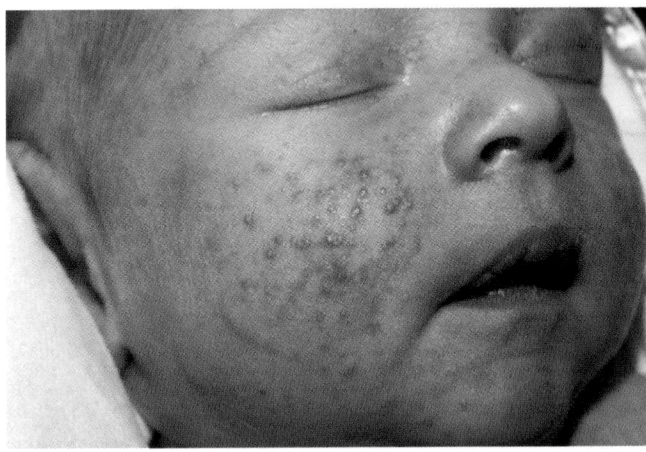

Figure 156.7 Acne neonatorum: Erythematous papules and papulopustules on the cheek. (Reprinted with permission from Paller, AS, Manicini AJ (eds.) *Hurwitz Clinical Pediatric Dermatology: A Textbook of Skin Disorders of Childhood and Adolescence* 3rd edn. Philadelphia, PA: Elsevier Saunders, 2006. © 2006 Saunders Inc., an affiliate of Elsevier Inc.)

exacerbations and remissions for the first 2 weeks of life then spontaneously resolves. The rash is asymptomatic. Testing is rarely necessary because of the distinct clinical picture. When the diagnosis is in question, a lesion can be scraped and contents smeared on a slide with Wrights or Giemsa stain to reveal sheets of eosinophils. Additionally, other pustular neonatal conditions lack the typical erythematous flare surrounding pustules. Parents should be reassured that no treatment is necessary for erythema toxicum neonatorum, and it will spontaneously resolve in a week or two.

Transient neonatal pustular melanosis

Transient neonatal pustular melanosis is very similar to erythema toxicum neonatorum but if it occurs it is always present at birth. It occurs primarily in African-American full-term infants. Lesions begin as small 2–10 mm superficial sterile pustules with a predilection for the forehead, nape, under the chin, neck, lower back, and shins (Fig. 156.6). Lesions can be diffuse and can be found occasionally on palms and soles. There is no surrounding erythema. Pustules last 1–2 days then rupture easily to leave a collarette of scale; they then become hyperpigmented brown macules resembling freckles and fade over months. Sometimes infants are born only with collarettes of scale, or the pustules are all removed when the vernix is wiped off at birth. Transient neonatal pustular melanosis is entirely benign and self-limited, and of unknown etiology. Pustule scrapings smeared on a slide with Wrights stain show neutrophils, rare eosinophils, and cellular debris.

Neonatal and infantile acne

Acne in the first few weeks of life (acne neonatorum) is also called neonatal cephalic pustulosis and lacks comedones but has small inflammatory papulopustules on the cheeks, chin, forehead, and scalp. It is unclear if this is a form of acne, or another papulopustular disorder of infancy. The condition spontaneously resolves without treatment.

Infants can develop an eruption of erythematous papules and pustules with open and closed comedones that closely resembles the acne vulgaris seen in adolescents (Fig. 156.7). The rash has a predilection for the cheeks, upper chest, and back. Onset is common at 2–3 months of age but rare before 4 weeks. Similar to adolescent acne, infantile acne is thought to be driven by androgens, levels of which are high in normal male and female infants for the first 6 months.

Treatment can be gentle washing with soap and water or mild topical benzoyl peroxide 2.5%. Larger papules and pustules that may scar can be treated with oral erythromycin. The condition usually clears by 12 months.

Salmon patches (nevus simplex)

Salmon patches (nevus simplex), also called "stork bites" when on the nape and "angel kisses" when on the glabella, are very common erythematous macules or patches composed of ectatic capillaries in the upper dermis covered by normal overlying skin. They are present in 70% of Caucasian newborns, nearly as many African-American and Latino babies, and 22% of Asian babies. They are common on the posterior neck, glabella, upper eyelids, and nasal regions. Most fade within a year or two, but nape or posterior scalp lesions can persist indefinitely. Lesions accentuate or even reappear with crying, breath-holding, straining, or exercise. Unlike port-wine stains, they are not associated with any syndromes.

Mongolian spots (dermal melanosis)

Mongolian spots are flat, poorly defined blue/black/grey/brown macules usually located over the lumbosacral area and buttocks of infants, occasionally found on the back, shoulders, or lower limbs. They occur in 90% of African-American and Native American babies, 80% of Asian babies, 70% of Hispanic babies, and approximately 10% of Caucasian babies. They are caused by an accumulation of spindle-shaped

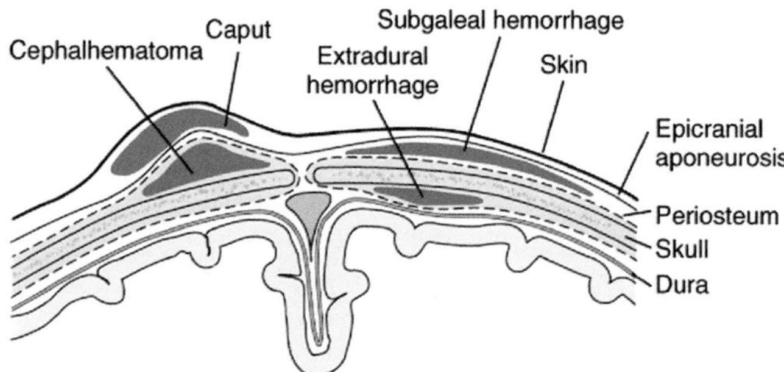

Figure 156.8 Sites of extracranial and extradural hemorrhages in the newborn: important tissue planes from skin to dura. (Reproduced with permission from Zitelli BJ, Davis HW *Atlas of Pediatric Physical Diagnosis* 5th edn. Philadelphia, PA: Mosby Elsevier, 2007. © 2007 Mosby Inc., an affiliate of Elsevier Inc.)

melanocytes deep in the dermis, probably arrested in embryonal migration. When this dermal melanosis occurs on the face around the eye it is called "nevus of ota", and on the shoulders or upper arms it is called "nevus of ito." Lesions on the lower back and buttocks usually resolve over several years or become markedly less prominent. Lesions elsewhere may not resolve, and nevus of ota is followed closely for its low risk of melanoma.

Cephalohematoma and caput succedaneum

Cephalohematoma and caput succedaneum are both swellings of the scalp following vaginal delivery. Cephalohematoma is a subperiosteal hematoma that does not cross the midline of the scalp, common over the parietal bone following vacuum-assisted delivery (Fig. 156.8). They may not be apparent for hours to days after birth, and overlying skin is normal. They normally reabsorb over weeks to months but can persist longer if they calcify. Occasionally (5–25%) they can be associated with an underlying linear skull fracture. Usually no treatment is necessary, but very large cephalohematomas can rarely cause hyperbilirubinemia, anemia, or even become infected. Caput succedaneum is a boggy scalp swelling, primarily edema from venous congestion in the scalp following a prolonged vaginal delivery. There can be associated petechiae and ecchymosis. The boggy edema usually crosses the midline, and reabsorbs over a few days.

Subcutaneous fat necrosis

Subcutaneous fat necrosis is a benign, self-limited disorder of term newborns that may be related to birth trauma or cold exposure. Lesions are firm, well-defined, red or purple plaques or nodules of subcutaneous fat necrosis that occur on the back, buttocks, cheeks, arms, or thighs in the first few days or weeks (Fig. 156.9). There may be no color change with deeper nodules. Lesions are single or multiple, and infants are usually healthy, vigorous, and feeding well, even if lesions are occasionally tender. Biopsy shows fat crystallization and necrosis. Subcutaneous fat necrosis is occasionally seen with ensuing

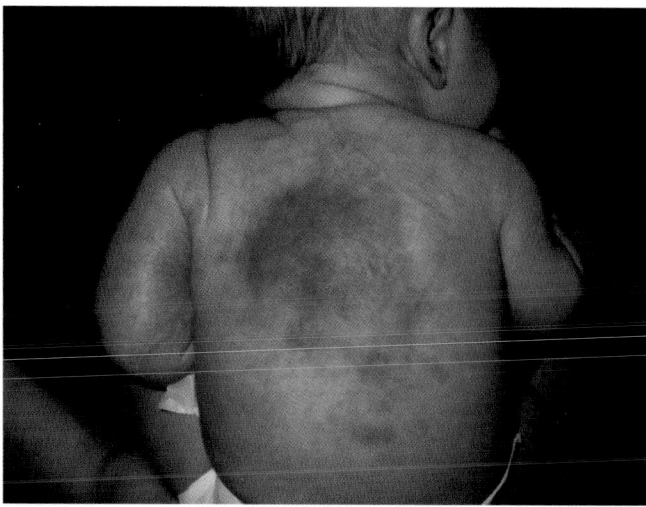

Figure 156.9 Subcutaneous fat necrosis. Confluent, indurated and well-demarcated subcutaneous nodules of fat on the back of a newborn. (Reproduced with permission from Kane KS, Lio PA, Stratigos AJ, Johnson RA (eds). *Color Atlas and Synopsis of Pediatric Dermatology*, 2nd edn. New York: McGraw Hill Medical 2009.)

hypercalcemia, and serum calcium levels should be checked and repeated weekly for infants with extensive disease. Infants should be followed for several months following delivery as onset of hypercalcemia can be delayed. Well-being of these infants helps to differentiate subcutaneous fat necrosis from sepsis or cellulitis. There is no specific therapy, and lesions usually resolve spontaneously. Rarely a lesion will liquefy, drain externally, and leave an atrophic scar with calcium deposits.

Infantile hemangioma

Infantile hemangiomas are benign vascular tumors formed of a proliferation of endotheial cells that undergo a period of rapid growth (often alarming to parents) and then spontaneously involute. They are noted in 1–3% of infants in the newborn period, rising to 10% of infants in the first year. They are more common in females than males, and somewhat more common in White races; they seem to have a predilection for the face and neck. There are three types of infantile hemangioma:

- superficial (50–60%): bright red, rubbery, sometimes partly blanching, raised papules/plaques that can have a lobulated surface
- deep (15%): partly compressible subcutaneous nodules often with bluish overlying skin with telangectasias
- combined (25–35%): features of both.

Hemangiomas in the "beard" distribution (jaw/lower cheek/anterior neck) have a high association with airway-impairing hemangiomas, which can cause hoarseness or stridor in the first few months of life; a high index of suspicion is warranted for these.

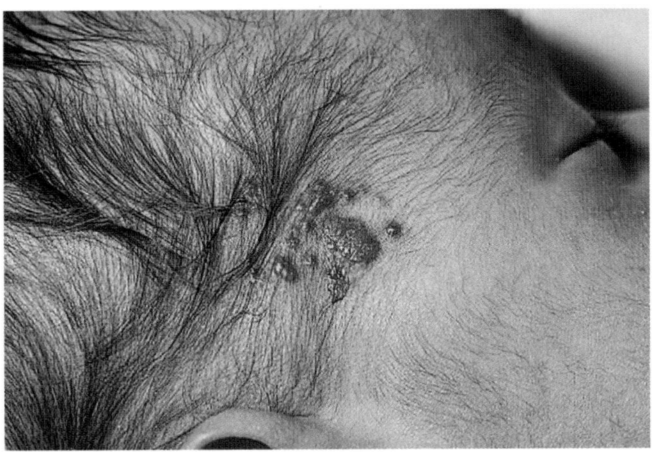

Figure 156.10 Neonatal herpes simplex. Grouped vesicles on an erythematous base on this 9-day-old infant. (Reproduced with permission from Weston WL, Lane AT, Morelli JG. *Color Textbook of Pediatric Dermatology*, 4th edn. Philadelphia, PA: Mosby Elsevier, 2007. © 2007 Elsevier Inc.)

Pustular or vesicular disease in the newborn

Infectious disease is responsible for many newborn skin findings, whether acquired congenitally, perinatally, or shortly after birth. Pustular or vesicular disease in the newborn is often benign, but distinguishing benign disease or even benign infection from serious infection is of paramount importance. Multiple systemic infections, bacterial, viral, and fungal, can cause widespread pustules and vesicles in neonates; differentiating well from ill infants is the most important clinical task.

Herpes simplex virus

In newborns, HSV causes vesicular lesions and requires a high index of suspicion as morbidity is significant and skin findings sometimes lag other systemic symptoms (Fig. 156.10).

Congenital or neonatal cutaneous candidiasis

Congenital or neonatal cutaneous candidiasis produces a widespread eruption of tiny erythematous papules and pustules with erythematous, scaly skin, including palms and soles; it is either present at birth or appears in the first week. It is acquired from maternal colonization and transmitted perinatally or during the birth process. Microscopy of pustule contents with KOH is diagnostic, and the placenta can also be examined for characteristic changes. In term healthy infants, this infection does not usually produce systemic symptoms and can be treated with topical nystatin, miconazole, or ketoconazole, along with close observation for any systemic spread. Congenital cutaneous candidiasis should be distinguished from systemic candidiasis, for which premature and low-birthweight infants are at special risk. Systemic candidiasis causes disseminated internal disease with signs of sepsis, including apnea, hyperglycemia, temperature instability, and hypotension; skin findings may be absent. Candidiasis can also be obtained in utero, usually in conjunction with instrumentation or foreign bodies and can produce benign cutaneous candidiasis in term infants as well as serious systemic disease in premature infants.

Pearls and pitfalls

Pearls

1. A range of well-defined neonatal dermatologic findings may be benign in etiology.
2. An assessment of the neonate's overall health status will aid in determining which rashes may be benign.
3. Close follow-up should be arranged for all neonates with a new, or unidentified, rash.

Pitfalls

1. Failure to consider HSV for vesicular lesions in a neonate.
2. Failure to provide strict return precautions for all neonates with a rash.

Selected references

Eitchenfield LF, Frieden IJ, Esterly NB. *Textbook of Neonatal Dermatology*. Philadelphia, PA: Saunders, 2001.

Mathes MD, Koerper M, Frieden I. A 6-month-old boy with an enlarging bruise on his back. *Pediatr Ann* 2006;**35**:441–443.

Paller AS, Mancini AJ. *Hurwitz Clinical Pediatric Dermatology, a Textbook of Skin Disorders in Childhood and Adolescence*. Philadelphia, PA: Elsevier Saunders, 2006.

Weston WL, Land AT, Morelli JG. *Color Textbook of Pediatric Dermatology*, 4th edn. Philadelphia, PA: Mosby Elsevier, 2007.

Chapter

157 Neonatal emergencies

J. Grace Park, Claire Turchi, Nikta Forghani, and Darrell M. Wilson

A Neonatal shock

Introduction

J. Grace Park

Neonates often present to the ED with one of a finite range of symptoms. However, a host of varying pathologies may be suggested by similar symptoms, making the workup challenging to the EP (Table 157.1). Sometimes, the infant will have a spectrum of symptoms (e.g., fever and respiratory distress) indicating the most probable diagnosis, but often the presenting signs are non-specific. While the initial approach is the same as in all resuscitation (establish and secure the ABCs), it is important to develop a neonatal differential diagnosis in order to address the underlying cause and provide definitive treatment. In this chapter, we discuss shock in the neonatal period, neonatal infection, and then proceed to an organ-system-based approach to neonatal emergencies. Neonatal conjunctivitis is discussed in Ch. 155.

The differential diagnosis of shock in the neonate includes sepsis, ductal-dependent congenital cardiac disease, inborn errors of metabolism, or congenital adrenal hyperplasia. Intracranial hemorrhage, abdominal surgical emergencies with circulatory collapse, and arrhythmias are more rare causes of neonatal shock.

Initial management of shock is identical regardless of etiology (Box 157.1). The ABCs and disability should be assessed and managed. A bedside glucose level should be checked and monitored hourly if found to be low (after repletion, of course). Initial laboratory analyses should include arterial or venous blood gases, CBC, electrolytes and anion gap, blood and urine cultures, lactate, ammonia, LFTs, and chest radiograph. Lumbar puncture should be performed only when the infant is stable enough to be manipulated; CSF should be sent for glucose, protein, cell counts, Gram stain, culture and HSV PCR.

Table 157.1. Neonatal manifestations of disease and their differential diagnosis

Symptom	Differential diagnosis
Fever	Sepsis, infection
Respiratory distress/ cyanosis	Infection (sepsis, pneumonia), congenital heart disease, respiratory tract anomalies, GI anomalies (tracheomalacia, choanal atresia, tracheoesophageal fistula), dehydration, hypoglycemia
Lethargy	Sepsis, dehydration, endocrine/metabolic disorders (hypoglycemia, IEM)
Crying	Infection, GI, cardiac, mechanical (hair tourniquet, corneal abrasion), trauma
Jaundice	Physiological change, jaundice of the newborn, hematologic disorders (hemolysis), infection (sepsis), dehydration
Vomiting	GI disorders (malrotation, NEC, pyloric stenosis), infection (sepsis), endocrine/ metabolic disorder (congenital adrenal hyperplasia)
GI bleeding	GI disorders (NEC, malrotation), hematologic disorders (hemorrhagic disease of the newborn)
Abdominal distension	Hirshsprung's disease, NEC, malrotation
Seizures	Infection (herpes encephalitis), endocrine/ electrolyte disorders (hypoglycemia, hypocalcemia), IEM, trauma, toxins, congenital neurologic or neurocutaneous syndromes
Shock	Sepsis, congenital adrenal hyperplasia, congenital heart disease, IEM, GI emergencies

IEM, inborn errors of metabolism; NEC, necrotizing enterocolitis.

Box 157.1. Management of shock

Initial stabilization

ABCs plus disability (and blood glucose).

Laboratory testing

- Arterial or venous blood gases.
- CBC.
- Electrolytes and anion gap.
- Blood and urine cultures.
- Lactate, ammonia, LFTs.
- Chest radiograph.
- CSF on stable infant testing for glucose, protein, cell counts, culture, Gram stain and HSV PCR.

Treatment

- Broad-spectrum antimicrobials
  - ampicillin
  - cefotaxime
  - gentamicin
  - acyclovir
  - other therapy
  - consider prostaglandin E_1 IV if a congenital heart lesion is suspected
  - consider steroids if congenital adrenal hyperplasia is suspected.

Early stabilization should include broad-spectrum antibiotics as well as acyclovir. If a congenital heart lesion is suspected (cyanosis, murmur, congestive heart failure, decreased femoral pulses), prostaglandin E_1 (prostacyclin) should be administered with the awareness that it can cause apnea requiring intubation.

If profound acidosis, hypoglycemia, hyperammonemia, or encephalopathy are detected, an inborn error of metabolism should be suspected (Ch. 168). Congenital adrenal hyperplasia will also present as shock – classically in a virilized female or male at ~2 weeks of age (discussed later in this chapter). Steroids should be given simultaneously with fluid resuscitation. Catastrophic intra-abdominal disease should present with some antecedent history of nausea, vomiting, or abdominal distension in addition to shock. Acidosis and shock should be corrected while surgical consults are being arranged.

B Infectious emergencies

J. Grace Park

The most common neonatal emergency is infection. Systemic bacterial infection occurs in 1–5/1000 neonates. The mortality rate can reach 15%. Infections are typically characterized as early or late onset. Early-onset disease usually occurs <7 days after birth and is characterized by non-specific symptoms or respiratory distress. Late-onset disease occurs at 7–30 days of life and can have a focal presentation. Infection is usually acquired perinatally and then spread hematogenously from the primary site of infection throughout the body. Neonates with infection may present in septic shock, respiratory failure, seizure, and altered mental status, or they may manifest initially with non-specific symptoms and signs, such as fever, temperature instability, feeding difficulties, or jaundice.

Since neonates have an immature immune system, limited interaction and communication skills, and recent exposure to maternal genital tract bacteria, any neonate presenting with a fever (>38.4°C), lethargy, irritability, or "not acting right" should have a full septic workup including CBC with differential, blood culture, CRP, urine analysis, urine culture, CSF glucose, protein, WBC, Gram stain, and culture. The infant should be admitted to hospital and started on broad-spectrum antibiotic therapy pending culture results. Of note, a neonate diagnosed with a localized infection such as otitis media, urinary tract infection, or cellulitis should still be admitted with a full workup and systemic antibiotics given the possibility of hemotogenous spread of a local infection. Box 157.2 outlines the empirical treatment for neonatal infection.

Box 157.2. Empiric treatment for neonatal infection

- Sepsis/meningitis: ampicillin, gentamicin or cefotaxime; acyclovir.
- *Chlamydia* or *B. pertussis* pneumonia:
  - erythromycin (40 mg/kg per day in three to four divided doses) or
  - azithromycin (10 mg/kg as a singe dose on day 1, followed by 5 mg/kg per day as a single dose on days 2 to 5).

Pathogens

Escherichia coli and group B streptococci are the most common causes of infection during the neonatal period. Group B streptococcal infection is most likely acquired perinatally and can manifest up to 3 months after birth. Other bacterial pathogens in newborns and infants include *Listeria* sp., *Streptococcus pneumoniae,* and *Haemophilus influenzae* serotype b. Typical antibiotic coverage includes IV ampicillin and gentamicin or cefotaxime. In the USA, fulminant herpes infection presenting with symptoms of septic shock and liver dysfunction is as common as group B streptococcal infection. Neonates presenting with fulminant sepsis within the first week of life should be empirically treated with acyclovir in addition to antibacterials pending culture results.

Meningitis

Neonates with meningitis usually do not exhibit neck rigidity or other signs of meningeal irritability; symptoms can be completely non-focal with fussiness and poor feeding. Any neonate with possible infection must have CNS infection ruled out. A neonate with a seizure must have a workup for HSV encephalitis and be presumptively treated with acyclovir.

Pneumonia

A chest radiograph should be obtained if an infant has any respiratory symptoms. The most common causes of bacterial pneumonia in neonates are group B streptococci and Gram-negative bacilli. *Bordetella pertussis* is worth mentioning because the fatality rate for infants is approximately 1%. Pertussis may cause paroxysms of cough accompanied by cyanosis and vomiting in an otherwise well-appearing infant. Neonates do not exhibit the characteristic whoop, and careful history is necessary to make the diagnosis. If pertussis is suspected, all infants <3 months old should be admitted for antibiotic therapy and monitoring. Complications include apnea, pneumonia, severe pulmonary hypertension and death. All ill contacts should also be given chemoprophylaxis.

Chlamydial pneumonia occurs after 2 weeks of age. The infection is acquired during birth from mothers with vaginal colonization of *Chlamydia* sp. The infants usually have a "staccato cough" as well as conjunctivitis in 50% of cases. Treatment for chlamydial or *B. pertussis* pneumonia is given in Box 157.2. Inability to eat, respiratory distress, and hypoxemia are criteria for hospitalization. Outpatients should be seen daily until symptoms resolve.

Common viral causes of pneumonia or bronchiolitis in otherwise well infants include respiratory syncytial virus, adenovirus, and parainfluenza virus. Young infants with early respiratory syncytial virus infection can present with apnea. Risk factors for apnea and the course of disease are not well understood. We recommend admission, workup for other causes of apnea (such as meningitis, head trauma), and monitoring.

Table 157.2. Spectrum of neonatal herpes simplex virus infection

Disease spectrum	Disseminated herpes	Localized HSV infection	Encephalitis
Time of onset	3–7 days	7–14 days	14–21 days
Clinical symptoms	Shock, liver failure	Vesicles skin, eye, mouth	Fever, lethargy, seizures
Mortality and morbidity	Mortality 57%; 20% of survivors with developmental delay	Mortality 0%	Mortality 15%; 60% of survivors with developmental delay

HSV, herpes simplex virus.

Pearls and pitfalls: infections

Pearls

1. Infection is the number one cause of neonatal emergencies; the neonate should be admitted and treated for infection while undertaking workup and considering other diagnoses.
2. Consider HSV infection in neonates with early-onset sepsis or with seizure and fever.
3. Congenital adrenal hyperplasia can present as shock in a male or virilized female.

Pitfalls

1. Failure to remember that localized infection in a neonate can be a cause or consequence of blood-borne spread of infection.
2. Failure to check a blood sugar in a lethargic neonate.
3. Failure to consider congenital causes of disease in the neonate.

Neonatal herpes infection

Infection with HSV in most often acquired perinatally from mothers who are not aware of acute primary infection. Infection can take on three forms: disseminated herpes (25%), CNS disease with or without skin lesions (30%), or limited skin-eyes-mouth (SEM) involvement (45%) (Table 157.2). Disseminated herpes manifests as systemic shock with liver failure usually in the first week of life. While skin lesions are typical (individual, grouped, or disseminated vesicles that eventually develop a crust and ulcerate), skin lesions are not seen in 20% of disseminated neonatal HSV. After 1–2 weeks of age, infants can present with localized vesicles classic of herpetic lesions particularly on the skin, eyes and mouth (SEM disease). If treated promptly, localized disease has no mortality; if not noticed, it can spread systemically. Herpes encephalitis presents at 2–3 weeks of age, often with a fever, lethargy, irritability, and/or seizures. Skin lesions are not seen in 30–40% of neonatal CNS disease.

All neonatal HSV disease should be treated with IV acyclovir 60 mg/kg daily divided q. 8 h; disseminated and CNS herpes should be treated for 21 days and SEM disease for 14 days. Any neonate presenting with fulminant sepsis or seizure within the first month of life should be treated with IV acyclovir and worked up for HSV encephalitis.

Conclusions

Neonates are at increased risk for infection, have decreased ability to fight infection, manifest limited signs and symptoms in response to infection, and have a high risk of morbidity and mortality. Any fever or localized infection warrants a full workup to exclude sepsis, including lumbar puncture, and hospitalization for empiric antibiotics pending culture results.

C Respiratory and cardiovascular emergencies

J. Grace Park

Congenital malformations responsible for respiratory distress in newborns include choanal atresia, tracheomalacia, tracheoesophageal fistula, and vascular rings. While these anomalies are often identified in the newborn nursery, these diagnoses should be considered in any infant with respiratory distress. For example, H-type tracheoesophageal fistula may present with recurrent pneumonia and respiratory distress after feedings.

Respiratory distress with stridor in neonates suggests congenital anomalies in the larynx and trachea such as webs, cysts, atresia, stenosis, clefts, or hemangiomas. Stridor worsening with crying, feeding, or increased activity suggests laryngomalacia or subglottic hemangioma. The latter should be strongly considered if the infant has hemangiomas noted in the "beard" distribution, as this portends a higher risk of an associated airway leision. (Lack of skin hemangioma however does not rule out airway hemangioma.) Laryngomalacia is the most common cause of stridor in the neonate. Stridor and feeding difficulties suggest vascular ring, laryngeal cleft, or tracheoesophageal fistula. Stridor with hoarseness or weak cry suggests unilateral or bilateral vocal cord paralysis. Be cautious in diagnosing a neonate with croup as other congenital diagnoses should be considered. Bilateral choanal atresia manifests with cyanosis while feeding and resolved with crying.

Other conditions to consider in infants with respiratory difficulty are neuromuscular disease associated with shallow breathing and compensatory increased respiratory rate. Possible neuromuscular disorders associated with respiratory difficulty include spinal cord lesions such as myelomeningocele, and peripheral nerve diseases such as Erb's palsy (secondary to macrosomia and phrenic nerve compromise), myasthenia gravis, metabolic disorders, myotonic dystrophy, and infantile botulism.

Cardiac problems can also cause respiratory distress (Ch. 14).

Diagnostic studies

Chest radiograph and CBC are warranted in a neonate with respiratory distress. A simple test to try to differentiate pulmonary from cardiac causes of respiratory distress is the hyperoxia oxygen test (p. 74).

Pearls and pitfalls: respiratory and cardiovascular emergencies

Pearls

1. In suspected ductal-dependent congenital heart disease, give prostaglandin E_1 in addition to antibiotics.
2. Consider congenital anomalies in a child who develops respiratory distress with feeding
3. Consider bilateral choanal atresia in a neonate who turns cyanotic with feeds and improves with crying.

Pitfalls

1. Failure to prepare for intubation in a child receiving prostaglandin.
2. Failure to consider pertussis in a coughing neonate.

Management

Patients should be placed on supplementary oxygen and symptoms and test results should guide further workup and treatment. In suspected ductal-dependent congenital heart disease, EPs should give prostaglandin E_1 (started at 0.05–0.1 μg/kg per min and titrated according to improvement in partial pressure of oxygen), in addition to antibiotics. Since prostaglandin E_1 can cause apnea, the EP should also be prepared to intubate a neonate receiving prostaglandin E_1.

Neonates with respiratory symptoms should be admitted for prompt workup of possible congenital anomalies unless symptoms are mild and very close follow-up can be arranged. Infants with stridor can be treated with racemic epinephrine to attempt to alleviate severe symptoms and should be admitted to the hospital for further evaluation.

D Gastrointestinal emergencies

J. Grace Park

Neonatal GI emergencies include: necrotizing enterocolitis (NEC), malrotation with mid-gut volvulus, and incarcerated hernia. Incarcerated inguinal hernias and intussusception (Ch. 66) are most common after 3 months of age.

Necrotizing enterocolitis

Necrotizing enterocolitis should be considered when an infant presents with one or more symptoms including feeding intolerance, vomiting, abdominal distention, or irritability. Bloody stools accompanying feeding intolerance, abdominal distention, and shock are late signs. Necrotizing enterocolitis usually affects premature infants, but term newborns make up 5–10% of overall infants developing NEC. Up to 12% of infants with a birth weight <1500 g develop NEC. The cause of

NEC is not completely understood but appears to be multifactorial (involving infection and hypoxic–ischemic insults leading to inflammation or injury to the bowel wall; this is followed by development of intramural air, necrosis, and perforation). The progression of bowel necrosis can lead to sepsis and death. The mortality rate is up to 33% of those developing the disease.

Necrotizing enterocolitis is associated with perinatal risk factors, including small for gestational age (SGA), younger maternal age, placental abruption, respiratory distress syndrome, the use of surfactant, and late initiation of enteral feeding. In full-term infants, a history of maternal diabetes or the presence of polycythemia seems to increase the risk of NEC.

Diagnostic studies

If NEC is suspected, a plain abdominal radiograph should be obtained looking for pneumatosis intestinalis (intramural air), portal venous air, or signs of obstruction. The classic radiograph findings include pneumatosis intestinalis and hepatic portal air. Free air in the abdomen may be seen if perforation has already occurred.

Management

Management comprises symptomatic treatment, including fluid resus citation, bowel rest, gastric decompression, systemic antibiotics, and parenteral nutrition. A pediatric surgeon should be consulted or a transfer arranged to an appropriate facility after stabilization. Broad-spectrum antibiotics include ampicillin, cefotaxime, and clindamycin or metronidazole to cover Gram-positive, Gram-negative, and anaerobic organisms (Box 157.3).

Box 157.3. Treatments for gastrointestinal emergencies

Necrotizing enterocolitis

1. Symptomatic treatments: bowel rest, gastric decompression.
2. Antibiotics
   - ampicillin (see Box 157.1)
   - cefotaxime (see Box 157.1)
   - clindamycin
     <1 week old (>2 kg): 15 mg/kg daily IV/IM divided q. 8 h
     1 week to 1 month old (>2 kg): 30 mg/kg daily IV/IM divided q. 6 h
   - metronidazole
     <7 days old (>1200 g): 7.5–15 mg/kg daily PO/IV divided q. 12–24 h
     neonates >7 days old (>1200 g): 15–30 mg/kg daily PO/IV divided q. 12 h

Malrotation

1. Stabilize patient with IV fluid and electrolyte replacement
2. Place nasogastric tube.
3. Order upper GI study.
4. Consult with surgery.

Pyloric stenosis

1. Assess possible dehydration and electrolyte imbalance.
2. Stabilize patient with IV fluid and electrolyte replacement to correct hypochloremia and hypokalemia.
2. Consult with surgery for pyloromyotomy.

Hirschsprung's disease

1. Symptomatic treatment.
2. Consult with surgery.

Malrotation

The incidence of malrotation and volvulus is 1 in 500 live births; 50% are diagnosed in the first month of life. Malrotation of the bowel is a congenital condition resulting from abnormal fixation of the mesentery of the bowel. The bowel has tendency to twist, causing volvulus. Since delayed diagnosis can cause ischemia of the bowel from complete volvulus, an infant with crying and bilious vomiting should have an immediate surgical evaluation. Delayed presentation or surgical correction results in an increased morbidity and mortality.

Diagnostic studies

A "double-bubble sign" in an upright film results from partial obstruction of the duodenum causing distension of the stomach and first part of the duodenum. The diagnostic test of choice is an upper GI radiographic series or ultrasound (Ch. 73).

Management

Management is outlined in Box 157.3.

Pyloric stenosis

Projectile vomiting of undigested milk immediately after feeding (in contrast to 20–30 min later in gastroesophageal reflux) occurs in infants with pyloric stenosis. The age of onset is usually at 2 to 5 weeks. The risk factors include firstborn males and family history of pyloric stenosis. The rate of incidence is 1 in 250 births, and the male to female ratio is 4:1. These infants are usually very hungry. The vomitus does not contain bile or blood and occurs soon after feeding. Examination of these infants is ideally carried out with the infant calm with an empty stomach. Prominent gastric waves may be seen going from the left to right. A firm olive mass may be best felt in calm infants by palpating under the liver edge at the mid-epigastrium. Signs of dehydration can present.

Diagnostic studies

The abdominal ultrasound is the diagnostic test of choice (Ch. 73). A pyloric length of ≥1.4 cm with ≥0.3 cm thickness of the circular muscle seen by ultrasound is diagnostic. Alternatively, the upper GI radiographic series can be carried out to look for a "string sign" in the pyloric channel. The upper GI series can also look for gastroesophageal reflux, malrotation, and antral web.

Pearls and pitfalls: gastrointestinal emergencies

Pearls

1. Neonates should pass a stool within the first 24 h of life.
2. Obtain an upper GI radiographic series if presented with a neonate with bilious vomiting.
3. A diagnostic workup should be performed for a neonate with abdominal distension.

Pitfalls

1. Failure to consider malrotation in a neonate with vomiting.
2. Failure to check a blood glucose in any seriously ill neonate.
3. Failure to consider necrotizing enterocolitis in a full-term infant.

Management

Management is outlined in Box 157.3.

Hirschsprung disease

Hirschsprung disease (congenital aganglionic megacolon) occurs in 1 in 5000 live births, with a male to female ratio of 4:1. Up to 75–80% involves rectum and sigmoid. It is a disease caused by the absence of ganglion cells along the distal intestine. Dysmotility of the segment with the absent ganglion cells results in functional obstruction. Classically, the infant does not pass a stool during the first 48 h of life; however, infants can present with short segment disease later in life. Symptoms include abdominal distention, constipation and increased fussiness. This disease effectively causes intestinal obstruction. Patients with a possible diagnosis should be admitted to hospital for workup. Surgery should be consulted for definitive repair, as well as for management of interim obstruction, volvulus, or enterocolitis.

E Neurologic emergencies

Claire Turchi

Neonatal seizures

Seizures are the most common manifestation of CNS pathology in neonates. However, because the brain is immature, organized epileptic activity is less common than in older children and symptoms can be very subtle, with apnea, sustained eye deviation, chewing or limb bicycling motion as possible presentations of seizures. Focal clonic movements are usually associated with an underlying structural lesion.

Seizures in neonates have multiple etiologies including:

- perinatal insults: hypoxic–ischemic encephalopathy
- intracranial infection
- congenital brain malformation, including neurocutaneous disease
- metabolic disturbances, including inborn errors of metabolism (hypoglycemia, hyponatremia, and hypocalcemia; see also Ch. 44, p. 212)
- trauma.

Neonatal seizures have high associated morbidity and mortality. Rates of mental retardation and cerebral palsy are 15–45% in survivors of neonatal seizures. The prognosis depends on the cause of the seizures. All neonates with seizure should be empirically treated with acyclovir and antibiotics, have a full laboratory workup including head CT and be admitted to the hospital.

Clinical presentation

Important history in neonates presenting with seizure includes prenatal history (possible congenital infection, anoxic event), birth history (possible maternal bacterial or HSV infection, perinatal hypoxic event), and family history (history of familial neurocutaneous disease, epilepsy). History of present illness should include birth weight and feeding patterns and presence or absence of associated symptoms. A previously healthy child with a sudden onset of lethargy and vomiting can indicate an inborn error of metabolism manifesting after initiation of new formula or diet that cannot be metabolized. Incorrectly prepared formula can cause hyponatremia and subsequent seizures. A female with ambiguous genitalia or a male with increased pigmentation could be a clue to congenital adrenal hyperplasia (CAH; see below).

All vital signs should be assessed including temperature, and the ABCs should be managed aggressively. Pay attention to signs of trauma including retinal hemorrhage (non-accidental trauma), head circumference, dysmorphic features (inborn errors of metabolism, congenital infection, or anomaly), bulging fontanelle (infection). A careful neurologic examination will look for increased or decreased muscular tone (inborn errors of metabolism, congenital disease) or possible focal lesions. Skin examination should include presence or absence of café au lait spots (neurofibromatosis), ash leaf spots (tuberous sclerosis), hemangiomata, or vesicles (neonatal herpes).

Diagnostic studies

Laboratory analyses should include rapid glucose, electrolytes including calcium, and CBC. A head CT should be obtained and a lumbar puncture for CSF evaluation.

Diagnosis and management

Management of the acute seizure is paramount (Box 157.4). Check a bedside glucose while first-line antiepileptics (benzodiazepine) are administered. Phenobarbital is the antiepileptic of choice in neonates.

Neonates with seizure should be evaluated by neurology and admitted to the hospital for further workup (electroencephalography or MRI), metabolic screens in some cases, observation and treatment.

Box 157.4. Treatment for neonatal seizures

1. Check a bedside glucose while first-line antiepileptics (benzodiazepines) are administered.
2. If hypoglycemia: dextrose 10% 8–10 ml IV push.
3. First-line therapy
   - lorazepam[a] 0.1 mg/kg IV or
   - diazepam[a] 0.2 mg/kg IV/0.5 mg/kg per rectum or
   - midazolam[a] 0.2 mg/kg IM.
4. Continued seizure
   - phenobarbital[a] 20 mg/kg IV
   - phenytoin 20 mg/kg IV.
5. Intractable seizures: consider pyridoxine 50–100 mg IV or IM in possible pyridoxine deficiency.

Note: Phenobarbital is the antiepileptic of choice in neonates.
[a]Anticipate respiratory depression and need for airway management.

Pearls and pitfalls: neurologic emergencies

Pearls

1. Hypocalcemia and hyponatremia are not uncommon causes of seizures in the neonate.
2. Consider pyridoxine in neonatal seizures recalcitrant to traditional treatment.

Pitfalls

1. Failure to consider and treat for neonatal herpes infection in a neonate with seizure.
2. Failure to check a bedside sugar in any seriously ill neonate.

F Endocrine emergencies

Nikta Forghani and Darrell M. Wilson

Neonatal endocrine emergencies are rare and can often be mistaken for more common disease processes such as sepsis. While these disease states are treated in an emergency similarly to adults, the EP who sees children and adults must maintain a high degree of suspicion to diagnose these disorders in neonates. This part of the chapter covers congenital adrenal hyperplasia, neonatal Graves' disease and hyperinsulinism.

Congenital adrenal hyperplasia

Congenital adrenal hyperplasia is the most common cause of primary adrenal insufficiency in neonates. Enzymatic defects in the steroid pathway lead to cortisol deficiency and variable effects on mineralocorticoid production (Fig. 44.1). Because of the implementation of newborn screening for CAH in many US states, most newborns with this disorder are now identified prior to the development of a clinical adrenal crisis. However, some infants will still present in salt-losing adrenal crisis.

Salt-losing adrenal crisis

More than 90% of CAH results from a deficiency of 21-hydroxylase, which prevents the conversion of 17-hydroxyprogesterone to 11-deoxycortisol. This is a critical step in the glucocorticoid pathway and, therefore, patients with a complete defect will be cortisol deficient. 21-Hydroxylase also catalyzes the conversion of progesterone to 11-deoxycorticosterone, a precursor to aldosterone, leading to impaired mineralocorticoid action. Patients with salt-losing CAH have both mineralocorticoid and glucocorticoid deficiency. Female infants with CAH usually have some virilization, often genital ambiguity, as cortisol deficiency leads to ACTH hypersecretion and adrenal stimulation, resulting in an accumulation of androgens. Male infants only have subtle signs of ACTH hypersecretion or androgen excess (hyperpigmentation or mild enlargement of genitalia, respectively) and the diagnosis is often missed until they present in adrenal crisis.

Fetal fluids and electrolytes are maintained by the placenta and mother's kidneys. Therefore, infants with salt loss present in adrenal crisis between the first and second week of life. Impaired aldosterone action leads to hyponatremia, hyperkalemia, and acidosis, eventually resulting in cardiovascular collapse and shock. In addition, since the infant is also cortisol deficient, they are unable to mount an appropriate stress response to the hypotension, leading to further collapse. Hypoglycemia is also often a concurrent finding.

Given the possible devastation of a delay in diagnosis, it is important to consider this diagnosis in any infant being evaluated for more common causes of shock, such as sepsis or dehydration, as infants with CAH will present with similar symptoms, including vomiting and lethargy.

Diagnostic studies

If an infant presents with either known or suspected CAH in adrenal crisis, obtaining electrolytes and a blood glucose is the most critical part of the evaluation. Ideally, point of care testing with electrolytes and blood sugar can quickly elucidate how critically ill the child is.

The diagnosis can be confirmed by measuring serum 17-hydroxyprogesterone, other androgens, aldosterone, cortisol, and plasma renin activity. However, since acute therapeutic management is so critical, saving and freezing 5 ml of serum in a red top tube can allow the diagnostic workup to be postponed until there is time to consult with a pediatric endocrinologist. Once corticosteroids or mineralocorticoid steroids have been started, they will interfere with the diagnostic workup, which is why obtaining an extra tube of serum is vital in these situations. If a patient is less critically ill and the practitioner has time to do an evaluation, ideally an ACTH stimulation test (Box 157.5) should be carried out to evaluate the response of the adrenal cortex to pharmacologic levels of ACTH.

Box 157.5. ACTH stimulation test

1. Administer 36 μg/kg (max. 250 μg) synthetic ACTH (Cortrosyn) IV/IM.
2. Draw a blood sample at baseline and at 30 min post-stimulation to measure cortisol, 17-hydroxyprogesterone, and other androgens.

Box 157.6. Suggested dosing for steroid replacement in congenital adrenal hyperplasia

1. Hydrocortisone:
   - infants and toddlers, 25 mg IV
   - small children, 50 mg IV
   - adolescents/adults, 100 mg IV.

   After the initial IV bolus, a stress dose of 100–150 mg/m^2 daily divided q. 6 h should be sufficient but can be re-evaluated after the initial presentation.
2. Mineralocorticoid:
   - fludrocortisone 0.1–0.2 mg orally then dosed twice a day.
3. If the patient is hyperkalemic or with ECG changes, it may be necessary to use insulin and glucose or a sodium–potassium exchange resin such as Kayexalate.

Management

Acute management initially includes fluid replacement. A 20-ml/kg normal saline bolus will not only aid in volume repletion but will also treat hyponatremia. Dextrose IV may also be necessary. After the initial bolus, IV fluids should be continued with dextrose containing 0.9% normal saline without potassium (D5NS). Adrenal insufficiency should be treated with parenteral glucocorticoids (Box 157.6). Although there are many options for glucocorticoid replacement, hydrocortisone is preferred (over prednisone or dexamethasone) as it is a more physiologic replacement of cortisol and also has cross-over mineralocorticoid activity, which can be helpful acutely. Body surface area is generally used to calculate adrenal replacement doses, but in an acute situation, doses in Box 157.6 are suggested.

Mineralocorticoid replacement is often necessary acutely (Box 157.6). If the patient is hyperkalemic, this should be treated. Any patient with suspected salt-losing adrenal crisis should be admitted; an infant with a new diagnosis of CAH should be admitted for stabilization and parental education unless completely stable.

Hypoglycemia

Although not all causes of neonatal hypoglycemia are related to endocrine deficiencies, it is certainly useful to assess hypoglycemia from an algorithmic standpoint in order to systematically exclude certain etiologies.

Pearls and pitfalls: congenital adrenal hyperplasia

Pearls

1. Consider congenital adrenal hyperplasia in any infant 1–2 weeks of age with vomiting, lethargy and shock.
2. Female infants will often be virilized.
3. Hydrocortisone should be used for glucocorticoid replacement.

Pitfalls

1. Failure to save a red top tube for diagnostics.
2. Failure to give bolus steroids if there is clinical suspicion of congenital adrenal hyperplasia.

1. Decreased availability of glucose
   - decreased intake: fasting, oro-motor dysfunction, illness
   - decreased absorption: acute diarrhea
   - inadequate glycogen reserves: prematurity, SGA, perinatal stress, defects in enzymes of glycogen synthetic pathways
   - ineffective glycogenolysis: defects in enzymes of glycogenolytic pathways
   - inability to mobilize glycogen: glucagon deficiency
   - ineffective gluconeogenesis: defects in enzymes of gluconeogenic pathway.
2. Increased use of glucose
   - hyperinsulinism: infant of diabetic mother, SGA, congenital hyperinsulinism
3. Diminished availability of alternative fuels
   - decreased or absent fat stores: prematurity, SGA
   - inability to oxidize fats: enzymatic defects in fatty acid oxidation
4. Complex mechanisms
   - sepsis/shock
   - adrenal insufficiency
   - growth hormone deficiency
   - hypopituitarism.

Hypoglycemia is defined as serum glucose <50 mg/dl in neonates and children.

Pathophysiology

In neonates and children, most problems with hypoglycemia are related to adaptation to the fasting state. In this state, a careful balance is maintained through multiple hormones and their effects on the body's own ability to maintain blood sugar through gluconeogenesis and glycogenolysis. In neonates and children, in comparison to adults, glucose homeostasis is limited not only because there are smaller stores of liver glycogen and muscle protein but also because there are large demands for glucose consumption for the larger brain in relation to body mass. The brain preferentially uses glucose as its energy substrate, although it can also use ketones (acetoacetate and β-hydroxybutyrate), which are released by the liver as the end products of fatty acid oxidation. Therefore, lipolysis, the release of fatty acids, and eventual production of ketone bodies by the liver is another important mechanism for adaptation to the fasting state.

Insulin and the counter-regulatory hormones (cortisol, growth hormone, glucagon, and epinephrine) serve to control the above processes. In a fasting state, insulin levels should be suppressed as it serves to inhibit all of the above mechanisms. If insulin levels remain high (as in hyperinsulinism), the child will have very little defense against a fasting state and will present early after starting to fast with symptoms of hypoglycemia. These patients will present early in the neonatal period as they will not be able to tolerate even a few hours without exogenous glucose. Also, as insulin suppresses lipolysis, they will not be ketotic.

Transient neonatal hypoglycemia

Neonates are particularly susceptible to hypoglycemia because of their immature or impaired fasting systems. Up to 10% of normal neonates with appropriate size for gestational age can develop severe hypoglycemia (glucose <30 mg/dl) when the first feeding is delayed for 6 h after birth. Premature, SGA, or ill neonates are even more prone to hypoglycemia as their metabolic demands may be high and their ability to overcome periods of fasting is diminished. In addition, infants with significant perinatal stress (birth asphyxia, intrauterine growth retardation, sepsis) can develop stress-induced hyperinsulinism, which can be persistent for weeks to months. Impaired adrenal function caused by sepsis is also a well-recognized mechanism for hypoglycemia in an ill infant.

Infants of diabetic mothers are also susceptible to a transient hyperinsulinism as a result of prenatal hyperglycemia. Often these infants exhibit an abnormally vigorous insulin response to glucose, reflective of intrauterine maintenance of hyperglycemia. Clinically, these infants are macrosomic and plethoric. The hypoglycemia usually presents in the first few hours of life and only persists for a few days, although in severe cases, it may need to be treated for a few weeks.

Hyperinsulinism

Intrinsic mutations of the islet cell can lead to insulin overproduction. Distinguishing features include profound hypoglycemia despite frequent feeding, high glucose needs (>10 mg/kg per min), and macrosomia. If hyperinsulinism is suspected, the infant should be very closely monitored and endocrinology should be consulted to direct diagnostic and therapeutic management after initial glucose stabilization.

Laboratory studies

The laboratory evaluation for these patients is reflective of the pathophysiologic mechanisms for development of hypoglycemia. If possible, a blood sample (5 ml in a red top tube) should be drawn and refrigerated before treatment is initiated. The components of the critical sample are listed in Box 157.7. In addition, the first voided urine after the episode should be quickly evaluated for ketones, as the presence or absence of ketones is a critical factor in the diagnostic workup. The urine should also be sent to the laboratory for toxicologic evaluation and organic acids.

Management

Initial treatment for hypoglycemia involves using a rapid bolus of dextrose (2.5–5 ml/kg 10% dextrose or 1–2 ml/kg 25% dextrose). An infusion of 10% dextrose should then be initiated at a rate of 8–10 mg/kg per min to maintain the blood sugar above 70 mg/dl. If a glucose infusion rate >12 mg/kg per min is required, there should be increased suspicion for hyperinsulinism. We generally do not recommend use of glucocorticoids in acute hypoglycemia as the effects on blood sugar can be delayed, unless the patient has underlying adrenal insufficiency.

Box 157.7. Blood sample for acute hypoglycemia

Primary sample

- Serum blood glucose.
- Insulin.
- Cortisol.
- Growth hormone.
- Free fatty acids.
- Urine ketones, serum ketones (acetoacetate, β-hydroxybutyrate).

Secondary sample

- Lactate.
- Pyruvate.
- Ammonia.
- Acylcarnitine profile.
- Serum amino acids.
- Urine organic acids.
- Urine toxicology screen.

Pearls and pitfalls: hypoglycemia

Pearls

1. Hypoglycemia in a neonate is glucose <50 mg/dl.
2. The etiology of hypoglycemia in a neonate is based on presence or absence of acidosis and ketones.

Pitfalls

1. Failure to promptly treat hypoglycemia in the neonate.
2. Failure to draw 5 ml blood into a red top tube for later workup of hypoglycemia.
3. Failure to send first voided urine for ketones, toxicology, and organic acids.

Graves' disease

Pathophysiology

Although neonatal Graves' disease is a very rare disorder, if untreated, it can lead to lifelong mental retardation and can even be life threatening. Its incidence is estimated at 1:25 000 neonates. Transplacental transfer of thyrotropin receptor-stimulating antibodies stimulates the fetus' thyroid gland. It is important to remember that even mothers who have had thyroidectomies or radioactive iodine in the past for treatment of their Graves' disease will have antibodies, which can lead to neonatal disease. Since the condition relates to the presence of maternally derived antibodies, it will eventually resolve, typically by 1–3 months of life. In exceedingly rare cases, neonatal hyperthyroidism is not associated with maternal Graves' disease and is not transient.

Clinical presentation

The timing of symptoms is dependent on whether the mother is taking antithyroid medication at the time of the delivery. Since these drugs also cross the placenta, the baby can be euthyroid or even hypothyroid at the time of delivery. As the infant's antithyroid medication levels decline, they will develop hyperthyroid symptoms, generally a few days after delivery. Infants can present as late as a few weeks of life. When the mother is not taking antithyroid medication, infants can have symptoms that can be detected in utero, or at birth.

Typical clinical manifestations in neonates include tachycardia, irritability, and poor weight gain despite hyperphagia, as well as goiter. Other clinical findings specific to neonates that can be present at birth include low birth weight, prematurity, microcephaly, and frontal bossing.

Laboratory studies

The laboratory evaluation for a baby with suspected neonatal Graves' disease includes measuring blood thyroid-stimulating hormone (TSH), free or total thyroxine (T_4), and total triiodothyronine (T_3). In neonatal Graves' disease, expected results include a very low or undetectable TSH, and a high T_4 or free T_4 and T_3 values. It is important to interpret the T_4 and T_3 levels using normal neonatal values, which are higher than in older children and adults.

Management

Treatment of neonatal Graves' disease includes antithyroid medication. Methimazole inhibits the synthesis of new thyroid hormone by blocking the oxidation of iodine in the thyroid gland. The dose is 0.5–1 mg/kg per day divided TID. If the neonate is very symptomatic, iodine (Lugol's solution) is used at a dose of 1 drop PO every 8 h. High concentrations of iodine paradoxically inhibit thyroid hormone release rapidly. Significant results can be witnessed within the first few days of therapy with iodine, which can be helpful while the methimazole is starting to take effect. It is important to use Lugol's solution 2–3 h after methimazole is given to avoid providing a substrate for more thyroid hormone synthesis. Finally, if an infant is very symptomatic from a cardiovascular standpoint (tachycardia, hypertension), a beta-blocker such as propranolol can be used. Heart failure must be excluded before using beta-blockers as they are contraindicated in this situation. Infants with symptomatic neonatal Graves' disease should be hospitalized and closely monitored initially. Once the symptoms abate after the initiation of treatment, they can be treated as outpatients with very close follow-up to avoid overtreatment and hypothyroidism.

Acknowledgements

The authors of this chapter would like to thank Vlad Ianus, MD for his input.

Pearls and pitfalls: Graves' disease

Pearls

1. Any mother with current or a history of Graves' disease is susceptible for having a child with neonatal Graves' disease.
2. Neonates with Graves' disease can be symptomatic at birth, but can also present after 2 weeks of life depending on maternal factors.

Selected references

Aspelund G, Langer JC. Current management of hypertrophic pyloric stenosis. *Semin Pediatr Surg* 2007;**16**:27–33.

Buckingham B. The hyperthyroid fetus and infant. *NeoReviews* 2000;**1**:103–109.

de Lorijn F, Boeckxstaens GE, Benninga MA. Symptomatology, pathophysiology, diagnostic work-up, and treatment of Hirschsprung disease in infancy and childhood. *Curr Gastroenterol Rep* 2007;**9**:245–253.

Escobedo M. Moving from experience to evidence: changes in US Neonatal Resuscitation Program based on International Liaison Committee on Resuscitation Review. *J Perinatol* 2008;**28**(Suppl. 1): S35–S40.

Fleisher G. *Endocrine Emergencies. Textbook of Pediatric Emergency Medicine.* Philadelphia, PA: Lippincott Williams & Wilkins, 2005.

Hsu SC. Perinatal calcium metabolism: physiology and pathophysiology. *Semin Neonatol* 2004;**9**:23–36.

Kahler S. Metabolic disorders associated with neonatal hypoglycemia. *NeoReviews* 2004;**5**:e377–e381.

Levine L. Congenital adrenal hyperplasia. *Pediatr Rev* 2000;**21**:159–171.

Pollack ES. Pediatric abdominal surgical emergencies. *Pediatr Ann* 1996;**25**:448–457.

Schulman D. Adrenal insufficiency: still a cause of morbidity and death in childhood. *Pediatrics* 2007;**119**:e484–e494.

Singh J. The investigation of hypocalcemia and rickets. *Arch Dis Childhood* 2003;**88**:403–407.

Sperling M. *Pediatric Endocrinology*, Philadelphia, PA: Saunders, 2008.

Styne D. *Pediatric Endocrinology*. Philadelphia, PA: Lippincott Williams & Wilkins, 2004.

Srinivasan PS, Brandler MD, D'Souza A. Necrotizing enterocolitis. *Clin Perinatol* 2008;**35**:251–272.

Section

27

Special populations: adolescents

Chapter

158 The approach to the adolescent patient

Sophia Yen and Stephanie Cooper

Introduction

The top three causes of mortality in adolescents are injuries (often related to substance abuse), homicide, and suicide. The HEADSS (home, education, activity, drugs, sex, suicide) assessment was developed to investigate the psychosocial history of the adolescent to prevent morbidity and mortality (Box 158.1). Approximately 75% of adolescents present themselves each year to the medical system. However, many of those visits may be to the ED or urgent care department. Therefore, a HEADSS assessment should be carried out on each adolescent every time they present to the medical system. This assessment can help to guide their clinical management. For example, knowing that a teenager has oral sex ensures that the EP will check for gonorrhea when they present with a sore throat. Similarly the differential diagnosis of abdominal pain might be broadened to include pelvic inflammatory disease, overdose, or abuse if concerns were elicited during the HEADSS assessment.

Performing the HEADSS screen

The HEADSS assessment is best carried out with the parent/guardian out of the room.

The home and education sections can be carried out with the parent present. Performing the "parent-ectomy," or removing the parents from the room, can be a bit tricky. When asking the parent to leave to discuss confidential matters with an adolescent, tell the parent "Your son/daughter is growing up. They might end up in the ER without you and they need to be able to interact with physicians without you. So, what we are going to talk about is confidential. However, if your son/daughter tells me they are hurting themselves, someone is hurting them, or they are going to hurt someone, I will *definitely* tell you." By stating these ground rules up front if the adolescent later says they are acutely suicidal, homicidal, or being sexually or physically abused, you have already established reasons to break confidentiality.

An important part of the HEADSS assessment is making the adolescent think through who they would talk to if they were upset, sad, depressed, suicidal, or in need of anything in an emergency situation (Box 158.1). If they choose you as their person to talk to, refer them to the social worker because they need more options than an EP. Do not accept boyfriend/girlfriend as the only answer, as that is the person who is most

Box 158.1. The HEADSS (home, education, activity, drugs, sex, suicide) assessment

Home. Who lives with you? How many siblings do you have? Do you live with mom during the weekdays, dad on weekends? What city or part of town do you live in?

Education. Where do you go to school? What grade are you in? How do your grades compare this year to last year? What are your goals after you graduate college?

Activities/abuse. What do you like to do for fun? Do you have a small group of friends, a large group of friends? Male or females or mixed? Do you have a best friend? Do you have access to a gun? Have you ever been arrested? Are you safe? Has anyone ever hit you, kicked you? Has anyone touched you sexually in a way you didn't want?

Drugs. Do you smoke cigarettes? Do you smoke marijuana? Drink alcohol? Do Ectasy? Heroin? Crack? Meth? If you get all "no"s, ask if they have friends that use these substances and how they react when offered.

Sex. Are you interested in men, women or both? Have you had oral, vaginal, or anal sex? Some, none, or all? What percentage of the time do you use condoms 0%, 30%, 70%? If they respond, 100%, ask "Has the condom ever popped, slipped off? For some people the penis goes in/out and then condom on before ejaculation. Do you ever do that?" What types of birth control have you tried? Do you know about emergency contraception? What is it? How does it work? Where can you get it? How soon do you take it?

Suicide. Have you ever thought of hurting yourself or killing yourself? Have you ever cut yourself on purpose? Who would you talk to if you were sad? Your family, a teacher, a religious counselor, a doctor?

A Practical Guide to Pediatric Emergency Medicine: Caring for Children in the Emergency Department, ed. N. Ewen Amieva-Wang (associate eds. Jamie Shandro, Aparajita Sohoni, and Bernhard Fassl). Published by Cambridge University Press.

likely to have conflict with the adolescent and possibly trigger suicidal ideation. It is important to identify another person as their back-up confidante.

Clinical tips

Use the HEADSS screen on all adolescents presenting to the ED, regardless of their chief complaint. Give the patient multiple choice questions to speed up the interview if needed. For example, instead of asking, "What percentage of the time do you use condoms?" ask, "What percentage of the time do you use condoms: 0%, 10%, 30%?" Never give 100% as an answer choice. If they answer 100% on their own, see Box 158.1 for further questions to clarify their use of protection during sexual intercourse. Treat the ED visit as an opportunity to screen for health and behavior risks and potentially offer safer alternatives or interventions as needed, thus preventing a myriad of serious issues, such as unplanned pregnancies, sexually transmitted infections, and self-harm.

Pearls and pitfalls

Pearls

1. Take time to interview the adolescent without parents present.
2. Use the HEADSS screen (home, education, activity, drugs, sex, suicide) for all adolescents presenting to the ED.
3. Avoid open-ended questions; however, giving options when asking questions will make the interview go more quickly if time is limited.

Pitfalls

1. Failure to deal openly with adolescent patients. Do not promise absolute confidentiality; be up front about the need to report if they are hurting themselves, someone is hurting them, or they are going to hurt someone else.
2. Accepting the EP as the sole confidante for an adolescent patient. A social worker should be involved to help the patient to find other, more consistent sources of support within their community.

Chapter 159

Medicolegal considerations

Rebecca Gudeman and Sophia Yen

Introduction

This chapter will cover the following questions:

- What services can adolescents receive without parental consent?
- Who may consent for a patient's care when neither parent is available?
- When may providers share healthcare information with a parent?
- What are the EP's obligations to adolescent patients under the Health Insurance Portability and Accountability Act 1996 (HIPPA)?

The AAP has a number of policy recommendations that are relevant to ED clinicians treating children (Box 159.1).

Consent

With rare exception, healthcare providers must have valid informed consent from the patient or the patient's legal representative before they provide any medical service. True emergencies are one of the rare exceptions to this rule; however, many of the health complaints that pass through the ED do not qualify as true emergencies and healthcare providers must get consent before providing treatment. Even in true emergencies, however, law and ethics demand that practitioners attempt to get consent before providing treatment whenever possible.

The EP must understand who may consent for a minor's health care in the range of situations they may see. In most cases, when a patient is a minor (under 18 years old in most states), a parent or legal guardian must consent for care on the minor's behalf. Because most children arrive at the ED accompanied by a parent or legal guardian, obtaining the appropriate consent is usually not a barrier to providing care.

In some cases, however, the minor's consent is necessary to provide treatment. In others, parental consent is necessary but the minor arrives in the ED unaccompanied.

Box 159.1. Challenging cases

A teenager presents with abdominal pain, without the parent

Do you need parental permission to see the patient in the USA?

That depends on whether there is concern for a sexually transmitted disease (STD). If the chief complaint is "I think I might have an STD or pelvic inflammatory disease," then start the encounter as a confidential minor consent case. But if it is vague, "I have pain," then tell the patient that you need parental consent to diagnose the problem. If it is a possible emergency situation (e.g., ectopic pregnancy, ovarian torsion, testicular torsion) then perform the evaluation under the emergency clause.

A parent brings teenager in for drug testing

The US state law often requires minor consent for such tests. In all cases, discuss the concept of patient assent. The standard clinician response here is "We don't test people against their will. If you aren't looking for a specific drug, then what will you do if the test comes back negative, because the test can only catch things within a certain window and it doesn't test everything? Will that be enough to allay your fears? If you think that your son/daughter is doing drugs, then the key is communication and trust." And then refer the family to psychological care and/or social work.

A minor must be admitted for pelvic inflammatory disease or ectopic pregnancy

The parents want to know why the minor needs hospitalization and the minor the does not authorize the EP to explain the underlying condition.

In such a case, tell the minor "I will never lie for you. So, we can tell your parents that you are here for an infection in your abdomen or we can tell them about the pelvic inflammatory disease. I would prefer to tell them about PID, because if they start asking questions, then I will have to say 'Your daughter has rights to confidential care for pregnancy, STDs, mental health. I need her permission to discuss this further.' And then you will have to face your parents alone. Or we can tell them together now or I can tell them without you with your permission."

A Practical Guide to Pediatric Emergency Medicine: Caring for Children in the Emergency Department, ed. N. Ewen Amieva-Wang (associate eds. Jamie Shandro, Aparajita Sohoni, and Bernhard Fassl). Published by Cambridge University Press.

Minor consent

In every US state, minors may consent to certain healthcare on their own accord.

The great majority of states allow minors to give their own consent for the treatment of:

- sexually transmitted diseases
- alcohol and drug abuse services
- diagnosis, prevention, and treatment of pregnancy (i.e., pregnancy tests, prenatal care, and contraception).

Many states also allow minors to consent to mental healthcare and sexual assault treatment. In addition, in many states, minors who have reached certain stages in life, such as marriage, parenthood, or emancipation, may consent for their own care as if they were an adults. In most states, emancipation is a legal status granted by a court, although in many states minors are "emancipated" if they are married or in the armed forces. Each state's emancipation and minor consent laws are slightly different, and many contain age limits or preconditions. Know the specifics of your state law. Often, if state law allows minors to consent to their own care, it also allows them to refuse that care and precludes others from consenting to that care on their behalf.

Unaccompanied minors

While most minors arrive in the ED with a parent or legal guardian, some arrive on their own. Others arrive accompanied by a caretaker who does not have legal authority to consent to medical care on the minor's behalf. When minors arrive in the ED unaccompanied, the EP must identify who has the legal right to consent to the particular care the minor seeks and must attempt to get appropriate consent. If consent is not available or cannot be obtained in a reasonable period, the EP must determine whether his or her state's emergency consent exception applies or if the minor may consent under "minor consent" services.

Confidentiality

Confidentiality should be addressed with minors and their caretakers prior to interviewing the minor alone. The physician should make it clear to all parties that there are times when confidentiality will be upheld as well as times when it will be breached. Confidentiality may be breached in life-threatening emergencies, when the patient may do harm to themselves or others, or in cases of abuse.

Federal and state laws protects the confidentiality of medical information and medical records. Generally, these laws prevent the release of personal healthcare information without authorization, but most include exceptions that allow providers to release personal information without authorization in special circumstances, for example for billing purposes or to report child abuse or certain other harms. In some situations, these laws prohibit parental access to a minor's records. Personnel in the ED need to know what information they may and may not share with parents of adolescent patients.

Parental access and minor privacy

Federal HIPAA regulations establish that generally parents have a right to review and to control access to their children's medical information. However, there are two important exceptions to this rule. First, federal HIPAA regulations allow providers to refuse parental access to a minor's medical information if the provider believes providing that information to parents is not in the best interests of the minor and either the minor may be endangered or the minor may be subject to abuse if parents are given access. In addition, many states have laws that allow providers to refuse parents access to their children's medical information under similar circumstances. Know your state law on this issue.

Second, the general rule changes when parents want access to medical information about "minor consent" care. Some state laws provide that if the minor consented for his or her own care, providers cannot give parents access to the related medical information without first obtaining the minor's consent. In these cases, providers can only share personal health information with a parent if the minor patient signs a HIPAA compliant authorization. If state law does not address whether parents may access "minor consent" records, the federal HIPAA regulations state that a licensed healthcare professional has discretion to decide, in the exercise of professional judgement, whether or not to share that information with the parents.

Why confidentiality is critical

Protecting adolescent confidentiality in certain circumstances encourages teenagers to seek treatment for conditions they may want to keep private from parents. Nothing in these laws prevents teenagers from involving parents in healthcare decision making, which most adolescents do.

In situations where parental notification might deter adolescents from seeking these essential health services, states have determined that protecting the minor's confidentiality is more important than promoting parental control and family autonomy. Many provider organizations support providing adolescents with access to confidential health services such as the American Medical Association, the AAP, the American College of Physicians, and the American Public Health Association.

Making parental involvement or notification mandatory drastically reduces the likelihood that minors will seek timely treatment. In a survey of suburban adolescents, only 45% of adolescents surveyed would seek care for depression if parental notification was required, and $<20\%$ would seek care related to birth control, sexually transmitted diseases, or drug use if parental notice was mandated. A teenager, struggling with sexual health concerns or drug and alcohol abuse, may not share concerns with a parent for fear of disapproval or violence. The parent or relative may be the source or focus of the teenager's emotional or physical problems. Additionally, some

Box 159.2. Consent: policy recommendations

1. Healthcare providers for adolescents should become familiar with their state and local laws and institutional policies regarding consent and the definition of emergency.
2. Both EDs and clinics should develop practical written guidelines regarding consent. These policies should be based on the nature of the practice and local or state law.
3. When another adult is acting in place of a parent for a child (*in loco parentis*), the physician should document the situation in the medical record, including attempts to obtain verbal or written consent from a parent.
4. Barriers to effective medical care of children should be removed. No evaluation of a life-threatening or emergency condition of a child should be delayed because of a perceived problem with consent or payment authorization. Decisions regarding the emergency nature of treatment should be made on the basis of that evaluation.

Adapted from the policy of the American Academy of Pediatrics, *Consent for Medical Services for Children and Adolescents.*

Pearls and pitfalls

Pearls

1. Get parental consent when possible and appropriate.
2. The great majority of states allow minors to give their own consent for the treatment of sexually transmitted diseases, alcohol and drug abuse services and diagnosis, prevention, and treatment of pregnancy.
3. Do not promise absolute confidentiality; instead, explain circumstances in which information will be shared (abuse, self-harm, or harm to others).

Pitfalls

1. Failure to know the state laws.
2. Failure to follow state reporting laws if alerted to a case of self-harm, abuse, or harm to others.
3. Failure to provide medical care for true emergencies because of delays in obtaining consent.

teenagers wish to have their confidentiality protected because they value their privacy and autonomy.

Child abuse reporting

Child abuse reporting is an exception to confidentiality. Every state has child abuse reporting laws that mandate certain professionals to report cases of confirmed or suspected abuse and neglect to specified authorities. However, each state has different definitions of abuse and, therefore, of what must be reported. It is critical to understand what must be reported in your state in order to provide appropriate care to patients. Box 159.1 outlines a number of such challenging cases in consent and confidentiality.

Selected references

American Academy of Pediatrics. Policy Statement RE9309: consent for medical services for children and adolescents. *Pediatrics* 1993;**92**:290–291.

Baren JM. Ethical dilemmas in the care of minors in the emergency department. *Emerg Med Clin North Am* 2006;**24**:619–631.

Committee on Bioethics, American Academy of Pediatrics. Informed consent, parental permission, and assent in pediatric practice. *Pediatrics* 1995;**95**:314–317.

Jacobstein CR, Baren JM. Emergency department treatment of minors. *Emerg Med Clin North Am* 1999;**17**:341–352, x.

Marks A, Malizio J, Hoch J, *et al.* Assessment of health needs and willingness to utilize healthcare resources of adolescents in a suburban population. *J Pediatr* 1983;**102**:456–460.

Neinstein LS. Consent and confidentiality laws for minors in the western United States. *West J Med* 1987;**147**:218–224.

Extra resources on consent and confidentiality

Policy

American Academy of Pediatrics. Policy statement on consent for medical services for children and adolescents (RE9309). *Pediatrics* 1993;**92**:290–291.

State minor consent laws

Advocates for Youth. *Adolescent Access to Confidential Health Services 7/1997.* http://www.advocatesforyouth.org/PUBLICATIONS/iag/confhlth.htm#18 (accessed 5 June 2010).

Center on Adolescent Health and the Law. Chapel Hill, NC www.cahl.org (accessed 5 June 2010).

Guttmacher Institute. *Teenager's Access to Confidential Reproductive Health Services.* New York: Guttmacher Institute, 2005 http://www.guttmacher.org/pubs/tgr/08/4/gr080406.html (accessed 5 June 2010).

National Center for Youth Law. Oakland, CA. Tel (510) 835-8098 http://www.youthlaw.org/health/ (accessed 5 June 2010).

New York Civil Liberties Union. For New York. Reference Card: Minors' Rights to Reproductive Health Care in New York (2005) http://www.nyclu.org/ (accessed 5 June 2010).

Physicians for Reproductive Choice and Health. For Florida, Georgia, Illinois, Maine, Massachusetts, Missouri, New Jersey, New Mexico, Ohio, Pennsylvania. New York: Physicians for Reproductive

Choice and Health http://www.prch.org/resources/index.php?pid=120&tpid=3 (accessed 5 June 2010).

Physicians for Reproductive Choice and Health. Providing Confidential Reproductive Health Services to Minors (01/22/2008). New York: Physicians for Reproductive Choice and Health http://www.prch.org/resources/index.php?pid=119&tpid=9 (accessed 5 June 2010).

For confidentiality law

Center for Adolescent Health and the Law. Chapel Hill, NC www.cahl.org (accessed 5 June 2010).

Georgetown Health Privacy Project. Washington, DC: Georgetown Health Privacy Project http://www.healthprivacy.org/ (accessed 5 June 2010).

National Center for Youth Law. Oakland, CA. Teen Health Rights Initiative, www.teenhealthrights.org (accessed 5 June 2010).

For state child abuse reporting rules

National Center for Youth Law. Oakland, CA. Tel (510) 835–8098 http://www.youthlaw.org/health/ (accessed 5 June 2010).

Chapter 160

Emergency contraception

Sophia Yen

Introduction

Emergency contraception (EC) is an important consideration in the care of adolescent patients. Use of some EC pills has been shown to prevent ovulation and decrease the rate of unwanted pregnancy if they are taken within 120 h after unprotected intercourse or contraceptive failure.

Box 160.1. Emergency contraception options

- Plan B (levonorgestrel-only method): levonorgestrel 750 μg/pill; two pills by mouth as soon as possible after unprotected intercourse. Available in packs of two pills.
- Yuzpe method: 100 μg ethinylestradiol and 1 mg norgestrel (or 0.5 mg levonorgestrel) by mouth as soon as possible after unprotected intercourse and again 12 h after the first dose.

Indications and administration

Emergency contraception can be prescribed for any female patient who presents within 120 h of a contraceptive failure (broken condom, lapse in alternative contraception methods, sexual assault) or unprotected intercourse. The EC should be given as soon as possible after the event.

Based on the WHO recommendations, EC should be taken as 1.5 mg levonorgestrel as soon as possible after contraceptive failure or unprotected intercourse. The success is increased with decreased time interval between unprotected intercourse and medication administration. It taken within 120 h, if reduces a woman's chance of pregnancy by 60–90%.

In the USA, the EC pill called Plan B contains levonorgestrel only; the alternative regimen is called the Yuzpe method and comprises ethinylestradiol and norgestrel (or levonorgestrel) (Box 160.1). The pills in each method can be taken PO or intravaginally, although the latter is off-label.

The Yuzpe method has half the efficacy and twice the side effects of the Plan B method.

With the Yuzpe method, more frequent nausea and vomiting can occur. Premedication with antiemetics 30 min prior to each dose should be considered.

As of July 2009, Plan B is available over the counter for males or females 17 years of age and older. For those under 17, several states allow pharmacists to dispense EC without a prescription if the pharmacist signs up (Alaska, California, Hawaii, Maine, Massachusetts, New Hampshire, New Mexico, Vermont, Washington State). In these states, adolescents can call the pharmacy and ask specifically, "Do you have a pharmacist that will give out EC to a X-year-old without a prescription, right now?" (X is whatever the adolescent's age is).

Anticipatory guidance

Side effects, and their frequency, with Plan B (levonorgestrel only) include nausea (20%), dizziness (10%), and vomiting (5%). With the Yuzpe method, the side effects are the same, but the frequency is increased: nausea (50%), dizziness (17%), and vomiting (19%).

Since EC is not 100% effective, patients who would not choose to terminate a resultant pregnancy should be counseled to "act as if pregnant," meaning do as they would have done if the pregnancy were to result. This incident should be used as an opportunity to discuss long-term birth control.

Precautions

An EC pill should not be given to a woman who is known to be pregnant. However, there are no known teratogenic effects of EC. There is no evidence of a post-fertilization effect of EC pills and, in fact, evidence exists to the contrary.

Conclusions

Discuss EC with all adolescents – both male and female – and offer a prescription for future events. Regardless of the reason for their ED visit, EC information may be useful to adolescent patients in the future event of unprotected intercourse, sexual assault or contraceptive failure.

A Practical Guide to Pediatric Emergency Medicine: Caring for Children in the Emergency Department, ed. N. Ewen Amieva-Wang (associate eds. Jamie Shandro, Aparajita Sohoni, and Bernhard Fassl). Published by Cambridge University Press.

Pearls and pitfalls

Pearls

1. Emergency contraception pills can be given up to 120 h after unprotected intercourse or contraceptive failure to decrease the likelihood of unintended pregnancy.
2. Discuss long-term contraception options with patients who need emergency contraception.
3. Know the local availability of emergency contraception.

Pitfalls

1. Failure to discuss emergency contraception with male and female adolescents.
2. Using estrogen/progesterone pills for emergency contraception instead of just levonorgestrel-only emergency contraception pills.
3. Failure to discuss common side effects of emergency contraception: nausea, vomiting, and unscheduled bleeding.

Selected references

Davidoff F, Trussell J. The politics of doubt. *JAMA* 2006;**296**:1775–1778.

Task Force on Postovulatory Methods of Fertility Regulation. Randomised controlled trial of levonorgestrel versus the Yuzpe regimen of combined oral contraceptives for emergency contraception. *Lancet* 1998;**352**:428–433.

Office of Population Research, University of Princeton. States that allow minors direct access to emergency contraceptive without a prescription. http://ec.princeton.edu/questions/state-pharmacy-access-list.html (accessed 28 April 2010).

Selbst SM. Treating minors without their parents. *Pediatr Emerg Care* 1985;**1**:168–173.

Trussell J. Mechanism of action of emergency contraceptive pills. *Contraception* 2006;**74**:87–89.

World Health Organization. *WHO Fact sheet No 244: Emergency Contraceptive.* Geneva: World Health Organization http://www.who.int/mediacentre/factsheets/fs244/en/ (accessed 28 April 2010).

Chapter 161

Substance abuse

Stephanie Cooper

Introduction

The teenage years are frequently a time of experimentation and identity shifting. Influenced by their own curiosity, in tandem with other traits common to adolescence – impulsivity, invincibility, and peer pressure – many young adults use illicit substances use during their teenage years. For many teenagers, substance use is associated with "coming of age" regardless of race, culture, or socioeconomic status.

Substance use prevalence and health implications

Adolescent substance use represents an important public health challenge. In 2006, one-fifth of American adolescents aged 12 to 17 years used an illicit drug, one-third drank alcohol, and one-sixth smoked cigarettes. Adolescent substance abuse is fraught with sociocultural implications. School absenteeism is linked to drug use and recovery; in 2005, teenagers made up 8% of all admissions to publicly funded treatment facilities. Teen pregnancy, date rape, sexually transmitted infections, hazardous violent and sexual behaviors, and unintentional accidents and injuries are linked to teenage drug use. Adolescents who use illicit substances are also more prone to suicide and at risk of homicide. Clearly, teenage substance-use patterns have significant impact on individual health, psychological health, and non-intentional trauma and injuries.

Risk factors

Risk factors for teenage substance use include low self-esteem, minimal supervision of activities, fractured adult–adolescent relationship(s), same-sex orientation, and an unstable home environment. Family history of substance abuse also may contribute to a culture of accepting teen substance use.

Warning signs

Significant pattern changes in friendships and school performance may signal that a teenager is doing drugs. This may manifest as diminished interest in school activities, lower grades, and hanging out with a new crowd of friends.

Screening

All children should be screened for substance use and abuse.

The CAGE questions are often used in adults to identify alcohol problems, but other screening questions may be more age appropriate in younger patients. The CRAFFT mnemonic is one of the recommended screening tools for adolescents (Box 161.1). This tool has a high sensitivity for detecting children likely to benefit from treatment if more than two questions are answered as Yes.

General management

While a complete review of the management of each substance is beyond the scope of this chapter, the EP should be familiar

Box 161.1. The CRAFFT screening tool for problems associated with substance use in younger people

C: Have you ever ridden in a **car** driven by someone (including yourself) who was high or had been using alcohol or drugs?
R: Do you ever use alcohol or drugs to **relax**, feel better about yourself, or fit in?
A: Do you ever use alcohol or drugs while you are by yourself (**alone**)?
F: Do you ever **forget** things you do while using alcohol or drugs?
F: Do your family or **friends** ever tell you that you should cut down on your drinking or drug use?
T: Have you ever gotten into **trouble** while you were using alcohol or drugs?

A Practical Guide to Pediatric Emergency Medicine: Caring for Children in the Emergency Department, ed. N. Ewen Amieva-Wang (associate eds. Jamie Shandro, Aparajita Sohoni, and Bernhard Fassl). Published by Cambridge University Press.

with a general approach to the adolescent patient who is either using/abusing or actively intoxicated with the substances reviewed below. Whereas for some substances, such as nicotine and marijuana, information regarding cessation may be the only intervention needed, the EP should also be ready to treat adolescents actively under the influence of other substances. The general approach should consist of:

- ABCs (as always)
- Fingerstick glucose level (in any patient with a suspected toxicologic ingestion)
- ECG (to document normal intervals and normal sinus rhythm)
- aspirin and acetaminophen levels (because of the possibility to treat these potentially lethal co-ingestions).

Specifics regarding the management of a known ingestion of "recreational" drugs of abuse are briefly covered below. The management of each patient will be individual, and the EP should consult the poison control center for any case of intoxication in an adolescent patient (1-800-411-8080) (see also Ch. 138).

Abused substances

Tobacco

Prevalence

Data from the National Survey on Drug Use and Health indicates that tobacco use is widespread among American teenagers. Everyday, an estimated 4000 youth aged 12 to 17 years try their first cigarette: 50% of high school students have tried cigarette smoking, with 20% reporting current cigarette use. Prevalence of current cigarette use is higher among White and Hispanic teenagers than Black youth. Nationwide, 8% of students reported use of smokeless tobacco, and 14% had smoked cigars or cigarillos. Among high school students who were current smokers, 50% reported attempting to quit tobacco within the past year.

Health effects of tobacco use by teenagers

In all people, cigarette smoking is correlated with coronary artery disease, chronic pulmonary disease, and lung cancer. In young people, cigarette smoking greatly augments the risk of lung cancer, as the risk of pulmonary malignancy increases with pack-year exposure.

Teenagers with asthma who are active smokers experience higher rates of severe asthma and severe rhinoconjunctivitis compared with non-smoking teenagers with asthma. Compared with non-smoking adolescents with known asthma, teenagers who smoke are more likely to experience recurrent wheezing, other asthma i-associated symptoms, and recurrent eczema.

Second-hand smoke significantly threatens the pulmonary health of teenagers and children. An estimated 6 million youth are exposed to second-hand smoke daily. Second-hand smoke can trigger new cases of asthma, worsen existing cases, and cause decline in lung function.

Alcohol

Prevalence

Although alcohol consumption by people <21 years of age is illegal in the USA, people aged 12 to 20 years drink 11% of all alcohol in America. Much of this alcohol is consumed in a binge pattern (more than five drinks in one sitting). Nationwide surveys report that 75% of students aged 12 to 17 years had consumed at least one alcoholic beverage; 45% were current alcohol drinkers (at least one drink in the past month), with 26% reporting occasional binge drinking. Prevalence of current alcohol use was higher among White and Hispanic youth than Black teenagers. In 2005, almost 150 000 youth presented to EDs for alcohol-related illnesses and injuries.

Risks related to teenager alcohol use

Alcohol-related motor vehicle crashes kill approximately 17 000 Americans annually. Almost a third of deaths among youth and young adults (ages 10–24 years) are in motor vehicle crashes. Despite campaigns against drunk driving, national data reveal that 10% of high school students acknowledged driving under the influence of alcohol and 29% rode with a driver who had been drinking alcohol. Alcohol use is also linked to unintentional injuries such as falls, burns, and drowning.

Earlier age at first alcohol consumption has been linked to increased incidence of driving drunk and increased likelihood of suffering a motor vehicle crash related to excessive alcohol. In the National Youth Risk Surveillance Survey, 23% of high school students reported drinking alcohol before 13 years of age. Teenagers who begin drinking before age 15 years are five times more likely to develop alcohol dependence or abuse later in life than those who begin drinking at or after age 21.

Behavioral consequences of youth alcohol consumption include school absenteeism, poor grades, physical and sexual assault, and increased risk of suicide and homicide. Alcohol use is linked to unplanned and sometimes unprotected sexual activity.

Clinical presentation

Alcohol is a CNS depressant, causing disinhibition, decreased motor function, and impaired level of consciousness. At high concentrations, alcohol leads to autonomic dysfunction and, eventually, coma and death secondary to respiratory depression and cardiovascular collapse. Patients under the influence of alcohol may present with agitation, belligerence, garrulousness or slurred speech, drowsiness, and stupor. The EP should confirm that toxic alcohols or other agents have not been ingested (Ch. 138) and carefully monitor alcohol-intoxicated patients for worsening respiratory depression. Adolescents who are unaccustomed to binge drinking and present to the

ED acutely intoxicated should have a blood alcohol level tested; they should be hydrated and monitored closely for their ability to control their airway as well as for any signs of respiratory depression. These patients should incrementally recover over a period of hours and if not, should have a workup for other causes of ALOC.

Marijuana

Despite marijuana being an illegal substance, in the National Youth Risk Surveillance Survey, 38% of students reported using marijuana one or more times: 20% were current marijuana users, with males reporting higher use than females; 8% had tried marijuana before age 13 years.

Clinical presentation

Teenagers under the influence of marijuana may exhibit euphoria, visual distortion, drowsiness, and increased appetite, although paranoia, panic, and psychotic episodes may also occur. Marijuana alters time and distance perception and may contribute to motor vehicle crashes. Observation in a darkened room with minimal stimuli can help the patient to recover from marijuana intoxication.

Cocaine

The NIH reported that, nationwide, 7% of adolescents had used cocaine in any form (crack, powder, freebase), with 3% reporting current use. Approximately 1 in 10 people who use cocaine gradually become heavy users. Cocaine use has been linked to risk-taking behaviors. In a study of cocaine-related fatalities in New York City, one-third were from direct toxicity; the remainder were from suicide, homicide, falls, and motor vehicle crashes.

Clinical presentation

Cocaine causes release of catecholamines and blocks their reuptake. Consequently, cocaine can cause cardiovascular effects such as tachycardia, hypertension, and increased myocardial oxygen consumption. Vasospasm of coronary arteries, caused by increased local serotonin levels, can lead to myocardial infarction. For these reasons, even teenage patients presenting with chest pain in the context of cocaine use should be taken seriously. Beta-blockers are contraindicated in cocaine patients because of the risk of unopposed alpha agonist stimulation. Also, cocaine is frequently used in combination with alcohol, which may significantly increase the risk of sudden death.

Patients may also present with "crack lung" – a hypersensitivity pneumonitis that develops after heavy cocaine smoking. So called "crack-lung" consists of the constellation of chest pain, cough with hemoptysis, dyspnea, bronchospasm, fever, diffuse alveolar infiltrates without effusions, and pulmonary and systemic eosinophilia.

Neurologic sequelae of cocaine use include agitation and psychomotor stimulation. After the cocaine high, a "crash" may ensue, in which the patient has profound somnolence and ennui from catecholamine depletion. Pregnant women who use cocaine should be assessed for the possibility of abruptio placenta, preterm labor, and spontaneous abortion.

The agitation and adrenergic stimulation associated with cocaine use is best treated with benzodiazepines such as lorazepam (0.05–0.1 mg/kg IV/IM/PO).

Heroin

Among youth aged 12–17 years, 2% reported a history of heroin injection in the National Youth Risk Surveillance Survey. Prevalence was higher among males than females, and among Hispanics than Whites or Blacks. The Drug Abuse Warning Network (DAWN) chronicled a doubling of adolescent heroin ER visits between 1995 and 2002.

Clinical presentation

Heroin users may present with decreased mental status, respiratory depression, and pupillary constriction. Dermatologic cues of heroin use include track marks from venous injection, or abscesses resulting from infected skin popping/IM injection. Heroin withdrawal symptoms include nausea, vomiting, abdominal pain, piloerection, and yawning.

Sequelae of heroin use include serious to severe skin infections such as methicillin-resistant *Staphylococcus aureus* (MRSA), celluliti, and necrotizing fasciitis. Heroin users may also present with soft tissue infections caused by rare bacteria; for example wound botulism from *Clostridium botulinum*, tetanus from *Clostridium tetani*, and sepsis/myonecrosis from *Clostridia* spp. have been linked to black-tar heroin use. Dirty needles can lead to bacteremia, which can progress to life-threatening endocarditis. Unintentional overdose deaths may result from respiratory depression and hypoxia.

For respiratory depression and hypoxia, administer naloxone (0.01 mg/kg IV/IM/SC every 2 to 3 min to desired degree of reversal).

Methamphetamine

Overall, 4% of students aged 12 to 17 years had ever used methamphetamines, although the use of "meth" is becoming more widespread. Methamphetamine is popular among young people since it is relatively cheap, and produces a high that lasts longer than cocaine. Methamphetamine-related ED visits are most commonly due to mental health, traumatic, dermatologic, and dental complaints.

Clinical presentation

Methamphetamine blocks reuptake of catecholamines (dopamine, norepinephrine). Consequently, patients may present with tachycardia, diaphoresis, agitation, anxiety, and acute psychosis. Complications of methamphetamine use include rhabdomyolysis, acute renal failure, seizures, coronary ischemia, ventricular arrhythmias, coma, and cerebrovascular accident.

The agitation and adrenergic stimulation associated with methamphetamine use is best treated with benzodiazepines such as lorazepam (0.05–0.1 mg/kg IV/IM/PO).

On physical examination, clinicians may observe "meth mouth," a pattern of severe dental caries widespread among chronic methamphetamine users. Meth mouth is caused by dry mouth, bruxism, extended periods of poor oral hygiene, and a carbohydrate-rich diet.

Methamphetamine frequently creates delusions of parasitosis, and users engage in repeated "skin picking." Combined with unhygienic environments, repeated skin picking predisposes to MRSA skin infections.

Associated risks

Because of methamphetamine's effect of heightened arousal and decreased inhibition, its use has been linked to increased sexual risk behaviors. Among US high school students, heavy methamphetamine users, compared with infrequent users, were over four times more likely to report engaging in sexual intercourse before age 13 years, having sex with multiple partners, and having been/gotten someone pregnant. Among men who have sex with men, methamphetamine use correlates with sexual practices that increase risk of HIV infection such as decreased condom use and increased number of sexual partners. Heterosexual methamphetamine users have increased rates of syphilis and gonorrhea: diseases, which are considered markers of unprotected sex. In addition, IV methamphetamine users are at risk for hepatitis B and C, as well as other infectious diseases acquired IV.

MDMA (Ecstasy)

Prevalence

Nearly 6% of US high school students report using MDMA (3,4-methylenedioxymethamphetamine) one or more times. It is a popular drug among youth and is most commonly used in the cohort aged 16–25 years, frequently in the setting of raves (all night dance parties, typically in hot, enclosed venues). Visits to the ED for MDMA complications have increased voluminously since the late 1990s, with some cities experiencing a 200% to 500% increase in MDMA-related presentations.

Clinical presentation

MDMA is an amphetamine derivative that causes massive catecholamine and serotonin release. Autonomic hyperactivity secondary to the amphetamine-mediated catecholamine and serotonin surge leads to tachycardia, hypertension, and hyperthermia. Clinicians should also watch for dehydration, rhabdomyolysis, acute renal failure, altered mental status, hyponatremia, seizures, and serotonin syndrome (a constellation of hyperthermia, altered mental status, autonomic instability, and increased muscle tone/rigidity). The hyponatremia associated with MDMA can be acute and severe. MDMA can exacerbate or unmask underlying cardiac arrhythmias and has been noted to cause cardiovascular collapse (ventricular fibrillation and asystole).

Hallucinogens

Prevalence

Hallucinogenic drugs include LSD (lysergic acid diethylamide; "acid") mushrooms, phencyclidine (PCP), and mescaline, among other plant-based and designer substances. Nationwide, 8% of high school students aged 12 to 17 years have used a hallucinogenic substance one or more times.

Clinical presentation

Patients high on hallucinogens may present to the ED with acute psychosis or agitation. Patients who have taken LSD may manifest signs of mydriasis, tachycardia, and tachypnea. Ingestion of PCP may trigger dissociative behavior, and patients may present to the ED after scenarios such as trying to walk in traffic, or with acute traumatic injuries after "trying to fly." In tandem with altered behavior, rotatory and vertical nystagmus is almost pathognomonic for PCP ingestion.

Gamma-hydroxybutyrate

Prevalence

Gamma-hydroxybutyrate (GHB) is a fatty acid molecule first identified in 1960. Early use focused on the anesthetic (anterograde amnesia) and sedative properties of the compound, resulting in marketing as an agent for insomnia. The body-building properties of the drug also led to its fame as a dietary supplement and body-building agent. The CNS depressant effects, combined with amnesia, resulted in the use of this compound for sexual assault. This resulted in the compound becoming a Schedule I drug in the USA, except for when used to treat patients with cataplexy, in which case a central pharmacy system is used to distribute the drug. Street names for GHB include Fantasy, liquid ecstasy, salty water, and Georgia Home Boy, amongst others. Various precursors of GHB, such as gamma-butyrolactone and 1,4-butanediol, are found in industrial solvents. The reported incidence and prevalence of GHB use is difficult to assess given that urine sample confirmatory testing is rarely ordered because of the 7–10 days required to get the final result. What is known is that GHB is used by adolescents as well as adults, and that there is a slightly higher prevalence of use in gay and bisexual men.

Clinical presentation

The effects of GHB are dose dependent. Low doses (10 mg/kg) usually produce amnesia, hypotonia, and euphoria. Mid-range doses (20–30 mg/kg) have been reported to cause somnolence within 15 min. Higher doses (50 mg/kg) cause coma and loss of consciousness, combined with respiratory depression and even respiratory arrest. When combined with alcohol, the results are additive, resulting in significant depressed consciousness even with moderate uses of both substances. Toxicity is usually diagnosed clinically – specifically when the patient awakens suddenly from a comatose state with completely normal level of functioning. Patients can also awaken into a hyperactive state of arousal. Addiction (tolerance and dependence) to GHB has been reported in frequent/cyclical users.

Inhalants

Prevalence

Nationwide, 13% of youth age 12 to 17 years reported sniffing glue or inhaling aerosols, paints or sprays for the purposes of getting high (National Youth Risk Surveillance Survey). Inhalants are low cost and readily accessible over the counter, contributing to their abuse potential among youth. Inhalation may occur via sniffing (directly inhaling the volatile compound), huffing (saturating a rag with solvent such as gasoline and placing it over the nostrils and mouth), or bagging (deep inhalations from a plastic bag filled with spray paint or another propellant). The typical inhalant user is a young male of lower socioeconomic background.

Clinical presentation

Inhaled hydrocarbons can have deleterious impacts on the CNS and cardiopulmonary system. Hydrocarbons easily cross the blood–brain barrier, causing disorientation, disinhibition, and euphoria. Slurred speech, impaired gait, drowsiness, and hallucinations may ensue.

Inhalants can precipitate cardiac arrhythmias and cause sudden cardiac death. Hydrocarbons sensitize the myocardium to catetcholamine surge, possibly leading to coronary artery spasm and myocardial infarction. Asphyxiation deaths secondary to plastic-bag suffocation have been noted. Interestingly, direct pulmonary injury from inhaled hydrocarbons has not been documented. In the USA, inhalant use caused 12% of deaths reported to poison control centers in the cohort aged 13–19 years.

Prescription drugs

Among US adolescents, 7% reported using prescription narcotics that were either purchased illicitly or prescribed for other people. Changing sociocultural behaviors are influencing patterns of prescription drug ingestion. Teenagers may ingest several unlabelled prescription pills at one time; the medications may act synergistically or may have contradictory effects. "Pharm parties" – in which multiple drugs are placed in a bowl and then the "trail mix" is passed around for youth to "graze" – can result in complex toxidromes with confusing clinical presentations. Particularly dangerous combinations include ecstasy and methamphetamine, and GHB and benzodiazepines.

Role of clinicians

Although most primary care physicians endeavor to ask teenage patients about drug and alcohol use, the extent of adolescent substance use is frequently underestimated. Adolescents are more likely to disclose substance use when interviewed without parents present.

The clinician in the ED has a unique opportunity to interface with adolescents during times of crisis. Substance-using youth frequently present to the ED in states of psychological distress, physiologic extremis, or with unintentional injury and trauma. Consequently, EPs may be the first adults to witness teenagers' drug and/or alcohol abuse and addiction. The "teachable moments" in the emergency setting provide a unique opportunity for patient education, intervention, and prevention regarding adolescent substance use.

Pearls and pitfalls

Pearls

1. The ED visit is a key "teachable moment" for addressing substance abuse and providing appropriate interventions and education.
2. Adolescent patients should be interviewed without parents present to screen for substance use.
3. Use of the "CRAFTT" questionnaire can identify adolescents who require, and may benefit from, an intervention or treatment.

Pitfalls

1. Failure to ask adolescents about substance abuse.
2. Failure to exclude a medical etiology for behavioral disturbances suspicious for drug abuse.
3. Failure to screen for associated risks of adolescent substance abuse: suicidality, abuse, injuries, and sexually transmitted infections.

Selected references

Annesi-Maesano I, Oryszczyn MP, Raherison C, *et al.* Increased prevalence of asthma and allied diseases among active adolescent tobacco smokers after controlling for passive smoking exposure. A cause for concern? *Clin Exp Allergy* 2004;**34**:1017–1023.

Berk W, Henderson WV. Alcohols. In Tintinalli JE, Kelen GD, Stapczynski JS (eds.) *Emergency Medicine: A Comprehensive Study Guide*. New York: McGraw-Hill, 2004, pp. 1064–1065.

Bernstein J, Adlaf E, Paglia-Boak A, for the Research Group on Drug Use. *Drug Use in Toronto 2004*. Toronto: Research Group on Drug Use, 2004 www.toronto.ca/health/rgdu/pdf/drug_use_in_toronto_2004.pdf (accessed 28 April 2010).

Boghdadi MS, Henning RJ. Cocaine: pathophysiology and clinical toxicology. *Heart Lung* 1997;**26**:466–483.

Brown PD, Ebright JR. Skin and soft tissue infections in injection drug users. *Curr Infect Dis Rep* 2002;**4**:415–419.

Centers for Disease Control and Prevention. Methamphetamine use and HIV risk behaviors among heterosexual men: preliminary results from five northern California counties, December 2002–November 2003. *MMWR Morb Mort Wkly Rep* 2006;**55**:273–277.

Centers for Disease Control and Prevention. *Quick Stats: Underage Drinking*. Atlanta, GA: Centers for Disease Control and Prevention, 2010 http://www.cdc.gov/alcohol/quickstats/underage_drinking.htm (accessed 28 April 2010).

Centers for Disease Control and Prevention. *Tobacco Use and the Health of Young People*. Atlanta, GA: Centers for Disease Control and Prevention, 2010 http://www.cdc.gov/HealthyYouth/tobacco/facts.htm (accessed 28 April 2010).

Cohen AL, Shuler C, McAllister S, *et al.* Methamphetamine use and methicillin-resistant *Staphylococcus aureus* skin infections. *Emerg Infect Dis* 2007;**13**:1707–1713.

Derlet RW, Heischober B. Methamphetamine. Stimulant of the 1990s? *West J Med* 1990;**153**:625–628.

Devlin RJ, Henry JA. Clinical review: major consequences of illicit drug consumption. *Crit Care* 2008;**12**:202.

Eaton DK, Kann L, Kinchen S, *et al.* Youth risk behavior surveillance: United States, 2007. *MMWR Surveill Summ* 2008;**57**:1–131.

Eisner MD, Wang Y, Haight TJ, *et al.* Secondhand smoke exposure, pulmonary function, and cardiovascular mortality. *Ann Epidemiol* 2007;**17**:364–373.

Flowers NT, Naimi TS, Brewer RD, *et al.* Patterns of alcohol consumption and alcohol-impaired driving in the United States. *Alcohol Clin Exp Res* 2008;**32**:639–644.

Forrester JM, Steele AW, Waldron JA, Parsons PE. Crack lung: an acute pulmonary syndrome with a spectrum of clinical and histopathologic findings. *Am Rev Respir Dis* 1990;**142**:462–467.

Hendrickson RG, Cloutier R, McConnell KJ. Methamphetamine-related emergency department utilization and cost. *Acad Emerg Med* 2008;**15**:23–31.

Hingson R, Heeren T, Levenson S, Jamanka A, Voas R. Age of drinking onset, driving after drinking, and involvement in alcohol related motor-vehicle crashes. *Accid Anal Prev* 2002;**34**:85–92.

Hingson RW, Heeren T, Winter MR. Age at drinking onset and alcohol dependence: age at onset, duration, and severity. *Pediatrics* 2006;**160**:739–746.

Kane J. Hydrocarbon inhalation injury. *Emedicine* June 2008 http://www.emedicine.com/ped/TOPIC2790.HTM (accessed 28 April 2010).

Kimura AC, Higa JI, Levin RM, *et al.* Outbreak of necrotizing fasciitis due to *Clostridium sordellii* among black-tar heroin users. *Clin Infect Dis* 2004;**38**:e87–e91.

Klasser GD, Epstein J. Methamphetamine and its impact on dental care. *J Can Dent Assoc* 2005;**71**:759–762.

Marzuk PM, Tardiff K, Leon AC. Fatal injuries after cocaine use as a leading cause of death among young adults in New York City. *N Engl J Med* 1995;**332**:1753–1757.

Mclaughlin CR, Daniel J, Joost TF. The relationship between substance use, drug selling, and lethal violence in 25 juvenile murderers. *J Forensic Sci* 2000;**45**:349–353.

National Institute on Drug Abuse. *Cocaine Abuse and Addiction*. Bethesda, MD: National Institutes of Health, National Institute on Drug Abuse, 1999.

Office of Applied Studies. *The OAS Report. A Day in the Life of American Adolescents: Substance Use Facts*. Washington, DC: Department of Health and Human Services, 2007 www.oas.samhsa.gov/2k7/youthFacts/youth.pdf (accessed 28 April 2010).

Pelkonen M, Marttunen M. Child and adolescent suicide: epidemiology, risk factors, and approaches to prevention. *Paediatr Drug* 2003;**5**:243–265.

Salomonsen-Sautel S, Van Leeuwen JM, *et al.* Correlates of substance use among homeless youths in eight cities. *Am J Addict* 2008;**17**:224–234.

Springer AE, Peters RJ, Shegog R, White DL, Kelder SH. Methamphetamine use and sexual risk behaviors in USA high school students: findings from a national risk behavior survey. *Prev Sci* 2007;**8**:103–113.

Substance Abuse and Mental Health Services Administration. *Drug Abuse Warning Network: Amphetamine and Methamphetamine Emergency Department Visits 1995–2002.* Rockville, MD: Substance Abuse and Mental Health Services Administration, Office of Applied Studies Substance Abuse and Mental Health Services Administration, 2002.

Substance Abuse and Mental Health Services Administration. *Drug Abuse Warning Network, 2005: National Estimates of Drug-Related Emergency Department Visits.* [DAWN Series D-29, DHHS Publication No. (SMA) 07-4256, 2007.] Rockville, MD: Substance Abuse and Mental Health Services Administration, Office of Applied Studies, 2007.

Weekes A. Substance abuse: cocaine. *eMedicine* March 2008 http://www.emedicine.com/ped/TOPIC2666.HTM#ref5 (accessed 28 April 2010).

Wilson CR, Sherritt L, Gates E, Knight JR. Are clinical impressions of adolescent substance use accurate? *Pediatrics* 2004;**114**:e536–e540.

Wu LT, Pilowsky DJ, Schlenger WE. Inhalant abuse and dependence among adolescents in the United States. *J Am Acad Child Adolesc Psychiatry* 2004;**43**:1206–1214.

Section

28

Special populations: children with special healthcare needs

Expert reviewers: Jin S. Hahn, Dorsey M. Bass, Michael S. B. Edwards, and Anna Messner

Chapter 162

Practical approach to medically complex children

Bernhard Fassl and Nancy Murphy

Introduction

Special healthcare needs are found in a large percentage of US children. In 1998 alone, 18% of US children (12.6 million) qualified as having special healthcare needs. Hospitalizations and emergency care use are common in this population because of the fragile nature of their medical condition. Improved survival of children with very low birth weight and children with chronic conditions will increase the proportion of children with complex medical conditions (medically complex children [MCC]).

Encounters with such MCC are among the most difficult tasks for EPs. Unfamiliarity with pediatric chronic conditions and the complexity of interrelated medical issues present a unique challenge. In addition, there is no unifying and precise definition. The term MCC used in this chapter includes all of the following groups of children with special healthcare needs.

Technology-dependent children. Children who are dependent on devices to compensate for the loss of a vital body function to avert death or further disability.

Neurologically impaired children. These children form the single largest group of MCC (85%), with cerebral palsy the largest diagnostic subgroup by far. These children often have multiple other medical problems indirectly related to their underlying illness, such as cerebral palsy, aspiration events, or seizures. Seizure disorder is the second most common group of MCC (8%).

Medically fragile children. Children with underlying conditions that predispose them to more frequent and severe illnesses.

A sudden deterioration in these children is generally related to:

- progression/complication of the underlying disease
- device-related complications in technology-dependent children
- intercurrent illnesses complicating or exacerbating chronic conditions.

Table 162.1 outlines common issues in these children.

This chapter is designed to aid the clinician in the recognition of emergency care specific differences regarding history, physical examination, complexity of medical assessment, and medical decision making for MCC. Strategies include:

- a family centered approach to patient care – listen to the parents (Box 162.1)
- familiarity with differences in presentation of MCC
- specifics in the emergency care for categories of chronic pediatric conditions.

Issues related to other MCC populations are discussed in other chapters of this section: children with congenital heart disease (Ch. 14), inborn errors of metabolism (Ch. 168), neoplasms/chemotherapy (Ch. 80). We also specifically address common "gizmo" malfunctions in technology-dependent children (Ch. 169).

Regardless of the underlying condition, a MCC commonly presents with one or a combination of the following chief complaints:

- respiratory distress
- seizures
- unexplained fever
- irritability
- feeding intolerance, nausea, vomiting, abdominal distention
- increased spasticity.

Over 40% of admissions are for respiratory tract infections and distress; 20% are for seizures with associated infections, and 13% are for feeding problems. One inciting event often is responsible for a cascade of conditions. For example, a neurologically impaired child with gastroesophageal reflux and aspiration may present with fever, irritability, respiratory distress, and seizures exacerbated by fever and G-tube leakage.

To ED clinicians, encounters with MCC are among the most difficult patient–physician interactions. Many clinicians, particularly those with little exposure to MCC, are concerned about sharing their decision-making authority with the family, thus leaving an impression that specific family concerns were left poorly addressed. This chapter outlines an approach to MCC *regardless* of the underlying medical condition. The basis for providing optimal care is a family-centered approach to evaluation and decision making.

A Practical Guide to Pediatric Emergency Medicine: Caring for Children in the Emergency Department, ed. N. Ewen Amieva-Wang (associate eds. Jamie Shandro, Aparajita Sohoni, and Bernhard Fassl). Published by Cambridge University Press.

Table 162.1. Examples of children with medically complex conditions

Category	Examples	Common issues
Technology dependent	Short gut syndrome and parenteral feeding dependence, respiratory failure and tracheostomy/ventilator dependency	Central line infections/thrombosis, feeding intolerance, total parenteral nutrition-induced liver damage
Neurologically impaired	Cerebral palsy, congenital infections, traumatic brain injuries, hydrocephalus, epilepsy, CNS malformation	Aspiration of food, seizures, CSF shunt malfunction, spasticity, severe gastroesophageal reflux
Medically fragile children	Congenital heart disease	Heart failure, respiratory distress
	Nephrotic syndrome	Fever, peritonitis
	Cystic fibrosis	Pulmonary exacerbations
	Muscular dystrophies	Respiratory insufficiency or failure Respiratory distress, cough, fever
	Neoplasms	Fever, neutropenia
	Immunosuppression	Immunosuppressant drug side effects
	Inborn errors of metabolism	Altered level of consciousness, seizure, dehydration

Assessment

History

Reason for the visit. The MCC may present to a clinician with a multitude of acute and chronic problems. The first step in history taking is to *elicit the main reasons for the visit* (i.e., what changed that urgent evaluation was required). The clinician needs to know

- What do I need to pay special attention to?
- What is different from the patient's baseline?
- What is the caretaker's concern for today's visit?

Take an organ system-based history. This can provide an overview of all acute and chronic issues. For example, a toddler with cerebral palsy (25-week premature child), epilepsy, and G-tube dependency presents with respiratory distress. In this case, an organ-based history and examination will provide information about the pulmonary status of the child (presence of bronchopulmonary dysplasia, history of aspiration), cardiac status (presence of a patent ductus arteriosus), neurologic status (intraventricular hemorrhage and seizures), nutritional status (G-tube use and oral feedings, presence of a fundoplication, constipation) and so on. This organ-based outline of problems will help the clinician to formulate a plan for diagnosis and treatment. This example shows how the approach allows the physician to distinguish an emergency from other active, non-urgent problems and provides a framework for further testing and management.

Create documentation based on the organ-based history. Identify acute and chronic issues for each organ system and incorporate chronic medical issues into the decision making process. For example,

- in a patient with spina bifida and vesicoureteral reflux with chronic kidney damage, a CT with IV contrast is problematic
- a patient with seizure disorder should not receive carbapenem antibiotics (particularly imipenem) as they lower the seizure threshold.

Medication history. Documentation of active, as needed, and recently started/discontinued medications provides information about potential drug adverse effects, drug interactions, appropriateness of drug prescribed, drug allergies, and idiosyncratic reactions (Table 162.2).

Physical examination

A child with a medically complex condition will often have abnormalities on baseline examination and can be hard to assess. Documentation of physical examination findings should include:

- changes from baseline findings as described by the family (i.e. "the patient has intercostal retractions, according to the caretaker this is the patient's baseline")
- mental status with reference to baseline status.

Medical decision making

Laboratory and radiological studies. Decisions about testing should be shared between parents and physicians. Specific questions and needs of the family identified in the history will influence the provider's decision making about testing.

Organ system-based information gathered in the examination. This approach should be used as the basis for developing a care plan but all decisions should be made in the recognition of the parent as disease expert and

Box 162.1. Family-centered care

Medically complex children (MCC) and their families are experienced consumers of ED and in-hospital care. Children whose medical issues have broad implications for family life are ideally cared for with a family-centered approach. Maintaining respect for families with MCC even if the belief system of the provider and family are different is important. The concept of family-centered care as described by the AAP includes:

- physician recognition of key family members
- recognition of family values and beliefs
- shared decision making between medical providers and family.

Clinical pearl. The importance of regarding parents of MCC as expert allies in the medical decision-making process cannot be overemphasized. Parents can provide meaningful and unique information and should be regarded as experts in the child's condition. They aid the clinician with:

- interpretation of physical signs, such as the degree of respiratory distress ("that's much more than her baseline secretions"), fever ("the last time she spiked to 39 degrees, she had bacteria in her blood")
- interpretation of laboratory and radiological studies ("the right upper lobe infiltrate is present on every chest radiograph")
- help in deciding about treatments ("the last time she turned blue, they found it was seizures").

Three specific questions that may aid the clinician in better understanding the family, while also making the family feel more involved and understood, are:

- What do you think might be causing your child to have (chief complaint)?
- Do you have any thoughts on what tests or evaluations might be helpful?
- Are there any treatments or medications that you think might be helpful to your child?

Table 162.2. Common medication-related medical problems

Effect	Example
Adverse drug effects	Excessive sedation or agitation with phenobarbital Pancreatitis/hepatitis with valproic acid Extrapyramidal symptoms (oculogyric crisis) with metoclopramide Blood dyscrasias and Stevens–Johnson syndrome with phenytoin Anticholinergic side effects with glycopyrrolate (Robinul) Antiepileptic medications
Drug interactions	Phenobarbital, phenytoin and carbamazepine induce cytochrome P450-mediated metabolism, which affects other antiepileptic drug levels Valproic acid inhibits hepatic enzymes and elevates lamotrigine levels
Drug levels appropriate	Antiepileptic medication (phenobarbital, phenytoin, valproic acid) in presentation with seizures Tacrolimus in a child after transplant Digoxin
Recently discontinued medications	Abrupt cessation of baclofen can cause agitation and seizures Cessation of clonidine can cause sympathetic overactivity with hypertension

with inclusion of the parent in the decision-making process. This aids in ensuring that:

- the patient's/family's needs are not left unaddressed
- there is appropriate understanding of the plan

Interdisciplinary care coordination. Many MCC are followed by multiple specialists. The EP should:

- communicate with specialists in their area of expertise (i.e., worsening seizures in a MCC should be treated in consultation with the patient's neurologist)
- communicate the child's medical plan to the primary care physician.

Responsibilities of the EP caring for the MCC. These include:

- recognizing and treating critical conditions such as septicemia/shock/respiratory failure promptly
- identifying conditions that warrant hospital admission
- initiating treatment of acute conditions
- maintaining and/or modifying treatments for chronic conditions (e.g., non-invasive modes of ventilation should be attempted first in a child with neuromuscular disease to avoid later problems of weaning post-extubation)
- being aware of disease-specific complications if a child has an intercurrent illness (e.g., fever and vomiting in a child with an organic acidemia indirectly worsens the metabolic status of the child and requires urgent intervention in addition to rehydration to avoid complete metabolic decompensation)
- identifying the underlying cause of the sudden deterioration is often not possible in ED as this will require a series of tests after hospital admission.

The comprehensive care plan. Decisions about further testing and treatments at the ED should be discussed with the parent. Suggestions from parents or the regular physician(s) are extremely valuable to the care plan and should not be regarded as intrusion into the ED treatment plan. A comprehensive plan that outlines all medical problems and therapeutic interventions is typically maintained by primary care or medical home providers. The focused care plan based on the ED encounter should encompass urgent problems by organ system, with reference to active and past issues and relevant therapeutic interventions. A copy of the focused care plan should be given to the family and kept in a central location in the medical record for access by other providers.

Pearls and pitfalls

Pearls

1. When caring for children with complex medical conditions, caregiver history and comparison of present vital signs with baseline values are the most important for recognizing a critically ill child.
2. Parents and caregivers should be regarded as expert allies in the medical decision-making process.
3. Carbapenem (i.e., imipenem) antibiotics should not be administered to a patient with a seizure disorder as these antibiotics can lower the seizure threshold.

Pitfalls

1. Failure to diagnose serious bacterial illnesses in a child with a complex medical condition.
2. Failure to obtain urine analysis and blood cultures as part of the routine evaluation of a child with a complex medical condition and a fever.

Selected references

Newacheck PW, Strickland B, Shonkof JP, *et al.* An epidemiologic profile of children with special health care needs. *Pediatrics* 1998;**102**:117–123.

Wegner J, Power EJ, Fox H. *Technology Dependent Children: Hospital Versus Home Care.* Philadephia, PA: Lippincott for the Office of Technology Assessment Task Force, 1988.

Chapter 163

Neurologically impaired children

Bernhard Fassl and Nancy Murphy

Introduction

Neurologically impaired children form the biggest subgroup within the grouping of medically complex children (MCC). Common conditions resulting in neurologically impaired children include:

- prematurity-related brain damage: periventricular leukomalacia, grade III and IV intraventricular hemorrhage
- birth asphyxia, intrauterine insult
- infectious and neoplastic brain damage
- neurotoxic encephalopathy in children with inborn errors of metabolism: amino acidopathies, fatty acid oxidation defects, lysosomal storage diseases
- children after accidental and non-accidental head injuries
- children with genetic syndromes: trisomy 18,4p deletion syndrome

Neurologically impaired children commonly have a multitude of active and chronic medical conditions making evaluation and management challenging in the ED. Neurologically impaired children usually present with one of the following chief complaints:

- respiratory distress
- unexplained fever
- worsening seizures
- nausea, vomiting, feeding intolerance
- increased spasticity.

Table 163.1 provides an overview of common causes at presentation and suggested workup.

The child with cerebral palsy

Cerebral palsy consists of a heterogeneous group of clinical syndromes that are characterized by motor and postural dysfunction. It ranges in severity, depending on the severity and degree of abnormalities in the developing brain. The main causes of cerebral palsy are static encephalopathies related to perinatal events (intraventricular hemorrhage, anoxia, in utero strokes), acquired injuries to the developing brain (meningitis, congenital infections), and congenital malformations of the brain (disorders of neuronal migration).

Although the primary insult to the developing brain in cerebral palsy is static, manifestations of the neurologic condition may change or worsen over time.

Manifestations

Spastic cerebral palsy. There are features of upper motor neuron disease characterized by spastic hypertonia, hyperreflexia, extensor plantar responses and clonus:

- spastic diplegia typically affects prematurely born children with periventricular leukomalacia; the lower limbs are affected predominantly, although upper limb impairments and other developmental delays may be present
- spastic quadriplegia is the most severe form of spastic cerebral palsy; children usually have intellectual disabilities, visual impairments, dysphagia and seizures
- spastic hemiplegia affects one side, usually more severely in the upper than lower limb; it is usually caused by perinatal stroke (internal carotid artery occlusion).

Dyskinetic cerebral palsy. This usually affects term infants with birth asphyxia. Dyskinetic syndromes are characterized by varying degrees of athetosis, chorea, and dystonia.

Ataxic cerebral palsy. There is a cerebellar or sensory origin of the cerebral palsy and this form is often found in children with congenital malformations of the developing brain.

Associated conditions

There are intellectual disabilities in 65% of children with cerebral palsy. Epilepsy occurs in up to 50%; other common conditions include behavioral problems, developmental delays, and impairments of vision and hearing. There are a number of other less-obvious but nonetheless clinically important associated conditions.

Respiratory effects. Pneumonia can occur secondary to problems with oropharyngeal incoordination, reflux, aspiration, chronic lung fibrosis, bronchopulmonary dysplasia, and scoliosis. Pneumonia is a major cause of decreased life expectancy in children with cerebral palsy.

A Practical Guide to Pediatric Emergency Medicine: Caring for Children in the Emergency Department, ed. N. Ewen Amieva-Wang (associate eds. Jamie Shandro, Aparajita Sohoni, and Bernhard Fassl). Published by Cambridge University Press.

Table 163.1. Evaluation algorithm for neurologically impaired children presenting to the emergency department

Presenting signs	Common clinical conditions	Testing/workup to consider
Respiratory distress, increased secretions, increased oxygen requirement	Respiratory tract infections, asthma, aspiration of food, aspiration of mucous secretions, atelectasis, pulmonary embolism	Chest radiograph: new infiltrates, atelectasis, heart size Blood gas analysis Tracheal secretion for Gram stain and culture
Seizures	Seizure disorder worsened by intercurrent infection, subtherapeutic antiepileptic medication levels, food–drug interactions, change in formulation, change in route of delivery, CSF shunt malfunction/infection, progression of underlying disease	Measure antiepileptic drug level Head CT: particularly if CSF shunt present If febrile: obtain CSF through lumbar puncture or shunt tap after head CT Neurology/neurosurgery consultation
Fever	Infections: urinary tract, vesico-ureteral reflux, central line, shunt, septicemia, viral	CBC Blood culture Urine analysis, microscopy, culture Viral testing[a] Consider CSF studies in children with shunts
Nausea, vomiting, feeding intolerance	Gastroesophageal reflux disease, constipation and fecal impaction, malposition of enteral feeding devices, paralytic ileus and feeding intolerance, G-tube leakage secondary to febrile illness, superior mesenteric artery syndrome, CSF shunt malfunction	Abdominal radiograph: stool mass, ileus, free air Upper GI series: malrotation, volvulus, reflux Dye study of feeding device Head CT and shunt series
Irritability and increased spasticity	Intercurrent illness, CSF shunt malfunction, constipation, esophagitis/gastritis, reflux disease, sleep deprivation, cessation of spasmolytic medication, urinary retention	Medication history: particularly recently added/discontinued medications Abdominal radiograph: stool masses Abdominal/bladder ultrasound: urinary retention Head CT and shunt series in children with CSF shunts

[a]Depending on availability of testing and seasonality of viral illnesses.

Musculoskeletal effects. The high muscle tone has effects on growing bones. While cerebral palsy is non-progressive, the effects of muscle imbalance are progressive and cause growth dysfunction:

- bracing is usually used to correct the abnormal posture of the ankle and foot
- hip subluxation and dysplasia occur because the flexors and adductors of the hips overpower the extensors and abductors as a result of spasticity and contractures
- severe pain may occur particularly with a change in posture.

Progressive scoliosis. Back pain, neck pain, chest deformity and respiratory insufficiency follow the increase in side curvature of the spine.

Growth failure. Inadequate intake of calories and micronutrients restricts growth.

Osteopenia. Pathologic fractures can occur.

Urinary disorders. Neurogenic bladder with urinary retention, recurrent urinary tract infections, renal and bladder stones can all occur.

Gastrointestinal system. Children with cerebral palsy are prone to:

- constipation: abdominal distention, feeding intolerance, nausea, vomiting, irritability, and pain.
- gastroesophageal reflux disease: pain, chronic aspirations, gastritis, esophagitis, anemia, tooth erosion
- swallowing disorders: chronic aspiration.

Superior mesenteric artery syndrome. This is caused by intermittent or functional obstruction of the duodenum. It may present as recurrent vomiting.

Management

Basic knowledge of common treatment interventions in children with CP is essential while evaluating an affected patient.

Table 163.2. Antiepileptic medications

	Common side effects	Drug interactions
Carbamazepine	Aplastic anemia, SJS, allergic rash	PB, PHT, FEL, primidone lower CBZ levels INH, calcium channel blockers, macrolides elevate CBZ levels CBZ raises or lowers PHT levels CBZ reduces efficacy of oral contraceptives
Phenytoin/ fosphenytoin	Ataxia, osteoporosis, nausea, vomiting, rash, blood dyscrasias, vitamin K and folate deficiency	PHT lowers levels of CBZ, ETX, FEL, primidone, PB CBZ PB may raise or lower PHT levels VPA raises PHT levels PHT interacts with warfarin, steroids, immunosuppressants, furosemide PHT reduces efficacy of oral contraceptives
Oxcarbazepine	Allergic rash, hyponatremia	OXC reduces efficacy of oral contraceptives
Lamotrigine	Rash, SJS	VPA significantly increases LTG levels and risk of serious rash Enzyme-inducing antiepileptics such as CBZ, PB, and PHT lower LTG levels by 40–50%
Zonisamide	Dizziness, headache, somnolence, SJS	CBZ, PB, PHT and VPA reduce levels of ZNS ZNS does not affect other drugs
Ethosuximide	GI side effects, bone marrow suppression, SJS, microscopic hematuria	ETX raises levels of PHT VPA lowers and raises levels of ETX
Phenobarbital	Cognitive and behavioral: sedation, cognitive slowing, agitation, paradoxical hyperkinesis	VPA, FEL, PHT increase PB levels Rifampin decreases PB levels PB lowers levels of CBZ, VPA, diazepam, warfarin, steroids, immunosuppression, furosemide PB reduces efficacy of oral contraceptives
Valproic acid	Hepatitis and pancreatitis (particularly child <2 years with polytherapy), sedation	VPA raises levels of PHT, PB, CBZ, LTG, FEL VPA levels are increased by FEL and clobazepam
Vigabatrin	Drowsiness, agitation, double vision	VGB lowers levels of PHT by 25%
Tiagabin	Dizziness, tremor, mood	TGB lowers levels of VPA
Felbamate	Insomnia, hepatic failure (rare), aplastic anemia	VPA raises levels of FEL, PHT VPA reduces levels of CBZ
Topiramate	Ataxia, somnolence, cognitive slowing, pruritus, weight loss	PHT, CBZ, VPA lower TOP levels
Levetiracetam	Somnolence, dizziness, headaches	No significant interactions
Ketogenic diet[a]	Dehydration during initiation phase, GI complaints (nausea, vomiting, diarrhea); ketogenic diet predisposes to metabolic acidosis; metabolic complications (hyponatremia, hypomagnesemia, hypoproteinuria, hyperuricemia); renal stones occur in <5% of patients; rare but life-threatening pancreatitis and cardiomyopathy	Children on ketogenic diet usually have low glucose levels (50–60 mg/dl) and have elevated anion gap Avoid using lactated Ringer's solution; try to avoid dextrose 5%; use normal saline if at all possible

CBZ, carbamazepine; ETX, ethosuximide; FEL, felbamate; INH, isoniazid; LEV, levetiracetam; LTG, lamotrigine; OXC, oxcarbazepine; PB, phenobarbital; PHT, phenytoin/fosphenytoin; SJS, Stevens–Johnson syndrome; TGB, tiagabin; TOP, topiramate; VGB, vigabatrin; VPA, valproic acid; ZNS, zonisamide.
[a]Induces ketosis, which is thought to have a direct antiepileptic effect.

Botulinum toxin

Injection of botulinum toxin A into the spastic muscles blocks the presynaptic release of acetycholine and decreases muscle tone by limiting muscle contraction. Botulinum toxin therapy is indicated in children with spasticity that limits function, causes pain, or contributes to orthopedic deformities. Injections may be repeated every 3–6 months as needed.

Table 163.3. Common examples of neuromuscular diseases in children

Location of defect	Disease
Anterior horn cell disease	Spinal muscular atrophy (SMA) I, II, III
Generalized childhood peripheral neuropathy	Guillain–Barré syndrome, acute intermittent porphyria, hereditary neuropathies, giant axonal neuropathies, metabolic diseases (Refsum disease, metachromatic leukodystrophy), toxins (lead, arsenic, mercury)
Diseases of the neuromuscular junction	Myasthenia gravis, botulism, tick paralysis
Myopathies	Muscular dystrophies: Duchenne (skeletal, cardiac muscle, mental retardation), Becker (skeletal and cardiac muscle), myotonic (elongated face, myotonia, mental retardation, cataract, cardiac conduction defect), congenital (mitochondrial encephalomyopathies), Kearns Sayre syndrome, MERRF syndrome, MELAS syndrome, defects of carnitine cycle and beta oxidation (MCAD), defects of glycogen metabolism (glycogen storage diseases, lactate dehydrogenase deficiency, aldolase deficiency), endocrine (hypothyroidism), inflammatory (dermatomyositis, polymyositis, viral myositis)

MCAD, medium chain acyl CoA dehydrogenase deficiency; MELAS, mitochondrial myopathy, encephalopathy, lactic acidosis, and stroke; MERRF, myoclonic epilepsy with ragged red fibers.

Complications are rare but include:
- fever after injection (up to 3 days)
- weakness and temporary loss of muscle function (up to 2 weeks)
- respiratory failure and death due to unintentional overdose or intravascular injection.

Benzodiazepines

Benzodiazepines produce muscle relaxation through increasing the affinity of gamma-aminobutyrate (GABA) at its ion channel receptors, thereby increasing presynaptic inhibition. Complications include:
- sedation, weakness
- respiratory depression
- dependence and tolerance after long-term use; withdrawal if abruptly discontinued.

Baclofen

Baclofen binds to the GABA-B receptor on the terminals of the primary afferent fibers suppressing release of excitatory neurotransmitters and thus reducing spasticity. Baclofen can be administered orally or intrathecally through an implanted pump and catheter system. Common side effects and complications are:
- systemic baclofen:
  - confusion, sedation, hypotonia
  - ataxia, paresthesiae
  - nausea
  - *if discontinued abruptly*: seizures, severe spasticity, hallucinations
- intrathecal baclofen:
  - catheter-related complications (disconnections, migration out of the intrathecal space, breaks), occur in up to 10–20% of patients
  - disruption of intrathecal baclofen delivery (catheter failure, pump failure, empty drug reservoir), leading to progressive worsening spasticity, sustained muscle contractions, rhabdomyolysis, seizures, and if untreated, death in extreme cases
  - overdose of intrathecal baclofen (programming errors, dosage changes), leading to lethargy, hypotonia, and respiratory insufficiency; history should suggest a refill or reprogramming of the pump in the past 1 to 2 days
  - infections: pump pocket, catheter site or meningitis
  - CSF leaks, seromas at the pump or catheter site generally occur within the first few weeks following implantation or revision.

Hyperosmolar enemas

In severe constipation, hyperosmolar enemas are used for disimpaction.

The child taking multiple seizure medications

Seizures are a common problem in neurologically impaired children and many children require multiple antiepileptic medications to control their seizures. Interactions between these medications complicate evaluation and management of the child who presents to the ED. Table 163.2 provides an overview of most commonly used antiepileptic medications, their side effects, and drug interactions.

The child with neuromuscular disease

Diseases involving the neuromuscular system are usually identified on the basis of the site of the primary pathologic manifestation such as anterior horn cell, peripheral nerve, neuromuscular junction, and skeletal muscle (Table 163.3).

The long term prognosis in children with neuromuscular disease is dependent on the underlying condition and ranges from fatal in early childhood (spinal muscular atrophy type I) to full recovery (infant botulism).

The EP should take following clinical considerations into account while providing care to a child with neuromuscular disease.

Minor respiratory illnesses. These may quickly result in respiratory failure. As there are no reliable physical signs of respiratory distress, a blood gas analysis (arterial or capillary) should be performed without delay.

Chronic hypercarbia. Many children with neuromuscular disease have chronic hypercarbia with a normal blood pH at baseline. An elevated carbon dioxide reading must be interpreted in the context of the presence or absence of respiratory acidosis.

Non-invasive ventilation (continuous/bilevel positive airway pressure). This is preferred in children with neuromuscular disease and respiratory failure. Once intubated and ventilated, extubation may become extremely difficult.

Bulbar dysfunction. This is common in some neuromuscular diseases: botulism, some forms of Guillain–Barré syndrome, dermatomyositis. These children are at risk for aspiration. A swallow evaluation should be performed to ensure safety of oral feedings.

Cardiac problems. Heart conduction defects and cardiomyopathies are common in muscular dystrophies and metabolic myopathies.

Pearls and pitfalls

Pearls

1. Aspiration of food and mucus are major causes of respiratory worsening in a neurologically impaired child with respiratory distress.
2. In a neurologically impaired child with seizures, intercurrent illnesses may have lowered the seizure threshold and caused a "breakthrough seizure."
3. Signs of respiratory distress such as retractions or accessory muscle use may be absent in children with neuromuscular diseases.

Pitfalls

1. Failure to evaluate vital signs carefully, and in comparison to the patient's baseline vital signs from past visits.
2. Failure to consider infection in any neurologically impaired child with indwelling catheters or shunts.
3. Failure to involve parents in decision making regarding the medical workup.

Selected references

Mahon M, Kibirige MS. Patterns of admission for children with special needs to the pediatric assessment unit. *Arch Dis Child* 2004; **89**:165–169.

Newacheck PW, Strickland B, Shonkoff JP *et al.* An epidemiologic profile of children with special health care needs. *Pediatrics* 1998;**102**:117–123.

Wegner J, Power EJ, Fox H. *Technology Dependent Children: Hospital Versus Home Care*. Philadephia, PA: Lippincott for the US Office of Technology Assessment Task Force, 1988.

Chapter

164 Graduate from the neonatal intensive care unit

Bernhard Fassl and Nancy Murphy

The medically complex premature infant

Survival rates of the smallest and youngest premature infants have continued to improve with technologic advances. In the AAP data for 2002–2003, neonatal survival of infants born at 23 weeks ranged from 10 to 30%; it was 26–52% at 24 weeks of gestation and 54–76% at 25 weeks of gestation. Of the surviving infants, 30–50% have moderate to severe disability. The EP will encounter these children after hospital discharge. Common medical issues in children with a history of prematurity include:

- respiratory problems: bronchopulmonary dysplasia, oxygen dependence, airway hyperreactivity
  - children born before 32 weeks of gestation qualify for palivizumab (Synagis) administration monthly to prevent respiratory syncytial virus infection in a vulnerable population; this has only a moderate effect on preventing severe disease, and such infections are common despite adequate coverage with palivizumab
- CNS problems: intraventricular hemorrhage, periventricular leukomalacia: cerebral palsy, hydrocephalus, seizure disorder, CNS shunts
- visual impairment: retinopathy of prematurity, occipital cortical damage
- hearing impairment
- global developmental delay
- feeding difficulties:
  - inability to protect the airway during feeding
  - dysphagia with G-tube feeding dependence
  - severe gastroesophageal reflux disease:
  - constipation
- technology malfunction: CNS shunts, G-tubes, tracheostomy.

Selected reference

American Academy of Pediatrics. *Committee on Fetus and Newborn.* http://www.aap.org/visit/cmte17.htm (accessed 29 April 2010).

Severe gastroesophageal reflux

Indications for treating a child with severe gastroesophageal reflux include poor weight gain, pain, or interference with normal activities. Common initial choices are ranitidine 1 mg/kg per dose given BID in combination with a proton pump inhibitor (lansoprazole) and a promotility agent. Metoclopramide is the most commonly used promotility agent but has been associated with severe dystonic reactions and oculogyric crisis. Erythomycin at 5 mg/kg per dose given QID can be used as an alternative but is associated with development of pyloric stenosis if given to young infants.

Pearls and pitfalls

Pearls

1. Aspiration of food and mucus are major causes of respiratory worsening in a child from neonatal intensive care with respiratory distress.
2. Intercurrent illnesses can lower the seizure threshold and cause a "breakthrough seizure."
3. Signs of respiratory distress such as retractions or accessory muscle use may be absent in children with neuromuscular diseases.
4. Children born before 32 weeks of gestation should be receiving palivizumab monthly after discharge.

Pitfalls

1. Failure to evaluate vital signs carefully, and in comparison to the patient's baseline vital signs from past visits.
2. Failure to consider infection in any child with indwelling catheters or shunts.
3. Failure to involve parents in decision making regarding the medical workup.

A Practical Guide to Pediatric Emergency Medicine: Caring for Children in the Emergency Department, ed. N. Ewen Amieva-Wang (associate eds. Jamie Shandro, Aparajita Sohoni, and Bernhard Fassl). Published by Cambridge University Press.

Chapter 165

Short gut syndrome and parenteral feeding dependence

Bernhard Fassl and Nancy Murphy

Introduction

Short gut syndrome is the result of extensive loss of small bowel in early childhood. The most common causes are necrotizing enterocolitis of prematurity, with subsequent bowel necrosis, and intestinal malrotation and volvulus with bowel necrosis. Because there is a reduction in small intestine surface area available for food absorption most children with short gut syndrome are dependent on parenteral nutrition for a significant amount of time. This requires long-term central line placement.

Clinical presentation

The EP is usually confronted with three clinical scenarios.

Fever. Central line infections are exceedingly common in short gut syndrome. Prompt evaluation should include a blood culture obtained centrally and peripherally, a CBC and CRP. Empiric antibiotics should cover *Staphylococcus aureus*, *Staphylococcus epidermidis* and include Gram-negative bacteria such as *Escherichia coli* and *Klebsiella* and *Pseudomonas* spp. Common treatment combinations include piperacillin/tazobactam and gentamicin or vancomycin and cefotaxime.

Swelling of the neck, face or upper extremity. Superior vena cava syndrome is a common complication of long-term indwelling catheters. Prompt recognition of the condition, removal of the catheter, and institution of anticoagulation are the mainstays of treatment.

Worsening jaundice. Children dependent on total parenteral nutrition experience bile stasis with subsequent liver damage. Liver enzyme elevations are common. Children who present with progressive jaundice should be evaluated for sudden changes in serum liver enzyme elevation (addition of other medications may have caused additional hepatotoxicity) and coagulopathy. A PT prolongation is most indicative of liver synthetic dysfunction.

A Practical Guide to Pediatric Emergency Medicine: Caring for Children in the Emergency Department, ed. N. Ewen Amieva-Wang (associate eds. Jamie Shandro, Aparajita Sohoni, and Bernhard Fassl). Published by Cambridge University Press.

Chapter 166 Cystic fibrosis

Bernhard Fassl

Introduction

Cystic fibrosis (CF) is a chronic multisystem disorder characterized by recurrent endobronchial infections, progressive obstructive pulmonary disease, and pancreatic insufficiency with intestinal malabsorption.

Cystic fibrosis is the result of an autosomal recessive genetic defect in the gene for the cystic fibrosis transmembrane conductance regulator (CFTR; a cyclic AMP-mediated chloride channel). The gene is found on chromosome 7. The malfunction in CFTR causes abnormal chloride ion transport on the apical surface of epithelial cells in exocrine gland tissues, leading to abnormally viscous secretions. Over 1500 mutations have been identified; the most common mutation is ΔF508, which results in deletion of a single phenylalanine residue at amino acid 508 of CFTR.

Epidemiology

Worldwide incidence of CF varies from 1 per 377 live births in parts of England (1 in 2400 in the UK as a whole) to 1 per 90 000 Asian live births in Hawaii. Whites are most often affected, at a rate of approximately 1 per 3500 births. Incidence is also high for Hispanics, at a rate of 1 per 9500 live births, but CF is quite rare in native Asians and Africans (<1 per 15 000 births).

Diagnosis

Cystic fibrosis is diagnosed through the **sweat chloride test.** Sweat chloride values >60 mEq/l are diagnostic, while values <30 mEq/l are within the normal range. Values between 30 and 60 mEq/l are equivocal and may represent heterozygous carriers or may be suspicious of occult disease. The diagnosis of CF is confirmed through genetic testing of known mutations.

Commonly affected organs

Cystic fibrosis is a multiorgan disease (Table 166.1) but not all organs are affected equally in all patients. Some patients have symptoms predominantly in certain organ systems and lack of involvement of others. Although CF is known as a disease that mainly affects the lungs, some patients have a remarkably low degree of lung disease while exhibiting all the signs of pancreatic dysfunction.

Clinical presentation

Known cystic fibrosis

Table 166.2 provides an overview of common presentations of patients with known CF.

Suspected cystic fibrosis

Suspicion of cystic fibrosis is often raised by the EP. The following is a list of presenting signs that warrant further evaluation for CF and specialist referral:

- neonate with conjugated or prolonged hyperbilirubinemia
- neonate with meconium ileus or delayed passage of stool after birth (>24 h)
- infant with significant hyponatremia
- infant with rectal prolapse
- child with "asthma," recurrent wheezing, and poor weight gain or signs of intestinal malabsorption
- child with recurrent sino-pulmonary infections
- child with digital clubbing
- child with evidence of chronic lung disease or bronchiectasis on chest radiograph.

Table 166.3 gives the incidence of presenting signs in CF.

Selected problems

Respiratory distress

Respiratory distress is the most common presentation of a patient with CF to the ED. Bacterial colonization/overgrowth of pathogens that colonize the lungs in CF are common, resulting in a pulmonary exacerbation of CF lung disease. Exacerbations are more common in children with poor

A Practical Guide to Pediatric Emergency Medicine: Caring for Children in the Emergency Department, ed. N. Ewen Amieva-Wang (associate eds. Jamie Shandro, Aparajita Sohoni, and Bernhard Fassl). Published by Cambridge University Press.

Table 166.1. Organ system effects of cystic fibrosis

Organ system	Complication	Presentation
Lung disease	Lung colonization with bacteria and fungi, recurrent pneumonia, bronchiectasis, allergic bronchopulmonary aspergillosis	Repeated infections, hemoptysis, digital clubbing, pneumothorax, wheezing
Sinus disease	Chronic sinusitis, nasal polyps	Recurrent sinus infections
Pancreas exocrine	Food malabsorption, malabsorption of fat-soluble vitamins (A, D, E, K), pancreatitis	Failure to thrive, greasy foul-smelling stool, rickets, visual disturbances, coagulopathy
Pancreas endocrine	Cystic fibrosis related diabetes mellitus	Glucose intolerance, diabetes mellitus
Intestinal	Meconium ileus, distal ileal obstruction syndrome, rectal prolapse, intussusception, colonic strictures, appendicitis	Emesis (often bilious), intestinal obstruction, delayed passage of stool after birth, colicky RLQ pain (presentation resembling appendicitis), constipation
Hepatobiliary	Bile stasis, focal biliary cirrhosis, gallstones	Conjugated neonatal hyperbilirubinemia and jaundice, impaired liver function, RUQ abdominal pain
Reproductive	Delayed puberty, azoospermia and infertility (95% of males, 20% females)	
Sweat gland, electrolytes	Excessive sodium and chloride losses	Hyponatremia (particularly in small infants), hyponatremic seizures or coma

Table 166.2. Common presentations of patients with known cystic fibrosis

Presenting sign	Common causes	Suggested workup
Respiratory distress	Exacerbation of chronic lung disease, pneumonia (bacterial, viral, fungal, mycobacterial)	Chest radiograph Induced sputum culture, viral testing of sputum, acid-fast bacilli stain and mycobacterium culture
Hemoptysis	Bronchopulmonary dysplasia (minor), hemoptysis (common in advanced disease)	Chest CT angiogram For severe hemoptysis: hematocrit, prothrombin time, partial thromboplastin time
Wheezing	Intercurrent viral illness, reactive airway disease, allergic bronchopulmonary aspergillosis	Chest radiograph Induced sputum culture, viral testing of sputum Spirometry, screen for aspergillosis
Conjugated hyperbilirubinemia	Bile stasis	LFTs, liver ultrasound
Seizures, mental status change	Severe hyponatremia resulting from intestinal, dermal, and pulmonary salt losses	Electrolyte panel Renal function testing
Emesis, abdominal pain	Meconium ileus, distal intestinal obstruction syndrome, pancreatitis	Abdominal radiograph Surgery consultation

adherence to chronic treatment regimens. These recurrent pneumonias contribute to the worsening of the overall lung function and formation of bronchiectatic changes.

It is important to determine whether bronchospastic findings are present at the time of presentation. Airway reactivity and asthma-like symptoms are common in patients with CF and require treatment with bronchodilators and possibly a steroid burst. Allergic bronchopulmonary aspergillosis is a disease that needs to be considered in all children with CF and wheezing.

Diagnostic studies

The initial evaluation in the ED should include:

- chest radiograph to determine presence of new pulmonary infiltrates

Table 166.3. Incidence of gastro intestinal presenting signs in cystic fibrosis

	Incidence (%)
Liver disease	20–50
Distal ileal obstruction syndrome	2–47
Biliary disease, gallstones	30
Rectal prolapse	20
Meconium ileus	10–20
Appendicitis	1–2
Intussusception	1
Pancreatic complications	0.5
Colonic strictures	Rare

- induced sputum culture, fungal culture, acid-fast bacilli stain, and mycobacterial culture
- viral testing of sputum if seasonally indicated: influenza, respiratory syncytial virus, parainfluenza, adenovirus, human metapneumovirus
- review of chronic CF medications and compliance with chest clearance measures (chest physiotherapy, vest treatment)
- additional testing as indicated according to the patient's condition: blood gas analysis, CBC.

Management

Antibiotic choice is complicated by the fact that the bacteria that colonize the lungs of patients with CF are usually resistant to treatments of choice for community-acquired pneumonia. Common pathogens in sputum samples of children admitted for CF exacerbations include *Pseudomonas aeruginosa*, *Staphylococcus aureus* (both methicillin resistant and sensitive), *Escherichia coli*, *Burkholderia cepacia*, *Stenotrophomonas maltophilia*, and other mostly Gram-negative bacteria.

The difference in the microbial spectrum alters the choice of empiric antibiotic coverage. If the last available sputum culture result is available, the EP should review this to decide about empiric initial antibiotic coverage. Commonly used initial antibiotic combinations include tobramycin and ticarcillin/clavulanic acid or ceftazidime and tobramycin.

Disposition

The decision about the need for hospital admission should be made in conjunction with the family and the CF specialist. Common indications for admission include:

- oxygen requirement
- significant respiratory distress, impending respiratory decompensation
- need for IV antibiotic coverage
- poor compliance with chronic medications.

Abdominal pain

A child with CF who presents with abdominal pain, distention, or vomiting presents a diagnostic challenge. CF predisposes children to a number of conditions, such as bowel obstruction and intussusception.

Diagnostic studies

In view of the difficulty in diagnosing the GI conditions in patients with CF and severe colicky abdominal pain, the initial ED evaluation should include

- abdominal radiograph: signs of bowel obstruction
- LFTs, amylase, lipase
- contrast enema to exclude intussusception; this may also relieve obstruction in distal intestinal obstruction syndrome or reduce the intussusception
- if contrast enema is unsuccessful, ultrasound or CT should be performed to look for other causes.

Management: distal ileal obstruction syndrome

Episodes of small bowel obstruction may occur in older children and adults. These have been termed "meconium ileus equivalent" or distal ileal obstruction syndrome. The obstruction occurs in up to 15% of adults with CF. Normally it can be managed conservatively. Treatment involves rehydration and the use of oral gastrograffin or *N*-acetylcysteine.

Meconium ileus

Meconium ileus is the presenting problem in 10–20% of newborns with CF and is virtually pathognomonic for disease.

Pearls and pitfalls

Pearls

1. Neonates with delayed passage of stool, rectal prolapse, hyponatremia, or children with recurrent respiratory infections and failure to gain weight appropriately should be referred for testing for cystic fibrosis.
2. Consider allergic bronchopulmonary aspergillosis in all children with cystic fibrosis and wheezing.
3. If available, the most recent sputum culture results should be used to guide selection of antibiotics during a cystic fibrosis respiratory exacerbation.

Pitfalls

1. Failure to consider cystic fibrosis in a child with poor weight gain and failure to thrive.
2. Failure to consider ileus/obstruction/intussusception in the workup of a child with cystic fibrosis and abdominal pain.
3. Failure to take any respiratory symptom, or change in respiratory status, seriously in a child with cystic fibrosis.

All CF mutations predispose to the development of meconium ileus. Meconium ileus can be categorized as either simple or complicated. Complicated meconium ileus includes those with volvulus, atresia, perforation, or giant cystic peritonitis.

Diagnostic studies

Abdominal radiograph is likely to show several loops of dilated small bowel without air–fluid levels; and possibly a soap bubble appearance in the RLQ, the so-called Neuhauser sign. Complicated meconium ileus may present with large bowel dilatation and air–fluid levels. Perforation or giant cystic meconium peritonitis calcifications are often noted. Most babies then undergo barium enema to confirm the diagnosis.

Management

The initial management of a neonate with abdominal distention and other features of obstruction includes fluid resuscitation, nasogastric tube insertion, and antibiotic administration. Gastrograffin enemas are the treatment of choice in simple meconium ileus. The iatrogenic perforation rate is approximately 5%. All neonates with complications and those with two unsuccessful enemas require operative intervention. The surgical management options for meconium ileus are varied and include (1) enterotomy/appendectomy with irrigation, (2) enterostomy with/without resection, and (3) resection with primary anastomosis. Infants with CF who present with meconium ileus (MI) and survive beyond 6 months have the same prognosis as any patient with CF, although they are at greater risk of developing distal intestinal obstruction syndrome in later life.

Chapter 167

Genetic disease in the pediatric emergency department

Alan F. Rope

Introduction

With the advancement of modern medicine and increased understanding of human genetics, an increased number of children with known genetic syndromes will present to the ED. This chapter gives a brief definition of terminology, describes important co-morbid features associated with specific syndromes and then describes common presentations of children with different syndromes.

Terminology

Anomaly. An irregularity of structure, the etiology of which is unspecified, with no indication as to whether it is a malformation or a deformation.

Malformation. Implies that the structure was made incorrectly because of an intrinsic process.

Deformation. Implies that the structure was programmed to be made correctly but was altered by external factors.

Sequence. A non-random pattern of anomalies that can be explained by a single disruption of morphogenesis, which subsequently caused a cascade of effects.

Syndrome. A non-random pattern of anomalies that can be attributed to an identifiable etiology or demonstrates a recognizable pattern of inheritance.

Association. A non-random pattern of anomalies that occurs without an identifiable etiology or heritability being established.

Catabolism. In this context refers to the physiologic process of breaking down larger molecules into smaller molecules with the primary goal of releasing stored energy in situations when metabolic demand exceeds exogenous caloric supply.

Clinical presentation

Table 167.1 give the co-morbid features and common presentations for a number of genetic disorders.

Co-morbid features of syndromic anomalies

General features

Disorders of growth are common, with growth failure being most likely (this can occur in the well-nourished state). Many syndromes have a higher lifetime incidence of endocrine dysregulation. Presentations may be insidious as in hypothyroidism and growth hormone deficiency, or more dramatic as with adrenal insufficiency or hypocalcemia. In syndromic patients, the following are always worthy of consideration:

- airway compromise
- infection of the respiratory and/or urinary tracts
- electrolyte and/or endocrine imbalance
- cardiovascular decompensation
- another congenital anomaly (one anomaly should increase suspicion for another).

Neurologic features

Because more than half of the >25 000 genes in humans are required for normal brain development and function, there is a high likelihood for various neurologic sequelae including hypotonia, dysautonomia, seizures, and mental retardation. Individuals with a chronic neuropathic state are at a greater risk for aspiration pneumonias, chronic lung disease, a high pain tolerance and an inability to perceive or communicate symptoms of illness. It is also important to remember that these individuals are more likely to have psychiatric disturbance and have many factors increasing their vulnerability to abuse.

Cardiac features

Many syndromes have associated cardiovascular anomalies, some of which are not congenital and represent a dynamic process. Hypoxia, cardiogenic shock, arrhythmia, pulmonary and systemic hypertension, and vascular integrity in the case of connective tissue disorders are all possible complications of cardiovascular anomalies.

A Practical Guide to Pediatric Emergency Medicine: Caring for Children in the Emergency Department, ed. N. Ewen Amieva-Wang (associate eds. Jamie Shandro, Aparajita Sohoni, and Bernhard Fassl). Published by Cambridge University Press.

Table 167.1. Features of genetic disorders

Genetic disorder	Co-morbid features	Common presentations
Trisomy 21 (Down syndrome)	Congenital heart disease: ventricular septal defect	Congestive heart failure
	Pulmonary hypertension	Respiratory distress, shock, cyanosis
	Severe constipation	Abdominal pain
	Cervical instability	Neck pain with trauma
Trisomy 13 and 18	Central apnea	Apnea, ALTE
	Aspiration pneumonia	Respiratory distress
	Congenital heart disease	Congestive heart failure, respiratory distress, shock, cyanosis
Velocardiofacial syndrome (DiGeorge/22q11DS)	Congenital heart disease: ventricular septal defect, conotruncal defects	Congestive heart failure, respiratory distress, shock, cyanosis
	Hypocalcemia	Tetany, seizures
	Respiratory tract infection	Respiratory distress
	Behavioral decompensation	
Williams syndrome	Congenital heart disease: supravalvular aortic stenosis	Congestive heart failure, respiratory distress, shock, cyanosis
	Hypercalcemia	Fussiness
	Failure to thrive	
	Infantile inconsolabilty	
Turner syndrome	Coarctation of aorta	Congestive heart failure
	Bicuspid aortic valve	Hypertension
	Failure to thrive	
Neurofibromatosis type 1	Pain and deficits associated with CNS tumors, chronic pain, migraine headaches	Headaches, neurologic deficits
Tuberous sclerosis	Seizure disorder	Seizures
	Renal angiomyolipomas	Hematuria
	Cardiac rhabdomyomas	Cardiac arrest outflow tract obstruction
Marfan syndrome	Mitral valve prolapse	Congestive heart failure, respiratory distress, shock, cyanosis
	Aortic dissection	Sudden onset chest pain with radiation to back
Ehlers–Danlos syndrome(s)	Visceral perforation	Acute abdomen
	Arterial rupture, abdominal aortic aneurysm/rupture, aortic dissection	Hypotension and shock, chest pain
Achondroplasia	Obstructive hydrocephalus, spinal cord compression at the foramen magnum	Headache, ALTE, neurologic deficits
Hurler and Hunter syndromes (mucopolysaccharidosis I and II)	Acquired hydrocephalus	Headache, ALTE, neurologic deficits
	Cardiac involvement	Congestive heart failure
	Lung infiltration, airway obstruction	Respiratory distress
Prader–Willi syndrome	Failure-to-thrive	As infant; later obesity
	Obstructive apnea	Apnea, snoring
	Behavioral decompensation	
	Developmental delay	

Table 167.1. *(cont.)*

Genetic disorder	Co-morbid features	Common presentations
Angelman syndrome	Seizure disorder	Seizures
	Aspiration	Respiratory distress
	Developmental delay	
Rett syndrome	Seizure disorder	Seizures
	Aspiration	Respiratory distress
	Failure to thrive	
	Developmental delay	

ALTE, acute life-threatening event.

Gastrointestinal features

There can be feeding problems leading to aspiration and/or malnutrition, gastroesophageal reflux, delayed gastric emptying, and constipation.

Genitourinary features

Even in non-syndromic individuals, anomalies of the genitourinary system are relatively common, but they are even more so within this cohort. Renal malformation and/or dysplasia and vesicourethral reflux can lead to frequent urinary tract infections and electrolyte disturbances.

Eyes, nose, and throat

Otitis media, palate anomalies and airway accessibility and instability should always be a consideration.

Presentations associated with difficult intubation include conditions with the Robin anomaly, Goldenhar/oculo–auriculo–vertebral association, Beckwith–Wiedemann syndrome, and advanced storage disease (Hurler, Hunter, Pompe syndromes).

Careful intubation (because of the potential for spinal cord injury) is required in Down syndrome, achondroplasia, and other skeletal dysplasias.

Pearls and pitfalls

Pearls

1. Intubating a child with a genetic syndrome is frequently complex, and the EP should be prepared with a difficult airway set-up.

Pitfalls

1. Failure to consider the presence of anomalies in one organ system because of the known anomalies in another.
2. Failure to consider cardiac abnormalities in the patient with respiratory distress.

Chapter 168

Inborn errors of metabolism

Renata C. Gallagher and Carol L. Greene

Introduction

Inborn errors of metabolism (IEM) are a heterogeneous group of diseases. Most are single enzyme or transport protein defects that result in a block of a biochemical pathway. The biochemical block may result in elevations of toxic metabolites or in deficiencies of important compounds. The consequences may include hypoglycemia, hyperammonemia, metabolic acidosis, developmental delay, and/or organ dysfunction (liver, kidney, heart). While each individual defect is rare, the overall incidence of these disorders is greater than 1 in 3000. It is crucial that EPs are familiar with the signs and symptoms of these disorders and the need for rapid triage, evaluation, and treatment. Delay in evaluation and management may result in irreversible neurologic damage or death.

Overview of disorders

Tables 168.1 and 168.2 give an overview of metabolic disorders and their related clincial symptoms.

Amino acid disorders

Amino acid disorders have variable presentations. Phenylketonuria causes mental retardation and is not associated with systemic illness, while maple syrup urine disease may cause progressive neurologic symptoms through elevated leucine levels. Tyrosinemia type 1 may cause liver and kidney failure, and classic homocystinuria is associated with skeletal findings (long fingers, scoliosis), seizures, and thrombosis. Amino acid disorders can be diagnosed by plasma amino acid analysis and urine organic acid analysis.

Organic acidurias

Most organic acidurias are also the result of a block in amino acid (protein) metabolism. After the amine group has been removed, the compound is an organic acid. Specific biochemical blocks, therefore, result in characteristic elevations of organic acids. These organic acids can themselves be harmful and can cause secondary metabolic derangements: hypoglycemia, hyperammonemia, lactic acidosis, neutropenia, and ketonuria. In the newborn period, the marked secondary elevation of ammonia can make these disorders difficult to distinguish from urea cycle disorders.

If there is significant acidosis with elevated anion gap in the first several days of life, it is crucial to send for ammonia and lactate analysis, and urine for organic acid analysis, to evaluate for an organic acid metabolism disorder.

Organic acidurias can be diagnosed by urine organic acid analysis and plasma acylcarnitine profile.

Urea cycle disorders

The urea cycle functions to rid the body of waste ammonia, a product of amino acid metabolism. A deficiency of any of the enzymes of the urea cycle can result in hyperammonemia. Urea cycle disorders may present at any age, as some enzyme deficiencies may be mild, and female carriers of ornithine transcarbamylase deficiency may have a late-onset presentation. Severe disorders present in the first 2–5 days of life with progressive neurologic symptoms, including obtundation, vomiting, and seizures.

It is critical to specifically order a serum ammonia measurement in anyone with unexplained altered mental status, seizures, vomiting, or progressive neurologic symptoms.

The most common urea cycle defect (ornithine transcarbamylase deficiency) is X-linked. There may be a family history of neonatal male deaths. These disorders can often be diagnosed by the combination of plasma amino acid analysis and urine orotic acid analysis. Definitive diagnosis may require enzyme assay or DNA sequencing.

Fat metabolism

Fat is an important source of energy that is used by the liver for ketone production and by the heart and skeletal muscle for energy production. Therefore, disorders of fat metabolism are associated with three distinct clinical presentations:

- hepatic presentation manifests with hypoglycemia in conjunction with inappropriately low ketones; there may

A Practical Guide to Pediatric Emergency Medicine: Caring for Children in the Emergency Department, ed. N. Ewen Amieva-Wang (associate eds. Jamie Shandro, Aparajita Sohoni, and Bernhard Fassl). Published by Cambridge University Press.

Table 168.1. Overview of metabolic disorders.

	Amino acid disorders	Organic acidurias	Urea cycle disorders	Carbohydrate metabolism disorders	Fat metabolism disorders
Pathology	Elevation of one or more amino acids, or side-products	Accumulation of abnormal organic acids, secondary elevations of ammonia, lactate, ketones	Hyperammonemia	Abnormal metabolism of glycogen, galactose, fructose, or production of glucose; resulting in hypoglycemia, or toxicity of abnormal sugars	Inability to fully utilize fat for energy, may result in cardiomyopathy (long-chain defects), skeletal myopathy, hypoketotic hypoglycemia
Examples	Phenylketonuria, maple syrup urine disease, homocystinuria tyrosinemia	MMA, PA, IVA, GA1	Ornithine transcarbamylase deficiency, carbamylphosphate synthase 1 deficiency, citrullinemia type 1, argininosuccinate lyase deficiency	GSD1, HFI, galactosemia	Medium-chain, very-long-chain, long-chain 3-hydroxyacyl-CoA dehydrogenase deficiency; carnitine transporter deficiency
Onset/ presentation	Variable onset and symptoms (see text)	MMA, PA, IVA may present with neonatal or later-onset metabolic acidosis, hypoglycemia, hyperammonemia; GA1 classically presents with dystonia after an illness at 6 months to 2 years	Neonates present in the first few days of life with poor feeding progressing to seizures and coma; older individuals may present with seizures, vomiting, hallucinations	GSD1 may present in infancy with hypoglycemia and acidosis; galactosemia may present with liver and kidney dysfunction; HFI presents after fructose has been introduced	May present with hypoglycemia at 6–18 months of age when the nighttime feeding interval is increased; cardiomyopathy may be early or late; rhabdomyolysis with stress or infection
Routine laboratories	Elevated homocysteine in homocystinuria otherwise unremarkable	Metabolic acidosis, with increased anion gap, hyperammonemia, ketosis, hypoglycemia, neutropenia in MMA, PA, IVA	Hyperammonemia, respiratory alkalosis, absence of marked ketosis or acidosis; liver dysfunction/failure in some cases	Hypoglycemia, lactic acidosis, elevated uric acid and triglycerides in GSD1a; liver and kidney dysfunction in galactosemia; renal Fanconi syndrome in HFI; reducing substances in urine in HFI and galactosemia	Hypoketotic hypoglycemia, elevated creatine phosphokinase, elevated lactate, metabolic acidosis, mild hyperammonemia, liver dysfunction
Biochemical laboratories	Abnormal plasma amino acids with characteristic elevations; abnormal urine organic acids in some disorders	Abnormal urine organic acid analysis, abnormal acylcarnitine profile	Characteristic pattern of plasma amino acids; elevated urine orotic acid in some disorders	No specific abnormalities on screening laboratories, specialized testing required	Abnormal acylcarnitine profile, abnormal urine organic acid analysis, abnormal carnitine panel (total and free)

GA1, glutaric aciduria type 1; GSD1, glycogen storage disease type 1; HFI, hereditary fructose intolerance; IVA, isovaleric aciduria; MMA, methylmalonic aciduria; PA, propionic aciduria.

Table 168.2. Association of inborn errors of metabolism and clinical symptoms

Progressive neurologic deterioration	Hypoglycemia	Organ dysfunction[a]
Urea cycle defect (hyperammonemia)	Fatty acid oxidation or carnitine cycle disorder	Cardiomyopathy (fatty acid oxidation disorders, carnitine cycle disorders, organic acidurias, glycogen storage disease, lysosomal storage diseases, mitochondrial energy metabolism disorders)
Maple syrup urine disease (leucine encephalopathy)	Glycogen storage disease	Liver failure (fatty acid oxidation disorders, urea cycle disorders, tyrosinemia, hereditary fructose intolerance, galactosemia, mitochondrial energy metabolism disorders, peroxisomal disorders)
Organic acidemia (hyperammonemia)	Gluconeogenesis defect	Renal tubular acidosis (glycogen storage disease type 1, mitochondrial energy metabolism disorders, tyrosinemia, galactosemia, hereditary fructose intolerance)

[a]Lysosomal storage diseases, mitochondrial energy metabolism disorders, and peroxisomal disorders are not otherwise addressed in this chapter as specific management is limited and diagnostic evaluation is complex. It is important to provide glucose and monitor for acidosis in a child with a known or suspected mitochondrial disorder.

also be mild metabolic acidosis, elevated AST and ALT, and hyperammonemia (Reye-like syndrome)

- cardiac presentation manifests with cardiomyopathy and is also associated with arrhythmias
- muscular presentation manifests with cramps and rhabdomyolysis.

These disorders are often the result of a deficiency of one of the enzymes of the fatty acid oxidation cycle, which generates ketones from fat in the mitochondria. Some individuals have a defect in the carnitine cycle. This prevents fat from entering fatty acid oxidation as carnitine is required to shuttle fat across the mitochondrial membranes. A classic presentation of medium-chain acyl-CoA dehydrogenase deficiency, the most common fatty acid oxidation disorder, is of lethargy and hypoketotic hypoglycemia during mild intercurrent illness at 6–18 months of age. At this time, feedings are less frequent and illness is more common; this may result in decreased appetite and intake. Fatty acid oxidation and carnitine cycle disorders are diagnosed by plasma acylcarnitine profile, total and free serum carnitine levels, and urine organic acid analysis. Urine acylglycines may be a useful adjunct test. Definitive diagnosis may require further studies.

Carbohydrate metabolism

Carbohydrate disorders include glycogen storage diseases, which may result in hypoglycemia, as well as galactosemia, and hereditary fructose intolerance, in which toxic metabolites accumulate as by-products of blocked galactose or fructose metabolism. The most common glycogen storage disease, type 1a, is associated with lactic acidosis, hypoglycemia, failure to thrive and "cherubic" facies. Galactosemia may present in the first weeks of life with indirect hyperbilirubinemia, elevated transaminases and liver dysfunction/failure. *Escherichia coli* sepsis may occur more commonly in individuals with galactosemia. Hereditary fructose intolerance does not manifest until fructose enters the diet. Disorders of gluconeogenesis such as fructose-1,6-bisphosphatase deficiency (not a disorder of fructose metabolism) present with acidosis and hypoglycemia.

Clinical presentation

There are three situations in which children with inborn errors of metabolism will present to the ED:

- individuals who have unrecognized inborn errors of metabolism
- individuals with known diagnoses and current or impending decompensation
- those referred for evaluation of abnormal newborn screens.

History

The majority of inborn errors are inherited in an autosomal recessive manner. Siblings may also be affected, and there may be a history of a previous sibling death. Some disorders are more common in certain ethnic groups.

Although these results are usually not available to the ED, it is important to emphasize that a normal newborn screen does *not* rule out an inborn error. Newborn screening for inborn errors of metabolism is not uniform throughout the country. Not all inborn errors are on the screening panel; not all forms of all disorders that are screened for are detected, and there may be false-negative results. Any child with symptoms suggestive of an inborn error should have appropriate diagnostic testing regardless of their newborn screen result. Finally, in severe inborn errors, neonates may present symptomatically in the first few days of life before the results of the newborn screen have been obtained.

Physical examination

Some individuals will present to the ED with decompensation and will not have a known diagnosis. Inborn errors of metabolism may present at any age, but severe defects of urea cycle, amino acid, organic acid, fat, or carbohydrate metabolism generally present in the first few days or weeks of life.

There are two peaks in presentation. The first is typically just after birth after a period of normal behavior and feeding during which the abnormal metabolites accumulate sufficiently to cause symptoms. The second peak is between 6 and 18 months of age, when feedings are less frequent and mild intercurrent illness is more common and may result in decreased appetite and intake.

Some individuals have a subacute, late-onset presentation. They may have pre-existing developmental delay, seizures, or hypotonia, with worsening of symptoms in illness. It is important to have a high index of suspicion for an inborn error of metabolism in children with abnormal development or an abnormal neurologic history. Often these children will be resuscitated and history, physical, and baseline laboratory values will prompt suspicion of, and further workup for, an inborn error of metabolism.

Individuals with a known inborn error should have a letter from their metabolic clinic that describes their disorder, outlines symptoms expected in illness, delineates the initial laboratory evaluation and management in illness, and includes contact information for the on-call metabolic physician. The metabolic physician should be contacted simultaneously with ED evaluation. It is important that the EP listens to the parents as they know the triggers and pattern of their child in a decompensation as well as measures that can help to reverse the process (See also Ch. 162).

Decompensation may be triggered by any of multiple factors, particularly intercurrent illness, stress, prolonged fasting, or dietary change.

Some individuals may be referred to the ED for evaluation for an abnormal newborn screen. In these cases, the metabolic clinic will recommend follow-up laboratory tests and request a clinical evaluation – for adequacy of feeding, alertness, presence of tachypnea, and jaundice. The likelihood of a true abnormal result varies with the specific disorder, the metabolic clinic can provide guidance regarding this.

Diagnostic studies

If there is unexplained altered mental status, blood sugar and ammonia should be rapidly measured. A blood gas is indicated if there is tachypnea or respiratory distress. Recommendations for laboratory testing are given in Tables 168.3 and 168.4. Initial test results may prompt further evaluation for an inborn error if the patient does not have a known diagnosis. For example, a primary respiratory alkalosis is a hallmark of neonatal-onset urea cycle disorders; ammonia stimulates the respiratory center, and a serum ammonia level should be obtained. Anion gap metabolic acidosis, particularly when the acidosis is severe in a neonate, suggests an organic aciduria or a primary lactic acidosis; it is important to check ammonia, lactate and urine organic acids. Hypoglycemia with low urine ketones and elevated AST and ALT suggests a fat metabolism disorder.

In some cases, the diagnostic elevations of compounds in blood or urine are seen only in illness and may not be present when the patient is stable on the ward the next morning. The EP is presented with a unique opportunity to aid in diagnosis by ensuring that metabolic laboratory tests are ordered (Table 168.4).

Often tests cannot be ordered immediately; in this case urine and plasma should be obtained and frozen, if possible prior to initiating treatment, but this should not delay treatment.

Table 168.3. Recommended laboratory tests for diagnosis and treatment of a child with known or suspected inborn error of metabolism at the emergency department

Test	Evaluate for
Glucose	Hypo/hyperglycemia
Electrolytes/BUN and creatinine	Acidosis/anion gap/renal function
Calcium	Hypocalcemia
LFTs including bilirubin	Liver dysfunction/cholestasis
Urinalysis	Ketones, reducing substances
Lactate	Lactic acidemia
CBC	Marrow suppression/infection
Ammonia	Hyperammonemia
Blood gas	Acid–base status
Creatine phosphokinase	Rhabdomyolysis
Prothrombin time/partial thromboplastin time	Liver dysfunction, disseminated intravascular coagulation
Amylase/lipase	Pancreatitis
Uric acid	Elevation
Triglycerides	Elevation
Homocysteine	Elevation

Table 168.4. Specific biochemical tests used in evaluation of known or suspected inborn errors of metabolism

Test	Evaluate for
Plasma amino acids	Amino acid disorders, urea cycle defects
Urine organic acids	Organic acid and fat metabolism disorders
Urine orotic acid	Urea cycle defects
Plasma acylcarnitine profile	Fat metabolism and organic acid disorders
Plasma total and free carnitine	Carnitine transporter deficiency, renal tubulopathy
Urine acylglycines	Organic acid and fat metabolism disorders

Box 168.1. Algorithm for acute treatment of known or suspected inborn error of metabolism

1. Follow recommended ED protocol if provided by metabolic clinic in known inborn errors.
2. Contact metabolic physician urgently for symptomatic hyperammonemia or severe neonatal metabolic acidosis.
3. Stop possibly harmful precursors: protein (amino acid disorders, organic acidemias, urea cycle disorders), fat (fatty acid oxidation and carnitine cycle disorders) and galactose and fructose (if possible galactosemia or hereditary fructose intolerance).
4. Provide 10% dextrose and appropriate electrolytes at 1.5× maintenance.
5. Correct electrolyte abnormalities and acidosis without the use of boluses if possible as cerebral edema may be present.
6. Provide carnitine at 25–400 mg/kg daily (organic acid or fat metabolism disorder).
7. Provide vitamin cofactors if proven or suspected responsiveness.

Urine is frozen as a 2–5 ml sample and plasma as a 2–5 ml sample in a green top (ethylenediaminetetracetic acid [EDTA]) tube. As these test results will usually return within 1–2 weeks in a non-urgent situation and will not be available to help with acute diagnosis in the ED, the primary care physician should be alerted to follow them up. However, if there is hyperammonemia or severe unexplained acidosis, the metabolic service should be contacted urgently, and test results will be expedited.

Management

After initial resuscitation according to the standard ABCs, the goal for a patient with a known or suspected inborn error is early intervention and prevention of further decompensation and severe sequelae (Box 168.1). Hypoglycemia should be treated with 25% dextrose 1 ml/kg IV push followed by maintenance glucose. A precipitating illness should be identified and treated. Broad-spectrum antibiotics should be given if there is a possibility of bacterial infection.

The initial treatment for disorders of the urea cycle, amino acid and fat metabolism consists of stopping the harmful exogenous precursors, protein or fat, and providing glucose to supply approximately half to two-thirds of daily calories, given as 10% dextrose with ¼ to ½ normal saline at 1.5× maintenance. It is important to correct electrolyte imbalances and acidosis. Note that cerebral edema may be present in a decompensation in these disorders; therefore, rapid correction and overhydration should be avoided. Correction of acidosis can be facilitated by supplying bicarbonate or acetate in the IV fluid as part of the maintenance electrolyte requirement. The administration of bicarbonate as a bolus is controversial. Reversing catabolism, which results in the breakdown of endogenous offending precursors, is critical to management of these disorders; therefore, glucose infusion should be maintained. If there is hyperglycemia, insulin can be administered to maintain glucose levels between 120 and 170 mg/dl; insulin also promotes anabolism. The starting dose is 0.05 U/kg per h. Calories may also be given in the form of intralipids for individuals with urea cycle, amino acid, or organic acid disorders at 2–3 g/kg daily. Intralipids should be administered cautiously in known fatty acid oxidation disorders under the guidance of a metabolic physician. Potentially harmful sugars, galactose and fructose, should be withheld if galactosemia or hereditary fructose intolerance is a possibility, and dextrose should be given as indicated if there is hypoglycemia.

Specific treatment is outlined in Table 168.5. Some disorders are vitamin responsive (e.g., vitamin B_{12}-responsive methylmalonic acidemia), and vitamin co-factors, if administered routinely to a patient with a known or suspected inborn error, should be continued. Individuals with organic acid and fat metabolism disorders are often prescribed carnitine; this overcomes the secondary deficiency of free carnitine and promotes excretion of abnormal acids as carnitine conjugates. The regimen may be summarized as the four "Cs".

The 4Cs: provide calories, administer carnitine, supply co-factors, and cut the harmful precursors.

If hyperammonemia is significant and/or there is poor tolerance of oral medications, the ammonia-scavenging medications used to treat a child with a urea cycle defect should be administered IV, only in consultation with a metabolic physician. Arginine IV is also used in many urea cycle defects if there is marked hyperammonemia. If the ammonia level is >300 μmol/l and rising, the patient should be evaluated for possible hemodialysis. Hemodialysis may also be indicated for marked acidosis or markedly elevated plasma leucine in maple syrup urine disease.

The same principles and use of medications apply for an individual with suspected diagnosis of an inborn error. Crucial in the case of marked acidosis and/or hyperammonemia in a patient with a possible diagnosis of an inborn error of metabolism is urgent contact with a metabolic center, and appropriate rapid metabolic testing, with the goal of achieving a diagnosis within 24 h. Transfer to a tertiary care facility may be indicated for appropriate evaluation and management.

Disposition

A child with a possible inborn error of metabolism should not be discharged until stabilized, laboratory studies have been obtained, or serum and urine sent for future studies, and follow-up has been arranged (Table 168.6). Children with known disorders will be evaluated and stabilized in the ED and transferred to an ICU, the ward, or discharged to home, as indicated by consultation with a metabolic specialist, the severity of their symptoms, and their tolerance of their home regimen.

Table 168.5. Common medications used in the treatment of specific inborn errors

Indication	Medication	Dose	Administration	Precautions
Hyperammonemia	Sodium benzoate and sodium phenylacetate (Ammunol)	250 mg/kg	Loading dose IV over 90 min, maintenance dose over 24 h	Central line, sodium overload, dilute in 25 ml/kg 10% dextrose, *do not reload*, hypokalemia, vomiting
Hyperammonemia	Arginine HCl	200–600 mg/kg	Loading dose IV over 90 min, maintenance dose over 24 h	Central line, hyperchloremia, acidosis
Organic acid or fat metabolism disorder	Carnitine	25–400 mg/kg daily	IV or PO, may be given IV continuous	
Methylmalonic acidemia	Hydroxocobalamin (vitamin B_{12})	1 mg	IM, IV, or SC	Hydroxo derivative preferred over cyano
Maple syrup urine disease	Thiamine	50–150 mg	PO or IV	
Multiple acyl-CoA dehydrogenase deficiency[a]	Riboflavin	100 mg	PO	
Multiple carboxylase deficiency[b]	Biotin	10 mg	PO	

[a]Combined fat metabolism and organic acid disorder.
[b]Multiple organic acid disorder.

Table 168.6. Factors to consider in decisions concerning patient disposition

Factor	High-risk features
Unexplained altered mental status	Possible inborn error of metabolism, consider admission for evaluation and diagnosis
Intercurrent illness in an individual with a known diagnosis	Hyperammonemia, metabolic acidosis, organ dysfunction, persistent emesis with intolerance of metabolic medications and formula, decreased oral intake, parental concern
Unexplained hypoglycemia	Recurrent episode, glucose <20 mg/dl, elevated ammonia, elevated creatine phosphokinase, elevated liver enzymes, rhabdomyolysis, elevated lactate, elevated ketones
Medical co-morbidities	Pancreatitis, cardiomyopathy, renal Fanconi syndrome, liver dysfunction
Access to metabolic center	Great distance or limited transportation

If there is markedly altered mental status, severe acidosis, or moderate hyperammonemia then admission to the neonatal or pediatric ICU is indicated. Transfer may be required if local metabolic services are not available, or if hemodialysis is indicated and not available.

Conclusions

Symptoms of inborn errors of metabolism are non-specific and may mimic sepsis, intestinal obstruction, or infection, emphasizing the importance of a high index of suspicion for these disorders. Patients with known diagnoses are at risk of metabolic decompensation with even mild intercurrent illness. These children may appear well in triage but can decompensate over hours. Expedient evaluation and early institution of appropriate therapy may prevent severe sequelae, including irreversible neurologic damage or death. Contact with a metabolic center is crucial for optimal evaluation and management of a child with a known or suspected inborn error of metabolism, and is crucial if hyperammonemia is identified, or if severe metabolic acidosis with elevated anion gap is identified in an infant. The New England Consortium of Metabolic Physicians has delineated protocols for emergency management of individuals with disorders identified on newborn screen; there is also a protocol for neonatal hyperammonemia (http://newenglandconsortium.org/for-professionals/acute-illness-protocols/). These should only be implemented under the guidance of a specialist.

Pearls and pitfalls

Pearls

1. Inborn errors of metabolism may present at any age; however, severe cases generally present in the newborn period and may mimic other conditions such as sepsis or intestinal obstruction.
2. An inborn error may be suggested by neurologic symptoms in conjunction with laboratory findings of hyperammonemia, hypoglycemia, or metabolic acidosis with anion gap.
3. A normal newborn screen does not rule out an inborn error of metabolism.

Pitfalls

1. Failure to recognize the potential for rapid decompensation in an individual with an inborn error of metabolism.
2. Failure to order a bedside glucose and ammonia level in a patient with unexplained altered mental status, seizures, or vomiting.
3. Failure to provide glucose and hydration to a patient with a suspected inborn error of metabolism.

Selected references

American College of Medical Genetics. *Newborn Screening ACT Sheets and Confirmatory Algorithms.* Bethesda, MD: American College of Medical Genetics, 2009, http://www.acmg.net/resources/policies/ACT/condition-analyte-links.htm (accessed 29 April 2010).

Burlina A, Bonafé L, Zacchello F. Clinical and biochemical approach to the neonate with a suspected inborn error of amino acid and organic acid metabolism. *Semin Perinatol* 1999;**23**:162–173.

Calvo M, Artuch R, Macià E, *et al.* Diagnostic approach to inborn errors of metabolism in an emergency unit. *Pediatr Emerg Care* 2000;**16**: 405–408.

Claudius I, Fluharty C, Boles R. The emergency department approach to newborn and childhood metabolic crisis. *Emerg Med Clin North Am* 2005;**23**:843–883, x.

Kwon K, Tsai V. Metabolic emergencies. *Emerg Med Clin North Am* 2007;**25**:1041–1060, vi.

New England Consortium of Metabolic Programs. *Acute Illness Protocols, 2009.* Boston, MA: New England Consortium of Metabolic Programs, http://newenglandconsortium.org/for-professionals/acute-illness-protocols/ (accessed May 2010).

Ogier de Baulny H. Management and emergency treatments of neonates with a suspicion of inborn errors of metabolism. *Semin Neonatol* 2002;7:17–26.

Prietsch V, Lindner M, Zschocke J, Nyhan W, Hoffmann G. Emergency management of inherited metabolic diseases. *J Inherit Metab Dis* 2002;**25**:531–546.

Saudubray J, Nassogne M, de Lonlay P, Touati G. Clinical approach to inherited metabolic disorders in neonates: an overview. *Semin Neonatol* 2002;7:3–15.

University of Washington. *GeneReviews*. Seattle: University of Washington, www.genereviews.org (accessed 29 April 2010).

Weiner DI. Pediatrics, inborn errors of metabolism. *eMedicine* March 2009 http://emedicine.medscape.com/article/804757-overview (accessed 29 April 2010).

Zand D, Brown K, Lichter-Konecki U, *et al.* Effectiveness of a clinical pathway for the emergency treatment of patients with inborn errors of metabolism. *Pediatrics* 2008;**122**:1191–1195.

Zschocke J, Horrmann G. *Vademecum Metabolicum: Manual of Metabolic Pediatrics,* 2nd edn. Friedrichsdorf: Milupa, 2004.

Chapter 169

Tutorial: Gizmos

Tamara D. Simon, Bryan L. Stone, Jay Riva-Cambrin, and Ginny Curtin

A Cerebrospinal fluid shunts

Tamara D. Simon and Jay Riva-Cambrin

Cerebrospinal fluid is produced principally by the choroid plexus; approximately 0.3 ml/h per kg body weight. It circulates from the lateral ventricles, through the foramen of Monro to the third ventricle; it then flows through the aqueduct of Sylvius to the fourth ventricle; finally it flows through the foramina of Lushka and Magendie to the subarachnoid space, where it is reabsorbed by arachnoid villi and arachnoid granulations into the dural venous sinuses (Fig. 169.1).

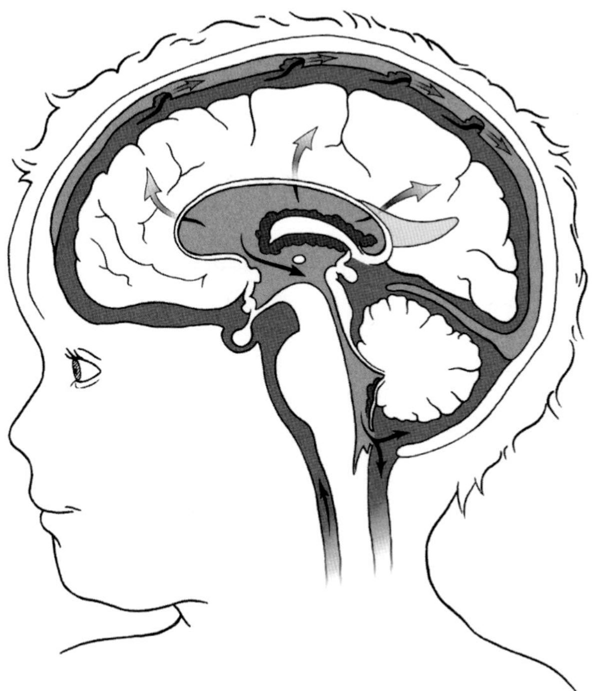

Figure 169.1 Cerebrospinal fluid circulatory pathway. The solid arrows show the major pathway of flow. The broken arrows show additional pathways. (Courtesy of Lynne Larson and the Hydrocephalus Association.)

Hydrocephalus develops when there is an increase in CSF production, a decrease in CSF absorption (rare), or obstruction to flow (most commonly). A CSF shunt allows for the relief of hydrocephalus and the prevention of increased intracranial pressure in a variety of medical conditions, including, but not limited to, tumors, congenital anomalies, post-traumatic hemorrhage, intraventricular hemorrhage, and post-infectious obstruction. Obstruction can occur anywhere within the CSF circulatory pathway, although it more commonly occurs in the passageways connecting the ventricles as well as where the CSF exits the fourth ventricle. This obstruction causes non-communicating hydrocephalus – a blockage of CSF flow.

Anatomy of a shunt

The CSF shunt is composed of three principal components: the proximal catheter, the valve/reservoir, and the distal catheter. The name of each type of shunt corresponds to the anatomical location of each end of the system. The most common shunt type is the ventriculoperitoneal (VP) shunt. The proximal catheters are placed most commonly in the lateral ventricles but can also be located in the fourth ventricle, subdural space, and inside intracranial cysts. The proximal catheter exits the skull through a burr hole and is then secured to a valve with or without a reservoir. The reservoir is a small chamber filled with CSF used, if necessary, to tap the shunt for bacterial culture, to infuse drugs, or to externally monitor intracranial pressure. The reservoir is frequently (but not always) part of the valve and is palpable over the convexity of the skull. The valve is a one-way valve system that allows drainage of CSF at a predetermined pressure differential and may be separate or integrated into the distal catheter. There are a multitude of valve types and adjuncts, including antisiphon devices to prevent overdrainage and programmable valves to adjust pressure settings. The distal catheter is subcutaneously tunneled and placed most commonly into the peritoneal space. Table 169.1 outlines the symptoms of shunt malfunction or infection.

A Practical Guide to Pediatric Emergency Medicine: Caring for Children in the Emergency Department, ed. N. Ewen Amieva-Wang (associate eds. Jamie Shandro, Aparajita Sohoni, and Bernhard Fassl). Published by Cambridge University Press.

Table 169.1. Age-based symptoms of shunt malfunction or infection

Infants	Toddlers	Children and adults	All ages
Head enlargement	Head enlargement	Headache	Vomiting
Full, tense fontanelle	Headache	Vision problems	Irritability, fatigue, sleepiness
Prominent scalp veins	Loss of developmental milestones	Personality change	Swelling along the shunt tract
Downward deviation of eyes (see Fig. 113.3, p. 531)		Loss of coordination or balance	Infection
Less interest in feeding		Decline in academic performance	Fever
			Redness along shunt tract

Complications with shunts

Table 169.2 outlines the potential complications with a CSF shunt and their management in ED. Neurosurgical consultation is warrented when shunt malfunction or an infection is identified. Perforation of hollow viscus, abdominal pseudocyst, intussusception, omental cyst torsion, volvulus around catheter, and abdominal pseudocyst are rare complications.

B Gastrostomy tubes

Tamara D. Simon and Bryan L. Stone

Gastrostomy tubes (G tubes; Fig. 169.2) allow for enteral feedings for children with swallowing dysfunction, esophageal atresia, esophageal burns or strictures, craniofacial abnormalities, chronic malabsorption, and failure to thrive.

Placement of a gastrostomy tube

G tubes are placed either using a percutaneous endoscopic technique (PEG, by GI or pediatric surgery) or surgically in conjunction with Nissen fundoplication (by pediatric surgery).

Nissen fundoplication is a surgical procedure in which the stomach is wrapped around the lower esophageal sphincter. This procedure is believed to reduce the risk of aspiration in high-risk patients, including those with neurological conditions and chronic pulmonary disease.

Jejunostomy tubes (J tubes) are also believed to reduce aspiration risk or bypass a dysfunctional stomach in high-risk patients. Patients with J tubes receive feeds continuously, rather than bolus feeds. These are often placed as extensions to G tubes by interventional radiologists or as tubes placed directly into the jejunum surgically.

Regardless of the method by which a G tube is placed (i.e., PEG or surgically), the stomach and anterior abdominal wall is punctured, a feeding catheter is inserted, and a gastrocutaneous fistula forms. The gastrocutaneous fistula matures between 2–4 weeks and 3 months after creation. Often a long feeding tube is placed initially, and then replaced with a low profile "button" after the stoma matures. However, some surgeons/GI specialists place G tube buttons in the immediate postoperative period. The G tube is held in place by internal and external bumper guards and/or (initially) sutures.

Complications of gastrostomy tubes

Table 169.3 outlines the complications and emergency management of G tubes. Complications of gastrostomy tubes with Nissen fundoplications (after the immediate postoperative period) include:

- gas-bloating syndrome: 30% of adults
- gagging, retching, food refusal, abdominal distention caused by difficulty belching, delayed gastric emptying after vagal trauma, tendency to swallow saliva and air
- dysphagia: 20% of adults
- dumping syndrome: wide swing in glucose caused by massive discharge of food into the duodenum
- operative failures: 5% of adults.

Complications of jejunostomy tubes include:

- migration of tube into stomach
- reflux of feeds/medications
- surgically placed direct J tubes can lead to volvulus.

Consider studies to assess the nature of the problem: dye study, abdominal radiographs, upper GI radiographic series, or endoscopy.

With complications, consult the G tube nurse, the gastroenterologist or surgeon who originally placed the G tube, and/or the interventional radiologist.

C Feeding pumps

Tamara D. Simon and Bryan L. Stone

Feeding pumps allow children who otherwise cannot tolerate oral or intermittent bolus tube feeds to receive enteral feeds and medications. They can be used both with temporary nasogastric tubes and nasojejunal tubes, as well as G tubes and J tubes. A J tube would require continuous pump feeding as bolus volumes are not tolerated in the relatively small jejunum.

Feeding pumps come with a feeding formula reservoir bag with an integral tube threaded through the pump mechanism that delivers the formula. Generally the rate for the flow of the formula is set and is indicated on a LED screen, and most pumps are programmable in advance. Alarms indicate when flow ceases or when there is no longer formula. Most pumps

Table 169.2. Complications with a shunt and emergency management

Complication	Symptoms/signs	Emergency management
Shunt malfunction		
Most common complication, seen in 30–40% of shunt procedures and 67% of patients with shunts Usually caused by simple obstruction with debris, fibrosis, or choroid plexus/ parenchymal occlusion of the proximal catheter (75%) Valve obstruction, kinking, knotting, disconnection, breaking or migration of distal catheter is less common (25%) Also caused by infection, inadequate drainage, or overdrainage	Highly variable signs and symptoms. Most predictive symptoms include vomiting, lack of fever, and parental suspicion	*Shunt series:* (plain radiographs of skull, neck, chest, abdomen used to detect disconnections, kinks, and migration of catheters; proximal and distal catheters are radiopaque, some reservoirs are radiolucent *Head CT*: location of proximal catheter tip and size of ventricles (*comparison with a prior study is critical*) *Ultrasound*: less common; used for children with an open fontanelle; radionucleotide clearance where radionucleotide is injected into the shunt reservoir and observed as it flows proximally and distally *Pumping shunt reservoir*: of little use and is not recommended *Tapping the shunt*: can assess function; is also used to analyze CSF for infection Hospitalization generally required
Shunt infection		
Second most common complication, seen in 8–15% of shunt procedures Increased risk in children under 1 year of age, or a short duration from shunt procedure (1–3 months) Most common organisms include: *Staphylococcus aureus*, *Staphylococcus epidermidis*, Gram-negative rods, pathogens that more commonly cause meningitis	Highly variable signs and symptoms; in children with VP shunts, may have abdominal pain, peritonitis, wound erythema, and drainage	*Tapping the shunt*: assesses shunt function and diagnoses shunt infection; pitfalls abound and experience is needed; consult neurosurgery *Clean reservoir*: 23-gauge butterfly needle (± manometer) is inserted into reservoir; opening pressure, rate of flow, closing pressure, and CSF sample is obtained; CSF should be sent for culture (aerobic and anaerobic), Gram stain, protein, glucose, cell count Hospitalization generally required
Slit-ventricle syndrome		
Found radiographically in 50–60% of patients, only symptomatic in 11–37%, requires treatment in 6–7% Overdrainage of CSF leads to collapse of ventricles, blocking fenestrations in proximal catheter, leading to increased ICP	Intermittent symptoms similar to shunt malfunction are the rule, until ICP rises and ventricles re-expand Some patients are position-sensitive and lying down increases ICP	Head CT: diagnosed when head CT shows small or slit-like ventricles in the face of signs and symptoms of shunt malfunction and/or increased ICP Hospitalization generally required
Proximal catheter obstruction		
	Medical signs of increased ICP include hypertension, bradycardia	Treat increased ICP: elevate head of bed; hyperventilation; diuretics (acetazolamide, mannitol); ventricular puncture through burr hole or open fontanelle Hospitalization generally required
Inguinal hernia		
Increased abdominal fluid increases intra-abdominal pressure, converting a potential into a clinical hernia	Pain and fullness (intermittent or constant) in the Inguinal area	
Migration of distal catheter tip		
Through abdominal incision, through neck incision, into mediastinum, thoracic cavity, umbilicus		*Shunt series*: plain radiographs of skull, neck, chest, abdomen used to detect disconnections, kinks, and migration of catheters; proximal and distal catheters are radiopaque, reservoirs are radiolucent

ICP, intracranial pressure; VP, ventriculoperitoneal.

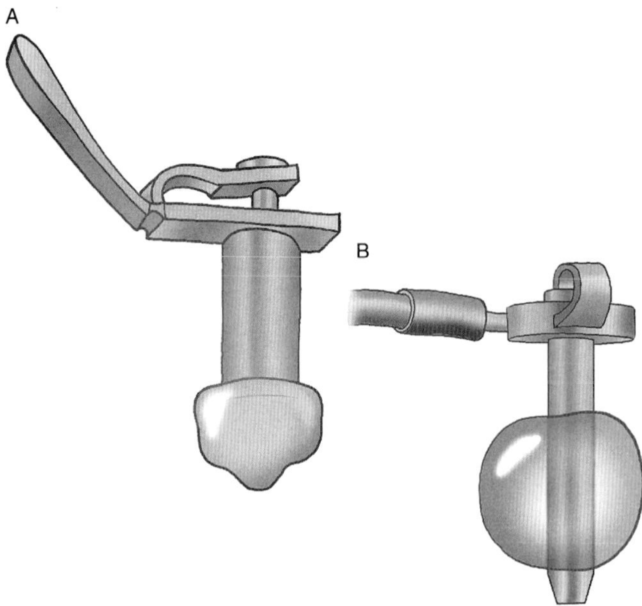

Figure 169.2 Types of gastrostomy tube: (A) button; (B) MIC-Key. (Copyright N. Ewen Amieva-Wang.)

have batteries that are rechargeable, and pumps are designed to be portable. The home health company that provides the pump is an excellent resource when pumps malfunction. If possible, transition to bolus feeds should be considered as this eliminates the need for a pump.

D Tracheostomy tubes

Tamara D. Simon, L. Bryan Stone, and Ginny Curtin

Tracheostomy tubes are used in children for many different reasons, including upper airway obstruction secondary to vocal cord paralysis or subglottic stenosis, risk of chronic aspiration, and the need for prolonged mechanical ventilation. This section discusses some basic concepts of tracheostomies in children and the major complications of tracheostomy that the EP must be able to manage.

Placement of a tracheostomy tube

In children, tracheostomy tubes are always placed surgically. They are placed at the level of the second or third tracheal rings. Children are discharged from the hospital only after the stoma has matured (approximately 1 week after placement) and the tracheostomy tube is able to be taken out and replaced by the caretaker. Tubes are usually changed for cleaning by the caretaker once a week for small children and at least once a month in older children. Ideally, caregivers are educated in tracheostomy care and given a kit with supplies including replacement tubes, one of the same size and another one half a size smaller.

Historically, tracheal tube sizing was esoteric and required a conversion chart. Since the late 1990s, conventions in sizing have become standardized. At present, most tracheostomy tubes are sized according to the tube inner diameter, similar to endotracheal tube sizing. The only important exception is the Jackson tube, a metal tracheostomy tube that is often used in developing world settings (Table 169.4). If the tracheostomy tube size is not known, the endotracheal tube size indicated on length-based resuscitation tapes can be used. Note that neonatal tracheostomy tubes are similarly sized in diameter to other tubes, however they are shorter than pediatric tracheostomy tubes.

The largest suction catheter which can fit easily into the tube should be used. While catheter sizes are usually in "French," the millimeter size should also be indicated on the packaging.

While details of tracheostomy tubes vary, they have three main parts: cannula, neck flange, and hub. The cannula is the curved tube that is inserted into the stoma. (Older children may have tracheal tubes with an inner cannula, which allows for ease of cleaning.) The neck flange sits against the child's neck and allows for the tube to be secured. The hub is a 15-mm connector that attaches directly to the ventilator or bag-valve mask (this universal connector may not be available in older tubes). An obturator usually comes with the tube and is inserted in the lumen of the tube to guide the tube during insertion (Fig. 169.3).

Patients should know the size of tracheostomy tube they are using and should always have a replacement tube with them. While the dimensions and type of tube often depend on the indication for tracheostomy placement, in the emergency setting any appropriately sized tracheostomy or even endotracheal tube can be used as a temporizing measure.

Complications of tracheostomies

Table 169.5 gives the complications and emergency management of tracheostomies. Figure 169.4 shows how the tube is inserted.

E Genitourinary conduits

Tamara D. Simon and Bryan L. Stone

Genitourinary conduits are used when the normal urinary structures are being bypassed or the bladder is removed and an opening is made in the urinary system to divert urine. The flow of urine is diverted through an opening in the abdominal wall. A neurogenic bladder results in a need for urinary diversion. The most common etiologies are myelomeningocele, followed by trauma and genitourinary malformations.

Anatony of a genitourinary conduit

Continent urinary diversion, most commonly, the Mitrofanoff, describes a procedure for making a continent supra-pubic conduit into any reservoir for self-catheterization. It requires a narrow tube, the commonest source of which is the appendix or, alternatively, a ureter, Fallopian tube, or length of tailored intestine. The tube is buried in the wall of the conduit in a tunnel

Table 169.3. Complications and emergency management of gastrostromy tubes

Complication	Symptoms/signs	Emergency management
Wound infection		
Occurs in 20% of patients	Purulent, bloody, cellulitic skin, yellow-brown discharge is normal	*Superficial*: easily treated, clean area with antiseptic, apply topical antibiotics *Cellulitis*: systemic antibiotics needed, watch for necrotizing fasciitis *Hospitalization*: consider *Prevention*: avoid occlusive dressings
Hemorrhage		
	Small, self-limited bleeding at placement; bleeding remote from the time of placement, consider ulcers, granulation tissue, or erosion of the gastric mucosa	Mucosal injury can range from gastritis to perforation of stomach; often occurs in gastric wall opposite the G tube from inappropriate suctioning of the gastrostomy (gravity drainage only)
Tube obstruction		
Most common cause of tube malfunction Most often caused by formula/medicines coagulating in acidic pH; common culprits are crushed pills, particularly sustained release; proteinaceous material		*Flushing*: gently with 5 ml warm water in 5 ml syringe; instill and pull back up five times; smaller syringes create more pressure; if successful, flush tube again to ensure patency *Pancreatic enzymes*: if flushing with water unsuccessful, try solution of pancreatic enzymes; crush 1 Viokase 8 (pancrelipase) and 325 mg sodium bicarbonate into fine powder; mix with 5 ml warm water, instill in 10 ml syringe, wait 5 min; attempt to flush with 5 ml or smaller syringes; can repeat above for 30 min *Other solutions*: carbonated liquids, meat tenderizer, and/or milking the tube *If unable to clear blockage*: notify GI/surgery that feeding tube cannot be cleared *Prevention*: flushing before and after feeds and medication administration
Tube dislodgement		
Determine maturity of fistula; conservatively consider the fistula immature if <6 weeks since surgical placement or <12 weeks since percutaneous placement For immature stomas, the stoma relies on the apposition of skin and gastric mucosa; gastric layer closes faster than skin. Almost anything can be used to keep stoma patent, and the stomach is not sterile. Mature stomas close in 24–48 h If necessary, a NG tube can be inserted and stoma permitted to close		*Immature stomas*: gently place a small Foley; *if any resistance* is felt, remove the Foley and consult surgery or GI *immediately*; complications include detachment of stomach from abdominal wall, development of false tract, peritonitis, pneumoperitoneum, and/or air embolism *Mature stomas*: replace with the same size and type of tube or button; if size not known, a measuring device can be used. If a replacement G tube is not immediately available, leave a taped Foley catheter in place If the fistula has almost closed, consult surgery/GI and insert a NG tube *To dilate a stoma*: successively larger tubes (Foleys) can be placed every 30 min; this should be performed in conjunction with GI; do not dilate with a hemostat *Contrast study*: recommended after all G tube replacements to rule out intraperitoneal placement[a]

Table 169.3. (cont.)

Complication	Symptoms/signs	Emergency management
Tube cracking or fracture		
		Remove original: (a) balloon-tip (MIC-Key) after deflating balloon; (b) mushroom or collapsible-wing tip with gentle traction or, if necessary, cut tip at external surface of wall and push into stomach for later excretion or removal by endoscopy *Replace tube with balloon tip (MIC-Key)*: clean site and select proper replacement; test new button by inflating and deflating balloon with water or saline looking for 360 degree inflation; lubricate tube with water soluble jelly; gently insert in stoma perpendicular to abdominal wall 3 cm beyond balloon; reinflate balloon with water or saline (3–5 ml for infants, 5–7 ml for children); check gastric placement (see below) and apply gentle traction pulling balloon against gastric mucosa; the button should lie flat against abdomen *Replace tube with mushroom and collapsible-wing tips*: insert obturator into open sides of tip to distend tip before placing in stoma; with tip distended, tube is inserted into stoma perpendicular to abdominal wall with steady pressure until flush with abdominal wall; once fully inserted, obturator is removed; check gastric placement (see below); the button should lie flat against abdomen *Check gastric placement*: check pH of aspirate (<5), color of aspirate; if no aspirate obtained, inject 5 ml air and aspirate again; also reposition patient
Leakage around wallx		
Occurs in 10% of patients May be caused by: clogged tube, deterioration of tube (*check balloon*), or stoma that is enlarged through external traction on the tube	Looks like formula	*Leakage alone*: stoma adhesive powder and Maalox/Aquaphor solution *Stoma is too big*: Sorbsan around the site if the stoma is too big; alternatively change size of G tube button
Granulation tissue formation		
May accumulate on abdominal wall Recurrences are frequent	Tissue bleeds easily, causes discharge, irritation, and discomfort; check for prolapse (pinker, regular color) which does not respond to silver nitrate (i.e., does not turn gray)	*Clean*: remove secretions or crusts from site; apply water-soluble jelly to normal tissue in 5-cm circle surrounding granulation; silver nitrate stick can be used to cauterize tissue once daily for 7–10 days (up to 3 weeks) until granuloma is gone *Medicate*: apply triamcinolone cream TID for 2 weeks (wait 1 h if after silver nitrate)
Tube migration		
Can migrate down the intestinal tract or up the esophagus. Downward migration can cause obstruction or even perforation. Upward migration can cause aspiration		Contact pediatric GI/pediatric surgery if this is diagnosed

NG, nasogastric
[a]Use 20–50 ml (based on child size) of undiluted water-soluble contrast material, which is pushed a few seconds prior to the radiograph.

Table 169.4. Conversion chart for Jackson tracheostomy tube sizing

Inner diameter (mm)	Jackson	Suction (Fr)
3.0	00	6
3.5	0	6–8
4.0	1	6–8
4.5	2	8
5.0	3	8–10
5.5	4	10
6.0	5	10

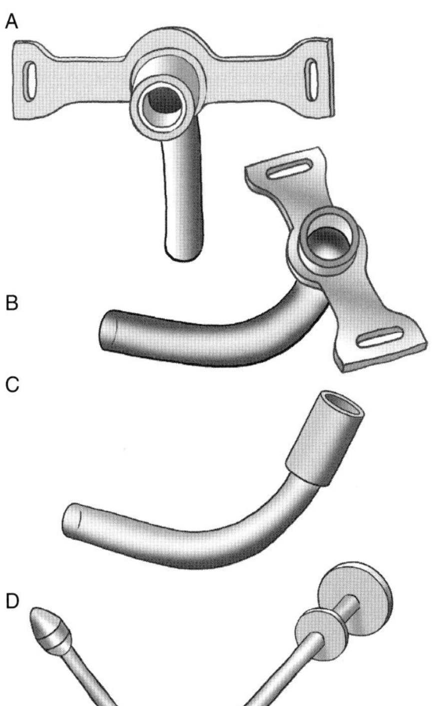

Figure 169.3 Tracheostomy tube. (A) Assembled with inner cannula in place. (B) Outer cannula. (C) Inner cannula (note in children an inner cannula is often not used). (D) Obturator. If the tracheostomy tube is rigid at the distal end, an obturator is necessary to pass the cannula to reduce the risk of tissue damage. (Copyright N. Ewen Amieva-Wang.)

approximately 5 cm long. Patients perform intermittent catheterization three to five times a day to empty the bladder.

Non-continent urinary diversions are less common and involve connecting the ureters to a segment of intestine and then bringing the intestine to the surface of the abdomen. The child then wears an ostomy bag into which the urine continuously drains.

Patients may be prone to urinary tract infections as a result of the intermittent catheterization. In addition, up to 30% of patients have conduit complications, particularly stenosis at the skin level and persistent leakage, which require surgical revision and/or repeated dilation. Rarer complications include intestinal occlusion from volvulus and adhesions.

F Gastrointestinal conduits

Tamara D. Simon

Gastrointestinal conduits are also used in children with neurogenic bowel caused by myelomeningocele and, less commonly, genitourinary malformations and trauma.

Anatomy of a gastrointestinal conduit

The antegrade continence enema technique maintains bowel continence while assisting with defecation timing and prevention of constipation. A conduit is constructed between the skin and the proximal large bowel using the appendix, large bowel, or small bowel (Monti tube); some surgeons create a valve at the base. Enemas can then be delivered via a catheter, promoting regular continent bowel function.

Non-continent bowel diversions include colostomy creation with drainage into a colostomy bag attached to the skin.

Complications include stenosis and, more rarely, peritonitis.

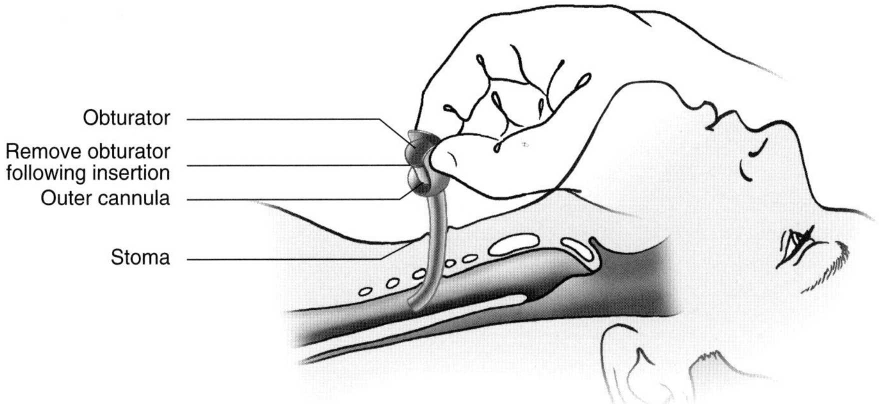

Figure 169.4 Insertion of tracheostomy cannula into airway through a tracheal stoma. (Copyright N. Ewen Amieva-Wang.)

Table 169.5. Complications of tracheostomies and emergency management

Complication	Description	Emergency management
Dislodgment or decannulation of tube	Usually families replace themselves; they will come to the ED if they are unable to replace	*Replacement*: attempt briefly to replace with the same size and model tracheostomy tube;[a] if this is not possible, a tube one size smaller should be promptly used; remove inner cannula if one is present and insert obturator into the lumen of the new tube; apply water-soluble lubricant while extending the patient's neck using shoulder roll; insert the tube into the stoma in smooth, curved motion, no resistance should be felt; remove obturator *Fixing new tube*: secure the tube with tapes so that the neck flange is against the child's neck. *If delay in replacing the tube*: oral BMV can be performed if there is no airway obstruction (the tracheostomy hole must be covered); if unable to place smaller tracheal tube or BVM, a suction catheter can be inserted as a temporizing measure
Obstruction of tube	Tracheostomies can accumulate dried secretions, which narrow the cannula lumen and make occlusion with mucus or other debris easier, or can create ball-valve obstruction; this occurs in spite of regular maintenance and care, including suctioning Humidification of air is critical in prevention	*Suction*: attempt suctioning using the largest catheter available that can fit inside the tube; suction only to the length of the tracheostomy tube (deep suctioning can cause trauma to the airway); there is no evidence that suctioning with saline is useful. *If respiratory distress continues*: replace with a new tracheostomy tube (see above)
Infection	Peritracheal cellulitis Lower respiratory tract infections present with change in quality, quantity, odor, and color of secretions. Risk factors include weak cough, decreased ciliary action, and direct access to trachea Recurrent tracheitis/ bronchitis	*Peritracheal cellulitis*: treat with oral antibiotics and local wound care; can be complicated by mediastinitis Check chest radiograph: consider broad-spectrum coverage for pathogens that colonize the tracheostomy (including *Staphylococcus aureus*, *Pseudomonas* sp., and *Candida albicans*); consider hospitalization
Hemorrhage	Most common cause is aggressive suctioning with abrasion of the tracheal mucosa; to avoid this, do not suction beyond the end of the tracheal tube and keep area humidified The risk of catastrophic bleeding from tracheal erosion into an artery exists but is rare	ENT assessment: identify the cause of bleeding; if suspected, the patient should be promptly managed in the OR

[a]If the same model is not available, use an appropriately sized tube which can be changed later.

Selected references

American Thoracic Society. ATS guidelines: care of the child with a chronic tracheostomy. *Am J Respir Crit Care Med* 2000;**161**:297–308.

American Urological Association Foundation. *Pediatric Conditions.* Linthicum, MD: American Urological Association Foundation http://www.urologyhealth.org/pediatric/index.cfm?cat=03&topic=145 (accessed 29 April 2010).

Aronson BS, Yeakel S, Ferrer M, *et al.* Care of the laparoscopic Nissen fundoplication patient. *Gastroenterol Nurs* 2001;**24**:231–239.

Cameron JL. *Current Surgical Therapy*, 7th edn. St. Louis, MO: Mosby Elsevier, 2001, pp. 1411–1412.

Di Lorenzo C, Orenstein S. Fundoplication: friend or foe? *J Pediatr Gastroenterol Nutrit* 2002;**34**:117–124.

Garton HJ, Piatt JH. Hydrocephalus. *Pediatr Clin North Am* 2004;**51**: 305–325.

Liard A, Sequier-Lipsyzc E, Mathiot A, Mitrofanoff P. The Mitrofanoff procedure: 20 years later. *J Urol* 2001; **165**:2394–2398.

Teoh DL. Tricks of the trade: assessment of high-tech gear in special needs children. *Clin Pediatr Emerg Med* 2002;**3**:62–75.

Washington K. *G Tube Care Handout.* Denver, CO: Special Care Clinic, Children's Hospital, Denver.

Woodhouse CRJ. The mitrofanoff principle for continent urinary diversion. *World J Urol* 1996; **14**:99–104.

Section

29

Special tutorials

Chapter

170 Radiology atlas

Bo Yoon Ha and Beverley Newman

Update on ALARA: restricting radiation dosage

Imaging with CT is an essential part of modern medical management. With all applications of ionizing radiation, the ALARA principle – as low as reasonably achievable – is an important goal.

Medical imaging is responsible for approximately 30–50% of population radiation exposure in the USA. Of this, CT accounts for 17% of medical imaging but 75% of medical irradiation: 11% of CT scans are performed in children and approximately 33% of those are in children <10 years of age. An average CT scan is equivalent in dose to approximately 50–100 chest radiographs although low-dose techniques can considerably reduce this.

There is increasing concern for cancer induction by ionizing radiation, particularly in children. The data are somewhat controversial and the overall cancer risk is small: <0.5% over baseline for lifetime cancer mortality risk (20%). Children, particularly infants, and females more than males, have greater organ sensitivity to radiation. Certain organs, including the breast, thyroid, and gonads, are particularly sensitive. With similar delivered radiation doses there is increased organ exposure in children because there is less peripheral tissue to attenuate the X-ray beam. Cancer risk is cumulative with multiple exposures and individuals exposed in childhood have a longer time for radiation effects to manifest.

As CT is a digital technology, unlike plain film radiographs, excessive radiation dose does not result in overexposed or poor quality images. While 40 to 70% reduction of typical adult CT doses will often produce quality diagnostic scans in children, there is an unfortunate tendency to apply adult practices and protocols in children, particularly in environments where care is shared.

The following should be considered when ordering imaging studies, particularly those that entail higher doses of ionizing radiation such as CT.

- What is the clinical question to be answered, so that the study can be tailored to provide the information needed?
- Can ultrasound or MR be used as an appropriate substitute for a CT study?
- Can the location be limited?
- Are specific pediatric protocols provided? (Note: Imagegently.com is a website sponsored by the Society for Pediatric Radiology and the American College of Radiology that provides information on how to adapt adult imaging protocols to lower dose studies in children).

The radiologist should pay attention to optimizing imaging parameters such as the kilovoltage peak (kVp), the milliampere-seconds (mAs), the gantry cycle time, pitch, and detector collimation to keep radiation doses ALARA. The use of protective shields (e.g., for the breast) may further help in reducing dose to vulnerable sites. Many newer CT scanners provide suggested pediatric protocols and features such as automodulation of the amperage (changing the milliamperes during a scan based on tissue thickness and shape).

Imaging with CT and other radiographic methods has much to offer diagnostically and should not be withheld when necessary because of radiation exposure fears. All medical professionals need to consider and balance the accompanying benefits and risks.

This chapter is not an attempt at exhaustive coverage of the emergency conditions that affect children but rather an overview of some of the more common entities that are likely to be encountered in the pediatric emergency setting and their typical radiographic appearances.

Imaging of the chest

The thymus

One of the most important features of pediatric chest radiographs is the variable appearance of the thymus, particularly in

A Practical Guide to Pediatric Emergency Medicine: Caring for Children in the Emergency Department, ed. N. Ewen Amieva-Wang (associate eds. Jamie Shandro, Aparajita Sohoni, and Bernhard Fassl). Published by Cambridge University Press.

children <3 years. The normal thymus is often seen as a prominent smooth soft tissue density in the antero-superior mediastinum on the frontal chest radiograph, located in the retrosternal area on the lateral view (Fig. 170.1A,B). Normal thymus is the most frequent cause of apparent widening of the mediastinum, raising concern for a mediastinal mass. Typical features such as the wave sign, sail sign, or notch in the cardiac border are helpful to differentiate normal thymus from a mediastinal mass. Smooth borders, anterior location, and lack of mass effect on adjacent structures are useful in allaying concerns (Fig. 170.1C). Review by an experienced pediatric radiologist will often prevent unnecessary additional imaging.

Ultrasound or CT will be indicated if plain radiographic findings are confusing or complex or an underlying chest mass is suspected. Ultrasound is particularly useful for the evaluation of thymus, cystic mass, or pleural effusion.

Viral bronchiolitis

Viral bronchiolitis is typically seen in young infants <2 years of age and is most often caused by respiratory syncytial virus. Diffuse lower airway inflammation, bronchospasm, and increased secretions result in bilateral hyperinflation (partial airway obstruction with air trapping) and patchy atelectasis (focal complete airway obstruction) on chest radiographs (Fig. 170.2). In an individual patient, it may be difficult to

A

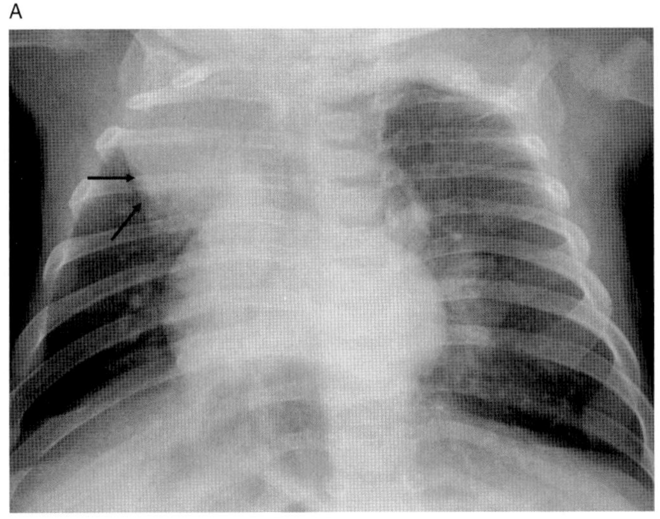

B

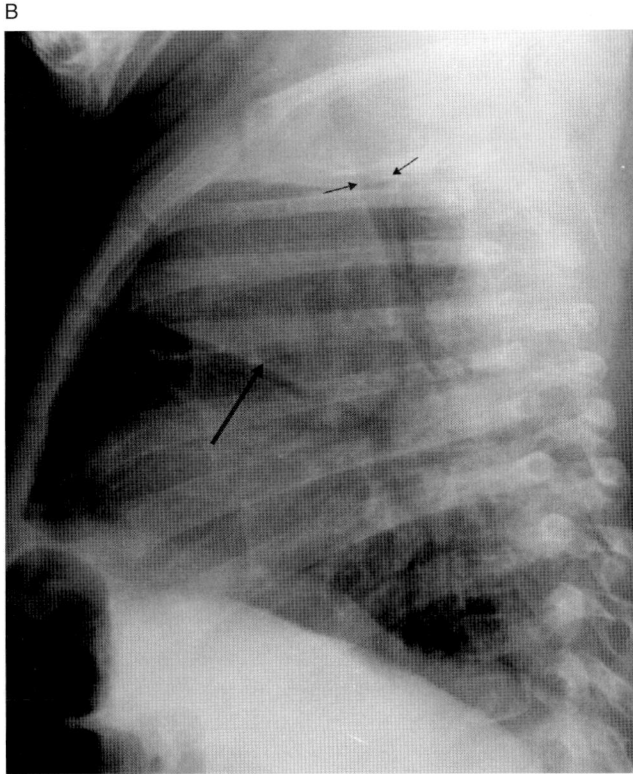

C

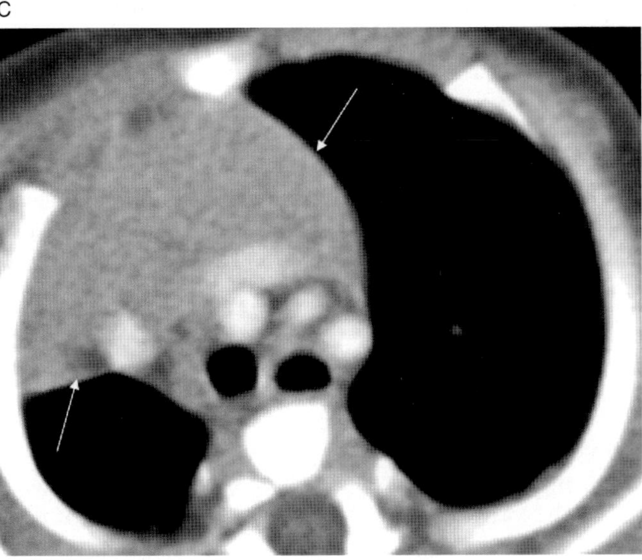

Figure 170.1 Normal thymus in a 6-month-old boy. (A,B) Chest radiograph shows the thymic sail sign (frontal-arrows) to the right and anteriorly in the superior mediastinum. There is a sharp inferior border with the minor fissure (lateral long arrows). Note the normal airway (lateral small arrows). (C) CT shows normal homogeneous thymus with smooth borders in the anterosuperior mediastinum and no mass effect on adjacent structures (arrows).

A

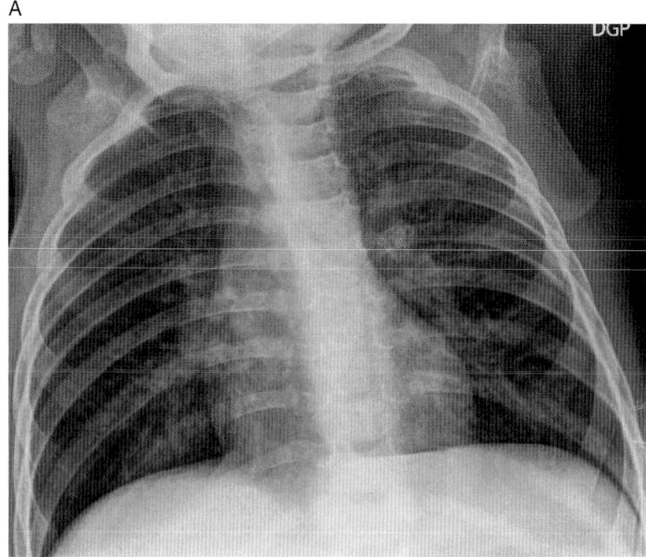

B

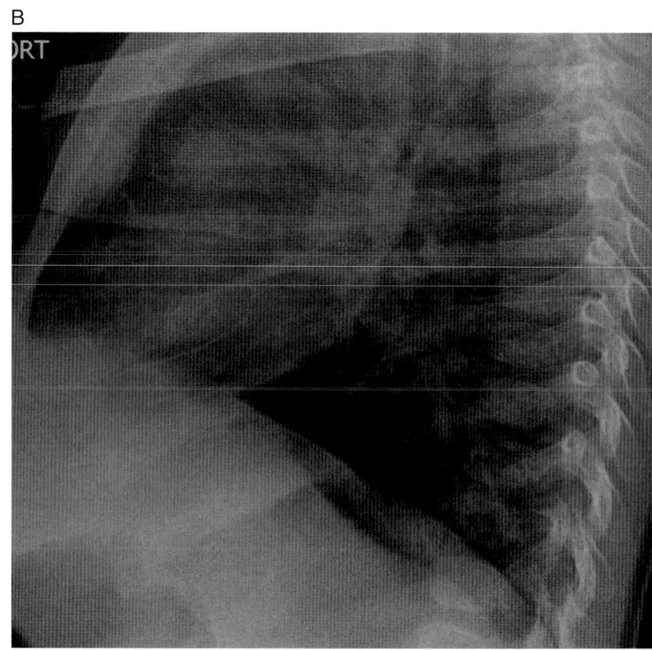

Figure 170.2 Viral bronchiolitis presenting with cough in an 11-month-old girl. Chest radiographs demonstrate diffuse peribronchial thickening and mild hyperinflation, seen as flattening of the diaphragm and air anterior to the heart. This is better appreciated on the lateral view.

differentiate focal atelectasis (typically central and linear) from patchy bronchopneumonia (raising concern for bacterial infection). Treatment decisions tend to be made based on clinical history and examination and further imaging workup is not needed in most cases.

Pneumonia

The role of imaging in patients with clinical suspicion of pneumonia is confirmation or exclusion of pneumonia, characterization, evaluation of extent and complications, and demonstration of other possible pathology. Features of imaging help in differentiation of viral, bacterial, and other causes.

Viral infection. Viral lower airway disease is most common in preschool children; it usually has the radiographic features of bronchiolitis or bronchitis (i.e., hyperinflation, peribronchial thickening, and subsegmental atelectasis). Hyperinflation is often better appreciated on the lateral chest radiograph. Viral pneumonia is interstitial in location, producing diffuse reticulonodular or hazy infiltrates.

Bacterial pneumonia. This is more common in older children and manifests with focal peripheral air space consolidation (Fig. 170.3). The distribution could be subsegmental, segmental or lobar. Pleural effusion is frequently associated. A round appearance of consolidation is quite common, particularly in children <8 years of age.

Mycoplasma pneumonia. This is a very common cause of pneumonia in school-age children, with a variable radiographic appearance spanning that of both viral and bacterial infection. In younger children or more indolent infection, reticulonodular perihilar infiltrates or patchy nodular opacities are most common. A more focal consolidative pattern is seen in older children or more acute clinical presentation (Fig. 170.4).

Additional imaging is rarely required in pneumonia in childhood. Indications include suspected complication, inadequate treatment response, to assist with anticipated surgery, complex clinical scenario (e.g., immunosuppressed patient or suspected unusual organism), chronic or recurrent infection, and suspected underlying mass or anatomic abnormality.

Ultrasound is often adequate to assess the presence, size, and degree of loculation of pleural effusions. Careful consideration should be given to the risks and benefits when ordering CT examinations for pulmonary infection. The imaging is optimally performed with administration of IV contrast; the lack of natural tissue contrast in children makes non-contrast CT evaluation very difficult.

Foreign body

The bronchus is the most common site for airway foreign body. The vast majority of airway foreign bodies are non-radiopaque and so imaging findings reflect the consequences of disturbed aeration secondary to their presence. Chest radiographs may be normal or show only subtle abnormality. The key radiographic finding is asymmetric aeration secondary to

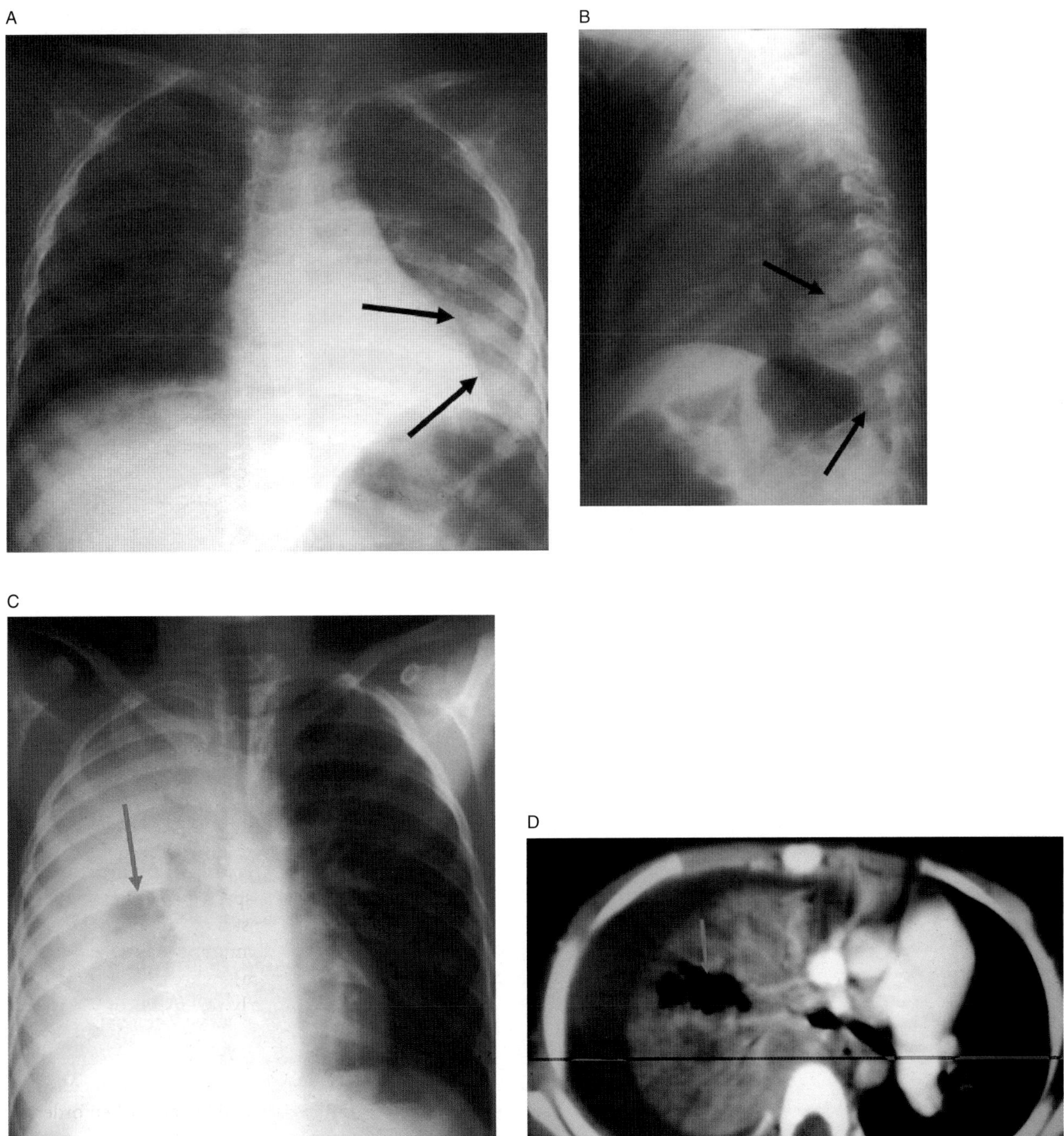

Figure 170.3 Penumococcal infection. (A,B) Pneumococcal pneumonia in a 5-year-old child. Frontal chest radiograph demonstrates air space consolidation in the left lower lobe with preservation of the left heart border (arrows); there is opacity overlying the spine on the lateral view (arrows). (C–E) Pneumococcal empyema in a 12-year-old patient. (C) Chest radiograph demonstrates almost complete opacification of the right hemithorax with irregular lucency in the right mid lung (arrow). It is uncertain whether the opacified hemithorax reflects fluid, atelectasis, or consolidated lung. (D) Contrast-enhanced CT clearly differentiates the large pleural effusion from the heterogeneously enhancing lung parenchyma containing an irregular air-filled cavity, findings suggesting necrotizing pneumonia and possible empyema. (E) Longitudinal ultrasound demonstrates multiple septations within the fluid, not well seen on CT, confirming a likely empyema rather than reactive effusion. Sc, subcutaneous tissue; s, spine; l, liver.

air trapping or atelectasis on the affected side (Fig. 170.5). Oligemia, consolidation, or other secondary complications such as pneumothorax or pneumomediastinum are additional findings on plain chest radiographs.

Particularly when regular frontal and lateral views are normal or questionable, it is useful to demonstrate a lack of change in lung volume on the affected side during different phases of the respiratory cycle. Inspiratory and expiratory films are used for this purpose in cooperative patients. Alternatively, bilateral decubitus views or fluoroscopic examination is used when children are unable to hold their breath.

One of the most common foreign bodies is a swallowed coin. A coin can become lodged either in the trachea or esophagus; the location is easily confirmed by chest radiographs. Respiratory symptoms from a foreign body in the esophagus may be subacute or chronic as a result of secondary tracheal compression by the inflammatory reaction around the impacted foreign body. This is best visualized on the lateral chest radiographic view (Fig. 170.6).

E

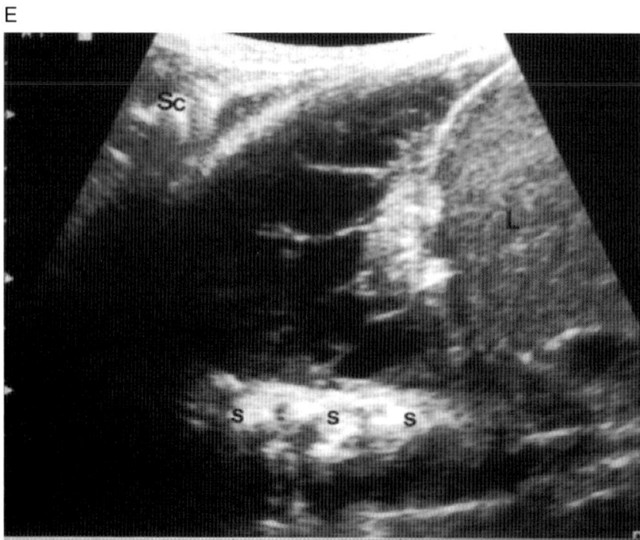

Figure 170.3 *(cont.)*

Croup

Radiographic findings in croup are characteristic in association with concomitant clinical features. Subglottic edema produces loss of the normal rounded lateral convex shouldering of the subglottic tracheal airway on the frontal plain film of the neck. This radiologic feature is called the "inverted V" or "church steeple" sign (Fig. 170.7).

Epiglottitis

Epiglottitis is now rarely seen because of the widespread implementation of vaccination for the most common causative agent *Hemophilus influenzae* type b.

Lateral plain film of the neck shows enlargement of the epiglottis and thickening of the aryepiglottic folds (Fig. 170.8). There is often reflex distention of the pharynx.

A

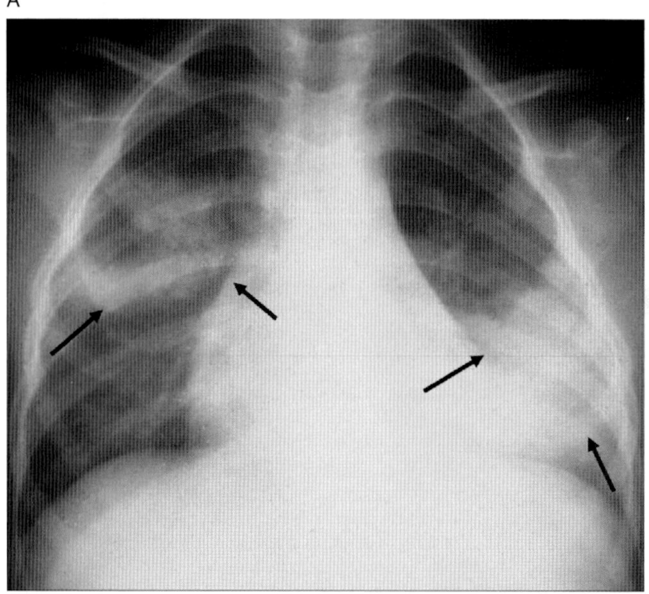

B

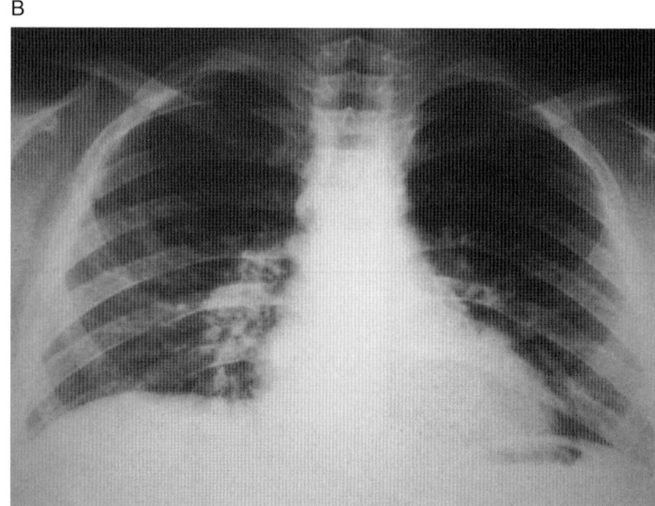

Figure 170.4 Variable pattern of *Mycoplasma* pneumonia. (A) Frontal chest radiograph in a 7-year-old child shows patchy air space consolidation in both lungs (arrows). (B) Frontal chest radiograph in a 4-year-old child shows reticulonodular infiltrates in bilateral perihilar and lower lobes.

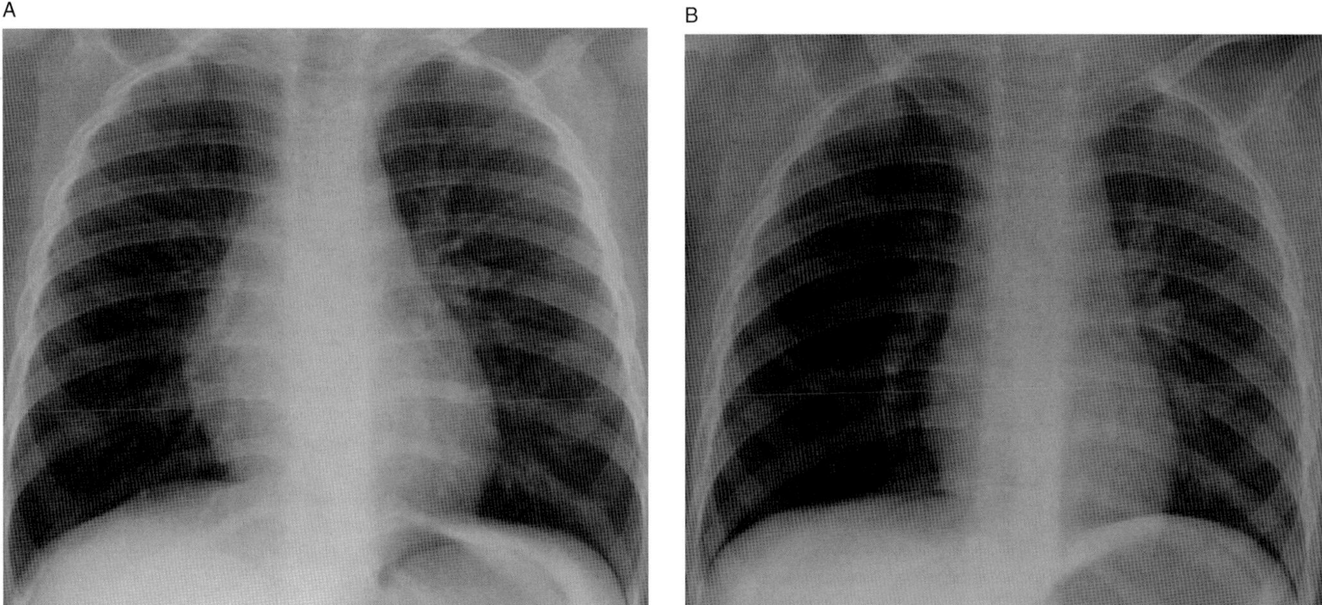

Figure 170.5 Right-sided bronchial foreign body in a 2-year-old girl presenting with wheezing. (A) Inspiratory radiograph. (B) Partially expiratory radiograph. Persistent hyperinflation and oligemia can be seen on the right side, indicative of partial right bronchial obstruction. Note the shift of heart towards the left on the expiratory view because of partial deflation of the left lung.

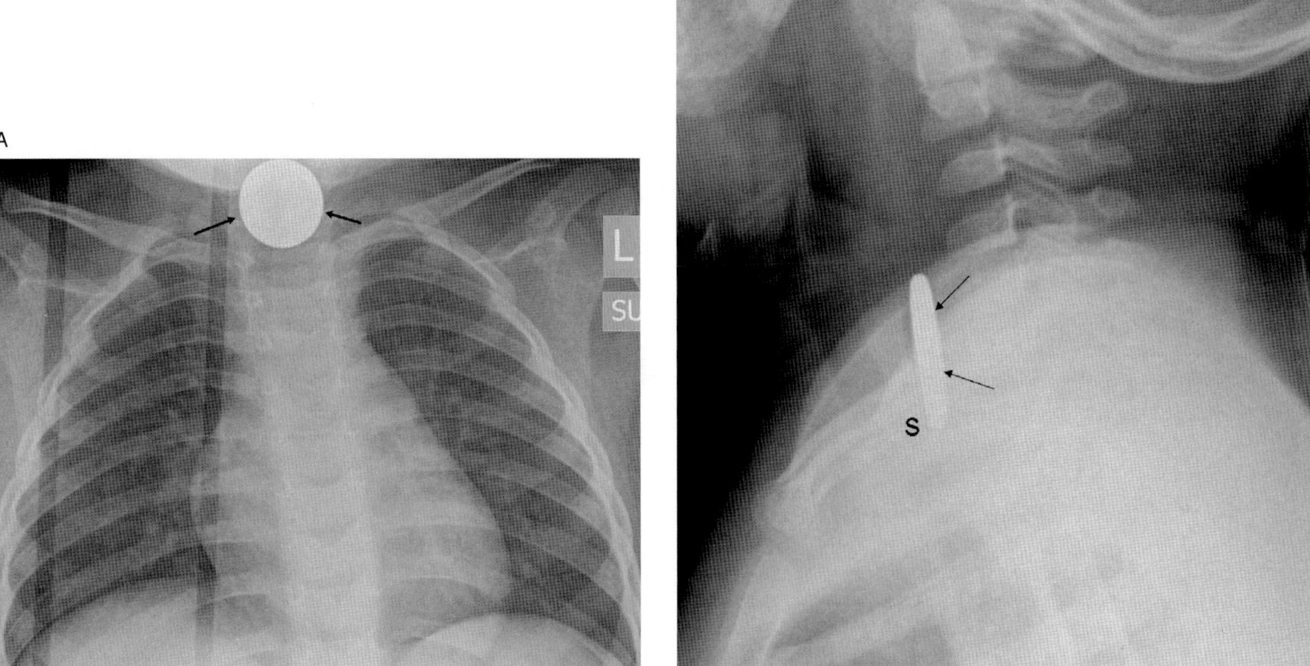

Figure 170.6 Chest radiographs in a 2-year-old boy with a coin lodged in the esophagus (A) Frontal view, where the coin is flat-on. (B) Lateral view with the coil edge-on (arrows). Soft tissue thickening between the trachea and the esophagus on the lateral view suggests subacute or chronic inflammatory reaction (S). The tracheal air column is focally narrowed in this location.

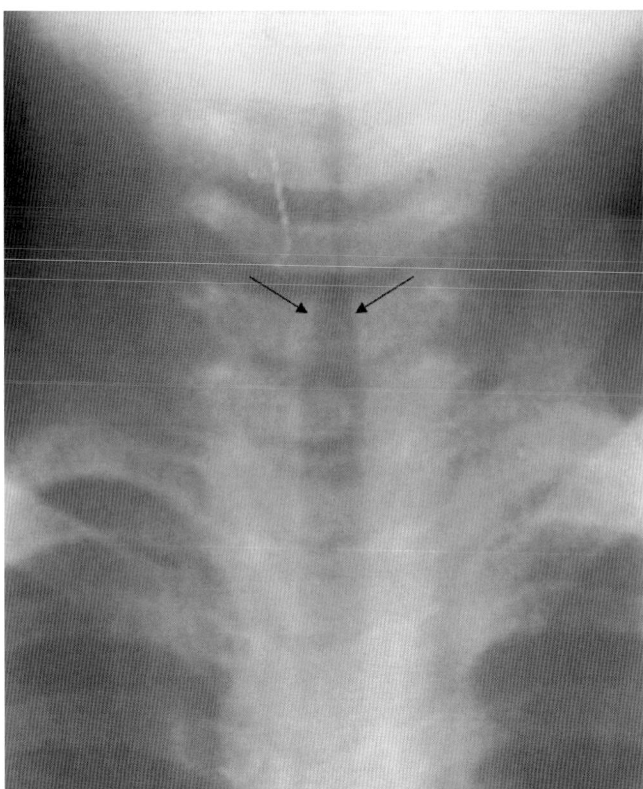

Figure 170.7 Croup. The frontal radiograph of the neck shows a "steeple sign" with the loss of the normal rounded lateral convex shouldering of the subglottic airway as a result of subglottic edema (arrows).

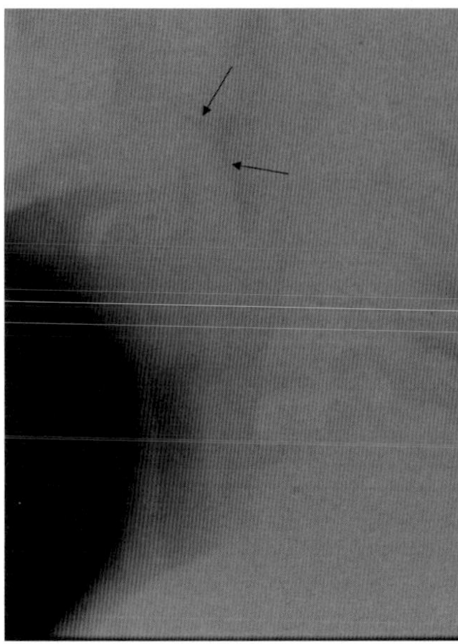

Figure 170.8 Epiglottitis. The lateral radiograph of the neck shows marked enlargement of the epiglottis and thickening of the aryepiglottic folds (arrows).

Imaging of the abdomen

Gastrointestinal conditions

A useful acronym in assessing plain abdominal radiographs is "stones, bones, gas, mass". It is useful to localize the GI tract, including stomach, rectum, and colon, which are relatively more fixed and commonly contain air. In children as opposed to adults, air is frequently present in small bowel loops also (Fig. 170.9). Solid abdominal viscera such as liver, spleen, kidneys, and bladder (if filled) can be assessed. Osseous structures, lung bases, and diaphragms should also be evaluated.

Often a single supine plain film of the abdomen will suffice. The value of additional films, including lateral, cross-table lateral, or upright views, would depend on the clinical situation, being most useful to evaluate obstruction or free air. Ultrasound is an excellent modality for delineating normal abdominal organs and pathologic processes in children if patients are not extremely obese. Ultrasound is usually a fast and readily available imaging modality in the ED setting and has the advantage of lack of exposure to ionizing radiation. However considerable expertise is required to perform high-quality sonographic imaging in children.

Indications for abdominal CT include:

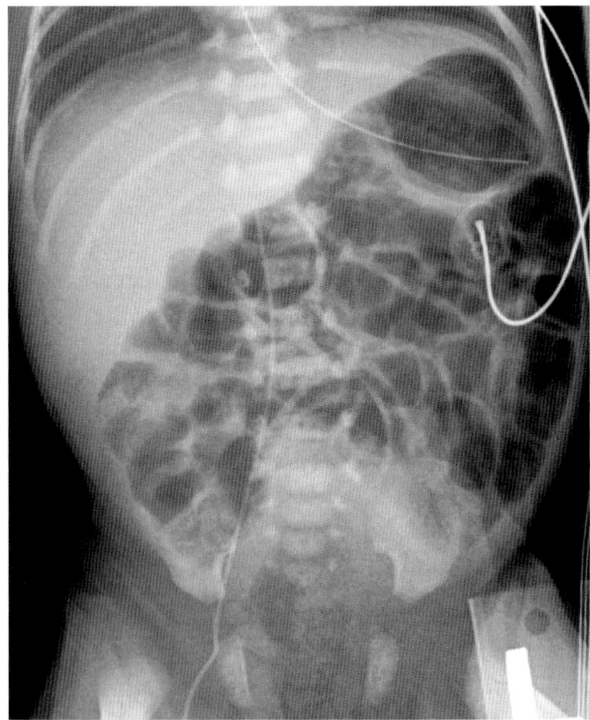

Figure 170.9 Normal abdominal radiograph in a 9-day-old infant shows air visible throughout the small and large bowel.

- obese patients where ultrasound is limited
- ultrasound does not provide definitive answers and there is ongoing clinical concern
- the clinical question is unlikely to be answered by ultrasound.

Intussusception

A paucity of bowel gas on the right side of the abdomen accompanied by a soft tissue mass opacity on an abdominal radiograph is highly suggestive of intussusception (Fig. 170.10A). However, a normal abdominal radiograph does not definitively exclude intussusception. Other findings may include small bowel obstruction, pneumatosis, and bowel perforation.

Ultrasound is highly accurate in diagnosing and excluding intussusception, and also allows unnecessary contrast enemas to be avoided. On ultrasound, the mass visualized is composed of alternating rings of hyperechoic mucosa and hypoechoic edematous wall of the intussusceptum (Fig. 170.10B). This is known as the "donut sign" in the transverse plane and "pseudo kidney sign" in the longitudinal plane. An underlying lead point can occasionally be visualized and color Doppler imaging may be helpful in assessing for bowel hyperemia/ischemia.

While ultrasound has been utilized along with hydrostatic reduction for intussusception, most pediatric departments approach intussusception reduction fluoroscopically utilizing air or water-soluble contrast, with a success rate of approximately 80–90% (Fig. 170.10C). Prior to attempting an intussusception reduction, the patient should be clinically stable, have IV access, and no free air on abdominal radiographs. The family should be informed of the risks and benefits of the reduction procedure and the child should be accompanied by a nurse or physician for monitoring in the fluoroscopic suite.

Appendicitis

Findings in appendicitis on plain film include normal bowel gas pattern, general or focal ileus, appendicolith, spinal splinting, apparent obstruction, or abscess with mass effect.

With ultrasound imaging, the inflamed appendix measures more than 6 mm in transverse diameter in most cases. Graded compression displaces adjacent bowel loops and differentiates the non-compressible inflamed appendix from compressible normal bowel loops (Fig. 170.11A,B). An echogenic appendicolith with posterior shadowing may be visualized. There is often appendiceal and periappendiceal hyperemia on color Doppler imaging. Perforation and abscess formation can be identified by the presence of periappendiceal fluid, intraperitoneal fluid, or a mixed echoic mass in the RLQ or pelvis. Perforation may be missed since the decompressed appendix is sometimes difficult to evaluate and an abscess can be mistaken for air-filled bowel. The normal appendix may not be visualized on ultrasound, creating difficulty with definitely excluding appendicitis. However, particularly in girls, other pathology (e.g., ovarian) may be found to explain the clinical symptoms.

The preferred imaging modality is CT if the result of abdominal ultrasound is negative or equivocal and the clinical findings warrant further evaluation. Imaging with CT is highly accurate, sensitive, and specific in diagnosing appendicitis and the complications thereof (Fig. 170.11C,D). In children, IV contrast use is essential; both oral and rectal contrast are used in some centers.

Hypertrophic pyloric stenosis

Ultrasound has become the imaging examination of choice to confirm or exclude pyloric stenosis in a vomiting infant. On ultrasound, the hypertrophic muscular layer is hypoechoic, and the mucosa is hyperechoic. Normal pyloric muscle thickness in the transverse plane should not exceed 3 mm and the length of the pyloric canal is normally <15 mm (Fig. 170.12). Additional supportive imaging features of pyloric stenosis may include a distended stomach with retained food/fluid and failure of the pylorus to open during the examination. When ultrasound findings are equivocal, an upper GI radiographic series can be obtained to differentiate pyloric stenosis from other diagnostic considerations, although it is often appropriate to follow the child clinically and repeat the ultrasound in a few days if symptoms persist and pyloric stenosis is still the clinical concern.

Malrotation and mid-gut volvulus

Upper GI radiographic series is the diagnostic modality of choice for malrotation, demonstrating the abnormally positioned duodenojejunal junction (Fig. 170.13A). The normal duodenum crosses the spine with the duodenojejunal junction located posteriorly and to the left of the spine at the same level or superior to the duodenal bulb. In questionable cases, small bowel follow-through may be helpful to assess the position of the cecum.

When mid-gut volvulus is present, the upper GI series demonstrates malrotation, a dilated obstructed proximal duodenum, and a corkscrew appearance of the mid/distal duodenum/ jejunum (Fig. 170.13B).

On ultrasound or CT, malrotation is characterized by reversal of the normal positions of the superior mesenteric artery and vein. With volvulus there may be a mass-like swirling pattern of bowel around the superior mesenteric vessels.

Genitourinary conditions

Ovarian torsion

Ovarian torsion is an uncommon cause of abdominal pain in pediatric patients, best evaluated by ultrasound in the emergency setting. Gray scale ultrasonographic images are important in evaluating ovarian torsion, with demonstration of increased heterogeneous echotexture in an enlarged ovary with multiple peripheral follicular cysts (Fig. 170.14A). Various imaging appearances can be seen with differing degrees of internal hemorrhage, edema, or infarction.

Doppler and color Doppler images can show absence or asymmetrically decreased ovarian arterial flow (Fig. 170.14B, C). Color Doppler imaging for analyzing ovarian torsion is generally helpful but may be confusing and not entirely reliable. There are documented cases of surgically proven ovarian torsion in which color Doppler imaging showed normal arterial flow at the time of imaging.

A

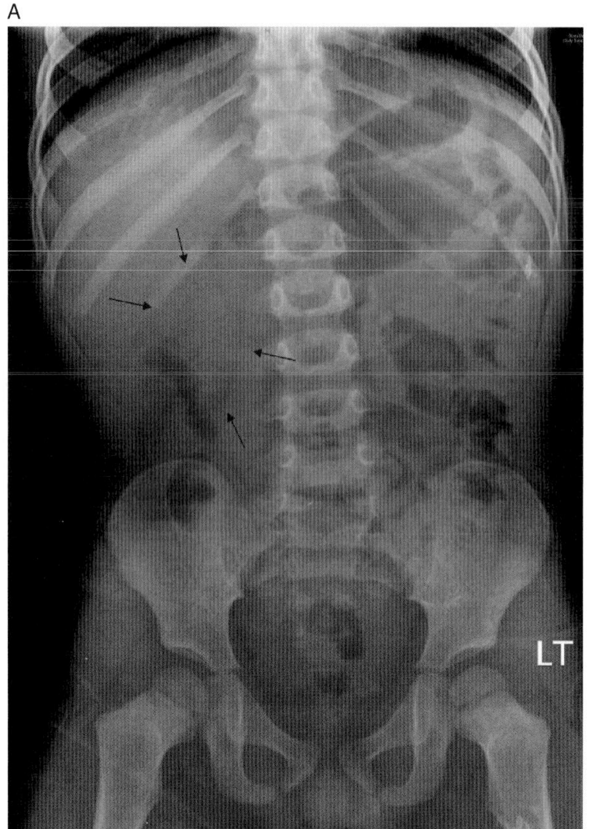

B

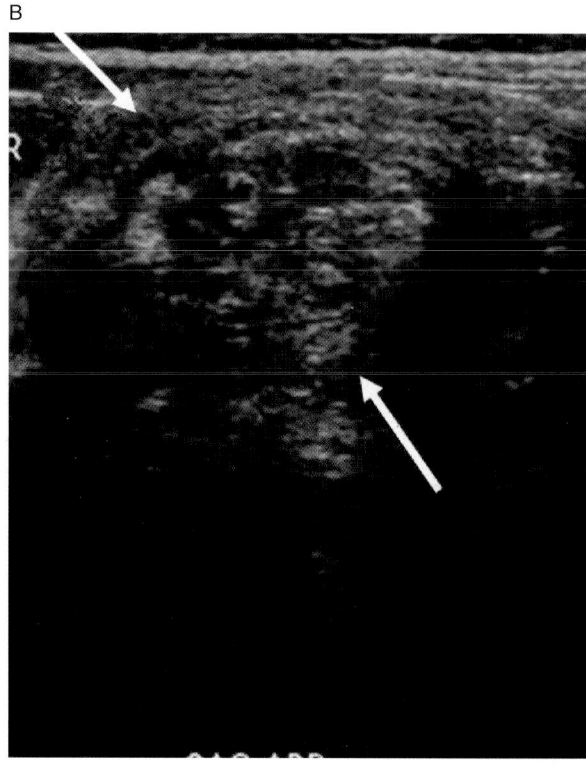

C

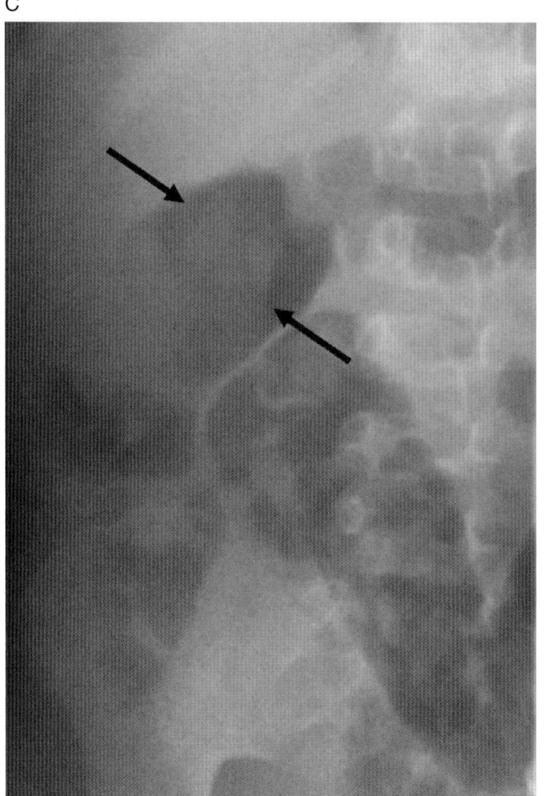

Figure 170.10 Intussusception in a 2.5-year-old girl presenting with crampy abdominal pain. (A) Abdominal radiograph shows a paucity of bowel gas in the RUQ with soft tissue fullness (arrows). (B) Ultrasound shows a RUQ mass composed of alternating rings of hyperechoic mucosa and hypoechoic edematous wall (arrows). (C) Fluoroscopy shows an intraluminal mass of the intussusception at the splenic flexure during air reduction (arrows).

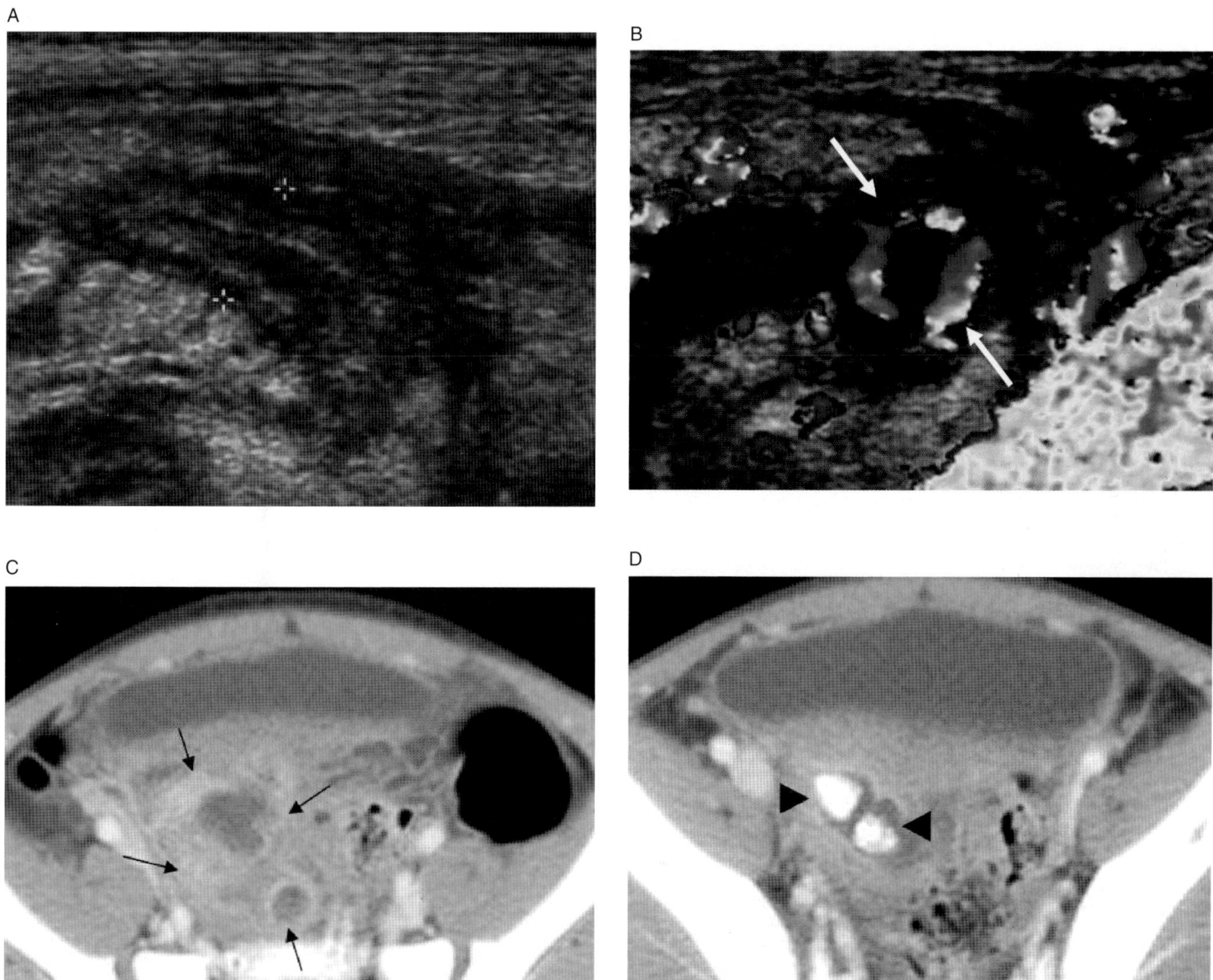

Figure 170.11 Appendicitis. (A–C) A 4-year-old boy presenting with abdominal pain. (A) Longitudinal ultrasound shows the non-compressible inflamed and thick-walled appendix measuring more than 6 mm in diameter (calipers). (B) There is marked hyperemia of the appendix on color Doppler imaging in transverse view (arrows) (C,D) Perforated appendix in an 11-year-old boy presenting with fever and abdominal pain. (C) CT shows marked RLQ inflammatory change and several peripheral rim-enhancing abscesses (arrows).(D) Two extruded appendicoliths can be seen with CT behind the bladder (arrowheads) and surrounded by fluid.

Testicular torsion

Testicular torsion is one of the most common causes of an acute painful scrotum in children. Prompt diagnosis and treatment are crucial because preservation of the testis is unlikely when torsion is not relieved within 6 to 10 h. Ultrasound is the key imaging modality for diagnosing testicular torsion, thus expediting appropriate surgical exploration. The affected testis could be normal in size or enlarged, with normal to heterogeneous hypoechogenicity depending on the progression of ischemia, venous congestion, and infarction (Fig. 170.15A).

Doppler and color Doppler ultrasound are essential for the diagnosis, with demonstration of absent or asymmetrically decreased flow (Fig. 170.15B). In addition, the spermatic cord should be examined to visualize the actual torsed cord. Occasionally, the testis can spontaneously detorse; in such cases Doppler imaging may show reactive hyperemia on the affected side, mimicking epididymitis.

Acute epididymitis

Acute epididymitis is the most common acute scrotal pathology in children. The cause is mostly bacterial, but viral (e.g., mumps) etiology is not uncommon. Ultrasound shows the enlarged epididymis with variable hypo- or hyperechogenicity (Fig. 170.16A). It is most often accompanied by a reactive hydrocele and scrotal wall thickening. The diagnosis can be

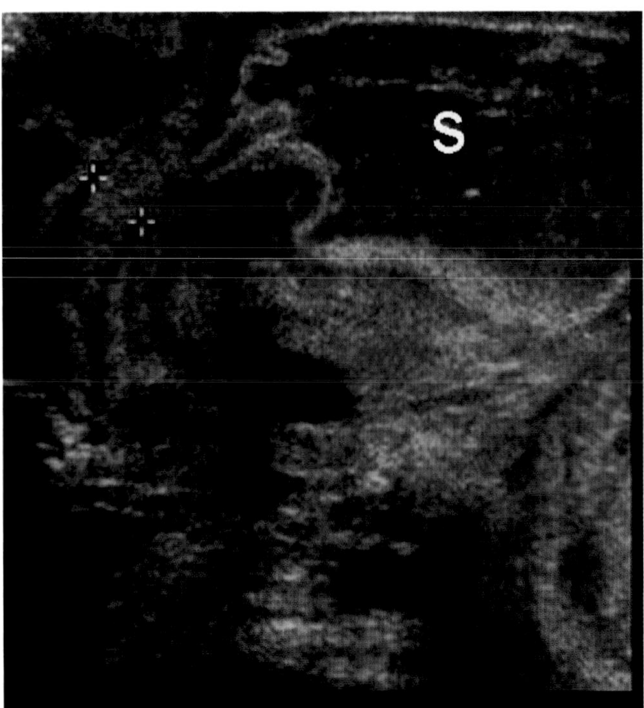

Figure 170.12 Hypertrophic pyloric stenosis in an 1-month-old boy presenting with projectile non-bilious vomiting. Ultrasound shows thickening of the pyloric muscle (5 mm) and elongated curved pyloric channel, which measured 2.3 cm in length. (S, stomach).

supported by increased flow on color Doppler imaging (Fig. 170.16B).

In most cases, the testis appears normal. However, these testes could be hyperemic, with infection producing epididymo-orchitis, or there could be decreased testicular Doppler flow as a result of compression by the inflamed and edematous epididymis, producing testicular ischemia.

Testicular appendage torsion

Torsion of the testicular appendage is a common cause of acute scrotal pain, particularly in prepubertal boys. Sonographically the testicular appendage is seen as a small hyper- or hypoechoic avascular mass adjacent to the superior testis or epididymis (Fig. 170.17). There may be a reactive hydrocele and epididymal and testicular hypoechogenicity and hyperemia. An infarcted appendage typically ultimately shrinks in size and may calcify or become one or more scrotoliths.

Imaging of the musculoskeletal system

Bones in children are more porous and have a greater propensity to deform prior to breaking. This plasticity frequently results in incomplete fractures, such as bowing fracture, buckle fracture, and greenstick fracture (Fig. 170.18).

A

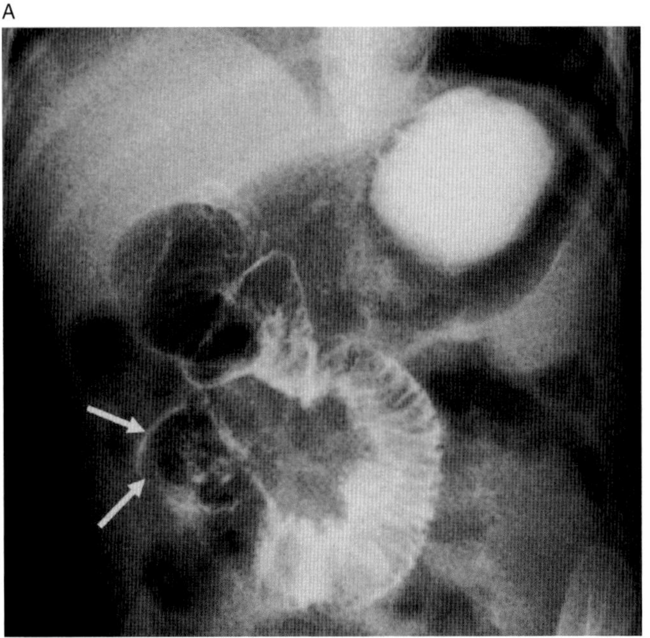

B

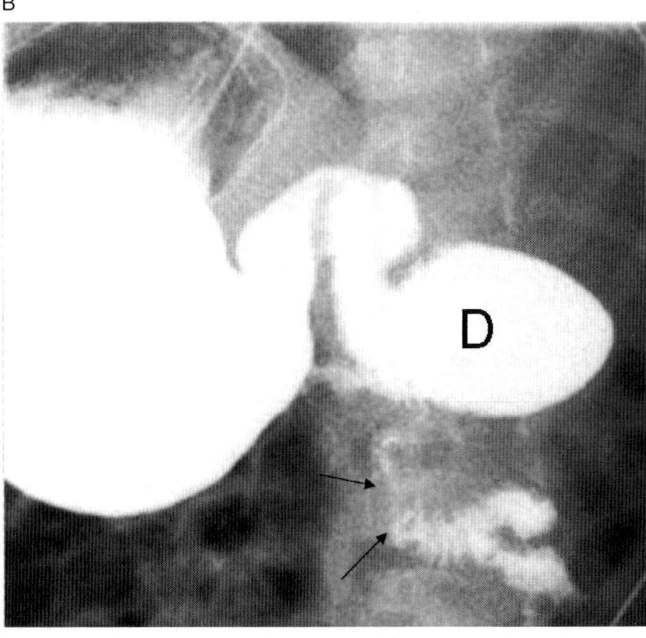

Figure 170.13 (A) Small bowel malrotation in a 21-month-old boy presenting with emesis. On UGI, there is no obstruction, but an abnormal duodenojejunal junction that fails to cross the spine to the left side and right-sided proximal jejunal loops (arrows). (B) Malrotation and mid-gut volvulus in a 19-month-old boy presenting with bilious emesis. The UGI shows a dilated obstructed proximal duodenum (D) and malrotation, with a corkscrew appearance of the distal duodenum/proximal jejunum suggesting volvulus (arrows).

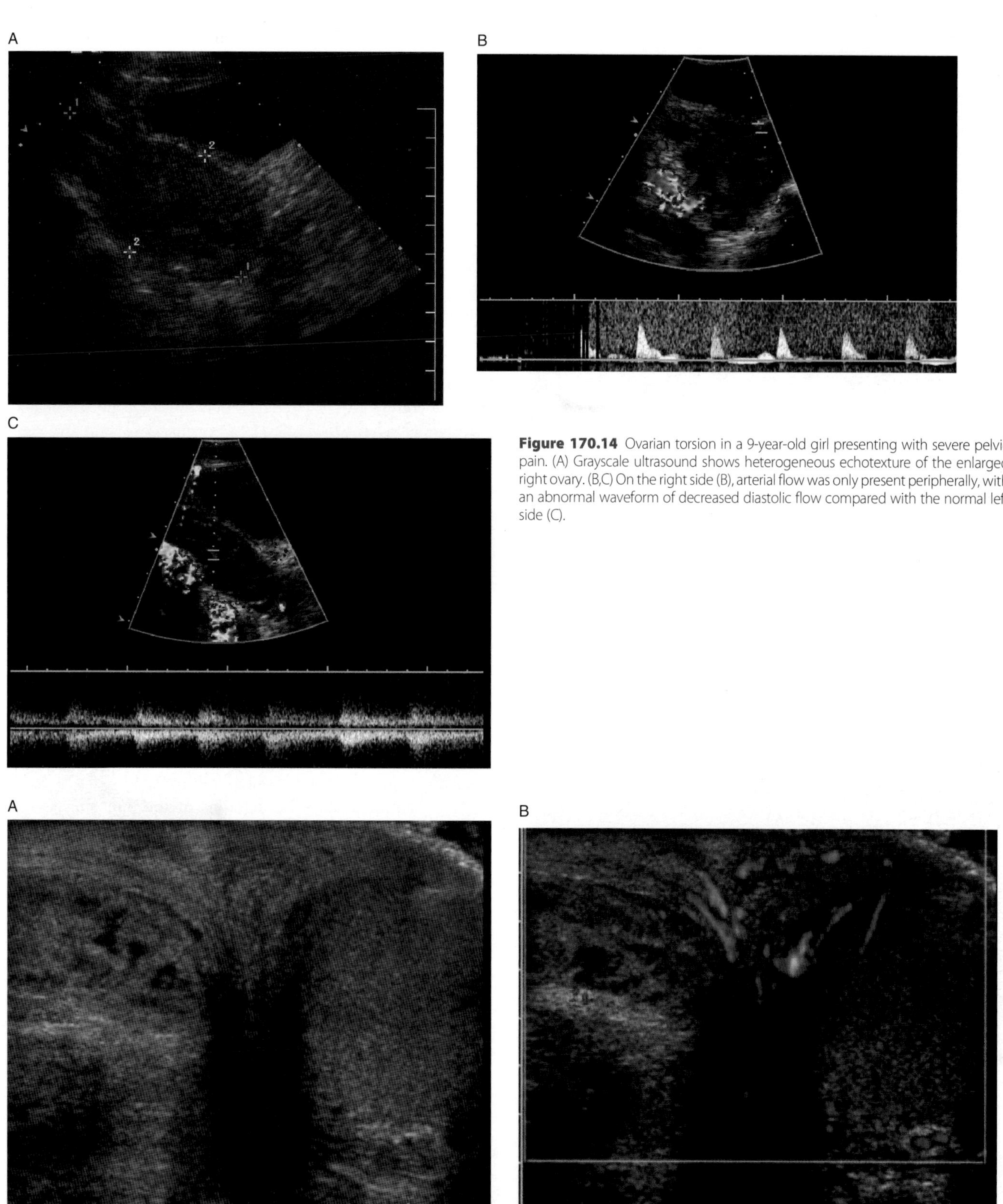

Figure 170.14 Ovarian torsion in a 9-year-old girl presenting with severe pelvic pain. (A) Grayscale ultrasound shows heterogeneous echotexture of the enlarged right ovary. (B,C) On the right side (B), arterial flow was only present peripherally, with an abnormal waveform of decreased diastolic flow compared with the normal left side (C).

Figure 170.15 Testicular torsion in a 15-year-old boy presenting with a 3-day history of scrotal pain. (A) Grayscale ultrasound shows an enlarged right testis with heterogeneous hypoechogenicity. (B) Color Doppler ultrasound shows an absence of intratesticular flow on that side.

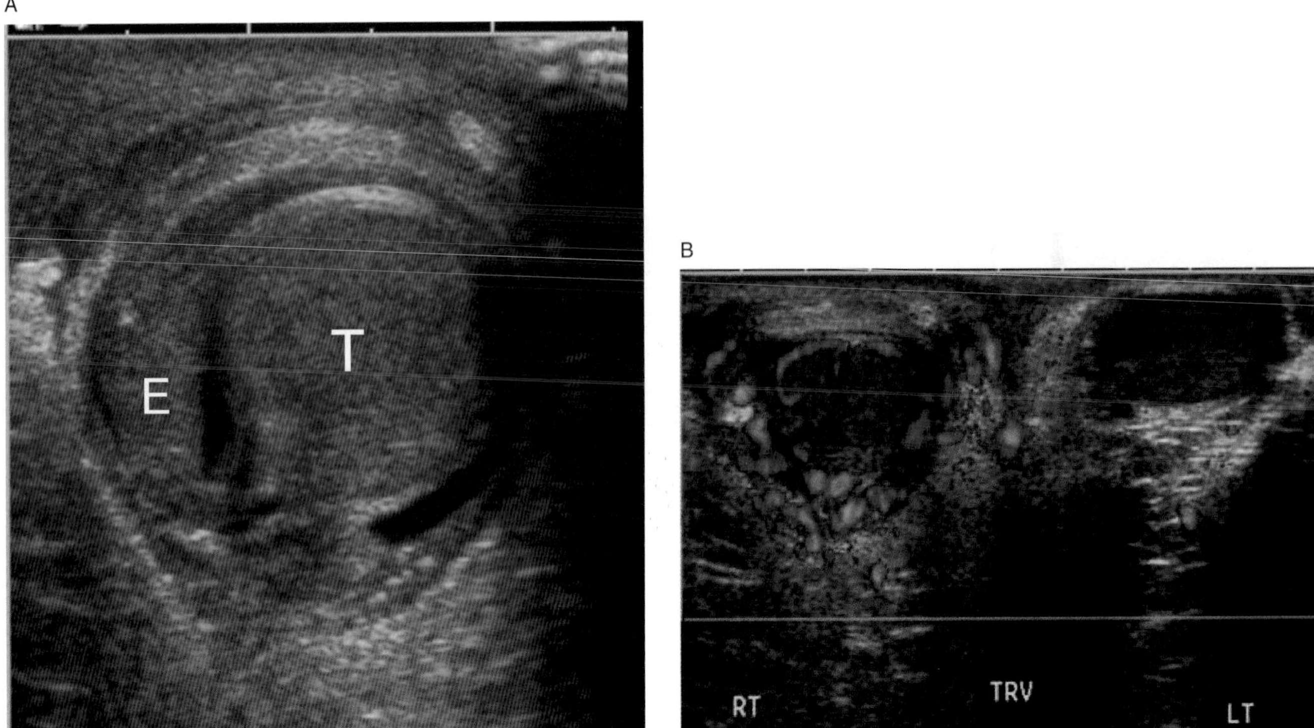

Figure 170.16 Epididymitis in a 6-year-old boy presenting with a 5-day history of scrotal pain and fever. (A) Ultrasound shows the enlarged right epididymis (E) with small reactive hydrocele and scrotal wall thickening T_1 testis. (B) There was increased epididymal, peritesticular, and scrotal flow on the right side as seen with color Doppler imaging. Normal arterial flow was preserved within the testis (not shown).

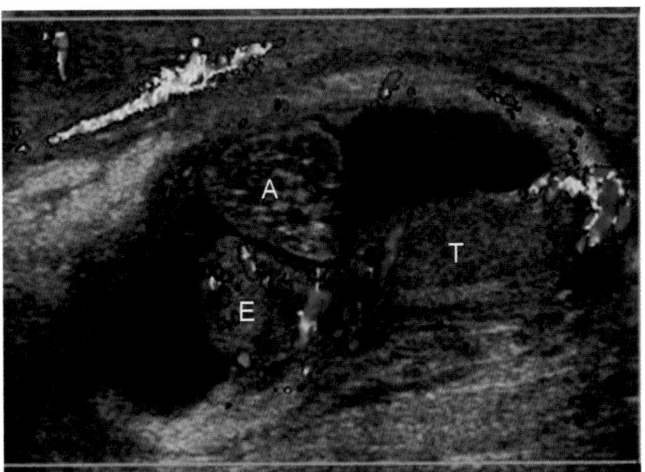

Figure 170.17 Testicular appendage torsion in a 13-year-old boy presenting with a 6-day history of scrotal pain. Ultrasound shows a heterogeneous avascular mass adjacent to the superior testis with reactive hydrocele. A, appendage; E, epididymis; T, testis.

Another characteristic of the pediatric skeleton is the presence of unfused physes, a site of relative weakness and, therefore, prone to fracture. In fact, approximately 20% of fractures in children involve the physis. The standard description of physeal fractures is based on the Salter–Harris classification.

The healing process in pediatric fractures is very rapid and usually complete without residual deformity in most cases.

It is helpful to have radiographs of the opposite normal side or prior films for comparison, particularly for complex joints such as the elbow. Knowledge of the normal appearance of ossification centers is important in the interpretation of fractures. The ossification centers of the elbow appear in a predictable order readily remembered by the acronym CRITOE (capitellum [C], radial head [R], internal [medial] epicondyle [I], trochlea [T], olecranon [O], and external [lateral] epicondyle [E]) (Fig. 170.19).

Commonly encountered fractures are outlined below based on anatomical location.

Forearm

The forearm is the most common location for fracture, often with more than one co-existent fracture:

- distal radial buckle fracture plus fracture of the ulnar styloid process
- Monteggia's fracture: proximal ulnar fracture with radial head dislocation (Fig. 170.20)
- Galeazzi's fracture: distal radial fracture with ulnar dislocation at the wrist.

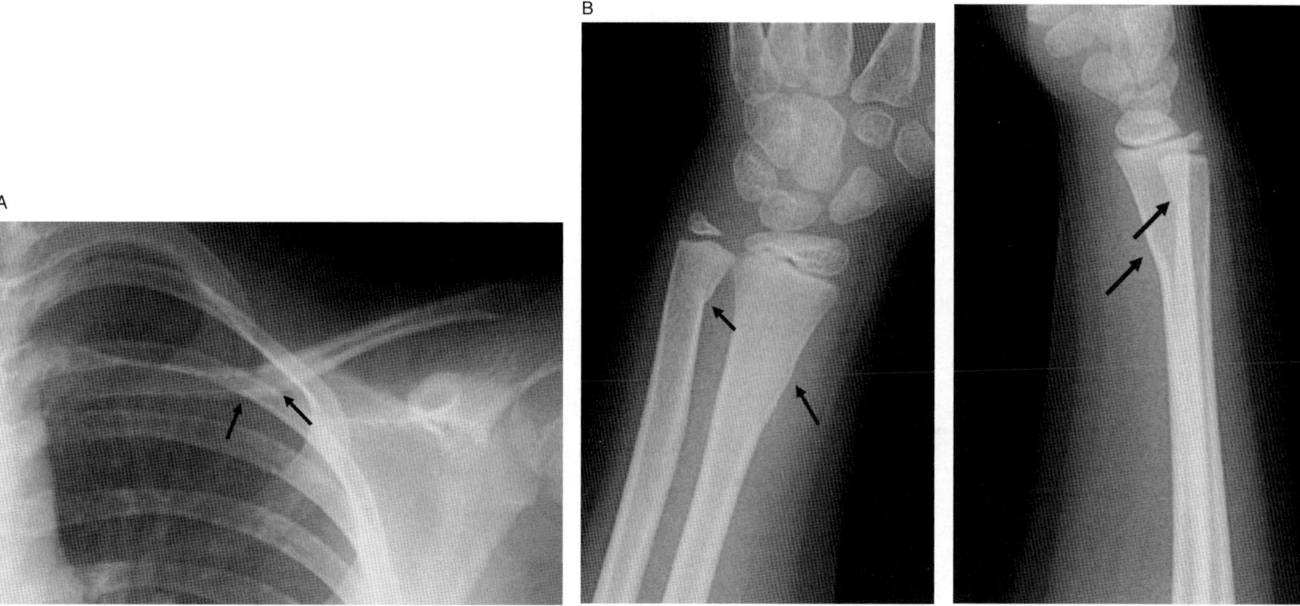

Figure 170.18 Fractures. (A) Bowing fracture of the clavicle in an 1-year-old girl. Plain radiograph shows inferior bowing of the left mid clavicle (arrows) with no cortical infraction. (B,C) Buckle fractures of the distal radius and ulna in an 8-year-old girl. There is buckling of the cortex of the radial and volar aspects of the distal radial and ulnar metaphyses on frontal and lateral views (arrows).

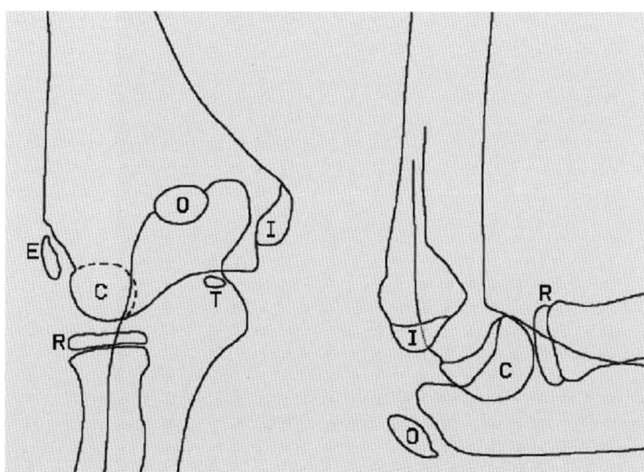

Figure 170.19 The order of appearance of ossification centers of the elbow, remembered with the mnemonic CRITOE: capitellum (C), radial head (R), internal (medial) epicondyle (I), trochlea (T), olecranon (O), and external (lateral) epicondyle (E).

Elbow

Supracondylar fracture

The supracondylar fracture is the most common fracture of the pediatric elbow. Typically, posterior displacement of the distal humeral fragment is appreciated radiographically by the loss of the normal relationship of the anterior humeral line bisecting the capitellum. Joint effusion is shown as an elevated anterior fat pad and abnormally visible posterior fat pad (Fig. 170.21A,B).

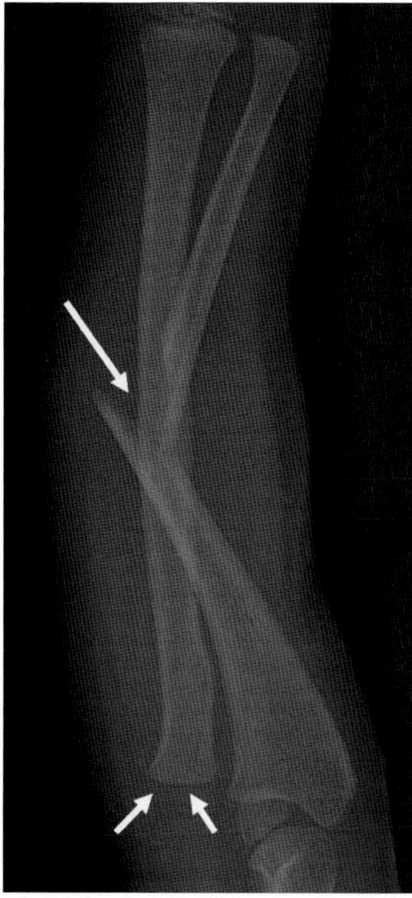

Figure 170.20 Monteggia's fracture in a 4-year-old girl. There is a mid-l ulnar diaphyseal fracture (arrow) with proximal radial head dislocation anteriorly (small arrows).

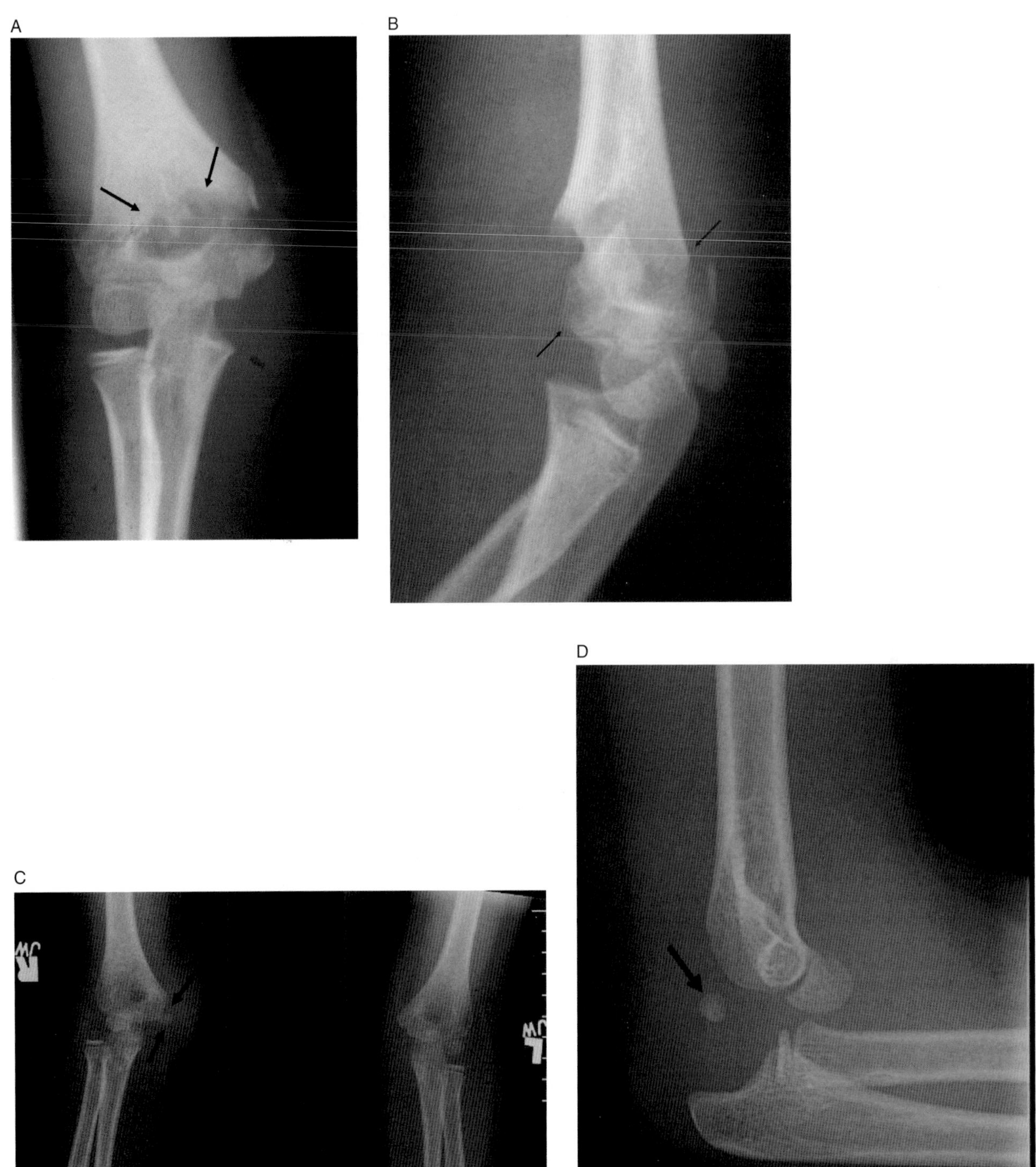

Figure 170.21 Fractures. (A,B) Supracondylar fracture in 8-year-old girl. Plain frontal radiograph shows the supracondylar fracture (arrows) with posterior displacement of the distal humerus seen on the lateral view (arrows) and a large joint effusion. (C,D) Avulsion fracture of the medial epicondyle of the humerus in a 6-year-old girl. Plain lateral radiograph shows the displaced avulsed medial epicondyle within the joint (arrows) compared with the normal left side. On the lateral view (D) complete right elbow dislocation is evident, only subtly seen on the frontal view (C).

Avulsion fracture of the medial epicondyle

An avulsion fracture can occur at the medial epicondyle of the humerus: The medial epicondyle of the humerus usually ossifies by 7 years and is fused by 16 years. With a non-displaced avulsion fracture, the medial epicondyle appears separated from the distal humerus. A comparison view of the contralateral side is often helpful (Fig. 170.21C,D). When the avulsed fragment is displaced into the joint, the unexpected absence of the medial epicondyle (remember CRITOE) should prompt a careful review of the radiographs.

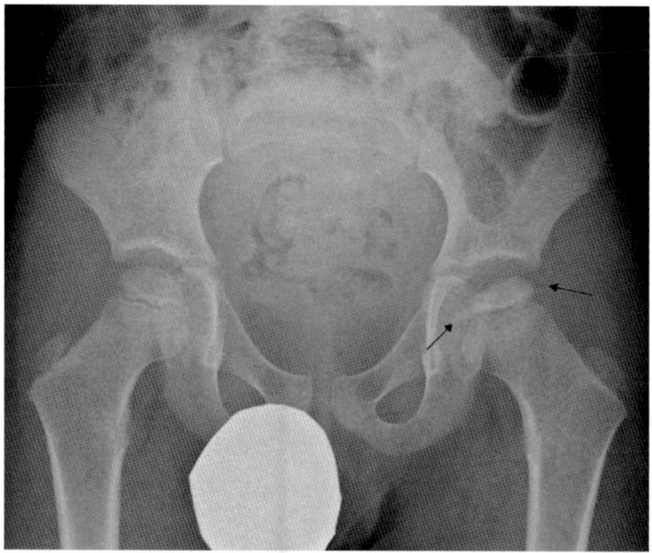

Figure 170.22 Legg–Calvé–Perthes disease. Frontal radiograph shows widening of the left hip joint space and a sclerotic flattened irregular left femoral head (arrows).

Hip

Legg–Calvé–Perthes disease

Early radiographic findings in Legg–Calvé–Perthes disease include widening of the joint space, asymmetrically irregular ossified femoral epiphyses, and subchondral linear lucency (Fig. 170.22). Later findings include fragmentation, sclerosis, and collapse of the femoral head. At different stages of disease, MRI may be useful to assess the degree and extent of disease.

Slipped capital femoral epiphysis

Posteromedial slippage of the femoral epiphysis can be seen on frontal or frog leg views. This finding can be very subtle on the frontal view. A line drawn tangential to the lateral cortex of the femoral metaphysis on the frog leg lateral view normally bisects a portion of femoral epiphysis; if the epiphysis is medial to this line, it is displaced. Other radiologic findings of widening of the physis and indistinctness of the metaphyseal side of the physis can also be suggestive of a slipped capital femoral epiphysis (Fig. 170.23)

Hip joint effusion

The presence of a hip joint effusion in a child with hip pain may be important. Asymmetric widening of the joint space can sometimes be appreciated on radiographs but may be very subtle. Ultrasound of the anterior hip joint is an easy and reliable method of evaluating the presence and amount of joint fluid, guiding in the decision to tap the joint for diagnostic and therapeutic purposes.

Child abuse

A skeletal survey and brain CT need to be obtained to evaluate fracture, soft tissue injury, or intracranial hemorrhage in cases of

A

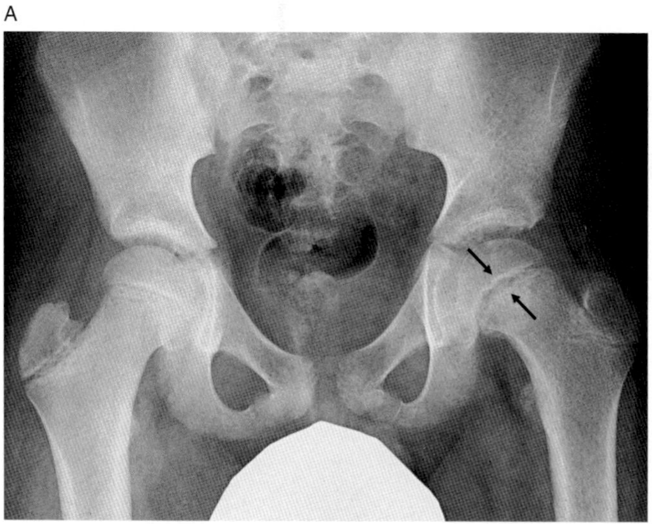

B

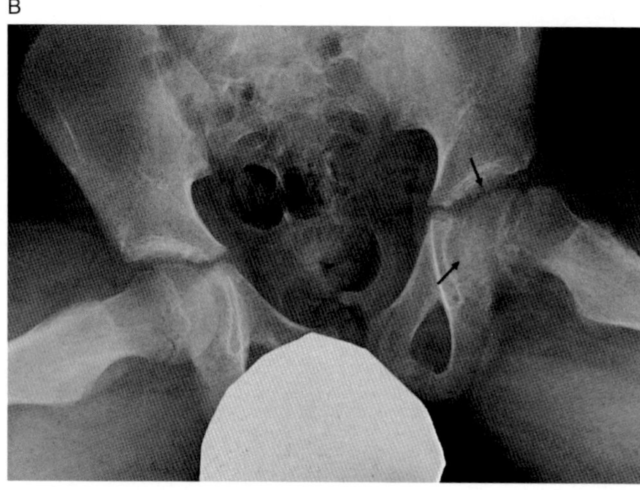

Figure 170.23 Slipped capital femoral epiphysis in a 12-year-old boy presenting with hip pain. (A) On the frontal view, there is subtle widening of the left femoral physis (arrows). (B) Frog lateral view demonstrates posteromedial slippage of the left femoral epiphysis (arrows).

suspected child abuse. Imaging findings suggesting non-accidental trauma include multiple fractures of different ages at different body sites; metaphyseal corner fractures; and fractures of posterior ribs, scapula, spinous process of vertebra, or sternum.

Rickets, and other metabolic disorders associated with multiple fractures can sometimes mimic child abuse.

Selected references

Frush DP. Review of radiation issues for computed tomography. *Semin Ultrasound CT MR* 2004;**25**:17–24.

Goske MJ, Applegate KE, Boylan J, *et al. The Image Gently Campaign: working together to change practice. AJR Am J Roentgenol* 2008;**190**:273–274.

Siegel MJ. *Pediatric Sonography.* Philadelphia, PA: Williams & Wilkins, 2001.

Slovis TL (ed.). *Caffey's Pediatric Diagnostic Imaging*. St. Louis, MO: Mosby, 2008.

Swischuk LE. *Emergency Imaging of the Acutely Ill or Injured Child.* Philadelphia, PA: Williams & Wilkins, 1994.

Swischuk LE. Emergency pediatric imaging: current status and update. *Semin Ultrasound CT MR* 2007;**28**:158–168.

Chapter 171

Pediatric emergency medicine pharmacy

Sandra Leigh Bardas and Carolyn Nguyen

Introduction

Medication often plays an important role in pediatric ED visits. Most medications are either not labeled or inadequately labeled for pediatric use. The lack of safety and efficacy information leads to both over- and underdosing. There are often inconsistent dosing recommendations for therapeutically equivalent products. Treatment is guided by experience with adults coupled with principles in pediatric physiology, and psychopharmacology. Parents often have questions about drug administration: route, timing, and association with food. This section will review basic principles for determining the pediatric appropriate dosage – clinical pearls for common medications used for children in the ED (Table 171.1). The chapter also presents recipes for magic mouthwash, information about the worst tasting medications, those with the most alcohol, and an analgesia equivalency table.

Age-specific factors

There are a number of factors specific to various ages that should be considered when determining dosages:

- preterm and fullterm infants:
  - immature renal and hepatic systems
  - immature blood–brain barrier
  - protein binding, especially displacement of bilirubin from albumen
  - increased transdermal absorption
  - susceptibilities to retinopathy
  - quicker induction and emergence from anesthesia
  - oral absorption unpredictable
  - gastric emptying faster
- infants and toddlers:
  - oral absorbtion more predictable
  - gastric emptying slower
  - drug clearance faster than adult
  - CNS effects on psychomotor skills
- children:
  - gastric emptying slower than adult
  - drug clearance rate faster than adult
  - CNS active drugs can impact psychomotor skills
- adolescents:
  - hormonal changes influence disease (asthma, migraines)
  - compliance issues
  - experimentation with substances (tobacco, alcohol, recreational drugs).

Determining dosage

In general, pediatric medications should be administered using weight-based dosing. When deciding a weight-based dosage, use the following guidelines:

- Broselow Color-Coded Tape:
  - length-based determination of body weight may be unreliable in certain ethnic populations
  - tape must be aligned correctly with the patient, red is at the head
  - verify units of scale, kilograms versus pounds
- lean body or surface area (BSA; mathematically derived)
  - BSA most accurate for drug dosages, but dose by BSA few drugs, mainly chemotherapy.
- dosing adjustments need to be made in renal or liver failure
  - consider enterohepatic recycling of medications in children with elevated bilirubin levels
- in general, do not exceed the adult dose, even with weight-based dosing.

The most up-to-date reference for pediatric dosing is given at http://www.fda.gov/cder/pediatric/index.htm.

Analgesic ceiling effect

The analgesic ceiling effect is the dosage of drug beyond which there is no additional analgesic benefit but great risk of increased adverse reactions and potential for increased costs.

Acetaminophen. This is safe and effective for mild pain but inadequate for severe pain.

A Practical Guide to Pediatric Emergency Medicine: Caring for Children in the Emergency Department, ed. N. Ewen Amieva-Wang (associate eds. Jamie Shandro, Aparajita Sohoni, and Bernhard Fassl). Published by Cambridge University Press.

Table 171.1. Clinical pearls regarding common medications used for children in the emergency department

Medication or medication class	Pearl
Acetaminophen	Do not dose by volume because of the a wide potential for differences in strengths; always dose by drug weight
Amoxicillin and clavulanic acid (Augmentin)	Dosage formulations are not additive; not equivalent to extended release tablet since the amount of clavulanic acid does not increase in proportion to the amoxicillin content; may be administered with food (except high-fat foods) to lessen GI effects; causes GI upset and diarrhea
Azithromycin	May be given with or without food
Cephalosporins	Cefazolin, cefepime, cefotaxime, cefoxitin, ceftazidime, and cefuroxime can be used in those <1 month of age *Cephalexin* (Keflex): first generation, PO, administer on an empty stomach (i.e., 1 h prior to, or 2 h after meals); administer with food if GI upset occurs *Cefotetan*: second generation; IM/IV; hemolytic anemia is three-fold higher relative to other cephalosporins; do not use in children, use cefoxitin instead *Cefotaxime*: third generation; IM/IV; adjust for renal function; use in place of ceftriaxone in hyperbilirubinemic neonates; use cefixime (Suprax), cefpodoxime (Vantin) for PO form. *Ceftriaxone*: third generation; IM/IV; do not use in neonates, use cefotaxime instead; no change in renal impairment
Charcoal, activated	Chocolate or fruit syrup may be mixed with charcoal to increase palatability and will not decrease efficacy; do not use sorbitol for more than first dose and not in children <1 year or with fructose intolerance; if given with sorbitol, doses should be limited to prevent excessive fluid and electrolyte losses; administer as soon as possible after ingestion, preferably given within 1 h for greatest effect; do not mix with milk
Clindamycin	90% of clindamycin HCl is rapidly absorbed orally, so remember reduce PO dose; IV dose is about two to three times higher than PO dose; oral solution does not taste good, so may mix with fruit syrup to increase palatability; can use for <1 month old
Cough and cold Preparations	Cough and cold preparations pose risks when given to children under 6 years of age and have no associated benefit
Dexamethasone	Long-acting corticosteroid; elixir contains benzoic acid (metabolite of benzyl alcohol) dexamethasone Intensol contains 30% alcohol, so use injection solution 10 mg/ml (preservative free) to give orally to avoid high alcohol content; IV formulations may contain sulfites
Diazepam	Injections and rectal gel contain benzoic acid, benzyl alcohol. and sodium benzoate; not recommended in neonates; high doses of oral solution may cause diarrhea because of the polyethylene glycol and propylene glycol content; to minimize this effect, use crushed tablets as a substitution for oral solution; can use undiluted
Griseofulvin	Take with fatty meals to increase absorption; avoid exposure to sunlight
Histamine H_2 antagonists (famotidine [Pepcid], ranitidine [Zantac], nizatidine [Axid], cimetidine)	These drugs are considered to be therapeutically interchangeable; formulary decisions and pricing usually determine the choice *Cimetidine* may be given PO/IM/IV; it has the most drug interactions and needs to be given the most frequently
Ondansetron	Round off the dose to minimum of half a tablet for the oral disintegrating tablet (ODT) form since ODT tablets can melt easily; typical PO/IV dose is 0.1–0.15 mg/kg for nausea/vomiting
Sulfamethoxazole and trimethoprim	Oral suspension may contain alcohol ≤0.5% and propylene glycol; can give PO or IV; do not give IM
Valproic acid and derivatives	Use of Depakote-ER in pediatric patients <10 years of age is *not* recommended; do not confuse Depakote-ER with Depakote as erroneous substitution of Depakote (delayed release tablets) for Depakote-ER has resulted in toxicities; only Depakote-ER is intended for once daily administration

Ibuprofen. The analgesic ceiling is reached at low doses but higher doses provide anti-inflammatory activity. However, anti-inflammatory action is not equivalent to analgesia.

Opioids. There is no analgesic ceiling for pure opioids but there is a ceiling for the mixed agonist–antagonist opioids and partial agonist opioids. Unlike pure opioids, they are poor choices for severe pain since they can exacerbate acute pain by precipitating a withdrawal syndrome. The dosing of combinations of opioids with acetaminophen or NSAIDs will be limited by their analgesic ceiling.

Table 171.2 gives guidelines for analgesic dosing. Doses should be titrated to pain relief or prevention. Opioid-naive patients should be started at lower doses. Patients with prior opioid exposure may require higher doses and/or shorter intervals.

Medication formulations

Taste

The worst-tasting medications are:

- acetylcysteine
- charcoal
- clarithromycin
- clindamycin
- dexamethasone
- prednisolone.

Alcohol content

Liquid medications with high alcohol content (alcohol is used for drug solubility and as a preservative) include:

- acetaminophen/codeine (7%)
- acetaminophen/hydrocodone (7%)
- dexamethasone intensol (30%)
- promethazine (7%)
- ranitidine (7.5%)
- theophylline (20%)
- prednisone intensol (30%).

Recipes

Pediatric Magic Mouthwash

1. Equal parts of diphenhydramine liquid and an aluminum/magnesium antacid such as Maalox or Mylanta.
2. Triple mix (originally developed for radiation stomatitis):
   - Maalox/Mylanta 50 ml
   - viscous lidocaine 30 ml
   - diphenhydramine liquid 20 ml.

Pediatric enema

Warm water 300 ml plus magnesium citrate 200 ml, plus glycerin 100 ml; or 30 ml lactulose with 30 ml magnesium citrate.

Table 171.2. gives guidelines for analgesic dosing

Drug	Dosing ranges in children	Comments
Strong opioids		
Morphine	IV dosing Infants <3 months are more prone to respiratory depression and reactions to sodium metabisulfite *Neonates*: 0.05–0.2 mg/kg per dose q. 4 h *Infants and children*: 0.05–0.2 mg/kg per dose q. 2–4 h *Adolescents*: 2.5–5 mg q. 2 h, q. 3 h or q. 4 h (start at lower doses)	Smaller and more frequent dosing is preferable to larger and less frequent dosing in acute pain management *Renal disease*: CrCL 10–50 ml/min, use 75% of normal dose; CrCL <10 ml/min, use 50% of normal dose *Liver disease*: excessive sedation may occur Histamine release may cause local reaction
Fentanyl	IV dosing *Neonates and infants*: 0.5–2 μg/kg dose every 2–4 h *18–36 months*: 2–3 μg/kg every 30–60 min *1–12 years*: 1–2 μg/kg per dose every 30–60 min	All doses should be titrated to analgesia with monitoring of vital signs *Renal disease*: doses may need to be adjusted Transdermal patches are indicated only for patients who are opioid tolerant (take routine, round-the-clock opiates); remove old patch before applying a new patch; heat sources (including fever) may increase the serum concentrations from transdermal patches Do not confuse fentanyl transdermal patches with fentanyl iontophoretic transdermal systems Because of the higher bioavailability of fentanyl in the buccal tablet, the dosage of the lozenge and the buccal tablet are not equivalent on microgram basis Minimal histamine release
Hydromorphone (Dilaudid)	IV dosing (IM, SC have variable absorption) *Young children*: 0.015 mg/kg per dose q. 3–6 h *Older children*: start with 0.2–0.6 mg per dose	Significant differences between PO and IV dosing.

Table 171.2. *(cont.)*

Drug	Dosing ranges in children	Comments
Methadone	IV/IM dosing 0.05–0.1 mg/kg dose with dosing interval to increase with repeated doses	Parenteral dose is one-half oral dose. Due to variable half-life, slow titration advised Vigilance during treatment initiation and titration needed because of the long elimination half-life, QT prolongation, possible severe respiratory depression and incomplete cross-tolerance with other opioids *Renal disease*: CrCL <10 ml/min, use 50–75% of normal dose *Hepatic disease*: avoid in severe disease
Oxycodone (ingredient in Percocet and Oxycontin)	*Children*: oral prompt release 0.05–0.15 mg/kg per dose *Oral extended release*: requirement is established using prompt release formulation, q. 12 h	Note cumulative dosage when combined with acetaminophen Do not crush sustained-release formulations Extended release formulation not intended for PR use
Weak opioids		
Codeine	*IM/PO*: 0.05–0.1 mg/kg per dose *Antitussive dose for children 2–12*: 0.25 mg/kg per dose, not to exceed a total daily dose of 1.5 mg/kg	Note cumulative dosage when combined with acetaminophen Not recommended as antitussive for children <2 years
Hydrocodone (ingredient in Vicodin, Norco, and Lortab)	PO 0.135 mg/kg per dose not to exceed *<2 years*: 1.25 mg as single dose *2–12 years*: 5 mg as single dose *Adolescent*: 10 mg as single dose	Note cumulative dosage when combined with acetaminophen
Non-steroidal anti-inflammatory drugs		
Ibuprofen (Motrin, Advil)	5–10 mg/kg/dose, not to exceed 40 mg/kg daily *Juvenile rheumatoid arthritis*: up to 12.5 mg/kg/dose, not to exceed 2400 mg daily	Observe all NSAID precautions Use with caution in patients with cardiovascular, GI, renal or hepatic disease; use with caution in those receiving anticoagulants
Ketorolac (Toradol)	Children 2–16 years *IM*: 1 mg/kg per dose not to exceed 30 mg *IV*: 0.05 mg/kg per dose not to exceed 15 mg	Observe all NSAID precautions Drug has high potential for GI bleed Maximum combined duration of treatment for both parenteral and oral forms is 5 days Supplement with low-dose opioids for breakthrough pain
Naproxen (Naprosyn, Aleve)	*Children <2 years*: 5–7 mg/kg per dose (may be higher in inflammatory disease) *Maximum long-term daily dose*: 1250 mg as naproxen base	Observe all NSAID precautions
Non-narcotic analgesic		
Acetaminophen (Tylenol)	*PO*: 10–15 mg/kg per dose every 4–6 h not to exceed 5 doses in 24 h *PR*: first dose 35–50 mg/kg; maintenance dose is 20 mg/kg per dose q. 6 h; round off to standardized doses	Be sure to account for acetaminophen in combination products Overdosage can cause hepatic toxicity Potential for toxicity is increased with concurrent administration of CYP450 enzyme-inducing drugs

CrCL, creatinine clearance; PR, per rectum.

Earwax removal

Docusate solution for impacted ear wax. Use docusate oral solution (sugar free) 10 mg/ml. Place one to four drops into the external ear canal. Tilt head or apply cotton to allow liquid to loosen material. Gently irrigate ear canal with warm water to remove the loosened wax.

Selected references

Lexi-Comp. Online 2008. http://online.lexi.com/crlsql/servlet/crlonline (accessed November 2008).

Micromedex. Online 2008. http://www.thomsonhc.com (accessed November 2008).

Phelps SJ, Hak EB, Crill CM. *Pediatric Injectable Drugs*, 8th edn. Bethesda, MD: American Society of Health-System Pharmacists, 2007.

Taketoma CK, Hodding JH, Kraus DM. *Pediatric Dosage Handbook*, 15th edn. Hudson, OH: Lexi-Comp, 2008.

Appendix

Table 1. Glasgow Coma Scale in adult with child modification

Sign	Adult	Child modification (< 2 years)	Points
Eye opening (4 possible)	None	None	1
	Open to command	Open to sound	2
	Open to pain	Open to pain	3
	Open spontaneously	Open spontaneously	4
Verbal (5 possible)	None	None	1
	Incomprehensible sounds	Moans to pain	2
	Inappropriate words	Cries to pain	3
	Confused	Cries, irritable	4
	Oriented	Age appropriate	5
Motor (6 possible)	None	None	1
	Abnormal extension to pain (decerebrate posturing)	Abnormal extension to pain (decerebrate posturing)	2
	Abnormal flexion to pain (decorticate posturing)	Abnormal flexion to pain (decorticate posturing)	3
	Withdraws to pain	Withdraws to pain	4
	Localizes pain	Localizes pain (withdraws to touch)	5
	Obeys commands	Spontaneous movements	6

Ventilator settings

Rate (breaths/min): newborn 30–40; child 20–25; adolescent 15
Positive end-expiratory pressure: 4–5 cmH_2O
Inspiration to expiration: 1:2 with inspiration time 0.5–1 s
Weight adjustment:

- < 10 kg: pressure-limited starting with inspiration pressure of 20 cmH_2O
- > 10 kg: volume-preset ventilator with tidal volume of 8–10 ml/kg (peak inspiratory pressure, 20–30 cmH_2O)

Anaphylaxis

Immediate treatment

- Epinephrine (1:1000): 0.01 ml/kg (max. 0.5 ml) IM/SQ, 3 doses q. 5 min
- Diphenhydramine: 1–2 mg/kg IV/IM (max. 50 mg)
- Hydrocortisone: 5 mg/kg IV (max. 100 mg)
- Famotidine: 0.2–0.4 mg/kg IV (max. 20 mg)

Bronchospasm

- Albuterol nebulizer 0.03 ml/kg (max. 1 ml) q. 20 min

Hypotension

- Epinephrine infusion 0.1 μg/kg per min (max. 1.5 μg/kg per min)

Status asthmaticus

Bronchodilation

Albuterol nebulizer: 0.03 ml/kg (max. 1.0 ml) q. 20 min ×3
Albuterol continuous nebulizer: 0.1 ml/kg per h (max. 3 ml/h)
Ipratropium nebulizer: < 12 years, 250 μg; > 12 years, 500 μg ×3 with albuterol

Table 2. Rapid sequence intubation (RSI)

	Methods
Pre-oxygenation	Oxygenate to 100% for 3 min
Pre-medication	Atropine 0.02 mg/kg (min. 0.1 mg, max. 1 mg; always use for patients < 5 years old and before second dose of succinylcholine)
	Lidocaine 1 mg/kg for elevated intracranial pressure
	Vecuronium 0.01 mg/kg defasciculating dose
Sedation	Etomidate 0.2–0.6 mg/kg IV
	Ketamine 0.5–2 mg/kg IV
	Thiopental 3–5 mg/kg IV
Paralysis	Succinylcholine 2 mg/kg IV
	Vecuronium 0.1 mg/kg IV
	Rocuronium 0.6–1.2 mg/kg IV
Endotracheal tube size	Uncuffed, 4 + age (years)/4; cuffed is 0.5–1.0 size smaller

Steroid
Prednisone: 1–2 mg/kg PO (max. 60 mg)
Dexamethasone: 0.2 mg/kg PO or IM
Methylprednisolone: 2 mg/kg IV (max. 125 mg)
Additional therapies
Magnesium sulfate: 40 mg/kg (max. 4 g) IV over 30 min
Epinephrine: (1:1000) 0.01 ml/kg (max. 0.3 ml) SQ
Terbutaline: 0.01 ml/kg (max. 0.25 ml) SQ
Terbutaline drip: 2–10 μg/kg IV load then 0.4 μg/kg per/min
If intubating, consider rapid sequence intubation with ketamine + (atropine + midazolam) or etomidate

Status epilepticus

Lorazepam: 0.05–0.1 mg/kg (max. 4 mg) slow IV ×2
No IV access: use rectal diazepam 0.5 mg/kg (max. 20 mg)
Fosphenytoin: 20 mg/kg slow IV over 10–15 min or IM
Phenobarbital: 20 mg/kg IV
Consider pentobarbital coma: load 10–15 mg/kg over 1–2 h, then 1 mg/kg per h

Hypoglycemia

Glucose 0.5–1 g/kg (2–4 ml/kg D25 or 1–2 ml/kg D50)
Glucagon 30–50 μg/kg (max. 1 mg) IV/IM/SQ

Hyperkalemia

If ECG changes: 10% calcium chloride 0.20–0.25 ml/kg IV over 2–5 min
Sodium bicarbonate: 1–2 mEq/kg IV over 5–10 min
K^+ 6–7 mEq/l: Kayexalate 1 g/kg in sorbitol
$K^+ > 7$ mEq/l: glucose 0.5–1.0 g/kg with regular insulin (1 unit/5 g glucose) over 30 min

Treatment of burns

Calculate estimated percentage of total body surface area burnt (Lund and Browder chart)
Fluid replacement:

- 4 ml/kg for every 1% total body surface area affected, plus maintenance fluids
- administer half over first 8 h, remainder over next 16 h

Goal urine output:

- < 30 kg body weight: 1–2 ml/kg per h
- > 30 kg body weight: 0.5–1 ml/kg per h

Index

Page numbers in **bold** indicate illustrations.
Page numbers in *italics* indicate tables.
In either case there is usually accompanlying information in the text, but this is not always the case.